MW00844493

Digestive System Tumours

WHO Classification of Tumours Editorial Board

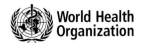

World Health Organization

Suggested citation
WHO Classification of Tumours Editorial Board. Digestive system tumours.
Lyon (France): International Agency for Research on Cancer; 2019.
(WHO classification of tumours series, 5th ed.; vol. 1).
http://publications.iarc.fr/579.

Sales, rights, and permissions
Print copies are distributed by WHO Press, World Health Organization, 20 Avenue Appia, 1211 Geneva 27, Switzerland
Tel.: +41 22 791 3264; Fax: +41 22 791 4857; email: bookorders@who.int; website: http://whobluebooks.iarc.fr

To purchase IARC publications in electronic format, see the IARC Publications website (http://publications.iarc.fr).

Requests for permission to reproduce or translate IARC publications – whether for sale or for non-commercial distribution – should be submitted
through the IARC Publications website (http://publications.iarc.fr/Rights-And-Permissions).

Second print run (5000 copies)

Updated corrigenda can be found at http://publications.iarc.fr

IARC Library Cataloguing-in-Publication Data
Digestive system tumours / WHO Classification of Tumours Editorial Board. – 5th edition.

(World Health Organization classification of tumours)

1. Digestive System Neoplasms – pathology
2. Digestive System Neoplasms – genetics

I. WHO Classification of Tumours Editorial Board II. Series

ISBN 978-92-832-4499-8   (NLM Classification: WI 149)

The WHO classification of digestive system tumours presented in this book reflects the views of the WHO Classification of Tumours Editorial Board that convened at the International Agency for Research on Cancer, Lyon, France, 3–5 July 2018.

The WHO Classification of Tumours Editorial Board

For the complete list of all contributors and their affiliations, see pages 551–556.

For the complete list of all contributors and their affiliations, see pages 551–556.

WHO Classification of Tumours
Digestive System Tumours

Edited by	The WHO Classification of Tumours Editorial Board
IARC Editors	Dilani Lokuhetty
	Valerie A. White
	Reiko Watanabe
	Ian A. Cree
Epidemiology	Ariana Znaor
Project Assistant	Asiedua Asante
Assistants	Anne-Sophie Hameau
	Laura Brispot
Technical Editor	Jessica Cox
Database	Alberto Machado
	Katherine Lloyd
Layout	Meaghan Fortune
Printed by	Maestro Gestion D'Edition
	69100 Villeurbanne, France
	Printed in Italy
Publisher	International Agency for Research on Cancer (IARC)
	150 Cours Albert Thomas
	69372 Lyon Cedex 08, France

Contents

List of abbreviations   x

Foreword   xi

1 Introduction to tumours of the digestive system   13
General introduction   14
Classification of neuroendocrine neoplasms
of the digestive system   16
TNM staging of well-differentiated neuroendocrine tumours
of the gastrointestinal tract   20

2 Tumours of the oesophagus   23
WHO classification of tumours of the oesophagus   24
TNM staging of tumours of the oesophagus   25
Introduction   28
Benign epithelial tumours and precursors
Squamous papilloma   30
Barrett dysplasia   32
Squamous dysplasia   36
Malignant epithelial tumours
Adenocarcinoma of the oesophagus and
oesophagogastric junction NOS   38
Adenoid cystic carcinoma   44
Adenosquamous and mucoepidermoid carcinomas   46
Squamous cell carcinoma NOS   48
Undifferentiated carcinoma   54
Neuroendocrine neoplasms   56

3 Tumours of the stomach   59
WHO classification of tumours of the stomach   60
TNM staging of carcinomas of the stomach   61
Introduction   64
Gastritis and metaplasia: precursors of gastric neoplasms   65
Benign epithelial tumours and precursors
Fundic gland polyps   67
Hyperplastic polyps   69
Dysplasia   71
Intestinal-type adenoma   76
Foveolar-type adenoma   79
Pyloric gland adenoma   81
Oxyntic gland adenoma   83
Malignant epithelial tumours
Adenocarcinoma   85
Squamous cell carcinoma   96
Adenosquamous carcinoma   98
Undifferentiated carcinoma   100
Gastroblastoma   102
Neuroendocrine neoplasms   104

4 Tumours of the small intestine and ampulla   111
WHO classification of tumours of the small intestine
and ampulla   112
TNM staging of carcinomas of the small intestine   113
TNM staging of carcinomas of the ampulla of Vater   114
Introduction   116
Benign epithelial tumours and precursors
Non-ampullary adenoma   118
Ampullary adenoma   121
Malignant epithelial tumours
Non-ampullary adenocarcinoma   124
Ampullary adenocarcinoma   127
Neuroendocrine neoplasms   131

5 Tumours of the appendix   135
WHO classification of tumours of the appendix   136
TNM staging of adenocarcinomas of the appendix   137
Introduction   140
Epithelial tumours
Serrated lesions and polyps   141
Mucinous neoplasm   144
Adenocarcinoma   147
Goblet cell adenocarcinoma   149
Neuroendocrine neoplasms   152

6 Tumours of the colon and rectum   157
WHO classification of tumours of the colon and rectum   158
TNM staging of carcinomas of the colon and rectum   159
Introduction   162
Benign epithelial tumours and precursors
Serrated lesions and polyps   163
Conventional adenoma   170
Inflammatory bowel disease–associated dysplasia   174
Malignant epithelial tumours
Adenocarcinoma   177
Neuroendocrine neoplasms   188

7 Tumours of the anal canal   193
WHO classification of tumours of the anal canal   194
TNM staging of tumours of the anal canal and perianal skin   195
Introduction   196
Benign epithelial tumours and precursors
Inflammatory cloacogenic polyp   198
Condyloma   200
Squamous dysplasia (intraepithelial neoplasia)   202
Malignant epithelial tumours
Squamous cell carcinoma   205
Adenocarcinoma   208
Neuroendocrine neoplasms   212

8 Tumours of the liver and intrahepatic bile ducts   215
WHO classification of tumours of the liver and
intrahepatic bile ducts   216
TNM staging of tumours of the liver   217
TNM staging of tumours of the intrahepatic bile ducts   218
Introduction   220
Benign hepatocellular tumours
Focal nodular hyperplasia of the liver   221
Hepatocellular adenoma   224
Malignant hepatocellular tumours and precursors
Hepatocellular carcinoma   229
Hepatoblastoma   240
Benign biliary tumours and precursors
Bile duct adenoma   245
Biliary adenofibroma   248
Mucinous cystic neoplasm of the liver and biliary system   250
Biliary intraepithelial neoplasia (see Ch. 9)
Intraductal papillary neoplasm of the bile ducts
(see Ch. 9)
Malignant biliary tumours
Intrahepatic cholangiocarcinoma   254
Combined hepatocellular-cholangiocarcinoma and
undifferentiated primary liver carcinoma   260
Hepatic neuroendocrine neoplasms   263

9 **Tumours of the gallbladder and extrahepatic bile ducts** 265
WHO classification of tumours of the gallbladder and
   extrahepatic bile ducts 266
TNM staging of tumours of the gallbladder 267
TNM staging of tumours of the perihilar bile ducts 268
TNM staging of tumours of the distal extrahepatic bile duct 269
Introduction 270
Benign epithelial tumours and precursors
   Pyloric gland adenoma of the gallbladder 271
   Biliary intraepithelial neoplasia 273
   Intracholecystic papillary neoplasm 276
   Intraductal papillary neoplasm of the bile ducts 279
   Mucinous cystic neoplasm of the liver and biliary system
      (see Ch. 8)
Malignant epithelial tumours
   Carcinoma of the gallbladder 283
   Carcinoma of the extrahepatic bile ducts 289
   Neuroendocrine neoplasms of the
      gallbladder and bile ducts 292

10 **Tumours of the pancreas** 295
WHO classification of tumours of the pancreas 296
TNM staging of carcinomas of the pancreas 297
Introduction 298
Benign epithelial tumours and precursors
   Acinar cystic transformation 300
   Serous neoplasms 303
   Intraepithelial neoplasia 307
   Intraductal papillary mucinous neoplasm 310
   Intraductal oncocytic papillary neoplasm 315
   Intraductal tubulopapillary neoplasm 317
   Mucinous cystic neoplasm 319
Malignant epithelial tumours
   Ductal adenocarcinoma 322
   Acinar cell carcinoma 333
   Pancreatoblastoma 337
   Solid pseudopapillary neoplasm 340
Neuroendocrine neoplasms
   Introduction 343
   Non-functioning pancreatic neuroendocrine tumours 347
   Functioning neuroendocrine tumours
      Insulinoma 353
      Gastrinoma 355
      VIPoma 357
      Glucagonoma 359
      Somatostatinoma 361
      ACTH-producing neuroendocrine tumour 363
      Serotonin-producing neuroendocrine tumour 365
   Neuroendocrine carcinoma 367
   MiNENs 370

11 **Haematolymphoid tumours of the digestive system** 373
WHO classification of haematolymphoid tumours
   of the digestive system 374
Introduction 376
Site-specific haematolymphoid tumours
   Extranodal marginal zone lymphoma of mucosa-
      associated lymphoid tissue (MALT lymphoma) 378
   Duodenal-type follicular lymphoma 383
   Enteropathy-associated T-cell lymphoma 386
   Monomorphic epitheliotropic intestinal T-cell lymphoma 390
   Intestinal T-cell lymphoma NOS 393
   Indolent T-cell lymphoproliferative disorder of the GI tract 395
   Hepatosplenic T-cell lymphoma 397
   EBV+ inflammatory follicular dendritic cell sarcoma 399
Haematolymphoid tumours occurring with some frequency
   in the digestive system
   Diffuse large B-cell lymphoma 402
   Follicular lymphoma 406
   Mantle cell lymphoma 408
   Burkitt lymphoma 411
   Plasmablastic lymphoma 415
   Posttransplant lymphoproliferative disorders 417
   Extranodal NK/T-cell lymphoma 420
   Systemic mastocytosis 423
   Langerhans cell histiocytosis 426
   Follicular dendritic cell sarcoma 428
   Histiocytic sarcoma 430

12 **Mesenchymal tumours of the digestive system** 433
WHO classification of mesenchymal tumours
   of the digestive system 434
TNM staging of gastrointestinal stromal tumours 435
Introduction 436
Gastrointestinal stromal tumour 439
Adipose tissue and (myo)fibroblastic tumours
   Inflammatory myofibroblastic tumour 444
   Desmoid fibromatosis 446
   Solitary fibrous tumour 448
   Lipoma 450
   Inflammatory fibroid polyp 452
   Plexiform fibromyxoma 454
Smooth muscle and skeletal muscle tumours
   Leiomyoma 456
   Leiomyosarcoma 458
   Rhabdomyosarcoma 460
Vascular and perivascular tumours
   Haemangioma 462
   Epithelioid haemangioendothelioma 466
   Kaposi sarcoma 468
   Angiosarcoma 471
   Glomus tumour 473
   Lymphangioma and lymphangiomatosis 475
Neural tumours
   Schwannoma 477
   Granular cell tumour 479
   Perineurioma 481
   Ganglioneuroma and ganglioneuromatosis 483
Tumours of uncertain differentiation
   PEComa, including angiomyolipoma 485
   Mesenchymal hamartoma of the liver 488
   Calcifying nested stromal-epithelial tumour of the liver 490
   Synovial sarcoma 492
   Gastrointestinal clear cell sarcoma / malignant
      gastrointestinal neuroectodermal tumour 494
   Embryonal sarcoma of the liver 497

13 Other tumours of the digestive system   499
　WHO classification of other tumours of the digestive system   500
　Mucosal melanoma   502
　Germ cell tumours   504
　Metastases   506

14 Genetic tumour syndromes of the digestive system   511
　Introduction   512
　Lynch syndrome   515
　Familial adenomatous polyposis 1   522
　GAPPS and other fundic gland polyposes   526
　Other adenomatous polyposes   529
　Serrated polyposis   532
　Hereditary diffuse gastric cancer   535
　Familial pancreatic cancer   539
　Juvenile polyposis syndrome   542
　Peutz–Jeghers syndrome   545
　Cowden syndrome   547
　Other genetic tumour syndromes   550

Contributors   551

Declaration of interests   557

IARC/WHO Committee for ICD-O   558

Sources   559

References   567

Subject index   625

Previous volumes in the series   635

List of abbreviations

3D	three-dimensional
ABC	activated B cell
ACRG	Asian Cancer Research Group
ADP	adenosine diphosphate
AJCC	American Joint Committee on Cancer
ATP	adenosine triphosphate
CI	confidence interval
CIMP	CpG island methylator phenotype
CNS	central nervous system
CSF	cerebrospinal fluid
CT	computed tomography
dMMR	mismatch repair–deficient
DNA	deoxyribonucleic acid
EBER	EBV-encoded small RNA
EBV	Epstein–Barr virus
EC cell	enterochromaffin cell
ECL cell	enterochromaffin-like cell
EHBD	extrahepatic bile duct
EMVI	extramural vascular invasion
ER	estrogen receptor
EUS	endoscopic ultrasonography
FDC	follicular dendritic cell
FDG PET	18F-fluorodeoxyglucose positron emission tomography
FISH	fluorescence in situ hybridization
FNA	fine-needle aspiration
FNCLCC	Fédération Nationale des Centres de Lutte Contre le Cancer
GCB	germinal-centre B cell
GI tract	gastrointestinal tract
GPC3	glypican-3
GS	glutamine synthetase
H&E	haematoxylin and eosin
HBV	hepatitis B virus
HCV	hepatitis C virus
HIV	human immunodeficiency virus
HPV	human papillomavirus
IARC	International Agency for Research on Cancer
ICD-11	International Classification of Diseases, 11th Revision
ICD-O	International Classification of Diseases for Oncology
IEL	intraepithelial lymphocyte
Ig	immunoglobulin
IMVI	intramural vascular invasion
InSiGHT	International Society for Gastrointestinal Hereditary Tumours
IQ	intelligence quotient
JGCA	Japanese Gastric Cancer Association
kb	kilo base pair
M:F ratio	male-to-female ratio
MALT	mucosa-associated lymphoid tissue
MF pattern	mass-forming pattern
MRI	magnetic resonance imaging
mRNA	messenger ribonucleic acid
MSI	microsatellite instability
MSS	microsatellite stability
N:C ratio	nuclear-to-cytoplasmic ratio
NK cell	natural killer cell
NSAID	non-steroidal anti-inflammatory drug
PAS	periodic acid–Schiff
PASD	periodic acid–Schiff with diastase
PCR	polymerase chain reaction
PET	positron emission tomography
PET-CT	positron emission tomography–computed tomography
PI pattern	periductal infiltrating pattern
PR	progesterone receptor
RNA	ribonucleic acid
SCNA	somatic copy-number alteration
SDH	succinate dehydrogenase
SEER Program	Surveillance, Epidemiology, and End Results Program
SNP	single nucleotide polymorphism
TACE	transarterial chemoembolization
TCGA	The Cancer Genome Atlas
TNM	tumour, node, metastasis
TRG	tumour regression grade
UICC	Union for International Cancer Control
UV	ultraviolet

Foreword

The WHO Classification of Tumours, published as a series of books (also known as the WHO Blue Books), is an essential tool for standardizing diagnostic practice worldwide. The WHO classification also serves as a vehicle for the translation of cancer research into practice. The diagnostic criteria and standards these books contain are underpinned by evidence evaluated and debated by experts in the field. About 200 authors and editors participate in the production of each book, and they give their time freely to this task. I am very grateful for their help; it is a remarkable team effort.

This first volume of the fifth edition of the WHO Blue Books incorporates several important changes to the series as a whole. For example, this is the first WHO Blue Book to be led by an editorial board. The WHO Classification of Tumours Editorial Board is composed of standing members nominated by pathology organizations and expert members selected on the basis of informed bibliometric analysis. The diagnostic process is increasingly multidisciplinary, and we are delighted that several radiology and clinical experts have already joined us to address specific needs. The editorial board also includes a patient representative.

The most conspicuous change to the format of the books in the fifth edition is that tumour types common to multiple systems are dealt with together – so there are separate chapters on haematolymphoid tumours and mesenchymal tumours. There is also a chapter on genetic tumour syndromes. Genetic disorders are of increasing importance to diagnosis in individual patients, and the study of these disorders has undoubtedly informed our understanding of tumour biology and behaviour over the past 10 years. The inclusion of a chapter dedicated to genetic tumour syndromes reflects this importance.

We have attempted to take a more systematic approach to the multifaceted nature of tumour classification; each tumour type is described on the basis of its localization, clinical features, epidemiology, etiology, pathogenesis, histopathology, diagnostic molecular pathology, staging, and prognosis and prediction. Where appropriate we have also included information on macroscopic appearance and cytology, as well as essential and desirable diagnostic criteria. This standardized, modular approach is in part to ready the books to be accessible online, but it also enables us to call attention to areas in which there is little information, and where serious gaps in our knowledge remain to be addressed.

The organization of the WHO Blue Books content now follows the normal progression from benign to malignant – a break with the fourth edition, but one we hope will be welcome.

The volumes are still organized on the basis of anatomical site (digestive system, breast, soft tissue and bone, etc.), and each tumour type is listed within a taxonomic classification that follows the format below, which helps to structure the books in a systematic manner:

- Site; e.g. stomach
- Category; e.g. epithelial tumours
- Family (class); e.g. adenomas and other premalignant neoplastic lesions
- Type; e.g. adenoma
- Subtype; e.g. foveolar-type adenoma

The issue of whether a given tumour type represents a distinct entity rather than a subtype continues to exercise pathologists, and it is the topic of many publications in the scientific literature. We continue to deal with this issue on a case-by-case basis, but we believe there are inherent rules that can be applied. For example, tumours in which multiple histological patterns contain shared truncal mutations are clearly of the same type, despite the differences in their appearance. Equally, genetic heterogeneity within the same tumour type may have implications for treatment. A small shift in terminology as of this new edition is that the term "variant" in reference to a specific kind of tumour has been wholly superseded by "subtype", in an effort to more clearly differentiate this meaning from that of "variant" in reference to a genetic alteration.

The WHO Blue Books are much appreciated by pathologists and of increasing importance to cancer researchers. The new editorial board and I certainly hope that the series will continue to meet the need for standards in diagnosis and to facilitate the translation of diagnostic research into practice worldwide. It is particularly important that cancers continue to be classified and diagnosed according to the same standards internationally so that patients can benefit from multicentre clinical trials, as well as from the results of local trials conducted on different continents.

Dr Ian A. Cree

Head, WHO Classification of Tumours Group
International Agency for Research on Cancer

June 2019

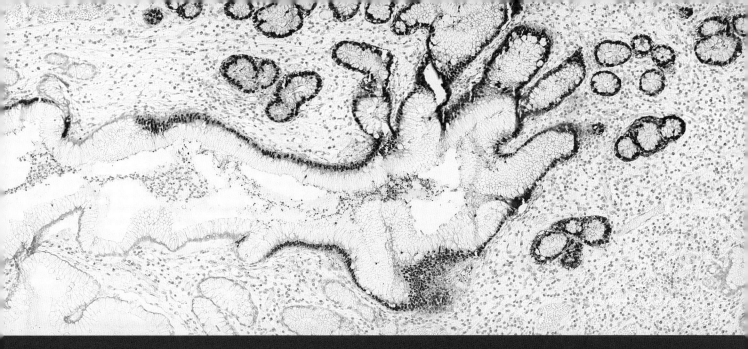

1

Introduction to tumours of the digestive system

Edited by: Washington MK

General introduction
Classification of neuroendocrine neoplasms of the digestive system

Introduction to tumours of the digestive system

Odze RD
Cree IA
Klimstra DS
Nagtegaal ID

Paradis V
Rugge M
Schirmacher P

The WHO classification of digestive system tumours presented in this volume of the WHO Classification of Tumours series' fifth edition reflects important advancements in our understanding of tumours of the digestive system. For the first time, certain tumour types are defined as much by their molecular phenotype as their histological characteristics; however, histopathological classification remains the gold standard for diagnosis in most instances. The WHO Classification of Tumours series is designed to be used worldwide, including those settings where a lack of tissue samples or of specific technical facilities limits the pathologist's ability to rely on molecular testing.

Since the publication of the fourth-edition digestive system tumours volume in 2010 {379}, there have been important developments in our understanding of the etiology and pathogenesis of many tumours. However, the extent to which this new information has altered clinical practice has been quite variable. For some of the tumours described in this volume, there is little molecular pathology in clinical use, despite the fact that we now have a more detailed understanding of their molecular pathogenesis. A tumour's molecular pathology, as defined for the purposes of this publication, concerns the molecular markers that are relevant to the tumour's diagnosis, biological behaviour, outcome, and treatment, rather than its molecular pathogenesis. The role of molecular pathology is expanding. For some tumour entities, molecular analysis is now essential for establishing an accurate diagnosis. Some of these analyses require investigation of somatic (acquired) genetic alterations, gene or protein expression, or even circulating tumour markers. For certain tumour types, specific analytical tests are needed to predict prognosis or tumour progression, and these tests are carefully outlined in this volume. In the following paragraphs, we have summarized some of the more notable changes since the fourth edition. More detailed descriptions can be found in the introductions to the chapters on each main tumour category and/or in the tumour-specific sections themselves. In instances where the editorial board determined that there was insufficient evidence of the diagnostic or clinical relevance of new information about a particular tumour entity, the position held in the fourth edition has been maintained as the standard in the current volume.

There has been substantial progress in our understanding of the development of oesophageal neoplasia and the sequential neoplastic progression from inflammation to metaplasia (Barrett oesophagus), dysplasia, and ultimately adenocarcinoma. This process is initially driven by gastro-oesophageal reflux disease, which leads to reprogramming of cell differentiation and proliferation in the oesophagus.

The molecular pathway of cancer progression in the stomach is less clear. Most so-called epidemic gastric cancers are now considered to be inflammation-driven, and their etiology is characteristically environmental – usually related to *Helicobacter pylori* infection. It is because of this infectious etiology that gastric cancer is included among the limited number of highly lethal but preventable cancers. Chronic gastric inflammation leads to changes in the microenvironment (including the microbiome) that result in mucosal atrophy/metaplasia, which may progress to neoplasia after further molecular alterations. Metaplastic changes in the upper GI tract are well recognized as early cancer precursors, but their precise molecular mechanisms and the exact role of the progenitor cells in the oncogenic cascade are still subjects of intense investigation.

The pathogenesis of precursor lesions is less clear in oesophageal squamous carcinogenesis than in gastric carcinogenesis. Environmental factors are believed to play an important role, but the mechanisms of neoplastic change as a result of specific factors, such as tobacco use and alcohol consumption, are poorly understood. For example, HPV infection was initially believed to play a key role in squamous carcinogenesis, but recent evidence suggests that there is no such association in most cases of oesophageal squamous cell carcinoma. This finding contrasts with our current knowledge of the etiology and pathogenesis of anal squamous lesions, in which HPV infection does appear to play an important etiological role, driving genetic alterations similar to those seen in cervical cancer.

The pathogenesis of adenocarcinomas of the intestines (the small and large bowel and the appendix) is now much better delineated than it was a decade ago. The introduction of population-based screening for colorectal cancer has laid the foundation for a better understanding of neoplastic precursor lesions and the molecular pathways associated with each type of tumour. For example, our knowledge of the molecular pathways and biological behaviour of conventional adenomas and serrated precursor lesions, including the recently renamed sessile serrated lesion (formerly called sessile serrated polyp/adenoma), has grown rapidly in the past decade, and this has enabled clinicians to provide tailored, evidence-driven screening and surveillance programmes. Our understanding of appendiceal tumours has also improved. For example, we now know that many tumours of the appendix develop via neoplastic precursor lesions similar to those in the small and large intestines, and the biological potential and molecular pathways of appendiceal tumours are therefore much better appreciated. The recently renamed goblet cell adenocarcinoma (formerly called goblet cell carcinoid/carcinoma) of the appendix is a prime example of a tumour whose biological potential and histological characteristics have been better described, resulting in improvements in the pathological approach to these tumours.

For some rare tumours, distinctive driver mutations have been identified, for example, the characteristic *MALAT1-GLI1* fusion gene in gastroblastoma and *EWSR1* fusions in gastrointestinal clear cell sarcoma and malignant gastrointestinal neuroectodermal tumour. In both examples, demonstration of the fusion gene is now required for the diagnosis.

One particularly important change in the fifth edition is in the classification of neuroendocrine neoplasms (NENs), which occur in multiple sites throughout the body. In this volume, NENs are covered within each organ-specific chapter, including the chapter on tumours of the pancreas, where detailed sections describing each functioning and non-functioning subtype are provided. Previously, these neoplasms were covered in detail only in the volume on tumours of endocrine organs {1936}. The general principles guiding the classification of all NENs are presented in a separate introduction to this topic (Classification of neuroendocrine neoplasms of the digestive system, p. 16). To consolidate our increased understanding of the genetics of these neoplasms, a group of experts met for a consensus conference at the International Agency for Research on Cancer (IARC) in November 2017 and subsequently published a paper in which they proposed distinguishing between well-differentiated neuroendocrine tumours (NETs) and poorly differentiated neuroendocrine carcinomas (NECs) in all sites where these neoplasms arise {2717}. Genomic data have also led to a change in the classification of mixed NENs, which are now grouped into the conceptual category of "mixed neuroendocrine–non-neuroendocrine neoplasms (MiNENs)". Mixed adenoneuroendocrine carcinomas (MANECs), which show genetic alterations similar to those of adenocarcinomas or NECs, rather than NETs, probably reflect clonal evolution within the tumours, which is a rapidly growing area of interest. The study of these mixed carcinomas may also lead to an improved understanding of other facets of clonality in tumours of the digestive system and other parts of the body.

Unfortunately, mixed tumours in other anatomical sites (e.g. oesophageal adenosquamous carcinoma and mucoepidermoid carcinoma, as well as hepatic carcinomas with mixed hepatocellular and cholangiolar differentiation) also remain subjects of uncertainty. The relative importance of the various lineages of differentiation within these neoplasms remains unknown. It is also uncertain how these neoplasms develop and how they should be treated clinically. These issues are a matter of debate because hard evidence is lacking, but improvements in the pathological criteria and classification of these neoplasms should help to standardize the diagnostic approach and facilitate better clinical and genomic research.

There are certain terms in current day-to-day use about which many pathologists continue to disagree. The editorial board carefully considered our current understanding of carcinogenesis pathways when considering the use of specific terms and definitions. In general, the overall consensus was that established terms, definitions, and criteria should not be changed unless there was strong evidence to support doing so and the proposed changes had clinical relevance. For some tumours, our understanding of the progression from normal epithelium to metastatic carcinoma remains inadequate. For example, in certain tumours the line between benign and malignant can be ambiguous, and in some cases the distinction is more definitional than biological. These are some of the many areas of tumour biology that need to be more fully investigated in the future.

In the fifth edition, the terminology for precursors to invasive carcinoma in the GI tract has been standardized somewhat, although the terms "dysplasia" and "intraepithelial neoplasia" are both still considered acceptable for lesions in certain anatomical locations, in acknowledgement of their ongoing clinical acceptance. For example, the term "dysplasia" is preferred for lesions in the tubular gut, whereas "intraepithelial neoplasia" is preferred for those in the pancreas, gallbladder, and biliary tree. For all anatomical sites, however, a two-tiered system (low-grade vs high-grade) is considered the standard grading system for neoplastic precursor lesions. This has replaced the three-tiered grading scheme previously used for lesions in the pancreatobiliary system {267}. The term "carcinoma in situ" continues to be strongly discouraged in clinical practice for a variety of reasons, most notably its clinical ambiguity. This term is encompassed by the category of high-grade dysplasia / intraepithelial neoplasia. Genomic findings have helped to determine that some tumours, such as pancreatic intraductal neoplasms (i.e. intraductal oncocytic papillary neoplasm and intraductal tubulopapillary neoplasm) are distinct from pancreatic intraductal papillary mucinous neoplasms, and these tumours are now classified as separate entities. Additional clinical and genomic information has also helped in the identification of carcinoma subtypes that are distinct enough to warrant separate classification.

Many refinements of the fourth-edition classification have been made concerning liver tumours, supported by novel molecular findings. For example, a comprehensive picture of the molecular changes that occur in common hepatocellular carcinoma has recently emerged from large-scale molecular profiling studies. Meanwhile, several rarer hepatocellular carcinoma subtypes, which together may account for 20–30% of cases, have been defined by consistent morphomolecular and clinical features, with fibrolamellar carcinoma and its diagnostic DNAJB1-PRKACA translocation being one prime example. Intrahepatic cholangiocarcinoma is now understood to be a distinct entity with two very specific subtypes: a large duct type, which resembles extrahepatic cholangiocarcinoma, and a small duct type, which shares etiological, pathogenetic, and imaging characteristics with hepatocellular carcinoma. The two subtypes have very different etiologies, molecular alterations, growth patterns, and clinical behaviours, exemplifying the conflict between anatomically and histogenetically/pathogenetically based classifications. Clinical research and study protocols will need to incorporate these findings in the near future. Also supported by molecular findings, the definition of combined hepatocellular-cholangiocarcinoma and its distinction from other entities have recently become clearer. Cholangiolocellular carcinoma is no longer considered a subtype of combined hepatocellular-cholangiocarcinoma, but rather a subtype of small duct intrahepatic cholangiocarcinoma, meaning that all intrahepatic carcinomas with a ductal or tubular phenotype are now included within the category of intrahepatic cholangiocarcinoma. A classic example of morphology-based molecular profiling leading to a new classification based on a combination of biological and molecular factors is the classification of hepatocellular adenomas, which has gained a high degree of clinical relevance and has fuelled the implementation of refined morphological criteria and molecular testing in routine diagnostics.

In this fifth-edition volume, haematolymphoid tumours and mesenchymal tumours that occur in the GI tract, some of which are very distinctive, have been grouped together in their own separate chapters, to ensure consistency and avoid duplication. The importance of genetic tumour syndromes has also been highlighted in this edition by their inclusion in a dedicated chapter, consolidating the increased knowledge of these disorders in a way that we hope will be helpful to all readers.

Classification of neuroendocrine neoplasms of the digestive system

Klimstra DS
Klöppel G
La Rosa S
Rindi G

General characteristics of NENs

Neuroendocrine neoplasms (NENs) can arise in most epithelial organs of the body and include many varieties, with widely differing etiologies, clinical features, morphological and genomic findings, and outcomes. Historically, NENs of the various anatomical sites have been classified separately, and although the various classification systems have shared some common features {1630}, differences in terminology and classification criteria between organ systems have caused considerable confusion. In 2018, WHO published a uniform classification framework for all NENs {2717}, based on a consensus conference held in November 2017. The key feature of this new, common classification is the distinction between well-differentiated neuroendocrine tumours (NETs), which were previously designated carcinoid tumours when occurring in the GI tract, and poorly differentiated neuroendocrine carcinomas (NECs), which share with NETs the expression of neuroendocrine markers but are now known not to be closely related neoplasms. The morphological classification of NENs into NETs and NECs is supported by genetic evidence, as well as by clinical, epidemiological, histological, and prognostic differences.

NETs are graded as G1, G2, or G3 on the basis of proliferative activity as assessed by mitotic count and the Ki-67 proliferation index {3431}. Mitotic counts are to be expressed as the number of mitoses/2 mm^2 (equalling 10 high-power fields at 40× magnification and an ocular field diameter of 0.5 mm) as determined by counting in 50 fields of 0.2 mm^2 (i.e. in a total area of 10 mm^2), although it is recognized that an accurate rate may not be possible to determine when only a small sample is available. The Ki-67 proliferation index value is determined by counting at least 500 cells in the regions of highest labelling (hotspots), which are identified at scanning magnification. In the event that the two proliferation indicators suggest different grades, the higher grade is assigned; generally, when there is discordance, it is the Ki-67 proliferation index that indicates the higher grade {2096}. NECs are considered high-grade by definition. The current classification and grading system is largely based on the 2017 WHO classification of neoplasms of the neuroendocrine pancreas {1936}, which formally introduced the concept that well-differentiated neoplasms could be high-grade {272}. In earlier classifications of both pancreatic and gastrointestinal NENs, the G3 category was considered to be synonymous with poor differentiation (i.e. NEC). However, after the publication of data related to pancreatic NETs (PanNETs), it became clear that NETs of other organs can also have a proliferative rate in the G3 range {3256}, justifying the extension of the pancreatic classification system in the current edition of the WHO classification to NENs occurring throughout the GI tract.

The rationale for a sharp separation of NETs and NECs into different families comes from a variety of sources. Although they share neuroendocrine differentiation based on immunolabelling for chromogranin A and synaptophysin, most NETs are morphologically distinct from NECs, which are subtyped as small cell NEC (SCNEC) and large cell NEC (LCNEC). NETs have an organoid architecture (e.g. nests, cords, and ribbons), uniform nuclear features, coarsely stippled chromatin, and minimal necrosis. NECs have a less nested architectural pattern, often growing in sheets, and they have either tightly packed fusiform nuclei with finely granular chromatin (SCNEC) or more-rounded, markedly atypical nuclei, sometimes with prominent nucleoli (LCNEC); necrosis is usually abundant. NETs may show grade progression, either within an individual tumour at presentation or between different sites of disease (e.g. primary vs metastasis) during the course of tumour progression. The presence of

Table 1.01 Classification and grading criteria for neuroendocrine neoplasms (NENs) of the GI tract and hepatopancreatobiliary organs

Terminology	Differentiation	Grade	Mitotic count[a] (mitoses/2 mm^2)	Ki-67 index[a]
NET, G1		Low	< 2	< 3%
NET, G2	Well differentiated	Intermediate	2–20	3–20%
NET, G3		High	> 20	> 20%
NEC, small cell type (SCNEC)	Poorly differentiated	High[b]	> 20	> 20%
NEC, large cell type (LCNEC)			> 20	> 20%
MiNEN	Well or poorly differentiated[c]	Variable[c]	Variable[c]	Variable[c]

LCNEC, large cell neuroendocrine carcinoma; MiNEN, mixed neuroendocrine–non-neuroendocrine neoplasm; NEC, neuroendocrine carcinoma; NET, neuroendocrine tumour; SCNEC, small cell neuroendocrine carcinoma.

[a]Mitotic counts are to be expressed as the number of mitoses/2 mm^2 (equalling 10 high-power fields at 40× magnification and an ocular field diameter of 0.5 mm) as determined by counting in 50 fields of 0.2 mm^2 (i.e. in a total area of 10 mm^2); the Ki-67 proliferation index value is determined by counting at least 500 cells in the regions of highest labelling (hotspots), which are identified at scanning magnification; the final grade is based on whichever of the two proliferation indexes places the neoplasm in the higher grade category. [b]Poorly differentiated NECs are not formally graded but are considered high-grade by definition. [c]In most MiNENs, both the neuroendocrine and non-neuroendocrine components are poorly differentiated, and the neuroendocrine component has proliferation indexes in the same range as other NECs, but this conceptual category allows for the possibility that one or both components may be well differentiated; when feasible, each component should therefore be graded separately.

both low-grade and high-grade components within an individual NET provides strong evidence that the high-grade component remains a well-differentiated neoplasm. In contrast, NECs do not commonly arise in association with NETs, but instead arise from precursor lesions that typically give rise to non-neuroendocrine carcinomas of the respective organs, such as adenomas in the colorectum or squamous dysplasia in the oesophagus. NECs may also contain non-neuroendocrine carcinoma elements such as adenocarcinoma or squamous cell carcinoma. Mixed neoplasms in which both components (neuroendocrine and non-neuroendocrine) are substantial (each accounting for ≥ 30% of the neoplasm), are classified into the general category of mixed neuroendocrine–non-neuroendocrine neoplasms (MiNENs), and they only exceptionally contain a well-differentiated (NET) component in addition to the non-neuroendocrine neoplasm. Emerging genomic data have provided further evidence that NETs and NECs are unrelated. In the pancreas in particular, frequent mutations in *MEN1*, *DAXX*, and *ATRX* are entity-defining for well-differentiated NETs {1463} and are not found in poorly differentiated NECs, which instead have mutations in *TP53*, *RB1*, and other carcinoma-associated genes {3632,1681,1682}. Sporadic PanNETs are also associated with germline mutations in the DNA repair genes *MUTYH*, *CHEK2*, and *BRCA2* {3500}. Even the G3 NETs of the pancreas retain the mutation profile of other well-differentiated neoplasms, providing a means to distinguish G3 NETs from NECs in challenging cases {3055,3253}. Genomic comparisons of NETs and NECs of other gastrointestinal sites are still emerging. NECs of these sites share frequent *TP53* and *RB1* mutations with NECs of the pancreas (and lung) {3577,1450}, but extrapancreatic NETs generally lack frequent recurrent mutations {233,961}, reducing the value of genomic analysis for diagnostic purposes, although extrapancreatic NETs do share abnormalities in chromatin remodelling pathways with their pancreatic counterparts.

There are also data supporting the distinction between G3 NETs and NECs from a clinical perspective. The common response of NECs to platinum-containing chemotherapy (which is dramatic in the case of SCNECs) led to the standard use of these regimens for the treatment of NECs of diverse anatomical origins {3153}. However, it was recognized that a subset of patients, probably patients who in fact had G3 NETs, failed to respond but paradoxically survived longer than the others {3104}. Alternative approved therapies are available for some subsets of NETs {1716}; therefore, there is a clinical need to distinguish NETs from NECs within the high-grade category.

One difference between the current WHO classification and the fourth-edition classification of tumours of the pancreas concerns the assignment of a grade for NECs. Previously, all NECs were graded G3, like high-grade NETs. The current proposal is not to assign a grade to NECs (they are all high-grade by definition), in order to avoid confusion about neoplasms within the G3 category.

The recently published proposal for a uniform classification of NENs {2717} is now formally adopted in this WHO classification of tumours arising throughout the entire GI tract and in the hepatopancreatobiliary organs. The terminology and grading criteria are presented in Table 1.01). The specific features of NETs, NECs, and MiNENs of individual organs are described in each organ's respective chapter. It is important to remember that despite the use of uniform terminology, there are important organ-specific differences among NENs in terms of hormonal function, clinical presentation, prognosis, morphology, and genomics; the current classification system is intended to standardize the approach to diagnosis and grading, but not to replace the key additional information to be included in pathological diagnoses reflecting the unique features of each NEN.

Well-differentiated NENs: NETs

Neuroendocrine tumours (NETs) are well-differentiated epithelial neoplasms with morphological and immunohistochemical features of neuroendocrine differentiation, most typically showing organoid architecture, uniform nuclei, and coarsely granular chromatin. NETs can be low-grade (G1), intermediate-grade (G2), or high-grade (G3).

NETs are a broad family of related neoplasms that can arise in any organ in the GI tract and hepatopancreatobiliary system. Former terms include "carcinoid tumour" and (for pancreatic tumours) "islet cell tumour" and "pancreatic endocrine neoplasm". The well-differentiated nature of NETs means that the neoplastic cells bear a strong resemblance to non-neoplastic neuroendocrine cells, usually including strong immunoexpression of general neuroendocrine markers (chromogranin A and synaptophysin) along with variable expression of specific peptide hormones. The morphological features of NETs are highly varied, and some organ-specific subtypes have characteristic histological patterns (see the individual sections in each organ's respective chapter). However, NETs generally display characteristic architectural patterns including nests, cords, and ribbons. Gland formation by the neoplastic cells is common, especially in the ileum and pancreas, as well as in a subset of appendiceal and duodenal NETs. The nuclei often contain coarsely clumped chromatin, giving rise to the classic salt-and-pepper appearance, but some NETs show more diffusely granular chromatin and others have prominent nucleoli. The cytoplasm may show intense granularity, reflecting abundant neurosecretory granules that are oriented towards the vascular pole of the cells. Most NETs have a low proliferative rate, defined in the fourth-edition digestive system tumours volume by a mitotic count of < 20 mitoses/2 mm² and a Ki-67 proliferation index of < 20% {379}. Although the mitotic count is indeed found to be within this range in almost all cases, it is now clear that some NETs, in particular those arising in the pancreas, have a Ki-67 proliferation index of > 20%, and values as high as 70–80% have been observed in some cases. Therefore, the Ki-67 proliferation index alone cannot be used to conclusively distinguish NETs from neuroendocrine carcinomas (NECs).

An important clinical distinction among NETs relates to their hormonal functionality. Functioning NETs are defined as those associated with characteristic clinical syndromes related to the abnormal production of hormones by the neoplasm. Clinically non-functioning NETs may also produce hormones, which can be detected in the serum or in the tumour cells using immunohistochemistry, but the hormones do not result in clinical symptoms. The nomenclature for functioning NETs often includes the name of the specific hormone causing the syndrome (insulinoma, gastrinoma, glucagonoma, etc.). The pancreas gives rise to the greatest variety of functioning NETs (see *Functioning pancreatic neuroendocrine tumours*, p. 353). Functioning gastrin-producing NETs (gastrinomas) typically occur in the duodenum, and NETs that cause carcinoid syndrome usually arise in the ileum. Most gastric NETs are non-functioning, although the conditions associated with hypergastrinaemia (including gastrinomas themselves) can induce NETs composed of enterochromaffin-like (ECL) cells in the oxyntic mucosa of the stomach. NETs of the bile ducts, liver, and colorectum are also usually non-functioning. Another characteristic feature of NETs is the expression of somatostatin receptors (in particular, abundant SSTR2), which can be detected by immunohistochemistry or using functional radiographical imaging, such as octreoscan and 68Ga-DOTATOC/DOTATATE/DOTANOC PET-CT. NETs are usually not detectable by FDG PET, with the exception of rare high-grade examples. Another distinctive clinical feature of NETs is their indolent natural history. Although all NETs are considered to be malignant neoplasms, early-stage NETs of all anatomical sites have a low risk of metastasis if they are entirely removed. Larger or higher-grade NETs can metastasize and are difficult to treat, but survival for many years is still possible, even in advanced stages.

The uniformity of the classification and grading system for gastroenteropancreatic NETs presented in this volume should not be interpreted as suggestive that NETs are a homogeneous group of closely related neoplasms; this is far from the case. Each organ gives rise to different types of NETs, with different functionality, different histological features, and different genomic underpinnings. Certain types of NETs (e.g. pancreatic and duodenal) occur commonly in patients with multiple endocrine neoplasia type 1 and are associated with frequent somatic mutations in *MEN1*, whereas other NETs (e.g. ileal and rectal) are not associated with this syndrome or with mutations in *MEN1*. There are also prognostic differences among NETs of different sites. These distinctive clinical features mean that the surgical and medical treatment of NETs is highly dependent on the site of origin. Attempts to determine the origin of NETs presenting with distant metastases can involve both radiographical and pathological techniques (e.g. immunohistochemistry for site-specific transcription factors {3674}).

Poorly differentiated NENs: NECs

Neuroendocrine carcinomas (NECs) are poorly differentiated epithelial neoplasms with morphological and immunohistochemical features of neuroendocrine differentiation. NECs can be small cell NEC (SCNEC), which displays fusiform nuclei with finely granular chromatin, scant cytoplasm, and nuclear moulding, or large cell NEC (LCNEC), which has round nuclei, sometimes with prominent nucleoli, and moderate amounts of cytoplasm. All NECs are high-grade neoplasms.

Like neuroendocrine tumours (NETs), NECs can arise in most sites within the gastroenteropancreatic system and may be pure or mixed with variable amounts of adenocarcinoma, squamous cell carcinoma, or other components. Previously, the term "neuroendocrine carcinoma" was also used for well-differentiated NETs with evidence of malignant behaviour (i.e. metastasis), but in the current classification the term "carcinoma" is reserved for poorly differentiated neoplasms. NECs are generally subclassified as SCNEC or LCNEC; however, this distinction can be challenging at some sites within the GI tract {2995}. NECs are considered to be high-grade by definition, with a mitotic count of > 20 mitoses/2 mm^2 and a Ki-67 proliferation index of > 20%. In most instances, these thresholds are substantially exceeded; however, NECs may occasionally have a Ki-67 proliferation

index of 20–50%, especially after exposure to chemotherapy, so the Ki-67 proliferation index cannot be used to conclusively distinguish a NEC from a G3 NET {3253}. Necrosis is commonly extensive. Demonstration of neuroendocrine differentiation is necessary to confirm the diagnosis of NEC. For the diagnosis of LCNEC, expression of either synaptophysin or chromogranin A must be present. The exact extent and intensity of staining required for the diagnosis have not yet been explicitly defined, but more than scattered positive cells should be present, and the morphology should also be suggestive of neuroendocrine differentiation.

NECs are somewhat more homogeneous among different sites of origin than are NETs. The morphological patterns overlap, as do the genomic alterations, which include common mutations in *TP53* and *RB1*. Additional organ-specific mutations that typify non-neuroendocrine carcinomas of the same site may also be found {3632,3587}. NECs lack mutations in the genes most commonly involved in the pathogenesis of NETs.

NECs are highly aggressive neoplasms, usually even more so than the more common types of carcinoma to arise at the same site. Advanced stage at presentation is common; therefore, chemotherapy is often the primary therapeutic approach, and it may be the initial treatment choice even for surgically resectable cases {3153}. Considerable evidence supports the treatment of extrapulmonary SCNEC with a platinum-containing regimen; anecdotal evidence of responses to similar regimens in LCNECs has promoted the widespread practice of treating all NECs with platinum-containing regimens, but there are no randomized clinical trials showing superior efficacy compared with the alternative regimens used for non-neuroendocrine carcinomas. Defining the molecular basis for responsiveness to platinum remains an area of active investigation.

Mixed neoplasms: MiNENs

Mixed neuroendocrine–non-neuroendocrine neoplasms (MiNENs) are mixed epithelial neoplasms in which a neuroendocrine component is combined with a non-neuroendocrine component, each of which is morphologically and immunohistochemically recognizable as a discrete component and constitutes ≥ 30% of the neoplasm.

Most epithelial neoplasms in the GI tract and hepatopancreatobiliary system are classified as either pure glandular or squamous neoplasms (or their precursors) or pure neuroendocrine neoplasms (NENs). Glandular (and to a lesser extent squamous) neoplasms may have a minor population of interspersed neuroendocrine cells that can be identified by immunohistochemistry, but this finding does not affect the classification. Less commonly, epithelial neoplasms are composed of quantitatively considerable neuroendocrine and non-neuroendocrine cell populations. Previously, when each component represented ≥ 30% of the neoplasm, these mixed neoplasms were classified under the category of "mixed adenoneuroendocrine carcinoma (MANEC)". However, in recognition that the non-neuroendocrine component may not be adenocarcinoma, and to reflect the possibility that one or both components may not be carcinoma, the current term for this category is "mixed neuroendocrine–non-neuroendocrine neoplasm (MiNEN)". MiNEN is regarded as a conceptual category of neoplasms rather than a specific diagnosis. Different types of MiNENs arise in different sites throughout the gastroenteropancreatic system,

Box 1.01 Specific subtypes of mixed neuroendocrine–non-neuroendocrine neoplasms (MiNENs) of the GI tract and hepatopancreatobiliary organs

Oesophagus and oesophagogastric junction
• Mixed SCC-NEC (SCNEC or LCNEC)
• Mixed adenocarcinoma-NEC (SCNEC or LCNEC)
• Mixed adenocarcinoma-NET {1249}

Stomach
• Mixed adenocarcinoma-NEC (SCNEC or LCNEC)
• Mixed adenocarcinoma-NET {1758,1754}

Small intestine and ampulla
• Mixed adenocarcinoma-NEC (SCNEC or LCNEC)

Appendix
• Mixed adenocarcinoma-NEC (SCNEC or LCNEC)
• Mixed adenocarcinoma-NET

Colon and rectum
• Mixed adenocarcinoma-NEC (SCNEC or LCNEC)
• Mixed adenocarcinoma-NET

Anal canal
• Mixed SCC-NEC (SCNEC or LCNEC)

Liver
• Mixed hepatocellular carcinoma–NEC
• Mixed cholangiocarcinoma-NEC

Gallbladder and bile ducts
• Mixed adenocarcinoma-NEC (SCNEC or LCNEC)

Pancreas
• Mixed ductal carcinoma–NEC (SCNEC or LCNEC)
• Mixed ductal adenocarcinoma–NET
• Mixed acinar cell carcinoma–NEC (distinct components)
• Mixed acinar cell carcinoma–ductal carcinoma–NEC (distinct components)

LCNEC, large cell neuroendocrine carcinoma; NEC, neuroendocrine carcinoma; NET, neuroendocrine tumour; SCC, squamous cell carcinoma; SCNEC, small cell neuroendocrine carcinoma.

and each should be diagnosed using site-specific terminology that reflects the nature of the components. Box 1.01 lists the specific neoplasms that are included in the MiNEN category, by anatomical site.

For a neoplasm to qualify as MiNEN, both components should be morphologically and immunohistochemically recognizable. The presence of neuroendocrine differentiation in the neuroendocrine component should be confirmed by immunolabelling for synaptophysin and/or chromogranin. In MiNENs arising in the GI tract and hepatopancreatobiliary system, both components are usually carcinomas; therefore, the neuroendocrine component is usually poorly differentiated neuroendocrine carcinoma (NEC) and can be either large cell NEC (LCNEC) or small cell NEC (SCNEC). Rarely, the neuroendocrine component of a MiNEN may be well differentiated. NENs can arise in association with carcinoma precursors such as adenomas of the tubular GI tract or intraductal or cystic neoplasms of the pancreas. However, neoplasms in which the non-neuroendocrine component consists solely of a precursor (preinvasive) neoplasm are not considered MiNENs. Similarly, independent neuroendocrine and non-neuroendocrine neoplasms arising in the same organ should not be classified as MiNEN, even if they abut one another (true collision tumours), because the MiNEN category applies only to neoplasms in which the two components are presumed to be clonally related. Carcinomas previously treated with neoadjuvant therapy should not be considered MiNENs either, unless the diagnosis of MiNEN is established based on a pretreatment specimen, because the neuroendocrine morphology exhibited by some treated carcinomas may not have the same prognostic significance as that seen in a de novo component of NEC {2996,2993}.

By arbitrary convention, each component should constitute ≥ 30% of a neoplasm for the neoplasm to be included in the MiNEN category; the presence of focal (< 30%) neuroendocrine differentiation may be mentioned in the diagnosis (in particular when the component is poorly differentiated) but does not affect the diagnostic categorization. However, an important consideration is the finding of focal (< 30%) SCNEC associated with a non-neuroendocrine neoplasm. Because of the clear clinical significance of SCNEC, even minor components should be mentioned in the diagnosis. When feasible, the two components of MiNENs should be graded individually; some data suggest that the grade of the neuroendocrine component correlates with prognosis {2163}. The non-neuroendocrine component should be classified as adenocarcinoma, acinar cell carcinoma (in the pancreas), squamous cell carcinoma, or any other definable tumour category as appropriate. In general, MiNENs composed of an adenocarcinoma with a NEC component, for which the designation MANEC can be retained, show poor prognosis (overlapping with that of pure NEC), independent of the non-neuroendocrine component {2163}. MiNENs composed of adenocarcinoma and neuroendocrine tumour (NET) have been reported, but their prognostic significance requires further study {1758,1754}. The intensity and degree of the immunolabelling of the neuroendocrine component for synaptophysin and chromogranin A should be documented.

TNM staging of well-differentiated neuroendocrine tumours of the gastrointestinal tract

Well-Differentiated Neuroendocrine Tumours of the Gastrointestinal Tract

Rules for Classification

This classification system applies to well-differentiated neuroendocrine tumours (carcinoid tumours and atypical carcinoid tumours) of the gastrointestinal tract, including the pancreas. Neuroendocrine tumours of the lung should be classified according to criteria for carcinoma of the lung. Merkel cell carcinoma of the skin has a separate classification.

High-grade (Grade 3) neuroendocrine carcinomas are excluded and should be classified according to criteria for classifying carcinomas at the respective site.

Well-Differentiated Neuroendocrine Tumours (G1 and G2) – Gastric, Jejunum/Ileum, Appendix, Colonic, and Rectal

Regional lymph nodes
The regional lymph nodes correspond to those listed under the appropriate sites for carcinoma.

TNM Clinical Classification
Stomach
T – Primary Tumour

TX	Primary tumour cannot be assessed
T0	No evidence of primary tumour
T1	Tumour invades mucosa or submucosa and 1 cm or less in greatest dimension
T2	Tumour invades muscularis propria or is more than 1 cm in greatest dimension
T3	Tumour invades subserosa
T4	Tumour perforates visceral peritoneum (serosa) or invades other organs or adjacent structures

Note
For any T, add (m) for multiple tumours.

N – Regional Lymph Nodes

NX	Regional lymph nodes cannot be assessed
N0	No regional lymph node metastasis
N1	Regional lymph node metastasis

M – Distant Metastasis

M0	No distant metastasis	
M1	Distant metastasis	
	M1a	Hepatic metastasis only
	M1b	Extrahepatic metastasis only
	M1c	Hepatic and extrahepatic metastases

Stage

Stage	T	N	M
Stage I	T1	N0	M0
Stage II	T2,T3	N0	M0
Stage III	T4	N0	M0
	Any T	N1	M0
Stage IV	Any T	Any N	M1

TNM Clinical Classification
Duodenal/Ampullary Tumours
T – Primary Tumour

TX	Primary tumour cannot be assessed
T0	No evidence of primary tumour
T1	*Duodenal:* Tumour invades mucosa or submucosa and 1 cm or less in greatest dimension *Ampullary:* Tumour 1 cm or less in greatest dimension and confined within the sphincter of Oddi
T2	*Duodenal:* Tumour invades muscularis propria or is more than 1 cm in greatest dimension *Ampullary:* Tumour invades through sphincter into duodenal submucosa or muscularis propria, or more than 1 cm in greatest dimension
T3	Tumour invades the pancreas or peripancreatic adipose tissue
T4	Tumour perforates visceral peritoneum (serosa) or invades other organs

Note
For any T, add (m) for multiple tumours.

N – Regional Lymph Nodes

NX	Regional lymph nodes cannot be assessed
N0	No regional lymph node metastasis
N1	Regional lymph node metastasis

M – Distant Metastasis

M0	No distant metastasis	
M1	Distant metastasis	
	M1a	Hepatic metastasis only
	M1b	Extrahepatic metastasis only
	M1c	Hepatic and extrahepatic metastases

Stage

Stage	T	N	M
Stage I	T1	N0	M0
Stage II	T2,T3	N0	M0
Stage III	T4	N0	M0
	Any T	N1	M0
Stage IV	Any T	Any N	M1

The information presented here has been excerpted from the 2017 *TNM classification of malignant tumours*, eighth edition (408,3385A). © 2017 UICC. A help desk for specific questions about the TNM classification is available at https://www.uicc.org/tnm-help-desk.

TNM Clinical Classification
Jejunum/Ileum
T – Primary Tumour
TX   Primary tumour cannot be assessed
T0   No evidence of primary tumour
T1   Tumour invades mucosa or submucosa and 1 cm or less in greatest dimension
T2   Tumour invades muscularis propria or is greater than 1 cm in greatest dimension
T3   Tumour invades through the muscularis propria into subserosal tissue without penetration of overlying serosa (jejunal or ileal)
T4   Tumour perforates visceral peritoneum (serosa) or invades other organs or adjacent structures

Note
For any T, add (m) for multiple tumours.

N – Regional Lymph Nodes
NX   Regional lymph nodes cannot be assessed
N0   No regional lymph node metastasis
N1   Less than 12 regional lymph node metastasis without mesenteric mass(es) greater than 2 cm in size
N2   12 or more regional nodes and/or mesenteric mass(es) greater than 2 cm in maximum dimension

M – Distant Metastasis
M0   No distant metastasis
M1   Distant metastasis
     M1a   Hepatic metastasis only
     M1b   Extrahepatic metastasis only
     M1c   Hepatic and extrahepatic metastases

Stage

Stage			
Stage I	T1	N0	M0
Stage II	T2,T3	N0	M0
Stage III	T4	Any N	M0
	Any T	N1,N2	M0
Stage IV	Any T	Any N	M1

TNM Clinical Classification
Appendix
T – Primary Tumour[a]
TX   Primary tumour cannot be assessed
T0   No evidence of primary tumour
T1   Tumour 2 cm or less in greatest dimension
T2   Tumour more than 2 cm but not more than 4 cm in greatest dimension
T3   Tumour more than 4 cm or with subserosal invasion or involvement of the mesoappendix
T4   Tumour perforates peritoneum or invades other adjacent organs or structures, other than direct mural extension to adjacent subserosa, e.g., abdominal wall and skeletal muscle[b]

Notes
[a] High-grade neuroendocrine carcinomas, mixed adenoneuroendocrine carcinomas and goblet cell carcinoid, are excluded and should be classified according to criteria for classifying carcinomas.
[b] Tumour that is adherent to other organs or structures, macroscopically, is classified T4. However, if no tumour is present in the adhesion, microscopically, the tumour should be classified as pT1–3 as appropriate.

N – Regional Lymph Nodes
NX   Regional lymph nodes cannot be assessed
N0   No regional lymph node metastasis
N1   Regional lymph node metastasis

M – Distant Metastasis
M0   No distant metastasis
M1   Distant metastasis
     M1a   Hepatic metastasis only
     M1b   Extrahepatic metastasis only
     M1c   Hepatic and extrahepatic metastases

pTNM Pathological Classification
The pT and pN categories correspond to the T and N categories.

pN0   Histological examination of a regional lymphadenectomy specimen will ordinarily include 12 or more lymph nodes. If the lymph nodes are negative, but the number ordinarily examined is not met, classify as pN0.

pM – Distant Metastasis*
pM1   Distant metastasis microscopically confirmed

Note
* pM0 and pMX are not valid categories.

Stage

Stage			
Stage I	T1	N0	M0
Stage II	T2,T3	N0	M0
Stage III	T4	N0	M0
	Any T	N1	M0
Stage IV	Any T	Any N	M1

TNM Clinical Classification
Colon and Rectum
T – Primary Tumour

TX   Primary tumour cannot be assessed
T0   No evidence of primary tumour
T1   Tumour invades lamina propria or submucosa or is no
      greater than 2 cm in size
    T1a   Tumour less than 1 cm in size
    T1b   Tumour 1 or 2 cm in size
T2   Tumour invades muscularis propria or is greater than 2 cm
      in size
T3   Tumour invades subserosa, or non-peritonealized pericolic
      or perirectal tissues
T4   Tumour perforates the visceral peritoneum or invades other
      organs

Note
For any T, add (m) for multiple tumours.

N – Regional Lymph Nodes

NX   Regional lymph nodes cannot be assessed
N0   No regional lymph node metastasis
N1   Regional lymph node metastasis

M – Distant Metastasis

M0   No distant metastasis
M1   Distant metastasis
    M1a   Hepatic metastasis only
    M1b   Extrahepatic metastasis only
    M1c   Hepatic and extrahepatic metastases

pTNM Pathological Classification
The pT and pN categories correspond to the T and N categories.

pM – Distant Metastasis*

pM1   Distant metastasis microscopically confirmed

Note
* pM0 and pMX are not valid categories.

Stage

Stage			
Stage I	T1	N0	M0
Stage IIA	T2	N0	M0
Stage IIB	T3	N0	M0
Stage IIIA	T4	N0	M0
Stage IIIB	Any T	N1	M0
Stage IV	Any T	Any N	M1

Well-Differentiated Neuroendocrine Tumours – Pancreas (G1 and G2)

Rules for Classification
This classification system applies to well-differentiated neuroendocrine tumours (carcinoid tumours and atypical carcinoid tumours) of the pancreas.
 High-grade neuroendocrine carcinomas are excluded and should be classified according to criteria for classifying carcinomas of the pancreas.

Regional Lymph Nodes
The regional lymph nodes correspond to those listed under the appropriate sites for carcinoma.

TNM Clinical Classification
Pancreas
T – Primary Tumour[a]

TX   Primary tumour cannot be assessed
T0   No evidence of primary tumour
T1   Tumour limited to pancreas,[b] 2 cm or less in greatest
      dimension
T2   Tumour limited to pancreas[b] more than 2 cm but less than
      4 cm in greatest dimension
T3   Tumour limited to pancreas,[b] more than 4 cm in greatest
      dimension or tumour invading duodenum or bile duct.
T4   Tumour invades adjacent organs (stomach, spleen, colon,
      adrenal gland) or the wall of large vessels (coeliac axis or
      the superior mesenteric artery)

Notes
[a] For any T, add (m) for multiple tumours.
[b] Invasion of adjacent peripancreatic adipose tissue is accepted but invasion of adjacent organs is excluded.

N – Regional Lymph Nodes

NX   Regional lymph nodes cannot be assessed
N0   No regional lymph node metastasis
N1   Regional lymph node metastasis

M – Distant Metastasis

M0   No distant metastasis
M1   Distant metastasis
    M1a   Hepatic metastasis only
    M1b   Extrahepatic metastasis only
    M1c   Hepatic and extrahepatic metastases

Stage

Stage			
Stage I	T1	N0	M0
Stage II	T2,T3	N0	M0
Stage III	T4	N0	M0
	Any T	N1	M0
Stage IV	Any T	Any N	M1

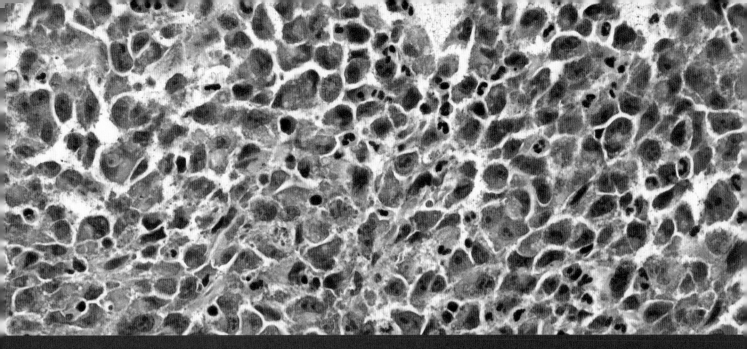

2

Tumours of the oesophagus

Edited by: Odze RD, Lam AK, Ochiai A, Washington MK

Benign epithelial tumours and precursors
  Squamous papilloma
  Barrett dysplasia
  Squamous dysplasia
Malignant epithelial tumours
  Adenocarcinoma of the oesophagus and oesophagogastric junction NOS
  Adenoid cystic carcinoma
  Adenosquamous and mucoepidermoid carcinomas
  Squamous cell carcinoma NOS
  Undifferentiated carcinoma
  Neuroendocrine neoplasms

WHO classification of tumours of the oesophagus

Benign epithelial tumours and precursors

8052/0	Squamous cell papilloma NOS
8060/0	Squamous papillomatosis
8148/0	Oesophageal glandular dysplasia (intraepithelial neoplasia), low grade
8148/2	Oesophageal glandular dysplasia (intraepithelial neoplasia), high grade
8077/0	Oesophageal squamous intraepithelial neoplasia (dysplasia), low grade
8077/2	Oesophageal squamous intraepithelial neoplasia (dysplasia), high grade

Malignant epithelial tumours

8140/3	Adenocarcinoma NOS
8200/3	Adenoid cystic carcinoma
8430/3	Mucoepidermoid carcinoma
8560/3	Adenosquamous carcinoma
8070/3	Squamous cell carcinoma NOS
8051/3	Verrucous squamous cell carcinoma
8074/3	Squamous cell carcinoma, spindle cell
8083/3	Basaloid squamous cell carcinoma
8020/3	Carcinoma, undifferentiated, NOS
8082/3	Lymphoepithelioma-like carcinoma
8240/3	Neuroendocrine tumour NOS
8240/3	Neuroendocrine tumour, grade 1
8249/3	Neuroendocrine tumour, grade 2
8249/3	Neuroendocrine tumour, grade 3
8246/3	Neuroendocrine carcinoma NOS
8013/3	Large cell neuroendocrine carcinoma
8041/3	Small cell neuroendocrine carcinoma
8154/3	Mixed neuroendocrine–non-neuroendocrine neoplasm (MiNEN)
8045/3	Combined small cell–adenocarcinoma
8045/3	Combined small cell–squamous cell carcinoma

These morphology codes are from the International Classification of Diseases for Oncology, third edition, second revision (ICD-O-3.2) {1378A}. Behaviour is coded /0 for benign tumours; /1 for unspecified, borderline, or uncertain behaviour; /2 for carcinoma in situ and grade III intraepithelial neoplasia; /3 for malignant tumours, primary site; and /6 for malignant tumours, metastatic site. Behaviour code /6 is not generally used by cancer registries.

This classification is modified from the previous WHO classification, taking into account changes in our understanding of these lesions.

TNM staging of tumours of the oesophagus

Oesophagus

(ICD-O-3 C15) Including Oesophagogastric Junction (C16.0)

Rules for Classification

The classification applies only to carcinomas and includes adenocarcinomas of the oesophagogastric/gastroesophageal junction. There should be histological confirmation of the disease and division of cases by topographic localization and histological type. A tumour the epicentre of which is within 2 cm of the **oesophagogastric junction** and also extends into the oesophagus is classified and staged using the oesophageal scheme. Cancers involving the oesophagogastric junction (OGJ) whose epicentre is within the proximal 2 cm of the cardia (Siewert types I/II) are to be staged as oesophageal cancers.

The following are the procedures for assessing T, N, and M categories.

T categories	Physical examination, imaging, endoscopy (including bronchoscopy), and/or surgical exploration
N categories	Physical examination, imaging, and/or surgical exploration
M categories	Physical examination, imaging, and/or surgical exploration

Anatomical Subsites

1. Cervical oesophagus (C15.0): this commences at the lower border of the cricoid cartilage and ends at the thoracic inlet (suprasternal notch), approximately 18 cm from the upper incisor teeth.
2. Intrathoracic oesophagus
   a) The upper thoracic portion (C15.3) extending from the thoracic inlet to the level of the tracheal bifurcation, approximately 24 cm from the upper incisor teeth
   b) The mid-thoracic portion (C15.4) is the proximal half of the oesophagus between the tracheal bifurcation and the oesophagogastric junction. The lower level is approximately 32 cm from the upper incisor teeth
   c) The lower thoracic portion (C15.5), approximately 8 cm in length (includes abdominal oesophagus), is the distal half of the oesophagus between the tracheal bifurcation and the oesophagogastric junction. The lower level is approximately 40 cm from the upper incisor teeth
3. Oesophagogastric junction (C16.0). Cancers involving the oesophagogastric junction (OGJ) whose epicentre is within the proximal 2 cm of the cardia (Siewert types I/II) are to be staged as oesophageal cancers. Cancers whose epicentre is more than 2 cm distal from the OGJ will be staged using the Stomach Cancer TNM and Stage even if the OGJ is involved.

Regional Lymph Nodes

The regional lymph nodes, irrespective of the site of the primary tumour, are those in the oesophageal drainage area including coeliac axis nodes and paraesophageal nodes in the neck but not the supraclavicular nodes.

TNM Clinical Classification

T – Primary Tumour

TX	Primary tumour cannot be assessed
T0	No evidence of primary tumour
Tis	Carcinoma in situ/high-grade dysplasia
T1	Tumour invades lamina propria, muscularis mucosae, or submucosa
	T1a Tumour invades lamina propria or muscularis mucosae
	T1b Tumour invades submucosa
T2	Tumour invades muscularis propria
T3	Tumour invades adventitia
T4	Tumour invades adjacent structures
	T4a Tumour invades pleura, pericardium, azygos vein, diaphragm, or peritoneum
	T4b Tumour invades other adjacent structures such as aorta, vertebral body, or trachea

N – Regional Lymph Nodes

NX	Regional lymph nodes cannot be assessed
N0	No regional lymph node metastasis
N1	Metastasis in 1 to 2 regional lymph nodes
N2	Metastasis in 3 to 6 regional lymph nodes
N3	Metastasis in 7 or more regional lymph nodes

M – Distant Metastasis

M0	No distant metastasis
M1	Distant metastasis

pTNM Pathological Classification

The pT and pN categories correspond to the T and N categories.

pN0   Histological examination of a regional lymphadenectomy specimen will ordinarily include 7 or more lymph nodes. If the lymph nodes are negative, but the number ordinarily examined is not met, classify as pN0.

pM – Distant Metastasis*

pM1   Distant metastasis microscopically confirmed

Note
* pM0 and pMX are not valid categories.

Stage and Prognostic Group – Carcinomas of the Oesophagus and Oesophagogastric Junction*

Squamous Cell Carcinoma
Clinical Stage

	T	N	M
Stage 0	Tis	N0	M0
Stage I	T1	N0,N1	M0
Stage II	T2	N0,N1	M0
	T3	N0	M0
Stage III	T1,T2	N2	M0
	T3	N1,N2	M0
Stage IVA	T4a,T4b	N0,N1,N2	M0
	Any T	N3	M0
Stage IVB	Any T	Any N	M1

Pathological Stage

	T	N	M
Stage 0	Tis	N0	M0
Stage IA	T1a	N0	M0
Stage IB	T1b	N0	M0
Stage IIA	T2	N0	M0
Stage IIB	T1	N1	M0
	T3	N0	M0
Stage IIIA	T1	N2	M0
	T2	N1	M0
Stage IIIB	T2	N2	M0
	T3	N1,N2	M0
	T4a	N0,N1	M0
Stage IVA	T4a	N2	M0
	T4b	Any N	M0
	Any T	N3	M0
Stage IVB	Any T	Any N	M1

Adenocarcinoma
Clinical Stage

	T	N	M
Stage 0	Tis	N0	M0
Stage I	T1	N0	M0
Stage IIA	T1	N1	M0
Stage IIB	T2	N0	M0
Stage III	T2	N1	M0
	T3,T4a	N0,N1	M0
Stage IVA	T1–T4a	N2	M0
	T4b	N0,N1,N2	M0
	Any T	N3	M0
Stage IVB	Any T	Any N	M1

Pathological Stage

	T	N	M
Stage 0	Tis	N0	M0
Stage IA	T1a	N0	M0
Stage IB	T1b	N0	M0
Stage IIA	T2	N0	M0
Stage IIB	T1	N1	M0
	T3	N0	M0
Stage IIIA	T1	N2	M0
	T2	N1	M0
Stage IIIB	T2	N2	M0
	T3	N1,N2	M0
	T4a	N0,N1	M0
Stage IVA	T4a	N2	M0
	T4b	Any N	M0
	Any T	N3	M0
Stage IVB	Any T	Any N	M1

Pathological Prognostic Group

Group	T	N	M	Grade	Location
Group 0	Tis	N0	M0	N/A	Any
Group IA	T1a	N0	M0	1,X	Any
Group IB	T1a	N0	M0	2–3	Any
	T1b	N0	M0	Any	Any
	T2	N0	M0	1	Any
Group IIA	T2	N0	M0	2–3,X	Any
	T3	N0	M0	Any	Lower
	T3	N0	M0	1	Upper, middle
Group IIB	T3	N0	M0	2–3	Upper, middle
	T3	N0	M0	Any	X
	T3	N0	M0	X	Any
	T1	N1	M0	Any	Any
Group IIIA	T1	N2	M0	Any	Any
	T2	N1	M0	Any	Any
Group IIIB	T2	N2	M0	Any	Any
	T3	N1,N2	M0	Any	Any
	T4a	N0,N1	M0	Any	Any
Group IVA	T4a	N2	M0	Any	Any
	T4b	Any N	M0	Any	Any
	Any T	N3	M0	Any	Any
Group IVB	Any T	Any N	M1	Any	Any

Pathological Prognostic Group

Group	T	N	M	Grade
Group 0	Tis	N0	M0	N/A
Group IA	T1a	N0	M0	1,X
Group IB	T1a	N0	M0	2
	T1b	N0	M0	1,2,X
Group IC	T1a,T1b	N0	M0	3
	T2	N0	M0	1,2
Group IIA	T2	N0	M0	3,X
Group IIB	T1	N1	M0	Any
	T3	N0		Any
Group IIIA	T1	N2	M0	Any
	T2	N1	M0	Any
Group IIIB	T2	N2	M0	Any
	T3	N1,N2	M0	Any
	T4a	N0,N1	M0	Any
Group IVA	T4a	N2	M0	Any
	T4b	Any N	M0	Any
	Any T	N3	M0	Any
Group IVB	Any T	Any N	M1	Any

Note
* The AJCC publishes prognostic groups for adenocarcinoma and squamous cell carcinoma after neoadjuvant therapy (categories with the prefix "y").

Tumours of the oesophagus: Introduction

Lam AK
Ochiai A
Odze RD

This chapter describes benign and malignant oesophageal tumours of epithelial differentiation and their precursor lesions. The ICD-O topographical coding for the anatomical sites covered in this chapter is presented in Box 2.01. The most common benign lesion, squamous papilloma, is addressed in a dedicated section. Throughout this fifth edition of the series, precursor lesions are typically described in separate sections from malignant tumours – a change from the fourth edition. The decision to make this change was based on the considerable expansion of our understanding of the biological and pathological features of precursor lesions and their relevance to clinical practice.

There are two main types of precursor lesions in the oesophagus: Barrett dysplasia and squamous dysplasia. Over the past 10 years or so, we have seen an important shift from surgery towards ablation for the treatment of Barrett oesophagus in patients with high-grade dysplasia. The same shift may eventually occur in the treatment of low-grade dysplasia, but this is currently a controversial issue. Therefore, the two-tiered (low-grade vs high-grade) system remains clinically useful for the time being, but this may change if ablation becomes the standard treatment for low-grade dysplasia as well. Regardless, we now have a much better understanding of the molecular pathways and pathological characteristics of carcinogenesis in Barrett oesophagus and its precursor lesions. The two most common types of dysplasia – intestinal and foveolar (gastric-type) – are now far better understood in terms of their pathological characteristics, biological behaviours, and clinical associations than a decade ago, but their distinction from non-neoplastic regenerative lesions remains a challenge and requires further research. Sampling error remains an issue of concern in surveillance programmes, but the increasing use of brush sampling and cytology-based diagnosis in the surveillance of Barrett oesophagus has already resulted in substantial improvements in the detection of goblet cells and dysplasia within both general and high-risk patient populations. There is ongoing controversy regarding the definition of Barrett oesophagus in different parts of the world: in the USA, goblet cells are an essential criterion for diagnosis, whereas this feature is not considered essential in Asian and European countries.

Squamous dysplasia remains a less well understood form of neoplasia in the oesophagus and a topic of disagreement between pathologists in different parts of the world. It is an uncommon entity, except in areas with high incidence of oesophageal squamous cell carcinoma where screening programmes are in place. One notable change since the fourth edition of this volume is that there is now wider agreement that a two-tiered grading system is preferable (because it is more reproducible and clinically more relevant) than a three-tiered system. However, oesophageal squamous dysplasia's pathological features and their variability, as well as the molecular characteristics, remain areas in need of further research.

Box 2.01 ICD-O topographical coding for the anatomical sites covered in this chapter

C15 Oesophagus
  C15.0 Cervical oesophagus
  C15.1 Thoracic oesophagus
  C15.2 Abdominal oesophagus
  C15.3 Upper third of the oesophagus
  C15.4 Middle third of the oesophagus
  C15.5 Lower third of the oesophagus
  C15.8 Overlapping lesion of the oesophagus
  C15.9 Oesophagus NOS

C16 Stomach
  C16.0 Oesophagogastric junction
  C16.0 Overlapping lesion of the digestive system

The two most common types of malignant epithelial tumours of the oesophagus are adenocarcinoma and squamous cell carcinoma. Subtypes of these entities have become better understood in recent years, and these new insights are covered in the tumours' respective sections. The incidence of these two types of oesophageal carcinomas varies in different parts of the world, and there have been improvements in our understanding of the reasons for this, such as certain environmental and dietary factors. One important change is that for patients who have not received neoadjuvant chemoradiation, the TNM staging criteria for these two carcinomas are now different. In recent years, neoadjuvant chemoradiotherapy has become a mainstay in the treatment of oesophageal carcinomas; as a result, there is increasing awareness of the effects of therapy on the morphology and molecular biology of carcinomas and their regression patterns, which are now incorporated into staging systems in recognition of their clinical relevance. For both squamous cell carcinoma and adenocarcinoma of the oesophagus, the two-tiered grading system for tumour differentiation is now strongly recommended.

In this fifth-edition volume, adenocarcinomas of the oesophagus and of the oesophagogastric junction are discussed together in a single section, because recent data suggest that these tumours share many etiological, histological, and biological features. However, readers should be aware of a change in the definition of adenocarcinoma of the oesophagogastric junction, which now includes any adenocarcinoma whose epicentre is within 2 cm of the junction.

There have recently been important advances in oesophageal carcinoma treatment related to the development of immunotherapy and targeted therapy. For example, ERBB2 (HER2) status is now considered a useful predictor of response to anti-ERBB2 therapy in adenocarcinoma of the oesophagogastric junction.

A subject of continued confusion is the definition and diagnostic criteria of mixed tumours, such as adenosquamous and mucoepidermoid carcinomas. These are rare tumours, but our poor understanding of their biological characteristics is mainly due to the lack of well-defined diagnostic criteria and lack of understanding of their pathogenesis. For example, there is controversy as to whether these two carcinomas are histological subtypes of squamous cell carcinoma or adenocarcinoma, although they seemingly arise in both conditions (at various rates in different parts of the world). Some may also arise from the oesophageal gland ducts, but it is unclear how such cases differ from those that arise from the mucosal epithelium.

Undifferentiated carcinoma is a tumour that lacks squamous, glandular, or neuroendocrine differentiation. In this fifth-edition volume, undifferentiated carcinoma is now considered a distinct entity rather than a subtype of squamous cell carcinoma.

Neuroendocrine neoplasms (NENs) of the oesophagus are uncommon. They are now classified according to the same criteria used for NENs in the pancreas and other parts of the GI tract. These classification criteria are described in more detail in the introductory section *Classification of neuroendocrine neoplasms of the digestive system* (p. 16).

Oesophageal squamous papilloma

Lam AK

Definition
Squamous papilloma of the oesophagus is a benign oesophageal epithelial polyp composed of squamous epithelium, usually with a papillary growth pattern.

ICD-O coding
8052/0 Squamous cell papilloma NOS

ICD-11 coding
2E92.0 & XH50T2 Benign neoplasm of oesophagus &
   Squamous cell papilloma

Related terminology
None

Subtype(s)
Squamous papillomatosis (8060/0)

Localization
In a large US series, 58% of squamous papillomas were located in the lower oesophagus {2502}. In Asian populations, squamous papilloma is more frequently found in the middle oesophagus. In a series from Taiwan, China, slightly more than half (54%) of squamous papillomas were located in the middle oesophagus {3594}.

Clinical features
Most patients with squamous papilloma are asymptomatic. Endoscopically, squamous papilloma appears as a small white exophytic growth with vessels crossing on a wart-like surface {3594}.

Epidemiology
Squamous papilloma is uncommon. The prevalence in endoscopic series ranges from 0.01% to 0.45% {705}. In a large endoscopy series from north-eastern France, the M:F ratio was 1.3:1 {705}. In many other populations, squamous papilloma is more common in females (with M:F ratios ranging from 0.2:1 to 0.8:1) {3594,3195}. Squamous papilloma typically presents in middle age (median age: 50 years) {705}. Squamous papillomatosis may present in paediatric {3050} or elderly {927} patients. Approximately 30 cases have been reported in the English-language literature {927,3050}.

Etiology
The causes of squamous papilloma include chronic mucosal irritation, HPV infection, and genetic syndromes. Chronic mucosal irritation can result from chemical factors (e.g. gastro-oesophageal reflux, alcohol consumption, cigarette smoking, and caustic injury) or mechanical factors (e.g. minor trauma, variceal sclerotherapy, self-expandable metal stents, chronic food impaction, nasogastric intubation, and bougie-assisted

oesophageal dilation) {705}. The etiological role of gastro-oesophageal reflux in squamous papilloma may explain why these lesions are frequently located in the lower oesophagus {705}. The observed prevalence of HPV infection in patients with squamous papilloma is as high as 87.5% in some series {705}. Squamous papillomatosis may occur in patients with focal dermal hypoplasia (also known as Goltz–Gorlin syndrome) {2540,313,1533} or angioma serpiginosum {347}; both genetic disorders are rare genodermatotic conditions that affect the X chromosome.

Pathogenesis
Chronic mucosal irritation or HPV infection leads to mucosal injury. The resulting hyperregenerative responses stimulate proliferation of the squamous mucosa, resulting in squamous papilloma. Oesophageal papillomas are hypothesized to be related to the high incidence of early-onset gastro-oesophageal reflux in focal dermal hypoplasia {1074}.

Macroscopic appearance
Macroscopically, squamous papillomas usually have a white, elevated, warty surface. The papillomas are often small (median diameter: 3 mm) {705}, but giant squamous papillomas have been reported {3196}.

Histopathology
Microscopic examination reveals a papillary proliferation of squamous epithelium with a fibrovascular core of lamina propria. Scattered vacuolated cells with morphological features of koilocytes are often seen. No atypical nuclear features and no viral inclusions are present. The proliferation patterns of squamous epithelium are most often exophytic {2408}, but they can also be endophytic or spiked. Rarely, dysplasia has been reported in squamous papilloma {705,2701}.

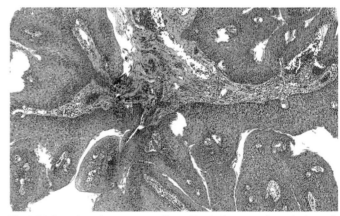

Fig. 2.01 Oesophageal squamous papilloma. Exophytic pattern of growth; the papillary fibrovascular core is surrounded by hyperplastic squamous epithelium with parakeratosis.

Squamous papilloma should be differentiated from fibrovascular polyp, which is typically located in the upper oesophagus and covered by stratified squamous epithelium, without papillary proliferation {1131}. Squamous papilloma must also be differentiated from squamous cell carcinoma, by excluding invasion.

Cytology
Not clinically relevant

Diagnostic molecular pathology
Not clinically relevant

Essential and desirable diagnostic criteria
Essential: papilloma consisting of squamous epithelium with fibrovascular cores.

Staging (TNM)
Not clinically relevant

Prognosis and prediction
Squamous papilloma does not recur after resection. Squamous cell carcinoma has been rarely reported to be associated with squamous papilloma or squamous papillomatosis {705,1465}.

Barrett dysplasia

Odze RD

Definition
Barrett dysplasia is defined by a morphologically unequivocal neoplastic epithelium without invasion, occurring in an area of metaplastic columnar epithelium in the oesophagus.

ICD-O coding
8148/0 Oesophageal glandular dysplasia (intraepithelial neoplasia), low grade

8148/2 Oesophageal glandular dysplasia (intraepithelial neoplasia), high grade

ICD-11 coding
DA23.1 Dysplasia of Barrett epithelium

2E92.0 & XH3K13 Benign neoplasm of oesophagus & Oesophageal glandular dysplasia (intraepithelial neoplasia), low-grade

2E60.1 & XH36M5 Carcinoma in situ of oesophagus & Oesophageal glandular dysplasia (intraepithelial neoplasia), high-grade

Related terminology
Low-grade Barrett dysplasia
Not recommended: glandular dysplasia.

High-grade Barrett dysplasia
Not recommended: columnar dysplasia.

Subtype(s)
None

Localization
Barrett dysplasia is restricted to metaplastic oesophageal mucosa.

Clinical features
There are no distinct clinical, radiological, or serological manifestations of dysplasia in Barrett oesophagus. Patients typically present because of the underlying Barrett oesophagus, with symptoms such as gastro-oesophageal reflux disease. Dysplasia may be visible endoscopically, appearing as a flat, plaque-like or irregular area of mucosa distinct from the surrounding non-dysplastic Barrett oesophagus {1073}. Mucosal abnormalities such as ulceration, plaques, nodules, and strictures are associated with an increased risk of cancer.

Epidemiology
The risk factors for dysplasia in Barrett oesophagus are similar to those for oesophageal adenocarcinoma (see Box 2.02, p. 39). Dysplasia develops mainly in patients who have metaplastic intestinal-type epithelium characterized by the presence of goblet cells {2966,3306}. However, neoplasia can also develop in mucosa without goblet cells {2787}. The true risk of neoplasia development in non-goblet columnar epithelium is unknown.

Etiology
See *Adenocarcinoma of the oesophagus and oesophagogastric junction NOS* (p. 38).

Pathogenesis
Cancer in Barrett oesophagus develops via sequential progression from inflammation to metaplasia, dysplasia, and ultimately carcinoma. As a result of chronic gastro-oesophageal reflux disease, the squamous epithelium converts to columnar epithelium, which is initially of the cardia type and devoid of goblet cells; it later develops goblet cell metaplasia and eventually dysplasia. Dysplasia has been shown to develop from clones of epithelium without goblet cells; both dysplasia and cancer have been shown to develop in patients without goblet cells anywhere in the oesophagus, and even in patients with short-segment columnar metaplasia. Dysplasia develops and progresses as a result of the accumulation of multiple genetic and epigenetic alterations, many of which occur before the onset of dysplasia {3539,3122}. Many of the molecular events, in particular those that occur early, are related to alterations of the cell-cycle regulatory genes, apoptosis, cell signalling, and adhesion pathways {3539,3122,822}. Late changes in Barrett oesophagus–associated neoplasia include widespread genomic abnormalities, losses and gains in chromosome function, and (most importantly) DNA instability characterized by an increased 4N (tetraploid) cell fraction and aneuploidy. Dysplasia shows an increased Ki-67 proliferation index, which is typically highest in the bases of the crypts, but it may also be high in the surface epithelium in high-grade dysplasia. Other abnormalities include mutations in *PCNA*, *CCND1*, *TP53*, *IGF2BP3*, and *AMACR* {3122,822,3444,3742}. A more complete description of the molecular abnormalities in Barrett oesophagus is provided in the section *Adenocarcinoma of the oesophagus and oesophagogastric junction NOS* (p.38).

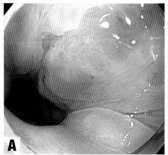 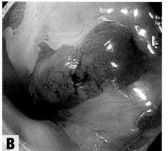

Fig. 2.02 High-grade Barrett dysplasia. **A** White-light endoscopy reveals a 2 cm tongue of Barrett oesophagus, with a focus of high-grade dysplasia appearing as a slightly irregular and plaque-like area of mucosa with slight loss of vascular pattern and congestion. **B** The focus of dysplasia is best visualized with narrow-band imaging, which helps delineate the area of abnormality.

Macroscopic appearance

Not clinically relevant

Histopathology

Histologically, the two most common types of dysplasia are intestinal and foveolar; the latter is also referred to as non-intestinal dysplasia or gastric-type dysplasia {2278}. Rarely, dysplasia may have a serrated pattern of growth. A mixture of intestinal and foveolar dysplasia is not uncommon. Intestinal dysplasia is composed of columnar cells with intestinal differentiation, including goblet cells and enterocyte-like cells.

Like inflammatory bowel disease, dysplasia can be classified as negative, indefinite, or positive (either low-grade or high-grade) according to the system proposed in 1988 by Reid et al. {2679}; however, many pathologists instead use the modified Vienna classification of dysplasia {2886} (see Table 2.01, p. 34).

Low-grade dysplasia shows cytological abnormalities but little or no architectural atypia. The cells show elongation, nuclear enlargement, hyperchromasia, and stratification, but they largely retain their nuclear polarity. Stratification is typically limited to the basal portion of the cell cytoplasm. Goblet cells vary from few to numerous, generally decreasing in number with increasing grade of dysplasia.

High-grade dysplasia shows a greater degree of cytological atypia, often along with architectural abnormalities. The cells show markedly enlarged nuclei (as large as 3–4 times the size of lymphocytes), full-thickness nuclear stratification in the base and surface epithelium, marked nuclear pleomorphism, irregular nuclear contours, and substantial loss of polarity. Mitoses are usually increased in number in the surface epithelium, and atypical mitoses are common. Intraluminal necrosis may be present. In some cases, the dysplastic nuclei may be irregularly shaped and show a more rounded configuration, with vesicular nuclei and prominent nucleoli; this is more common in foveolar dysplasia. The crypts in high-grade dysplasia may show variability in size and shape, may appear crowded, and/or may contain marked budding or angulation. Back-to-back gland formation and cribriforming are not uncommon. The diagnosis of high-grade dysplasia can be established in the presence of either high-grade cytological or architectural aberrations alone, but most cases show a combination of both.

Foveolar (non-intestinal) dysplasia typically shows few, if any, goblet cells; instead, it is characterized by prominent cytoplasmic mucin. The cells are more uniformly columnar and are typically composed of a single layer. They have small or slightly enlarged, round to oval, basally located nuclei without stratification or pleomorphism. In some cases, the nuclei may be pencil-shaped. High-grade foveolar dysplasia shows cells with a markedly increased N:C ratio and more-irregular nuclear contours, often with an open chromatin pattern, prominent nucleoli, and an increased mitotic count. Some cases may also show

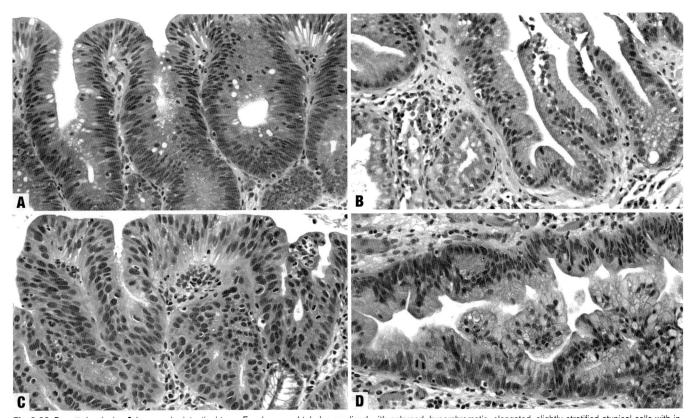

Fig. 2.03 Barrett dysplasia. **A** Low-grade, intestinal type. Evenly spaced tubules are lined with enlarged, hyperchromatic, elongated, slightly stratified atypical cells with increased numbers of mitoses and a lack of surface maturation. **B** Low-grade, foveolar type. The dysplastic epithelium shows mildly to moderately enlarged, hyperchromatic, round to oval-shaped nuclei, with slight stratification and increased numbers of mitoses but no goblet cells; the cytoplasm is mucinous. **C** High-grade, intestinal type. Compact crypts with markedly enlarged, oval to elongated, hyperchromatic nuclei with multiple nucleoli, showing full-thickness stratification, increased numbers of mitoses, loss of polarity, and pleomorphism. **D** High-grade, foveolar type. Markedly atypical epithelium composed of enlarged, hyperchromatic, elongated, irregularly shaped nuclei, with pleomorphism, full-thickness stratification, loss of polarity, and increased numbers of mitoses; the cytoplasm is mucinous but somewhat depleted.

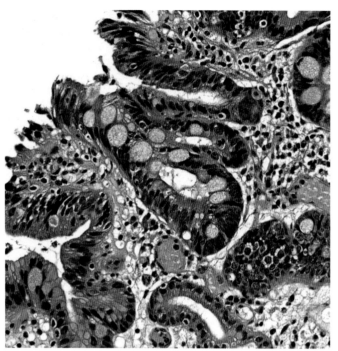

Fig. 2.04 Barrett dysplasia with intestinal metaplasia. Intestinal-type low-grade dysplasia with multiple goblet cells.

Cytology

Cytology is increasingly used as an adjunct to biopsy in the diagnosis of Barrett oesophagus and associated neoplasms. In general, the degree of atypia depends on the grade of dysplasia, although well-accepted criteria for diagnosing low-grade and high-grade dysplasia on cytology samples have not been established {3512}. The observed sensitivity of cytology in the diagnosis of low-grade dysplasia is as low as 31% in some studies {2806}, but the cytological diagnosis of high-grade dysplasia is more accurate – comparable to diagnosis using mucosal biopsy samples, with a reported sensitivity of 82% and specificity as high as 95% {2806,1721}. Cytologically, dysplasia shows some of the atypical features of malignancy, such as cellular diffusion, haphazard arrangement of cells, an increased N:C ratio, nuclear enlargement, hyperchromasia, nuclear membrane irregularity, and chromatin aberration (either clumping or clearing). The periphery of the cell groups is often irregular. In high-grade dysplasia, the cells are more discohesive, with a higher N:C ratio and moderate to markedly enlarged atypical nuclei.

Diagnostic molecular pathology

Not clinically relevant

Essential and desirable diagnostic criteria

Essential: unequivocal neoplastic alteration of the epithelium, without invasion.

Note: Unequivocal neoplastic alteration (dysplasia) most often consists of cells with enlarged hyperchromatic elongated, pleomorphic, and stratified nuclei with increased numbers of mitoses, lack of surface maturation, and loss of polarity. Architecturally, the neoplastic epithelium may show glands of abnormal size and shape, with branching, increased complexity, and/or a back-to-back pattern of growth with little or no intervening lamina propria when the dysplasia is of high grade.

Staging (TNM)

Not clinically relevant

Prognosis and prediction

In various studies, the observed rates of progression of low-grade dysplasia to high-grade dysplasia or cancer range from

stratification of the nuclei. Foveolar dysplasia may develop in fields of metaplastic columnar mucosa without goblet cells.

Like inflammatory bowel disease, dysplasia can sometimes be detected at an early stage, when it is still restricted to the bases of the crypts; such cases are referred to as crypt dysplasia {1945}. Crypt dysplasia most often shows low-grade cytological features, but some cases can show high-grade cytological changes as well.

Immunohistochemistry using antibodies to p53, AMACR, and IMP3 is sometimes useful for differentiating between non-dysplastic and dysplastic epithelium, but the results are variable and of mixed value {2136}. For example, one of the problems with p53 immunohistochemistry is that a non-mutant pattern does not exclude dysplasia.

Table 2.01 The Vienna and Reid classifications of dysplasia in Barrett oesophagus

Vienna	Reid
Negative for neoplasia/dysplasia	Negative for dysplasia
Indefinite for neoplasia/dysplasia	Indefinite for dysplasia
Non-invasive low-grade neoplasia (low-grade adenoma/dysplasia)	Low-grade dysplasia

Non-invasive high-grade neoplasia
  High-grade dysplasia
  Non-invasive carcinoma (carcinoma in situ)
  Suspicious for invasive carcinoma
	High-grade dysplasia

Invasive neoplasia
  Intramucosal adenocarcinoma
  Submucosal carcinoma or beyond
	Adenocarcinoma
	Intramucosal adenocarcinoma
	Invasive adenocarcinoma

3% to 23% {2752,2976}, undoubtedly as a result of interobserver variability. In one meta-analysis, the pooled annual incidence rate of progression to adenocarcinoma was 0.5% for adenocarcinoma alone and 1.7% for either high-grade dysplasia or adenocarcinoma {3049}. In some studies, as many as 55% of high-grade dysplasias have been found to progress to cancer during 5 years of follow-up, and high-grade dysplasia is associated with a cancer incidence of ≥ 6% per year {2976,2680}. In a recent European study, the risk of progression to adenocarcinoma associated with low-grade dysplasia was 5 times that associated with no dysplasia {732}. Progression rates for both low-grade and high-grade dysplasia have been shown to correlate with the number of pathologists who agree on the diagnosis {3120}. In one study, 15 of 25 patients (60%) with a dysplastic lesion associated with a nodule were diagnosed with oesophageal cancer {451}. A similarly strong association has been observed between adenocarcinoma and polypoid dysplasia, ulceration, or stricture formation {3307,2204}. Other markers of progression that have been evaluated include p53, p16, and DNA content abnormalities {941,3742,1549}. Several studies have shown a positive association between aberrant p53 expression and an increased risk of neoplastic progression {3742,1549}. Genomic instability is also a useful marker of progression {941}.

Oesophageal squamous dysplasia

Takubo K
Fujii S

Definition
Squamous dysplasia of the oesophagus is an unequivocal neoplastic alteration of the oesophageal squamous epithelium, without invasion.

ICD-O coding
8077/0 Oesophageal squamous intraepithelial neoplasia (dysplasia), low grade
8077/2 Oesophageal squamous intraepithelial neoplasia (dysplasia), high grade

ICD-11 coding
2E92.0 & XH3Y37 Benign neoplasm of oesophagus &
 Oesophageal squamous intraepithelial neoplasia (dysplasia), low-grade
2E60.1 & XH9ND8 Carcinoma in situ of oesophagus &
 Oesophageal squamous intraepithelial neoplasia (dysplasia), high-grade

Related terminology
None

Subtype(s)
None

Localization
Squamous dysplasia can occur anywhere in the oesophagus, and it is likely to follow the distribution of squamous cell carcinoma.

Clinical features
Patients at high risk of oesophageal squamous cell carcinoma are usually followed using a combination of Lugol's chromoendoscopy and narrow-band imaging {1376}. With Lugol's iodine, low-grade dysplasia appears as an unstained or weakly stained area; high-grade dysplasia is consistently unstained {2971}.

Features associated with neoplastic disease include large size, non-flat appearance, positive pink-colour sign, and multiplicity of distinct iodine-unstained lesions {3706}. On narrow-band imaging, dysplastic lesions appear as areas of brownish discolouration {2268,2220}. Abnormalities on narrow-band imaging reflect the invasion depth of intramucosal carcinoma and changes of intrapapillary capillary loops {2477}.

Epidemiology
The reported prevalence of oesophageal squamous dysplasia varies from 3% in some parts of the world to as high as 38% in the countries with the highest prevalence of oesophageal squamous cell carcinoma, such as China and the Islamic Republic of Iran {1148}. In series from China, the most common grade of squamous dysplasia was mild, followed by moderate and severe {1148}. Most patients are asymptomatic; however, larger areas of dysplasia or erosion, as well as coexisting squamous cell carcinoma, can cause symptoms such as dysphagia and bleeding. The prevalence and sex distribution of squamous dysplasia mirror those of squamous cell carcinoma. Squamous dysplasia is most common among patients in the fifth and sixth decades of life {3518}.

Etiology
The risk factors for oesophageal squamous dysplasia are similar to those for oesophageal squamous cell carcinoma (see Box 2.03, p. 48).

Pathogenesis
Overexpression of p53 and hypermethylation of CDKN2A (*P16INK4a*) have been reported in squamous dysplasia {3266}.

Macroscopic appearance
Squamous dysplasia can appear as a small, superficial or flat lesion.

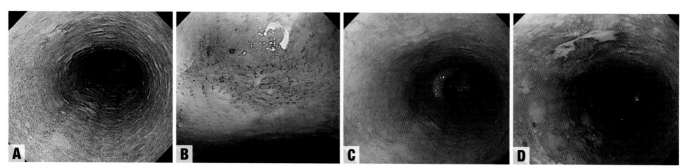

Fig. 2.05 Oesophageal squamous dysplasia. **A** On low-magnification endoscopy with narrow-band imaging, the lesion appears as a brownish area about 10 mm in size on the front left wall, 30 cm from the incisors. **B** On high-magnification endoscopy with narrow-band imaging, the intrapapillary capillary loops are mildly irregular and the mucosa between them is brightly coloured. **C** On white-light endoscopy, the lesion appears as a flat, slightly depressed lesion with mild redness. **D** On Lugol's chromoendoscopy, the lesion is positive for the pink-colour sign – it is well demarcated and unstained.

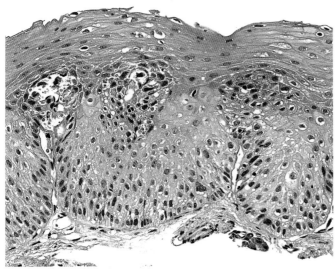

Fig. 2.06 Low-grade oesophageal squamous dysplasia. There is expansion of the basal cell layer, with mild nuclear pleomorphism.

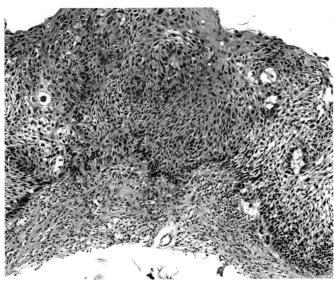

Fig. 2.07 High-grade oesophageal squamous dysplasia. There is full-thickness dysplasia, with severe nuclear pleomorphism.

Histopathology

The diagnosis of squamous dysplasia requires the presence of both cytological and architectural atypia. Cytological atypia is characterized by nuclear atypia, including enlargement, pleomorphism, hyperchromasia, loss of polarity, and overlapping. Architectural atypia is characterized by abnormal epithelial maturation.

The grading of squamous dysplasia is controversial; there are two main systems in use. Pathologists in some countries use a system with three tiers (mild, moderate, and severe). In other countries, pathologists use a two-tiered (low-grade vs high-grade) system, and this is the grading system currently recommended by the WHO Classification of Tumours Editorial Board. Low-grade dysplasia is defined as dysplasia involving only the lower half of the epithelium, with only mild cytological atypia. High-grade dysplasia is diagnosed when more than half of the epithelium is involved or when severe cytological atypia is present (regardless of the extent of epithelial involvement). High-grade dysplasia includes the group of lesions also termed "carcinoma in situ" in Japan and other parts of Asia {3224}.

Cytology

Oesophageal balloon cytology screening, which is based largely on the size of the squamous cell nuclei, has been proposed for the early detection of squamous dysplasia in China {3518}.

Diagnostic molecular pathology

Not clinically relevant

Essential and desirable diagnostic criteria

Squamous dysplasia
Essential: cytological atypia (nuclear atypia: enlargement, pleomorphism, hyperchromasia, loss of polarity, and overlapping); architectural atypia (abnormal epithelial maturation).

Low grade
Essential: involvement of only the lower half of the epithelium, with only mild cytological atypia.

High grade
Essential: involvement of more than half of the epithelium or severe cytological atypia (regardless of the extent of epithelial involvement).

Staging (TNM)

Not clinically relevant

Prognosis and prediction

In a study population of Chinese patients with biopsy-proven oesophageal squamous dysplasia, over a follow-up period of 3.5 years, clinically diagnosed oesophageal squamous cell carcinoma developed in 5% of the patients with mild dysplasia, 27% with moderate dysplasia, and 65% with severe dysplasia {726}; after 13.5 years, these proportions increased to 24%, 50%, and 74%, respectively {3511}. In parts of the world with high incidence of squamous cell carcinoma, such as China, detection of squamous dysplasia by screening and early treatment of the disease hold promise for the prevention of progression to squamous cell carcinoma {3266}.

Adenocarcinoma of the oesophagus and oesophagogastric junction NOS

Lam AK
Kumarasinghe MP

Definition

Adenocarcinoma of the oesophagus and oesophagogastric junction NOS is an oesophageal epithelial malignancy with glandular or mucinous differentiation.

ICD-O coding

8140/3 Adenocarcinoma NOS

ICD-11 coding

2B70.0 Adenocarcinoma of oesophagus
2B71.0 Adenocarcinoma of oesophagogastric junction

Related terminology

None

Subtype(s)

None

Localization

Nearly all adenocarcinomas occur in the lower oesophagus and the oesophagogastric junction. It can sometimes be difficult to distinguish an oesophageal adenocarcinoma from a proximal gastric tumour. Ideally, the oesophagogastric junction should be defined endoscopically (by either the most proximal gastric fold or the distal end of the palisade vessels); however, this information is not always available. Complicating the issue further, changes in Barrett oesophagus can distort the landmarks used to identify the oesophagogastric junction. In the current pathological staging system, oesophagogastric junction adenocarcinoma is defined as having its epicentre within 2 cm of the oesophagogastric junction and extending into the oesophagus {1770}. Rarely, adenocarcinomas can occur in the middle or upper third of the oesophagus {1772}. Such cases most likely develop from mucosal glands, submucosal glands, or ectopic columnar epithelium in the oesophagus (also known as inlet patches or ectopic gastric mucosa {1492,2460}. Fewer than 50 cases of upper oesophageal adenocarcinoma coexisting with ectopic gastric glands have been reported in the literature {2460}.

Clinical features

The most common symptoms at presentation are dysphagia, reflux, weight loss, and pain {3370}. Less common symptoms are nausea, vomiting, anaemia, and dyspepsia. The diagnosis of oesophageal adenocarcinoma is confirmed by endoscopic biopsy. EUS can be used to determine the extent of local involvement of the carcinoma, as well as perioesophageal lymph node metastasis. EUS staging is less accurate for pT1 adenocarcinomas, because of the presence of duplicated muscularis mucosae {926}. Suspicious lymph nodes can be sampled with EUS-guided FNA. Radiological imaging (CT, PET-CT, or MRI) is essential for staging (to identify any distant metastases) and important for the assessment of response to neoadjuvant therapy {1167}.

Epidemiology

The global incidence rate of oesophageal adenocarcinoma is 0.7 cases/100 000 person-years (1.1 in men and 0.3 in women) {192}. The incidence of oesophageal adenocarcinoma is highest in North America, northern and western Europe, Australia, and New Zealand, which together account for 46% of all cases

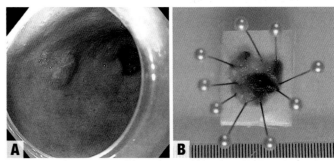

Fig. 2.08 Early oesophageal adenocarcinoma. **A** An example detected by endoscopy. **B** A specimen removed by endoscopic resection.

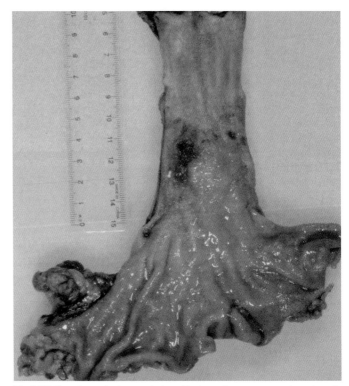

Fig. 2.09 Oesophageal adenocarcinoma. Macroscopic appearance of an example presenting as ulcerative growth; note the mucosal changes adjacent to the adenocarcinoma, constituting dysplasia and Barrett oesophagus.

Box 2.02 Risk factors for oesophageal adenocarcinoma

Gastro-oesophageal reflux disease (GORD)
- GORD is the single most important risk factor.
- The risk in individuals with heartburn for ≥ 30 years was found to be 6.2 times that in individuals without heartburn.
- The risk in patients with Barret oesophagus is 10–55 times the risk in the general population {3305}.

Obesity
- Abdominal obesity is strongly associated with an increased risk of GORD because of the mechanical effect {3305}.
- Obesity might also increase the risk of Barrett oesophagus and oesophageal adenocarcinoma independent of GORD {3305}; this may be related to the adipokines (e.g. leptin) and proinflammatory cytokines (e.g. insulin-like growth factors).
- An increase in physical activity may reduce the risk of oesophageal adenocarcinoma, although it is unclear whether weight loss is associated with reduced risk {2626}.

Male sex
- The M:F ratio peaks among individuals aged 50–54 years and then decreases.
- Higher ratios of circulating androgen to estrogen are noted in patients with oesophageal adenocarcinoma {2576}.
- Estrogen might protect against (and androgen might promote) the development of oesophageal adenocarcinoma {2626}.

Smoking
- In addition to being a carcinogen, smoking can relax the lower oesophageal sphincter, which may increase GORD.
- Smoking increases the risk of Barrett oesophagus and oesophageal adenocarcinoma, although the association is not as strong as that of other risk factors {3305,2626}.

***Helicobacter pylori* infection**
- *H. pylori* infection is inversely associated with risk of oesophageal adenocarcinoma {3305,2626}; a possible mechanism is reduced volume and acidity of gastric juice in atrophic gastritis after infection.

Antireflux therapies
- The preventive role of antireflux therapies is questionable {652}.
- It is unlikely that antireflux medications (proton-pump inhibitors) prevent the progression of oesophageal adenocarcinoma; in fact, long-term use of proton-pump inhibitors has been associated with increased risk {432}.
- Antireflux surgery (fundoplication) may be more preventive than antireflux medications.

Medications
- NSAIDs (including acetylsalicylic acid) and statins have shown inverse associations with the development of oesophageal adenocarcinoma {3305,2626}, but large controlled clinical trials are needed to confirm the protective effect of these drugs.

Dietary factors
- The consumption of dietary fibre, vegetables, vitamins, minerals, meat (in particular red meat), and fats has been associated with different risks of reflux oesophagitis, Barrett oesophagus, and oesophageal adenocarcinoma {1772}; however, these associations require confirmation in larger population studies {2626}.

worldwide. The rate of increase in incidence over the past four decades is the highest of any cancer, especially in high-income countries {652}. In some parts of Asia, such as Israel and Singapore, there has also been a small increase in the incidence of oesophageal adenocarcinoma {2773}. Less than 1% of oesophageal adenocarcinomas occur in patients aged < 40 years {192}. The mean patient age at presentation of the cancer is in the seventh decade of life {3370}. Oesophageal adenocarcinoma predominantly occurs in men, with an M:F ratio of 4.4:1 {192}; the incidence among men is 3–9 times that among women. The time trend of increasing incidence is roughly the same in both sexes. The M:F ratio of incidence is higher in high-incidence regions, such as North America (7.6:1), Oceania (6.2:1), and Europe (6.0:1). The male predominance in oesophageal adenocarcinoma is greater than in oesophageal squamous cell carcinoma or Barrett oesophagus {3370}.

Etiology

Like many cancers, oesophageal adenocarcinoma is associated with advanced age. This carcinoma is most often seen in white populations. Risk factors for oesophageal adenocarcinoma include gastro-oesophageal reflux disease, obesity, and male sex. Other modulating factors include smoking, *Helicobacter pylori* infection, antireflux therapies, medications, and dietary factors (see Box 2.02 for more details). Approximately 7% of cases of Barrett oesophagus and oesophageal adenocarcinoma are familial {652}; genome-wide association studies

have identified loci (detected by SNPs) and germline mutations associated with increased risk for both entities. These loci often

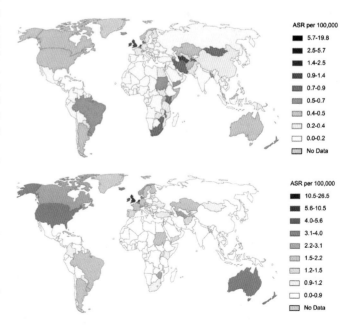

Fig. 2.10 Estimated age-standardized incidence rates (ASRs; World), per 100 000 person-years, of oesophageal adenocarcinoma in women (**top**) and men (**bottom**) in 2012.

encode transcription factors {3305}. Larger studies are needed to validate the potential use of these loci in screening for family members affected by Barrett oesophagus or oesophageal adenocarcinoma.

Pathogenesis

In response to the effects of acid/biliary reflux of gastric and intestinal contents and dysbiosis (microbial imbalance), stem cell and/or progenitor cells in the basal portion of the gastro-oesophageal epithelium are reprogrammed to columnar cell lineage {3758,2626}. The reparative epithelium develops into non-goblet columnar epithelium (proximal gastric type). Over time, this epithelium follows one of two lines of differentiation: either a gastric pathway (parietal and chief cells) or an intestinal pathway (goblet and Paneth cells) {2626}. The intestinal pathway, with goblet cells, characterizes Barrett oesophagus. Recent studies have shown that early Barrett neoplasia is always associated with intestinal metaplasia {108}. Barrett oesophagus may progress through dysplasia to adenocarcinoma. The genetic and epigenetic changes of progression from Barrett oesophagus have been studied for decades {1399,1832,1831}. Mutations of some genes (*TP53* and *SMAD4*) occur in a stage-specific manner and are restricted to high-grade dysplasia and adenocarcinoma {3539,2759}.

In recent years, next-generation sequencing techniques have given rise to global projects involving whole-genome sequencing of oesophageal adenocarcinoma {2585}. These projects have revealed key gene pathways and mutations involved in pathogenesis {2923,915}, identified novel genes {822}, and shown that the genomic landscapes of prechemotherapy and postchemotherapy samples of oesophageal adenocarcinoma are similar {2385}. There are currently no clinical applications for these comprehensive but complex data, but clinically relevant and diagnostically useful prognostic and predictive markers may emerge in the future. Data from The Cancer Genome Atlas (TCGA) also suggest that oesophageal adenocarcinoma strongly resembles gastric carcinoma with chromosomal instability {475}.

Macroscopic appearance

Oesophageal adenocarcinomas often present in advanced stages and appear as stricturing, polypoid, fungating, ulcerative, or diffuse infiltrating lesions. In earlier stages, adenocarcinomas may appear as irregular plaques. Early-stage carcinomas may present as small nodules or may not be detected on endoscopy. Adjacent to the carcinoma, there may be irregular tongues of reddish mucosa (resembling a salmon patch) that represent Barrett oesophagus and reflux changes and that contrast with the greyish-white colour of the squamous-lined oesophageal mucosa.

Histopathology

Oesophageal adenocarcinoma shows gastric, intestinal, and mixed (hybrid) lineage, evidenced by a combination of morphological and immunohistochemical features {1565,426}. The mucosa adjacent to the adenocarcinoma may show Barrett dysplasia and intestinal metaplasia (Barrett oesophagus). Oesophageal adenocarcinomas can be classified as having tubular, papillary, mucinous, and signet-ring cell patterns. Only limited evidence of the relevance of these patterns is available; therefore, patterns are described rather than subtypes. A mixture of these patterns is often seen. The tubular pattern is most

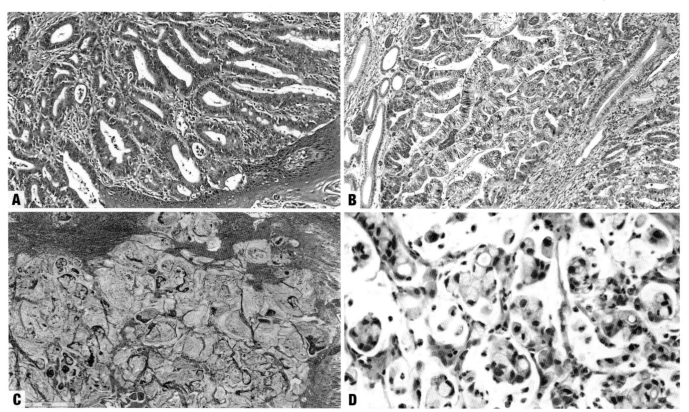

Fig. 2.11 Oesophageal adenocarcinoma. **A** Tubular pattern. **B** Papillary pattern. **C** Mucinous pattern. **D** Signet-ring cell pattern.

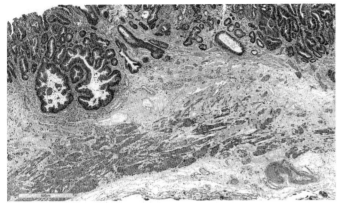

Fig. 2.12 Oesophageal adenocarcinoma. An example in Barrett oesophagus with a double layer of muscularis mucosae.

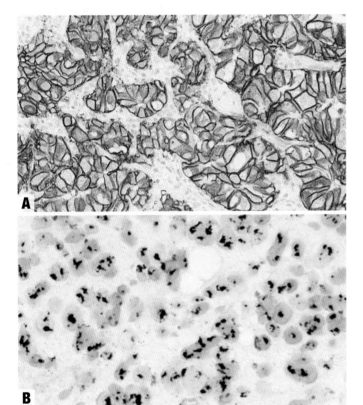

Fig. 2.13 Oesophageal adenocarcinoma. **A** Immunohistochemistry indicates an ERBB2 (HER2) immunoscore of 3+ for this tumour; note the lateral membrane and basolateral membrane staining. **B** Silver in situ hybridization (SISH) confirms the presence of *ERBB2* (*HER2*) amplification; the black dots represent amplified *ERBB2* signals and the red dots diploid CEP17 signals. FISH can also be used to confirm *ERBB2* amplification, but many authorities recommend SISH over FISH for testing upper GI tract adenocarcinomas.

common. It is characterized by irregular, single or anastomosing tubular glandular structures lined by a layer of single or stratified malignant epithelium; neoplastic glands often show variable amounts of intracellular mucin production and may show dilatation {1771}. The papillary pattern is characterized by papillae, with rare cases showing micropapillary architecture {1191}. The mucinous pattern generally shows carcinoma cells floating in abundant extracellular mucin. Pure mucinous carcinomas are rare, with isolated reports of mixed mucinous and signet-ring

cell patterns {3669,613,3767}. The signet-ring cell pattern shows cells resembling signet rings, with large intracellular mucin vacuoles that displace the nuclei to the periphery. The presence of signet-ring cells in oesophageal adenocarcinoma is associated with worse clinical outcome. Pure signet-ring cell carcinomas are extremely rare. The reported prevalence of the signet-ring cell pattern in oesophageal adenocarcinoma varies; the highest reported relative prevalence is 7.61% {3709,3696}. However, the criteria for diagnosis in these reports appear to be inconsistent. The poorly cohesive non–signet-ring cell pattern appears to be uncommon in the oesophagus.

Therapy effect

About half of all oesophageal adenocarcinomas are treated with preoperative chemoradiation, which causes morphological changes in the carcinomas, adjacent non-neoplastic tissue, and metastatic lymph nodes. In patients with complete response or substantial partial response to preoperative chemoradiation, the lesion may become smaller or even invisible. On cut section, lesions may also appear as irregular white scars with fibrosis. Mucinous change after preoperative chemoradiation is common in oesophageal adenocarcinoma. Histological examination may reveal cytoplasmic changes in the malignant cells (e.g. vacuolation, oncocytic changes, and neuroendocrine changes), as well as the presence of tumour giant cells. Mitoses are uncommon, but nuclear changes (including hyperchromasia, pyknosis, karyorrhexis, enlargement, and irregularity) are frequent findings. Many of the tumour cells on the mucosal surface may disappear. The carcinoma site shows fibrosis, inflammation, and granulation tissue. Residual carcinoma may appear as isolated cells or cell clusters in the stroma with reaction to chemoradiation. Stromal reactions include fibrosis; dystrophic calcification; necrosis; inflammation; mucinous degeneration (acellular mucin lakes); the presence of foamy or haemosiderin-laden macrophages, foreign body giant cells, and cholesterol clefts; and reactive change in fibroblasts, glands, and vessels {3294,1771,1786}.

Invasion

Invasive features such as tumour budding (defined as the presence of detached, isolated groups of 1–5 cells) and perineural invasion may be detected in oesophageal adenocarcinoma {3293}. These features often correlate with each other, as well as with high tumour grade, advanced tumour stage, and worse survival.

Grading

The grading of oesophageal adenocarcinoma affects its staging {1770}. In the eighth edition of the American Joint Committee on Cancer (AJCC) cancer staging manual, grade 1 (well-differentiated) is defined as adenocarcinoma with > 95% of the carcinoma composed of well-formed glands. Grade 2 (moderately differentiated) is adenocarcinoma with 50–95% of the carcinoma demonstrating glandular formation. Grade 3 (poorly differentiated) is adenocarcinoma with < 50% of the carcinoma demonstrating glandular formation {1770}.

Immunohistochemistry and histochemistry

Oesophageal adenocarcinoma has a consistent cytokeratin expression pattern of CK7+, CK19+, and CK20– {3258}, which does not distinguish it from gastric adenocarcinoma {812}. PAS, Alcian blue, and mucicarmine are histochemical stains that may identify mucin in poorly differentiated adenocarcinoma.

Differential diagnosis
It can be difficult to distinguish a poorly differentiated adenocarcinoma from a poorly differentiated squamous cell carcinoma in a biopsy of a lower oesophageal tumour. Squamous cell carcinomas are strongly positive for CK5/6, p63 (often > 75% positive), and p40 (which is more specific than p63), whereas adenocarcinomas are strongly positive for CK7 (often > 75% positive) and negative for squamous markers. The diagnosis of undifferentiated carcinoma should be considered for cases with an equivocal immunohistochemical pattern and no morphologically identifiable squamous or glandular features. Some poorly

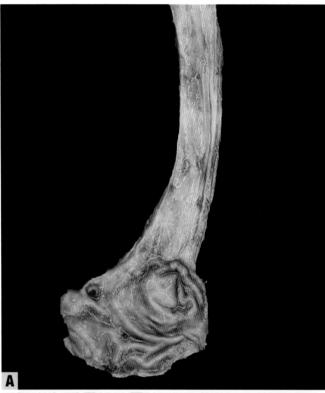

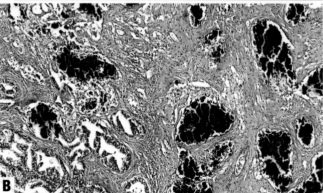

Fig. 2.14 Oesophageal adenocarcinoma. **A** Macroscopic appearance after neoadjuvant chemotherapy. **B** An example previously treated with preoperative chemoradiation, showing clear-cell change in the adenocarcinoma and calcification and foamy macrophages in the stroma.

differentiated adenocarcinomas may show neuroendocrine differentiation {3515}; such cases are more resistant to chemoradiation. Preoperative chemoradiation can potentially complicate diagnosis in two ways. Firstly, it can be difficult to distinguish the mucinous component of oesophageal adenocarcinoma from acellular mucin pools after neoadjuvant chemoradiotherapy {613}; cytokeratin staining to identify the carcinoma cells within the mucin may be helpful in some instances. Secondly, treatment-associated alterations of non-neoplastic epithelia may include cytoplasmic and nuclear changes that mimic changes in carcinoma cells. Atrophic and metaplastic glands may also present diagnostic pitfalls {1786}.

Cytology
The use of cytology for oesophageal tumour detection is increasing {2415}. Malignant glandular epithelial elements suggest the presence of an adenocarcinoma, whereas malignant squamous elements suggest squamous cell carcinoma. A mixture of cytologically malignant squamous and glandular cells should prompt suspicion for adenosquamous or mucoepidermoid carcinoma.

Diagnostic molecular pathology
Not clinically relevant

Essential and desirable diagnostic criteria
Essential: evidence of glandular or mucinous differentiation within an invasive tumour.
Desirable: immunohistochemistry (may be necessary to demonstrate differentiation towards adenocarcinoma in poorly differentiated lesions).

Staging (TNM)
There are two pathological staging systems in the eighth edition of the AJCC cancer staging manual: one for adenocarcinoma not previously treated with neoadjuvant therapy (pTNM) and the other for adenocarcinoma after adjuvant therapy (ypTNM) {1770,2707}. In the ypTNM classification, stage grouping is not affected by tumour grade or histological type. In early-stage carcinomas, grade (either G1–2 or G3) is an important parameter for determining stage. In patients who have received adjuvant therapy, the survival differences among pathological stage groups are less pronounced {1770,2707}.

An adenocarcinoma in the upper GI tract that infiltrates the lamina propria or muscularis mucosae without invasion of the submucosa is defined as intramucosal adenocarcinoma (pT1a). Endoscopic resection with or without radiofrequency ablation is the standard of treatment for early (pT1) oesophageal adenocarcinomas that do not show adverse pathological features {251}. Adverse pathological features include submucosal invasion (pT1b) to a depth > 500 μm, poor differentiation, lymphovascular invasion, and margin involvement {2966}. The presence of duplicated and distorted muscularis mucosae, which is a consistent finding in Barrett oesophagus, may lead to misinterpretation of the depth of invasion of carcinoma {1720}.

Regional lymph nodes are commonly the first sites of spread. The current staging system for oesophageal adenocarcinoma depends on the number of positive lymph nodes and therefore relies on extensive lymph node sampling. Patients who have received neoadjuvant therapy need more-extensive sampling,

Table 2.02 The Mandard and Becker systems for assessing the tumour regression grade (TRG) of carcinoma after neoadjuvant therapy {2036,1786}

Mandard	Becker
TRG 1: Absence of residual cancer, with fibrosis extending through the various layers of the oesophageal wall (complete regression)	**TRG 1a:** No carcinoma present
TRG 2: Rare residual cancer cells scattered through the fibrosis	**TRG 1b:** < 10% carcinoma present
TRG 3: An increase in the number of residual cancer cells, but fibrosis still predominates	**TRG 2:** 10–50% carcinoma present
TRG 4: Residual cancer outgrowing fibrosis	**TRG 3:** > 50% carcinoma present
TRG 5: Absence of regressive changes	

because the lymph nodes may undergo atrophy and become impalpable. Regression of metastases can occur in lymph nodes. Careful examination and step sectioning of cases that show fibrosis or other reactive changes may identify small metastatic foci. Approximately half of all patients with high-stage oesophageal adenocarcinoma have distant lymph node or organ metastases at initial presentation. The carcinoma may metastasize to peritoneum, liver, lung, bone, brain, and adrenal gland {505,3618}. The liver is the most common site of distant spread.

Prognosis and prediction

The most important parameter for predicting the prognosis of patients with oesophageal adenocarcinoma is pathological stage. Other pathological factors associated with survival include tumour size, histological features (grading, lymphovascular invasion, perineural invasion, and budding), and histological subtype. Other prognostic determinants are treatment-related, such as type of surgery and clearance of surgical margins. A few studies have suggested that adenosquamous and mucoepidermoid carcinomas may be more aggressive than conventional oesophageal carcinomas {1777,1139,3697,887}. After neoadjuvant chemoradiotherapy, the survival of patients with adenocarcinoma depends on the response to therapy. Tumour regression grade (TRG) and lymph node downstaging after neoadjuvant therapy are associated with improved disease-free survival {2377}. The amount of residual carcinoma determines the TRG. The most common method of assessing TRG in oesophageal adenocarcinoma is the Mandard system {1786,2376}, which divides tumour regression into five grades based on the proportion of viable tumour tissue relative to fibrosis. The four-tiered Becker

system is favoured by some authors for pathological assessment because of its better reproducibility {1786}; this system depends on the proportion of residual cancer cells present (see Table 2.02 for more details).

Trastuzumab, an antibody targeting the human EGFR family member ERBB2 (HER2), is approved for the treatment of advanced or metastatic adenocarcinoma of the oesophagogastric junction in combination with other chemotherapeutic agents (cisplatin and capecitabine/fluorouracil). Lower oesophageal adenocarcinoma should also be responsive to this therapy {1684}. Amplification of the *ERBB2* gene (demonstrated by in situ hybridization) and the resulting overexpression of the ERBB2 (HER2) protein (demonstrated by immunohistochemistry) in oesophageal adenocarcinoma are predictive of response to ERBB2-targeted therapy. The algorithm for ERBB2 testing in oesophageal adenocarcinoma varies across organizations; some recommend performing both immunohistochemistry and in situ hybridization, whereas many others recommend in situ hybridization only in the event of equivocal (2+) immunohistochemical findings. The ERBB2 immunoscore is defined as 0, 1+ (faint), 2+ (weak to moderate), or 3+ (strong) on the basis of membrane staining {1684}. Oesophagogastric adenocarcinomas that are positive for ERBB2 often show basolateral or lateral membrane staining (unlike breast carcinomas, which often show complete membrane staining) {1098}.

The immuno-oncology agent pembrolizumab has shown promising early results for the treatment of advanced and metastatic oesophagogastric junction adenocarcinoma {2589,3543}. High microsatellite instability and PDL1 overexpression are potential biomarkers for the response of oesophageal adenocarcinoma to immunotherapy {2967}.

Oesophageal adenoid cystic carcinoma

Lam AK

Definition

Adenoid cystic carcinoma of the oesophagus is a malignant oesophageal epithelial tumour of glandular differentiation with epithelial and myoepithelial cells in true glandular and pseudoglandular lumina arranged in cribriform, tubular, or solid architecture.

ICD-O coding

8200/3 Adenoid cystic carcinoma

ICD-11 coding

2B70.Y & XH4302 Other specified malignant neoplasms of oesophagus & Adenoid cystic carcinoma

Related terminology

None

Subtype(s)

None

Localization

These carcinomas are most often located in the middle third of the oesophagus {2871,3779}.

Clinical features

The most common symptom is dysphagia. Endoscopy and EUS are used to confirm the diagnosis and determine the extent of disease; the carcinoma appears as a protruding/elevated or ulcerative lesion. Radiological evaluation (CT, MRI, or PET) is used to determine the clinical staging of the carcinoma.

Epidemiology

Oesophageal adenoid cystic carcinoma is uncommon, with only slightly more than 100 reported cases {2871,3779,2578}. Approximately half of these cases are from Asian populations {2871,3779,1118}. Adenoid cystic carcinoma constitutes about 0.1% of all oesophageal malignancies {1525}. It is more common in men, with an M:F ratio of 3.5:1 to 5:1 {2871,3779,2578}, and it most often occurs in the seventh decade of life (mean patient age: 65 years; range: 36–84 years) {2871,2578}.

Etiology

Unknown

Pathogenesis

Unknown

Macroscopic appearance

Macroscopically, adenoid cystic carcinoma is either protruding or ulcerative {2871,3779,1118}. In the early stage, it often located in the submucosa, with the mucosa still intact. The lesions have a mean size of 56 mm {867}, but they can be highly variable in size {3714,2083}.

Histopathology

Adenoid cystic carcinoma consists of a mixture of epithelial and myoepithelial cells in a variety of cribriform, tubular (glandular), or solid patterns. The cribriform pattern is characterized by tumour cells forming cystic lumina, which contain either basophilic glycosaminoglycans that are Alcian blue–positive (true glands) or hyalinized basal lamina material that are PASD-positive (pseudoglands). In both the cribriform and tubular patterns, the glands are lined by inner epithelial and outer myoepithelial cells, whereas the solid pattern shows no lumina. Perineural infiltration and lymphovascular permeation are common {2871}. Adenoid cystic carcinoma can coexist with squamous cell carcinoma or with dysplasia / carcinoma in situ {535}. The myoepithelial cells in adenoid cystic carcinoma are positive for p63, S100, SMA, and calponin. The epithelial cells are positive for cytokeratin, CEA, and KIT (CD117) {3779,3274}. Basaloid squamous cell carcinoma may be considered in the differential diagnosis, because it often has a pseudoglandular pattern similar to that of adenoid cystic carcinoma {1890}. However, adenoid cystic carcinoma rarely has squamous cells, central necrosis, or prominent mitotic figures, and basaloid squamous cell carcinoma is negative for SMA and S100.

Cytology

The cytological appearance of adenoid cystic carcinoma arising in the oesophagus has not been documented in the literature.

Diagnostic molecular pathology

Not clinically relevant

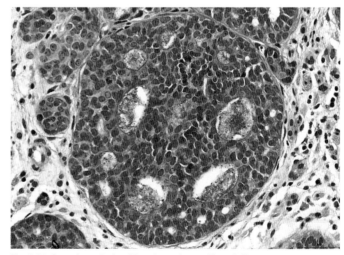

Fig. 2.15 Oesophageal adenoid cystic carcinoma. The cribriform pattern.

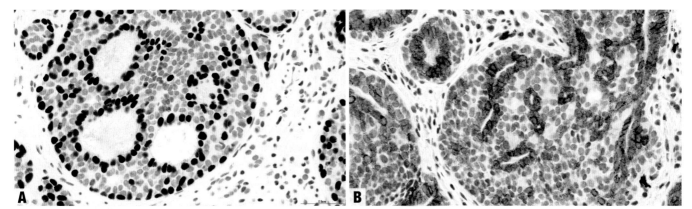

Fig. 2.16 Oesophageal adenoid cystic carcinoma. **A** p63 staining highlights the myoepithelial cells. **B** KIT staining highlights the luminal cells.

Essential and desirable diagnostic criteria

Essential: the distinctive histological pattern described above (diagnostic in most instances); immunohistochemistry and/ or re-biopsy (in the case of small biopsies showing basaloid differentiation).

Staging (TNM)

The staging of oesophageal adenoid cystic carcinoma follows that of oesophageal adenocarcinoma.

Prognosis and prediction

Prognosis depends on pathological stage. In Japanese series, half of the cases consisted of cancer limited to the submucosal layer, with only rare lymph node metastasis {2871}. In other populations, there is high incidence of metastasis to lymph nodes, liver, lung, and brain. The prognosis is poor, with a 1-year survival rate of 23% {2578}.

Oesophageal adenosquamous and mucoepidermoid carcinomas

Brown IS
Ohashi K

Definition

Adenosquamous carcinoma of the oesophagus is an oesophageal neoplasm composed of separate malignant squamous and glandular components. Mucoepidermoid carcinoma of the oesophagus is an oesophageal neoplasm composed of an admixture of malignant epidermoid, intermediate, and mucous cells.

ICD-O coding

8560/3 Adenosquamous carcinoma
8430/3 Mucoepidermoid carcinoma

ICD-11 coding

2B70.Y & XH7873 Other specified malignant neoplasms of oesophagus & Adenosquamous carcinoma
2B70.Y & XH1J36 Other specified malignant neoplasms of oesophagus & Mucoepidermoid carcinoma

Related terminology

None

Subtype(s)

None

Localization

Adenosquamous carcinoma arises most commonly in the middle oesophagus {582,2348}, although a predominance of lower oesophageal cases was observed in one recent series {3697}. Mucoepidermoid carcinoma occurs most commonly in the middle and lower oesophagus {581}.

Clinical features

The clinical features are similar to those of conventional adenocarcinoma or squamous cell carcinoma of the oesophagus.

Epidemiology

These are rare tumours. Adenosquamous carcinoma presents at a median patient age of 60 years and affects males 5 times as often as females {582,2348}. Mucoepidermoid carcinoma accounts for < 1% of primary oesophageal carcinoma and occurs most commonly in males, at a median patient age of 58 years {581}.

Etiology

The risk factors are similar to those associated with conventional squamous cell carcinoma.

Pathogenesis

Adenosquamous and mucoepidermoid carcinomas of the oesophagus are of uncertain origin. The best evidence is for an origin from a stem cell {581,1777}, probably from the oesophageal duct, giving rise to biphasic differentiation {3429}, similar to the pathogenesis of other adenosquamous carcinomas. It has also been suggested that these tumours are simply primary squamous cell carcinomas from which a subpopulation has undergone diverging glandular differentiation {3764}, or primary adenocarcinomas showing squamous differentiation {2500,1773,1777}. There is also a rare possibility that the pattern of adenosquamous carcinoma could be the result of a collision of two separate primary carcinomas (one glandular and one squamous). On balance, an origin from oesophageal submucosal glands is favoured, supported by the common embryology of oesophageal and salivary glands and the occasional restriction of the tumour to the oesophageal submucosa, but further evidence is needed. At other sites, notably the salivary glands, mucoepidermoid carcinomas have defined molecular characteristics that include translocations resulting in fusion genes, which are not found in adenosquamous carcinomas {852}.

Macroscopic appearance

The macroscopic appearance is similar to that of squamous cell carcinoma.

Histopathology

The histology of these lesions in their pure forms differs considerably, but intermediate forms also appear to exist, and these should probably be designated as adenosquamous carcinomas. Pure mucoepidermoid carcinomas arising from submucosal glands are extremely rare.

Adenosquamous carcinoma shows an admixture of distinct components of both adenocarcinoma and squamous cell carcinoma. Generally, the proportions of these components are not relevant, although the Japanese Classification of Esophageal Cancer {1428} requires ≥ 20% of either component for the diagnosis; otherwise the tumour is classified according to the primary component alone. Any degree of differentiation can

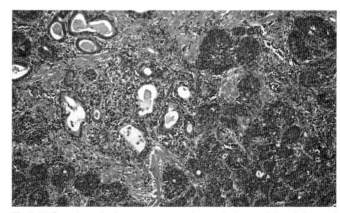

Fig. 2.17 Oesophageal adenosquamous carcinoma. A characteristic admixture of malignant squamoid cell and glandular components.

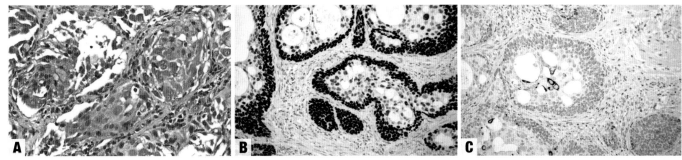

Fig. 2.18 Oesophageal mucoepidermoid carcinoma. **A** A characteristic admixture of malignant squamoid cells and mucin-containing cells. **B** p63 staining highlights the squamous component. **C** CK7 staining highlights the mucin-producing cells.

be exhibited by the squamous areas, which may include areas with no clear keratinization or intercellular bridges {582}. The adenocarcinoma component is typically tubular or glandular, with evidence of intracellular or extracellular mucin production. Single mucinous cells within squamous nests are more typical of mucoepidermoid carcinoma. The squamous and glandular elements can be intimately intermixed or can show apparent geographical separation. In general, the squamous elements are superficially located and the glandular elements are deeper in the tumour.

Mucoepidermoid carcinoma of the oesophagus, like its salivary gland counterpart, is composed of glands and nests of malignant squamoid cells and admixed mucin-containing epithelial cells. Rare examples are associated with prominent sclerosis with lymphoid tissue and eosinophils {2129}.

Cytology
The cytology of these lesions is challenging, but a mixture of cytologically malignant squamous and glandular cells should prompt suspicion for adenosquamous or mucoepidermoid carcinoma.

Diagnostic molecular pathology
Not clinically relevant

Essential and desirable diagnostic criteria
Adenosquamous carcinoma
Essential: distinct squamous and adenocarcinomatous components; absence of intermediate cells; true glandular or mucous cell differentiation.
Note: The presence of adenoid or microcystic changes within squamous foci of otherwise pure squamous cell carcinoma is not sufficient for the diagnosis.

Mucoepidermoid carcinoma
Essential: intermediate cells; mixed glandular and squamous cells; true glandular or mucous cell differentiation.

Staging (TNM)
There is no definitive evidence for whether the staging of these tumours should follow that of squamous cell carcinoma or adenocarcinoma.

Prognosis and prediction
There have not been enough studies to determine the prognosis of these carcinomas compared with more-common oesophageal carcinomas. The results of a few studies suggest that adenosquamous and mucoepidermoid carcinomas may be more aggressive than conventional squamous cell carcinoma {1777,1139,3697,887}.

Oesophageal squamous cell carcinoma NOS

Brown IS
Fujii S
Kawachi H
Lam AK
Saito T

Definition
Oesophageal squamous cell carcinoma NOS is a malignant oesophageal epithelial neoplasm displaying squamous cell differentiation characterized by keratinocyte-type cells with intercellular bridges and/or keratinization.

ICD-O coding
8070/3 Squamous cell carcinoma NOS

ICD-11 coding
2B70.1 Squamous cell carcinoma of oesophagus

Related terminology
Spindle cell squamous cell carcinoma
Acceptable: sarcomatoid carcinoma; carcinosarcoma; pseudosarcomatous squamous cell carcinoma; polypoid carcinoma; squamous cell carcinoma with a spindle cell component.

Box 2.03 Risk factors for oesophageal squamous cell carcinoma

Low socioeconomic status
- Low socioeconomic status has been found to be associated with increased risk in multiple studies, even when confounding variables (e.g. tobacco use and alcohol consumption) were controlled for {8}.

Tobacco use
- Tobacco use (smoking or chewing) remains the most important risk factor in high-income countries {865,3386,8}; it is a much weaker factor in high-incidence areas.
- Risk is dependent on both intensity and duration of use.
- Cessation is associated with decreasing risk after 5 years and a return to the baseline risk level of a lifelong non-smoker after 10–20 years.
- Tobacco-specific nitrosamines and polycyclic aromatic hydrocarbons are believed to be the main carcinogenic substances {8}.

Alcohol consumption
- Alcohol consumption has been causally linked to oesophageal squamous cell carcinoma {8}.
- Consumption of > 3 drinks per day is associated with a risk almost 5 times that in individuals who consume ≤ 1 drink per day {3386}.
- The mechanism of carcinogenesis remains uncertain, but acetaldehyde, a metabolite of ethanol, is a known carcinogen able to cause DNA abnormalities and structural and functional alterations to protein {8}.
- There is good indirect evidence for a role of acetaldehyde. *ALDH2* and *ALDH1A1* mutations, which are found almost exclusively in eastern Asian populations, lead to the accumulation of acetaldehyde following the consumption of alcohol. These mutations are associated with a dose-dependent increase in risk of oesophageal squamous cell carcinoma. For example, heterozygous and homozygous *ALDH2* mutations, respectively, are associated with risks 4 times and 13 times that in individuals without *ALDH2* mutation {1247}.

Drinking very hot beverages
- Drinking very hot beverages appears to be an important risk factor in Uruguay, southern Brazil, northern Argentina, the United Republic of Tanzania, and the Islamic Republic of Iran {3386,8}.

Dietary factors
- Diets high in fruits and vegetables are associated with a reduction of risk (a 10–25% reduction in patients who smoke) {8}.
- Pickled vegetables are associated with increased risk, possibly explained by the generation of carcinogenic mycotoxins and presence of nitrosamine compounds {8}.
- There is also limited evidence that some micronutrients may affect risk; the best evidence suggests a protective effect of selenium and riboflavin in high-risk populations {8}.

Increased body mass index
- Increased body mass index is associated with lower risk {3386,8}, but the mechanism underlying this association in unknown.

Genetic factors
- Several genetic diseases are associated with increased risk; the best characterized are tylosis, a keratosis disorder caused by an autosomal dominant mutation in *RHBDF2* at 17q25.3 (> 90% of patients develop oesophageal squamous cell carcinoma by the age of 65 years) {3386,346}, and Fanconi anaemia {8}.

Associated medical conditions
- Plummer–Vinson syndrome, related to deficiencies in iron, riboflavin, and other vitamins
- Achalasia
- Radiotherapy to the chest area
- Caustic ingestion injury {3386,8}

Unlikely to be a risk factor: HPV infection
- HPV DNA has been identified in oesophageal squamous cell carcinoma cells.
- In most cases, the virus appears to be an innocent bystander; viral integration and transcription is uncommon {475}.
- The current consensus is that HPV infection is unlikely to be a substantial risk factor for the development of oesophageal squamous cell carcinoma {8}.

Box 2.04 Summary of key genetic abnormalities identified in oesophageal squamous cell carcinoma

Genes that regulate cell cycle
- The most important genetic abnormality appears to be *TP53* mutation, which is found in 59–93% of all cases {3099,1917,1008,3756}. In most cases, this is a key driver mutation developing at the stage of intraepithelial neoplasia (preinvasive carcinoma).
- Mutations in other cell-cycle regulatory genes, such as *CDKN2A* (*P16*), *RB1*, *NFE2L2*, *CHEK1*, and *CHEK2*, have also been identified {3099,1917,1008}, as have amplifications of cell-cycle regulatory genes (*CCND1*, *CDK4*, *CDK6*, and *MDM2*).

Genes that control cell differentiation
- *NOTCH1* and *NOTCH3* mutations are detected in as many as 28% of cases {1008}.

EGFR (HER1) signalling pathway
- EGFR overexpression, reported in 59.6–76% of cases, is an adverse prognostic factor {2420}.
- Mutations and/or amplifications in RAS and AKT family oncogenes are seen in at least 75% of cases {3099}.

Epigenetic factors
- DNA methylation, chromatin modification, RNA editing, and loss of genomic imprinting are relatively common in oesophageal squamous cell carcinoma {2420,1918}.
- Promoter hypermethylation–related silencing of *CDKN2A* leads to overexpression of p53 {3204}.

Inherited factors
- Tylosis, an autosomal dominant disorder caused by a missense mutation in *RHBDF2*, results in overactivation of the EGFR signalling pathway {346}.
- Fanconi anaemia, an autosomal recessive disorder, affects the Fanconi anaemia pathway, which is normally active in DNA repair {2199}.

Copy-number alterations and structural rearrangements
- Chromosome aneuploidy (in particular, gains in chromosomes 3, 10, 12, and 20) is common in oesophageal squamous cell carcinoma {1918}.
- Copy-number alterations result from mutations and amplifications of genes as described above {1918}.

Other genetic abnormalities
- SNPs, including *TP53* polymorphisms {3099}, have been detected in patients with oesophageal squamous cell carcinoma.
- A common somatic mutation signature in oesophageal squamous cell carcinoma is G:C→A:T transitions; interestingly, this is a typical mutation signature induced by acetaldehyde {2420}.

Subtype(s)

Verrucous squamous cell carcinoma (8051/3); squamous cell carcinoma, spindle cell (8074/3); basaloid squamous cell carcinoma (8083/3)

Localization

Squamous cell carcinoma is located most commonly in the middle third of the oesophagus, followed by the lower third {3197,3010,140}. In a large Japanese series, slightly more than half (55%) of squamous cell carcinomas occurred in the middle oesophagus, 32% in the lower oesophagus, and 14% in the upper oesophagus {140}. Similarly, in a series from Hong Kong SAR, China, about half (49%) of the tumours were located in the middle oesophagus, 41% in the lower oesophagus, and 10% in the upper oesophagus {1774}.

Clinical features

The most common clinical symptom is dysphagia, which usually indicates advanced disease. Chest pain, painful swallowing, and weight loss can also be presenting symptoms {865}. Upper oesophageal tumours may be associated with hoarseness due to recurrent laryngeal nerve involvement. Early-stage disease is generally asymptomatic and discovered incidentally. Any persistent ulceration or refractory stricture in the oesophagus should arouse concern for malignancy.

The gold standard for diagnosis is upper GI tract endoscopy and biopsy for histological analysis, with or without brushings for cytological examination. Image-enhanced endoscopy (e.g. narrow-band imaging) and chromoendoscopy may help identify early-stage lesions by highlighting an abnormal vascular pattern or iodine negativity associated with neoplasia {2420,2041}. Evolving techniques such as confocal endomicroscopy may facilitate better targeting of biopsies {2041}. EUS is useful for evaluating the depth of invasion into the oesophageal wall and may reveal regional lymph node metastasis; however, it is unreliable in diffusely infiltrating disease. Endoscopic mucosal resection or endoscopic submucosal dissection is the best procedure for determining depth of invasion in superficial disease. CT and FDG PET are useful for staging more-advanced disease and response after chemoradiation {865,2420}.

Epidemiology

Oesophageal squamous cell carcinoma is the sixth leading cause of cancer-related death worldwide {923}. There is marked geographical variation in the incidence of disease both among regions and even within individual countries. The highest incidence rates (> 50 cases/100 000 person-years) are found in the Asian oesophageal cancer belt, which stretches from eastern to central Asia. Intermediate rates (10–50 cases/100 000 person-years) are observed along the Indian coast of Africa, in southern Brazil and Uruguay, and in parts of the Caribbean {923,3386}. The incidence of oesophageal squamous cell carcinoma (now < 10 cases/100 000 person-years) has been decreasing in North American and European countries over the past few decades, whereas the incidence of oesophageal adenocarcinoma has been increasing. Even within high-incidence countries, there is marked variation. For example, the rate is much lower in the southern provinces of China than in the north-east. Overall, oesophageal squamous cell carcinoma is more common in males, who account for 69% of cases {923}. This male predominance is more pronounced in North American and European countries, where males are at least 4 times as likely as females to develop the disease. In high-incidence countries such as China and the Islamic Republic of Iran, the male predominance is less pronounced. The median patient age at diagnosis is in the seventh decade of life, and most patients

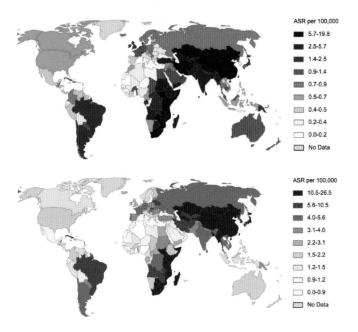

ASR per 100,000
- ■ 5.7–19.8
- ■ 2.5–5.7
- ■ 1.4–2.5
- ▥ 0.9–1.4
- ▨ 0.7–0.9
- ▤ 0.5–0.7
- ▦ 0.4–0.5
- ▨ 0.2–0.4
- □ 0.0–0.2
- ▥ No Data

ASR per 100,000
- ■ 10.5–26.5
- ■ 5.6–10.5
- ■ 4.0–5.6
- ■ 3.1–4.0
- ▨ 2.2–3.1
- ▤ 1.5–2.2
- ▦ 1.2–1.5
- □ 0.9–1.2
- □ 0.0–0.9
- ▥ No Data

Fig. 2.19 Estimated age-standardized incidence rates (ASRs; World), per 100 000 person-years, of oesophageal squamous cell carcinoma in women (**top**) and men (**bottom**) in 2012.

present in their fifth to eighth decade {1778}. Multiple squamous cell carcinomas can occur in the oesophagus and other parts of the aerodigestive tract (e.g. the oral cavity and oropharynx); this finding is related both to the common exposure of these regions to risk factors such as tobacco smoke and to the rich lymphatic networks in the oesophagus {1775,1779}.

Etiology
The etiology of oesophageal squamous cell carcinoma is multifactorial and heavily dependent on the population being studied. The main risk factors are presented in Box 2.03 (p. 48).

Pathogenesis
Oesophageal squamous cell carcinoma develops by stepwise progression, with accumulating genetic abnormalities driving progression from histologically normal squamous mucosa to low-grade intraepithelial neoplasia (dysplasia) to high-grade intraepithelial neoplasia and finally to invasive squamous cell carcinoma. *TP53* mutation is a key early driver mutation {1918}. Genetic changes identified at the intraepithelial neoplasia stage include aneuploidy, copy-number alterations, changes related to the amplification of genes such as *EGFR*, and the silencing of genes such as *CDKN2A* due to promoter hypermethylation {1918}. The specific mutations required for the invasion beyond the basement membrane that is characteristic of invasive squamous cell carcinoma are still unknown. Acquisition of invasive and migratory capability via epithelial–mesenchymal transition is important. *EIF5A2* amplification has been shown to be a factor in inducing this phenotype {1893}. The key genetic abnormalities identified in oesophageal squamous cell carcinoma {2420,8} are summarized in Box 2.04 (p. 49).

Macroscopic appearance
Squamous cell carcinoma often presents at an advanced pathological stage with an ulcerative mass. The most useful macroscopic classification, illustrated in Fig. 2.20, has been provided by the Japan Esophageal Society {1427}.

Histopathology
Grading
Squamous cell carcinoma has both vertical and horizontal growth of neoplastic squamous epithelium beyond the basement membrane. Grading is based on the degree of cytological atypia, mitotic activity, and presence of keratinization. A three-tiered system (grades 1, 2, 3) is commonly applied; however, a two-tiered system (grade 1–2 vs grade 3) may be clinically relevant, because the pathological distinction between grade 1 and grade 2 often shows high interobserver variation.

Grade 1 (well-differentiated) squamous cell carcinoma contains enlarged cells with abundant eosinophilic cytoplasm and keratin pearl production. Cytological atypia is minimal and the mitotic count is low. The invasive margin is pushing and the cells remain well ordered.

Grade 2 (moderately differentiated) squamous cell carcinoma has evident cytological atypia and the cells are less ordered. Mitotic figures are easily identified. There is usually surface parakeratosis, but keratin pearl formation is infrequent.

Grade 3 (poorly differentiated) squamous cell carcinoma consists predominantly of basal-like cells forming nests, which may show central necrosis. The tumour nests consist of sheets or pavement-like arrangements of tumour cells with occasional parakeratotic or keratinizing cells.

Therapy effects
Most patients with advanced oesophageal squamous cell carcinoma are treated with combined preoperative chemotherapy and radiotherapy. This usually induces progressive changes in both the tumour cells and the peritumoural stroma, with macroscopic tumour regression. Cellular changes include nuclear enlargement or shrinkage, nuclear vacuolation, apoptosis, and necrosis. Keratin released from the dying cells may accumulate, undergo dystrophic calcification, and elicit a surrounding giant cell reaction. A neutrophilic or chronic inflammatory cell response may be seen. There is fibrosis and sometimes stromal elastosis. Regional vessels typically show arteriosclerosis.

The extent of tumour regression is an important prognostic factor. It is graded on histological examination by comparing the amount of residual tumour with the amount of therapy-induced fibrosis. The most widely used method of assessing tumour regression grade (TRG) is the Mandard system (see Table 2.02, p. 43) {2036,2708}. Another system relies on the estimated percentage reduction in tumour volume, with < 10% residual tumour constituting a good prognostic finding {244}. Pathological complete response (i.e. complete or nearly complete tumour eradication) is the primary goal of preoperative therapy.

Subtypes
Verrucous squamous cell carcinoma {2461,76,3341} is a subtype often arising in the setting of chronic irritation, oesophagitis, or previous oesophageal injury. Therefore, most cases are identified in the lower third of the oesophagus, as a protuberant mass. Association with HPV51 and HPV11 has been demonstrated in

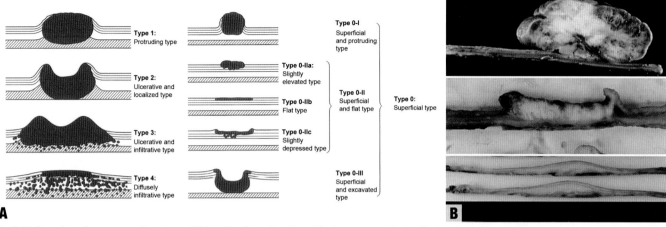

Fig. 2.20 Oesophageal squamous cell carcinoma NOS. **A** The Japan Esophageal Society macroscopic classification of squamous cell carcinoma of the oesophagus. **B** Macroscopic appearance on cut surface of examples classified according to the Japan Esophageal Society classification as type 0–1: superficial and protruding type (**top**), type 2 (advanced): ulcerative and localized type (**middle**), and type 4 (advanced): diffusely infiltrative type (**bottom**).

some cases. The tumour comprises exceedingly differentiated squamous cells with minimal cytological atypia, minimal mitotic activity, and surface papillary projections. Keratinization occurs abruptly, with no intervening granular cell layer, and cup-like collections of keratin are present at the base of the papillary structures. The invasive front is characterized by broad bulbous pushing projections. The tumour is slow-growing, and metastases are uncommon.

Spindle cell squamous cell carcinoma typically has a polypoid growth pattern. Microscopically, there is a biphasic pattern of neoplastic squamous epithelium and spindle cells. Squamous elements are typically well to moderately differentiated

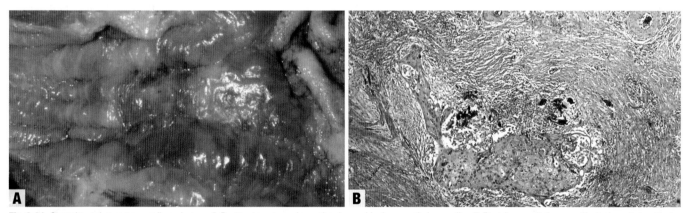

Fig. 2.21 Oesophageal squamous cell carcinoma. **A** Posttreatment specimen showing residual mucosal abnormality. **B** Postchemoradiotherapy effect, characterized by tumour shrinkage, surrounding fibrosis, keratin collections with dystrophic calcification, chronic inflammation, and arteriosclerosis.

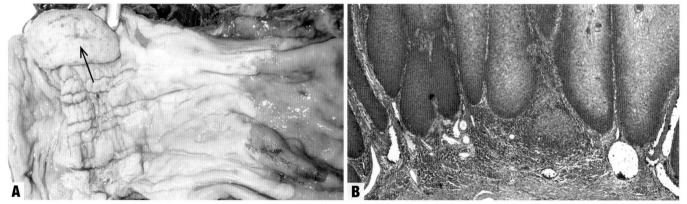

Fig. 2.22 Oesophageal verrucous squamous cell carcinoma. **A** The typical fungating appearance (arrow). **B** The well-differentiated cells, cup-like keratin, and pushing pattern of infiltration typical of this subtype.

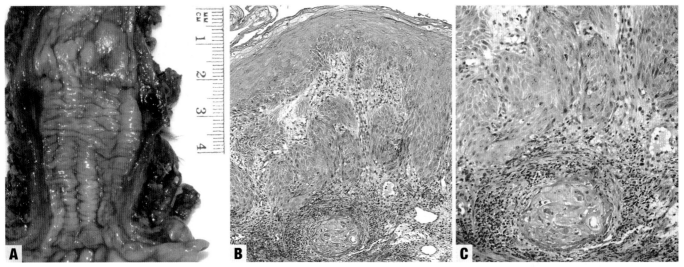

Fig. 2.23 Oesophageal squamous cell carcinoma. **A** Macroscopic appearance of a mid-oesophageal mass. **B** A well-differentiated example; note the submucosal invasion by clusters of malignant squamous cells. **C** A higher-power view of an infiltrating malignant squamous cell cluster.

or may occasionally be carcinoma in situ alone. The spindle cell component is a high-grade malignancy, which may show osseous, cartilaginous, or skeletal muscle differentiation {1412,2662,1428}. Although these tumours tend to be large, the prognosis is sometimes better than that of conventional squamous cell carcinoma of the same size, primarily because of the intraluminal rather than deeply invasive growth.

Basaloid squamous cell carcinoma shows a marked male predominance and accounts for approximately 5% of all oesophageal cancers {1890,293,2846}. Unlike similar tumours in the oropharynx, oesophageal basaloid squamous cell carcinoma has no association with HPV infection {293}. The tumours show a solid or nested growth pattern of basaloid cells, sometimes with central comedonecrosis and occasionally with pseudoglandular or cribriform formations. The tumour morphology has been confused with rare primary adenoid cystic carcinoma {1890}. Exclusion of high-grade neuroendocrine carcinoma (NEC) by immunohistochemistry is often required. Areas of squamous cell carcinoma in situ or conventional invasive squamous cell

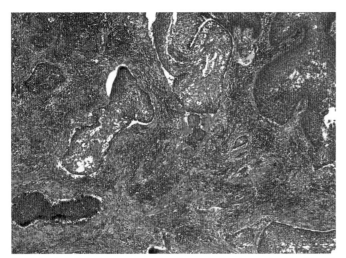

Fig. 2.24 Oesophageal squamous cell carcinoma. An invasive, moderately differentiated example arising in the middle oesophagus of a patient with achalasia.

carcinoma are relatively common. The tumour is highly aggressive, with a worse prognosis than conventional squamous cell carcinoma, although the difference is often not statistically significant {3341}.

Differential diagnosis
In small biopsy specimens, it may be difficult to differentiate conventional squamous cell carcinoma from other subtypes of squamous cell carcinoma, as well as from undifferentiated carcinoma or adenocarcinoma (see *Adenocarcinoma of the oesophagus and oesophagogastric junction NOS*, p. 38).

Cytology
Cytological sampling using directed mucosal brushings and blind sampling using techniques such as the Cytosponge procedure are cost-effective for screening in high-risk populations and facilitate primary diagnosis of early squamous neoplasia {775}.

Diagnostic molecular pathology
At present, no molecular tests are required. See the *Pathogenesis* subsection above for further information on the molecular abnormalities present in this tumour type.

Essential and desirable diagnostic criteria
Essential: histological evidence of vertical and horizontal growth of neoplastic squamous epithelium, with definite evidence of invasion.

Staging (TNM)
Oesophageal squamous cell carcinoma should be staged using the eighth editions (2017) of the Union for International Cancer Control (UICC) TNM classification {408} and the American Joint Committee on Cancer (AJCC) cancer staging manual {127}. Depth of invasion provides a clinically relevant division of oesophageal squamous cell carcinoma into superficial (or early) disease versus advanced (or late) disease. Superficial disease is invasion restricted to the mucosa and submucosa. It has a low risk of regional lymph node metastasis and is curable

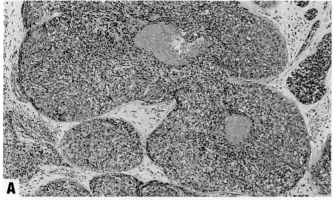

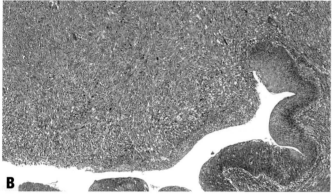

Fig. 2.25 Oesophageal squamous cell carcinoma. **A** Oesophageal basaloid squamous cell carcinoma. Rounded nests of basaloid cells with central necrosis. **B** Oesophageal spindle cell squamous cell carcinoma. Spindle-cell features and dysplasia in the squamous epithelium.

by local resection if submucosal invasion is < 200 μm deep {3224}. Advanced disease is invasion beyond the muscularis propria, with a high risk of regional or systemic metastasis. Superficial disease, which accounts for as many as 35% of all cases in Japan, is associated with a 5-year survival rate of approximately 85%. The 5-year survival rate with advanced disease is < 10–15% {3197}.

Prognosis and prediction
The most important prognostic factor is staging, which is used to determine the most appropriate treatment regimen for a given patient. Despite the frequent overexpression of EGFR (HER1) in squamous cell carcinoma, targeted therapy against this protein has failed to improve survival. There is a potentially promising role for immune checkpoint inhibitors as novel therapies in advanced disease {1852,2967}.

Oesophageal undifferentiated carcinoma

Kawachi H
Saito T

Definition
Undifferentiated carcinoma of the oesophagus is a malignant oesophageal epithelial tumour that lacks definite microscopic features of squamous, glandular, or neuroendocrine differentiation.

ICD-O coding
8020/3 Carcinoma, undifferentiated, NOS

ICD-11 coding
2B70.Y & XH1YY4 Other specified malignant neoplasms of oesophagus & Carcinoma, undifferentiated, NOS

Related terminology
None

Subtype(s)
Lymphoepithelioma-like carcinoma (8082/3)

Localization
This carcinoma is most often located in the lower oesophagus or the oesophagogastric junction {3063}.

Clinical features
The most common symptom is progressive dysphagia, followed by gastro-oesophageal reflux, weight loss, and anaemia {3063}.

Epidemiology
The reported relative prevalence varies widely, from 0.18% to 4% of oesophageal carcinomas {2709,3427}; this apparent variation is probably related to the lack of diagnostic criteria. In reported US series, patients ranged in age from 39 to 84 years (mean: 65.5 years) and were predominantly male {3063}.

Etiology
Unknown

Pathogenesis
Undifferentiated carcinoma most likely results from the dedifferentiation of squamous cell carcinoma or adenocarcinoma of oesophageal epithelial origin. In the largest study of undifferentiated carcinomas to date, 12 of 16 cases (75%) were associated with Barrett oesophagus, and some of those carcinomas contained focal glandular differentiation {3063}.

Macroscopic appearance
The tumours are exophytic, with raised edges, and they are centred in either the oesophagus or the oesophagogastric junction {3063}. In most cases, there are central areas of depression and ulceration.

Histopathology
The tumour cells form variably sized nests and sheet-like arrangements. The cells are medium-sized to large, with poorly defined amphophilic to slightly eosinophilic cytoplasm imparting a syncytial-like appearance. Cytologically, the nuclei are oval and vesicular. Large pleomorphic nuclei and multinucleated giant cells mimicking osteoclasts or rhabdoid cells are occasionally found {3063}.

Lymphoepithelioma-like carcinoma {3273} is considered to be a distinct subtype of undifferentiated carcinoma. Most reported cases have been from Japan and clinically resemble conventional squamous cell carcinoma {611,2305}. This subtype is characterized by a sheet-like arrangement of large epithelioid cells with prominent nucleoli and indistinct cell borders. The tumour is surrounded by a characteristic inflammatory infiltrate that is rich in lymphocytes and plasma cells. Unlike

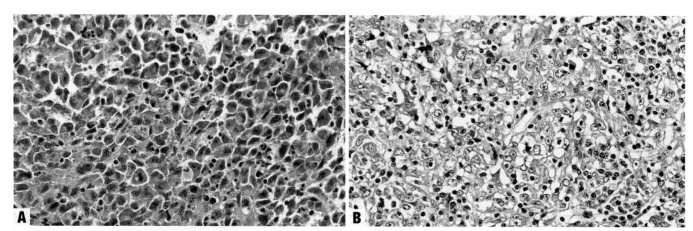

Fig. 2.26 Oesophageal undifferentiated carcinoma. **A** The nuclei of the tumour cells are pleomorphic; rhabdoid cells are occasionally found. **B** The lymphoepithelioma-like carcinoma subtype is characterized by sheet-like arrangement of large epithelioid cells with prominent nucleoli and indistinct cell borders; a characteristic inflammatory infiltrate rich in lymphocytes and plasma cells surrounds the tumour.

similar tumours located in the head and neck region, lymphoep-ithelioma-like carcinoma of the oesophagus is only occasionally positive for EBV {3273}.

When present, cytokeratin positivity may help exclude non-epithelial neoplasms such as melanoma, lymphoma, and sarcoma. Other immunohistochemical markers are recommended for distinguishing undifferentiated carcinoma from neuroendo-crine carcinoma (NEC; chromogranin A, synaptophysin, and CD56), poorly differentiated squamous cell carcinoma (p63 and p40), and poorly differentiated adenocarcinoma (mucins).

Cytology

Undifferentiated carcinoma consists of malignant cells without evidence of differentiation.

Diagnostic molecular pathology

Not clinically relevant

Essential and desirable diagnostic criteria

Essential: malignant cells without evidence of differentiation by histology; equivocal immunohistochemistry.

Staging (TNM)

The staging of oesophageal undifferentiated carcinoma follows that of oesophageal squamous cell carcinoma.

Prognosis and prediction

In a US series, most undifferentiated carcinomas were detected at an advanced stage; the prognosis was poor, with a 1-year survival rate of 25% {3063}.

Oesophageal neuroendocrine neoplasms

Scoazec JY
Rindi G

Definition

Neuroendocrine neoplasms (NENs) of the oesophagus are oesophageal epithelial neoplasms with neuroendocrine differentiation, including well-differentiated neuroendocrine tumours (NETs), poorly differentiated neuroendocrine carcinomas (NECs), and mixed neuroendocrine–non-neuroendocrine neoplasms (MiNENs) – an umbrella category including mixed adenoneuroendocrine carcinoma (MANEC).

ICD-O coding

8240/3 Neuroendocrine tumour NOS
8246/3 Neuroendocrine carcinoma NOS
8154/3 Mixed neuroendocrine–non-neuroendocrine neoplasm (MiNEN)

ICD-11 coding

2B70.Y & XH55D7 Other specified malignant neoplasms of oesophagus & Neuroendocrine carcinoma, well-differentiated
2B70.Y & XH0U20 Other specified malignant neoplasms of oesophagus & Neuroendocrine carcinoma NOS
2B70.Y & XH9SY0 Other specified malignant neoplasms of oesophagus & Small cell neuroendocrine carcinoma
2B70.Y & XH0NL5 Other specified malignant neoplasms of oesophagus & Large cell neuroendocrine carcinoma
2B70.Y & XH7YE3 Other specified malignant neoplasms of oesophagus & Combined small cell carcinoma

Related terminology

Acceptable: carcinoid; well-differentiated endocrine tumour/carcinoma; poorly differentiated endocrine carcinoma; mixed exocrine-endocrine carcinoma; mixed adenoneuroendocrine carcinoma.

Subtype(s)

Neuroendocrine tumour, grade 1 (8240/3); neuroendocrine tumour, grade 2 (8249/3); neuroendocrine tumour, grade 3 (8249/3); large cell neuroendocrine carcinoma (8013/3); small cell neuroendocrine carcinoma (8041/3); combined small cell–adenocarcinoma (8045/3); combined small cell–squamous cell carcinoma (8045/3)

Localization

NENs typically occur in the lower oesophagus, often in association with metaplastic Barrett mucosa or (rarely) ectopic gastric mucosa. NECs can also occur in the middle and even upper oesophagus {2066,1319}.

Clinical features

Dysphagia, pain, weight loss, asthenia, and sometimes melaena are the most common presenting symptoms {2188,882,2884}. Some NETs are discovered incidentally {1249,634}. Metastatic NETs may present with carcinoid syndrome {2188}. NECs may be associated with paraneoplastic syndromes {141}. On endoscopy, NETs usually appear as polypoid or nodular submucosal masses, < 2 cm in diameter {1249,634}, whereas NECs are large, infiltrative, and ulcerated {2884}.

Epidemiology

Oesophageal NENs are exceedingly rare {2188,882,2884}. They account for 0.04–1% of all gastroenteropancreatic NENs overall {2188,2884,3371}, but figures as high as 5% have been reported in some countries {882}. The incidence is higher in males than in females (M:F ratio: 6:1), with a predominance in the sixth and seventh decades of life (mean patient age: 56 years) {2188,2884,2187}.

Etiology

The etiology is unknown. The presence of endocrine cells in the submucosal glands of the lower oesophagus or in Barrett

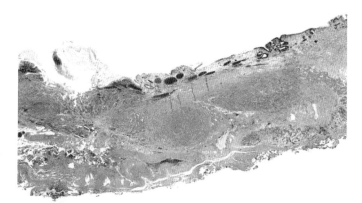

A

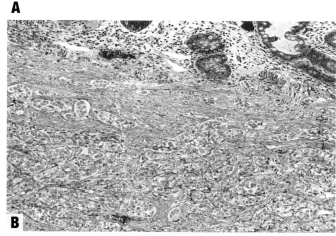

B

Fig. 2.27 Well-differentiated oesophageal neuroendocrine tumour (NET). **A** Low magnification of an endoscopic resection specimen from a case arising in Barrett mucosa. **B** High magnification of a tumour of the lower oesophagus arising in Barrett mucosa with intestinal metaplasia.

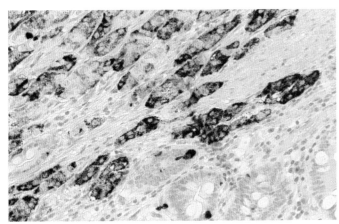

Fig. 2.28 Serotonin-producing oesophageal neuroendocrine tumour (NET). Serotonin expression in a well-differentiated NET of the lower oesophagus arising in Barrett mucosa with intestinal metaplasia (indirect immunoperoxidase staining).

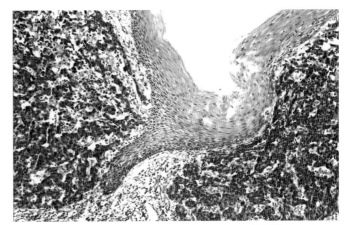

Fig. 2.29 Oesophageal large cell neuroendocrine carcinoma (LCNEC).

mucosa {3265} might explain the predominance of NENs in the lower oesophagus {1249,518}. NECs might be associated with alcohol consumption and/or heavy smoking {3371,518}.

Pathogenesis

A recent study of 55 oesophageal NECs {3508} showed a high rate of inactivating mutations in *TP53* and *RB1* – as are seen in most cases of small cell NEC (SCNEC) – as well as in three other genes: *NOTCH1*, *FAT1*, and *FBXW7*. Also reported were recurrent mutations in three genes not known to be involved in oesophageal or neuroendocrine tumorigenesis: *PDE3A*, *PTPRM*, and *CBLN2*.

Macroscopic appearance

NETs are usually small lesions. In a systematic review of 19 cases, the mean tumour size was 2.4 cm {2650}. NECs are often large, bulky, deeply infiltrative tumours. They may be exophytic or ulcerated {1319}.

Histopathology

NET: Fewer than 50 cases of oesophageal NETs have been reported in the literature. They showed the typical features of well-differentiated NENs. The growth pattern may be insular or cribriform. The tumours consist of medium-sized cells with a low N:C ratio, abundant cytoplasm, and a small ovoid nucleus with dispersed chromatin containing small nucleoli. Variable amounts of well-vascularized stroma are present. Focal necrosis may be seen. Neuroendocrine differentiation is confirmed by the expression of chromogranin A and synaptophysin. Various hormones have been detected by immunohistochemistry, including serotonin, (entero)glucagon, PP, gastrin, and calcitonin {1249,935,2870}. VMAT2 expression, suggestive of an enterochromaffin-like (ECL) cell–like phenotype, has been described in some cases {518,1647}. Grading information is rarely available, especially for cases reported in the older literature, but most cases can be retrospectively graded as G1–2.

NEC: These tumours account for > 90% of all oesophageal NENs {882}. They are subtyped as small cell NEC (SCNEC) and large cell NEC (LCNEC); the relative proportion of LCNEC varies across studies, from 12% to 62% {2066,1319,2995}. Like other NECs, oesophageal NECs usually show solid, rosette-like or palisading patterns; necrosis is frequent and often extensive. Mitotic activity is consistently brisk. SCNECs are characterized by small to medium-sized cells with a high N:C ratio, scant basophilic cytoplasm, and elongated nuclei containing finely dispersed chromatin without well-formed nucleoli. LCNECs are characterized by medium-sized to large cells with basophilic cytoplasm and large ovoid nuclei containing large nucleoli. Neuroendocrine differentiation should be confirmed by immunohistochemistry. Synaptophysin expression is a consistent feature, whereas chromogranin A expression, present in about 60% of cases, is usually focal and faint {1319}. TTF1 is positive in about 70% of cases {1319}. The main differential diagnosis is basaloid squamous cell carcinoma, which usually shows immunohistochemical evidence of squamous cell differentiation, including expression of p63, p40, and CK5/6 {618}; however, p63 is not fully discriminant, because it may be detected in some oesophageal NECs {1319}.

MiNEN: Oesophageal MiNENs usually consist of poorly differentiated NEC and either squamous cell carcinoma or adenocarcinoma (in Barrett mucosa or ectopic gastric mucosa) {3371}. Rare collision tumours combining an apparently well-differentiated component and adenocarcinoma have also been reported in Barrett mucosa {1249}.

Collision tumours: Collision tumours do not meet the definition of MiNENs.

Grading: Oesophageal NENs are graded using the same system used for other gastroenteropancreatic NENs.

Cytology

There are no specific cytological features.

Diagnostic molecular pathology

Not clinically relevant

Essential and desirable diagnostic criteria

Essential: morphological criteria suggestive of neuroendocrine differentiation (must be confirmed by the immunohistochemical demonstration of specific lineage markers, e.g. chromogranin A or synaptophysin).

Staging (TNM)

Unlike for NETs occurring at other gastrointestinal sites, there is no TNM staging system specifically for oesophageal NET. The staging of oesophageal NEC and MiNEN follows that of oesophageal carcinomas.

Prognosis and prediction

Despite reports to the contrary in older literature, the prognosis of oesophageal NETs appears to be good, mainly depending on tumour size and extent of dissemination. The influence of tumour grade cannot be assessed, because only very limited data are available. Metastatic dissemination is rare {634}. The overall survival time ranges from 1 to 23 years. In contrast, the prognosis of NECs is very poor. Metastatic dissemination is frequent at diagnosis. The median overall survival time ranges from 8 to 15 months; most patients die within 2 years of diagnosis. The presence of distant metastases seems to be the strongest adverse prognostic factor {2066}. There is no statistically significant difference in survival between LCNEC and SCNEC {2066}. Prognosis apparently depends on the Ki-67 proliferation index {2164}. MiNENs might have a better prognosis than pure NECs; the median survival time is about 20 months {2066}, and prognosis is based on the Ki-67 proliferation index of the NEC component {2163}.

There is no consensus on the optimal treatment for oesophageal NENs {2884}. Small NETs (< 1–1.5 cm in size) without evidence of locoregional metastasis can be successfully treated by endoscopic resection. Larger tumours require surgery; adjuvant chemotherapy has been used in metastatic cases. The treatment of NECs and MiNENs is commonly based on chemotherapy with platinum salts. Tumours with only locoregional extension can be treated by a combination of surgery, chemotherapy, and even radiotherapy {2066}.

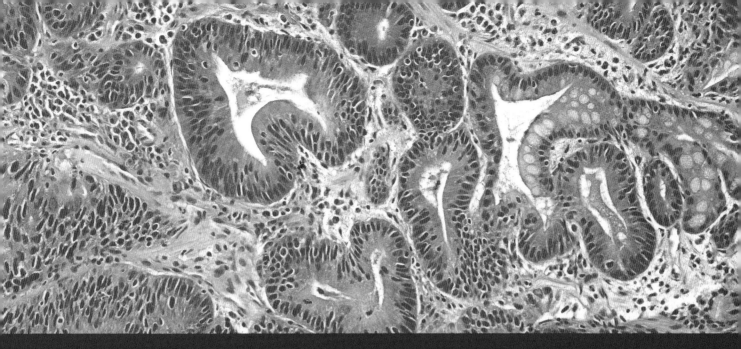

3

Tumours of the stomach

Edited by: Fukayama M, Rugge M, Washington MK

Gastritis and metaplasia: precursors of gastric neoplasms
Benign epithelial tumours and precursors
   Fundic gland polyps
   Hyperplastic polyps
   Dysplasia
   Intestinal-type adenoma
   Foveolar-type adenoma
   Pyloric gland adenoma
   Oxyntic gland adenoma
Malignant epithelial tumours
   Adenocarcinoma
   Squamous cell carcinoma
   Adenosquamous carcinoma
   Undifferentiated carcinoma
   Gastroblastoma
   Neuroendocrine neoplasms

WHO classification of tumours of the stomach

Benign epithelial tumours and precursors

8148/0   Glandular intraepithelial neoplasia, low grade
8148/2   Glandular intraepithelial neoplasia, high grade
8213/0*   Serrated dysplasia, low grade
8213/2*   Serrated dysplasia, high grade
       Intestinal-type dysplasia
       Foveolar-type (gastric-type) dysplasia
       Gastric pit/crypt dysplasia
8144/0*   Intestinal-type adenoma, low grade
8144/2*   Intestinal-type adenoma, high grade
       Sporadic intestinal-type gastric adenoma
       Syndromic intestinal-type gastric adenoma
8210/0*   Adenomatous polyp, low-grade dysplasia
8210/2*   Adenomatous polyp, high-grade dysplasia

Malignant epithelial tumours

8140/3   Adenocarcinoma NOS
8211/3   Tubular adenocarcinoma
8214/3   Parietal cell carcinoma
8255/3   Adenocarcinoma with mixed subtypes
8260/3   Papillary adenocarcinoma NOS
8265/3   Micropapillary carcinoma NOS
8430/3   Mucoepidermoid carcinoma
8480/3   Mucinous adenocarcinoma
8490/3   Signet-ring cell carcinoma
8490/3   Poorly cohesive carcinoma
8512/3   Medullary carcinoma with lymphoid stroma
8576/3   Hepatoid adenocarcinoma
       Paneth cell carcinoma
8070/3   Squamous cell carcinoma NOS
8560/3   Adenosquamous carcinoma
8020/3   Carcinoma, undifferentiated, NOS
8014/3   Large cell carcinoma with rhabdoid phenotype
8022/3   Pleomorphic carcinoma
8033/3   Sarcomatoid carcinoma
8035/3   Carcinoma with osteoclast-like giant cells
8976/1*   Gastroblastoma
8240/3   Neuroendocrine tumour NOS
8240/3   Neuroendocrine tumour, grade 1
8249/3   Neuroendocrine tumour, grade 2
8249/3   Neuroendocrine tumour, grade 3
8153/3   Gastrinoma NOS
8156/3   Somatostatinoma NOS
8241/3   Enterochromaffin-cell carcinoid
8242/3   ECL-cell carcinoid, malignant
8246/3   Neuroendocrine carcinoma NOS
8013/3   Large cell neuroendocrine carcinoma
8041/3   Small cell neuroendocrine carcinoma
8154/3   Mixed neuroendocrine–non-neuroendocrine neoplasm (MiNEN)

These morphology codes are from the International Classification of Diseases for Oncology, third edition, second revision (ICD-O-3.2) {1378A}. Behaviour is coded /0 for benign tumours; /1 for unspecified, borderline, or uncertain behaviour; /2 for carcinoma in situ and grade III intraepithelial neoplasia; /3 for malignant tumours, primary site; and /6 for malignant tumours, metastatic site. Behaviour code /6 is not generally used by cancer registries.

This classification is modified from the previous WHO classification, taking into account changes in our understanding of these lesions.

* Codes marked with an asterisk were approved by the IARC/WHO Committee for ICD-O at its meeting in April 2019.

TNM staging of carcinomas of the stomach

Stomach

(ICD-O-3 C16)

Rules for Classification

The classification applies only to carcinomas. There should be histological confirmation of the disease. Cancers involving the oesophagogastric junction (OGJ) whose epicentre is within the proximal 2 cm of the cardia (Siewert types I/II) are to be staged as oesophageal cancers. Cancers whose epicentre is more than 2 cm distal from the OGJ will be staged using the Stomach Cancer TNM and Stage even if the OGJ is involved.

Changes in this edition from the seventh edition are based upon recommendations from the International Gastric Cancer Association Staging Project.[1]

The following are the procedures for assessing T, N, and M categories.

T categories	Physical examination, imaging, endoscopy, and/or surgical exploration
N categories	Physical examination, imaging, and/or surgical exploration
M categories	Physical examination, imaging, and/or surgical exploration

Anatomical Subsites

1. Cardia (16.0)
2. Fundus (C16.1)
3. Corpus (C16.2)
4. Antrum (C16.3) and pylorus (C16.4)

Regional Lymph Nodes

The regional lymph nodes of the stomach are the perigastric nodes along the lesser and greater curvatures, the nodes along the left gastric, common hepatic, splenic, and coeliac arteries, and the hepatoduodenal nodes.

Involvement of other intra-abdominal lymph nodes such as retropancreatic, mesenteric, and para-aortic is classified as distant metastasis.

TNM Clinical Classification

T – Primary Tumour

TX	Primary tumour cannot be assessed
T0	No evidence of primary tumour
Tis	Carcinoma in situ: intraepithelial tumour without invasion of the lamina propria, high-grade dysplasia
T1	Tumour invades lamina propria, muscularis mucosae, or submucosa
T1a	Tumour invades lamina propria or muscularis mucosae
T1b	Tumour invades submucosa
T2	Tumour invades muscularis propria
T3	Tumour invades subserosa
T4	Tumour perforates serosa (visceral peritoneum) or invades adjacent structures[a, b, c]
T4a	Tumour perforates serosa
T4b	Tumour invades adjacent structures[a, b]

Notes

[a] The adjacent structures of the stomach are the spleen, transverse colon, liver, diaphragm, pancreas, abdominal wall, adrenal gland, kidney, small intestine, and retroperitoneum.
[b] Intramural extension to the duodenum or oesophagus is classified by the depth of greatest invasion in any of these sites including stomach.
[c] Tumour that extends into gastrocolic or gastrohepatic ligaments or into greater or lesser omentum, without perforation of visceral peritoneum, is T3.

N – Regional Lymph Nodes

NX	Regional lymph nodes cannot be assessed
N0	No regional lymph node metastasis
N1	Metastasis in 1 to 2 regional lymph nodes
N2	Metastasis in 3 to 6 regional lymph nodes
N3	Metastasis in 7 or more regional lymph nodes
N3a	Metastasis in 7 to 15 regional lymph nodes
N3b	Metastasis in 16 or more regional lymph nodes

M – Distant Metastasis

M0	No distant metastasis
M1	Distant metastasis

Note

Distant metastasis includes peritoneal seeding, positive peritoneal cytology, and omental tumour not part of continuous extension.

pTNM Pathological Classification

The pT and pN categories correspond to the T and N categories.

pN0   Histological examination of a regional lymphadenectomy specimen will ordinarily include 16 or more lymph nodes. If the lymph nodes are negative, but the number ordinarily examined is not met, classify as pN0.

pM – Distant Metastasis*

pM1   Distant metastasis microscopically confirmed

Note
* pM0 and pMX are not valid categories.

Clinical Stage

Stage 0	Tis	N0	M0
Stage I	T1,T2	N0	M0
Stage IIA	T1,T2	N1,N2,N3	M0
Stage IIB	T3,T4a	N0	M0
Stage III	T3,T4a	N1,N2,N3	M0
Stage IVA	T4b	Any N	M0
Stage IVB	Any T	Any N	M1

Pathological Stage*

Stage 0	Tis	N0	M0
Stage IA	T1	N0	M0
Stage IB	T1	N1	M0
	T2	N0	M0
Stage IIA	T1	N2	M0
	T2	N1	M0
	T3	N0	M0
Stage IIB	T1	N3a	M0
	T2	N2	M0
	T3	N1	M0
	T4a	N0	M0
Stage IIIA	T2	N3a	M0
	T3	N2	M0
	T4a	N1,N2	M0
	T4b	N0	M0
Stage IIIB	T1,T2	N3b	M0
	T3,T4a	N3a	M0
	T4b	N1,N2	M0
Stage IIIC	T3,T4a	N3b	M0
	T4b	N3a,N3b	M0
Stage IV	Any T	Any N	M1

Note
* The AJCC publishes prognostic groups for after neoadjuvant therapy (categories with the prefix "y").

Reference

1   Sano T, Coit D, Kim HH, et al. for the IGCA Staging Project. Proposal of a new stage grouping of gastric cancer for TNM classification: International Gastric Cancer Association Staging Project. Gastric Cancer 2017; 20: 217-225.

Note: Gastric neuroendocrine tumours (NETs) are staged using the NET-specific TNM staging system, which is presented in Chapter 1 (p. 20).

Tumours of the stomach: Introduction

Rugge M
Fukayama M

Epithelial malignancies can occur in any gastric compartment (cardia, corpus, or antrum) {1600,1338}. Siewert's classification {3040,1355} includes gastric cardia adenocarcinoma among the cancers of the oesophagogastric junction, whereas the eighth edition of the Union for International Cancer Control (UICC) TNM classification {408} specifies that any cancer whose epicentre is > 2 cm distal from the oesophagogastric junction (i.e. into the proximal stomach) should be staged using the system for stomach cancer, even if the oesophagogastric junction is involved. The ICD-O topographical coding for the anatomical sites covered in this chapter is presented in Box 3.01.

Proliferative gastric epithelial lesions include non-neoplastic (benign) polyps, non-invasive neoplastic lesions (dysplasia and adenomas), and carcinoma; their epidemiology varies according to geography, ethnicity, infectious agents, lifestyle factors, and medication use. Gastric cancer (GC) is the most prevalent epithelial malignancy, and *Helicobacter pylori*–associated gastritis is the primary pathogenic factor involved in its development {3162,2031}. Inflammation-associated GC is preceded by Correa's cascade: a sequence of epithelial phenotypic and genotypic changes (metaplasia and dysplasia) that can ultimately result in invasive cancer {674}. Therefore, the treatment of longstanding gastritis and gastric atrophy, metaplasia, and dysplasia is an essential part of any clinicopathological strategy for the secondary prevention of GC {1486,2819,3693}.

Both gastric precancerous lesions and GCs are associated with a spectrum of genetic and epigenetic abnormalities {2483}. Some uncommon GCs have molecular profiles associated with heritable tumour syndromes (see *Genetic tumour syndromes of the digestive system*, p. 511). Somatic mutations may occur in proliferative and preinvasive lesions (e.g. mutations of *CTNNB1*

Box 3.01 ICD-O topographical coding for the anatomical sites covered in this chapter

C16 Stomach
C16.0 Cardia NOS
C16.1 Fundus of the stomach
C16.2 Body of the stomach
C16.3 Gastric antrum
C16.4 Pylorus
C16.5 Lesser curvature of the stomach NOS
C16.6 Greater curvature of the stomach NOS
C16.8 Overlapping lesion of the stomach
C16.9 Stomach NOS

in fundic gland polyps {2935}, *GNAS* in pyloric gland adenomas {2079}, and *TP53* in high-grade dysplasia and adenocarcinoma {908,2167}.

Molecular profiling has also provided a new framework for GC classification {2960,61,3661,476,1540}. The key (epi) genetic molecular abnormalities associated with the four GC subtypes (EBV-positive, microsatellite-unstable, genomically stable, and chromosomally unstable) proposed by The Cancer Genome Atlas (TCGA) Research Network and the Asian Cancer Research Group (ACRG) are described in Table 3.05 (p. 94) {1512,1851,476,692,3021}. Specific somatic molecular alterations have been linked to rare subtypes of GC, gastroblastoma {1083,3106}, and rhabdoid carcinoma {46}. *ERBB2* (*HER2*) amplification identifies GC subtypes susceptible to molecularly targeted therapy {237,3406,1098}; therefore, in high-income countries, oncology diagnostics may include clinical sequencing {756,1710}. However, at its core, the clinical management of GC still relies on traditional histology and pTNM staging (see *Gastric adenocarcinoma*, p. 85).

Gastritis and metaplasia: precursors of gastric neoplasms

Rugge M

Atrophic gastritis and gastric cancer (GC)

In the gastric mucosa, longstanding inflammation can promote phenotypic changes: fibrosis of the lamina propria (replacing glandular loss) and/or metaplastic transformation of the native glands (mucosecreting or oxyntic). These changes result in mucosal atrophy (i.e. the loss of glands appropriate to the native anatomy of the gastric compartment) {791,2784,2801}. The definition of mucosal atrophy encompasses both disappearance and metaplastic (intestinal and/or pseudopyloric) transformation of the native glands. Mucosal atrophy (of any histological subtype) results in functional changes affecting the production of acid and the secretion of pepsinogens and gastrin {675,676, 2792,2785,3708,3693,2791,718,1338,3182,1763,2161,3728}. Pepsinogen and gastrin serology may be used for non-invasive assessment of gastric atrophy (and, by extension, GC risk). The severity and topography (antral or oxyntic) of atrophy are both related to the etiology of the inflammation. Worldwide, the most common pathogenic factor for gastric atrophy is *Helicobacter pylori* infection, followed by autoimmune conditions (possibly triggered by *H. pylori* infection in some cases) {2599,3162,2338, 2789,2799,125,2796}. Although the term "atrophic gastritis" technically applies only to cases featuring both atrophy and inflammation, in practice it is usually considered equivalent to the term "atrophic gastropathy".

Metaplastic atrophy in gastric glands

Any metaplastic transformation of the native gastric glands qualifies as metaplastic atrophy. Both intestinal metaplasia and pseudopyloric metaplasia (also called spasmolytic polypeptide–expressing metaplasia) have been associated with increased GC risk {3107}. Well-established evidence links intestinal metaplasia to the intestinal subtype of GC; a direct role of pseudopyloric metaplasia in the histogenesis of GC is more debated {1061,2639,1225}. Pseudopyloric metaplasia features the same morphology and TFF2 expression seen in pyloric-type

glands {3640}. Pseudopyloric metaplasia may also undergo further changes towards intestinalization. Intestinal metaplasia is defined as the replacement of native gastric epithelium by intestinal-type epithelium, including both goblet cells and columnar mucin-rich cells. There are two subtypes of intestinal metaplasia: the small-intestinal type and the colonic type. Intestinal metaplasia can also be subtyped, on the basis of mucin histochemistry, as type I (complete, small-intestinal type, sialomucin-secreting) or type II or III (incomplete, colonic type, further subclassified according to the expression of particular sialomucins and/or sulfomucins). Type III intestinal metaplasia is the most prone to neoplastic transformation {1437,938}. Because of the direct correlation between extensive intestinalization and sulfomucin-rich intestinal metaplasia, the topographical extent of intestinal metaplasia is assumed to be a reliable indicator of GC risk {854,1866,2790,521}. Immunohistochemistry shows that complete intestinal metaplasia expresses intestinal mucins and has reduced expression of the gastric mucins EMA (MUC1), MUC5AC, and MUC6. Incomplete intestinal metaplasia coexpresses gastric mucins and MUC2 {1576}.

Histological staging of gastritis

Gastric mucosal atrophy is the cancerization field of non-syndromic GCs. The Operative Link on Gastritis Assessment (OLGA) staging system defines five stages of gastritis with increasing cancer risk (stages 0–IV), based on atrophy scores {2793,2794,2797} (see Table 3.01). International guidelines for the secondary prevention of GC use the OLGA staging system to distinguish between low-risk (stage 0–II) and high-risk (stage III–IV) gastritis {2031,3162}. An alternative staging system, the Operative Link on Gastric Intestinal Metaplasia Assessment (OLGIM) system, focuses on intestinal metaplasia scores alone {491}. Gastritis staging facilitates patient-tailored surveillance programmes {2797,2788,787,2791}. Recent evidence supports a correlation between gastritis stage (high-risk vs

Table 3.01 The Operative Link on Gastritis Assessment (OLGA) staging system for gastritis, including the atrophy scores to be applied to both the mucosecreting and oxyntic compartments

Atrophy score		Corpus biopsy specimens			
0: No atrophy in any of the specimens obtained from the same compartment		Overall atrophy score as assessed in the biopsy samples obtained from the oxyntic mucosa			
1: Atrophy involving 1–30% of the specimens obtained from the same compartment					
2: Atrophy involving 31–60% of the specimens obtained from the same compartment		Score 0	Score 1	Score 2	Score 3
3: Atrophy involving > 60% of the specimens obtained from the same compartment	**Score 0**	Score 0	Stage I	Stage II	Stage II
Antrum biopsy specimens Overall atrophy score as assessed in the biopsy samples obtained from both the antrum and the angularis incisura	**Score 1**	Stage I	Stage I	Stage II	Stage III
	Score 2	Stage II	Stage II	Stage III	Stage IV
	Score 3	Stage III	Stage III	Stage IV	Stage IV

low-risk) and gastric serology (i.e. pepsinogen I/II and gastrin positivity). This correlation can be clinically exploited in combined strategies for the secondary prevention of GC {53,2785}.

Gastric dysplasia

Gastric epithelial dysplasia was originally defined as a precancerous lesion of the gastric glands involving three (variably expressed) histological changes: epithelial atypia, abnormal differentiation, and disorganized mucosal architecture {2227,2795,219,2792}. Gastric dysplasia (also called intraepithelial neoplasia) is now defined as an unequivocal neoplastic lesion (depressed, flat, or elevated) without evidence of stromal invasion. Lesions showing different combinations of the histological changes associated with the dysplastic phenotype were traditionally grouped into various grades {2781}. Currently, dysplasia is graded dichotomously as either low-grade or high-grade, and the degree of dedifferentiation has been consistently shown to directly correlate with GC risk. Various classifications have been proposed for the histological phenotypes occurring along the histological spectrum of gastric carcinogenesis (see Table 3.02, p. 72). Each classification reflects its specific nosological orientation (biological, clinical, or therapeutic) {3182,2783,1024,3143,2885,2886,793,1430}. Regardless of differences in nosological focus, pathologists around the world agree on the neoplastic character of gastric dysplasia, which is supported by its dedifferentiated morphology, its molecular deregulation, and its strong association with (and high-risk of progression to) cancer.

Fundic gland polyps

Genta RMG

Definition
Fundic gland polyps (FGPs) are benign gastric epithelial lesions consisting of hyperplastic expansion of the deep epithelial compartment of the oxyntic mucosa.

ICD-O coding
None

ICD-11 coding
DA44.1 Fundic gland polyp of stomach

Related terminology
Acceptable: Elster's cysts.

Subtype(s)
None

Localization
FGPs arise exclusively in the oxyntic mucosa.

Clinical features
These polyps are usually asymptomatic, discovered as incidental findings on endoscopy {504,2968,3100}. When FGPs are found in young patients (especially when the polyps are numerous, e.g. ≥ 20), a polyposis syndrome must be considered. When FGPs are associated with duodenal adenomas, a familial polyposis syndrome should be strongly suspected, and colonoscopy is recommended {2968}.

Epidemiology
These are the most common type of polyps detected at oesophagogastroduodenoscopy. They may occur at any age and have a distinct female predominance {1025}. In a large pathology study in the USA, FGPs were diagnosed in 7.2% of patients who had an oesophagogastroduodenoscopy and constituted 70–90% of all gastric polyps submitted for histopathological evaluation {3100}. Individuals with familial polyposis syndromes are typically younger than the average patient with FGPs (mean age: 40 years) {2968}.

Etiology
They may occur sporadically or as part of several polyposis syndromes, including familial adenomatous polyposis and gastric adenocarcinoma and proximal polyposis of the stomach (GAPPS) {326}. When first discovered, these polyps were believed to be hamartomatous; however, their association with proton-pump inhibitor use, confirmed in several studies {3336,2061}, suggests that mechanisms in the sporadic setting can be related to the suppression of acid secretion by proton-pump inhibition as part of their pathogenesis. FGPs are inversely related to *Helicobacter pylori* gastritis: < 1 in 200 patients with *H. pylori* gastritis have FGPs {504,2968}.

Pathogenesis
The polyps result from hyperplasia and dilatation of oxyntic glands. Sporadic FGPs are devoid of *APC* mutations but can have mutations in *CTNNB1* (encoding β-catenin). Epigenetic alterations involving methylation of CpG islands play a role in the development of some FGPs with a proton-pump inhibitor effect {16}. *CTNNB1* mutation is seen in 64–91% of sporadic FGPs without dysplasia {15,2935}. Dysplastic FGPs may harbour *APC* mutations, typically together with wildtype *CTNNB1* {18}. Familial adenomatous polyposis–associated FGPs feature biallelic *APC* mutations and wildtype *CTNNB1* {15}.

Macroscopic appearance
FGPs occur as multiple small polyps (typically < 5 mm).

Histopathology
FGPs typically show dilated oxyntic glands, foveolar hypoplasia, and parietal hyperplasia. Polyp erosion can coexist with regenerative changes that may be misinterpreted as dysplasia.

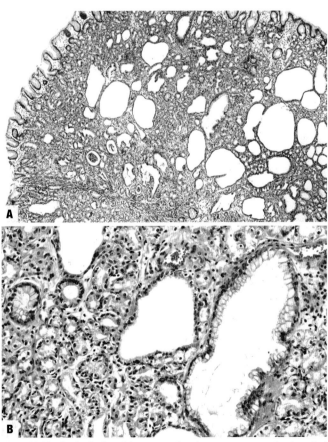

Fig. 3.01 Fundic gland polyp. **A** Low-power view; there are numerous closely packed fundic (oxyntic) glands with dilated glandular lumina. **B** High-power view; dilated glands are lined by flattened oxyntic gland cells or foveolar epithelium.

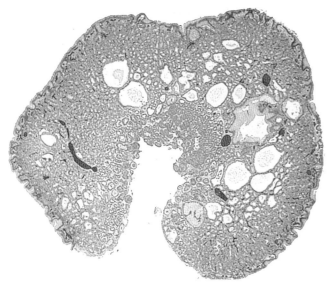

Fig. 3.02 Fundic gland polyp. Low-power view of a typical example; there are numerous dilated oxyntic glands lined by flattened parietal cells; there are also two dilated mucous glands lined by foveolar cells.

Dysplasia is rare in sporadic FGPs, but it is not uncommon in the syndromic setting (see *GAPPS and other fundic gland polyposes*, p. 526).

Cytology
Not clinically relevant

Diagnostic molecular pathology
Not clinically relevant

Essential and desirable diagnostic criteria
Essential: hyperplastic expansion of the deeper epithelial compartment of the oxyntic mucosa with dilatation of one or more oxyntic glands; parietal cell hyperplasia; foveolar hypoplasia.

Staging (TNM)
Not clinically relevant

Prognosis and prediction
Sporadic FGPs associated with proton-pump inhibitor therapy disappear when the therapy is discontinued. There have been no reliable reports of malignant transformation occurring in the sporadic setting. For information about the hereditary setting, see *GAPPS and other fundic gland polyposes* (p. 526).

Gastric hyperplastic polyps

Genta RMG

Definition
Hyperplastic polyps of the stomach are benign gastric epithelial lesions featuring elongated or tortuous (hyperplastic) foveolae and cystically dilated glands coexisting with inflammatory changes.

ICD-O coding
None

ICD-11 coding
DA44.0 Hyperplastic polyp of stomach

Related terminology
Acceptable: inflammatory polyp.

Subtype(s)
Polypoid foveolar hyperplasia; mucosal prolapse polyp; gastritis cystica polyposa (profunda)

Localization
Hyperplastic polyps are most frequently located in the antrum.

Clinical features
Hyperplastic polyps, which may be multiple, are typically asymptomatic. Bleeding due to superficial erosion(s) may result in iron-deficiency anaemia. Rarely, large polyps affecting the pyloric transit may result in obstruction or subobstruction {537,577}.

Epidemiology
Hyperplastic polyps show no sex predilection. They typically occur in the sixth or seventh decade of life (median age: 66 years), and most arise in the setting of longstanding gastritis. In a study involving 78 909 endoscopy patients in the USA, 6.4% of the patients had polypoid lesions; among the patients with polypoid lesions, the prevalence of hyperplastic polyps was 17% {504}. In a case–control study of 71 575 case subjects with gastric polyps and 741 351 control subjects without gastric polyps, the overall prevalence of hyperplastic polyps among all subjects was 1.79% (fundic gland polyps: 7.72%, gastric adenomas: 0.09%, and neuroendocrine tumours [NETs]: 0.06%). All types of gastric polyps showed a clear increase in prevalence with increasing age {2968,3100}. In a 2007 study of 153 Brazilian patients with at least one gastric polyp, hyperplastic polyps accounted for about 71% of the cases {2208}.

Etiology
The specific etiology is unknown. However, there is a strong association with chronic gastritis, including both postgastrectomy gastritis and *Helicobacter pylori* gastritis.

Pathogenesis
Hyperplastic polyps arise as a hyperproliferative response to tissue injury {792,2001,1675}. Mutation of *TP53* and overexpression of p53 are detected in foci of malignant transformation {3686,2834}.

Macroscopic appearance
Gastric hyperplastic polyps can occur as small dome-shaped polyps, generally < 1 cm in size, or as a large polyp, lobulated and pedunculated, with erosion.

Histopathology
Typical features include elongated, distorted, branching, and dilated hyperplastic foveolae lying in an oedematous, inflamed stroma, rich in vasculature. Small, haphazardly distributed smooth muscle bundles are present. Between 1% and 20% of hyperplastic polyps harbour dysplasia, and about 2% may have foci of carcinoma {3739}, especially when polyps are > 1 cm in size {3739,3686}.

Polypoid foveolar hyperplasia is a tiny polypoid lesion (< 10 mm) consisting of elongated pits without features of dilatation, and the lamina propria is either normal or only slightly swollen. Polypoid foveolar hyperplasia is regarded as a precursor of gastric hyperplastic polyps {1070}.

Gastric mucosal prolapse polyps are characterized by the presence of a glandular component along with thick-walled vessels and organized thick bundles of arborizing smooth muscle in the lamina propria. These polyps likely occur in the antrum and may have a different pathogenesis {1070}.

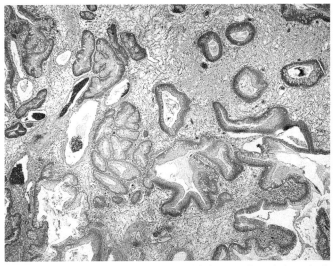

Fig. 3.03 Gastric hyperplastic polyp. Characteristic features of gastric hyperplastic polyps include irregularly shaped, haphazardly dilated foveolae in a background of a loose oedematous stroma, with variable numbers of inflammatory cells. The surface is frequently eroded.

Gastritis cystica polyposa (profunda) is a benign polypoid hyperplasia with cystic dilatation of the glands frequently extending into the submucosa. The lesions mostly occur as a linear arrangement along the stoma of Billroth II anastomosis {2968}.

Gastric hyperplastic polyps should be differentiated from other sporadic polyps (fundic gland polyps, adenomatous polyps) and polyps of gastric manifestation of polyposis (juvenile polyposis and Cowden syndrome) {2968}. Hamartomatous inverted polyp is a solitary polypoid lesion characterized by downgrowth of hyperplastic and cystic glandular components into the submucosa. The muscularis mucosae, continuous from the normal layer, demarcates the lesion {2556}.

Cytology
Not clinically relevant

Diagnostic molecular pathology
Not clinically relevant

Essential and desirable diagnostic criteria
Essential: a polyp consisting of elongated and tortuous (hyperplastic) foveolar epithelium; cystically dilated glands mixed with inflammatory changes.
Desirable: erosions, ulcerations, and (in some cases extensive) inflammation (expected features of these polyps).

Staging (TNM)
Not clinically relevant

Prognosis and prediction
Foci of dysplasia and adenocarcinoma have been reported in hyperplastic polyps > 10 mm in size {3739,3686}. If dysplasia or intramucosal carcinoma is found but the stalk is unaffected, the lesion can be considered completely removed and most likely cured.

Gastric dysplasia

Kushima R
Lauwers GY
Rugge M

Definition
Gastric dysplasia consists of unequivocal neoplastic changes of the gastric epithelium without evidence of stromal invasion.

ICD-O coding
8148/0 Glandular intraepithelial neoplasia, low grade
8148/2 Glandular intraepithelial neoplasia, high grade

ICD-11 coding
2E92.1 & XH6AF9 Benign neoplasm of stomach & Glandular intraepithelial neoplasia, low grade
2E60.2 & XH28N7 Carcinoma in situ of stomach & Glandular intraepithelial neoplasia, high grade

Related terminology
Acceptable: intraepithelial neoplasia.

Subtype(s)
Serrated dysplasia, low grade (8213/0); serrated dysplasia, high grade (8213/2); intestinal-type dysplasia; foveolar-type (gastric-type) dysplasia; gastric pit/crypt dysplasia

Localization
Dysplasia most frequently arises in the gastric antrum. However, in extensive metaplastic atrophy, dysplastic lesions may occur in any gastric compartment {2522,3400}. This topographical distribution is consistent with the localization of early differentiated-type gastric adenocarcinoma (51%, 40%, and 8% in the lower, middle, and upper thirds of the stomach, respectively) {1197}.

Clinical features
Dysplasia is mostly asymptomatic; symptoms are usually related to the patients' underlying disease. Bleeding, anaemia, or dyspepsia may result from large or ulcerated lesions.

Endoscopically, gastric dysplasia presents as a flat, depressed, or elevated (polypoid) lesion, along with erosion/ulcer and colour tone change. A diagnosis of dysplasia can be issued on target biopsies from mucosa showing these endoscopic abnormalities. Most definite dysplastic lesions, especially those with depressed and erythematous appearances on conventional endoscopy, are proved to be high-grade dysplasia (HGD) / intramucosal adenocarcinoma in the subsequently resected specimens {3182}. Magnifying endoscopy with narrow-band imaging may substantially improve the endoscopy assessment, which has made it possible to detect dysplastic lesions more accurately, paying attention to the structure of surface epithelium and subepithelial vessels {3685}.

Polypoid, elevated, or even flat dysplasias are also referred to as adenomas (intestinal and foveolar types; refer to the respective sections).

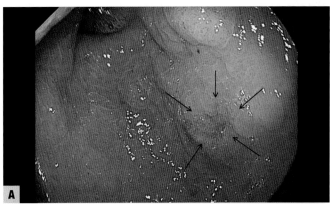
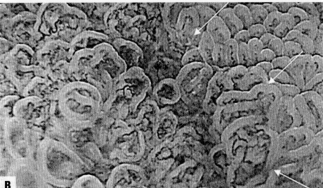

Fig. 3.04 Gastric dysplasia. **A** A slightly depressed and reddish area (arrows), 4 × 3 mm in size, in the antrum by conventional endoscopy with white light. **B** Narrow-band imaging of high-grade dysplasia (magnifying endoscopy); note the well-demarcated area with irregular microvascular and microsurface structures (arrows).

Epidemiology
Gastric dysplasia has a prevalence that mirrors that of gastric cancer (GC) and similarly shows a male predominance in most series. It also displays the same geographical disparity, with high incidence in part of Asia and much lower risk in North America and part of Europe. In the areas with high incidence, endoscopic screening identifies abnormalities of gastric mucosa in 10–15% of participants {1149}. Forceps biopsies demonstrate low-grade dysplasia (LGD) in 1–2% and HGD and adenocarcinoma in 4–6% of these lesions (in 0.1–0.2% and 0.4–0.5% of all participants, respectively). In the Republic of Korea, similar incidences were reported, with adenoma, early GC, and advanced GC identified in 0.43%, 0.21%, and 0.09%, respectively, of 40 821 participants over a period of 7 years {1515}.

Etiology
The pathogenetic risk factors of gastric dysplasia are similar to those of gastric adenocarcinoma.

Table 3.02 Classifications of the histological phenotypes involved in gastric carcinogenesis, each listing the categories in order of increasing risk of malignancy

Padova International	Vienna	Revised Vienna	Japanese Diagnostic Framework for Forceps Biopsy	WHO (2019)
Category 1: Negative for dysplasia	Category 1: Negative for dysplasia	Category 1: Negative for dysplasia	Group 1: Normal/non-neoplastic	Negative for dysplasia/IEN
Category 2: Indefinite for dysplasia	Category 2: Indefinite for dysplasia	Category 2: Indefinite for dysplasia	Group 2: Indefinite for neoplasia	Indefinite for dysplasia/IEN
Category 3.1: Low-grade dysplasia (low-grade NiN)	Category 3: Non-invasive low-grade neoplasia (low-grade adenoma/dysplasia)	Category 3: Low-grade adenoma/ dysplasia	Group 3: Adenoma	Low-grade dysplasia/IEN (low-grade adenoma/dysplasia)
Category 3.2: High-grade dysplasia (high-grade NiN)	Category 4: High-grade neoplasia 4.1: High-grade adenoma/ dysplasia 4.2: Non-invasive carcinoma 4.3: Suspicious for invasive carcinoma	Category 4: High-grade neoplasia 4.1: High-grade adenoma/ dysplasia 4.2: Non-invasive carcinoma 4.3: Suspicious for invasive carcinoma	Group 4: Suspicious for carcinoma	High-grade dysplasia/IEN (high-grade adenoma/dysplasia)
Category 4: Suspicious for invasive carcinoma		4.4: Intramucosal carcinoma	Group 5: Carcinoma (non-invasive or invasive)	
Category 5: Invasive adenocarcinoma	Category 5: Invasive neoplasia 5.1: Intramucosal carcinoma			Intramucosal invasive neoplasia (intramucosal carcinoma)

IEN, intraepithelial neoplasia; NiN, non-invasive neoplasia. References: {2783,2886,3143,1430}.

Pathogenesis

The molecular profiling of gastric dysplastic lesions may be partially biased by different criteria applied in the histological assessment of the dysplasia phenotype (see Table 3.02). Many of the molecular alterations seen in invasive GC (particularly intestinal-type) may also be detected in gastric dysplasia. These abnormalities include chromosomal instability, microsatellite instability (MSI), and CpG-island methylation {3161,2791}.

Functional loss of *TP53* is the main driver of gastric oncogenesis {692}. According to recent data {908}, *TP53* mutations and p53 overexpression are detected at high frequencies in HGD (40% and 40%, respectively) and intramucosal carcinoma (60% and 73%, respectively). *APC* mutations exist at high frequencies in LGD and HGD (~70%), but at low rates in intramucosal carcinoma (4–20%) {1826,2167}.

MSI is caused by abnormalities of the DNA mismatch repair system, including CpG-island methylation of the *MLH1* promoter {1316}. Dysplasia with the MSI-high phenotype shows increased numbers of gene mutations (enriched in indel type) {1912}. Among them, *RNF43* abnormalities are associated with both HGD and intramucosal carcinoma {1467,2167,2780}.

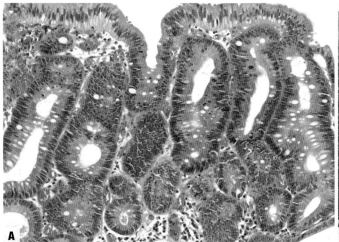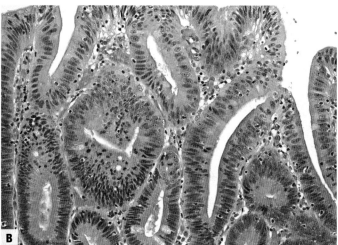

Fig. 3.05 Intestinal-type gastric dysplasia. **A** Low-grade dysplasia; note that tall columnar cells differentiate to intestinal-type cells, with elongated basically located nuclei. **B** High-grade dysplasia; note disoriented nuclei of tall columnar cells that differentiate to intestinal-type cells.

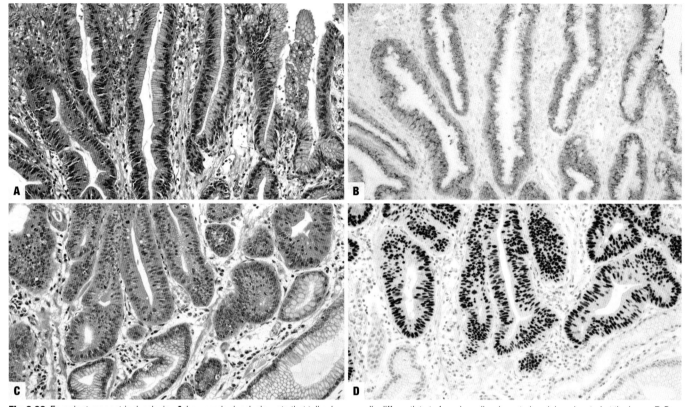

Fig. 3.06 Foveolar-type gastric dysplasia. **A** Low-grade dysplasia; note that tall columnar cells differentiate to foveolar cells; elongated nuclei are located at the base. **B** Dysplastic cells are immunohistochemically positive for MUC5AC. **C** High-grade dysplasia; note disorientation of the nuclei in tall columnar epithelial cells. **D** High-grade dysplasia; dysplastic cells immunohistochemically overexpress p53.

Macroscopic appearance

Gastric dysplasia presents as a flat, depressed, or elevated (polypoid) lesion.

Histopathology

Gastric dysplasia is associated with a risk of developing metachronous or synchronous gastric adenocarcinoma. Grading of gastric dysplasia is based on the Padova International {2783} and Vienna systems {2886}, using a two-tiered system

(LGD vs HGD), which has been proven to be relatively reproducible and clinically relevant {2781,2791}. Various classifications have been proposed for the histological phenotypes occurring along the histological spectrum of gastric carcinogenesis (see Table 3.02). Each classification reflects its specific nosological orientation (biological, clinical, or therapeutic) {3182,2783,1024, 3143,2885,2886,793,1430}. When surgical treatment is clinically considered, most international guidelines recommend obtaining a pretreatment second diagnostic opinion.

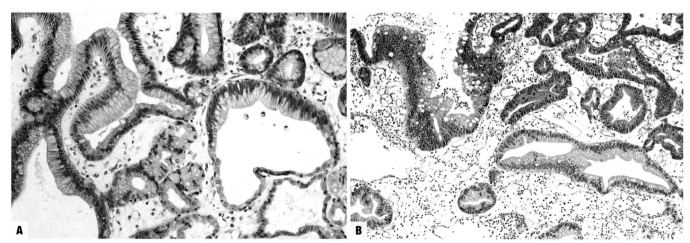

Fig. 3.07 Foveolar-type gastric dysplasia in polyps. **A** Low-grade dysplasia on the surface of a fundic gland polyp. **B** High-grade dysplasia and intramucosal adenocarcinoma arising in a hyperplastic polyp; foveolar-type and goblet cells are seen in a hybrid manner.

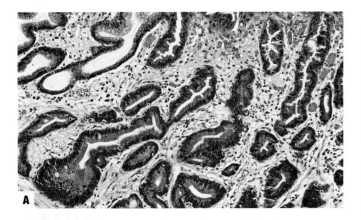

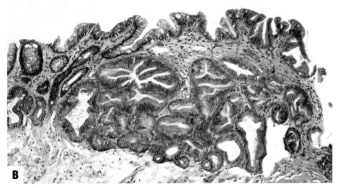

Fig. 3.08 Subtypes of dysplasia. **A** Crypt/pit dysplasia; dysplastic nuclear changes are limited to the gastric pits, with surface maturation showing a serrated profile. **B** Serrated dysplasia.

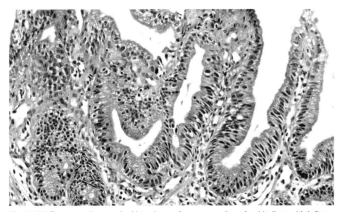

Fig. 3.09 Regenerative atypia. Note the surface maturation of epithelium with inflammatory background.

Typing

The two broad categories of dysplasia in the stomach are intestinal and foveolar (gastric) types {1732,13,3400}. However, many cases are mixed {2522}. Dysplasia occurs de novo or within pre-existing benign lesions such as fundic gland polyps and hyperplastic polyps.

Intestinal-type dysplasia consists of tubular, tubulovillous, or villous lesions lined by tall columnar cells. The nuclei are enlarged, elongated, stratified, and hyperchromatic. The cytoplasm is variably eosinophilic. Terminal differentiation towards absorptive-type cells, goblet cells, endocrine cells, or even Paneth cells is common. Intestinal-type dysplasia is immunoreactive for MUC2, CD10, and CDX2 {3363,2523}.

Foveolar-type dysplasia is usually characterized by tubulovillous epithelial fronds and/or serrated glandular structures lined by cuboidal to low columnar cells resembling gastric foveolar cells. The nuclei are round to oval and display variably prominent nucleoli. The cells present a pale eosinophilic cytoplasm due to the presence of apical neutral mucin and are immunoreactive for MUC5AC {17,2522}. MUC2-positive goblet cells are rarely observed, and MUC6-positive cells may be seen at the bottom of glands.

Grading

Dysplasia, regardless of the morphological type, is graded as either low-grade or high-grade, on the basis of degree of nuclear atypia (i.e. crowding, hyperchromasia, and stratification), mitotic activity, cytoplasmic differentiation, and architectural distortion. In LGD, unequivocal neoplastic cells show minimal architectural disarray and only mild to moderate cytological atypia. The nuclei are hyperchromatic, and they are elongated (cigar-shaped) in intestinal-type dysplasia and round to oval in foveolar-type. In both types, the nuclei maintain polarity and are basally located. The mitotic activity is mild to moderate. Relative preservation of the glandular architecture is characteristic of LGD.

HGD shows cuboidal to columnar cells with prominent cytological atypia, enlarged nuclei with a high N:C ratio, and commonly prominent amphophilic nucleoli. Loss of nuclear polarity and extension of atypical nuclei to the luminal surface is common. Mitoses (including atypical forms) are frequently detected. The glandular architecture is usually complex, showing marked distortion, including back-to-back glands. However, marked glandular crowding, budding, and cribriforming should prompt a diagnosis of intramucosal adenocarcinoma. Even if mild cytological atypia is observed, cases with marked structural atypia (e.g. variably sized and shaped glands) should be diagnosed as HGD {2827}. This category also includes carcinoma in situ. Overexpression of p53 is frequently observed in these lesions.

There is only limited consensus regarding the diagnostic criteria of gastric dysplasia and adenocarcinoma, especially between pathologists in Japan and those in North America, Europe, and the Republic of Korea {1804,1024,1731,1585}. Japanese pathologists establish the diagnosis of adenocarcinoma on the basis of cytoarchitectural atypia, irrespective of evidence of stromal invasion. In North America, Europe, and the Republic of Korea, pathologists primarily base the diagnosis on disruption of the basal membrane in conjunction with the spread of cancer cells into the lamina propria. In Japan, gastric non-invasive neoplastic lesions with high-grade cellular and/or architectural atypia are diagnosed as non-invasive carcinoma, whereas the same lesions would be classified as HGD by most pathologists in other countries {2937}.

Subtypes

Several subtypes of gastric dysplasia have been recognized, although their clinical implications are not fully understood.

Gastric pit/crypt dysplasia shows dysplasia at the basal portion of gastric pits. The glandular structures show maturation to the surface epithelial cells. It has been reported at the periphery of traditional neoplasia in 49–72% of cases, and it is believed to be an independent predictor of cancer progression {3018,1574,52}.

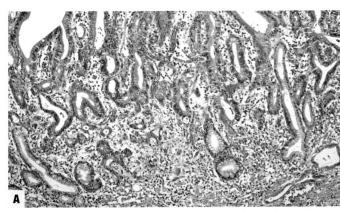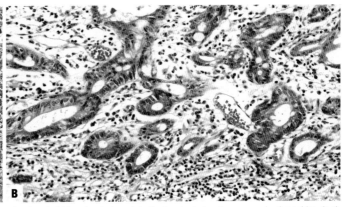

Fig. 3.10 Intramucosal invasive neoplasia / intramucosal adenocarcinoma. **A** Irregular glands, mimicking dysplasia or intestinal metaplasia, show excessive branching, budding, and single-cell infiltration in the deep mucosa; so-called very well differentiated carcinoma of intestinal type. **B** Intestinal-type tubules showing irregular (crawling) fusions.

Serrated dysplasia is characterized by its distinctive topography (pit region); it frequently features a micropapillary pattern, extending to the mucosal surface and exhibiting MUC5AC expression. This phenotype has also been reported as serrated adenoma and frequently coexists with adenocarcinoma {1740,2777}.

Differential diagnosis
The term "indefinite for dysplasia" does not identify a biological entity; it mostly represents a diagnostic label to be applied to questionable cases lacking the histological features required to reliably distinguish neoplastic/dysplastic phenotypes from non-neoplastic phenotypes (i.e. reactive or regenerative changes) {906}. The label "indefinite for dysplasia" is typically applied when dealing with small biopsy specimens featuring high-grade inflammation {2783,522}. The interpretative dilemma can be solved by evaluating serial histological sections and/or obtaining more-reliable biopsy samples after clearing the mucosal inflammation. Because of its cellular atypia and (even atypical) mitotic figures, regenerative atypia can be misinterpreted as dysplasia {522}; however, in non-dysplastic changes, cytoarchitectural alterations infrequently involve the mucosal surface {522}.

The term "intramucosal invasive neoplasia / intramucosal adenocarcinoma" refers to neoplasms that invade the lamina propria or muscularis mucosae. It is distinguished from HGD by distinct structural anomalies such as glandular crowding, excessive branching, and budding, irrespective of the presence or absence of desmoplastic reaction. Single-cell infiltration, trabecular growth, intraglandular necrotic debris, irregular (crawling) fusions, or small degenerative glands may be helpful findings {3391,2435}.

Cytology
Not clinically relevant

Diagnostic molecular pathology
Not clinically relevant

Essential and desirable diagnostic criteria
Essential: an unequivocal intraepithelial neoplastic lesion (non-polypoid or polypoid); no evidence of invasion; low-grade to high-grade cytological and structural changes; an intestinal and/or gastric phenotype {2786}.

Staging (TNM)
HGD and intramucosal invasive neoplasia / intramucosal adenocarcinoma correspond to pTis and pT1a, respectively.

Prognosis and prediction
Gastric dysplasia is associated with an increased risk of progression to invasive adenocarcinoma {2786,2791}. In a prospective centralized study involving only patients with an endoscopy follow-up > 12 months, the overall progression rate of LGD was 15% (progression to cancer: 9%). HGD progressed to invasive GC in 69% of the cases. Indefinite for dysplasia lesions only progressed to LGD (in 11% of the cases) {2782}. In a recent retrospective multicentre study, only 4.3% of LGD cases progressed to invasive carcinoma (median follow-up: 2.6 years). In 59% of the patients with HGD, GC was diagnosed histologically within 12 months of the initial diagnosis, but the natural history of HGD remained undetermined. Of the 16 patients who did not develop adenocarcinoma in 1 year, 11 had been treated with endoscopic resection and 2 progressed to GC {1880}.

Re-grading: Some studies have unequivocally demonstrated that biopsy-based histological diagnosis of dysplasia may be upgraded on the basis of the resection specimen. In a series of 78 biopsy-assessed HGD cases, the subsequent endoscopic submucosal dissection demonstrated submucosal infiltration and/or venous invasion in 3.8% and 1.3% of the cases, respectively {2827}. Among 293 patients with LGD, 18.7% of the endoscopic mucosal resection specimens featured HGD or GC {1604}.

Risk stratification: Histological grading (low-grade vs high-grade) is strongly related to the prognosis of gastric dysplasia {2782}. The clinical usefulness of ancillary markers is still under investigation. DNA content abnormality (aneuploidy or elevated 4N fraction, as assessed by flow cytometry) statistically significantly correlates with increasing grades of dysplasia and even with cancer progression {3546}. Other predictive biomarkers include immunohistochemistry for p53; target sequencing of *TP53*, *ARID1A*, *APC*, *ARID2*, and *RNF43* {908,2167}; MSI {1316}; and promoter methylation of p16 {3176}, but none of these are in clinical use.

Intestinal-type gastric adenoma

Montgomery EA
Sekine S
Singhi AD

Definition
Intestinal-type gastric adenoma (IGA) is a localized polypoid lesion consisting of dysplastic intestinalized epithelium.

ICD-O coding
8144/0 Intestinal-type adenoma, low grade
8144/2 Intestinal-type adenoma, high grade

ICD-11 coding
2E92.1 & XH3DV3 Benign neoplasm of stomach &
  Adenoma NOS

Related terminology
None

Subtype(s)
Sporadic intestinal-type gastric adenoma; syndromic intestinal-type gastric adenoma

Localization
They prevail in the gastric compartments where intestinal metaplasia is prevalent (60% in the distal stomach, including the angularis incisura) {17}.

Clinical features
Patients are usually older than 60 years and are asymptomatic. Extensive metaplastic atrophic gastritis mostly coexists. Recurrent bleeding of large adenomas may result in anaemia and/or haematochezia {17,485}.

Epidemiology
Adenomas (mostly intestinal-type adenomas) are the third most common gastric polyps, after hyperplastic and fundic gland polyps. In endoscopic series, the prevalence of IGA basically parallels that of gastric cancer (China: 3–10%, USA: < 1%) {485,504}.

Etiology
Any cause of gastric mucosa intestinalization is a risk factor. The etiology includes environmental agents (*Helicobacter pylori*), host-related factors (autoimmune gastritis), genetic syndromes (*APC* gene mutations), and epigenetic deregulation.

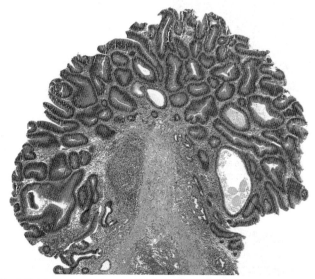

Fig. 3.11 Intestinal-type adenoma. This lesion resembles a colorectal tubular adenoma; note that the adjoining gastric mucosa shows chronic gastritis.

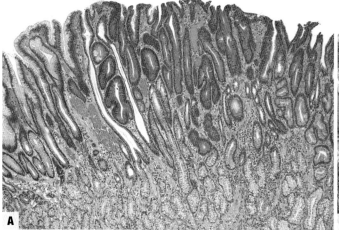
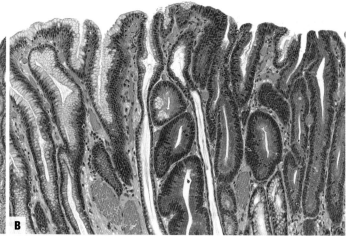

Fig. 3.12 Intestinal-type adenoma. **A** This antral lesion has an appearance similar to that of a colorectal adenoma with low-grade dysplasia; note the normal antral mucosa on the left side. **B** Note that the nuclei are elongated, similar to those of an intestinal tubular adenoma; there are few goblet cells at the right side of the lesion.

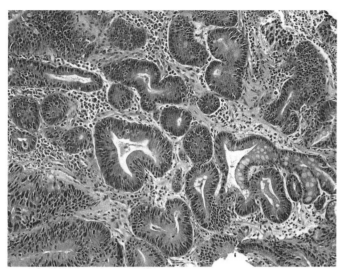

Fig. 3.13 Intestinal-type adenoma. This adenoma is accompanied by intestinal metaplasia on the right side and shows prominent tumour-infiltrating lymphocytes; a subset of such adenomas are microsatellite-unstable.

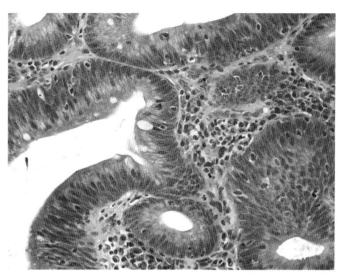

Fig. 3.14 Intestinal-type adenoma. Note the nuclear features; there is a goblet cell in the centre of the field.

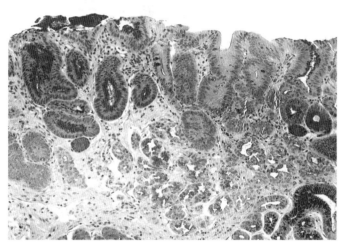

Fig. 3.15 Intestinal-type adenoma. PAS / Alcian blue staining of an antral adenoma from a patient with familial adenomatous polyposis; there is no intestinal metaplasia in the antral mucosa at the left, but a few goblet cells are highlighted in the adenoma.

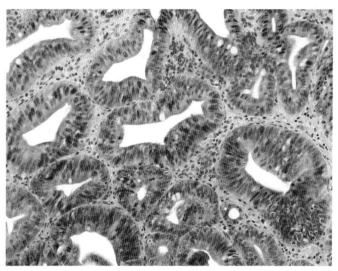

Fig. 3.16 Intestinal-type adenoma. An example located in the antrum in a patient with familial adenomatous polyposis; note the high-grade dysplasia and numerous goblet cells in the lesion.

Pathogenesis

The pathogenesis involves genetic and/or epigenetic deregulation promoting gastric intestinal metaplasia {907,2639,2528}. The molecular findings are somewhat analogous to those in colorectal adenomas. Lesions harbour mutations in *APC*, *KRAS*, *ERBB2*, and *ARID2* but not alterations in *CTNNB1*, and some cases (probably 20–30%) are microsatellite-unstable {17,1912}. Syndromic cases typically occur as part of familial adenomatous polyposis.

Macroscopic appearance

IGAs are usually solitary and < 2 cm in largest diameter {503}.

Histopathology

IGAs consist of proliferations of dysplastic tubules that form polyps. The same appearance in flat mucosa is termed dysplasia (intraepithelial neoplasia). The tubules are lined by columnar epithelium showing intestinal differentiation in the form of elongated nuclei akin to those in colorectal adenomas with variable contributions of Paneth and goblet cells. The background mucosa often shows intestinal metaplasia and flat dysplasia. In North American and European patients with familial adenomatous polyposis, the flat mucosa is usually normal, whereas Asian patients often have intestinalized surrounding mucosa {2286}. Dysplasia grading is consistent with that applied to any other dysplastic lesion.

In some IGAs (mostly arising in metaplastic atrophic gastritis), both intestinal and gastric differentiation (type) do coexist; these hybrid lesions carry a cancer risk higher than that of IGA featuring only intestinal commitment {2522,3400}. The hybrid phenotype has also been called foveolar dysplasia; note the difference between this and foveolar-type adenoma, as described elsewhere (p. 79).

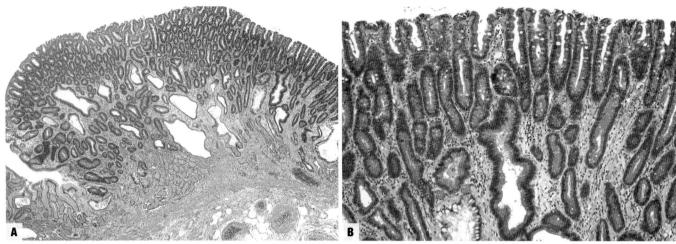

Fig. 3.17 Intestinal-type adenoma. **A** An elevated lesion consisting of proliferating dysplastic tubules, accompanied by dilated non-neoplastic glands below. **B** The tubules are lined by dysplastic columnar cells differentiating to goblet, absorptive, and Paneth cells; intestinal metaplasia is present at the lower left.

Cytology
Not clinically relevant

Diagnostic molecular pathology
Not clinically relevant

Essential and desirable diagnostic criteria
Essential: unequivocal neoplastic changes in a polypoid lesion consisting of gastric intestinalized glands; no evidence of invasion.

Staging (TNM)
If high-grade dysplasia is present, this is staged as pTis.

Prognosis and prediction
IGAs are more prone to progression than foveolar-type lesions {13}. Gastric cancer progression is most frequent in adenomas featuring both intestinal and gastric differentiation (hybrid type) {2522}. The gastric cancer risk of familial adenomatous polyposis adenomas is lower in North American and European patients than in Asian patients, probably because of the different prevalence of *H. pylori* infection {2413,3604,2286,2526,1410,1849}. Treatment is endoscopic resection.

Foveolar-type adenoma

Sekine S
Montgomery EA
Vieth M

Definition
Foveolar-type adenoma is an epithelial polyp consisting of neoplastic foveolar epithelium.

ICD-O coding
8210/0 Adenomatous polyp, low-grade dysplasia
8210/2 Adenomatous polyp, high-grade dysplasia

ICD-11 coding
2E92.1 & XH3DV3 Benign neoplasm of stomach & Adenoma NOS

Related terminology
Acceptable: foveolar-type gastric adenoma.

Subtype(s)
None

Localization
Foveolar-type adenomas mostly occur in the oxyntic gastric compartment (body/fundus) {13}.

Clinical features
Foveolar-type adenomas usually develop in otherwise healthy gastric mucosa (with no inflammation or atrophy/metaplasia) {13}. Sporadic cases are extremely rare and they have never been reported to progress to gastric cancer {3604}. The (more frequent) syndromic foveolar-type adenoma may occur in familial adenomatous polyposis (FAP) and gastric adenocarcinoma and proximal polyposis of the stomach (GAPPS); in both syndromes, foveolar-type adenomas may coexist with fundic gland polyposis, and their rate of cancer progression is consistently low {3604}.

Epidemiology
Sporadic foveolar-type adenomas are extremely rare. In a population studied in the USA, the ratio of sporadic foveolar-type adenoma to intestinal-type adenoma was < 0.25:1 {13}.

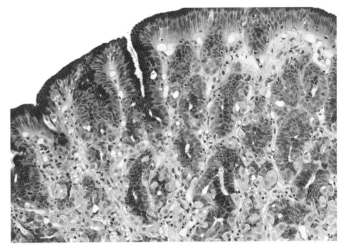

Fig. 3.18 Foveolar-type adenoma. This is a PAS / Alcian blue stain of an example that involves oxyntic mucosa without gastritis or intestinal metaplasia; the apical mucin cap, composed of gastric-type neutral mucin, is prominent.

Etiology
The etiology of sporadic lesions is unknown. For more information about syndromic foveolar-type adenoma, see the associated genetic disorders (e.g. *Familial adenomatous polyposis 1*, p. 522, and *GAPPS and other fundic gland polyposes*, p. 526).

Pathogenesis
Foveolar-type adenomas prevail in FAP, through biallelic *APC* inactivation. Limited data are available on the molecular underpinnings. Sporadic adenomas infrequently harbour mutations of *APC* and *KRAS*; mutations of *CTNNB1* (which encodes β-catenin) have never been reported {17,2079}. Conflicting results are available on the mismatch repair status {17,2079}. FAP-associated lesions show both somatic and germline *APC* mutations {14,1184}.

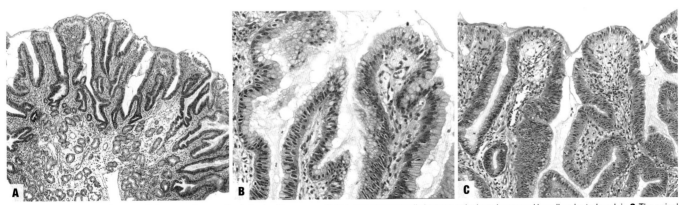

Fig. 3.19 Foveolar-type adenoma. **A** An example occurring in the fundic mucosa. **B** Columnar tumour cells have an apical mucin cap and basally oriented nuclei. **C** The apical mucin cap is less prominent, but still present, in this area.

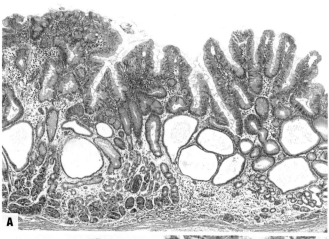

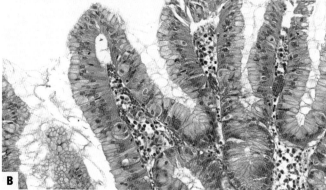

Fig. 3.20 Foveolar-type adenoma. **A** An example in a patient with familial adenomatous polyposis; the lesion mainly involves the superficial layer of fundic gland mucosa. **B** Papillary projections are lined by mildly dysplastic foveolar-type epithelial cells with mild nuclear stratification.

Macroscopic appearance
Sporadic foveolar-type adenomas are small, solitary polyps. In patients with FAP, foveolar-type adenomas usually coexist with multiple fundic gland polyps.

Histopathology
Both sporadic and syndromic foveolar-type adenomas consist of dysplastic columnar (foveolar-type) epithelia, with stratified/elongated nuclei. A distinctive apical cap of neutral (PAS-positive) mucins differentiates foveolar-type from pyloric gland adenomas. Most lesions show low-grade atypia. High-grade adenomas should be differentiated from invasive gastric cancer (cancer lesions feature more-pronounced superficial papillary architecture and more-severe glandular disarrangement) {1735}. Neoplastic cells feature strong/diffuse MUC5AC expression {590}, weak/focal MUC6 immunoreaction, and no expression of MUC2 or CDX2. However, the histological diagnosis primarily relies on H&E/PAS features rather than on immunophenotyping. Syndromic foveolar-type adenoma (FAP, in particular) is frequently associated with fundic gland polyps and pyloric gland adenomas {3604}. Foveolar-type adenomas may exhibit both intestinal and gastric-type differentiation; this hybrid phenotype carries a higher risk of cancer progression {2522,3400}.

Cytology
Not clinically relevant

Diagnostic molecular pathology
Not clinically relevant

Essential and desirable diagnostic criteria
Essential: polypoid growth of dysplastic columnar epithelia with a foveolar-cell phenotype, with a distinctive apical cap of neutral mucins.

Staging (TNM)
If high-grade dysplasia is present, this is staged as pTis.

Prognosis and prediction
Sporadic foveolar-type adenomas are usually solitary and low-grade, and they rarely coexist with longstanding gastritis. They convey negligible risk of malignant progression or of synchronous or metachronous gastric cancers {13,590}. A low risk of invasive cancer is associated with syndromic (FAP-associated) foveolar-type adenomas {590}.

Gastric pyloric gland adenoma

Sekine S
Montgomery EA
Vieth M

Definition
Pyloric gland adenoma (PGA) of the stomach is a gastric epithelial polyp consisting of neoplastic pyloric-type glands.

ICD-O coding
8210/0 Adenomatous polyp, low-grade dysplasia
8210/2 Adenomatous polyp, high-grade dysplasia

ICD-11 coding
2E92.1 & XH3DV3 Benign neoplasm of stomach & Adenoma NOS

Related terminology
Acceptable: pyloric gland tubular adenoma; pyloric gland intracystic papillary neoplasm.

Subtype(s)
None

Localization
PGAs arise in the gastric body or fundus {3474,590,625}.

Clinical features
Most PGAs occur in patients aged 60–70 years and coexist with atrophic/metaplastic changes of the oxyntic mucosa, as due to autoimmune and/or *Helicobacter pylori* gastritis {625,3474,590}. The female predominance reflects their association with autoimmune gastritis {3474,590}. Syndromic (familial adenomatous polyposis–associated) PGAs occur in patients younger than those harbouring sporadic PGAs {3604,1184,1135}. Unlike sporadic PGAs, syndromic PGAs are not associated with any inflammatory background and they may coexist with fundic gland polyps.

Epidemiology
PGAs account for no more than 3% of gastric epithelial polyps (excluding fundic gland polyps) {3474}.

Etiology
Sporadic cases are closely associated with atrophic (mostly autoimmune) gastritis. PGAs can be associated with columnar epithelial dysplasia all throughout the GI tract {3476}, or they can arise in polypoid syndromes, including familial adenomatous polyposis, gastric adenocarcinoma and proximal polyposis of the stomach (GAPPS), McCune–Albright syndrome {3602}, juvenile polyposis {1984}, and Lynch syndrome {1841}.

Pathogenesis
Pyloric gland metaplasia (wherever arising; i.e. the gastrointestinal and hepatobiliary tract) is the putative precursor lesion of PGA {590,3477,3474}. Both sporadic and familial adenomatous polyposis–associated PGAs consistently feature activating *GNAS* and/or *KRAS* mutations and inactivating *APC* mutations {2079,1184,1135}.

Macroscopic appearance
PGAs are polypoid lesions or masses with an average size of 2 cm (range: 0.3–10 cm) {3474,625}.

Histopathology
PGAs consist of closely packed pyloric-type glands, lined by cuboidal/low columnar epithelia. Large lesions may include dilated glands. Neoplastic cells feature a defined ground-glass appearance, with clear or lightly eosinophilic cytoplasm. The lack of a well-defined apical mucin cap distinguishes PGAs from foveolar-type adenomas. The nuclei (round to ovoid) are basally located, with inconspicuous nucleoli. High-grade PGAs consistently exhibit disturbed architecture, crowded nuclei, and loss of nuclear polarity. High-grade dysplasia is observed in 40–50% of cases, and it is easily recognizable by its high

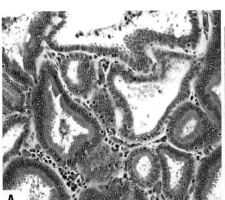 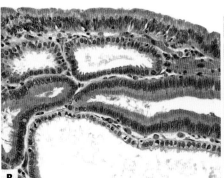 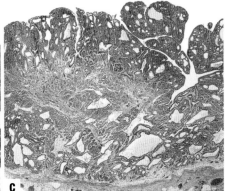

Fig. 3.21 Gastric pyloric gland adenoma. **A,B** High-power view. **C** Low-power view.

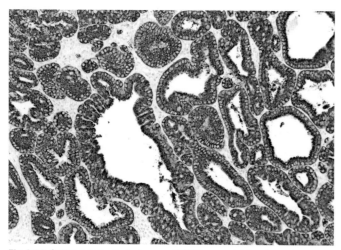

Fig. 3.22 Gastric pyloric gland adenoma. MUC6 immunostaining shows strong cytoplasmic labelling.

proliferation index. Adenocarcinoma (even focal) is observed in almost half of all cases {3475}; however, submucosal invasion does not exceed 10% {590,625}.

Consistent with their pyloric-type histological phenotype, PGAs express (variably) MUC6 {590,3475,625}. MUC5AC expression may involve the whole lesion (no restriction to the surface epithelium). Low-grade PGAs mostly feature diffuse MUC6 expression, with a surface coating of MUC5AC. As many as 10% of PGAs exhibit focal expression of MUC2 and/or CDX2 {3475}. Occasional expression of nuclear β-catenin has also been reported {1184}.

Cytology
Not clinically relevant

Diagnostic molecular pathology
Not clinically relevant

Essential and desirable diagnostic criteria
Essential: a polypoid proliferation of pyloric-type glands consisting of cuboidal/columnar cells with foamy, ground-glass cytoplasm; no well-formed apical mucin cap.

Staging (TNM)
If high-grade dysplasia is present, this is staged as pTis.

Prognosis and prediction
Because of the relatively high risk of high-grade dysplasia / gastric cancer, complete resection is mandatory. Progression to high-grade dysplasia / gastric cancer is more frequent in patients with autoimmune gastritis. The neoplastic risk increases with larger polyp size, tubulovillous architecture, and the mixed immunophenotype. Prognosis depends on any carcinomatous component; however, after endoscopic or surgical resection, the overall local recurrence rate is < 10% {625}.

Oxyntic gland adenoma

Yao T
Vieth M

Definition

Oxyntic gland adenoma (OGA) is a benign epithelial neoplasm composed of columnar cells with differentiation to chief cells, parietal cells, or both, with a high rate of progression to adenocarcinoma (submucosal invasion).

ICD-O coding

8210/2 Adenomatous polyp, high-grade dysplasia
8210/0 Adenomatous polyp, low-grade dysplasia

ICD-11 coding

2E92.1 & XH3DV3 Benign neoplasm of stomach & Adenoma NOS

Related terminology

Acceptable: gastric dysplasia of chief cell–predominant type; chief cell–predominant gastric polyps; oxyntic gland polyp/ adenoma.

Subtype(s)

None

Localization

OGA occurs predominantly in the upper third of the stomach (80%), mostly in non-atrophic oxyntic mucosa, similar to gastric adenocarcinoma of fundic-gland type (GA-FG) {297}.

Clinical features

OGAs occur most commonly in patients aged 60–70 years. In Japan, most tumours are identified during endoscopic screening; elsewhere, most patients present with reflux symptoms {3056,546}. Endoscopy reveals a polypoid, submucosal tumour or flat lesion with faded-whitish mucosa {3383,1842}. Vasodilatation or branched vessels may be visible on the tumour surface {3383,3315}.

Epidemiology

This is a rare neoplasm, but the exact incidence is unknown. Most cases of OGA and GA-FG have been reported from Japan, with only a few reports from North America and Europe {297}. The incidence of GA-FG is 1.6% of gastric adenocarcinoma {1227}, and the relative incidence of OGA to GA-FG is estimated to be about 0.5 {297}.

Etiology

The etiology is unknown, but there is no association with *Helicobacter pylori* infection {3383}. In one study from Australia, a history of acid reduction therapy was reported by 7 of 8 patients {546}.

Pathogenesis

A morphological continuum exists from OGA to GA-FG. However, there is ongoing discussion as to whether OGA should be regarded as an intramucosal component of GA-FG {297}.

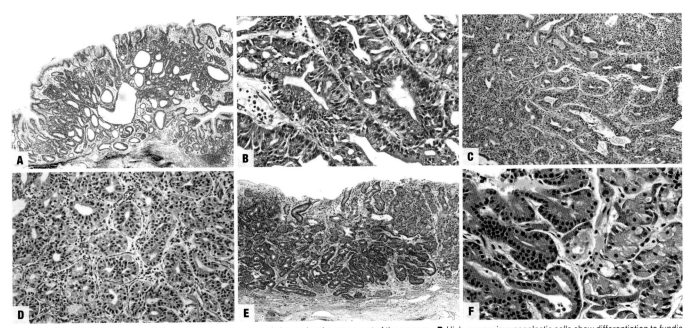

Fig. 3.23 Oxyntic gland adenoma. **A** Low-power view of an example located at the upper part of the mucosa. **B** High-power view; neoplastic cells show differentiation to fundic gland cells and parietal cells, mimicking oxyntic glands. **C** Note eosinophilic cells showing parietal cell differentiation. **D** Note the proliferation of chief cell–like cells. **E** Low-power view of oxyntic gland adenoma mainly occupying the deeper zone of the fundic mucosa; note the sharp border between neoplastic and non-neoplastic fundic glands. **F** High-power view of panel C; note the neoplastic glandular cells of immature type (left) compared with the non-neoplastic glandular cells (right).

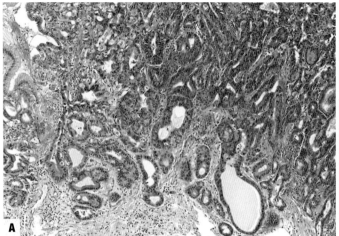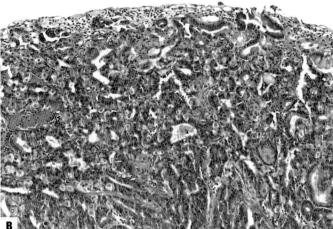

Fig. 3.24 Oxyntic gland adenoma. **A** With transition to submucosal invasive carcinoma. **B** With transition to carcinoma.

Missense or nonsense mutations in the genes of the WNT/β-catenin signalling pathway (*CTNNB1*, *APC*, *AXIN1*, and *AXIN2*) are relatively frequent in GA-FG (50%). These mutations, except for *CTNNB1* mutation, are also identified in OGA (30%). β-catenin nuclear labelling is low or non-existent in OGA {1842}, whereas high labelling (> 30%) is one of features of GA-FG (26%) {1227}. Mutation in *GNAS*, which is present in 19% of GA-FGs {2381,1734}, has not been investigated in OGA.

Macroscopic appearance
The size ranges from 3 to 18 mm and is < 10 mm in most cases.

Histopathology
OGA is composed of highly differentiated columnar cells with pale basophilic cytoplasm and mild nuclear atypia, mimicking the oxyntic (fundic) gland (mainly chief cell). The tumour may be situated in the upper portion of the mucosa, but it is mainly situated in deeper mucosa and covered by foveolar epithelium. The tumour consists of irregular architectures, such as tubular fusion and lateral expansion of glands. The differentiation to the components of oxyntic (fundic) gland is confirmed by immunohistochemistry, such as pepsinogen I (chief cell) and H+/K+ ATPase (parietal cell) {3384}. The predominant cell type is immature chief cells, positive for both pepsinogen I and MUC6. The Ki-67 proliferation index is low, but its distribution is irregular.

Some of the architectural patterns (e.g. clustered and solid glands and anastomosing cords) may be mistaken for a neuroendocrine tumour (NET) {546}. Although some lesions display weak to moderate positivity for synaptophysin and/or CD56, there is no chromogranin A positivity.

The tumour shows a pushing border against the muscularis mucosae in absence of desmoplasia. When the tumour shows invasion to the submucosa, it should be classified as GA-FG, a subtype of adenocarcinoma.

Cytology
Not clinically relevant

Diagnostic molecular pathology
Not clinically relevant

Essential and desirable diagnostic criteria
Essential: intramucosal proliferation of differentiated columnar cells with pale basophilic cytoplasm and mild nuclear atypia, mimicking the oxyntic (fundic) gland.
Desirable: immunohistochemically confirmed positivity for both pepsinogen I and MUC6.

Staging (TNM)
If high-grade dysplasia is present, this is staged as pTis.

Prognosis and prediction
There is a high (60%) risk of submucosal invasion (progression to malignancy).

Gastric adenocarcinoma

Carneiro F
Fukayama M
Grabsch HI
Yasui W

Definition
Adenocarcinoma of the stomach is a malignant epithelial neoplasm of the gastric mucosa, with glandular differentiation.

ICD-O coding
8140/3 Adenocarcinoma NOS

ICD-11 coding
2B72.0 & XH74S1 Adenocarcinoma of stomach & Adenocarcinoma NOS

Related terminology
None

Subtype(s)
Tubular adenocarcinoma (8211/3); parietal cell carcinoma (8214/3); adenocarcinoma with mixed subtypes (8255/3); papillary adenocarcinoma NOS (8260/3); micropapillary carcinoma NOS (8265/3); mucoepidermoid carcinoma (8430/3); mucinous adenocarcinoma (8480/3); signet-ring cell carcinoma (8490/3); poorly cohesive carcinoma (8490/3); medullary carcinoma with lymphoid stroma (8512/3); hepatoid adenocarcinoma (8576/3); Paneth cell carcinoma

Localization
The localization of these tumours varies geographically according to the incidence of gastric cancer (GC). In regions with high GC incidence (Asia, Central and South America, and eastern Europe), about 80% of cases are distal (occurring in the gastric body, antrum, and/or pylorus), with a relative predominance of antral-pyloric location. In northern Europe (including the United Kingdom) and the USA, 50–60% of GCs are located in the cardia and/or fundus, primarily because of the lower incidence of distal carcinoma in these parts of the world {920}. In contrast, the proportion of cardia/fundus cases in a study from the Republic of Korea was a relatively stable 5.9–7.1% over the 15-year period of 1999–2014. In Japan, the incidence of proximal GC has been increasing, with 18–22% of all GCs arising in the proximal stomach {3237,1539,1263}. A recent increase in GC arising in the corpus has also been observed in the USA and the Netherlands {469,1261}.

Clinical features
GC can be asymptomatic at early stages. At advanced disease stages, common symptoms include dysphagia, asthenia, indigestion, vomiting, weight loss, early satisfaction of appetite, and anaemia {112}.

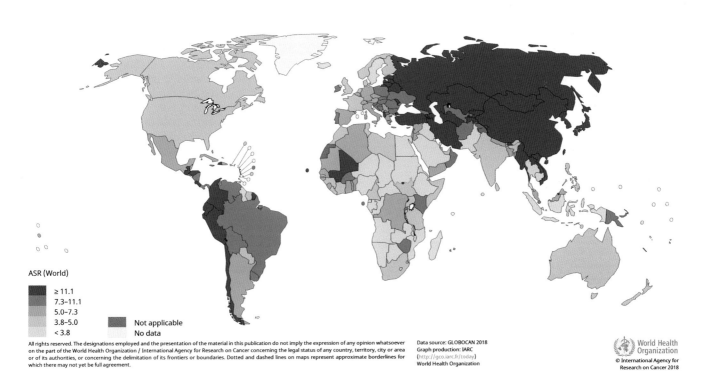

ASR (World)

≥ 11.1
7.3–11.1
5.0–7.3
3.8–5.0
< 3.8
Not applicable
No data

Data source: GLOBOCAN 2018
Graph production: IARC
(http://gco.iarc.fr/today)
World Health Organization

World Health Organization
© International Agency for Research on Cancer 2018

Fig. 3.25 Estimated age-standardized incidence rates (ASRs; World), per 100 000 person-years, of gastric cancer in 2018.

Endoscopic examination and forceps biopsies remain the gold standard method of diagnosing GC. Details of the mucosal surface can be evaluated by narrow-band imaging or chromoendoscopy in combination with magnifying endoscopy. Submucosal invasion can be suspected if mucosal abnormalities are seen, such as deep depression, irregular nodules, or an amorphous surface {3172}. Endoscopic mucosal resection and endoscopic submucosal dissection are used for staging and treatment of superficial lesions such as dysplasia or intramucosal carcinoma {2452,2586}.

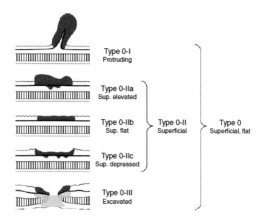

Fig. 3.26 Subclassification of early gastric carcinoma (type 0). Superficial (sup.) tumours with two or more components should have all components recorded in order of the surface area occupied, for example, "0-IIc III". See Box 3.03 for details.

For more-advanced cancers, staging is performed using EUS, contrast-enhanced CT, MRI, or FDG PET-CT {2924,497,622,1545}. EUS may also be useful to identify enlarged perigastric lymph nodes and, if necessary, to confirm metastasis by FNA. Staging laparoscopy is required to exclude peritoneal disease {1365}.

Epidemiology

Worldwide, GC is the third most common cause of cancer-related mortality {399}; despite its declining incidence {229}, > 1 million new cases were estimated worldwide in 2018 {399}. The incidence is highest in central and eastern Asia, eastern Europe, and South America {399}. In a studied population in the United Kingdom, 1 in 2 patients with GC presented with locally advanced disease {3639,109}. Laurén's 1965 classification {1798} divided GC into two main histological types: intestinal-type and diffuse-type. A decrease in the incidence of intestinal-type GC with a relative increase in the incidence of diffuse-type GC has been observed in some countries {2058}.

Etiology

GC is a multifactorial disease; 90% of cases are sporadic and the other 10% develop in a familial/hereditary setting. Environmental factors include *Helicobacter pylori* infection, EBV infection, tobacco smoking, and dietary factors (see Box 3.02) {1351,1921,229,2791,2316}.

Several subtypes of GC have been associated with specific etiologies and molecular mechanisms. Germline mutations and specific types of GC have been recognized, such as *CDH1* mutations in hereditary diffuse GC (see *Hereditary diffuse gastric cancer*, p. 535) and *APC* exon 1B mutations in gastric adenocarcinoma and proximal polyposis of the stomach (GAPPS) (see *GAPPS and other fundic gland polyposes*, p. 526).

Pathogenesis

H. pylori infection is thought to be responsible for most GCs, in particular non-cardia GCs {2031,3359,621}. Chronic infection of the gastric mucosa leads to atrophic gastritis and intestinal metaplasia in a stepwise progression known as Correa's cascade {674,2123}. Eradication of *H. pylori* reduces the risk of GC {1846}. However, the degree of risk reduction depends on the presence, severity, and extent of the atrophic damage at the time of eradication {3162,3003,2797,1846}. In patients with advanced stages of gastric atrophy, *H. pylori* eradication may no longer reduce the risk of neoplastic progression {2797}. Chronic *H. pylori* infection has been assumed to cause DNA mutations and epigenetic changes in epithelial cells of the stomach (field cancerization) {3014,3659,2483}. Infection with *cagA*-positive *H. pylori* strains is the strongest risk factor for the development of GC {1230,2159}. Infection with the most virulent *vacA* s1, m1, and i1 strains is associated with an increased risk of gastric adenocarcinoma, although the predictive value of *vacA* virulent genotypes, observed in the USA and Colombia, was not confirmed in some studies from eastern and southeastern Asia {2417,2159}. Genetic susceptibility is also involved, such as SNPs of inflammation-associated genes (*IL1B*, *TNF*) {1040}. Furthermore, autoimmune gastritis is considered a risk factor for GC in high-income countries {137}.

Multiple genetic and epigenetic alterations occur during gastric carcinogenesis and progression {3690,3691}. These include

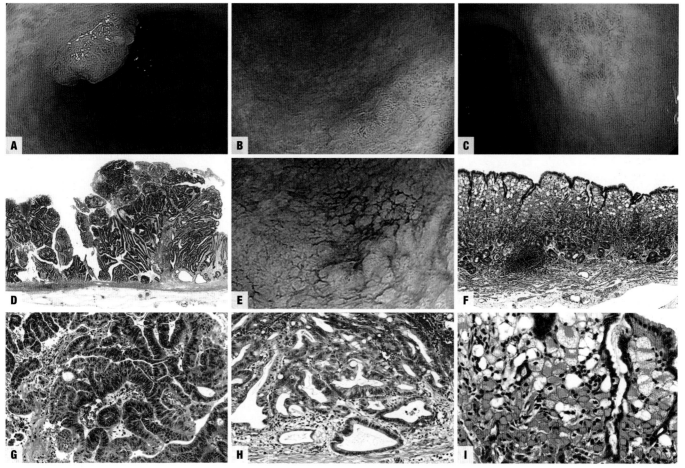

Fig. 3.27 Early gastric carcinoma. **A** Type 0-I, endoscopic features. A slightly reddish protruding lesion with irregular surface, 16 mm in size, located in the lesser curvature of the lower gastric body. **B** Type 0-IIc, endoscopic features. A reddish depressed lesion with irregular margins, 10 mm in size, located in the greater curvature of the lower gastric body. **C** Type 0-IIc, endoscopic features. A discoloured depressed lesion with irregular margins, 18 mm in size, located on the posterior wall of the gastric angle. **D** Type 0-I, histological appearance (low power). The tumour displays features of papillary adenocarcinoma. **E** Type 0-IIc, endoscopic features. In the same lesion shown in panel B, chromoendoscopy with indigo carmine enhances the surface irregularity, with clearer margins of the lesion. **F** Type 0-IIc, histological appearance (low power). The tumour displays features of signet-ring cell carcinoma. **G** Type 0-I, histological appearance (high power). **H** Type 0-IIc, histological appearance. The tumour displays features of tubular adenocarcinoma. **I** Type 0-IIc, histological appearance (high power).

genetic instability and abnormalities in oncogenes, tumour suppressor genes, growth factors, receptor tyrosine kinases, DNA repair genes, matrix degradation enzymes, cell-cycle regulators, and cell adhesion molecules. Genetic polymorphisms or variations, such as SNPs of *MUC1* and *PSCA*, are predisposing endogenous factors and appear to alter GC susceptibility as well as disease progression {3154,2811,3691,2107}. DNA methylation, histone modification, chromatin remodelling, and regulation by non-coding RNAs are important epigenetic alterations {1190,2483}. Advanced multiplatform genomic technology has recently identified potential molecular mechanisms underlying GC carcinogenesis {3234,605,1540,3467}.

Using high-throughput sequencing technology, several groups, including The Cancer Genome Atlas (TCGA) Research Network and the Asian Cancer Research Group (ACRG), have proposed genetic and epigenetic molecular classifications of GC {1851,476,692}.

TCGA has proposed a classification categorizing GC into four molecular subtypes: EBV-positive, microsatellite-unstable, genomically stable, and chromosomally unstable (see Table. 3.05, p. 94) {476,1540}. Most EBV-positive GCs are

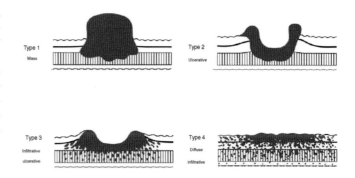

Fig. 3.28 Macroscopic types of advanced gastric cancer. **Type 1** (mass): polypoid tumours, sharply demarcated from the surrounding mucosa. **Type 2** (ulcerative): ulcerated tumours with raised margins surrounded by a thickened gastric wall with clear margins. **Type 3** (infiltrative ulcerative): ulcerated tumours with raised margins, surrounded by a thickened gastric wall without clear margins. **Type 4** (diffuse infiltrative): tumours without marked ulceration or raised margins; the gastric wall is thickened and indurated and the margin is unclear.

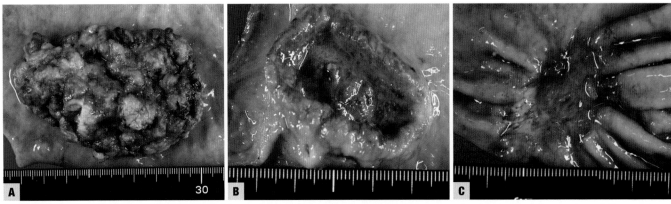

Fig. 3.29 Gastric adenocarcinoma. **A** Borrmann type I. A large polypoid and fungating tumour with broad base; the surface has a variegated appearance. **B** Borrmann type II. An ulcer-forming mass with elevated base in relation to the neighbouring mucosa, which appears as a thick wall surrounding the ulcer. **C** Borrmann type III. A large ulcer with a surrounding zone of infiltration; thick gastric folds fuse each other at the ulcer edge, indicating cancer infiltration.

histologically GC with lymphoid stroma or lymphoepithelioma-like, and display *PIK3CA* and *ARID1A* mutations, genome-wide hypermethylation, and amplification of the *CD274* (*PD-L1*) gene, an important immune checkpoint regulator {3234,2818,3021}. Microsatellite-unstable GCs are characterized by mutations or promoter methylation of mismatch repair genes, such as *MLH1*. Like EBV-positive GC, the microsatellite-unstable GC subtype exhibits global hypermethylation. Genomically stable GCs show predominantly diffuse-type histology and are characterized by a substantially lower frequency of genetic aberrations. However, mutations of *RHOA* or fusions involving RHO-family GTPase-activating proteins have been observed in a subset of genomically stable GC {1501}. GCs with chromosomal instability show mostly intestinal-type histology together with extensive DNA copy-number abnormalities, including amplification of receptor tyrosine kinase genes, such as *ERBB2*, *EGFR*, *MET*, and *FGFR2*. In routine pathology, immunohistochemistry of mismatch repair proteins (MLH1, etc.), p53, and E-cadherin combined with in situ hybridization for EBV-encoded small RNA (EBER) might allow molecular GC subtyping similar to the classification proposed by TCGA {1069,61,2960}.

ACRG proposed a classification of GC into four different subtypes: microsatellite-unstable, microsatellite-stable (MSS) with epithelial–mesenchymal transition gene signature, MSS and *TP53*-active, and MSS and *TP53*-inactive {692}.

Macroscopic appearance

Early gastric carcinomas can be macroscopically subclassified into three main types: 0-I, 0-II, and 0-III (see Fig. 3.26 and Box 3.03, p. 86) {1431,3172}. Advanced gastric carcinomas are macroscopically subclassified according to the Borrmann classification as localized growth with a fungating or ulcerated appearance or as infiltrative growth with or without ulceration. The term "linitis plastica" or "scirrhous carcinoma" is used when there is an abundant fibrous stroma reaction resulting in thickening and rigidity of the stomach wall {51}.

Histopathology

Intratumoural and intertumoural heterogeneity of the histological phenotype can be striking in GC and is most likely the reason for the many histopathological classification schemes for GC. The most commonly used classifications are those published by the Japanese Gastric Cancer Association (JGCA) {1430}, WHO, Nakamura et al. {2284}, and Laurén {1798}, which are compared in Table 3.03. Other classifications have been proposed by Ming {2169}, Mulligan {2242}, and Carneiro et al. {507}. Five main histological subtypes of gastric

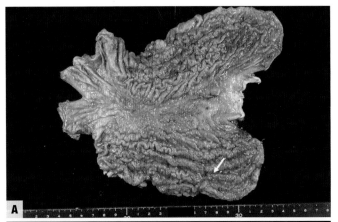

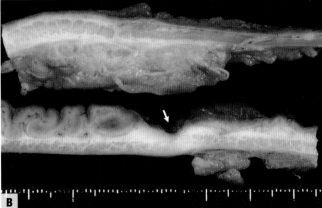

Fig. 3.30 Gastric adenocarcinoma, Borrmann type IV, an extreme example (linitis plastica). **A** Whole stomach with prominent gastric folds, which resemble hypertrophic gastric rugae; the waffle-like appearance of the folds indicates loss of extensibility due to scirrhous infiltration of cancer cells; note a small ulcer between large folds on the posterior wall (arrow). **B** On the cut surface, diffuse white streaks delineate the submucosa, muscularis propria, and subserosal layer; note a shallow ulcer in the centre of the lower slice (arrow; corresponds to the arrow in panel A).

Table 3.03 Comparison of the Laurén {1798}, Nakamura {2284}, Japanese Gastric Cancer Association (JGCA) {1430}, and WHO classifications of gastric cancer

Laurén (1965)	Nakamura et al. (1968)	JGCA (2017)	WHO (2019)
Intestinal	Differentiated	Papillary: pap Tubular 1, well-differentiated: tub1 Tubular 2, moderately differentiated: tub2	Papillary Tubular, well-differentiated Tubular, moderately differentiated
Indeterminate	Undifferentiated	Poorly 1 (solid type): por1	Tubular (solid), poorly differentiated
Diffuse	Undifferentiated	Signet-ring cell: sig Poorly 2 (non-solid type): por2	Poorly cohesive, signet-ring cell phenotype Poorly cohesive, other cell types
Intestinal/diffuse/indeterminate	Differentiated/undifferentiated	Mucinous	Mucinous
Mixed		Description according to the proportion (e.g. por2 > sig > tub2)	Mixed

Not defined	Not defined	Special type:
		Adenosquamous carcinoma
		Squamous cell carcinoma
		Undifferentiated carcinoma
		Carcinoma with lymphoid stroma
		Hepatoid adenocarcinoma
		Adenocarcinoma with enteroblastic
		   differentiation
		Adenocarcinoma of fundic gland type
			Other histological subtypes:
			Adenosquamous carcinoma
			Squamous cell carcinoma
			Undifferentiated carcinoma
			Carcinoma with lymphoid stroma
			Hepatoid carcinoma
			Adenocarcinoma with enteroblastic
			   differentiation
			Adenocarcinoma of fundic gland type
			Micropapillary adenocarcinoma

adenocarcinoma are recognized: tubular, papillary, poorly cohesive (including signet-ring cell and other subtypes), mucinous, and mixed adenocarcinomas.

Tubular adenocarcinoma: This is the most common subtype, with a relative frequency ranging from 45% in Europe {727} to 64% in a nationwide study in Japan {1429}. A much higher frequency (72.4%) has been reported in elderly patients in Japan {174}. This subtype is composed of dilated or slit-like branching tubules of variable diameter. Acinar structures may also be present. Individual neoplastic cells can be columnar, cuboidal, or flattened by prominent intraluminal mucin or cell debris. A clear cell subtype has been recognized with predilection for the cardia/oesophagogastric region {1032}. Tumours with solid structures and barely recognizable tubules are included in this category; they are classified as poorly differentiated tubular (solid) carcinoma, which corresponds to the designation "poorly 1 (solid type): por1" in the JGCA classification (see Table 3.03).

Papillary adenocarcinoma: This is a relatively rare subtype, accounting for 2.7–9.9% of GCs {1429,23}. This subtype usually shows an exophytic growth pattern and is histologically most commonly well differentiated, with elongated finger-like processes lined by columnar or cuboidal cells supported by fibrovascular connective tissue cores. Some tumours also contain tubules (tubulopapillary). Despite being a well-differentiated tumour with a pushing invading edge and frequent infiltration by inflammatory cells, papillary adenocarcinoma is associated with a higher frequency of liver metastasis and poor survival {3688,3723}.

Poorly cohesive carcinoma (PCC), including signet-ring cell carcinoma and other subtypes: PCCs account for 20–54% of GCs {3639,3076}, with higher frequencies reported in Japanese

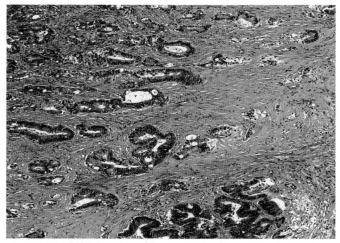

Fig. 3.31 Tubular adenocarcinoma. The tumour is composed of dilated tubules invading the muscle layer.

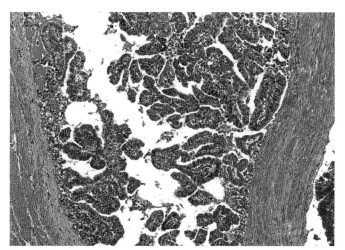

Fig. 3.32 Papillary carcinoma. The tumour consists of elongated finger-like processes with fibrovascular connective tissue cores, lined by columnar cells.

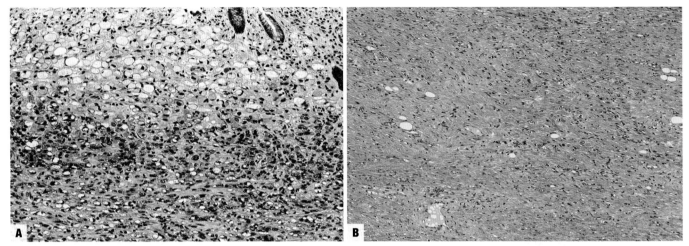

Fig. 3.33 Gastric adenocarcinoma. **A** Poorly cohesive carcinoma, signet-ring cell type. The tumour is composed predominantly of signet-ring cells; the neoplastic cells are larger at the superficial part of the mucosa. **B** Poorly cohesive carcinoma NOS (i.e. non–signet-ring cell type). The tumour consists of poorly cohesive cells of non–signet-ring cell type that invade the gastric wall widely, with marked desmoplasia.

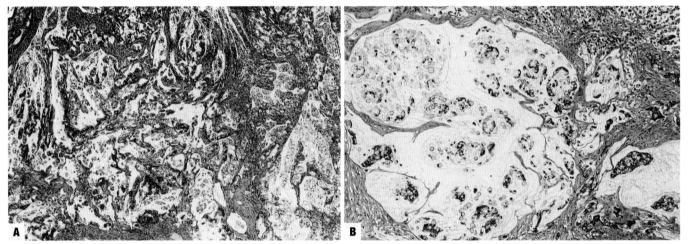

Fig. 3.34 Mucinous carcinoma. **A** Malignant glands are seen in extracellular mucinous pools. **B** Nests of signet-ring cells are present, floating in extracellular mucous.

patients {1547,3639}. PCCs are composed of neoplastic cells that are isolated or arranged in small aggregates without well-formed glands. PCCs can be of either signet-ring cell type or non–signet-ring cell type (PCC-NOS) {2052A}. Signet-ring cell type tumours are composed predominantly or exclusively of signet-ring cells, which are characterized by a central, optically clear, globoid droplet of cytoplasmic mucin with an eccentrically placed nucleus. Signet-ring cells may form a lace-like glandular or delicate microtrabecular pattern (especially in the mucosa). Other cellular subtypes (non–signet-ring cell type: PCC-NOS) include tumours composed of neoplastic cells resembling histiocytes or lymphocytes; others have deeply eosinophilic cytoplasm; some poorly cohesive cells are pleomorphic, with bizarre nuclei. A mixture of the different cell types can be seen, including few signet-ring cells {1737}. PCCs can be accompanied by marked desmoplasia, in particular when infiltrating into the submucosa or beyond. There is preliminary evidence suggesting lower sensitivity of signet-ring cell carcinomas to chemo(radio)therapy {2569,565}. A subgroup of *RHOA*-mutated GC {1501} consists of predominantly or exclusively PCC with limited tubular differentiation and a permeative growth pattern at the edge of the mucosa {3393}.

Mucinous adenocarcinoma: This subtype has been reported to account for 2.1–8.1% of GCs {1429,1079}. This tumour is composed of malignant epithelium and extracellular mucin pools, with the latter accounting for > 50% of the tumour area. Two main growth patterns can be seen: (1) recognizable glandular structures or tubules lined by columnar epithelium with interstitial mucin and (2) chains, nests, or single tumour cells (signet-ring cells can be seen) surrounded by mucin. Recent comprehensive genetic analysis demonstrated that the mutation profile of the latter type of mucinous adenocarcinoma is different than that of intestinal-type or diffuse-type GCs {2747}.

Mixed adenocarcinoma: The reported relative frequency of this subtype is 6–22% {3639,3076,3769}. These carcinomas display two or more distinct histological components: glandular (tubular/papillary) and signet-ring cell / poorly cohesive. Any distinct histological component should be reported. Mixed carcinomas appear to be clonal {516,3769}, and their phenotypic divergence has been attributed to somatic mutation in the gene encoding E-cadherin (*CDH1*), which is restricted to

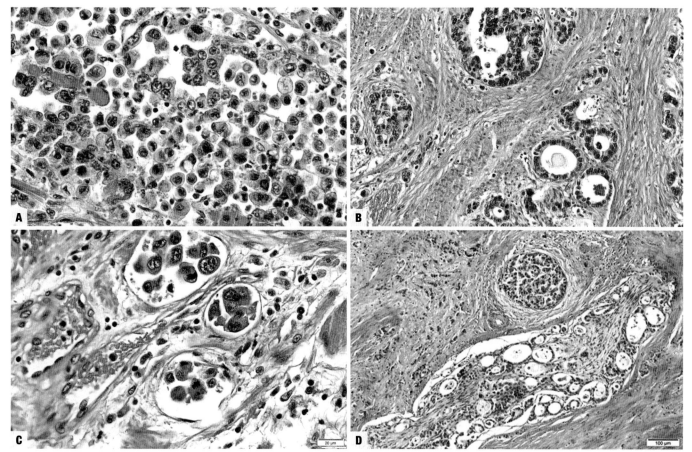

Fig. 3.35 Mixed carcinoma. **A** Poorly cohesive cell component. **B** Tubular component. **C** Lymphatic invasion by poorly cohesive cells. **D** Vascular and perineural invasion by the tubular component.

the signet-ring cell / poorly cohesive component {1991}. Available data suggest that patients with mixed adenocarcinomas have a poorer prognosis than those with only one component {3135,3769}.

Other and rare histological subtypes

Gastric (adeno)carcinoma with lymphoid stroma: This subtype has been reported to account for 1–7% of GCs {3536,1245}. It has also been referred to as lymphoepithelioma-like carcinoma and medullary carcinoma. The subtype is characterized by irregular sheets, trabeculae, ill-defined tubules, or syncytia of polygonal cells embedded within a prominent lymphocytic infiltrate, with intraepithelial lymphocytes {470,2252,1110}. In early-stage disease, gastric (adeno)carcinoma with lymphoid stroma shows a characteristic lace pattern with anastomosing or branching glandular structures {681}. The tumours are frequently localized in the proximal stomach or gastric stump, and they are more common in males. Reported rates of EBV infection in this subtype vary from 22.5% to 100% {1245,559,3513}, and the highest frequencies (> 80%) are detected by performing EBER in situ hybridization {1356,5,2252,594,1913}. A subset of gastric carcinomas with microsatellite instability (MSI) and/or mismatch repair deficiency has a similar histological phenotype but a different transcriptomic profile {1109}.

Hepatoid adenocarcinoma and related entities: Hepatoid adenocarcinoma is predominantly composed of large polygonal eosinophilic hepatocyte-like neoplastic cells. AFP can be detected by immunohistochemistry in the tumour cells, and also in the serum. Bile and PASD-positive intracytoplasmic eosinophilic globules can be observed. Other AFP-producing carcinomas include well-differentiated papillary or tubular-type adenocarcinoma with clear cytoplasm, adenocarcinoma with enteroblastic differentiation and yolk-sac tumour–like carcinoma {1371,892,69,220,3621}. More than one of these histological types often coexist. The reported frequencies of hepatoid

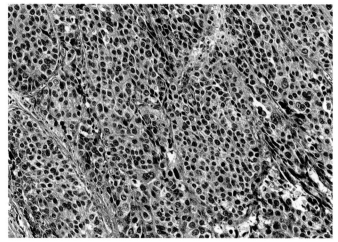

Fig. 3.36 Hepatoid adenocarcinoma. Sheets and cords of polygonal cells with abundant eosinophilic cytoplasm, closely resembling hepatocellular carcinoma.

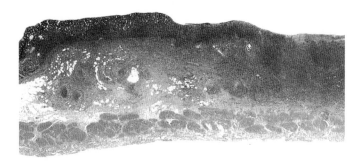

A

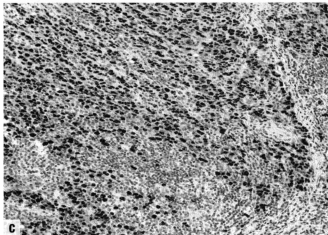

Fig. 3.37 Gastric carcinoma with lymphoid stroma (EBV-positive gastric cancer). **A** Low-power view of the tumour; note lymphoid follicles in the submucosa adjacent to the carcinomatous lesion. **B** Cancer cells forming small nests or fused glands, accompanied by abundant lymphocyte infiltration. **C** Nuclei of carcinoma cells are positive by in situ hybridization targeting EBV-encoded small RNA (EBER). Nuclei of infiltrating lymphocytes are negative.

carcinoma and AFP-producing carcinomas are 0.3–2% {3661,3397} and 2.6–5.4% {3661,562} of all GCs, respectively. Adenocarcinoma with enteroblastic differentiation is a tumour showing a tubulopapillary architecture composed of columnar neoplastic cells with clear cytoplasm, resembling early fetal gut epithelium. These types of tumours may express marker proteins of fetal gut, such as SALL4, claudin-6, and glypican-3 (GPC3) {3395,3396,3397,59}. SALL4 and claudin-6 immunohistochemistry are diagnostically useful in distinguishing hepatoid adenocarcinoma from hepatocellular carcinoma {3395}.

Micropapillary adenocarcinoma: This subtype is characterized by the presence of small clusters of tumour cells without fibrovascular cores protruding into clear spaces {2744}. This component, ranging between 10% and 90% of the entire tumour, accompanies tubular or papillary GCs. A pure invasive micropapillary carcinoma of the oesophagogastric junction has been reported {1191}. The micropapillary subtype has an unfavourable prognosis, and patients often have lymph node metastasis {866,3394,3757}.

Gastric adenocarcinoma of fundic-gland type: This subtype is assumed to develop from oxyntic gland adenoma, and it accounts for 1% of early GCs treated by endoscopic submucosal dissection {2181}. The characteristic oxyntic gland differentiation can be divided into three subcategories on the basis of the tumours' composition: chief cell–predominant (~99% of reported cases), parietal cell–predominant, and mixed phenotype {297}. Submucosal invasion is observed in 60% of cases {297}. Immunohistochemistry demonstrates positivity of both pepsinogen I and MUC6 {2464}. Some cells also show differentiation towards parietal cells (H+/K+ ATPase–positive) {3384}. This subtype of GC is slow-growing, and lymph node metastasis is extremely rare.

Rare subtypes encompass mucoepidermoid carcinoma {1198}, Paneth cell carcinoma {2454}, and parietal cell carcinoma {489}.

Grading

Grading applies primarily to tubular and papillary carcinomas and not to other GC subtypes. Thus, well-differentiated adenocarcinomas are composed of well-formed glands, whereas poorly differentiated carcinomas have poorly formed glands and may display solid areas or individual cells. Grading is preferably performed using a two-tiered system: low-grade (formerly well or moderately differentiated) versus high-grade (formerly poorly differentiated).

Tumour spread

GCs can spread by direct extension to adjacent organs, by lymphatic and/or haematogenous spread, and/or by serosal dissemination. Lymphovascular invasion should be systematically assessed; it is an indicator of biological aggressiveness and may be a prognostic factor for lymph node–negative GC {1827,1723}. Tubular/papillary carcinomas are more likely to give rise to liver metastases by haematogenous spread, whereas PCCs are more likely to involve the serosa. Mixed tumours exhibit the metastatic patterns of both types. Widespread tumour extension is particularly common in PCCs, which frequently show extensive spread on the serosal surface, well beyond the macroscopically visible tumour. Consequently, frozen section examination of longitudinal margins is desirable, particularly if the clearance is < 4 cm, to assess completeness of resection. If carcinoma penetrates the serosa, peritoneal implants generally flourish. Bilateral massive ovarian involvement (Krukenberg tumour) can result from transperitoneal or haematogenous spread. Pulmonary lymphangitic carcinomatosis and pulmonary tumour thrombotic microangiopathy may rarely develop in patients with GC {4,2168}.

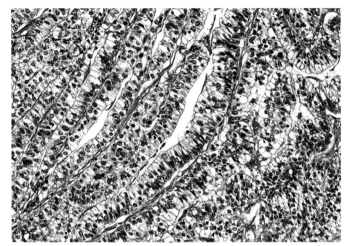

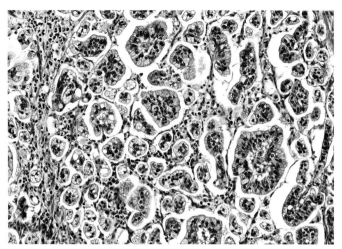

Fig. 3.38 Adenocarcinoma with enteroblastic differentiation. The glands consist of the columnar neoplastic cells characterized by glycogen-rich clear cytoplasm, reminiscent of fetal gut epithelium.

Fig. 3.39 Invasive micropapillary adenocarcinoma. The tumour clusters display the characteristic inside-out growth pattern, with the luminal pole of the cells present on the outer surface of the cluster.

Response to therapy

Neoadjuvant therapy may modify the histopathological appearance. Tumour response, which can vary from no detectable response to pathological complete response, can be assessed by tumour regression grade (TRG). Various methods have been proposed, including the Becker and Mandard systems {280,1786,3294,2036}, but there is no international consensus on which TRG system should be used.

Cytology

Peritoneal lavage cytology has been used for GC staging and monitoring adjuvant chemotherapy for GC {1420}. Abnormal cytology findings include irregularly shaped nuclei, high N:C ratio, increased chromatin, and anisonucleosis. The presence of a single signet-ring cell, > 5 cell clusters, or ≥ 50 isolated cancer cells in the peritoneal lavage is reported to affect the outcome of patients with R1 resection despite the absence of macroscopic peritoneal metastasis {1229}.

Diagnostic molecular pathology

Routine evaluation for MSI and PDL1 expression is not currently recommended, but gastric adenocarcinomas are good potential candidates for immunotherapy targeting the PD1/PDL1 axis, and these biomarkers are now under investigation in clinical trials.

Essential and desirable diagnostic criteria

Essential: evidence of invasion of the lamina propria or deeper layers by neoplastic glandular cells; immunohistochemistry (may be required for the characterization of some histological subtypes, as well as for small biopsies and metastases).

Desirable: ERBB2 (HER2) immunohistochemistry (required if anti-ERBB2 therapy is being considered).

Staging (TNM)

According to the eighth editions (2017) of the Union for International Cancer Control (UICC) TNM classification {408} and the American Joint Committee on Cancer (AJCC) cancer staging manual {127}, tumours involving the oesophagogastric junction

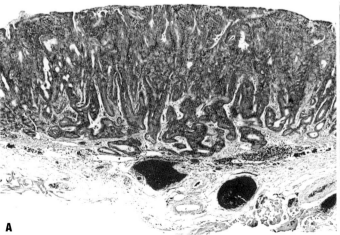

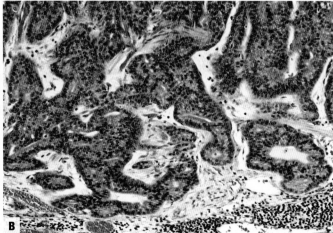

Fig. 3.40 Gastric adenocarcinoma of fundic-gland type. **A** Low-power view; note the submucosal invasion in the central portion of the tumour. **B** High-power view of the invasive carcinoma, which consists of neoplastic cells of immature fundic-gland type.

Table 3.04 Therapeutic recommendations for endoscopic treatment of gastric cancer based on histopathological examination of endoscopically resected specimens, from the 2018 Japanese Gastric Cancer Association (JGCA) treatment guidelines {1433}

Endoscopic treatment (EMR/ESD)			
Differentiated[a]		Undifferentiated[a]	
Vertical/deep margin (−) Lymphovascular infiltration (−) Any of following: • Intramucosal without ulcer, any size • Intramucosal with ulcer, diameter ≤ 3 cm • Submucosal, diameter ≤ 3 cm		Vertical/deep margin (−) Horizontal/lateral margin (−) Lymphovascular infiltration (−) Intramucosal without ulcer, diameter ≤ 2 cm	
Yes	No	No	Yes
Follow-up[b]	Surgery		Follow-up

EMR, endoscopic mucosal resection; ESD, endoscopic submucosal dissection.
[a]According to the Nakamura classification; see Table 3.03 (p. 89) for the corresponding 2017 JGCA and 2019 WHO classifications. [b]If the horizontal margin is positive, additional endoscopic treatment or surgery is required.

with an epicentre ≤ 2 cm into the proximal stomach are staged as oesophageal cancers; tumours with an epicentre located > 2 cm into the proximal stomach are staged as GCs, even if the oesophagogastric junction is involved. All tumours in the stomach that do not cross the oesophagogastric junction are staged as GC.

Prognosis and prediction
Prognostic factors

Stage: The pTNM staging system is currently the single most important factor for prognosis prediction in patients with GC. The 5-year survival rate in patients with pT1 (tumour invades the lamina propria, muscularis mucosae, or submucosa) and pN0 (no regional lymph node metastasis) GC is > 90% {2842}. Survival decreases in a stepwise fashion with increasing pT and pN category {2842}. The 5-year survival rate is 30% in patients with pT4b GC, 20% in those with pN3b GC, and 20% in patients with stage IIIC GC {2842}.

Histology: It has been suggested that histological phenotype may affect prognosis {3768,3657}. The Japanese recommendations for endoscopic treatment of GC are based on the size and histopathological characteristics of the lesion (see Table 3.04) {978,1433}. Detailed histopathological examination of the resected material is mandatory to identify even minute foci of submucosal invasion or other features that indicate the need for further treatment {1431}. Patients with PCC with abundant fibrous stroma (linitis plastica or scirrhous carcinoma) have the worst prognosis, with a 5-year survival rate of < 15% {2557,51,1962}.

Molecular profile: The recently identified molecular profiles are not only important to improve our understanding of driver alterations involved in gastric carcinogenesis, but may also help identify clinically relevant biomarkers and new potential therapeutic targets in the future.

Table 3.05 Key features of the four molecular gastric carcinoma subtypes proposed by The Cancer Genome Atlas (TCGA)

	EBV-positive	Microsatellite-unstable	Genomically stable	Chromosomally unstable
Relative frequency	9%	22%	20%	50%
Representative histology	Gastric carcinoma with lymphoid stroma	None	Diffuse type[a]	Intestinal type[a]
Methylation				
CpG island	CIMP	CIMP	Rare	Rare
MSI-high	Absent	All	Absent	Absent
CDKN2A	All	Frequent	Rare	Rare
MLH1	Absent	Frequent	Rare	Rare
Copy-number aberrations	Rare	Rare	Rare	Frequent
Genomic mutations/alterations	Rare	Frequent	Rare	Rare
TP53	Rare	Present	Rare	Frequent
CDH1	Absent	Rare	Present	Rare
PIK3CA	Frequent	Present	Rare	Rare
RHOA	Rare	Rare	Present	Rare
CLDN18-ARHGAP fusion	Absent	Rare	Present	Rare
ARID1A	Frequent	Present	Rare	Rare
RTK amplification	Rare	Rare	Rare	Frequent
RTK mutation	Rare	Frequent	Rare	Rare
CD274 (PD-L1) and PDCD1LG2 (PD-L2) amplification	Frequent	Rare	Rare	Rare

CIMP, CpG island methylator phenotype; MSI, microsatellite instability; RTK, receptor tyrosine kinase.
[a]The Laurén histological classification used by TCGA; see Table 3.03 (p. 89) for the corresponding 2017 Japanese Gastric Cancer Association (JGCA) and 2019 WHO classifications.

Established predictive biomarkers

ERBB2 (HER2): Anti-ERBB2 therapy benefits patients with unresectable or metastatic/recurrent ERBB2-positive GC, and ERBB2 testing is used to predict potential therapy response {1432}. ERBB2 status is assessed primarily by immunohistochemistry; if the findings are equivocal, *ERBB2* in situ hybridization is recommended {254}. The prognostic value of ERBB2 overexpression / *ERBB2* amplification has been demonstrated in some studies but not in others {1730,996,2231}.

Predictive biomarkers partly established and/or under development

Receptor tyrosine kinases: *EGFR* amplification has been suggested to be an independent prognostic factor in stage II/III GC {3278}. Similarly, c-MET status has been suggested to be an independent prognostic factor for unresectable or recurrent GC in patients who received standard chemotherapy {996}.

MSI and EBV: The prognosis of GC with EBV positivity or MSI / mismatch repair deficiency is better than that of cases that are EBV-negative or MSS / mismatch repair proficient {3781,2602,1329,2818,3021}. Therefore, histological recognition of GC with lymphoid stroma, EBV detection by EBER testing, and detection of hypermethylation of *MLH1* are biomarkers of good prognosis.

Cancer immunotherapy: Tumour mutation load, density of intratumoural CD8+ T-cell infiltrates, and PDL1 expression have been proposed as biomarkers of response to immune checkpoint blockade therapy {3324}. Among the four molecular subtypes proposed by TCGA, microsatellite-unstable GC with promoter methylation of mismatch repair genes is characterized by a high frequency of mutations, and among EBV-positive GCs, amplification and elevated expression of PDL1 is observed in 10–15% and 30–50%, respectively {476,3021,759A,2818,617A}. Therefore, these two molecular subtypes might be good potential candidates for immunotherapy targeting the PD1/PDL1 axis, which is currently under investigation in clinical trials.

Other predictive/prognostic biomarkers: A very large number of single gene marker studies have been published, including studies of EGF/TGF-α, VEGF-A, CD44, E-cadherin, MMP1, MMP7, MMP10, SPC18, and protocadherin B9 {3689,2469,2872,2239,3230}. Several comprehensive molecular profiles have been proposed to have prognostic value {575,3221,3658,2539,476,692}. Certain microRNA signatures have been associated with survival in GC {1892,3380,3761}. However, none has yet been introduced into clinical practice.

Gastric squamous cell carcinoma

Agaimy A

Definition
Squamous cell carcinoma of the stomach is a malignant gastric epithelial neoplasm showing squamous cell differentiation, characterized by keratinocyte-type cells with intercellular bridges and/or keratinization.

ICD-O coding
8070/3 Squamous cell carcinoma NOS

ICD-11 coding
2B72 & XH0945 Malignant neoplasm of stomach & Squamous cell carcinoma NOS

Related terminology
None

Subtype(s)
None

Localization
The upper, lower, and middle portions of the stomach are affected in decreasing order of frequency {380,1006}.

Clinical features
The clinical features are the same as those of other gastric cancers.

Epidemiology
Limited data are available. Primary gastric squamous cell carcinoma accounts for 0.04–0.07% of all gastric cancers, and < 100 cases have been reported {1006,380,3503}.

Etiology
Unknown

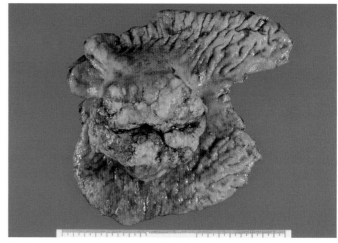

Fig. 3.41 Primary gastric squamous cell carcinoma. Gross appearance.

Pathogenesis
Various origins have been proposed, including via squamous cell metaplasia of gastric mucosa, from pluripotent stem cells, from ectopic squamous nests in the gastric mucosa, or from gastric carcinoma undergoing squamous metaplasia {3503,2456,60}.

Macroscopic appearance
The macroscopic appearance is the same as that of other gastric cancers.

Histopathology
The histology is similar to that of squamous cell carcinoma of the oesophagus (see *Oesophageal squamous papilloma*, p. 30) and other organs. The tumour shows uniform squamous cell differentiation and lack of any adenocarcinoma or other histology on thorough sampling. Sufficient sampling to exclude another

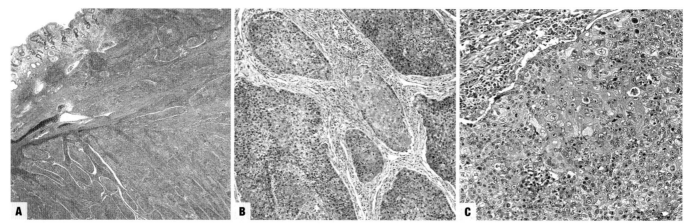

Fig. 3.42 Gastric squamous cell carcinoma. **A** Infiltrating gastric wall. **B** Showing infiltrating nests of malignant squamous cells with extensive areas of necrosis. **C** At high power.

component is mandatory, as is exclusion of metastasis from squamous cell carcinoma of another organ. Extension from lower oesophageal squamous cell carcinoma should be ruled out.

Cytology
Not clinically relevant

Diagnostic molecular pathology
No conclusive data are available.

Essential and desirable diagnostic criteria
None

Staging (TNM)
Gastric squamous cell carcinoma frequently presents at an advanced stage, which is associated with poor outcome. Spread to the liver is frequent in advanced disease.

Prognosis and prediction
Because of the rarity of this disease, no specific prognostic features have been identified. Disease stage at diagnosis is probably the main determinant of prognosis {2120}. Gastric squamous cell carcinoma seems to behave more aggressively than adenocarcinoma of the same disease stage {2120}.

Gastric adenosquamous carcinoma

Agaimy A

Definition

Adenosquamous carcinoma of the stomach is a primary gastric carcinoma composed of both glandular and squamous cell components, with the squamous cell component constituting ≥ 25% of the tumour.

ICD-O coding

8560/3 Adenosquamous carcinoma

ICD-11 coding

2B72 & XH7873 Malignant neoplasms of stomach & Adenosquamous carcinoma

Related terminology

None

Subtype(s)

None

Localization

Gastric adenosquamous carcinomas develop most commonly in the lower third, followed by the upper and middle third {916}. Extension from the most frequent oesophagogastric junction adenosquamous carcinoma should be excluded.

Clinical features

The clinical features of gastric adenosquamous carcinoma are similar to those of other types of gastric cancer {1431}. Most tumours present as large masses, with a mean size of 5 cm {2213,576,169}.

Epidemiology

Gastric adenosquamous carcinoma accounts for 0.25% of all gastric cancers {587}. Males are predominantly affected, with a mean age of 60 years {2213,576}.

Etiology

Unknown

Pathogenesis

Unknown

Macroscopic appearance

The macroscopic appearance is similar to that of other gastric cancers.

Histopathology

Gastric adenosquamous carcinoma is composed of an admixture of adenocarcinoma and squamous cell carcinoma in variable proportions. The squamous cell component should account for ≥ 25% of the tumour {2820}. The squamous cell component may show all cytological and architectural features

known to occur in conventional squamous cell carcinoma of the oesophagus and other sites. Mucin staining is useful for highlighting areas of glandular differentiation; p63/p40

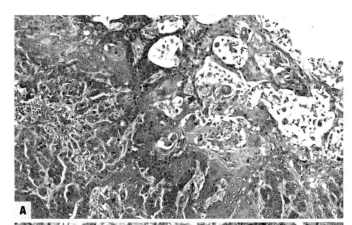

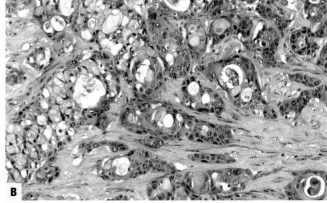

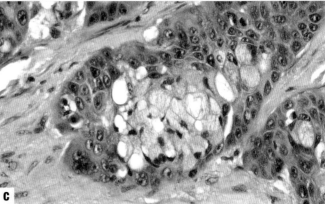

Fig. 3.43 Gastric adenosquamous carcinoma. **A** The superficial part may be indistinguishable from pure gastric squamous carcinoma. **B** Transition from pure squamous areas (right) to goblet cell–rich glandular areas (left). **C** Higher magnification showing goblet cell–like differentiation within squamous cell nests imparting a hybrid pattern.

immunohistochemistry may help determine the presence and extent of the squamous cell component.

Cytology
Not clinically relevant

Diagnostic molecular pathology
Not clinically relevant

Essential and desirable diagnostic criteria
Essential: True glandular or mucous cell differentiation.
Note: The presence of adenoid or microcystic changes within squamous foci of otherwise pure squamous cell carcinoma is not sufficient for the diagnosis.

Staging (TNM)
Tumour spread to regional nodes and to liver or peritoneum is common. Lymph node metastases are mostly from the adenocarcinoma component, but the squamous cell component or both components may be seen in the metastases.

Prognosis and prediction
Because of the rarity of disease and its generally aggressive nature, no specific prognostic features have been identified. Disease stage at diagnosis is the main prognostic determinant {2820}.

Gastric undifferentiated carcinoma

Agaimy A

Definition

Undifferentiated carcinoma of the stomach is a primary gastric carcinoma composed of anaplastic cells showing no specific cytological or architectural type of differentiation.

ICD-O coding

8020/3 Carcinoma, undifferentiated, NOS

ICD-11 coding

2B72 & XH1YY4 Malignant neoplasms of stomach & Carcinoma, undifferentiated, NOS

Related terminology

Acceptable: anaplastic carcinoma; pleomorphic carcinoma.
Not recommended: giant cell carcinoma.

Subtype(s)

Large cell carcinoma with rhabdoid phenotype (8014/3); pleomorphic carcinoma (8022/3); sarcomatoid carcinoma (8033/3); carcinoma with osteoclast-like giant cells (8035/3)

Localization

No specific localization within the stomach is observed, but diffuse involvement of more than one region is not uncommon.

Clinical features

Most patients present with a large ulcerated and extensively necrotic transmural fungating mass, which is often associated with extensive synchronous regional metastases. Most patients with initially localized disease develop widespread metastases shortly after diagnosis and surgery, and most patients die of their disease within 1 year {46,44}.

Epidemiology

Limited data are available. Undifferentiated rhabdoid carcinomas have been estimated to account for 0.1–0.3% of all gastric carcinomas and 5.6% of solid adenocarcinomas {3385,3398}.

Etiology

Unknown

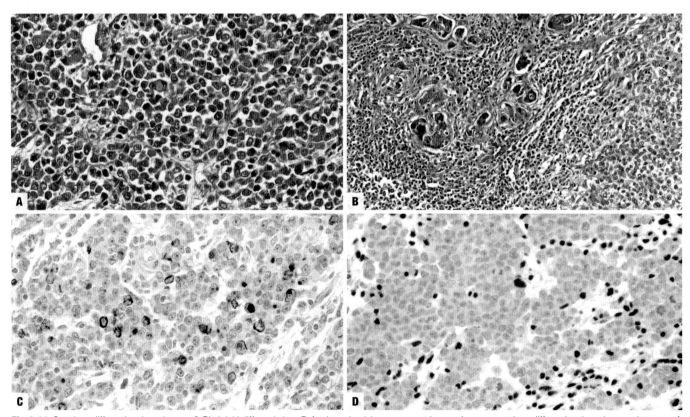

Fig. 3.44 Gastric undifferentiated carcinoma. **A** Rhabdoid differentiation. **B** A minor glandular component is seen in most gastric undifferentiated carcinomas that are sufficiently sampled. **C** Variable pancytokeratin expression. **D** Loss of SMARCB1 in rhabdoid gastric undifferentiated carcinoma.

Pathogenesis

The frequent presence of a variable glandular component or areas of transition to adenocarcinoma in otherwise undifferentiated tumours suggests an origin via dedifferentiation. In cases originating from other gastric cancer types via dedifferentiation, the genotype is essentially dictated by the clone of origin. In some cases, the undifferentiated phenotype is probably driven by various components of the SWI/SNF chromatin-remodelling complex; in particular, loss of SMARCB1 (INI1), SMARCA4, and ARID1A has been reported. In a subset of cases, SWI/SNF loss is superimposed on mismatch repair deficiency {46,44}.

Macroscopic appearance

The carcinoma is a large, ulcerated, necrotic, and usually transmural fungating mass, often with extensive regional lymph node involvement.

Histopathology

Anaplastic carcinoma is composed of diffuse sheets of anaplastic, large to medium-sized polygonal cells, with frequent pleomorphic tumour giant cells. A variable rhabdoid cell component is common and may be the predominant pattern; these cells frequently show binucleation or multinucleation. Other histological patterns that may be seen focally or as the dominant pattern include the spindled sarcomatoid pleomorphic pattern, undifferentiated carcinoma with osteoclast-like giant cells, and carcinoma with lymphoepithelioma-like features {1466,3567}. Depending on the extent of sampling, a glandular component may be observed and can vary from minimal to prominent. The stroma may be myxoid or mucinous, and it commonly contains mononuclear inflammatory cells. Immunohistochemistry, which is not specific, reveals variable expression of pancytokeratin. EMA staining may be helpful in keratin-poor examples. Vimentin is consistently expressed, frequently with a perinuclear dot-like pattern {46,44}. Gastric undifferentiated carcinoma should be distinguished from EBV-associated carcinoma with lymphoid stroma, aggressive lymphomas (including anaplastic large cell lymphoma), metastatic melanoma, germ cell neoplasms, PEComa, and other types of poorly differentiated sarcomas with an epithelioid large cell pattern.

Cytology

Gastric undifferentiated carcinoma contains malignant cells without evidence of differentiation.

Diagnostic molecular pathology

See *Gastric adenocarcinoma* (p. 85). ERBB2 (HER2) immunohistochemistry is recommended in all gastric carcinomas for which treatment is appropriate, but there are no specific recommendations.

Essential and desirable diagnostic criteria

Essential: malignant cells without histological evidence of differentiation; equivocal immunohistochemistry.

Staging (TNM)

See *Gastric adenocarcinoma* (p. 85).

Prognosis and prediction

Because of the rarity of this entity and its highly aggressive nature, no specific prognostic features have been identified. Disease stage at diagnosis might be prognostically relevant.

Gastroblastoma

Montgomery EA

Definition
Gastroblastoma is a biphasic tumour arising in the gastric muscularis propria (usually of the antrum), generally in boys and young men.

ICD-O coding
8976/1 Gastroblastoma

ICD-11 coding
None

Related terminology
None

Subtype(s)
None

Localization
Only 12 examples have been reported, all in the gastric muscularis propria {2138,3016,3556,1988,924,1083,3332}; 8 were antral, 2 were of the body, and 1 was of the fundus. The precise site of the last was not reported.

Clinical features
Most patients present with abdominal pain or epigastric pain, some with fatigue, and some with haematochezia {2138,3016, 3556,1988,924,1083,3332}. In some patients, a mass lesion is detected on physical examination. The reported tumours have ranged in size from 3.8 to 15 cm (mean: 7 cm; median: 6 cm).

Epidemiology
The reported patients with gastroblastoma have ranged in age from 9 to 56 years (mean: 24 years; median: 27 years). There appears to be a male predominance, with cases reported in 8 males and 4 females to date {2138,3016,3556,1988,924,1083,3332}.

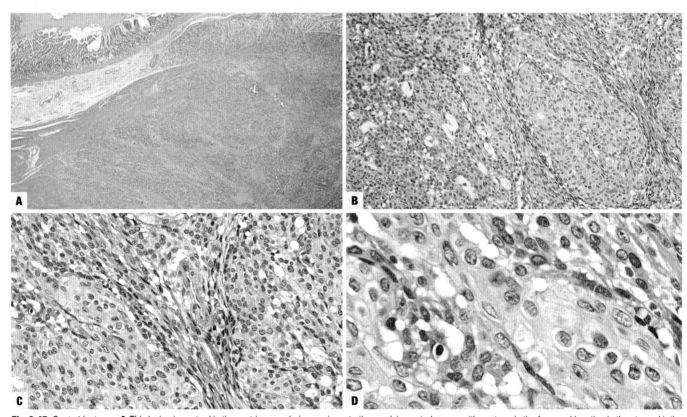

Fig. 3.45 Gastroblastoma. **A** This lesion is centred in the gastric muscularis propria; note the overlying antral mucosa (the antrum is the favoured location in the stomach); the tumour forms slightly plexiform lobules as it fills the muscularis propria. **B** There are epithelial nests with cords of spindle cells coursing diagonally from the upper left to the lower right of the image; note the uniform appearance of the cells. **C** This high-magnification image shows both the spindle cell and epithelial cell components of the neoplasm; the nuclei are small and the cytoplasm is pale. **D** This oil immersion H&E image shows the cytological features of gastroblastoma to full advantage; note the delicate nucleoli, which are only apparent at high magnification.

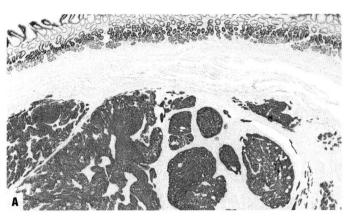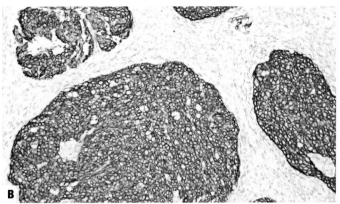

Fig. 3.46 Gastroblastoma. **A** The epithelial component of gastroblastoma expresses cytokeratin, but the spindle cell component does not (CAM5.2 immunostain). **B** Cytokeratin staining (CAM5.2) labels the epithelial cells but not the spindle cells.

Etiology
Unknown

Pathogenesis
Other than an association with a characteristic gene fusion (*MALAT1-GLI1* {1083}), the pathogenesis of these neoplasms is unknown. Somatic *MALAT1-GLI1* gene fusion is shared by some examples of plexiform fibromyxoma, which is also a neoplasm of the gastric muscularis propria {3106}. However, all reported cases of plexiform fibromyxoma are benign. Because gastroblastomas are biphasic, some examples have been tested for *SS18* fusions, which were not found {2138}, distinguishing these neoplasms from synovial sarcoma.

Macroscopic appearance
Gastroblastoma is centred in the muscularis propria of the stomach and grows in nodules, some with surrounding sclerosis.

Histopathology
Gastroblastoma shows a biphasic histology, consisting of uniform spindle cells and uniform epithelial cells arranged in nests. There are varying proportions of spindle and epithelial cells in any given neoplasm. The epithelial cells have scant pale cytoplasm, round nuclei, and inconspicuous nucleoli. The spindle cell component is monotonous and the cells are long and slender, often in a myxoid background. Areas of mineralization can be encountered. Mitoses are rare in most cases (with exceptions {2138}), and mitotic counts seem unrelated to outcome. On immunolabelling, the epithelial component expresses various pancytokeratins and shows focal labelling for CD56 and CD10, whereas the spindle cell component lacks expression of keratins, instead labelling for CD56 and CD10. Importantly, there is no expression of KIT, DOG1, CD34, SMA, desmin, synaptophysin, chromogranin, or S100.

Cytology
Not clinically relevant

Diagnostic molecular pathology
Demonstration of the *MALAT1-GLI1* fusion gene in tumour cells is required for the diagnosis of gastroblastoma.

Essential and desirable diagnostic criteria
Essential: biphasic histology, with spindle cells and nests of epithelial cells; *MALAT1-GLI1* fusion gene.

Staging (TNM)
Gastroblastoma is staged as gastric adenocarcinoma.

Prognosis and prediction
Most patients have had surgical resection of their neoplasms. Of 11 patients with available information, 7 have had uneventful follow-up for as long as 14 years (168 months), but the median reported follow-up is only 12 months. Liver metastases were reported in 2 patients at presentation (one of whom also had lymph node and peritoneal spread {1083}), lymph node metastases in one other patient {3556}, and local recurrence in another {3332}. No follow-up was available for the last {924}. Chemotherapy, tested in a limited number of cases, has been ineffective {2138,1083}. The number of reported cases is too low to define prognostic or predictive markers.

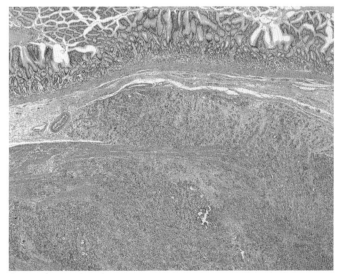

Fig. 3.47 Gastroblastoma. This lesion involves the muscularis propria of the antrum and forms nests that splay the smooth muscle bundles of the muscularis propria apart.

Gastric neuroendocrine neoplasms

La Rosa S
Rindi G
Solcia E
Tang LH

Definition

Neuroendocrine neoplasms (NENs) of the stomach are gastric epithelial neoplasms with neuroendocrine differentiation, including well-differentiated neuroendocrine tumours (NETs), poorly differentiated neuroendocrine carcinomas (NECs), and mixed neuroendocrine–non-neuroendocrine neoplasms (MiNENs) – an umbrella category including mixed adenoneuroendocrine carcinoma (MANEC).

ICD-O coding

8240/3 Neuroendocrine tumour NOS
8246/3 Neuroendocrine carcinoma NOS
8154/3 Mixed neuroendocrine–non-neuroendocrine neoplasm (MiNEN)

ICD-11 coding

2B72.1 & XH55D7 Malignant neuroendocrine neoplasm of stomach & Neuroendocrine carcinoma, well-differentiated
2B72.1 & XH9LV8 Malignant neuroendocrine neoplasm of stomach & Neuroendocrine tumour, grade I
2B72.1 & XH7F73 Malignant neuroendocrine neoplasm of stomach & Neuroendocrine carcinoma, moderately differentiated
2B72.1 & XH0U20 Malignant neuroendocrine neoplasm of stomach & Neuroendocrine carcinoma NOS
2B72.1 & XH9SY0 Malignant neuroendocrine neoplasm of stomach & Small cell neuroendocrine carcinoma

Box 3.04 Subtypes of gastric neuroendocrine neoplasms (NENs)

Neuroendocrine tumour (NET) (8240/3)
Histamine-producing enterochromaffin-like–cell (ECL-cell) NET
Type 1 ECL-cell NET (8242/3)
Type 2 ECL-cell NET (8242/3)
Type 3 NET (8240/3)
G1 NET (8240/3)
G2 NET (8249/3)
G3 NET (8249/3)
Somatostatin-producing D-cell NET (8156/3)
Gastrin-producing G-cell NET (8153/3)
Serotonin-producing enterochromaffin-cell (EC-cell) NET (8156/3)
Neuroendocrine carcinoma (NEC) (8246/3)
Small cell neuroendocrine carcinoma (SCNEC) (8041/3)
Large cell neuroendocrine carcinoma (LCNEC) (8013/3)
Mixed neuroendocrine–non-neuroendocrine neoplasm (MiNEN) (8154/3)
Mixed adenocarcinoma-NEC, or mixed adenoneuroendocrine carcinoma (MANEC) (8244/3)
Mixed adenocarcinoma-NET (8244/3)

2B72.1 & XH0NL5 Malignant neuroendocrine neoplasm of stomach & Large cell neuroendocrine carcinoma
2B72.1 & XH6H10 Malignant neuroendocrine neoplasm of stomach & Mixed adenoneuroendocrine carcinoma
2B72.1 & XH7NM1 Malignant neuroendocrine neoplasm of stomach & Enterochromaffin cell carcinoid
2F70.1 & XH93H8 Neoplasms of uncertain behaviour of stomach & Gastrinoma NOS
2B72.1 & XH0GY2 Malignant neuroendocrine neoplasm of stomach & Gastrinoma, malignant

Related terminology

Acceptable: carcinoid; well-differentiated endocrine tumour/carcinoma; poorly differentiated endocrine carcinoma; mixed exocrine-endocrine carcinoma; composite carcinoid-adenocarcinoma.

Subtype(s)

See Box 3.04.

Localization

NETs occur in the stomach with a site-specific distribution according to tumour subtype. Enterochromaffin-like–cell (ECL-cell) NETs arise in the corpus/fundus, D-cell and G-cell NETs in the antrum, and enterochromaffin-cell (EC-cell) NETs in both the antrum and corpus/fundus {1760}. NECs and MiNENs can arise in any part of the stomach, but usually occur in the antral or cardiac regions {1760}.

Clinical features

Most gastric NETs do not cause specific symptoms or local tumour effects and are discovered during evaluation for underlying gastric conditions. Rarely, they are associated with secretory syndromes such as Zollinger–Ellison syndrome.
Histamine-producing ECL-cell NET: Type 1 ECL-cell NETs are associated with hypergastrinaemia due to chronic atrophic gastritis (often autoimmune, with antibodies against parietal cells and/or intrinsic factor), achlorhydria, hypergastrinaemia due to other causes, and (less frequently) macrocytic anaemia (pernicious anaemia). Type 2 ECL-cell NETs are associated with hypergastrinaemia due to duodenal or (rarely) pancreatic gastrinoma in multiple endocrine neoplasia type 1 and hypertrophic hypersecretory gastropathy. Type 3 NETs arise in normal oxyntic mucosa, with variable gastritis and nonspecific symptoms due to tumour growth or metastatic dissemination, including melaena, pain, and weight loss. Patients with extensive liver metastases may present with atypical carcinoid syndrome, characterized by cutaneous flushing, facial oedema, lacrimation, headache, and bronchoconstriction {2186}. The rare ECL-cell NETs related to an intrinsic defect in acid secretion from parietal cells are associated with hypergastrinaemia, achlorhydria, and parietal cell hyperplasia {9}. See Table 3.06

Table 3.06 Key clinicopathological features of gastric neuroendocrine tumour (NET) types 1, 2, and 3

Feature	Type 1 ECL-cell NET	Type 2 ECL-cell NET	Type 3 NET
M:F ratio	0.4:1	1:1	2.8:1
Relative frequency	80–90%	5–7%	10–15%
Hypergastrinaemia	Yes	Yes	No
Antral G-cell hyperplasia	Yes	No	No
Acid secretion	Low or absent	High	Normal
Background mucosa	Atrophic gastritis	Parietal cell hypertrophy/hyperplasia	No specific change
ECL-cell proliferations	Yes	Yes	No
Grading	G1 G2 (rare) G3 (exceptional)	G1 G2 (rare)	G1 (rare) G2 G3 (rare)
Staging	I–II: 95% III: 4% IV: 1%	I–II: 70% III: 20% IV: 10%	I–II: 38% III: 32% IV: 30%
Metastasis rate	1–3%	10–30%	50%
5-year survival rate	~100%	60–90%	< 50%

for a summary of key clinicopathological features of gastric histamine-producing ECL-cell NETs.

Serotonin-producing EC-cell NET: This rare tumour subtype is usually non-functioning, but it may be associated with the classic carcinoid syndrome symptoms of diarrhoea, flushing, tricuspid regurgitation, and asthma.

Gastrin-producing G-cell NET: These tumours are usually non-functioning, but a minority of cases may cause Zollinger–Ellison syndrome; the term "gastric gastrinoma" is used only for such functioning cases, and not for gastrin-expressing tumours in the absence of associated clinical manifestations.

NEC and MiNEN: These neoplasms present with nonspecific symptoms including dyspepsia and weight loss due to tumour growth and/or distant metastases. Ulcerated neoplasms may be associated with gastric bleeding, anaemia, and pain; large pyloric lesions may cause obstruction.

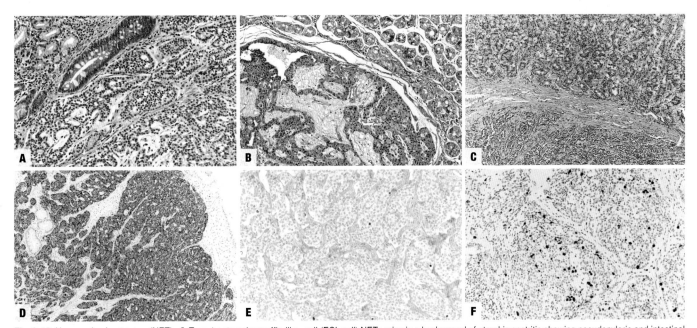

Fig. 3.48 Neuroendocrine tumour (NET). **A** Type 1 enterochromaffin-like–cell (ECL-cell) NETs arise in a background of atrophic gastritis showing pseudopyloric and intestinal metaplasia (upper-left corner); tumour cells form a microlobular architecture without necrosis and show monomorphic nuclei lacking nucleoli. **B** In type 2 ECL-cell NETs, peritumoural mucosa is not atrophic; this case is characterized by a proliferation of well-differentiated monomorphic cells with eosinophilic cytoplasm forming trabeculae and ribbons associated with extracellular mucoid-like material. **C** Type 3 NETs arise in normal oxyntic mucosa. **D** Immunohistochemical staining for VMAT2 shows strong and diffuse positivity in tumour cells of a type 1 ECL-cell NET. **E** Ki-67 immunohistochemical staining of a G1 type 3 NET. **F** Ki-67 immunohistochemical staining of a G2 type 3 NET.

Epidemiology

The incidence of gastric NENs has increased about 15-fold in recent years, probably as a result of the widespread use of endoscopy. In 2012, the estimated age-adjusted incidence rate in the USA was about 0.4 cases/100 000 person-years {716}, with a female predominance and a mean patient age at diagnosis of 64 years {3684,1807,1195}. Similar epidemiological characteristics have been reported for European cases {1760}. Although a female predominance is reported for gastric NETs overall, the specific age and sex distributions vary across the tumour subtypes. Of the ECL-cell NETs, type 1 is the most common; it accounts for about 80–90% of all ECL-cell NETs and is more frequent in females. Type 2 accounts for about 5–7% of ECL-cell NETs and shows no sex predilection. Type 3 NETs account for about 10–15% of all gastric NENs and are more frequent in males. Antral NETs are rare, accounting for about 5% of gastric NENs in one series {1753}. Gastric NECs account for about 21% of all gastric NENs, are more frequent in males, and account for 20.5% of all digestive NECs {1753,2164}. Gastric mixed cancers composed of adenocarcinoma and NEC (MANECs), although rare overall, account for about 20% of all digestive MANECs {2163}.

Etiology

Type 1 ECL-cell NETs are typically associated with autoimmune chronic atrophic gastritis (autoantibodies against parietal cells and intrinsic factor), but *Helicobacter pylori* infection has also been implicated in some cases. Type 2 ECL-cell NETs occur in the setting of multiple endocrine neoplasia type 1 subsequent to hypergastrinaemia occurring as a result of gastrinoma. There are no known etiological factors for type 3 NET {2720}. A few cases of ECL-cell NETs seem to be related to an intrinsic defect in acid secretion from parietal cells, probably due to abnormal proton pump activity {9,955}. No specific etiological factors have been identified for NECs or MiNENs, with the exception of the presence of Merkel cell polyomavirus in a rare case of primary gastric Merkel cell carcinoma {490}.

Pathogenesis

Histamine-producing ECL-cell NET: The pathogenesis of type 1 and type 2 ECL-cell NETs directly relates to unregulated gastrin stimulus {3179}. Potential cooperating factors include TGF-α and bFGF {369}. *MEN1* gene abnormality is required for the development of type 2 ECL-cell NET. Loss of heterozygosity for *MEN1* gene locus markers has also been identified, in 17–73% of type 1 ECL-cell NETs and 25–50% of type 3 NETs {369}. The pathogenesis of type 3 NET is unknown. Little information is available regarding genetic alterations in gastric NET. Loss of heterozygosity for markers at the chromosomal locus of the *MEN1* gene is the rule in type 2 ECL-cell NETs. *MEN1* gene loss of heterozygosity and/or mutations have also been demonstrated in about 30–40% of sporadic type 3 NETs. NETs with *CDKN1B* mutation and reduced p27 (p27Kip1) protein levels have been described in the setting of multiple endocrine neoplasia type 4 {2029,1834}. A family carrying an inactivating mutation of the *ATP4A* gene (which encodes the α-subunit of the gastric proton pump) has been reported to have developed ECL-cell NETs {955}.

NEC and MANEC: The pathogenesis of both NECs and high-grade MiNENs (MANECs) is unknown, but involves complex genetic factors. Few data are available. Gastric NECs show multiple chromosomal abnormalities involving cell-cycle regulatory genes, such as *TP53*, *RB1*, *FHIT*, *DCC*, and *SMAD4*. A direct comparison study showed that gastric NECs have a higher mutation rate and a different mutation profile than conventional gastric adenocarcinomas, with only 40 of 557 analysed genes

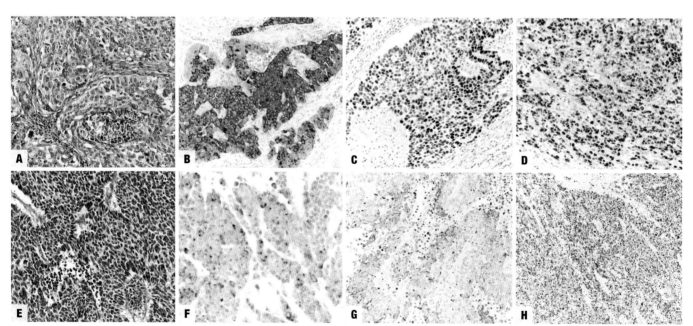

Fig. 3.49 Neuroendocrine carcinoma (NEC). **A** Large cell NEC (LCNEC) composed of large cells with dispersed chromatin and prominent nucleoli forming sheets with necrosis. **B** LCNEC. Immunohistochemical staining for chromogranin shows diffuse and strong cytoplasmic immunoreactivity. **C** LCNEC. Tumour cells are positive for p53. **D** LCNEC with a high Ki-67 proliferation index. **E** Small cell NEC (SCNEC) forming solid sheets of small cells with hyperchromic nuclei lacking nucleoli. **F** SCNEC. Immunohistochemical staining for chromogranin with a typical perinuclear dot-like pattern of immunoreactivity. **G** SCNEC. The epithelial nature of a NEC is demonstrated by the immunoreactivity for cytokeratin, which can be focal. **H** SCNEC with a high Ki-67 proliferation index.

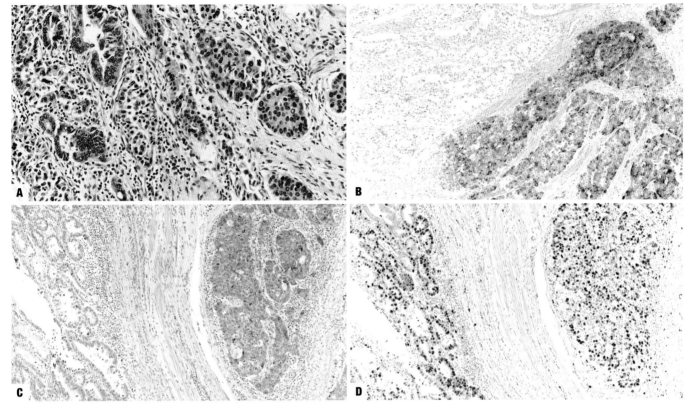

Fig. 3.50 Gastric mixed adenoneuroendocrine carcinoma (MANEC). **A** MANEC of the cardial region, composed of adenocarcinoma (left part of the image) and large cell neuroendocrine carcinoma (LCNEC; right part of the image). **B** Immunohistochemical staining for chromogranin shows diffuse and strong cytoplasm immunoreactivity in the neuroendocrine component, whereas it is negative in the adenocarcinoma. **C** The neuroendocrine component is also positive for synaptophysin. **D** High Ki-67 proliferation index of the neuroendocrine component is the most important prognostic marker of MANEC {2163}.

(7.2%) showing mutations in both tumour types {2022}. The vast majority (98.2%) of the 557 analysed genes were mutated in NECs only, including *SMAD4*, *PIK3CA*, *KRAS*, and *RB1* {2022}. *TP53* and *RB1* mutations can help distinguish NECs from G3 NETs, in which these genes are more frequently wildtype. The sparse data on gastric MANECs indicate that these neoplasms have features similar to those of NECs. The similarities in the chromosomal alteration patterns and mutation profiles of the two components of MANEC suggest a monoclonal origin {985,1588,2877,3486}.

Macroscopic appearance

Type 1 ECL-cell NETs are multiple in about 60% of cases and present as small (< 1 cm) polyps or nodules of the corpus/fundus mucosa {2715}. Type 2 ECL-cell NETs arise in the oxyntic mucosa and present as multiple lesions typically < 2 cm in size; the stomach mucosa may be thickened as a result of severe hypertrophic hypersecretory gastropathy. Type 3 NETs are usually single and large (~2 cm) {2715}. Gastrin-producing G-cell NETs are typically small, mucosal/submucosal proliferations located in the antral region, most frequently in proximity to the pylorus. Gastric NECs may form large fungating masses that deeply infiltrate the gastric wall. MANECs are similar in appearance to conventional gastric adenocarcinomas, often occurring as polypoid or ulcerating stenotic large masses, with a mean size of about 5 cm {1754}.

Histopathology

Histamine-producing ECL-cell NET

ECL-cell NETs usually show small microlobular and/or trabecular architecture without necrosis. They are composed of well-differentiated cells with abundant eosinophilic cytoplasm and monomorphic round nuclei that lack prominent nucleoli. Mitotic figures are scarce. In rare instances, NETs show a more solid structure, with large, disordered trabeculae and occasional spotty necrosis; these tumours are composed of larger cells with abundant cytoplasm and moderate to severe nuclear atypia, characterized by polymorphic, crowded nuclei and less-regularly distributed chromatin. Mitoses are numerous and sometimes atypical.

Type 1 ECL-cell NETs > 0.5 cm in size usually infiltrate beyond the muscularis mucosae; rare cases > 1 cm in size with muscularis propria invasion may produce metastases. Most cases are G1 or G2, with similar degrees of gastric wall invasion and metastatic spread, as well as similar outcome. Very rare G3 type 1 ECL-cell NETs have been described, accounting for 1.6% of all type 1 ECL-cell NETs in one series {3441}. The background mucosa is atrophic, with intestinal and pseudopyloric metaplasia and complex ECL-cell hyperplastic and dysplastic changes {3440,2721}. In the corresponding antral mucosa, gastrin-producing G-cell hyperplasia is usually observed, as the morphological counterpart of hypergastrinaemia {3440}. The vast majority of type 1 ECL-cell NETs are of low stage.

Type 2 ECL-cell NETs are mainly confined to the mucosa/submucosa when they are G1, but lymph node and distant

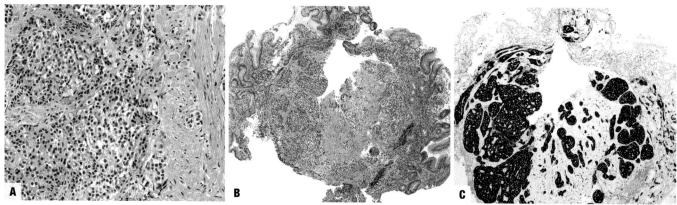

Fig. 3.51 Gastric neuroendocrine tumour (NET). A case of type 1 NET of stomach (**A**), associated with autoimmune gastritis; features of both can be well seen at low power (**B**). Corresponding synaptophysin staining (**C**) also reveals enterochromaffin-like cell (ECL cell) hyperplasia in the autoimmune gastritis part.

metastases are present in 30% and 10% of patients, respectively {2720,2714}. The background mucosa is hyperplastic and displays various types of hyperplastic and dysplastic ECL-cell proliferations {1760}.

Type 3 NETs range from G1 to G3, and they often deeply invade the gastric wall and develop lymph node and distant metastases. Type 3 NETs are often of high stage.

ECL-cell NETs related to an intrinsic defect in acid secretion from parietal cells are multiple lesions with features similar to those of type 1 and type 2 ECL-cell NETs. They also arise in association with hypergastrinaemia; the uninvolved mucosa shows distinctive changes of oxyntic gland hypertrophy and hyperplasia and associated hyperplastic/dysplastic ECL-cell proliferations. Oxyntic glands are frequently dilated, filled with inspissated material, and lined with parietal cells with swollen cytoplasm (either deeply eosinophilic or vacuolated with apical projection into the glandular lumen) {9,2455}. Similar to in type 1 ECL-cell NETs, the corresponding antral mucosa shows gastrin-producing G-cell hyperplasia. Regional lymph node metastases have been reported {9}.

Serotonin-producing EC-cell NET
Gastric EC-cell NETs have morphological features similar to those of ileal EC-cell NETs, including rounded nests of cells with peripheral palisading. The tumour cells are uniform, with intense eosinophilic cytoplasm.

Gastrin-producing G-cell NET and gastrinoma
Gastrin-producing G-cell NETs typically show a thin trabecular pattern and gyriform pattern, although some cases grow in more-solid nests. The tumour cells are uniform, with scant cytoplasm {1753}.

Somatostatin-producing D-cell NET
Somatostatin-producing D-cell NETs are composed of well-differentiated monomorphic cells that are positive for somatostatin.

NEC
Gastric NECs are composed of large, poorly formed trabeculae or sheets of poorly differentiated cells. They are subtyped as small cell NEC (SCNEC) and large cell NEC (LCNEC), which resemble their more common lung counterparts. LCNECs are composed of large cells with vesicular nuclei showing prominent

nucleoli and abundant eosinophilic cytoplasm. SCNECs are composed of neoplastic cells with scant cytoplasm and hyperchromatic nuclei without nucleoli. NECs typically have a mitotic count of > 20 mitoses/mm2, and the Ki-67 proliferation index is frequently > 60–70%, especially in SCNECs.

MiNEN
MANECs are MiNENs composed of adenocarcinoma associated with NEC. The presence of a solid or organoid structure with extensive necrosis, together with a very high mitotic count, may suggest the diagnosis of MANEC, which is confirmed by positive expression of neuroendocrine markers. The neuroendocrine component of MANEC often has a Ki-67 proliferation index > 55% {2163}. Mixed adenocarcinoma-NETs (both primary tumours and metastases) are composed of areas of tubular, papillary, or mucinous adenocarcinoma and areas of G1 or G2 NET. Cases of gastric mixed adenocarcinoma-NETs associated with autoimmune chronic atrophic gastritis have been described {1758,1754}.

Mixed adenoma-NET
Gastric mixed adenoma-NETs are rare tumours composed of tubular or tubulovillous adenoma associated with G1 or G2 NET. The neuroendocrine component is generally located in the deep central portion of the polyp, whereas the adenomatous component occupies most of the periphery {1758,1759}. These unusual tumours are not considered MiNENs at present.

Immunohistochemistry
Gastric NETs are positive for the general neuroendocrine markers synaptophysin and chromogranin A. In addition, all ECL-cell NETs are positive for VMAT2, HDC, and SSTR2A. They can also show scattered cells positive for serotonin, ghrelin, somatostatin, and α-hCG {2720,2508}. An ECL-cell phenotype cannot be demonstrated in all type 3 NETs; in addition to cases composed of ECL cells, this category also includes cases composed of uncharacterized cells lacking a specific phenotype. Some features, including the expression of SSTR2A and HDC, may be lost in rare G3 NETs. Gastric EC-cell NETs are positive for serotonin, SSTR2A, and CDX2. Gastrin-producing G-cell NETs are positive for gastrin and SSTR2A. Somatostatin-producing D-cell NETs are positive for somatostatin, chromogranin A, synaptophysin, and SSTR2A. Gastric NECs are positive for

synaptophysin, whereas chromogranin A may be absent or only focally expressed (with a typical perinuclear dot-like pattern). NEC, in particular SCNEC, may also be positive for TTF1 and ASH1L (ASH1).

Grading
Gastric NENs are graded using the same system used for other gastroenteropancreatic NENs.

Cytology
FNA is rarely performed on small gastric NETs because of their small size (and in many cases multiplicity); however, it can be useful for the diagnosis of submucosal nodules, as demonstrated in one study of patients with Zollinger–Ellison syndrome, in which NETs were successfully diagnosed in 11 of 12 cases {301}. Like at other anatomical sites, there is a uniform cell population with round nuclei and stippled chromatin. The cytology of gastric NECs is the same as that of other high-grade NECs.

Diagnostic molecular pathology
TP53 and *RB1* mutations can help distinguish NECs from G3 NETs, in which these genes are more frequently wildtype.

Essential and desirable diagnostic criteria
NET
Essential: a uniform population of cells with round nuclei and finely stippled chromatin; architectural patterns such as trabeculae, acini, nests, and ribbons; expression of synaptophysin and chromogranin A.

NEC
Essential: small cell carcinoma or large cell carcinoma pattern; sheets or trabeculae of poorly differentiated cells; high mitotic count and Ki-67 proliferation index.

Staging (TNM)
Gastric NETs are staged using the NET-specific Union for International Cancer Control (UICC) TNM staging system presented in Chapter 1 (p. 20). NEC and MiNEN are staged following the system used for adenocarcinomas.

Prognosis and prediction
The prognosis of gastric NENs largely depends on the tumour subtype {2720,2714,1753,3441}, grade, and stage; higher grade and stage are associated with increased morbidity. The prognosis of type 1 ECL-cell NETs is excellent, and that of type 3 NETs is substantially worse. Type 2 ECL-cell NETs have intermediate prognostic features, largely depending on the concurrent multiple endocrine neoplasia type 1–associated neoplasms. In type 1 ECL-cell NETs, staging parameters (e.g. size and wall invasion) seem to be more prognostically significant than grade {750,3441}. In type 3 NETs, both grade and stage are relevant {1753,750,3441}. Antral NETs are usually indolent, with an excellent prognosis {2720,2714,1753,1760}. Gastric NEC and MANEC have a poor prognosis, with survival time usually measured in months. In MANEC, the NEC component and its Ki-67 proliferation index drives the outcome, like in NEC {2720,2714,1753,2163,3441}.

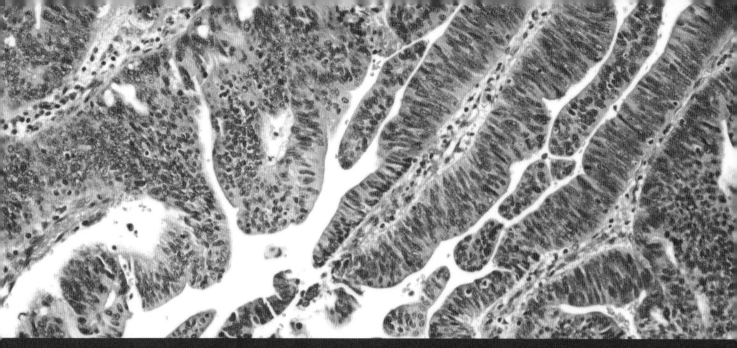

4

Tumours of the small intestine and ampulla

Edited by: Klimstra DS, Nagtegaal ID, Rugge M, Salto-Tellez M

Benign epithelial tumours and precursors
    Non-ampullary adenoma
    Ampullary adenoma
Malignant epithelial tumours
    Non-ampullary adenocarcinoma
    Ampullary adenocarcinoma
    Neuroendocrine neoplasms

WHO classification of tumours of the small intestine and ampulla

Benign epithelial tumours and precursors

8210/0*	Adenomatous polyp, low-grade dysplasia
8210/2*	Adenomatous polyp, high-grade dysplasia
8144/0*	Intestinal-type adenoma, low grade
8144/2*	Intestinal-type adenoma, high grade
8213/0*	Serrated dysplasia, low grade
8213/2*	Serrated dysplasia, high grade
8163/0	Non-invasive pancreatobiliary papillary neoplasm with low-grade dysplasia
8163/2	Non-invasive pancreatobiliary papillary neoplasm with high-grade dysplasia
	Intra-ampullary papillary-tubular neoplasm

Malignant epithelial tumours

8140/3	Adenocarcinoma NOS
8480/3	Mucinous adenocarcinoma
8490/3	Signet-ring cell carcinoma
8510/3	Medullary carcinoma NOS
8144/3	Adenocarcinoma, intestinal type
8163/3	Pancreatobiliary-type carcinoma
8211/3	Tubular adenocarcinoma
8240/3	Neuroendocrine tumour NOS
8240/3	Neuroendocrine tumour, grade 1
8249/3	Neuroendocrine tumour, grade 2
8249/3	Neuroendocrine tumour, grade 3
8153/3	Gastrinoma NOS
8156/3	Somatostatinoma NOS
8241/3	Enterochromaffin-cell carcinoid
8693/3	Extra-adrenal paraganglioma NOS
8246/3	Neuroendocrine carcinoma NOS
8013/3	Large cell neuroendocrine carcinoma
8041/3	Small cell neuroendocrine carcinoma
8154/3	Mixed neuroendocrine–non-neuroendocrine neoplasm (MiNEN)

These morphology codes are from the International Classification of Diseases for Oncology, third edition, second revision (ICD-O-3.2) {1378A}. Behaviour is coded /0 for benign tumours; /1 for unspecified, borderline, or uncertain behaviour; /2 for carcinoma in situ and grade III intraepithelial neoplasia; /3 for malignant tumours, primary site; and /6 for malignant tumours, metastatic site. Behaviour code /6 is not generally used by cancer registries.

This classification is modified from the previous WHO classification, taking into account changes in our understanding of these lesions.

* Codes marked with an asterisk were approved by the IARC/WHO Committee for ICD-O at its meeting in April 2019.

TNM staging of carcinomas of the small intestine

Small Intestine
(ICD-O-3 C17)

Rules for Classification
The classification applies only to carcinomas. There should be histological confirmation of the disease.

The following are the procedures for assessing T, N, and M categories.

T categories	Physical examination, imaging, endoscopy, and/or surgical exploration
N categories	Physical examination, imaging, and/or surgical exploration
M categories	Physical examination, imaging, and/or surgical exploration

Anatomical Subsites
1. Duodenum (C17.0)
2. Jejunum (C17.1)
3. Ileum (C17.2) (excludes ileocecal valve C18.0)

Note
This classification does not apply to carcinomas of the ampulla of Vater (see p. 114).

Regional Lymph Nodes
The regional lymph nodes for the duodenum are the pancreaticoduodenal, pyloric, hepatic (pericholedochal, cystic, hilar), and superior mesenteric nodes.

The regional lymph nodes for the ileum and jejunum are the mesenteric nodes, including the superior mesenteric nodes, and, for the terminal ileum only, the ileocolic nodes including the posterior caecal nodes.

TNM Clinical Classification
T – Primary Tumour

TX	Primary tumour cannot be assessed
T0	No evidence of primary tumour
Tis	Carcinoma in situ
T1	Tumour invades lamina propria, muscularis mucosae or submucosa
T1a	Tumour invades lamina propria or muscularis mucosae
T1b	Tumour invades submucosa
T2	Tumour invades muscularis propria
T3	Tumour invades subserosa or non-peritonealized perimuscular tissue (mesentery or retroperitoneum*) without perforation of the serosa
T4	Tumour perforates visceral peritoneum or directly invades other organs or structures (includes other loops of small intestine, mesentery, or retroperitoneum and abdominal wall by way of serosa; for duodenum only, invasion of pancreas)

Note
* The non-peritonealized perimuscular tissue is, for jejunum and ileum, part of the mesentery and, for duodenum in areas where serosa is lacking, part of the retroperitoneum.

N – Regional Lymph Nodes

NX	Regional lymph nodes cannot be assessed
N0	No regional lymph node metastasis
N1	Metastasis in 1 to 2 regional lymph nodes
N2	Metastasis in 3 or more regional lymph nodes

M – Distant Metastasis

M0	No distant metastasis
M1	Distant metastasis

pTNM Pathological Classification
The pT and pN categories correspond to the T and N categories.

pN0 Histological examination of a regional lymphadenectomy specimen will ordinarily include 6 or more lymph nodes. If the lymph nodes are negative, but the number ordinarily examined is not met, classify as pN0.

pM – Distant Metastasis*
pM1 Distant metastasis microscopically confirmed

Note
* pM0 and pMX are not valid categories.

Stage

Stage 0	Tis	N0	M0
Stage I	T1,T2	N0	M0
Stage IIA	T3	N0	M0
Stage IIB	T4	N0	M0
Stage IIIA	Any T	N1	M0
Stage IIIB	Any T	N2	M0
Stage IV	Any T	Any N	M1

Note: Neuroendocrine tumours (NETs) of the small intestine are staged using the NET-specific TNM staging system, which is presented in Chapter 1 (p. 20).

The information presented here has been excerpted from the 2017 *TNM classification of malignant tumours*, eighth edition (408,3385A). © 2017 UICC.
A help desk for specific questions about the TNM classification is available at https://www.uicc.org/tnm-help-desk.

Chapter 4

TNM staging of carcinomas of the ampulla of Vater

Ampulla of Vater

(ICD-O-3 C24.1)

Rules for Classification

The classification applies only to carcinomas. There should be histological confirmation of the disease.

The following are the procedures for assessing T, N, and M categories.

T categories	Physical examination, imaging, and/or surgical exploration
N categories	Physical examination, imaging, and/or surgical exploration
M categories	Physical examination, imaging, and/or surgical exploration

Regional Lymph Nodes

The regional lymph nodes are the same as for the head of the pancreas and are the lymph nodes along the common bile duct, common hepatic artery, portal vein, pyloric, infrapyloric, subpyloric, proximal mesenteric, coeliac, posterior and anterior pancreaticoduodenal vessels, and along the superior mesenteric vein and right lateral wall of the superior mesenteric artery.

Note

The splenic lymph nodes and those of the tail of the pancreas are *not* regional; metastases to these lymph nodes are coded M1.

TNM Clinical Classification

T – Primary Tumour

TX	Primary tumour cannot be assessed
T0	No evidence of primary tumour
Tis	Carcinoma in situ
T1a	Tumour limited to ampulla of Vater or sphincter of Oddi
T1b	Tumour invades beyond the sphincter of Oddi (perisphincteric invasion) and/or into the duodenal submucosa
T2	Tumour invades the muscularis propria of the duodenum
T3	Tumour invades pancreas or peripancreatic tissue
T3a	Tumour invades 0.5 cm or less into the pancreas
T3b	Tumour invades more than 0.5 cm into the pancreas or extends into peripancreatic tissue or duodenal serosa but without involvement of the celiac axis or the superior mesenteric artery
T4	Tumour with vascular involvement of the superior mesenteric artery or celiac axis, or common hepatic artery

N – Regional Lymph Nodes

NX	Regional lymph nodes cannot be assessed
N0	No regional lymph node metastasis
N1	Metastasis in 1 to 3 regional lymph nodes
N2	Metastasis in 4 or more regional lymph nodes

M – Distant Metastasis

M0	No distant metastasis
M1	Distant metastasis

pTNM Pathological Classification

The pT and pN categories correspond to the T and N categories.

pN0   Histological examination of a regional lymphadenectomy specimen will ordinarily include 12 or more lymph nodes. If the lymph nodes are negative, but the number ordinarily examined is not met, classify as pN0.

pM – Distant Metastasis*

pM1   Distant metastasis microscopically confirmed

Note

* pM0 and pMX are not valid categories.

Stage – Ampulla of Vater

Stage	T	N	M
Stage 0	Tis	N0	M0
Stage IA	T1a	N0	M0
Stage IB	T1b,T2	N0	M0
Stage IIA	T3a	N0	M0
Stage IIB	T3b	N0	M0
Stage IIIA	T1a,T1b,T2,T3	N1	M0
Stage IIIB	Any T	N2	M0
	T4	Any N	M0
Stage IV	Any T	Any N	M1

Note: Ampullary neuroendocrine tumours (NETs) are staged using the NET-specific TNM staging system, which is presented in Chapter 1 (p. 20).

Tumours of the small intestine and ampulla: Introduction

Salto-Tellez M
Rugge M

The mucosal surface of the small bowel covers > 90% of the digestive canal, but the overall prevalence of small bowel cancers among those of the tubular GI tract is < 5%. This prompts the assumption of a protective environment associated with enzymes specific to the small bowel {747}, or it may be related to the shorter time of transit of any (potential) dietary carcinogens.

The ICD-O topographical coding for the anatomical sites covered in this chapter is presented in Box 4.01. Overall, small bowel neoplasms are uncommon, with an incidence of 1.1–2.5 cases per 100 000 person-years {3629,171}. Most likely as a result of improvements in diagnostic procedures, the incidence of small bowel tumours is rising in North American and European countries; for example, the incidence in the United Kingdom more than doubled over the 25-year period of 1990–2015: from 1 to 2.5 cases per 100 000 person-years {2751}. The increasing incidence of neoplastic cases is mainly due to an increase in duodenal tumours {170}. Similarly, the relative frequencies of histological subtypes differ substantially across studies. An increased relative risk of small bowel cancer has been associated with a high level of alcohol consumption. Potential associations with dietary risk factors are currently equivocal. Industrial exposures have also been linked to small bowel cancer {1494,1493}.

The prevalence of cancer decreases progressively along the small bowel segments, from the duodenum (55–75%), to the jejunum (15–25%), to the ileum (10–15%) {2473}. Most duodenal cancers arise from the ampullary region. The prognosis of cancers arising deep within the ampulla (which have been termed "ampullary-ductal" carcinomas according to site/origin and are usually pancreatobiliary type by histology) differs from that of cancers originating from the duodenal surface of the ampulla (which have been termed "[peri]ampullary duodenal"

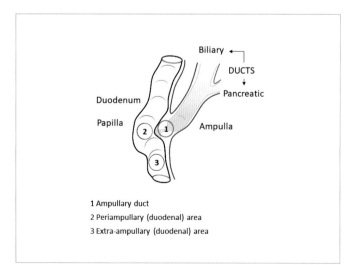

1 Ampullary duct
2 Periampullary (duodenal) area
3 Extra-ampullary (duodenal) area

Fig. 4.01 Basic structure of the ampulla.

carcinomas according to site/origin and are often intestinal type by histology), with 5-year survival rates of 29% and 52%, respectively {2449,43}. Upper small intestine carcinomas sometimes exhibit pancreatobiliary or gastric differentiation, which suggests their origin from submucosal glandular units.

Non-syndromic cancers are often related to two main pathological conditions: Crohn disease and coeliac disease. Longstanding Crohn disease is associated with adenocarcinoma, mainly arising in the distal ileum {198,2125}. Ileal Crohn cancers show both traditional histology and a lymphoepithelioma-like phenotype characterized by a high-density of tumour-infiltrating T lymphocytes {3438}. Coeliac patients (particularly of advanced age and/or with longstanding gluten enteropathy) are at increased risk of both non-Hodgkin lymphomas (enteropathy-associated T-cell lymphoma) and adenocarcinoma {400,309,424}.

Since the 2010 edition {379}, there have been some important changes in the taxonomy of neoplasia of the small bowel and ampulla. Following the nomenclature in lesions from pancreatic and biliary ducts, the term "intra-ampullary papillary-tubular neoplasm" is now used for preinvasive neoplasms (adenomas and non-invasive papillary neoplasms) occurring almost exclusively within the ampulla. Fundamentally, these are intra-ampullary versions of intraductal papillary neoplasms or intraductal tubulopapillary neoplasms of the pancreas and bile ducts. These lesions can have a variety of phenotypes, from gastric to intestinal to pancreatobiliary, but they are often mixed and often show a mixture of papillary and tubular growth patterns. For intestinal adenomas that arise (and grow) predominantly on the duodenal surface of the ampulla ("periampullary duodenum"), the term "adenoma" (of intestinal phenotypes) is retained, in parallel with the terminology used in the intestinal tract (see *Ampullary adenoma*, p. 121). In the section on small intestine adenoma (see *Non-ampullary adenoma*, p. 118), the term "pyloric gland adenoma" is also recognized as representing a separate entity, in order to harmonize the classification of lesions across many organs. In the section on ampullary adenocarcinoma (p. 127), we adopt the classification of ampullary carcinomas into four anatomically based subtypes, which also have some degree of histological correlation: intra-ampullary papillary-tubular neoplasm–associated carcinoma (carcinomas arising from intraluminal-growing preinvasive neoplasms), ampullary-ductal carcinoma (arising and growing along the walls of intra-ampullary ducts), (peri)ampullary-duodenal carcinoma (growing on the duodenal surface of the ampulla), and ampullary carcinoma NOS. This subdivision is driven by the anatomical complexity at that site and also affects the difficulty in tumour staging.

New information at the molecular level is incorporated throughout the chapter (when relevant), although the clinical importance of this information still requires further work for the most part.

Non-ampullary adenoma

Sekine S
Shia J

Definition
Non-ampullary adenoma is a polyp of the small intestine consisting of dysplastic glandular epithelium, which may show intestinal-type or pyloric gland differentiation.

ICD-O coding
8210/0 Adenomatous polyp, low-grade dysplasia
8210/2 Adenomatous polyp, high-grade dysplasia

ICD-11 coding
2E92.3 & XH3DV3 Benign neoplasm of other or unspecified parts of small intestine & Adenoma NOS
2E92.3 & XH8MU5 Benign neoplasm of other or unspecified parts of small intestine & Adenomatous polyp NOS

Related terminology
Not recommended: Brunner gland adenoma.

Subtype(s)
Intestinal-type adenoma, low grade (8144/0); intestinal-type adenoma, high grade (8144/2); serrated dysplasia, low grade (8213/0); serrated dysplasia, high grade (8213/2)

Localization
Adenomas occur throughout the small intestine, but predominantly in the duodenum and ampulla (ampullary adenomas are described separately) {2941}. Each histological subtype exhibits distinct distributions: intestinal-type adenomas develop anywhere in the small intestine, with the ampulla and periampullary duodenum being the most frequent sites; pyloric gland adenomas (PGAs) are mostly located in the proximal duodenum {3474,3477}.

Clinical features
Small intestine adenomas are usually small and solitary, and most are asymptomatic. Large adenomas can cause obstructive symptoms due to intussusception. Duodenal adenomas are endoscopically accessible, whereas adenomas in the jejunum and ileum are seldom detected before they cause obstructive symptoms or progress to invasive carcinoma {1023}. Because of the late presentation of jejunal and ileal adenomas (often after they have evolved into invasive carcinoma) and their associated acute clinical obstructive symptoms, surgery is the treatment of choice. The removal of duodenal polyps (ampullary or extra-ampullary) allows both surgical and endoscopic approaches.

Epidemiology
In general, adenomas of the small bowel are rarer than their colorectal counterparts. Several series have reported duodenal polyps to occur in as many as 4.6% of patients presenting for endoscopy, with the prevalence of sporadic non-ampullary adenomas being 0.3–0.5% {1986,1023,780}. The mean age of patients with

Table 4.01 The Spigelman classification of duodenal polyposis in familial adenomatous polyposis {3114}

Polyp feature	Allocated points		
	1	2	3
Number	1–4	5–20	> 20
Size (mm)	1–4	5–10	> 10
Histology	Tubular	Tubulovillous	Villous
Degree of dysplasia	Low (mild)	Low (moderate)	High (severe)

Correlation of points with stages:

Stage 0	0 points
Stage I	1–4 points
Stage II	5–6 points
Stage III	7–8 points
Stage IV	9–12 points

Note: Stages III and IV represent severe polyposis. Originally designed as a three-tiered dysplastic system (mild to severe), this table has been updated to include the preferred current two-tiered system {2002,2867}.

duodenal adenomas is 65 years, and there is a slight male predominance {2375}. The exact incidence of PGAs is unknown, but they are less frequent than intestinal-type adenomas.

Etiology
About 60% of non-ampullary adenomas occur in patients with familial adenomatous polyposis (FAP) {2375}, predominantly intestinal-type adenomas of the duodenum {454}; indeed, FAP often presents as duodenal polyposis, and the severity of polyposis has been linked to the risk of adenocarcinoma (see Table 4.01 {3114}. *MUTYH*-associated polyposis is also associated with an increased risk of duodenal adenomas {1341}. The other 40% of intestinal-type non-ampullary adenomas are sporadic. PGAs are associated with ectopic gastric mucosa, gastric foveolar hyperplasia, or Brunner gland metaplasia {2002}.

Pathogenesis
Non-ampullary intestinal-type adenoma is a precancerous lesion, and the model of the adenoma–carcinoma sequence {415} is predicted to involve the small intestine as well. At least a proportion of the adenomas show WNT/β-catenin activation {2375}. The precise molecular pathogenesis of PGAs is unknown, but there is a clear correlation of PGAs with gastric-type dysplasia, gastric foveolar metaplasia, and Brunner gland hyperplasia associated with gastric-type adenocarcinomas {3392,2002}. In addition, a common presence of *GNAS* and *KRAS* mutations in gastric foveolar metaplasia, gastric heterotopia, and adenocarcinoma of the duodenum {2078} has been established. Together, these facts strongly suggest a molecular

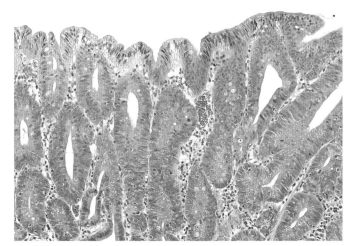

Fig. 4.02 Duodenal intestinal-type adenoma. This low-grade adenoma shows basal elongated nuclei; Paneth and goblet cells are intermingled.

pathogenetic pathway of duodenal cancer involving PGAs and the associated metaplastic and heterotopic changes.

Macroscopic appearance

The macroscopy of non-ampullary adenomas in the small bowel is similar to that of the counterpart adenomas in the colon and rectum. They are smooth, sometimes tan, sessile or pedunculated growths in the mucosa (for further characterization, see *Conventional colorectal adenoma*, p. 170). The number and size of the adenomas in the small bowel, particularly in the duodenal segment, may carry a certain prognostic value (see *Prognosis and prediction*, below). Duodenal adenomas in the setting of FAP are usually multiple, sessile, and predominantly located in the mucosal folds {697}.

Histopathology

Intestinal-type adenomas are the most common subtype in the small intestine, where most cases show a tubular or tubulovillous growth pattern and intestinal epithelial differentiation. Most intestinal-type adenomas have low-grade dysplasia and consist of tall columnar cells with elongated nuclei and inconspicuous nucleoli. Paneth, goblet, or endocrine cells may be prominent

in low-grade lesions {3369}. Adenomas with high-grade dysplasia are characterized by increased architectural complexity, nuclear stratification, and nuclear atypia. FAP-associated adenomas have the same histological features as sporadic lesions. Immunohistochemically, intestinal-type adenomas express markers of the intestinal epithelium, including CDX2 and MUC2, and they usually lack expression of EMA (MUC1) {3502}. Coexpression of CK7 and CK20 is common {3502}.

PGAs consist of closely packed pyloric-type glands lined by cuboidal to low columnar cells. Foamy, ground-glass cytoplasm is characteristic of this type of adenoma. The tumour cells have round and basally located nuclei with inconspicuous nucleoli. These lesions can be associated with gastric-type foveolar metaplasia or Brunner gland hyperplasia, and thus the terms "pyloric-type adenoma" and "Brunner gland adenoma" have been used in the literature. However, recent studies have identified PGAs in many organs {3474}, presumably associated with gastric heterotopia, and therefore the general term "PGA" is preferred. Their mutation profile, in both stomach and duodenum {2079}, exhibits a notable frequency of *GNAS* mutations, making them molecularly linked and distinct from other precursor lesions. Immunohistochemically, PGAs show MUC6 expression (usually extensive) and a variable extent of MUC5AC expression {590}.

Serrated lesions and polyps, similar to their colonic counterparts (see *Colorectal serrated lesions and polyps*, p. 163), are identifiable in the small intestine, frequently associated with dysplasia or adenocarcinoma {2002}.

Cytology

The cytopathological diagnostic features of duodenal intestinal-type adenomas have been described {662}, showing small sheets and clusters of elongated columnar cells with granular chromatin and one or more nucleoli, and/or features of high-grade dysplasia (HGD) with nuclear overlapping, loss of polarity, and coarse clumped chromatin. However, cytology cannot always differentiate between HGD and adenocarcinoma, providing no substantial improvement over biopsy diagnosis {3722}.

Diagnostic molecular pathology

There are no routinely used biomarkers of diagnostic or predictive value in non-ampullary adenomas.

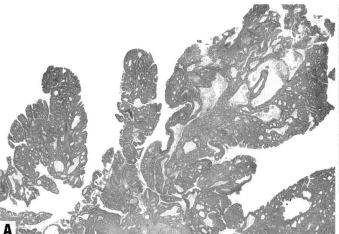
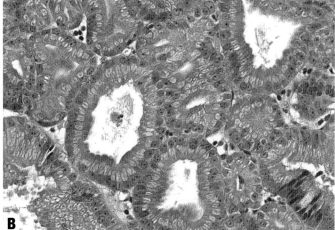

Fig. 4.03 Duodenal pyloric gland adenoma. **A** An example with a lobulated configuration and some dilated glands. **B** High-power magnification reveals the characteristic ground-glass cytoplasm and basal round nuclei.

Essential and desirable diagnostic criteria

Essential: sessile or pedunculated mucosal growth(s) in a non-ampullary location; a closely packed tubular, glandular, or tubulopapillary growth pattern with epithelial dysplasia; intestinal epithelial differentiation, pyloric gland differentiation, or a serrated growth pattern (for subtyping).

Note: The degree of dysplasia is determined on the basis of architectural complexity, nuclear stratification, and nuclear atypia.

Staging (TNM)

Adenomatous polyps with high-grade dysplasia are regarded as pTis.

Prognosis and prediction

The prognosis of non-ampullary adenomas, particularly those of intestinal type, mirror the prognosis of those in the large bowel {3125}, and like in the colon, the risk of developing invasive disease is related to the size of the adenoma, the villous component, and the presence of HGD {2572}. In sporadic cases, a multivariate analysis {2434} showed that large diameter (> 2 cm) in combination with the presence of HGD at first biopsy is an indicator of malignant progression. This natural history also dictates treatment: they should be endoscopically removed if possible, and larger lesions should be considered for surgical removal. The five-grade system by Spigelman et al. (Table 4.01, p. 118) grades the burden of duodenal adenomatosis and estimates of the risk of patients with FAP developing duodenal adenocarcinoma {3114,2002,2867}.

Ampullary adenoma

Sekine S
Shia J

Definition
Ampullary adenoma is a polyp consisting of dysplastic glandular epithelium within the anatomical duodenal ampulla, which may show intestinal or pancreatobiliary differentiation.

ICD-O coding
8210/0 Adenomatous polyp, low-grade dysplasia
8210/2 Adenomatous polyp, high-grade dysplasia

ICD-11 coding
2E92.2 & XH3DV3 Benign neoplasm of duodenum & Adenoma NOS
2E92.2 & XH8MU5 Benign neoplasm of duodenum & Adenomatous polyp NOS

Related terminology
None

Subtype(s)
Intestinal-type adenoma, low grade (8144/0); intestinal-type adenoma, high grade (8144/2); non-invasive pancreatobiliary papillary neoplasm with low-grade dysplasia (8163/0); non-invasive pancreatobiliary papillary neoplasm with high-grade dysplasia (8163/2); intra-ampullary papillary-tubular neoplasm

Localization
Adenomas occur on the duodenal surface of the ampulla, and intra-ampullary papillary-tubular neoplasms (IAPNs) occur within the intra-ampullary channel (i.e. the lumen of the distal ends of the common bile duct and the main pancreatic duct).

Clinical features
These neoplasms are often asymptomatic and incidentally discovered on endoscopy. Patients may present with symptoms related to obstruction of the biliary or pancreatic duct (jaundice) {610}. In rare instances, cholangitis or pancreatitis is caused by ampullary adenomas. Substantial weight loss in a patient with an ampullary lesion may be due to malignant transformation {2062}. Endoscopic approaches are increasingly used {2547}, but they carry a risk of complications {382,534}. Both complications and invasive components in endoscopic resections require surgical intervention. Surgical options are pancreatoduodenectomy (the Whipple procedure) and transduodenal ampullectomy {199}.

Epidemiology
In general, these neoplasms are rarer than their colorectal counterparts. Several series have reported duodenal polyps to occur in as many as 4.6% of patients presenting for gastroscopy. In autopsy series, the estimated prevalence of ampullary adenoma is 0.04–0.12% {2861,225,610}.

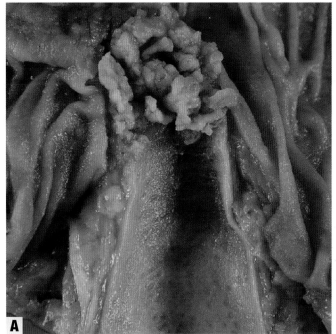

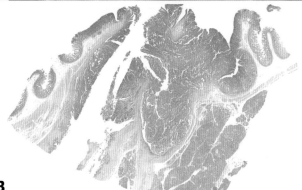

Fig. 4.04 Intra-ampullary papillary-tubular neoplasm. **A** This entity is characterized by an exophytic granular polypoid mass filling the intra-ampullary (very distal) end of the common bile duct but mostly sparing the duodenal mucosa. **B** Intra-ampullary papillary-tubular neoplasm–associated carcinoma. Low-power histological view.

Etiology
As discussed in the section on *Non-ampullary adenoma* (p. 118), more than half of small bowel neoplasms occur in the duodenum (most around the ampulla), suggesting that bile acids may be carcinogenic {312}. This topographical pattern is also observed in patients with familial adenomatous polyposis, who are genetically predisposed to developing small bowel adenomas (see also Chapter 14: *Genetic tumour syndromes of the digestive system*, p. 511) {3114}. In addition, population-based studies highlight the ampulla as part of a field effect with carcinogenic potential {1217}.

Chapter 4

Pathogenesis

Sporadic and familial adenomatous polyposis–related ampullary adenomas of the small bowel show similar molecular features, associated with the WNT signalling pathway, including *APC* and *KRAS* mutations {3502}. However, other mutations such as those in *BRAF* are rarer, as is mismatch repair deficiency {2079}. This mutation profile is consistent with the molecular background identified in a large percentage of ampullary adenocarcinomas of intestinal type (see *Ampullary adenocarcinoma*, p. 127).

Macroscopic appearance

The surface appearance of an ampullary adenoma is in many ways not dissimilar to its colorectal counterparts. However, careful macroscopic analysis may provide clues to predict malignancy. In particular, large size, a nodular appearance with erosion, evidence of fold convergence with the adjacent duodenum, and ductal dilatation (sometimes observed endoscopically) should alert the pathologist to potential foci of invasion in the biopsy or surgical specimen {1495,58,2002}.

Histopathology

In the previous edition, there were two subtypes of ampullary adenomas: intestinal-type and pancreatobiliary-type.

Intestinal-type adenomas are the most common type of adenomas of the ampullary duodenum. They mostly show a tubular or tubulovillous growth pattern. Most have low-grade dysplasia and consist of tall columnar cells with elongated nuclei and inconspicuous nucleoli. Paneth, goblet, or endocrine cells may be prominent in low-grade lesions {3369}. Adenomas with

high-grade dysplasia are characterized by an increased degree of architectural complexity, nuclear stratification, and nuclear atypia. Ampullary adenomas may extend from the papilla down to involve the biliary epithelium of the ampulla. At the periphery of the polypoid lesion, flat adenomatous changes may also extend into the common bile duct or periampullary ductules within the sphincter of Oddi. Familial adenomatous polyposis–associated adenomas have the same histological features as sporadic lesions. Immunohistochemically, intestinal-type adenomas express markers of the intestinal epithelium, including CDX2 and MUC2, and usually lack expression of EMA (MUC1) {3502}. Coexpression of CK7 and CK20 is common {3502}. Occasionally, pyloric gland adenomas also arise in the duodenal surface of the ampulla, and the characteristics of these rare cases seem to be very similar to those of the cases described in the stomach and non-ampullary duodenum.

Rarer non-invasive lesions with pancreatobiliary-type features have also been described. These exhibit a villous or papillary growth pattern and morphologically resemble pancreatobiliary-type intraductal papillary mucinous neoplasm of the pancreas {33}. Following the proposed nomenclature for preinvasive lesions in the pancreatic ducts {33} and biliary tract, the unified term "intra-ampullary papillary-tubular neoplasm (IAPN)" has been proposed for these lesions {2423}. IAPN is defined as a dysplastic, compact, exophytic lesion localized almost exclusively within the ampulla, growing predominantly within the ampullary channel, with minimal or no involvement of bile duct, pancreatic duct, or duodenal papilla. IAPN exhibits a spectrum of dysplastic grades (> 80% of cases exhibit a mixture of low-grade and high-grade dysplastic foci within the same lesion)

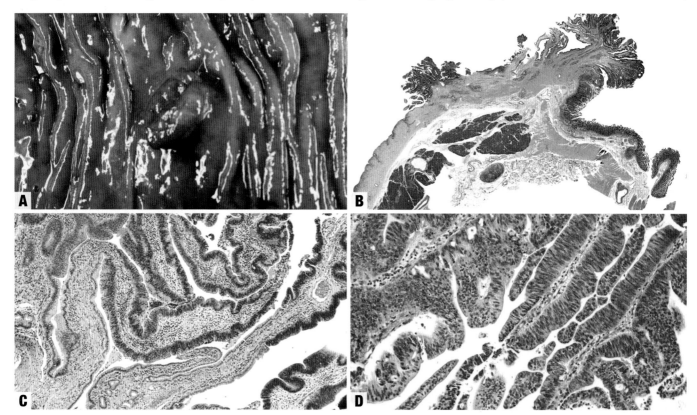

Fig. 4.05 Ampullary adenoma. **A** Gross appearance; note the exophytic mass protruding towards the duodenal lumen. **B** Scanning view. **C** Higher-power view of intestinal-type adenoma growing along biliary epithelium; the adenoma is low-grade in this region. **D** The adenoma shows high-grade dysplasia in this region.

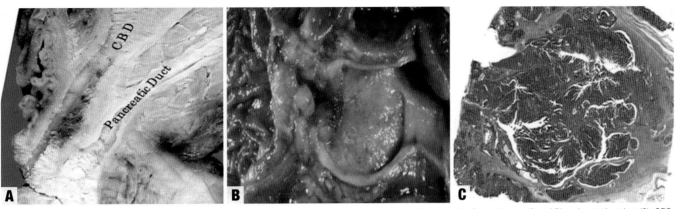

Fig. 4.06 Intra-ampullary papillary-tubular neoplasm (also described as non-invasive papillary neoplasm of the ampulla). Gross images (**A** and **B**) and scanning view (**C**). CBD, common bile duct.

and cell lineage differentiation (in 50% of cases there is coexistence of intestinal and pancreatobiliary differentiation). The immunohistochemistry profile of these lesions typically follows their differentiation lineage, with predominant MUC2 and CDX2 expression in the intestinal patterns and predominant expression of EMA (MUC1), MUC5AC, and MUC6 in the pancreatobiliary pattern; > 50% of cases coexpress CK7 and CK20.

Cytology

Most ampullary adenomas and IAPNs are accessible to conventional endoscopic biopsy, but brush cytology is occasionally obtained for deeper-seated intra-ampullary neoplasms {3137}. The cytological features of ampullary adenomas show a general preservation of architectural arrangement, with relatively scant dissociated malignant cells, but with cell clusters similar to those seen in confirmed invasive adenocarcinoma {3137}. A recent review of cytological diagnoses of ampullary adenomas confirmed these features and highlighted the validity of liquid-based cytology preparations to make this diagnosis {2043}.

Diagnostic molecular pathology

There are no routinely used molecular determinants of malignant transformation or therapeutic prediction in these lesions.

Essential and desirable diagnostic criteria

Essential: sessile or pedunculated mucosal growth at the ampulla; a tubular, tubulovillous, villous, or papillary growth pattern with dysplastic epithelial lining; intestinal or pancreatobiliary differentiation (for subtyping).
Note: The degree of dysplasia is determined on the basis of architectural complexity, nuclear stratification, and nuclear atypia.

Staging (TNM)

Adenomatous polyps with high-grade dysplasia are regarded as pTis. When ampullary adenoma or IAPN is accompanied by an invasive carcinoma, these neoplasms should be staged based on the invasive component. Their prognosis is related to the stage and subtype of the invasive component and is substantially better than with other lesions involving the ampulla {2423,43}.

Prognosis and prediction

Ampullary adenomas have a higher chance of malignant transformation than other duodenal adenomas {1023}. There is a high false negative rate on endoscopic biopsies {1584} because invasive carcinomas are often well hidden in the crevices of the lesions. Incomplete resection of adenomas is associated with a high risk of development of adenocarcinomas {2607,3213,2941}.

Invasive carcinomas commonly accompany IAPNs, which are found in about 75% of resected cases but can be subtle and easily missed, especially in biopsies or poorly dissected resection specimens. Pure, non-invasive IAPNs have 3-year and 5-year survival rates of 100% after successful removal.

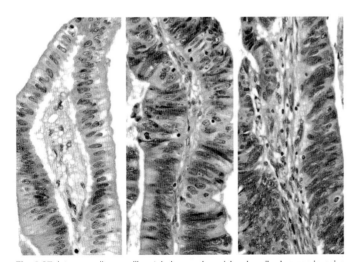

Fig. 4.07 Intra-ampullary papillary-tubular neoplasm (also described as non-invasive papillary neoplasm of the ampulla). An example showing varying grades of dysplasia: from low-grade (left panel) to high-grade (right panel).

Non-ampullary adenocarcinoma

Adsay NV
Nagtegaal ID
Reid MD

Definition

Non-ampullary adenocarcinoma is a malignant epithelial neoplasm of the small intestine showing glandular differentiation.

ICD-O coding

8140/3 Adenocarcinoma NOS

ICD-11 coding

2B80.20 Adenocarcinoma of small intestine

Related terminology

None

Subtype(s)

Mucinous adenocarcinoma (8480/3); signet-ring cell carcinoma (8490/3); poorly cohesive carcinoma (8490/3); medullary carcinoma NOS (8510/3)

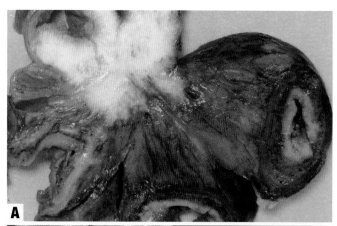

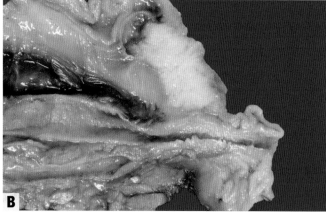

Fig. 4.08 Non-ampullary adenocarcinoma. **A** Small intestine adenocarcinoma causing complex adhesions to form between loops of bowel. **B** Extra-ampullary duodenal carcinoma. Note the plaque-like mass in the duodenum (in the region of the accessory ampulla), whereas the ampulla of Vater, common bile duct, and pancreatic duct are uninvolved; this was also verified on microscopy.

Localization

Non-ampullary tumours can occur anywhere in the GI tract between the pylorus and the ileocaecal valve. Ampullary adenocarcinomas are discussed separately (see *Ampullary adenocarcinoma*, p. 127). The duodenum is the most frequently involved segment, accounting for 55–82% of cases, followed by the jejunum and ileum {171}. Much of the increase in frequency reported in these tumours in the small bowel is due to an increase in duodenal tumours {629}, predominantly around the ampulla {2844}. For duodenal cancers occurring in the vicinity of the ampulla, the lack of ampullary involvement by gross and microscopic examination is the criterion to define non-ampullary duodenal cancers {3629,3392}.

Clinical features

The clinical presentation and diagnosis of small intestine adenocarcinomas is usually delayed, with cases presenting at advanced stages; lymph node involvement and/or distant metastases are reported in more than two thirds of all patients {707,3226}. The neoplasms are generally asymptomatic in their early stages, but occult bleeding may occur. The symptoms are relatively nonspecific: 66% of patients have abdominal pain when diagnosed. Small intestine adenocarcinoma is often a diagnosis of emergency, with occlusion reported in 40% of cases (more frequently in ileal and jejunal cases) and bleeding in 24% {707}. In cases presenting at later stages, complex adhesions between bowel loops are not infrequent. One of the largest clinical studies {707} showed upper endoscopy, surgery, small-bowel barium transit, and CT to be the main modalities for diagnosis.

Epidemiology

The incidence of small bowel cancer in general is 1.2–2.3 cases per 100 000 person-years {328}. The most common subtype, adenocarcinoma of the small intestine, accounts for 30–40% of all small bowel cancers {170}. They are, in any case, remarkably rare, accounting for < 3% of GI tract cancers {3565,1297,2496}. As a result of this incidence, 3600 new cases of small intestine adenocarcinoma are diagnosed annually in Europe {891} and 5300 in the USA, with 1100 related deaths {1722}.

The duodenum is the most common tumour site (> 50%), followed by the jejunum and ileum {328}. For a tumour in the distal small bowel, the possibility of a metastatic neoplasm, lymphoma, or neuroendocrine neoplasm (NEN) must be considered. The increasing incidence of small intestine adenocarcinoma is mainly due to the increase in duodenal tumours {2471,629}. Men are affected slightly more frequently than women {2907}, and the median patient age is in the early to mid-60s {2907,558}.

Small intestine adenocarcinomas share many characteristics with colorectal cancer, including a positive geographical correlation in incidence rates {1183}, whereas duodenal adenocarcinomas are slightly different in these associations {3629,3392}.

Etiology

Chronic inflammatory disorders (Crohn disease and coeliac disease), as well as other factors that expose the small intestine to non-native milieu (ileal conduits and reservoirs), are substantial risk factors for small intestine adenocarcinoma {3043,298,3357,1459}. The predilection for occurrence in the duodenum (particularly in the vicinity of the ampulla/pylorus) is attributable to exposure to acid and bile. Smoking, alcohol consumption, and specific diets have also been associated with small intestine adenocarcinoma {3611}.

Hereditary causes (see *Non-ampullary adenoma*, p. 118, *Ampullary adenoma*, p. 121, and Chapter 14: *Genetic tumour syndromes of the digestive system*, p. 511) are relatively common in the small bowel. Familial adenomatous polyposis primarily affects the extra-ampullary duodenum in > 50% of the cases, and seldom the ileum {1418}. Duodenal adenocarcinoma is the main cause of cancer-related death in patients with familial adenomatous polyposis who have undergone proctocolectomy {3449}. There is an association between small intestine adenocarcinoma and Lynch syndrome. In non-ampullary duodenal cancers, mismatch repair protein loss is seen at the same rate as in colon cancers {3629}. The small bowel has the highest relative risk (520) of cancer development in Peutz–Jeghers syndrome {1034}.

Pathogenesis

There is a strong association between distal small intestine adenocarcinoma and Crohn disease, with an incidence ratio between 27 and 33 {3490,1451}. In addition, inflammatory bowel disease–related colorectal cancer shares molecular markers with Crohn disease–related small intestine adenocarcinoma {3188}. A lower but statistically significant association (relative risk of 10 when compared with normal population) with coeliac disease has been documented in the literature {12404215,1294}.

Non-ampullary duodenal cancers are less commonly associated with an adenoma component than colorectal cancers. In addition, some are accompanied by background gastric-type epithelial alterations {3629,3392}. All of this suggests a gastric metaplasia–dysplasia–carcinoma sequence {3392,3313,614}, presumably induced by the local chemical factors, including acid.

Box 4.02 Molecular abnormalities described in small intestine adenocarcinoma

- *TP53* mutations {3557,116}
- Loss of E-cadherin, mutation of *CTNNB1* (encoding β-catenin) with nuclear localization {3557,351,173,2251}
- *SMAD4* and *KRAS* mutations and activation of the RAS/RAF/MAPK pathway {173,351}
- *IDH1, CDH1, KIT, FGFR2, FLT3, NPM1, PTEN, MET, AKT1, RET, ERBB2* (*HER2*), *NOTCH1*, and *ERBB4* mutations {116}
- *CHN2* downregulation through hypermethylation {116}

The molecular data on small intestine adenocarcinoma are limited {117}. The mutation landscape in small intestine adenocarcinoma is summarized in Box 4.02. Some of the biomarkers reported may be potential future druggable targets. Microsatellite instability (MSI) occurs in 5–35% of small intestine adenocarcinoma cases and is associated with a more favourable outcome {3629,2474,2598,2609}. Undifferentiated carcinomas with rhabdoid morphology are characterized by alterations of SMARC genes {44}.

Macroscopic appearance

The macroscopic examination is dictated by the likely clinical features and associations of this cancer: advanced stage at presentation {707}, as well as the etiological associations with Crohn disease, previous surgery or radiotherapy, polyposis syndromes, Meckel diverticulum, or intestinal duplications {2002}. These features, as well as the high chance of serosal involvement and the frequent extension to neighbouring abdominal organs, should be considered before gross dissection.

Tumours arising in the jejunum and ileum tend to be annular and constricting {404}. Those that arise in the duodenum have a polypoid component in about a third of cases, but a substantial proportion of cases show plaque-like growth {3629}.

Histopathology

Small intestine adenocarcinomas resemble their counterparts in the colon, but with a higher proportion of poorly differentiated tumours {1776} with glandular, squamous, and undifferentiated components {2002}. Therefore, reporting protocols require a histological characterization of small intestine adenocarcinoma

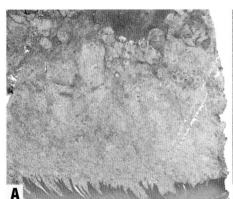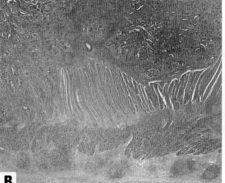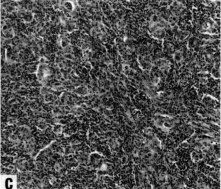

Fig. 4.09 Non-ampullary adenocarcinoma. **A** Mucinous adenocarcinoma. Transmural extension. **B** Adenocarcinoma. Crohn disease–like lymphocytic aggregates in a patient with no history of inflammatory bowel disease and no unequivocal evidence of Crohn disease in the resection specimen. **C** Poorly differentiated small intestine adenocarcinoma with abundant lymphocytic response; this case showed high levels of microsatellite instability.

as adenocarcinoma (not otherwise characterized), mucinous adenocarcinoma (> 50% mucinous), poorly cohesive cell carcinoma with or without signet-ring cells, medullary carcinoma, adenosquamous carcinoma, squamous cell carcinoma, mixed neuroendocrine–non-neuroendocrine neoplasm (MiNEN), or undifferentiated carcinoma.

Many of the less common varieties of small intestine adenocarcinoma are more common in the duodenum than in the jejunum or ileum. In addition, as indicated above, the subclassification mirrors the subtypes described in the colorectum (see *Colorectal adenocarcinoma*, p. 177, for further explanation).

Small intestine adenocarcinoma in the setting of Crohn disease tends to be predominantly distal jejunal or ileal {3624}. This can pose substantial diagnostic difficulties, because the diagnosis of Crohn disease is often not established before surgery {2002}, and many of the histological characteristics of Crohn disease can be mimicked by the transmural nature and associated inflammation. Pathologists should be alerted by the clinical risk factors recently proposed, which include longstanding history, younger-than-average age of onset, male sex, strictures and fistulae, and previous immunosuppressant use {841}. The confirmation or exclusion of concomitant Crohn disease may require sampling of multiple tissue blocks, within and away from the main lesion.

Duodenal adenocarcinomas, unlike distal small intestine adenocarcinomas, often have a spectrum of morphological patterns, with an immunophenotype closer to that of gastro-pancreatobiliary cancers. Upper gastrointestinal markers (CK7, EMA [MUC1], MUC5AC, and MUC6) are positive in half of the cases, and intestinal differentiation markers are present in about a third {3629,3392,591}. Establishing a diagnosis of primary small intestine adenocarcinoma versus the common colorectal cancer metastasis to the small bowel is important, because a metastasis can morphologically mimic a primary small intestine adenocarcinoma; furthermore, when they infiltrate into (and colonize) the mucosa, they often acquire a morphology closely simulating that of an adenoma with preneoplastic background {2982}. Partial expression of many other antibodies has been reported {171}, but no other immunohistochemical marker is used routinely.

Cytology

Cytopathological analysis (FNA or brushing) is seldom employed for small bowel tumours, with rare exceptions in the ampullary region in order to analyse an associated deep-seated lesion (see *Ampullary adenocarcinoma*, p. 127), and it is not generally used elsewhere in the small bowel. Studies reporting FNA applications in the peritoneum seldom include primary small bowel origin {1809}.

Diagnostic molecular pathology

MSI determination is required to evaluate a possible hereditary cause of small intestine adenocarcinoma, and it is also of use for selection for immunotherapy {1816}.

Essential and desirable diagnostic criteria

Essential: small intestine adenocarcinoma located in a non-ampullary region, with mainly glandular differentiation (rarely of other subtypes).

Staging (TNM)

Small intestine adenocarcinoma is pathologically staged according to the eighth edition (2017) of the Union for International Cancer Control (UICC) TNM classification {408}. Ampullary tumours, because of their unusual location, require a more detailed staging approach (see *Ampullary adenocarcinoma*, p. 127).

Prognosis and prediction

The overall survival associated with small intestine adenocarcinomas (when all areas are included) appears to be worse than that of colon {3629,20,3392,3750}. However, it is substantially better than for pancreatobiliary tract cancers {2756,2449,248}. The median survival time is approximately 40 months {558}. The number of lymph nodes retrieved and analysed is in itself a strong prognostic indicator, with a cut-off point of 8–10 lymph nodes to improve survival {2472}.

The early results in immunotherapy may improve overall survival in patients with high MSI (see *Diagnostic molecular pathology*, above).

Ampullary adenocarcinoma

Adsay NV
Reid MD

Definition

Ampullary adenocarcinoma is a malignant epithelial tumour of the small bowel, with its epicentre in the ampulla, showing glandular or mucinous differentiation.

ICD-O coding

8140/3 Adenocarcinoma NOS

ICD-11 coding

2B80.20 Adenocarcinoma of small intestine

Related terminology

None

Subtype(s)

Mucinous adenocarcinoma (8480/3); signet-ring cell carcinoma (8490/3); poorly cohesive carcinoma (8490/3); medullary carcinoma NOS (8510/3); adenocarcinoma, intestinal type (8144/3); pancreatobiliary-type carcinoma (8163/3); tubular adenocarcinoma (8211/3); adenosquamous carcinoma (8560/3); carcinoma, undifferentiated, NOS (8020/3)

Localization

The ampulla is the most common location for small intestinal adenocarcinoma {2844}, attributed to biliary and/or pancreatic effluents. To establish whether a tumour is of ampullary origin (and to exclude metastatic tumours from the immediately neighbouring regions of bile duct and pancreas), proper dissection of pancreatoduodenectomy specimens is crucial (to document that the epicentre of the cancer is in the ampulla). The bivalving approach {32}, with sectioning of the common bile duct and main pancreatic duct along the same plane as they enter the ampulla, allows demonstration of the specific localization of the tumour, as well as the further site-specific subclassification of ampullary tumours {43}.

Ampullary adenocarcinomas can arise from (and grow preferentially in) the various compartments of this small organ. (Peri)ampullary-duodenal carcinomas are those arising from the duodenal surface of the ampulla (often from an adenoma), and they characteristically form ulcerating or vegetating masses that are readily visible from the duodenal perspective. In (peri)ampullary-duodenal tumours, the orifice of the ampulla is typically engulfed eccentrically in the superior pole of the lesion.

In contrast, intra-ampullary carcinomas appear, from the duodenal view, as only subtle ulcers, mucosa-covered elevations, or granular material protruding from within the ampulla. These occur in two distinct subsets by localization: (1) arising from the intra-ampullary papillary-tubular neoplasm and characterized by a polypoid, nodular, or granular mass localized within the ampullary cavity, and (2) arising from the ampullary ducts, with a scirrhous constrictive and circumferential tumour localized on the walls of the ampullary ducts (the distal ends of the common bile duct and ampulla).

Ampullary carcinoma NOS is the diagnosis reserved for tumours clearly of ampullary origin but that cannot be placed into any of the three categories above, despite proper handling of the specimens and gross–microscopic correlation.

Clinical features

Unlike adenocarcinomas in other segments of the small intestine, ampullary adenocarcinomas are often detected at a relatively earlier stage because of the symptoms and signs caused by the obstruction of the biliary ducts, leading to cholestasis and related findings. For the subset of (peri)ampullary-duodenal cases, which often form ulcers, the initial presentation is

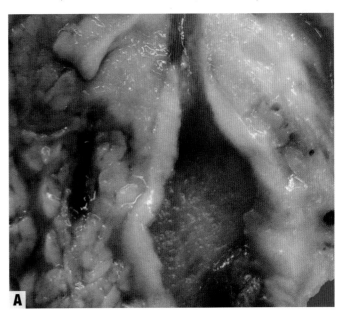

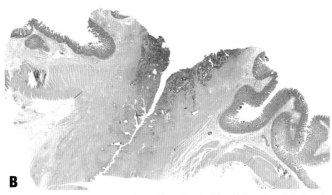

Fig. 4.10 Ampullary carcinoma of ampullary-ductal origin. **A** Note the relatively subtle scirrhous mass that circumferentially constricts the intra-ampullary duct, whereas the ampullary-duodenal mucosa is mostly spared. **B** Low-power histological view of carcinoma at the ampullary orifice.

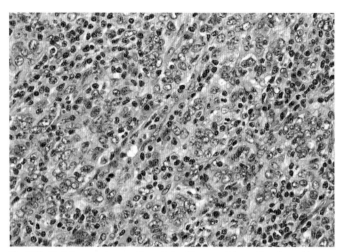

Fig. 4.11 Medullary carcinoma. Characterized by syncytial growth pattern of tumour cells; inflammatory cells are intermixed with large tumour cells, which contain overlapping nuclei with vesicular chromatin and prominent nucleoli.

often gastrointestinal bleeding with occult blood. Occasionally, pancreatic injury/insufficiency due to pancreatic outflow occlusion may also occur, but findings are typically related more to the bile duct obstruction {43,2421,2423,3226}. Close to half of the cases are found to have lymph node metastasis at resection {230}.

Epidemiology

Ampullary adenocarcinoma accounts for 6–9% of all periampullary malignancies. Approximately 15% of pancreatoduodenectomies are performed for ampullary cancers {43,230,2421,3138}. Men are affected slightly more frequently than women, and the median patient age is in the mid-60s {43,230,2423}.

Etiology

For the vast majority of ampullary adenocarcinomas, a specific etiology is not evident {43,2423,555}. Some of the inflammatory diseases (e.g. Crohn, coeliac) and previous surgical procedures, which have been documented as important predisposing factors for adenocarcinomas of other parts of the small bowel, account for only a small percentage of cases in the ampulla. Hereditary conditions such as familial adenomatous polyposis, Lynch syndrome, and Peutz–Jeghers syndrome are also relevant associations.

Pathogenesis

It is believed that the predilection of small bowel adenocarcinomas for occurrence in the ampullary region is attributable to exposure to bile and pancreatic products. The ampulla is also one of the common sites for familial adenomatous coli syndrome–related adenocarcinomas, although such cases account for a very small percentage of ampullary cancers. In addition, specific mutations and a gene expression signature with potential clinical significance have been described in this cancer (see *Prognosis and prediction*, below).

Macroscopic appearance

The macroscopic appearance of these carcinomas is dependent on the portion of the ampulla from which they derive.

Carcinomas arising from (and growing predominantly on) the (peri)ampullary duodenum typically present as large ulcerovegetating masses that are readily evident upon opening the duodenum and inspecting this region. Polypoid nodular components correspond to adenomas, and ulcerating areas (which can be hidden in the creases underneath the polypoid areas, and therefore missed by biopsies) often reveal invasive carcinomas. In (peri)ampullary-duodenal cancers, the ampullary orifice can be obscured and difficult to locate, but probes inserted into the proximal common bile duct often exit eccentrically and superiorly in this mass.

By definition, ampullary carcinomas arising from intra-ampullary papillary-tubular neoplasms have polypoid, nodular granular material filling the ampullary cavity. From the duodenal perspective, these neoplasms can present as mucosa-covered bulges, often with a centrally located dilated ampullary orifice, from within which granular nodular material may protrude to the duodenal lumen.

Carcinomas of ampullary duct origin are also "intra-ampullary", and they often appear, from the duodenal perspective, as mucosa-covered button-like elevations of the ampulla, some with subtle ulceration. Bivalving the ampulla typically reveals poorly defined sclerosing thickening of the intra-ampullary ducts leading to circumferentially constrictive lesions.

Histopathology

The vast majority of ampullary adenocarcinomas, regardless of site-specific classification, are gland-forming (tubular) adenocarcinomas {3629,558,2471}.

Historically, ampullary adenocarcinomas have been expected to fall into one of two broad histological categories: pancreatobiliary (see below and other chapters) or intestinal (colonic-type). However, about 40% of cases reveal mixed or hybrid phenotypes, which is also reflected in the immunoprofiles {3629,2683}. It also leaves a substantial number of cases with heterogeneous immunoprofiles {146,555,3628,2423}. This is not surprising considering the ampulla is a transitional region with distinctive cellular compartments, as well as its exposure to different etiopathogenic factors, along with the fact that small intestinal epithelium is not truly colonic, and ampullary ducts are not exactly identical to pancreatobiliary ducts. Nevertheless, panels of immunohistochemical stains including EMA (MUC1), MUC2, CDX2, and MUC5AC can aid in the classification of tubular-patterned adenocarcinomas as intestinal or pancreatobiliary type in a substantial proportion of cases {146,555,3628}.

Intestinal-type adenocarcinoma

These gland (tubule)-forming adenocarcinomas are morphologically similar to colon adenocarcinomas {2683}. The glands are lined by tall columnar cells with elongated, pseudostratified nuclei. Scattered goblet, Paneth, and neuroendocrine cells may be present {2683,2170,930}. A substantial proportion are associated with intestinal-type adenoma {2170,2340,3585}. In the ampullary region especially, some of these tumours exhibit other patterns and immunophenotypes different than those of true colonic intestinal-type adenocarcinomas (see below) {2683}.

Pancreatobiliary-type or gastric-type adenocarcinoma

Similar to pancreatic ductal, gallbladder, and extrahepatic biliary tract adenocarcinomas, this type is composed of relatively small glandular units widely separated by desmoplastic stroma. The epithelium is usually a single layer of cuboidal to low columnar cells, without substantial nuclear pseudostratification, but with more pleomorphism than in the intestinal-type {2683,43,3713}. Although tumours with gastric-like mucin (histologically and immunophenotypically) have been designated as gastric type {3628}, the two groups appear to be closely related and are often regarded as one group {3628,2423}.

Tubular adenocarcinoma with mixed features

Many carcinomas in the ampulla have ambiguous features that are difficult to classify definitively as pancreatobiliary or intestinal. These ambiguous/hybrid cases account for more than a third of all ampullary carcinomas {146,3629,2683,3628} and should be classified as tubular adenocarcinomas with mixed features, with the predominant pattern noted. Immunohistochemical studies using EMA (MUC1), MUC2, CDX2, CK20, and MUC5AC may be helpful in determining the predominant lineage {3629,2683,3628,146}.

Non-tubular patterns

In addition to the conventional adenocarcinoma types, most of which have a tubular pattern, carcinomas with non-glandular patterns can also occur in this region but are often associated with ordinary tubule-forming adenocarcinomas. In some cases, the non-tubular patterns may predominate and the tumours are classified accordingly. These are discussed below.

Mucinous adenocarcinoma

Mucinous adenocarcinoma (with > 50% stromal mucin deposition) is proportionally more common in the duodenum. In the ampulla, some degree of extracellular mucin deposition is seen in 15% of cases, with two thirds qualifying as mucinous adenocarcinoma {93}. The malignant epithelial strips and glands floating in mucin pools are often columnar with intestinal phenotype (also with diffuse CDX2 and MUC2 expression), making these cases closer to intestinal-type adenocarcinomas. Scattered signet-ring cells may be seen floating within the mucin but not infiltrating the stroma as individual cells or cords – an important distinction from true poorly cohesive cell carcinoma. Mucinous adenocarcinoma in the ampulla most commonly arises from adenomas of the ampullary duodenum but may also be seen in association with intra-ampullary tumours.

Poorly cohesive cell carcinoma

These tumours, which are relatively uncommon in the small bowel, often lack an adenomatous component {93,3504,3547}, are usually advanced at diagnosis, and behave more aggressively.

Medullary carcinoma

Medullary carcinomas akin to their colonic counterparts may occur in the small intestine, especially in the duodenum and ampulla {3629}. They constitute 3% of ampullary cancers and are characterized by large, nodular masses with pushing borders and syncytial growth, with associated inflammation. Like in the colon, they behave less aggressively despite their large size.

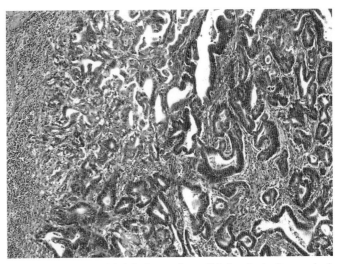

Fig. 4.12 Gland-forming (tubular) adenocarcinoma. Note the mixed pattern, predominantly intestinal type (right and lower) with transition to more gastropancreatobiliary phenotype in the upper left.

Adenosquamous carcinoma

Adenosquamous carcinoma is extremely rare. It accounts for 1% of all ampullary carcinomas {3097,1283,3672}. Adequate sampling often illustrates the glandular component. The squamous component exhibits squamous-type cytokeratins, along with p63 and p40. A pure squamous cell carcinoma should raise the possibility of metastasis.

High-grade neuroendocrine carcinoma (NEC) and mixed carcinomas

Poorly differentiated NECs (both small cell and large cell types) can arise in the small bowel, particularly the ampulla {2317,682,3164,3774}. Immunohistochemical confirmation of neuroendocrine differentiation with synaptophysin and chromogranin A is warranted, because other poorly differentiated malignant neoplasms may have neuroendocrine-like features (see *Small intestinal and ampullary neuroendocrine neoplasms*, p. 131).

Undifferentiated carcinoma

Undifferentiated carcinoma with osteoclast-like giant cells as described in the pancreas can occasionally occur in the small intestine, most often in the ampulla or duodenum {2248,1544,2407,2087}. Metastatic or direct involvement by a pancreatic or bile duct primary should be excluded {2248}. The giant cells in these tumours are conventional osteoclasts (histiocytic and non-neoplastic) and label positively for the histiocytic marker CD68. In contrast, the neoplastic mononuclear cells, which often have a sarcomatoid appearance, may be keratin-positive and often show a mutant p53 staining pattern {3555}.

Very rare examples of undifferentiated carcinomas with a distinct rhabdoid phenotype have been described in the ampulla and small intestine {44}. The tumours are typically large and show characteristic rhabdoid cells with abundant intracytoplasmic, eosinophilic rhabdoid bodies. The tumour cells are often dyscohesive and embedded in a myxoid matrix. Pleomorphic giant or spindle cell differentiation, as well as areas of glandular differentiation, may also be seen. Loss of nuclear immunostaining for SMARCB1 (INI1), a core subunit of the SWI/

SNF chromatin-remodelling complex, is characteristic. These tumours appear to have loss/coactivation of multiple members of the SWI/SNF family of proteins, including SMARCA4, SMARCA2, and/or SMARCB1, indicating an association between SWI/SNF deficiency and rhabdoid phenotype. Some have ARID1A abnormalities.

Cytology

For cases with a large adenomatous component and infiltrative areas deeper in the tissues, FNA may be informative, but it is seldom used, because most ampullary tumours are readily accessible by duodenal endoscopy rather than requiring FNA {3137}.

Diagnostic molecular pathology

Mutations in *KRAS* have been identified and show potential prognostic value, but they are of little diagnostic and no predictive value {2751,7148,1739}. More recently, a 92-gene signature has been postulated to have significant diagnostic concordance with the classification gold standard, and it has objective prognostic value, particularly in poorly differentiated cases {2475}. Microsatellite instability appears to be involved in about 15% of ampullary carcinomas, and immunohistochemical analysis for mismatch repair proteins may be helpful.

Essential and desirable diagnostic criteria

Essential: adenocarcinoma of ampullary origin with mainly glandular differentiation and rarely squamous, neuroendocrine, or sarcomatoid differentiation.

Staging (TNM)

Ampullary adenocarcinoma is pathologically staged according to the eighth edition (2017) of the Union for International Cancer Control (UICC) TNM classification {408}. However, because of the anatomical complexity of ampullary cancers, proper macroscopic examination and dissection of resection specimens is crucial in order to achieve proper staging {32}. Careful examination of any extension into the periduodenal soft tissues adjacent to the ampulla (where it is not cushioned by the pancreas) is critical, because carcinomas readily infiltrate into this region without first penetrating through the pancreas {30}.

Prognosis and prediction

Resected ampullary carcinomas have an overall 5-year survival rate of 45% {43,93,2402,2421}. Independent prognostic factors include patient age, lymph node metastasis, perineural and vascular invasion, margin status, tumour budding, and MUC5AC expression {3628}; size of invasive carcinoma, histological type, and grade appear to play a lesser role {43,230,2421}. Carcinomas of ampullary-ductal origin are often aggressive despite their small size; they are presumably typically pancreatobiliary-type and of advanced T stage due to their ready access to the soft tissue {43,2423}. Of note, the pancreatobiliary phenotype in ampullary carcinoma has a substantially better prognosis than its pancreatic counterpart (pancreatic ductal adenocarcinoma), and it is not an independent factor by itself when compared with intestinal phenotype {2683}. See the *Diagnostic molecular pathology* subsection above for discussion of the use of molecular tests with predictive therapeutic value.

Small intestinal and ampullary neuroendocrine neoplasms

Perren A
Basturk O
Bellizzi AM
Scoazec JY
Sipos B

Definition
Neuroendocrine neoplasms (NENs) of the small intestine and ampulla are duodenal, jejunal, and ileal epithelial neoplasms with neuroendocrine differentiation, including well-differentiated neuroendocrine tumours (NETs) and poorly differentiated neuroendocrine carcinomas (NECs). Mixed neuroendocrine–non-neuroendocrine neoplasms (MiNENs) have an exocrine component (typically adenocarcinoma) and a neuroendocrine component (typically NEC), each accounting for ≥ 30% of the neoplasm.

ICD-O coding
8240/3 Neuroendocrine tumour NOS
8246/3 Neuroendocrine carcinoma NOS
8154/3 Mixed neuroendocrine–non-neuroendocrine neoplasm (MiNEN)

ICD-11 coding
2B80.01 Neuroendocrine neoplasm of duodenum
2B80.01 & XH9LV8 Neuroendocrine neoplasm of duodenum & Neuroendocrine tumour, grade I
2B80.01 & XH7F73 Neuroendocrine neoplasm of duodenum & Neuroendocrine carcinoma, moderately differentiated
2B80.01 & XH0U20 Neuroendocrine neoplasm of duodenum & Neuroendocrine carcinoma NOS
2B80.01 & XH9SY0 Neuroendocrine neoplasm of duodenum & Small cell neuroendocrine carcinoma
2B80.01 & XH0NL5 Neuroendocrine neoplasm of duodenum & Large cell neuroendocrine carcinoma
2B80.01 & XH6H10 Neuroendocrine neoplasm of duodenum & Mixed adenoneuroendocrine carcinoma
2B80.01 & XH7NM1 Neuroendocrine neoplasm of duodenum & Other specified malignant neoplasms of colon & Enterochromaffin cell carcinoid
2B80.01 & XH93H8 Neuroendocrine neoplasm of duodenum & Gastrinoma NOS
2B80.01 & XH5VH0 Neuroendocrine neoplasm of duodenum & Somatostatinoma NOS
2B80.01 & XH2012 Neuroendocrine neoplasm of duodenum & Gangliocytic paraganglioma

Related terminology
Intestinal NET
Acceptable: carcinoid; well-differentiated endocrine tumour/carcinoma.

Intestinal NEC
Acceptable: poorly differentiated endocrine carcinoma; high-grade neuroendocrine carcinoma; small cell and large cell endocrine carcinoma.

Subtype(s)
Neuroendocrine tumour, grade 1 (8240/3); neuroendocrine tumour, grade 2 (8249/3); neuroendocrine tumour, grade 3 (8249/3); gastrinoma NOS (8153/3); somatostatinoma NOS (8156/3); enterochromaffin-cell carcinoid (8241/3); extra-adrenal paraganglioma NOS (8693/3); large cell neuroendocrine carcinoma (8013/3); small cell neuroendocrine carcinoma (8041/3)

Localization
More than 95% of duodenal NETs are located in part 1 or 2, with those in part 2 predominating in the ampullary region. Somatostatin-expressing NET and gangliocytic paraganglioma are located almost exclusively in the ampullary region. The vast majority of jejunoileal NETs are located in the distal ileum, with only 11% of jejunal origin; occasional enterochromaffin-cell (EC-cell) tumours arise in Meckel diverticula {445}. In the small intestine, NEC is almost exclusive to the ampullary region. Jejunoileal NEC is considered exceptional, with only very rare case reports {3276}.

Clinical features
Non-functioning NENs may become clinically apparent as a result of mass effect (e.g. intestinal obstruction, jaundice). Occasionally, small bowel or ampullary NETs are diagnosed because of symptoms referable to secretion of hormones (functioning tumours). The clinical features therefore differ according to localization and hormone production.

Ampullary NENs lead to obstructive jaundice and rarely to acute pancreatitis {3087}. Most duodenal NETs are clinically asymptomatic and detected incidentally by endoscopy, but gastrinomas, by definition, lead to Zollinger–Ellison syndrome, characterized by hypergastrinaemia, gastric hypersecretion, refractory peptic ulcer disease, and diarrhoea due to

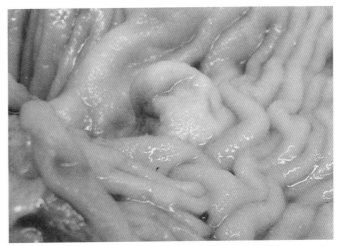

Fig. 4.13 Ileal neuroendocrine tumour (NET). Note the mucosal nodule with erosion of the mucosa.

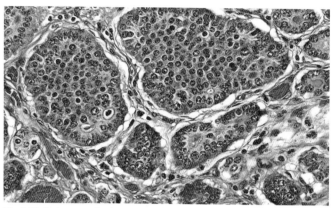

Fig. 4.14 Ileal neuroendocrine tumour (NET). A G1 NET showing packets of neuroendocrine cells separated by fibrovascular tissue.

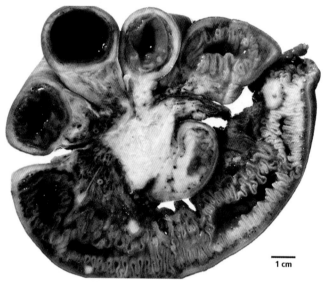

Fig. 4.15 Ileal neuroendocrine tumour (NET). A multifocal ileal NET with white/yellowish mural nodules and large mesenteric metastasis with sclerosis leading to ileus.

uncontrolled secretion of gastrin {2128}, the symptoms of which are often obscured by proton-pump inhibitor therapy. The somatostatinoma syndrome (diabetes mellitus, diarrhoea, steatorrhoea, hypohydria or achlorhydria, anaemia, and gallstones) is exceedingly rare {1009}.

Jejunal and ileal NETs may lead to intermittent abdominal pain consistent with intermittent obstruction or small bowel ischaemia. Carcinoid syndrome with diarrhoea, bronchospasms, flushing, and tricuspid valve fibrosis only occurs if liver metastases are present, and it is found in at most 10% of patients {2185}.

Epidemiology
The incidence of small intestinal NETs has risen steadily over the past 30 years, to 1.2 cases per 100 000 person-years clinically {716}. The prevalence in autopsy series is much higher {304}.

Etiology
The etiology of sporadic small intestinal NETs is unknown. A substantial minority of duodenal NENs arise in the setting of

a hereditary cancer predisposition syndrome. Patients with multiple endocrine neoplasia type 1 develop multiple duodenal gastrinomas {3439}. About 10% of ampullary, somatostatin-expressing tumours arise in the setting of neurofibromatosis type 1 {2693}. Rare activating mutations of *EPAS1* (encoding HIF2α) lead to duodenal somatostatin-expressing tumours in combination with paraganglioma and polycythaemia {833}. As many as 5% of patients with a jejunoileal NET have an affected first-degree relative; however, the genetic basis is essentially unknown. *IPMK* mutations were identified in one family, but the same gene was found to be wildtype in 32 other families with ≥ 2 jejunoileal NETs {2929}.

Pathogenesis
The pathogenesis of sporadic NET of the small intestine and the ampullary region is poorly understood. About one third of gastrinomas are associated with multiple endocrine neoplasia type 1 {803}; 46% of gastrinomas reveal allelic loss of the wildtype *MEN1* allele, indicating that other mechanisms frequently inactivate the wildtype allele. Allelic loss occurs at the same frequency in multifocal tiny lesions (300 µm), defining these as neoplasms, whereas hyperplastic G cells and D cells show retention of both alleles {154}. In multifocal familial jejunoileal NETs, multiple minute tumours develop from reserve EC cells expressing reserve intestinal stem-cell markers {2928}.

Macroscopic appearance
Duodenal and periampullary NETs are usually small (< 2 cm) polypoid lesions within the submucosa; only rarely are they large, infiltrating tumours. The average size is 0.8 cm for duodenal gastrin-producing NET {803} and 1.8 cm for somatostatin-producing (mainly) ampullary NET {1009}. Jejunoileal NETs are multifocal (2–100 tumours) in at least one third of cases {445,619}. Upper jejunal NETs are heterogeneous and may be large and locally invasive {627}. Lower jejunal and ileal NETs (including the rare cases occurring in Meckel diverticulum) present as mucosal/submucosal nodules with intact or slightly eroded mucosa. Deep infiltration of muscular wall and subserosa is frequent. Mesenteric lymph node metastases can lead to a strong desmoplastic reaction with retraction of the mesentery.

Histopathology
Small intestinal NETs are composed of uniform tumour cells with round to oval nuclei with finely granular chromatin typical of NETs in other sites. They usually show little pleomorphism. Gastrin-expressing G-cell NETs (duodenal) are typically arranged in trabeculae. Somatostatin-expressing D-cell NETs (ampullary) are tubuloglandular and may contain psammoma bodies. Serotonin-expressing EC-cell NETs (jejunoileal) are composed of nests of tumour cells with peripheral palisading, often with a minor component of pseudogland formation. In regions of sclerosis, the growth pattern may break down into single-file cells and small nests of cells.

Poorly differentiated NECs are high-grade carcinomas growing in sheets or poorly formed trabeculae or nests. Tumour cells are pleomorphic and may show large cell or small cell patterns. Some have a concurrent adenocarcinoma component (i.e. MiNEN). Some NETs arise in association with an adenoma.

Gangliocytic paraganglioma demonstrates triphasic histology, including neuroendocrine, Schwannian, and ganglion cell–like components.

Immunohistochemistry
NENs are characterized by the expression of keratins, peptide hormones and/or biogenic amines, and general neuroendocrine markers. Chromogranin A and synaptophysin are the recommended general neuroendocrine markers and strongly recommended for small cell NEC (SCNEC), large cell NEC (LCNEC), and MiNEN. Somatostatin-expressing NETs are less likely to express chromogranin A, and NECs are less likely to express either of the general neuroendocrine markers.

Ileal serotonin-producing EC-cell NETs and their metastases are positive for CDX2, and > 90% show positivity for SSTR2A {2505}. The demonstration of keratin expression is useful in the distinction of NETs from paraganglioma/phaeochromocytoma. NENs are more likely to express CK8 and CK18 (e.g. as demonstrated by keratin AE1/AE3 and CAM5.2 staining) than CK7.

Absent RB1 and aberrant p53 expression may be useful to support a diagnosis of NEC, especially in the differential with G3 NETs.

Hormone immunohistochemistry is useful in specific settings (e.g. gastrin in patients with Zollinger–Ellison syndrome, somatostatin in patients with tubuloglandular ampullary region tumours, serotonin to support the jejunoileal origin of a NET liver metastasis of occult origin).

SSTR2A immunohistochemistry may be useful to select patients with metastatic disease for somatostatin-analogue therapy or if somatostatin receptor scintigraphy is negative or unavailable.

Grading
Small intestinal and ampullary NENs are graded using the same system used for other gastroenteropancreatic NENs.

Cytology
Not clinically relevant

Diagnostic molecular pathology
No molecular data are available for sporadic duodenal and ampullary NENs. Small intestine NETs have a complex genomic landscape, including frequent large-scale chromosomal abnormalities (i.e. whole-chromosome/whole-arm), a low rate of somatic mutations, and a high rate of epigenetic changes {2365,3156}. About 60–90% of jejunoileal NETs show chromosome 18 deletion, detectable by array comparative genomic hybridization or FISH, even in early lesions {3510,1741}; however, there is no definitive evidence for driver genes in the regions involved, even if candidates have been proposed {840,2357}. Chromosome 14 gain is typically found in advanced lesions and metastatic sites, and it may be an adverse prognostic factor {139}. Other abnormalities (mainly on chromosomes 4, 5, 11, 14, 16, and 20) can be found at lower rates, especially in metastases

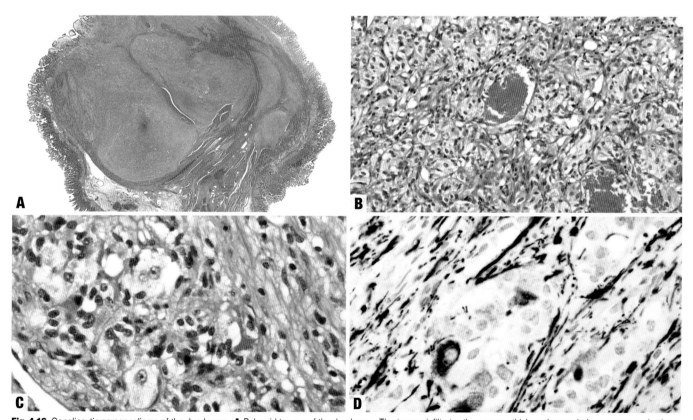

Fig. 4.16 Gangliocytic paraganglioma of the duodenum. **A** Polypoid tumour of the duodenum. The tumour infiltrates the mucosa, thickened muscularis mucosae, and submucosa. **B** In areas, the tumour looks like typical neuroendocrine tumour (NET), comprising packets and trabeculae demarcated by a delicate vasculature. **C** In areas, large cells with round nuclei, vesicular chromatin, and nucleoli (ganglion cells) are admixed with the NET (more chromatin-rich). In the right field, spindly Schwannian cells are seen. **D** The ganglion cells and their cell processes are highlighted by staining for neurofilament, whereas the NET cells are negative.

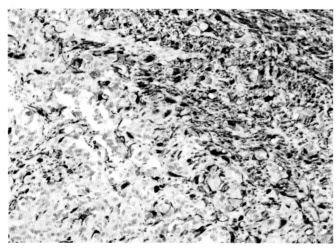

Fig. 4.17 Gangliocytic paraganglioma of the duodenum. S100 staining highlights the Schwannian cells. Some positive cells wrap around packets of neuroendocrine tumour (NET) cells, and might be sustentacular cells or Schwann cells.

{139,138}. Mutations of *CDKN1B* (which encodes p27) are found in ≤ 10% of ileal NETs {961,695}. Numerous other mutations, mainly involving the mTOR, PDGFR, EGFR (HER1), and TGF-β pathways, have been described, but only in individual cases or at very low rates {233,138}. Epigenetic changes appear to be very common; > 50% of ileal NETs are CpG island methylator phenotype, and substantial epigenetic dysregulation is found in 70–80% of tumours {1292,1529}. Three molecular subgroups with potential prognostic impact have recently been described: small intestinal NET with chromosome 18 loss (55%), which correlated with CpG island methylator phenotype negativity, *CDKN1B* mutation, and favourable prognosis; no whole-arm copy-number variation (19%), which correlated with CpG island methylator phenotype positivity and intermediate prognosis; and multiple whole-arm copy-number variations (26%), which correlated with poor prognosis {1529}.

Essential and desirable diagnostic criteria

NET
Essential: a uniform population of cells with round nuclei and finely stippled chromatin; architectural patterns include trabeculae, acini, nests, and ribbons; expression of synaptophysin and chromogranin A.

NEC
Essential: small cell carcinoma or large cell carcinoma pattern; sheets or trabeculae of poorly differentiated cells; high mitotic count and Ki-67 proliferation index.

Staging (TNM)
For well-differentiated NETs, an organ-based Union for International Cancer Control (UICC) staging system is in place, which is presented in Chapter 1 (p. 20). For NECs and MiNENs, the UICC staging system for the corresponding adenocarcinoma is used.

Prognosis and prediction
The 5-year and 10-year relative survival rates of patients with ampullary NETs have been reported as 82% and 71%, respectively {86}. Tumours that are < 2 cm or limited to the ampulla have a better prognosis {823,1345}. Although frequent, lymph node metastases do not appear to influence overall and disease-free survival rates {2015,1009,823,3671}. After curative resection, the liver is the most common site of metastasis {1345}.

Gangliocytic paragangliomas usually follow a benign course; however, occasional large neoplasms (> 2 cm) may spread to regional lymph nodes, and a rare patient has been found to succumb to the disease {453,1372}.

Gastrinomas associated with Zollinger–Ellison syndrome are prognostically less favourable than their non-functioning counterparts, having a higher frequency of metastases {3094}.

Patients with small intestine NETs often present with metastatic disease {972}, which has been estimated to occur in 35% of cases in large population-based studies {3684} and in > 60% of cases from larger referral centres {2218,2386,1817}. The most common metastatic sites are the locoregional lymph nodes and liver {972,127}. However, despite this advanced presentation at the time of diagnosis, most patients have prolonged survival due to the low proliferative rate. Patients with localized disease have a 5-year overall survival rate of 70–100%; in patients with distant metastases, the rate is 35–60% {2386,2038,1045}.

The results of studies assessing outcomes suggest that long-term recurrence rates are approximately 50% {1045,1817,779}. Patients with nodal metastasis, mesenteric involvement, lymphovascular invasion, or perineural invasion have a higher risk of recurrence {2038}.

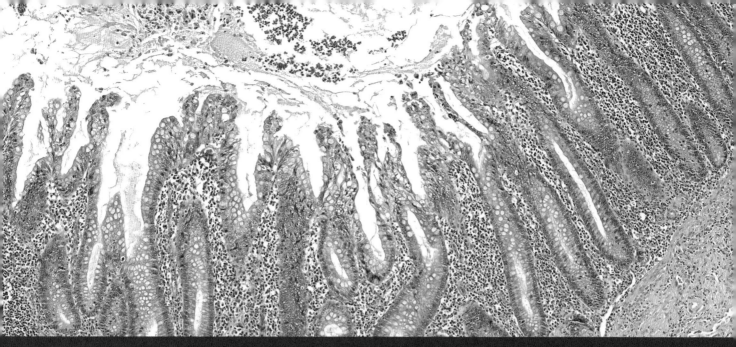

5

Tumours of the appendix

Edited by: Nagtegaal ID, Klimstra DS, Washington MK

Epithelial tumours
    Serrated lesions and polyps
    Mucinous neoplasm
    Adenocarcinoma
    Goblet cell adenocarcinoma
    Neuroendocrine neoplasms

WHO classification of tumours of the appendix

Epithelial tumours

	Hyperplastic polyp
	Sessile serrated lesion without dysplasia
8213/0*	Serrated dysplasia, low grade
8213/2*	Serrated dysplasia, high grade
8480/1	Low-grade appendiceal mucinous neoplasm
8480/2*	High-grade appendiceal mucinous neoplasm
8140/3	Adenocarcinoma NOS
8480/3	Mucinous adenocarcinoma
8490/3	Signet-ring cell adenocarcinoma
8020/3	Carcinoma, undifferentiated, NOS
8243/3*	Goblet cell adenocarcinoma
8240/3	Neuroendocrine tumour NOS
8240/3	Neuroendocrine tumour, grade 1
8249/3	Neuroendocrine tumour, grade 2
8249/3	Neuroendocrine tumour, grade 3
8152/3	L-cell tumour
8152/3	Glucagon-like peptide-producing tumour
8152/3	PP/PYY-producing tumour
8241/3	Enterochromaffin-cell carcinoid
8241/3	Serotonin-producing carcinoid
8246/3	Neuroendocrine carcinoma NOS
8013/3	Large cell neuroendocrine carcinoma
8041/3	Small cell neuroendocrine carcinoma
8154/3	Mixed neuroendocrine–non-neuroendocrine neoplasm (MiNEN)

_____

These morphology codes are from the International Classification of Diseases for Oncology, third edition, second revision (ICD-O-3.2) {1378A}. Behaviour is coded /0 for benign tumours; /1 for unspecified, borderline, or uncertain behaviour; /2 for carcinoma in situ and grade III intraepithelial neoplasia; /3 for malignant tumours, primary site; and /6 for malignant tumours, metastatic site. Behaviour code /6 is not generally used by cancer registries.

This classification is modified from the previous WHO classification, taking into account changes in our understanding of these lesions.

* Codes marked with an asterisk were approved by the IARC/WHO Committee for ICD-O at its meeting in April 2019.

TNM staging of adenocarcinomas of the appendix

Appendix
(ICD-O-3 C18.1)

Rules for Classification
The classification applies to adenocarcinomas of the appendix. Neuroendocrine carcinomas are classified separately (p. 20). There should be histological confirmation of the disease and separation of carcinomas into mucinous and non-mucinous adenocarcinomas.

Goblet cell carcinoids are classified according to the carcinoma scheme. Grading is of particular importance for mucinous tumours.

The following are the procedures for assessing T, N, and M categories.

T categories	Physical examination, imaging, and/or surgical exploration
N categories	Physical examination, imaging, and/or surgical exploration
M categories	Physical examination, imaging, and/or surgical exploration

Anatomical Site
Appendix (C18.1)

Regional Lymph Nodes
The ileocolic are the regional lymph nodes.

TNM Clinical Classification
T – Primary Tumour

TX	Primary tumour cannot be assessed
T0	No evidence of primary tumour
Tis	Carcinoma in situ: intraepithelial or invasion of lamina propria[a]
Tis (LAMN)	Low-grade appendiceal mucinous neoplasm confined to the appendix (defined as involvement by acellular mucin or mucinous epithelium that may extend into muscularis propria)
T1	Tumour invades submucosa
T2	Tumour invades muscularis propria
T3	Tumour invades subserosa or mesoappendix
T4	Tumour perforates visceral peritoneum, including mucinous peritoneal tumour or acellular mucin on the serosa of the appendix or mesoappendix and/or directly invades other organs or structures[b,c,d]
	T4a Tumour perforates visceral peritoneum, including mucinous peritoneal tumour or acellular mucin on the serosa of the appendix or mesoappendix
	T4b Tumour directly invades other organs or structures

Notes
[a] Tis includes cancer cells confined within the glandular basement membrane (intraepithelial) or lamina propria (intramucosal) with no extension through muscularis mucosae into submucosa.

[b] Direct invasion in T4 includes invasion of other intestinal segments by way of the serosa, e.g., invasion of ileum.

[c] Tumour that is adherent to other organs or structures, macroscopically, is classified cT4b. However, if no tumour is present in the adhesion, microscopically, the classification should be pT1, 2, or 3.

[d] LAMN with involvement of the subserosa or the serosal surface (visceral peritoneum) should be classified as T3 or T4a respectively.

N – Regional Lymph Nodes

NX	Regional lymph nodes cannot be assessed
N0	No regional lymph node metastasis
N1	Metastasis in 1 to 3 regional lymph nodes
	N1a Metastases in 1 regional lymph node
	N1b Metastases in 2–3 regional lymph nodes
	N1c Tumour deposit(s), i.e. satellites,* in the subserosa, or in non-peritonealized pericolic or perirectal soft tissue *without* regional lymph node metastasis
N2	Metastasis in 4 or more regional lymph nodes

Note
* Tumour deposits (satellites) are discrete macroscopic or microscopic nodules of cancer in the pericolorectal adipose tissue's lymph drainage area of a primary carcinoma that are discontinuous from the primary and without histological evidence of residual lymph node or identifiable vascular or neural structures. If a vessel wall is identifiable on H&E, elastic or other stains, it should be classified as venous invasion (V1/2) or lymphatic invasion (L1). Similarly, if neural structures are identifiable, the lesion should be classified as perineural invasion (Pn1).

M – Distant Metastasis

M0	No distant metastasis
M1	Distant metastasis
	M1a Intraperitoneal acellular mucin only
	M1b Intraperitoneal metastasis only, including mucinous epithelium
	M1c Non-peritoneal metastasis

The information presented here has been excerpted from the 2017 *TNM classification of malignant tumours*, eighth edition (408,3385A). © 2017 UICC. A help desk for specific questions about the TNM classification is available at https://www.uicc.org/tnm-help-desk.

Chapter 5

pTNM Pathological Classification

The pT and pN categories correspond to the T and N categories.

pN0   Histological examination of a regional lymphadenectomy specimen will ordinarily include 12 or more lymph nodes. If the lymph nodes are negative, but the number ordinarily examined is not met, classify as pN0.

pM – Distant Metastasis*

pM1   Distant metastasis microscopically confirmed

Note
* pM0 and pMX are not valid categories.

Stage

Stage					
Stage 0		Tis	N0	M0	
Stage 0		Tis(LAMN)	N0	M0	
Stage I		T1,T2	N0	M0	
Stage IIA		T3	N0	M0	
	IIB	T4a	N0	M0	
	IIC	T4b	N0	M0	
Stage IIIA		T1,T2	N1	M0	
	IIIB	T3,T4	N1	M0	
	IIIC	Any T	N2	M0	
Stage IVA		Any T	Any N	M1a	Any G
		Any T	Any N	M1b	G1
	IVB	Any T	Any N	M1b	G2,G3,GX
Stage IVC		Any T	Any N	M1c	Any G

Note: Neuroendocrine tumours (NETs) of the appendix are staged using the NET-specific TNM staging system, which is presented in Chapter 1 (p. 20).

Tumours of the appendix: Introduction

Washington MK
Nagtegaal ID

The most common tumours of the appendix are of epithelial and mesenchymal origin. Haematolymphoid tumours are rare at this site. Appendiceal neuroendocrine tumours (NETs) are common and often discovered incidentally (see *Appendiceal neuroendocrine neoplasms*, p. 152). The appendix is also the site of mucinous neoplasms, usually of low grade, which can generate abundant mucin that accumulates in the peritoneal cavity. Colorectal-type adenocarcinomas are relatively rare in the appendix; when they occur, they resemble their colorectal counterparts morphologically and genetically. The ICD-O topographical coding for the anatomical sites covered in this chapter is presented in Box 5.01.

In this fifth-edition volume, epithelial tumours of the appendix have been broadly classified as serrated lesions and polyps, mucinous neoplasms, adenocarcinomas, and neuroendocrine neoplasms (NENs), reflecting our current understanding of the behaviour and genetic findings associated with these lesions. The nomenclature for non-invasive lesions and polyps of the appendix now reflects that of their colorectal counterparts. The term "serrated lesion" is preferred to "serrated adenoma" or "serrated polyp". The term "hyperplastic polyp" is retained.

The term "low-grade mucinous neoplasm" is recommended for lesions formerly classified as mucinous tumour of uncertain malignant potential, mucinous cystadenocarcinoma, or

Box 5.01 ICD-O topographical coding for the anatomical sites covered in this chapter

C18 Colon
  C18.1 Appendix
  C18.8 Overlapping lesion of the colon

mucinous cystadenoma; this recommendation is based on growing consensus regarding the nomenclature for these lesions {511} and their inclusion in current TNM staging systems {408}. High-grade appendiceal mucinous neoplasm is now recognized as a subtype of appendiceal mucinous neoplasm.

Goblet cell carcinoid/carcinoma has been renamed goblet cell adenocarcinoma because of its composition predominantly of mucin-secreting cells and minor component of neuroendocrine cells. These tumours are staged according to the Union for International Cancer Control (UICC) system for appendiceal adenocarcinomas rather than with appendiceal NETs, because of their more-aggressive course.

The nomenclature for appendiceal NETs remains largely unchanged from the previous edition of this WHO classification, with the exception of the term "tubular NET", which was previously "tubular carcinoid". The grading system for appendiceal NETs has been revised to include G3 NETs, in alignment with the grading of other gastrointestinal NETs.

Appendiceal serrated lesions and polyps

Misdraji J
Carr NJ
Pai RK (Reetesh)

Definition
Appendiceal serrated lesions and polyps are mucosal epithelial polyps characterized by a serrated (sawtooth or stellate) architecture of the crypt lumen.

ICD-O coding
8213/0 Serrated dysplasia, low grade
8213/2 Serrated dysplasia, high grade
    Hyperplastic polyp
    Sessile serrated lesion without dysplasia

ICD-11 coding
2E92.4Y & DB35.0 Other specified benign neoplasm of the large intestine & Hyperplastic polyp of large intestine

Related terminology
Not recommended: diffuse mucosal hyperplasia; serrated adenoma; sessile serrated polyp/adenoma.

Subtype(s)
None

Localization
Serrated lesions and polyps can occur throughout the appendix.

Clinical features
Most serrated lesions and hyperplastic polyps (HPs) are incidental findings detected in appendices removed for other reasons. Large lesions may cause obstruction and lead to appendicitis, potentially complicated by rupture.

Epidemiology
Appendiceal serrated polyps occur in men and women with about equal frequency. Patients are generally older adults, in their sixth to eighth decade of life, although there is a wide age range {3679,2488}.

Etiology
Unknown

Pathogenesis
HPs and mucosal hyperplasia can be seen in postinflammatory reparative settings, including after an episode of acute appendicitis, in diverticular disease of the appendix, and in interval appendectomy. However, genetic alterations raise the possibility that some of these polyps are neoplastic. *KRAS* or *BRAF* mutations are found in some hyperplastic lesions {3679,2488}. *KRAS* mutations are frequent in serrated polyps of the appendix, particularly in serrated polyps with dysplasia. *BRAF* mutations are less common but have been found in a subset of serrated polyps {3679,2488}. These studies suggest that KRAS may be more biologically important in the appendix than BRAF,

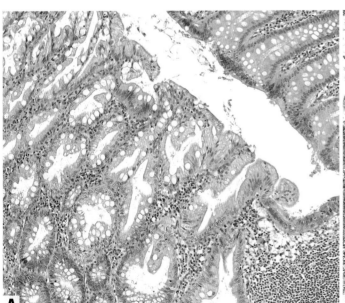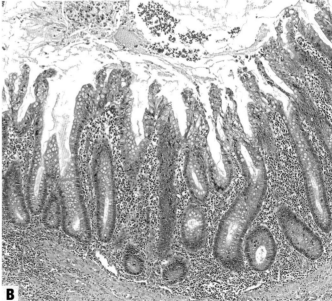

Fig. 5.01 Hyperplastic polyp of the appendix. **A** High-power view of a hyperplastic polyp (bottom) and adjacent normal crypts (right); the crypts in the hyperplastic polyp show serration of the luminal aspect of the crypt and no dysplasia. **B** The mucosa does not protrude above the surface, but the crypts show serrated profiles towards their luminal aspects.

Table 5.01 Histological and molecular features of appendiceal serrated lesions and polyps

Polyp type	Histological features			Molecular features	
	Crypts	Cytological dysplasia	Architecture	*KRAS* mutation	*BRAF* mutation
Hyperplastic polyp	Straight crypts with serration limited to luminal aspect of the crypt	Absent	Discrete polyp or circumferential mucosal involvement; villous growth uncommon	Often present	Rarely present
Serrated lesion without dysplasia	Distorted crypts with serration and crypt dilatation extending to crypt bases	Absent	Often with circumferential mucosal involvement; villous growth uncommon	Typically present	Rarely present
Serrated lesion with dysplasia	Distorted crypts with serration and crypt dilatation extending to crypt bases	Present	Often with circumferential mucosal involvement; villous growth variable	Typically present	Rarely present

and that the serrated pathway of carcinogenesis may have less relevance in the appendix than in the colon.

Macroscopic appearance

Serrated lesions may form a discrete polyp or may circumferentially involve the appendiceal mucosa.

Histopathology

In appendiceal HPs, similar to in colonic HPs, the affected mucosa shows elongated crypts with increased numbers of goblet cells or a mixture of goblet cells and columnar cells with smaller mucin vacuoles {1228,2625}. The luminal part of the crypts shows a serrated crypt profile. Cytological atypia is mild at most, generally in the deep crypts, and can be attributed to reactive changes. Cytological dysplasia is not present.

In serrated lesions without dysplasia, the mucosa demonstrates abnormal crypt proliferation with elongated and serrated crypt profiles. Serration and dilation extend to the crypt bases with abnormal shapes including L shapes and inverted T shapes. Varying degrees of villous architecture may be seen. There may be mild cytological atypia with dystrophic goblet

cells and possibly more mitotic figures than would be seen in an HP. Luminal mucin may be abundant {292,2776}.

In serrated lesions with dysplasia, dysplasia can take the form of conventional adenoma–like dysplasia, serrated dysplasia, or traditional serrated adenoma–like dysplasia, and multiple morphological patterns of dysplasia may be seen within a single polyp {3679}. The dysplastic component may be well demarcated from non-dysplastic areas of the serrated polyp. Conventional adenoma–like dysplasia usually develops a villous growth pattern with elongated, hyperchromatic nuclei with pseudostratification, increased mitoses, and apoptotic bodies, similar to in colorectal adenomas. Serrated dysplasia maintains the serrated architecture of the crypts, but the crypts are lined by cuboidal to low columnar cells with hyperchromatic enlarged nuclei, reduced cytoplasmic mucin, and increased mitoses. Traditional serrated adenoma–like dysplasia shows complex serration and villous growth, with the villi lined by tall columnar cells with eosinophilic cytoplasm. The nuclei are elongated and mildly hyperchromatic, but the degree of atypia is less than in conventional adenoma–like dysplasia. The villi may have abortive-type crypts along their lateral edges, which

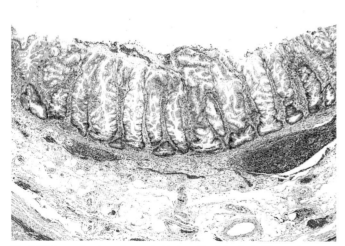

Fig. 5.02 Appendiceal sessile serrated lesion without dysplasia. The crypts are serrated and the base of the crypts shows abnormal architecture, with crypt dilatation and inverted T shapes.

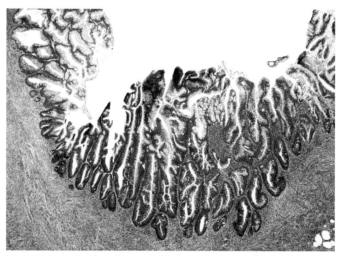

Fig. 5.03 Appendiceal sessile serrated lesion with adenoma-like dysplasia. In the centre of the field, the polyp shows hyperchromatic pseudostratified nuclei consistent with dysplasia, whereas at the sides of the image, the polyp is serrated but lacks cytological dysplasia.

has also been described in traditional serrated adenomas in the colorectum. The dysplasia can be classified as low-grade or high-grade.

Like serrated lesions and polyps, low-grade appendiceal mucinous neoplasms (LAMNs) can show serrated architecture, but they usually show areas with long filiform villi without serration. In contrast to LAMN, which often results in loss of the lamina propria and muscularis mucosae as well as mural fibrosis, serrated polyps retain the normal architecture of the appendix and typically have an intact muscularis mucosae and lamina propria. In addition, tumours with pushing invasion and submucosal fibrosis or dissemination to the peritoneum as pseudomyxoma peritonei are probably LAMNs and should not be classified as serrated polyps. Some tumours are heterogeneous, with areas resembling serrated polyp and other areas resembling LAMN; in such cases, the lesion is best classified as LAMN.

Cytology
Not clinically relevant

Diagnostic molecular pathology
Not clinically relevant

Essential and desirable diagnostic criteria
See Table 5.01.

Staging (TNM)
Not clinically relevant

Prognosis and prediction
Not clinically relevant

Appendiceal mucinous neoplasm

Misdraji J
Carr NJ
Pai RK (Reetesh)

Definition

Mucinous neoplasm of the appendix is an appendiceal neoplasm characterized by mucinous epithelial proliferation with extracellular mucin and pushing tumour margins.

ICD-O coding

8480/1 Low-grade appendiceal mucinous neoplasm
8480/2 High-grade appendiceal mucinous neoplasm

ICD-11 coding

2E92.4Y & XH0EK3 Other specified benign neoplasm of the large intestine & Mucinous cystic neoplasm with low-grade dysplasia
2E61.Y & XH81P3 Carcinoma in situ of other specified digestive organs & Mucinous cystic tumour with high-grade dysplasia

Related terminology

Not recommended: mucinous tumour of uncertain malignant potential; mucinous cystadenoma of the appendix; borderline tumour of the appendix; mucinous cystadenocarcinoma of the appendix.

Subtype(s)

None

Localization

Appendiceal mucinous neoplasm is a mucinous neoplasm occurring in the appendix.

Clinical features

Patients can present with features of appendicitis, with or without appendiceal perforation. The clinical presentations of patients with peritoneal dissemination may include progressive abdominal distention, new onset of an umbilical hernia, or a palpable mass on abdominal or pelvic examination. CT or ultrasound may show a soft tissue mass in the appendix that may appear fluid-filled. Curvilinear calcification of the wall increases specificity but is present in only about half of all cases.

Epidemiology

Appendiceal mucinous neoplasms tend to occur in adults in their sixth decade of life, but there is a wide age range. They occur in men and women with roughly equal frequency.

Etiology

Unknown

Pathogenesis

The vast majority of low-grade appendiceal mucinous neoplasms (LAMNs) have *KRAS* mutations {3737}, and the majority have *GNAS* mutations {2372,2077,1165,1932,2565,3053}. However, *GNAS* mutations are somewhat less common in high-grade mucinous tumours, suggesting that they may not arise from low-grade tumours {79,3053}. *GNAS* mutations may play a role in the abundant mucin production in these tumours {3053}. Mutations typical of colorectal carcinoma, such as *APC*, *TP53*, and *SMAD4* mutations, are not common in appendiceal mucinous neoplasms, and are more common in high-grade tumours {725,79,1932}. Other mutations have been described in a minority of cases, including mutations in *FAT4*, *SMAD2*, *AKT1*, *MET*, *JAK3*, *PIK3CA*, *STK11*, and *RB1* {1932,2565}. The mutation profile shows an excess of C→T transitions, suggesting that deamination of 5-methylcytosine is a mutational mechanism in these tumours {2565,79}. Microsatellite instability, *BRAF* mutations, and loss of DNA mismatch repair protein expression are not features of LAMN {3737,2174}.

Macroscopic appearance

The appendix may appear grossly unremarkable or demonstrate dilatation as a result of abnormal accumulation of mucin. Gross perforation with mucin extrusion may be evident. The wall may be attenuated, or markedly thickened and partially calcified.

Histopathology

The microscopic appearance of LAMN can take several forms. The classic pattern is replacement of the normal appendiceal mucosa by a filiform villous mucinous epithelial proliferation. The tumour cells tend to have tall cytoplasmic mucin vacuoles that compress the nucleus, creating a hypermucinous but cytologically bland appearance. Other tumours may show an undulating or scalloped appearance, with columnar epithelial cells with nuclear pseudostratification growing on fibrotic submucosal tissue. Some cases are characterized by an attenuated or flattened monolayer of mucinous epithelium. The degree of atypia is mild, resembling low-grade colonic dysplasia at most. The lymphoid tissue of the appendix is usually absent. The wall can have varying degrees of fibrosis, hyalinization, and calcification. The mucin can dissect through the structures of the appendix and extend to the peritoneal surface or cause rupture of the appendix. Intramural glandular epithelium protruding into or through the appendiceal wall and exhibiting a rounded, pushing pattern of invasion can occur. If an infiltrative pattern is observed, this qualifies as adenocarcinoma. Serosal involvement can consist of mucin at the surface, or it can consist of replacement of a portion of the appendix with a hyalinizing reaction with strips of low-grade mucinous epithelial cells associated with extracellular mucin {2486,2175,512}.

High-grade appendiceal mucinous neoplasm (HAMN) is rare. It shows histological features similar to those of LAMN, including subepithelial fibrosis, a broad pushing margin, broad-front pushing invasion, rupture, and peritoneal dissemination, but the neoplastic epithelium has unequivocal high-grade features {511}. Architecturally, the neoplastic epithelium may show

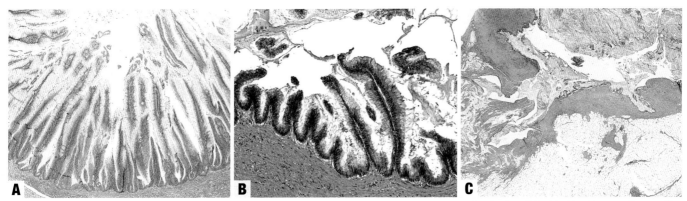

Fig. 5.04 Low-grade appendiceal mucinous neoplasm. **A** The appendiceal mucosa is replaced by a villous tumour with slender villi lined by bland hypermucinous epithelium. **B** The typical appearance, with slender villi lined by tall mucinous epithelial cells with low-grade cytological atypia. **C** Low-power view exhibiting a pushing margin; note that the tumour lines a jagged and fibrotic appendiceal wall but lacks infiltrative-type invasion. On the left, the tumour has perforated through the appendix, showing dissecting mucin with fibrosis and epithelial cells, consistent with localized pseudomyxoma peritonei.

micropapillary features, cribriforming, or piling up of the epithelial cells, but most often a single layer of cells is present. The epithelial cells in HAMNs have enlarged, hyperchromatic, and pleomorphic nuclei. Mitotic figures may be frequent, including atypical mitoses. There may be more single-cell necrosis of the epithelial cells or sloughing of necrotic epithelial cells into the lumen of the appendix.

Ruptured diverticular disease of the appendix often shows mucin extrusion onto the appendix surface and hyperplastic changes of the mucosa that are frequently misinterpreted as LAMN. Appendices with diverticular disease show mucosal alterations but maintained crypts separated by lamina propria, maintained lymphoid tissue, and often a Schwann cell proliferation in the lamina propria {1315}. Serrated polyps generally have complex serration and lack the filiform villous pattern or undulating pattern. Serrated polyps typically maintain the mucosal architecture of the appendix and are not associated with mucin dissection through the wall or pseudomyxoma peritonei. Mucinous adenocarcinoma shows at least focal destructive or infiltrative invasion characterized by pools of mucin with floating clusters or strips of epithelium, cribriform glands, or infiltrative glands with desmoplastic stromal response. Dissemination to the peritoneal cavity occurs in both HAMN and mucinous adenocarcinoma, and it should not be the sole factor in distinguishing the two.

Cytology
Not clinically relevant

Diagnostic molecular pathology
Not clinically relevant

Essential and desirable diagnostic criteria
LAMN
Essential: a filiform or villous mucinous epithelium with tall cytoplasmic mucin vacuoles and compressed bland nuclei or epithelial undulations/scalloping with columnar cells with nuclear pseudostratification (the mucinous epithelium could also be monolayered and attenuated, with only mild atypia); a broad pushing margin; various degrees of extracellular mucin (with absent lymphoid tissue), fibrosis, hyalinization, and calcification of the appendiceal wall.

Table 5.02 Histological criteria for grading appendiceal mucinous neoplasms and adenocarcinomas and their peritoneal metastases

Tumour grade[a]	Histological criteria	
	In the appendiceal primary tumour	**In the peritoneal metastasis**
1	Low-grade cytology with a pushing margin (low-grade appendiceal mucinous neoplasm)	Hypocellular mucinous deposits Neoplastic epithelial elements have low-grade cytology No infiltrative-type invasion
2	High-grade cytology with a pushing margin (high-grade appendiceal mucinous neoplasm) Invasive mucinous adenocarcinoma without a signet-ring cell component	Hypercellular mucinous deposits as judged at 20× magnification High-grade cytological features Infiltrative-type invasion characterized by jagged or angulated glands in a desmoplastic stroma, or a small mucin pool pattern with numerous mucin pools containing clusters of tumour cells
3	Signet-ring cell adenocarcinoma, with numerous signet-ring cells in mucin pools or infiltrating tissue	Mucinous tumour deposits with signet-ring cells[b]

[a]Generally, the grade of the appendiceal tumour and the peritoneal tumour are concordant. Rarely, they are discordant. In discordant cases, the grade of the appendiceal and peritoneal tumour deposits should be separately reported. The grade of the peritoneal tumour is likely to have a greater effect on prognosis than that of the appendiceal primary tumour. [b]The presence of signet-ring cells in peritoneal mucin may be prognostically significant even if they do not constitute 50% of the tumour. However, signet-ring cells floating in mucin may not have the prognostic significance of signet-ring cells infiltrating tissue. Signet-ring cells in mucin must be distinguished from degenerate tumour cells in the mucin (pseudo–signet-ring cells). In some cases of signet-ring cell adenocarcinoma, the primary appendiceal tumour may be a goblet cell adenocarcinoma.

HAMN

Essential: Histological features similar to those of LAMN, with the addition of micropapillary features, cribriforming, piling up of epithelial cells with high-grade features (i.e. enlarged, hyperchromatic, and pleomorphic nuclei; numerous atypical mitotic figures; single-cell necrosis; and sloughed necrotic epithelial cells in the lumen of the appendix).

Note: See also Table 5.02 (p. 145).

Staging (TNM)

According to the Union for International Cancer Control (UICC) staging system, LAMN and HAMN are considered in situ (pTis) if confined to the submucosa and muscularis propria. A tumour that extends into subserosa is staged as pT3. Tumours that perforate the serosa and involve the appendiceal serosa are considered pT4a. HAMN is staged using the same staging system as invasive appendiceal adenocarcinoma. Mucin and/or epithelial cells that involve peritoneal surfaces beyond the appendix are staged as pM1a if the mucin is acellular and pM1b if the mucin contains mucinous epithelial cells.

Prognosis and prediction

The prognosis of LAMN is highly stage-dependent, with tumours limited to the appendix having an excellent prognosis and those with peritoneal dissemination having a variable prognosis {512,3680,2486}. The prognosis in disseminated tumours depends on the grade of the peritoneal mucinous epithelium {2753,393}, the extent of disease, and the ability to achieve complete cytoreduction of macroscopically visible tumour within the abdomen {3720}. The addition of hyperthermic intraperitoneal chemotherapy (HIPEC) together with complete cytoreduction has increased survival {3163}.

HAMNs are rare, and there are limited data regarding their natural history when they are confined to the appendix. Currently, the management of patients with HAMNs confined to the appendix and the role of additional surgery are uncertain. HAMNs that have disseminated to the peritoneal cavity are likely to behave like other mucinous tumours that have spread to the peritoneum.

Appendiceal adenocarcinoma

Misdraji J
Carr NJ
Pai RK (Reetesh)

Definition

Appendiceal adenocarcinoma is a malignant glandular neoplasm characterized by invasion.

ICD-O coding

8140/3 Adenocarcinoma NOS

ICD-11 coding

2B81.0 Adenocarcinoma of appendix
2B81.1 Mucinous adenocarcinoma of appendix

Related terminology

Not recommended: mucinous cystadenocarcinoma.

Subtype(s)

Signet-ring cell adenocarcinoma (8490/3); mucinous adenocarcinoma (8480/3); carcinoma, undifferentiated, NOS (8020/3)

Localization

Appendiceal adenocarcinoma can occur anywhere along the appendix.

Clinical features

Patients usually present with appendicitis or abdominal pain, but they can also present with a palpable mass, obstruction, gastrointestinal bleeding, or symptoms attributable to metastases.

Epidemiology

Appendiceal adenocarcinomas typically affect patients in their fifth to seventh decade of life. In the USA, in both the SEER Program database and National Cancer Database (NCDB), there is a slight female predominance for mucinous adenocarcinoma (53–57% female) but a slight male predominance for non-mucinous adenocarcinoma (55% male). Surprisingly, signet-ring cell adenocarcinoma had a female predominance (62–64%). These sex differences were statistically significant {2470,196}.

Etiology

Unknown

Pathogenesis

Mucinous adenocarcinomas exhibit *KRAS* exon 2 mutations in 60–80% of cases {724,2379,1932,1046} and *GNAS* mutations in approximately 30–70% of cases {1046,2379,1932,3053}, resulting in *KRAS* co-mutation identified in 65–85% of cases with *GNAS* mutation {1046,3053}. The presence of these mutations does not affect survival in patients with disseminated intraperitoneal disease. *BRAF* mutations and microsatellite instability are rarely identified in mucinous adenocarcinoma {724,2379,1932,2395}. Non-mucinous adenocarcinoma can demonstrate high levels of microsatellite instability {3203}. The

pathogenesis of signet-ring cell adenocarcinoma is unknown; they less frequently harbour *KRAS* and *GNAS* mutations {724}.

Macroscopic appearance

The appendix may be dilated due to obstruction of the lumen. The tumour may be polypoid, ulcerative, or infiltrative, and appendiceal perforation may be evident.

Histopathology

Non-mucinous adenocarcinoma NOS shows irregular or jagged glands infiltrating the wall of the appendix, with a desmoplastic stromal response. Most cases have glands lined with columnar cells and some degree of extracellular mucin. The morphology may resemble colorectal adenocarcinoma, with glands lined with columnar cells containing hyperchromatic nuclei, as well as dirty necrosis (in intestinal-type cases). Rarely, the morphology resembles pancreatobiliary adenocarcinoma, with glands lined with columnar cells containing pale cytoplasm and irregular nuclei. Mucinous adenocarcinoma is a carcinoma with

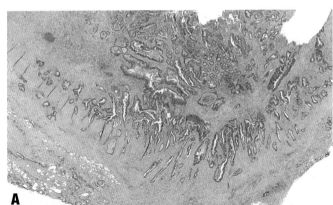

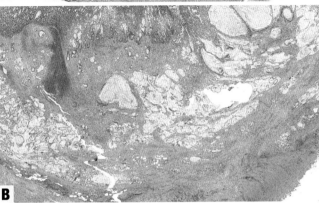

Fig. 5.05 Invasive adenocarcinoma of the appendix. **A** Low-power view; the tumour is composed of glands lined by columnar cells with hyperchromatic nuclei and luminal necrosis, identical to colorectal adenocarcinoma. **B** Mucinous adenocarcinoma, low-power view; the tumour is composed of infiltrating glands, with abundant extracellular mucin forming pools.

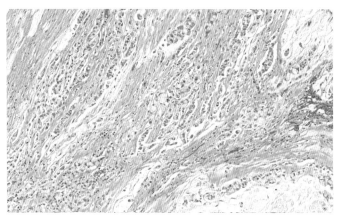

Fig. 5.06 Signet-ring cell adenocarcinoma of the appendix. Medium-power view shows infiltration of the wall of the appendix by mucinous cells as single cells in chains and ribbons. Extracellular mucin is often present and can be abundant. Unlike in high-grade goblet cell carcinoma, no low-grade goblet cell carcinoma component is present in this tumour.

extracellular mucin composing > 50% of the tumour. The mucin pools contain floating strips, glands, or clusters of mucinous epithelial cells. Signet-ring cell adenocarcinoma of the appendix resembles signet-ring cell tumours elsewhere; > 50% of the tumour consists of signet-ring cells, which may be present in large numbers in mucin pools or may invade tissue. Undifferentiated carcinomas of the appendix are rare. Their histology is analogous to that of undifferentiated carcinomas of the colorectum.

Mucinous tumours, including low-grade appendiceal mucinous neoplasm (LAMN), high-grade appendiceal mucinous neoplasm (HAMN), and mucinous adenocarcinomas, are graded according to a three-tiered grading system (Table 5.02, p. 145) {724}. Grade 1 tumours are LAMNs. Conventional mucinous adenocarcinomas qualify as grade 2. Tumours with unequivocal signet-ring cells qualify as grade 3. Non-mucinous adenocarcinomas are graded using a two-tiered grading system, similar to that for colorectal cancer.

LAMN can be distinguished from mucinous adenocarcinoma by the pattern of invasion. LAMN invades with a broad tumour front, with hyalinization and fibrosis of the underlying tissue. Mucinous adenocarcinoma generally shows more crowded, expansile mucin pools, which contain detached strips, glands, and clusters of atypical neoplastic cells. Like LAMN, HAMN can be distinguished from mucinous adenocarcinoma by the pattern of invasion. However, high-grade mucinous tumours are often at least focally invasive, which becomes apparent when the entire appendix is examined; therefore, examining the entire appendix is recommended when the differential diagnosis includes HAMN.

High-grade goblet cell adenocarcinomas can resemble signet-ring cell adenocarcinomas or other poorly differentiated adenocarcinomas. High-grade goblet cell adenocarcinomas have at least focal areas that are diagnostic of low-grade goblet cell adenocarcinoma.

Cytology
Not clinically relevant

Diagnostic molecular pathology
Molecular investigation may be warranted to underpin treatment, but there is insufficient evidence to make firm recommendations.

Essential and desirable diagnostic criteria
Essential: irregular malignant glands infiltrating the stroma (eliciting a desmoplastic response).
Note: The subtypes have specific morphological features (see *Histopathology*, above).

Staging (TNM)
Staging is performed according to the eighth edition of the TNM classification {408}. Tumour deposits, which are only considered in the absence of nodal metastases, categorize a tumour as N1c. The presence of distant metastases categorizes a tumour as M1a (intraperitoneal acellular mucin only), M1b (intraperitoneal metastases only, including mucinous epithelium), or M1c (non-peritoneal metastases).

Prognosis and prediction
The 5-year survival rate for patients with appendiceal carcinoma ranges from 19% to 55% {560,2374}. Patients with mucinous adenocarcinomas have a better outcome than those with non-mucinous adenocarcinomas {680,2374}. Histological grade has repeatedly been shown to be an independent prognostic factor in mucinous adenocarcinoma: grade 2 and 3 tumours have overall 5-year survival rates of 30–60% and 20–30%, respectively {724,2983,196}.

Appendiceal goblet cell adenocarcinoma

Misdraji J
Carr NJ
Pai RK (Reetesh)

Definition

Appendiceal goblet cell adenocarcinoma is an amphicrine tumour composed of goblet-like mucinous cells, as well as variable numbers of endocrine cells and Paneth-like cells, typically arranged as tubules resembling intestinal crypts.

ICD-O coding

8243/3 Goblet cell adenocarcinoma

ICD-11 coding

2B81 & XH4262 Malignant neoplasms of appendix & Goblet cell adenocarcinoma

Related terminology

Acceptable: goblet cell carcinoma.
Not recommended: goblet cell carcinoid; crypt cell carcinoma; microglandular carcinoma; adenocarcinoid.

Subtype(s)

None

Localization

Appendiceal goblet cell adenocarcinoma most often involves the distal appendix.

Clinical features

The tumour usually presents with symptoms of appendicitis or nonspecific abdominal pain, but it can also be found incidentally in appendices removed for other indications. The tumour may also present as an abdominal mass, particularly in women with metastatic disease to the ovaries.

Epidemiology

Males and females are affected equally, although in some series women outnumber men. Patients are adults aged 30–85 years, with a mean age of 50–60 years {3202,3255,3721}.

Etiology

Unknown

Pathogenesis

In one study, genetic profiling of goblet cell adenocarcinomas revealed mutations in genes in the WNT signalling pathway (*USP9X*, *NOTCH1*, *CTNNA1*, *CTNNB1*, and *TRRAP*) {1449}. Other studies have shown mutations in chromatin remodelling genes, including *ARID1A*, *ARID2*, *KDM6A*, and *KMT2D* (*MLL2*) {3545,1472}. A subset of cases have mutations in genes associated with gastric signet-ring cell adenocarcinomas, such as *CDH1* and *RHOA* {1472,3545}. Mutations in genes typical of colorectal adenocarcinoma (*KRAS*, *APC*, and *SMAD4*) are rare in goblet cell adenocarcinomas {3545,1449,1472,3124}. *TP53*

Table 5.03 The three-tiered grading system for goblet cell adenocarcinoma, based on the proportion of the tumour that consists of low-grade and high-grade patterns

Grade	Tubular or clustered growth (low-grade pattern)	Loss of tubular or clustered growth (any combination of high-grade patterns)
1	> 75%	< 25%
2	50–75%	25–50%
3	< 50%	> 50%

mutations may be found in high-grade goblet cell adenocarcinomas {2651,3255,1472}.

Macroscopic appearance

The appendix may be grossly normal or thickened, and the tumour is easily overlooked macroscopically. High-grade large tumours may appear infiltrative and indurated.

Histopathology

To be classified as a goblet cell adenocarcinoma, a tumour must demonstrate at least a component of classic low-grade goblet cell adenocarcinoma. The tumour usually involves the wall of the appendix circumferentially, without eliciting a stromal reaction. The classic low-grade tumour grows as tubules composed of goblet-like mucinous cells, variable numbers of endocrine cells, and Paneth-like cells with granular eosinophilic cytoplasm. Some tumour cell clusters lack lumina and appear as small groups of cohesive goblet-like cells. Mild architectural disarray or tubular fusion can be seen. Nuclear atypia is mild and mitoses are infrequent. Extracellular mucin is often present and sometimes abundant.

High-grade histological features include tumour cells infiltrating as single mucinous or non-mucinous cells, complex anastomosing tubules, cribriform masses, sheets of tumour cells, and large aggregates of goblet-like or signet-ring–like cells. In some cases, conventional adenocarcinoma may be seen, with irregular glands lined by columnar cells with malignant-appearing nuclei. Desmoplastic stromal response, high-grade cytological features, numerous mitoses with atypical mitotic figures, and necrosis may be present in high-grade areas.

Perineural invasion is common among all grades and is not prognostically significant. Lymphovascular invasion is more common in high-grade tumours.

Staining for chromogranin and synaptophysin highlights variable numbers of endocrine cells, but these stains are not required for diagnosis.

Goblet cell adenocarcinoma is graded using a three-tiered system, which is summarized in Table 5.03 {443,3202,3721}. High-grade tumours are characterized by loss of the tubular or clustered growth pattern; they may resemble signet-ring cell adenocarcinomas or other types of adenocarcinomas.

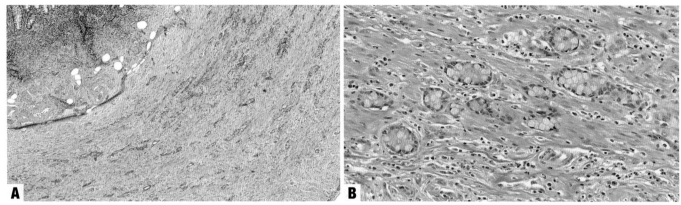

Fig. 5.07 Goblet cell carcinoma, grade 1. **A** Low-power view; the tumour infiltrates the muscularis propria of the appendix without eliciting a desmoplastic stromal response. The tumour is composed of clusters of cuboidal cells and goblet-like mucinous cells in discrete, clustered units. No high-grade growth is seen in this example. **B** High-power view of classic low-grade goblet cell carcinoma shows cohesive clusters of tumour cells with goblet-like mucinous cells resembling intestinal crypts.

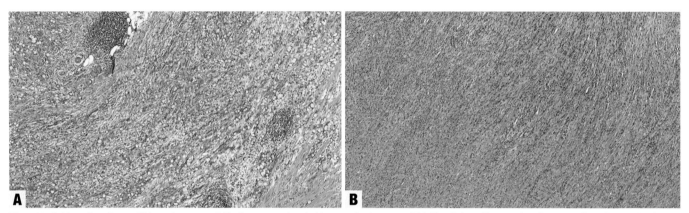

Fig. 5.08 Goblet cell carcinoma, high-grade pattern. **A** Medium-power view; in this example, the tumour is highly cellular, with streaming of tumour cells and loss of the discrete clustered units of low-grade goblet cell carcinoma. The grade of the tumour is determined by the percentage of tumour with high-grade growth. **B** In this high-grade area, the tumour is growing as linear arrays of single, highly atypical cells, with no attempt to form tubular or clustered groups. The overall grade of the tumour is determined by the tumour percentage that shows high-grade features.

Signet-ring cell adenocarcinoma shows widespread (> 50%) discohesive and disorganized growth of signet-ring cells with high-grade cytological features. Signet-ring cell adenocarcinoma differs from high-grade goblet cell adenocarcinoma by the absence of a recognizable low-grade goblet cell adenocarcinoma component. The term "mixed adenoneuroendocrine carcinoma" implies separate adenocarcinoma and high-grade neuroendocrine components, each of which constitutes ≥ 30% of the tumour. This term is best avoided in the context of goblet cell adenocarcinoma. Metastatic adenocarcinoma to the appendix can resemble goblet cell adenocarcinoma.

Cytology
Not clinically relevant

Diagnostic molecular pathology
Not clinically relevant

Essential and desirable diagnostic criteria
Low-grade goblet cell adenocarcinoma
Essential: tubules of goblet-like mucinous cells; endocrine and Paneth-like cells with granular eosinophilic cytoplasm, mild nuclear atypia, and infrequent mitoses (tubular fusion and small groups of cohesive goblet-like cells may also be seen); extracellular mucin (which may be abundant); circumferential involvement of the appendix wall by tumour cells, without a stromal reaction.

High-grade histological features
Essential: tumour cells infiltrating as single mucinous or non-mucinous cells, complex anastomosing tubules, cribriform masses, sheets, or large aggregates of goblet-like or signet-ring–like cells with high-grade cytological features, numerous mitoses with atypical mitotic figures, and necrosis (a conventional adenocarcinoma component is seen in some cases); desmoplastic stromal response.

Staging (TNM)

The staging of appendiceal goblet cell adenocarcinoma is identical to that of appendiceal adenocarcinomas (see *Appendiceal adenocarcinoma*, p. 147).

Prognosis and prediction

Prognosis depends on stage and tumour grade. Most patients with low-grade goblet cell adenocarcinoma present with stage I or II disease {3721,3202}, although as many as one third of patients with low-grade goblet cell adenocarcinomas presented with metastasis in one series {3255}. In contrast, 50–70% of high-grade goblet cell adenocarcinomas present with stage IV disease {3721,3202}. The most common sites of metastasis are the peritoneum, omentum, abdominal wall, and ovaries {3202,2685,3255}. Low-grade tumours have an overall survival time of 84–204 months. Intermediate-grade tumours have an overall survival time of 60–86 months. High-grade and disseminated tumours behave aggressively, with an overall survival time of 29–45 months {3202,3721,3255}. In one series, cytoreductive surgery and hyperthermic intraperitoneal chemotherapy (HIPEC) did not improve survival for patients with high-grade goblet cell adenocarcinoma {2637}.

Appendiceal neuroendocrine neoplasms

Couvelard A
Perren A
Sipos B

Definition

Neuroendocrine neoplasms (NENs) of the appendix are appendiceal epithelial neoplasms with neuroendocrine differentiation, including well-differentiated neuroendocrine tumours (NETs) and poorly differentiated neuroendocrine carcinomas (NECs). Mixed neuroendocrine–non-neuroendocrine neoplasms (MiN-ENs) are mixed epithelial neoplasms with a neuroendocrine component combined with a non-neuroendocrine component, each of which is morphologically and immunohistochemically recognizable as a discrete component and constitutes at least 30% of the neoplasm.

This section excludes goblet cell adenocarcinoma, which is no longer considered to be a subtype of NEN and is therefore discussed separately (see *Appendiceal goblet cell adenocarcinoma*, p. 149).

ICD-O coding

8240/3 Neuroendocrine tumour NOS
8246/3 Neuroendocrine carcinoma NOS
8154/3 Mixed neuroendocrine–non-neuroendocrine neoplasm (MiNEN)

ICD-11 coding

2B81.2 & XH55D7 Neuroendocrine neoplasms of appendix & Neuroendocrine carcinoma, well-differentiated
2B81.2 & XH9LV8 Neuroendocrine neoplasms of appendix & Neuroendocrine tumour, grade I
2B81.2 & XH7F73 Neuroendocrine neoplasms of appendix & Neuroendocrine carcinoma, moderately differentiated
2B81.2 & XH0U20 Neuroendocrine neoplasms of appendix & Neuroendocrine carcinoma NOS
2B81.2 & XH9SY0 Neuroendocrine neoplasms of appendix & Small cell neuroendocrine carcinoma
2B81.2 & XH0NL5 Neuroendocrine neoplasms of appendix & Large cell neuroendocrine carcinoma
2B81.2 & XH6H10 Neuroendocrine neoplasms of appendix & Mixed adenoneuroendocrine carcinoma
2B81.2 & XH7NM1 Neuroendocrine neoplasms of appendix & Enterochromaffin cell carcinoid
2B81.2 & XH7LW9 Neuroendocrine neoplasms of appendix & L-cell tumour
2B81.2 & XH7152 Neuroendocrine neoplasms of appendix & Glucagon-like peptide-producing tumour
2B81.2 & XH9ZS8 Neuroendocrine neoplasms of appendix & Pancreatic peptide and pancreatic peptide-like peptide within terminal tyrosine amide-producing tumour
2B81.2 Neuroendocrine neoplasms of appendix

Related terminology

NEN

Acceptable: carcinoid; well-differentiated endocrine tumour/carcinoma.

MiNEN

Acceptable: mixed adenoneuroendocrine carcinoma.

Subtype(s)

Neuroendocrine tumour, grade 1 (8240/3); neuroendocrine tumour, grade 2 (8249/3); neuroendocrine tumour, grade 3 (8249/3); L-cell tumour (8152/3); glucagon-like peptide-producing tumour (8152/3); PP/PYY-producing tumour (8152/3); enterochromaffin-cell carcinoid (8241/3); serotonin-producing carcinoid (8241/3); large cell neuroendocrine carcinoma (8013/3); small cell neuroendocrine carcinoma (8041/3)

Localization

Appendiceal NETs mainly occur in the tip of the appendix (in 67% of adult patients and 73% of paediatric patients) {2658,1214}. Appendiceal NECs have no specific preferential localization.

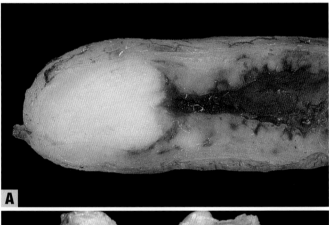

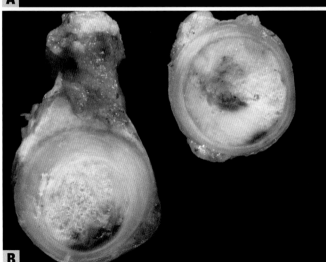

Fig. 5.09 Appendiceal neuroendocrine tumour (NET). **A** An example at the tip of the appendix, with typical yellow coloration. **B** An example infiltrating the mesoappendix.

Clinical features

There are no specific symptoms attributed to appendiceal NETs, which in 80% of cases are found incidentally after surgery for acute appendicitis {2658}. The association with carcinoid syndrome is extremely rare and is indicative of metastatic disease {2504,104,2219}. NECs often present with advanced disease, similar to other appendiceal carcinomas.

Epidemiology

A recent SEER Program database analysis classified appendiceal NET as the fifth most frequent gastrointestinal NET, after small intestine, rectum, pancreas, and stomach locations {716}. Appendiceal NETs present with an incidence of 0.15–0.6 cases per 100 000 person-years, with a slight female predominance and the highest incidence before the age of 40 years {716,2504,2219,2112}. However, epidemiological data may have some limitations, because some registries and databases have regarded these neoplasms to be benign and therefore not included, whereas others include goblet cell adenocarcinoma with the NETs {1309}. In a large recent review, appendiceal NETs were diagnosed in 1.86% of appendectomies between 2001 and 2015 {2553}. Appendiceal NETs frequently occur in children, and they have an excellent long-term outcome in this age group {1214,733}.

Etiology

Unknown

Pathogenesis

The pathogenesis of appendiceal NETs is largely unknown. They may arise from neuroendocrine cells within the mucosal crypts, but some evidence also suggests an origin from subepithelial neuroendocrine cells, particularly for enterochromaffin-cell (EC-cell) NETs, which commonly display S100-positive sustentacular-like cells surrounding the nests of neoplastic cells {1053}. Although molecular data are still limited, appendiceal NETs appear to lack mutational changes in common cancer-associated genes {3545}. Unlike in ileal NETs, chromosome 18 deletions are rare, although appendiceal NETs do show non-recurrent large copy-number changes in several other chromosomes.

Macroscopic appearance

Macroscopically, appendiceal NETs appear as well-demarcated yellowish (after formalin fixation) nodules. Because many small incidental NETs are not visible macroscopically, embedding of the entire tip of the appendix in two longitudinal pieces is recommended. Most appendiceal NETs are < 2 cm in diameter (52–62% are < 1 cm, 28–30% are 1–2 cm, and 8–19% are > 2 cm) {2658,2112}.

Histopathology

NET: Microscopically, EC-cell NETs are most common and consist of uniform polygonal tumour cells frequently arranged in large nests, often with peripheral palisading and glandular formations, similar to ileal EC-cell NETs. Mitoses are infrequent to absent and necrosis is uncommon. The tumours are associated with a fibrotic stromal response in most cases. The bulk of the tumour (even in small tumours) often lies in the deep muscular wall and subserosa {3140}. In the muscular wall, the nests

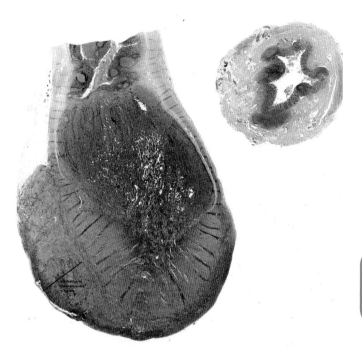

Fig. 5.10 Appendiceal neuroendocrine tumour (NET). A G1 NET, 15 mm in diameter, at the tip of the appendix, invading the mesoappendix.

can be replaced by small tumour cell ribbons. About one third of appendiceal NETs infiltrate the mesoappendix, including 50–82% that infiltrate the mesoappendix with a thickness of < 3 mm {2658,3484}. L-cell NET is a subtype of appendiceal NET composed of a different cell type. Incidental L-cell NETs show a distinct trabecular or glandular growth pattern. Similar to rectal L-cell NETs, they are formed by cells producing GLP-1 and other proglucagon-derived peptides. A rare subtype is tubular NET (formerly called tubular carcinoid), which must be distinguished from adenocarcinoma and goblet cell adenocarcinoma. Care must be taken not to misinterpret stromal retraction artefact as vascular invasion. The vast majority of both EC-cell and L-cell appendiceal NETs are G1 (86–91%) or G2 (9–14%) {2658,3484}. It is not required or mandatory to specify L-cell NET or EC-cell NET in pathological reports, because this has no prognostic value and no treatment consequences.

NEC: Appendiceal NECs are exceedingly rare and are morphologically identical to colonic NECs of either small cell or large cell type {3319,2658,3484}. They may arise in association with a glandular mucosal precursor lesion.

MANEC/MiNEN: The term "mixed adenoneuroendocrine carcinoma (MANEC)" has been previously used in the appendix to refer to goblet cell adenocarcinoma. These neoplasms are no longer considered to be a type of appendiceal NEN, but rather an adenocarcinoma subtype. True MiNENs of the appendix are rare and comparable to colonic MiNENs, showing a combination of a NEC and adenocarcinoma; they are diagnosed as mixed adenocarcinoma–large (or small) cell NEC.

Immunohistochemistry: Production of serotonin can be demonstrated by immunohistochemistry in EC-cell NETs, along with staining for chromogranin A and synaptophysin, and there are often S100-positive spindle cells surrounding the nests. L-cell NETs express chromogranin B rather than chromogranin A.

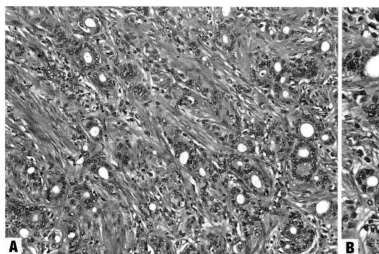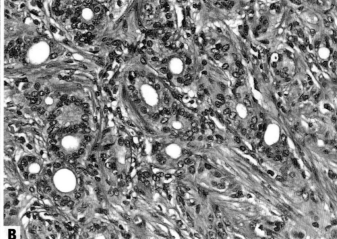

Fig. 5.11 Tubular neuroendocrine tumour (NET) of the appendix. **A** Low-power view. **B** High-power view.

Grading: Appendiceal NENs are graded using the same system used for other gastroenteropancreatic NENs.

Cytology

Cytological evaluation of appendiceal NETs is not performed, because most cases are incidental findings at appendectomy.

Diagnostic molecular pathology

Not clinically relevant

Essential and desirable diagnostic criteria

NET

Essential: a uniform population of cells with round nuclei and finely stippled chromatin; architectural patterns include trabeculae, acini, nests, and ribbons; expression of synaptophysin and chromogranin A or chromogranin B.

NEC

Essential: a small cell carcinoma or large cell carcinoma pattern; sheets or trabeculae of poorly differentiated cells; a high mitotic count and Ki-67 proliferation index.

Staging (TNM)

The staging of appendiceal NETs, which is presented in Chapter 1 (p. 20), has been modified in the eighth editions (2017) of the Union for International Cancer Control (UICC) TNM classification {408} and the American Joint Committee on Cancer (AJCC) cancer staging manual {127}. It is based mainly on tumour size and infiltration of serosa/mesoappendix. In this classification, the great majority of NETs are classified as pT3 due to invasion of the subserosa or mesoappendix. NECs, MiNENs, and goblet cell adenocarcinomas are staged using the parameters for appendiceal adenocarcinomas.

Prognosis and prediction

The value of follow-up data for appendiceal NETs is still a matter of debate for several reasons: most registry-based studies dated before 2010 are compromised by inconsistent coding of the neoplasms; also, institutional retrospective studies were small and provided limited long-term survival data. Most patients with appendiceal NET have an excellent outcome, the majority being cured by appendectomy. A recent SEER Program database study including 658 NETs found a 10-year survival rate of 92% {2112}, and institutional series show an even better prognosis of 97–99% {2553,3484}. Metastases occur in 1.4–8.8% of cases {385}, typically involving only regional lymph nodes. Liver and other distant metastases are rare. There is no clear evidence that microscopic lymph node metastases lead to decreased survival {733,1598}. The 5-year survival rate is 34% when there are distant metastases {2187}. Size is the most reliable indicator of metastatic potential. The risk of lymph node metastases is 0–11% in tumours < 1 cm, 18–44% in tumours 1–2 cm, and 30–86% in tumours > 2 cm {2254,2190,2112,1102 ,2240,2658}. The predictive size cut-off point for tumours considered to be at high risk of lymph node metastasis ranges from 1 cm {2112} to 2 cm {2658,2504}. Lymphatic invasion seems to be a weak risk factor for nodal metastasis {2658}. Data regarding mesoappendiceal fat invasion are contradictory. In the most recent European Neuroendocrine Tumor Society (ENETS) classification {2719}, invasion depth > 3 mm was considered an

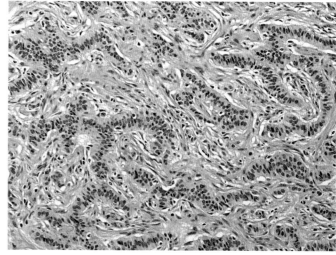

Fig. 5.12 L-cell neuroendocrine tumour (NET) of the appendix. Low-power view.

indication to perform an extended resection, but without clear data in the literature that validate this 3 mm limit as predictive of lymph node metastasis {2658}. However, both invasion of mesoappendix and invasion > 3 mm were reported to be associated with lower survival rates {3484}. Lastly, a grade of G1 or G2 was not reported to be a predictor of adverse outcome or lymph node metastasis {3484,2658}. There are therefore no established prognostic factors for survival of appendiceal NETs, and even the survival benefit of right hemicolectomy is unclear {2112,2658}.

Appendiceal NECs and MiNENs are high-grade malignant neoplasms, with a poor survival similar to that of their counterparts elsewhere in the GI tract.

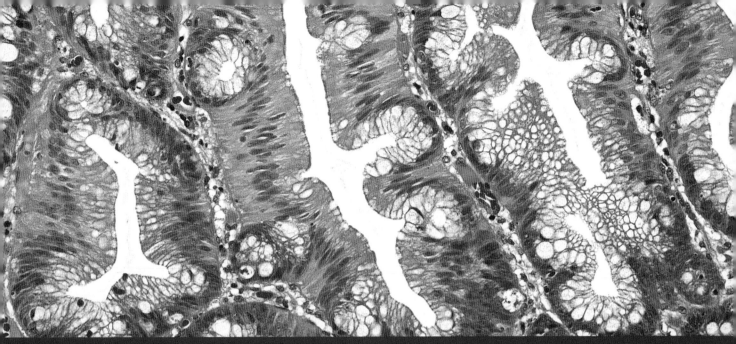

6

Tumours of the colon and rectum

Edited by: Nagtegaal ID, Arends MJ, Odze RD, Lam AK

Benign epithelial tumours and precursors
    Serrated lesions and polyps
    Conventional adenoma
    Inflammatory bowel disease–associated dysplasia
Malignant epithelial tumours
    Adenocarcinoma
    Neuroendocrine neoplasms

WHO classification of tumours of the colon and rectum

Benign epithelial tumours and precursors
8213/0*	Serrated dysplasia, low grade
8213/2*	Serrated dysplasia, high grade
8210/0*	Adenomatous polyp, low-grade dysplasia
8210/2*	Adenomatous polyp, high-grade dysplasia
8211/0*	Tubular adenoma, low grade
8211/2*	Tubular adenoma, high grade
8261/0*	Villous adenoma, low grade
8261/2*	Villous adenoma, high grade
8263/0*	Tubulovillous adenoma, low grade
8263/2*	Tubulovillous adenoma, high grade
	Advanced adenoma
8148/0	Glandular intraepithelial neoplasia, low grade
8148/2	Glandular intraepithelial neoplasia, high grade

Malignant epithelial tumours
8140/3	Adenocarcinoma NOS
8213/3	Serrated adenocarcinoma
8262/3*	Adenoma-like adenocarcinoma
8265/3	Micropapillary adenocarcinoma
8480/3	Mucinous adenocarcinoma
8490/3	Poorly cohesive carcinoma
8490/3	Signet-ring cell carcinoma
8510/3	Medullary adenocarcinoma
8560/3	Adenosquamous carcinoma
8020/3	Carcinoma, undifferentiated, NOS
8033/3*	Carcinoma with sarcomatoid component
8240/3	Neuroendocrine tumour NOS
8240/3	Neuroendocrine tumour, grade 1
8249/3	Neuroendocrine tumour, grade 2
8249/3	Neuroendocrine tumour, grade 3
8152/3	L-cell tumour
8152/3	Glucagon-like peptide-producing tumour
8152/3	PP/PYY-producing tumour
8241/3	Enterochromaffin-cell carcinoid
8241/3	Serotonin-producing tumour
8246/3	Neuroendocrine carcinoma NOS
8013/3	Large cell neuroendocrine carcinoma
8041/3	Small cell neuroendocrine carcinoma
8154/3	Mixed neuroendocrine–non-neuroendocrine neoplasm (MiNEN)

These morphology codes are from the International Classification of Diseases for Oncology, third edition, second revision (ICD-O-3.2) {1378A}. Behaviour is coded /0 for benign tumours; /1 for unspecified, borderline, or uncertain behaviour; /2 for carcinoma in situ and grade III intraepithelial neoplasia; /3 for malignant tumours, primary site; and /6 for malignant tumours, metastatic site. Behaviour code /6 is not generally used by cancer registries.

This classification is modified from the previous WHO classification, taking into account changes in our understanding of these lesions.

* Codes marked with an asterisk were approved by the IARC/WHO Committee for ICD-O at its meeting in April 2019.

TNM staging of carcinomas of the colon and rectum

Colon and Rectum
(ICD-O-3 C18–20)

Rules for Classification
The classification applies only to carcinomas. There should be histological confirmation of the disease.

The following are the procedures for assessing the T, N, and M categories.

T categories	Physical examination, imaging, endoscopy, and/or surgical exploration
N categories	Physical examination, imaging, and/or surgical exploration
M categories	Physical examination, imaging, and/or surgical exploration

Anatomical Sites and Subsites
Colon (C18)
1. Caecum (C18.0)
2. Ascending colon (C18.2)
3. Hepatic flexure (C18.3)
4. Transverse colon (C18.4)
5. Splenic flexure (C18.5)
6. Descending colon (C18.6)
7. Sigmoid colon (C18.7)

Rectosigmoid junction (C19)
Rectum (C20)

Regional Lymph Nodes
For each anatomical site or subsite the following are regional lymph nodes:

Caecum	ileocolic, right colic
Ascending colon	ileocolic, right colic, middle colic
Hepatic flexure	right colic, middle colic
Transverse colon	right colic, middle colic, left colic, inferior mesenteric
Splenic flexure	middle colic, left colic, inferior mesenteric
Descending colon	left colic, inferior mesenteric
Sigmoid colon	sigmoid, left colic, superior rectal (haemorrhoidal), inferior mesenteric and rectosigmoid
Rectum	superior, middle, and inferior rectal (haemorrhoidal), inferior mesenteric, internal iliac, mesorectal (paraproctal), lateral sacral, presacral, sacral promontory (Gerota)

Metastasis in nodes other than those listed here is classified as distant metastasis.

TNM Clinical Classification
T – Primary Tumour

TX	Primary tumour cannot be assessed
T0	No evidence of primary tumour
Tis	Carcinoma in situ: invasion of lamina propria[a]
T1	Tumour invades submucosa
T2	Tumour invades muscularis propria

T3	Tumour invades subserosa or into non-peritonealized pericolic or perirectal tissues
T4	Tumour directly invades other organs or structures[b,c,d] and/or perforates visceral peritoneum
	T4a Tumour perforates visceral peritoneum
	T4b Tumour directly invades other organs or structures

Notes

[a] Tis includes cancer cells confined within the mucosal lamina propria (intramucosal) with no extension through the muscularis mucosae into the submucosa.

[b] Invades through to visceral peritoneum to involve the surface.

[c] Direct invasion in T4b includes invasion of other organs or segments of the colorectum by way of the serosa, as confirmed on microscopic examination, or for tumours in a retroperitoneal or subperitoneal location, direct invasion of other organs or structures by virtue of extension beyond the muscularis propria.

[d] Tumour that is adherent to other organs or structures, macroscopically, is classified cT4b. However, if no tumour is present in the adhesion, microscopically, the classification should be pT1–3, depending on the anatomical depth of wall invasion.

N – Regional Lymph Nodes

NX	Regional lymph nodes cannot be assessed
N0	No regional lymph node metastasis
N1	Metastasis in 1 to 3 regional lymph nodes
	N1a Metastasis in 1 regional lymph node
	N1b Metastasis in 2 to 3 regional lymph nodes
	N1c Tumour deposit(s), i.e. satellites,* in the subserosa, or in non-peritonealized pericolic or perirectal soft tissue *without* regional lymph node metastasis
N2	Metastasis in 4 or more regional lymph nodes
	N2a Metastasis in 4–6 regional lymph nodes
	N2b Metastasis in 7 or more regional lymph nodes

Note

* Tumour deposits (satellites) are discrete macroscopic or microscopic nodules of cancer in the pericolorectal adipose tissue's lymph drainage area of a primary carcinoma that are discontinuous from the primary and without histological evidence of residual lymph node or identifiable vascular or neural structures. If a vessel wall is identifiable on H&E, elastic or other stains, it should be classified as venous invasion (V1/2) or lymphatic invasion (L1). Similarly, if neural structures are identifiable, the lesion should be classified as perineural invasion (Pn1). The presence of tumour deposits does not change the primary tumour T category, but changes the node status (N) to pN1c if all regional lymph nodes are negative on pathological examination.

The information presented here has been excerpted from the 2017 *TNM classification of malignant tumours*, eighth edition {408,3385A}. © 2017 UICC. A help desk for specific questions about the TNM classification is available at https://www.uicc.org/tnm-help-desk.

Chapter 6

M – Distant Metastasis

M0   No distant metastasis
M1   Distant metastasis
    M1a   Metastasis confined to one organ (liver, lung, ovary, non-regional lymph node(s)) without peritoneal metastases
    M1b   Metastasis in more than one organ
    M1c   Metastasis to the peritoneum with or without other organ involvement

TNM Pathological Classification

The pT and pN categories correspond to the T and N categories.

pN0   Histological examination of a regional lymphadenectomy specimen will ordinarily include 12 or more lymph nodes. If the lymph nodes are negative, but the number ordinarily examined is not met, classify as pN0.

pM – Distant Metastasis*

pM1   Distant metastasis microscopically confirmed

Note
* pM0 and pMX are not valid categories.

Stage

Stage	T	N	M
Stage 0	Tis	N0	M0
Stage I	T1,T2	N0	M0
Stage II	T3,T4	N0	M0
Stage IIA	T3	N0	M0
Stage IIB	T4a	N0	M0
Stage IIC	T4b	N0	M0
Stage III	Any T	N1,N2	M0
Stage IIIA	T1,T2	N1	M0
	T1	N2a	M0
Stage IIIB	T1,T2	N2b	M0
	T2,T3	N2a	M0
	T3,T4a	N1	M0
Stage IIIC	T3,T4a	N2b	M0
	T4a	N2a	M0
	T4b	N1,N2	M0
Stage IV	Any T	Any N	M1
Stage IVA	Any T	Any N	M1a
Stage IVB	Any T	Any N	M1b
Stage IVC	Any T	Any N	M1c

Note: Neuroendocrine tumours (NETs) of the colon and rectum are staged using the NET-specific TNM staging system, which is presented in Chapter 1 (p. 20).

The information presented here has been excerpted from the 2017 *TNM classification of malignant tumours*, eighth edition {408,3385A}. © 2017 UICC.
A help desk for specific questions about the TNM classification is available at https://www.uicc.org/tnm-help-desk.

Tumours of the colon and rectum: Introduction

Nagtegaal ID
Arends MJ
Odze RD

Colorectal cancer is the most common type of gastrointestinal cancer. This fact is reflected by the more extensive description of the molecular features and pathogenesis in this publication. The ICD-O topographical coding for the anatomical sites covered in this chapter is presented in Box 6.01.

Due to changes in lifestyle, the incidence of colorectal cancer is rising worldwide. The presence of recognizable precursor lesions and well-developed screening tests has led to a worldwide introduction of population screening over the past decade. This necessitates a more comprehensive description of those precursor lesions, including both serrated polyps and conventional adenomas, in this chapter.

There is now a better understanding of the different types of colorectal serrated pathway lesions and polyps (and their biological characteristics): hyperplastic polyps, sessile serrated lesions, and traditional serrated adenomas. The terminology used in this fifth edition is a change from the previous edition. For instance, sessile serrated polyp or adenoma (SSP/SSA) is now termed "sessile serrated lesion (SSL)", for a variety of reasons – most notably, because not all lesions that fall into this category are necessarily polypoid in appearance. In addition, to reflect the fact that some serrated lesions cannot always be classified reliably into one of the above three general categories after careful clinical/endoscopic and pathological evaluation, a fourth category has been added: unclassified serrated adenoma. For conventional adenomas, essential diagnostic criteria have been added. This chapter on colorectal tumours is linked to the chapter on genetic syndromes of polyposes and cancer susceptibility (Chapter 14: *Genetic tumour syndromes of*

Box 6.01 ICD-O topographical coding for the anatomical sites covered in this chapter

C18 Colon
C18.0 Caecum
C18.2 Ascending colon
C18.3 Hepatic flexure of the colon
C18.4 Transverse colon
C18.5 Splenic flexure of the colon
C18.6 Descending colon
C18.7 Sigmoid colon
C18.8 Overlapping lesion of the colon
C18.9 Colon NOS
C19 Rectosigmoid junction
C19.9 Rectosigmoid junction
C20 Rectum
C20.9 Rectum NOS

the digestive system, p. 511), which contains useful information about molecular carcinogenesis.

Carcinogenesis related to inflammatory bowel disease is described in a dedicated section (*Inflammatory bowel disease–associated dysplasia of the colorectum*, p. 174), which provides detailed information about pathogenesis and histopathology. In the section regarding colorectal cancer (*Colorectal adenocarcinoma*, p. 177), prognostic and predictive morphological and molecular features are described in detail. For colorectal neuroendocrine neoplasms (NENs), the classification has been updated and aligned with that of NENs in other parts of the GI tract.

Colorectal serrated lesions and polyps

Pai RK (Rish)
Mäkinen MJ
Rosty C

Definition
Colorectal serrated lesions and polyps are characterized by a serrated (sawtooth or stellate) architecture of the epithelium.

ICD-O coding
8213/0 Serrated dysplasia, low grade
8213/2 Serrated dysplasia, high grade

ICD-11 coding
DB35.0 Hyperplastic polyp of large intestine
2E92.4 & XH2F06 Benign neoplasm of the large intestine & Sessile serrated adenoma
2E92.4 & XH63V9 Benign neoplasm of the large intestine & Sessile serrated polyp
2E92.4 & XH9PD9 Benign neoplasm of the large intestine & Traditional sessile serrated adenoma

Related terminology
Note: Many terms have previously been used to describe sessile serrated lesion.
Not recommended: sessile serrated polyp; sessile serrated adenoma.

Subtype(s)
Hyperplastic polyp; hyperplastic polyp, microvesicular type; hyperplastic polyp, goblet cell–rich type; sessile serrated lesion; sessile serrated lesion with dysplasia; traditional serrated adenoma (8213/0); serrated adenoma, unclassified (8213/0)

Localization
The majority (75–90%) of hyperplastic polyps (HPs) – both microvesicular HPs (MVHPs) and goblet cell–rich HPs (GCHPs) – are found in the distal colon and rectum; sessile serrated lesions (SSLs) have a predilection for the proximal colon (70–80%), particularly SSLs with dysplasia (SSLDs) {3670,2624,317}. About 70% of traditional serrated adenomas (TSAs) occur in the distal colon and rectum {320}.

Clinical features
Most serrated polyps are asymptomatic and therefore an incidental finding at endoscopy. Because bleeding of serrated polyps is rare, and most serrated polyps are sessile, faecal blood–based screening and virtual colonoscopy are not effective screening methods {1362}.

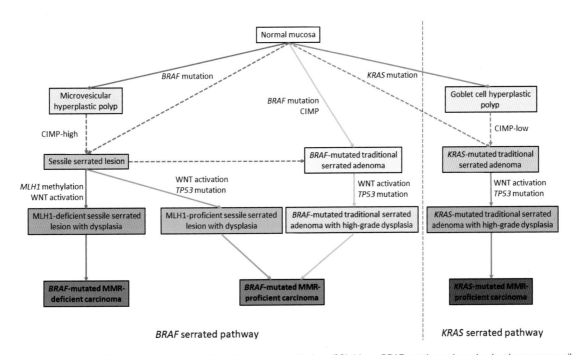

Fig. 6.01 Schematic representation of the serrated neoplasia pathway. Sessile serrated lesions (SSLs) have *BRAF* mutation and can develop de novo or possibly (dotted line) from microvesicular hyperplastic polyps (HPs). A key molecular event thought to precipitate the progression of SSL to malignancy is either *MLH1* methylation, secondary to high levels of CpG island methylator phenotype (CIMP), progressing to mismatch repair (MMR)-deficient colorectal carcinoma, or *TP53* mutation progressing to MMR-proficient colorectal carcinoma. Traditional serrated adenomas (TSAs) may develop de novo, possibly from SSL or from goblet cell HP (dotted lines). TSAs progress via the *BRAF* or *KRAS* pathway to high-grade dysplasia and MMR-proficient colorectal carcinoma. WNT signalling pathway activation occurs in all pathways through different mechanisms, at the transition to dysplasia.

Chapter 6

Table 6.01 Histological and molecular features of serrated polyps

Type	Histological features				Molecular features		
	Crypt architecture	Proliferation zone	Cytological features	Mucin type	*BRAF* mutation	*KRAS* mutation	CpG-island methylation
MVHP	Funnel-shaped crypts with serrations limited to upper two thirds	Located uniformly in the basal portion of crypts	Small basally located nuclei; no dysplasia	Mixed microvesicular and goblet cell	70–80%	0%	+
GCHP	Elongated crypts that resemble enlarged normal crypts; little to no serration	Located uniformly in the basal portion of crypts	Small basally located nuclei; no dysplasia	Goblet cell predominant	0%	50%	–
SSL	Horizontal growth along the muscularis mucosae, dilation of the crypt base (basal third of the crypt), and/or serrations extending into the crypt base	Proliferation may be abnormally located away from the crypt base, variable from crypt to crypt	Small basally located nuclei with occasional larger nuclei with inconspicuous nucleoli; no dysplasia	Mixed microvesicular and goblet cell	> 90%	0%	++
SSLD	Complex architecture in the dysplastic component (crypt crowding, complex branching, cribriforming, villous architecture)	Like in SSL, but with more proliferation in the dysplastic component	Varied morphological appearance of dysplastic component	Varied type	> 90%	0%	+++
TSA	Slit-like serrations; often ectopic crypts	Present within ectopic crypts and crypt bases	Elongated pencillate nuclei with nuclear stratification and cytoplasmic eosinophilia; may develop overt dysplasia	Occasional scattered goblet cells; rare goblet cell subtype has been described	20–40%	50–70%	+

GCHP, goblet cell–rich hyperplastic polyp; MVHP, microvesicular hyperplastic polyp; SSL, sessile serrated lesion; SSLD, sessile serrated lesion with dysplasia; TSA, traditional serrated adenoma.

Epidemiology

The reported frequency of serrated polyps in average-risk populations varies substantially, but SSLs and HPs probably account for about 10% and 30% of all colorectal polyps, respectively {317,1224,2601,2487,3117,723}.

Etiology

See *Colorectal adenocarcinoma* (p. 177).

Pathogenesis

As many as 30% of all colorectal carcinomas arise via the serrated neoplasia pathway {2401,2765}. SSL and TSA are known precursors to carcinoma, although HP, particularly proximal MVHP, is probably a precursor to SSL. GCHPs and some MVHPs may also give rise to TSA. The progression of SSL to carcinoma proceeds through the development of overt epithelial dysplasia (SSLD) as a result of progressive CpG-island methylation. Overt dysplasia and low levels of CpG methylation also occur in TSA during its progression to carcinoma.

The serrated pathway involves a sequence of genetic and epigenetic alterations that lead to the development of sporadic carcinomas with hypermethylation with or without microsatellite instability. Activating mutations of either *BRAF* (in MVHP, SSL, and TSA) or *KRAS* (in GCHP and TSA) are thought to initiate

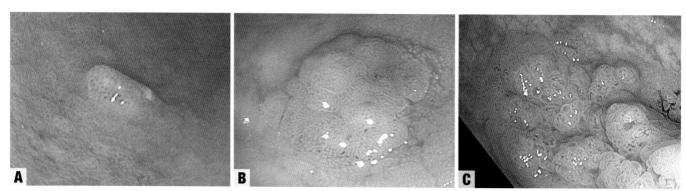

Fig. 6.02 Colorectal serrated lesions and polyps, endoscopic appearance. **A** Microvesicular hyperplastic polyp. A small polyp with well-defined margins and an open pit pattern. **B** Sessile serrated lesion. This lesion is large and has poorly defined margins. **C** Traditional serrated adenoma. A large lesion composed of a central, protruding polypoid mass with a coral-like appearance.

the development of serrated polyps and are mutually exclusive {320,3117,3560,2400}. Extensive methylation of various CpG islands within SSL leads to a CpG island methylator phenotype (CIMP) and is associated with the development of dysplasia and eventually invasive carcinoma {316}. *MLH1* promoter methylation is a critical step occurring in 75% of SSLDs, resulting in mismatch repair deficiency {316,1929}. The remaining 25% of SSLDs are mismatch repair–proficient and often harbour *TP53* mutations {316}. Alterations in the WNT signalling pathway also occur in the transition from SSL to overt dysplasia and carcinoma {370,1185,3663}.

TSA shows some differences from SSL, including more frequent alterations in *RNF43* and the presence of RSPO gene family fusions, both of which potentiate WNT signalling, as well as some degree of CIMP {320,3560,1185,2936,3347,2933}. *KRAS* and *BRAF* mutations occur with relatively equal frequencies in TSA, and approximately 10% of TSAs lack mutations in one of these genes {320,3560}. Low levels of CIMP with mismatch repair proficiency and *TP53* mutation are associated with *KRAS*-mutated TSA progression {320}. *BRAF*-mutated TSAs are more frequently associated with CIMP, and they progress to mismatch repair–proficient carcinoma with a poor prognosis {320}.

Macroscopic appearance

Distal HPs are usually small (< 5 mm) and appear as discrete mucosal elevations. Proximal HPs and SSLs are pale, poorly defined, sessile (Paris type Is) to flat (Paris type 0-IIa and type 0-IIb) lesions covered with a mucus cap and a rim of debris or bubbles imparting a cloud-like surface {3200,1200,3287}. They also tend to flatten during bowel inflation, making their detection challenging. Proximal TSAs may be flat, but TSAs are usually polypoid, broad-based lesions with a surface texture resembling a pinecone or coral pattern {320,3329,1181}.

Histopathology

Hyperplastic polyp

HPs are composed of superficial serrated epithelium and funnel-shaped, evenly spaced crypts with proliferative zones confined to crypt bases. The crypts do not show basal dilatation, substantial distortion, or submucosal misplacement, but individual crypt branching may occur. Epithelial serration in HPs is seen in the surface epithelium and the superficial part of the crypts {3328}. In well-oriented specimens, the diagnosis of MVHP is a diagnosis by exclusion, i.e. when the criteria of SSL are not met {317,3328,2699}. In MVHP, the epithelium matures early, and it is composed of microvesicular epithelial cells (with abundant cytoplasm containing fine apical vacuoles) and a variable number of goblet cells. Nuclei are small, round to oval, and basally located. Epithelial serrations are present in the surface epithelium and limited to the upper two thirds of the crypts, resulting in stellate lumina in cross-sectioned crypts, corresponding to the Kudo type II pit pattern {1712}. GCHPs are small, and their morphological alterations are often so subtle that they are easily overlooked as epithelial hyperplasia or reactive alteration. Most of the cells of the surface and crypt epithelium are goblet cells with small, uniform basal nuclei. In GCHPs, the crypts are taller and wider than in normal mucosa, and they show occasional branching or tortuosity. The epithelium shows slight serration that is confined to the surface epithelium and

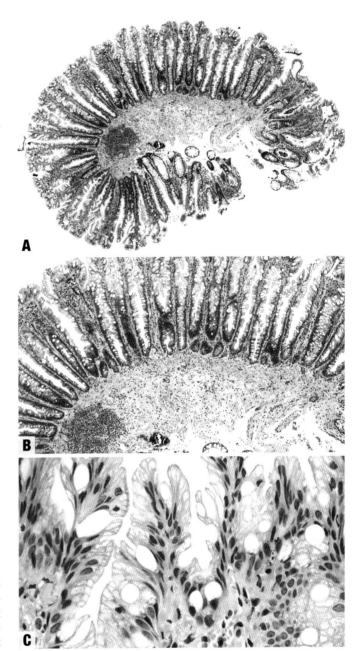

Fig. 6.03 Microvesicular hyperplastic polyp. **A** The serrated crypts are narrow and architectural features of sessile serrated lesion are absent. **B** In the same lesion, the crypts are straight and narrow, and they are lined by serrated epithelium. **C** The surface epithelium shows typical serration and is composed of a mixture of microvesicular and goblet cells; the basement membrane area beneath the surface epithelium is thickened.

crypt orifices. Cross-sectioned crypt lumina are round rather than stellate {317,3328}.

Sessile serrated lesion

The distinction of SSL from HP (particularly MVHP) and TSA is based mainly on architecture, although cytological features also play an important role {3329,3328}. Like MVHP, SSL has bland cytology and crypts with prominent serrations. SSLs contain a mixture of goblet cells and cells with microvesicular mucin droplets. The distinguishing feature of SSL is an overall distortion of

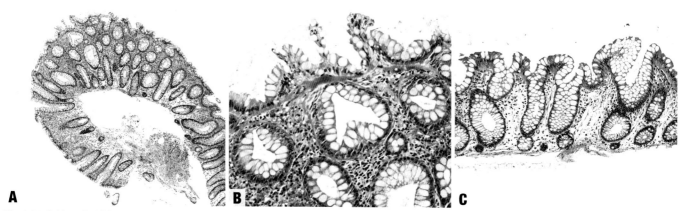

Fig. 6.04 Goblet cell–rich hyperplastic polyp. **A** At low power, the crypts are wider and taller than normal. **B** At high power, the crypts contain a large number of goblet cells with superficial serration. **C** A transition between normal colonic mucosa and the polyp is apparent in the right portion of the biopsy. Only subtle superficial serration is seen in this example.

the normal crypt architecture, probably resulting from alterations of the proliferative zone. Crypt architectural changes in SSL are defined as horizontal growth along the muscularis mucosae, dilation of the crypt base (basal third of the crypt), serrations extending into the crypt base (in contrast to superficial serrations in HP), and asymmetrical proliferation {317,3328}. These changes result in a type II open-shaped endoscopic Kudo pit pattern (type II-O) {1606}. The presence of at least one of these features defines an architecturally distorted crypt. Occasional branched crypts are seen, but the presence of branched crypts in a serrated polyp is not sufficient for the diagnosis of SSL, because crypt branching is also seen in HP. Importantly, the majority of SSL crypts lack abnormal architecture, and most crypts resemble those seen in MVHP. Recent studies have

indicated that the presence of ≥ 1 unequivocal architecturally distorted serrated crypt, as defined above, is sufficient for a diagnosis of SSL {317,2699,597}. The term "unequivocal" is important, because crypts with only subtle architectural abnormalities should not be regarded as diagnostic of SSL. Mild symmetrical dilatation of crypt bases is not sufficient for SSL diagnosis {904}. Crypts with mature cells, such as goblet cells, in the crypt base are also not diagnostic of SSL. Importantly, the size, location, and endoscopic appearance alone should not be used to make the diagnosis of SSL; rather, these may be considered adjunctive features that may favour the diagnosis for ambiguous cases or poorly oriented sections. Furthermore, SSL size as measured by endoscopy may not be accurate, especially given the difficulty in delineating the borders of these

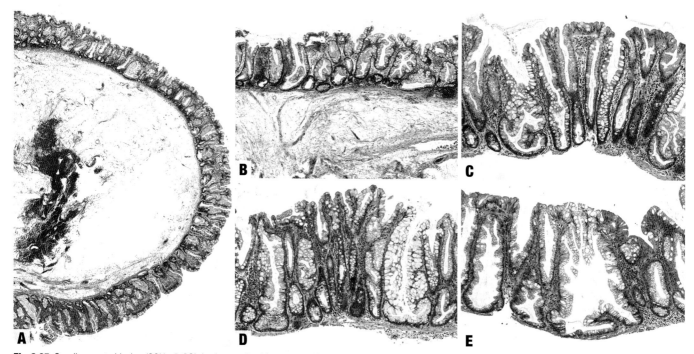

Fig. 6.05 Sessile serrated lesion (SSL). **A** SSL is characterized by many architecturally distorted serrated crypts. **B** Architecturally distorted serrated crypts with prominent basal crypt dilatation. **C** Architecturally distorted serrated crypts with deep crypt serrations and basal crypt dilatation with lateral growth along the muscularis mucosae. **D** Architecturally distorted serrated crypts with lateral growth along the muscularis mucosae. **E** Architecturally distorted serrated crypts with deep crypt serrations and lateral growth along the muscularis mucosae.

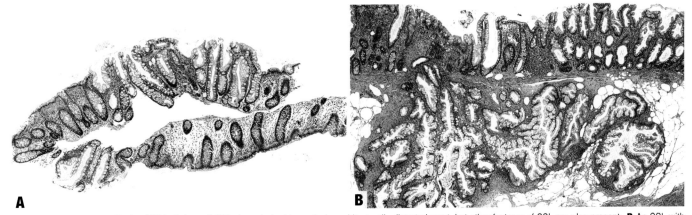

Fig. 6.06 Sessile serrated lesion (SSL). **A** A small SSL characterized by a single architecturally distorted crypt, but other features of SSL are also present. **B** An SSL with mucosal herniation of serrated crypts into the submucosa.

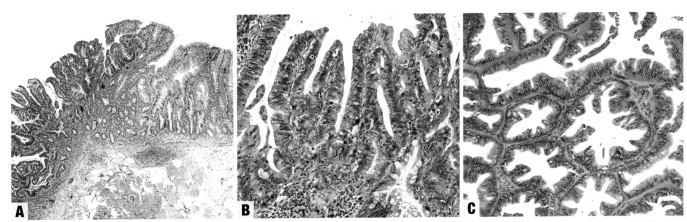

Fig. 6.07 Sessile serrated lesion (SSL) with dysplasia. **A** The dysplastic component on the left is sharply demarcated from the SSL on the right and shows partial villous architecture. **B** In the same lesion, there is nuclear pleomorphism, loss of nuclear polarity, mitotic figures, and amphophilic mucin-depleted cytoplasm. **C** The serrated dysplastic epithelium shows an irregular serrated or sawtooth pattern of growth lined by cells with hyperchromatic enlarged and slightly stratified nuclei and eosinophilic cytoplasm.

polyps, which results in a higher incidence of incomplete endoscopic resection {2601}. The presence of mucosal herniation is a diagnostic pitfall for SSL, because smooth muscle fibres may distort the crypt architecture {2487,1318}. Serrated crypts may herniate through the muscularis mucosae into the submucosa, often in association with lipomatous areas or lymphoid aggregates. The presence of mucosal herniation should not be confused with invasion, particularly when dysplasia is present.

Because the diagnosis of SSL is dependent predominantly on crypt architecture, well-oriented sections evaluating crypt bases are helpful. Deeper levels may be helpful in sections that are not well oriented {597}. Both SSL and MVHP have been associated with unusual stromal proliferation resembling perineurial cells. This stromal proliferation is probably a reactive phenomenon related to the adjacent serrated epithelium rather than a true stromal neoplasm, and it has no clinical significance {2489,872}.

Sessile serrated lesion with dysplasia
Dysplasia may develop in some SSLs as a transient step during progression to carcinoma {316}. The dysplastic component is usually sharply demarcated from the SSL and shows greater morphological heterogeneity than conventional adenomas. Architectural changes include villous architecture, crypt elongation, crowding of crypts with complex branching, cribriforming, and excessive or reduced luminal serration compared with the background SSL. Cytologically, cells can show intestinal dysplasia resembling dysplasia in conventional adenomas; serrated dysplasia with round atypical nuclei, prominent nucleoli, numerous mitoses, and eosinophilic cytoplasm; or (more rarely) subtle cytological atypia, including hypermucinous changes {532,1929}. Multiple morphological patterns of dysplasia often occur in a single polyp {1929}. Loss of MLH1 expression may help when the dysplastic changes are subtle; however, not all dysplastic patterns are MLH1-deficient {316,1929}. Stratification of dysplasia into low-grade vs high-grade is not recommended, because it may be difficult and not reproducible due to the heterogeneity of morphological changes and the lack of correlation with loss of MLH1 expression {2401,1929}.

Traditional serrated adenoma
TSA can present as large protuberant polyps predominant in the distal colorectum or as flat lesions predominant in the proximal colon {320,3560,1591}. The two most distinctive features of TSA are the slit-like serration, reminiscent of the narrow slits in the normal small intestinal mucosa, and the tall columnar cells with intensely eosinophilic cytoplasm and pencillate nuclei. Ectopic

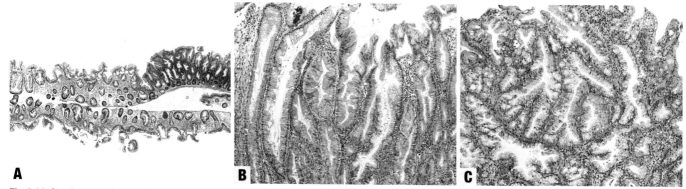

Fig. 6.08 Sessile serrated lesion (SSL) with dysplasia (SSLD). **A** At low power, the small flat area of dysplasia on the upper right is characterized by crypt crowding, reduced lamina propria, and eosinophilic cells. **B** The dysplastic cells have reduced mucin content with gastric foveolar differentiation. **C** In this case, the dysplastic crypts exhibit complex architecture with serration, crypt branching, and focal cribriforming.

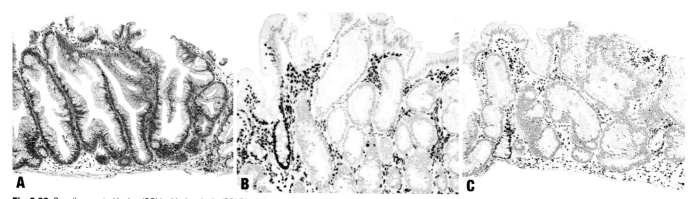

Fig. 6.09 Sessile serrated lesion (SSL) with dysplasia (SSLD). **A** In contrast with the non-dysplastic crypt on the right, the dysplastic area is characterized by crypt crowding and subtle cytological changes. **B** At higher power, the dysplastic area shows complete loss of MLH1 expression by immunohistochemistry. **C** Loss of MLH1 expression can help in the diagnosis of SSL with subtle dysplastic changes.

crypt formations, defined as epithelial buds not anchored to the muscularis mucosae, are always found along the sides of the villous projections of protuberant TSA, but they are rarely present in (and are not necessary for the diagnosis of) flat TSA {319}. Most TSAs contain only scattered goblet cells, although a mucin/goblet cell–rich TSA has been described {2265}. An adjacent precursor polyp, either an MVHP, GCHP, or SSL, is found in as many as 50% of TSAs {599}. Like in SSL, areas

of overt dysplasia can be found in TSA {320,1591,3346}. This superimposed dysplasia is described as either intestinal or serrated type, different from the senescent changes of typical TSA cells. No specific surveillance guidelines currently exist for this scenario, but these polyps probably represent more advanced lesions, and they should be reported separately when high-grade dysplasia is present {319}.

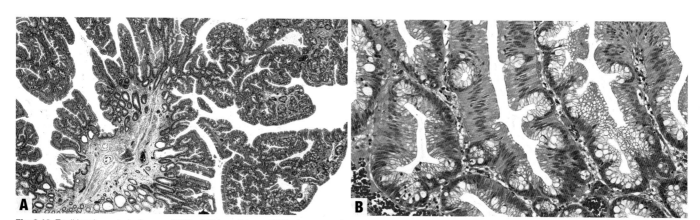

Fig. 6.10 Traditional serrated adenoma (TSA). **A** This protuberant TSA shows complex villiform projections and slit-like serration. **B** The cells lining the villi are predominantly tall and columnar, with abundant eosinophilic cytoplasm and centrally located oval nuclei with pseudostratification but no mitotic activity. Note the multiple ectopic crypt formations along the villi with differentiated goblet cells.

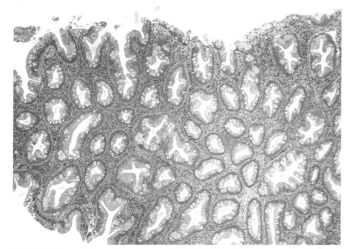

Fig. 6.11 Tangential sections often result in difficulties in the diagnosis of serrated lesions. Although irregularities in crypt shape and diameter are suggestive of a sessile serrated lesion, evaluation of deeper levels is warranted.

Unclassified serrated adenoma

Some dysplastic polyps with serrated architecture are difficult to classify as either TSA or SSLD. Included within this group are the recently described serrated tubulovillous adenomas {318,1928}.

Cytology

Not clinically relevant

Diagnostic molecular pathology

Not clinically relevant; see *Pathogenesis*, above.

Essential and desirable diagnostic criteria

See Table 6.01 (p. 164).

Staging (TNM)

Not clinically relevant

Prognosis and prediction

Small distal HPs have no substantial malignant potential and do not affect colonoscopic surveillance intervals. Index SSL, TSA, and large (≥ 1 cm) serrated polyp irrespective of histology increase the risk of large metachronous serrated polyp {134}. Large serrated polyp also increases the risk of colorectal carcinoma {2699,1259,1903,868}. Recommended follow-up intervals are based on low level of evidence and vary by country {2699,1903,837}. Synchronous conventional adenoma may affect surveillance intervals {2118}.

Conventional colorectal adenoma

Hamilton SR
Sekine S

Definition

Conventional colorectal adenoma is a benign, premalignant neoplasm composed of dysplastic epithelium. The descriptor "conventional" distinguishes this from lesions in the serrated pathway.

ICD-O coding

8210/0 Adenomatous polyp, low-grade dysplasia
8210/2 Adenomatous polyp, high-grade dysplasia

ICD-11 coding

2E92.4Y & XH7SY6 Other specified benign neoplasm of the large intestine & Tubular adenoma NOS

Related terminology

None

Subtype(s)

Tubular adenoma, low grade (8211/0); tubular adenoma, high grade (8211/2); villous adenoma, low grade (8261/0); villous adenoma, high grade (8261/2); tubulovillous adenoma, low grade (8263/0); tubulovillous adenoma, high grade (8263/2); advanced adenoma

Localization

Adenomas occur throughout the colorectum, from the ileocaecal valve to the anorectal junction.

Clinical features

Most patients with an uncomplicated adenoma are asymptomatic. Occult bleeding is common and serves as the basis for common screening tests {1796}. Symptoms and signs can occur with larger lesions, including evident bleeding, abdominal pain, and change in bowel habits. Rarely, distal large villous

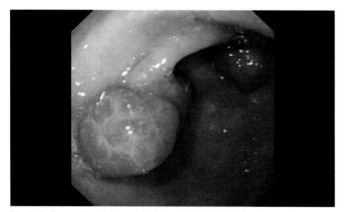

Fig. 6.12 Conventional adenoma. Endoscopic image of tubular villous adenoma on a stalk and a sessile tubular villous adenoma more proximally.

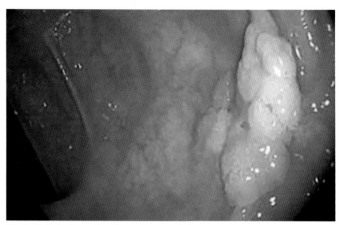

Fig. 6.13 Colonic sessile villous adenoma. Colonoscopic image; the polyp is broad-based and has a nodular surface.

adenomas can produce secretory diarrhoea with electrolyte imbalance (McKittrick–Wheelock syndrome) {465}.

At endoscopy or pathological specimen examination, adenomas can have a pedunculated, sessile protuberant, slightly elevated/flat, or depressed appearance. These characteristics influence the ease of detection by imaging and visualization. Magnification / high definition, dye sprays, modified light wavelengths, and colon dilation by insufflation or luminal fluid instillation are used to improve endoscopic detection rates. Removal of adenomas by snare polypectomy, endoscopic mucosal or submucosal resection, or surgery reduces the risk of colorectal adenocarcinoma.

Epidemiology

The epidemiological characteristics of conventional adenomas overlap with those of colorectal adenocarcinoma.

Etiology

The etiological characteristics of conventional adenomas overlap with those of colorectal adenocarcinoma.

Pathogenesis

Adenoma formation mostly involves change from normal colon mucosa epithelium to the benign precursor (adenoma), with the risk of further evolution to adenocarcinoma in a minority of adenomas. The transitions are associated with alterations to a small number of driver genes (mainly *APC*, *KRAS*, *SMAD4*, and *TP53*) {517,3316,3603,3613}, conferring growth advantages. Some of these genetic changes occur before morphologically identifiable tumour formation, in stem or progenitor cells {3317}.

The earliest changes involve aberrations of the WNT signalling pathway, most frequently altering APC function, usually by mutations that truncate the APC protein that reduces degradation of β-catenin allowing it to accumulate and dysregulate WNT signalling {3000}. Increased numbers of stem cells and loss of their hierarchy are evident as compared with non-neoplastic mucosa. The resultant altered morphology becomes recognizable histopathologically as dysplasia. Single crypt dysplasia (monocryptal adenomas, similar to dysplastic aberrant crypt foci in experimental models) shows abnormal epithelial proliferation of cells with altered differentiation and increased rate of crypt fission leading to formation of microadenomas with a few crypts containing dysplastic epithelium. Inherited (constitutional) *APC* pathogenic mutations cause familial adenomatous polyposis, in which large numbers of adenomas are seen (> 100 adenomatous polyps in classic familial adenomatous polyposis syndrome), including monocryptal adenomas and microadenomas (see *Familial adenomatous polyposis 1*, p. 522).

The enlargement of these to form small adenomas and eventually large adenomas (> 10 mm) occurs through accumulation of further molecular abnormalities affecting a small number of key signalling pathways. Activating mutations of the *KRAS* oncogene contribute to growth dysregulation through the MAPK signalling pathway {2428}. Abnormalities that disrupt the TGF-β growth inhibitory pathway are most commonly due to deletion (and some mutations) of *SMAD4* on chromosome 18. Abnormalities of the PI3K pathway, due to deletion or mutation of the tumour suppressor *PTEN* or activating mutations of the oncogene *PIK3CA* and others, inhibit apoptosis and promote neoplastic cell survival {1164,3619}. *TP53* alterations, most frequently by mutations at hotspot sites within the gene, deregulate p53 protein function (even one mutant *TP53* allele expressing mutated p53 polypeptide can deregulate a p53 tetramer containing other non-mutated p53 polypeptides), allowing the cell to survive substantial DNA damage and other cellular stresses, by inactivating the p53-mediated response to DNA damage that either triggers apoptotic cell death (via BAX and other proteins) or induces cell-cycle arrest, primarily through p21, to allow an opportunity for repair of small amounts of DNA damage {1180}.

As the adenoma expands in size, neoangiogenesis occurs to increase blood supply, and a tumour stroma develops including inflammatory and immune cells as well as stromal myofibroblasts within the surrounding lamina propria. A small subset of adenomas acquire defects in DNA mismatch repair genes, sporadically due to hypermethylation of the *MLH1* promoter, with a very small number of cases of inherited mutations in *MLH1* or *MSH2* (or rarely *MSH6*) in Lynch syndrome families, and these may evolve into defective mismatch repair adenocarcinomas (see *Lynch syndrome*, p. 515) {3735}. Population differences

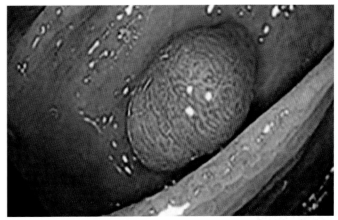

Fig. 6.15 Colonic villous adenoma. Colonoscopic image; the surface of the polyp has irregular ridges.

appear to influence the morphogenesis of adenomas, as evidenced by a higher frequency of flat and depressed adenomas among Asian patients.

Macroscopic appearance

Adenomas may have a pedunculated, sessile protuberant, slightly elevated or flat, or even depressed appearance. The size of the adenoma (largest dimension in mm) is important for defining its level of risk in screening programmes.

Histopathology
Subtyping of conventional adenomas
Three subtypes of conventional adenomas can be distinguished on the basis of their villosity or villousness. In tubular adenomas, the normal crypt architecture is largely conserved, with variable elongation of the crypts and an increase in the number of glands. The epithelium shows enlarged, hyperchromatic nuclei, with varying degrees of nuclear spindling and stratification and with loss of polarity. There is pseudostratification and loss of differentiation with decreased numbers of goblet and absorptive cells. A small villous component (< 25%) is acceptable in tubular adenomas. Tubular adenomas are the most common group of conventional adenomas detected during population screening {816,3775,1186,1339}. Villous structures resembling small intestinal villi in > 25% of the adenoma is generally required for the diagnosis of tubulovillous adenoma. If > 75% of the adenoma

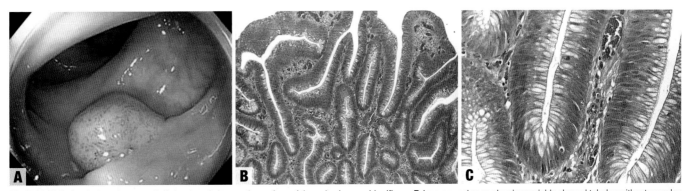

Fig. 6.14 Colonic tubular adenoma. **A** Colonoscopic image; the surface of the polyp has ovoid orifices. **B** Low-power image showing variably shaped tubules without complex architecture (no cribriform or solid areas), composed of cells with low-grade dysplasia with only mild or moderate nuclear enlargement and pleomorphism. **C** High-power image showing tubules lined by cells with mild or moderate nuclear enlargement and pleomorphism.

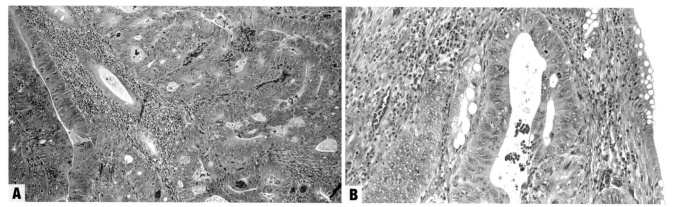

Fig. 6.16 Tubular adenoma with high-grade dysplasia. **A** Low-power image showing an area of high-grade dysplasia with more-complex cribriform architecture, including foci of near-solidity, composed of cells with nuclear enlargement and marked nuclear pleomorphism. **B** High-power image showing a focus of high-grade dysplasia that illustrates prominent nuclear atypia with marked pleomorphism and mitotic figures, in a partly cribriform gland that demonstrates arch and bridge formation.

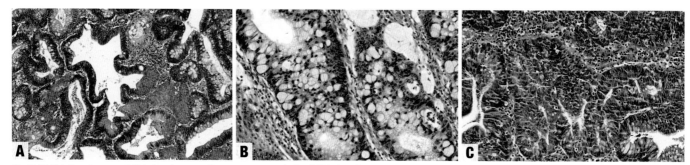

Fig. 6.17 Tubular adenoma. **A** Tubular adenoma with squamous metaplasia. **B** Tubular adenoma with clear-cell changes. **C** Tubular adenoma with Paneth cells and high-grade dysplasia.

has a villous architecture, it is commonly diagnosed as villous adenoma. Despite the poor intraobserver variability in subtyping conventional adenomas {3368,2463}, this approach is used clinically. By tradition, this is the manner in which adenomas are histologically characterized; however, the limited evidence behind this approach warrants further research.

Advanced adenomas

The term "advanced adenoma" has been coined for use in the international comparison of population screening programmes. This group of adenomas encompasses all adenomas with a size

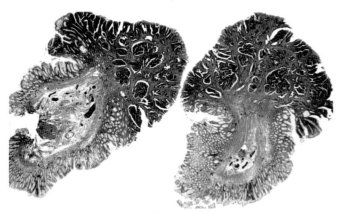

Fig. 6.18 Tubulovillous adenoma with invasive carcinoma. An ultra-low-power image of an example with high-grade dysplasia showing invasion into the smooth muscle in the head/neck region of the polyp by small clusters and single cells of adenocarcinoma.

> 10 mm, tubulovillous or villous architecture, and/or high-grade dysplasia (HGD) or intramucosal adenocarcinoma. The removal of advanced adenomas has the largest effect on cancer prevention, and it forms the basis of population screening. Advanced adenoma is associated with a high risk of synchronous or metachronous adenomas. The association with synchronous lesions indicates the need for a full colonoscopy in case of sigmoidoscopy screening programmes {205}, and the association with metachronous adenomas is the indication for more stringent surveillance in these patients {3576,414,816,204}.

Morphological subtypes

Rare morphological subtypes of conventional adenomas have been described. The most common is the Paneth cell–rich subtype. Paneth cells, which can be observed in as many as 20% of adenomas, are more common in proximal adenomas and in younger patients {1482,2004}. In < 0.1% of adenomas, squamous components are present, either as morules or as true squamous metaplasia, including keratinization {3382}. Clear cells are present in < 0.1% of adenomas {800}.

Grading of adenomas

For dysplasia grading of conventional adenomas, we use a two-tiered stratification into low-grade and HGD, although there is a high level of interobserver variability. HGD is characterized by marked complex glandular crowding and irregularity of glands, cribriform architecture, and intraluminal necrosis as architectural features. These can be observed at low magnification. For the diagnosis of HGD, these must be accompanied by cytological features of HGD, including substantial loss of cell polarity, markedly enlarged nuclei with prominent nucleoli, and a dispersed chromatin pattern, often with atypical mitotic figures {1105,2874}.

Pseudoinvasion (epithelial misplacement) and invasive cancer

Pseudoinvasion, sometimes called epithelial misplacement, represents prolapse of the adenomatous epithelium into the polyp head, stalk, or deeper, often accompanied by extracellular mucin, haemorrhage, and haemosiderin, indicating trauma from peristalsis and prolapse. These appearances can sometimes mimic malignancy. It can be difficult to distinguish pseudoinvasion (or epithelial misplacement), particularly in cases with HGD, from an early-stage T1 colorectal cancer. Such cases usually require histological review by more than one pathologist (often several) or referral to an expert panel of pathologists {1096,452,215,3428}.

Cytology

Cytopathology is not commonly used in the evaluation of colorectal adenomas.

Diagnostic molecular pathology

Not clinically relevant

Essential and desirable diagnostic criteria

Essential: a villous or polypoid lesion; dysplasia (low-grade or high-grade); histological subtype (tubular, tubulovillous, or villous); absence of true invasion.

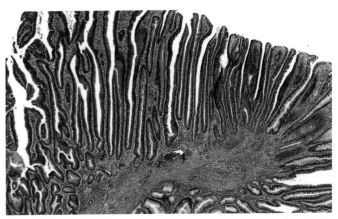

Fig. 6.19 An area of villous architecture within an adenoma.

Staging (TNM)

Polyps with high-grade dysplasia are pTis.

Prognosis and prediction

Most adenomas do not progress through the adenoma–carcinoma sequence, as evidenced by the high incidence of adenomas in populations relative to that of colorectal adenocarcinoma. The likelihood of carcinoma being present at the time of identification of an adenoma or developing subsequently is greater with higher number, larger size, higher proportion of villous architecture, and more extensive HGD.

Inflammatory bowel disease–associated dysplasia of the colorectum

Odze RD
Harpaz N

Definition

Colorectal dysplasia associated with inflammatory bowel disease (IBD) is an unequivocal neoplastic alteration of the intestinal epithelium that remains confined within the basement membrane in which it originated.

ICD-O coding

8148/0 Glandular intraepithelial neoplasia, low grade
8148/2 Glandular intraepithelial neoplasia, high grade

ICD-11 coding

DD7Y Other specified inflammatory bowel diseases
2E61.0 Carcinoma in situ of colon

Related terminology

Not recommended: dysplasia-associated lesion or mass.

Subtype(s)

None

Localization

In ulcerative colitis, most cases of dysplasia occur in the left or distal colon. The rectosigmoid alone accounts for 44–72% of dysplasia cases {1063,2805,624}, mirroring the localization of ulcerative colitis–associated colorectal cancers (CRCs). Dysplasia in Crohn disease is distributed more evenly throughout the colon and is present adjacent to cancer in > 80% of cases {3123,3067,3043}.

Clinical features

There are no specific signs or symptoms related to dysplasia in IBD. Elevated ulcerating and polypoid lesions may cause bleeding, but this is unusual until cancer has developed. Endoscopically, dysplasia is now classified according to the SCENIC classification as either visible or invisible lesions {1769}. Visible lesions are subclassified as either polypoid (pedunculated or sessile) or non-polypoid (superficial, flat, or depressed). The SCENIC classification also recommends that dysplasia be categorized according to its growth features, such as the presence or absence of ulceration, and the characteristics of the borders (distinct vs indistinct).

Epidemiology

Overall, < 1% of all CRC in the USA is associated with IBD. Cancer risk in ulcerative colitis and Crohn disease is roughly equivalent for patients who have equal lengths of colon involved {1452}. Two population-based studies show the relative risk of neoplasia in IBD to be 1.9–2.6 for Crohn disease and 2.4–2.7 for ulcerative colitis {310}. In a 2001 meta-analysis of 116 studies, the estimated risk of cancer in patients with ulcerative colitis was 2% after 10 years, 8.5% after 20 years, and 17.8% after 30 years {836}; however, in a later study from the United Kingdom, the risk of dysplasia and cancer in ulcerative colitis was lower (2.5%, 7.6%, and 10.8% at 20, 30, and 40 years, respectively) {2805}.

Features associated with an increased risk of dysplasia and/ or carcinoma in patients with ulcerative colitis include increased duration of disease, anatomical extent of disease, the presence or absence of primary sclerosing cholangitis, family history of CRC, early age of onset, and severity of endoscopic and histological inflammation {849,3080,201,2804}. The relative risk of dysplasia/cancer significantly increases after 8–10 years of disease. In a recent meta-analysis, a diagnosis of extensive colitis was associated with a 4.8-fold increase in risk of dysplasia or CRC {1453}. Primary sclerosing cholangitis develops in approximately 2–5% of patients with ulcerative colitis {3080}. In one meta-analysis, patients with primary sclerosing cholangitis and ulcerative colitis were found to have a 4-fold increased risk of dysplasia or cancer {3080}. Several studies have shown good correlation between severity of inflammation and risk of colorectal neoplasia {2804,1122}. In two studies from the USA, the risk of neoplasia increased with increasing inflammation score. The risk increased with the average activity over time rather than with single severe disease episodes {1122,2775}.

Etiology

IBD-associated carcinogenesis is thought to be due to sustained inflammation within the colorectum, along with a combination of genetic, immunological, infectious, and other environmental factors. Genetic factors include inheritance of one or more cancer susceptibility gene mutations or polymorphisms, which have been identified in some IBD-associated CRC cases {783}, although it is unknown whether this predisposes individuals to the formation of dysplasia in IBD or to progression from dysplasia to adenocarcinoma. The sustained inflammation is considered to contribute to tumour formation via both generation of reactive oxygen species that cause DNA mutations and ulcer-related regeneration of the epithelium acting as a tumour promoter that propagates mutated epithelial stem cells and progenitor cells, such as TP53-mutant cells that can spread along the length of the IBD bowel over time {1001}.

Pathogenesis

IBD-associated tumorigenesis is the product of a sustained inflammatory microenvironment. At the molecular level, it involves the induction of host responses to inflammation-related cellular damage that interact with tumorigenic transcription factors such as NF-κB through the direct or indirect effects of cytokines such as IL-1β, IL-6, and TNF-α, as well as matrix proteases and proangiogenic and antiapoptotic factors. The frequent multifocality of IBD-associated dysplasia of the colorectum and cancer reflects a field effect in which extensive regions of the mucosa are populated by epithelial clones that harbour aneuploidy or deleterious mutations and have the capacity to

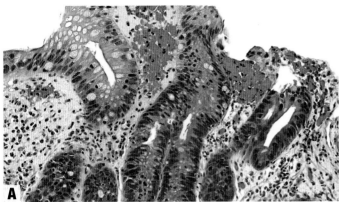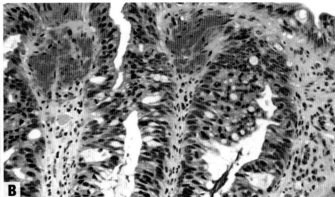

Fig. 6.20 Dysplasia, intestinal type. **A** Low-grade dysplasia. Slender, hyperchromatic, crowded nuclei are aligned along the cell bases and extend to the epithelial surface; goblet cells are sparse and their mucin vacuoles are frequently small. **B** High-grade dysplasia. Hyperchromatic, pleomorphic nuclei are stratified haphazardly within the cytoplasm.

expand and progress {226,279,820,1172}. The inflammatory environment promotes cellular damage from oxidative stress due to heightened production and accumulation of reactive oxygen species. These participate in the initiation and progression of neoplasia by generating mutagenic DNA adducts (accelerating cellular senescence) and potentiating immune reactions that further augment tissue damage. Reactive metabolites and carcinogens are also produced by the dysbiotic intestinal microbiota in IBD. Aneuploidy is promoted by telomere shortening resulting from oxidative DNA damage and accelerated epithelial cell turnover. Mutations of *TP53* are introduced by the mutagenic enzyme activation-induced cytidine deaminase in response to proinflammatory cytokines. Inflammation also promotes epigenetic DNA modifications that can disrupt critical homeostatic gene functions, including DNA-repair processes {324,2880,860,226}.

The progression of oncogenic mutations that accompanies the inflammation–dysplasia–carcinoma sequence in IBD differs from the classic paradigm of the sporadic adenoma–carcinoma sequence. Oncogenic mutations of *TP53* occur in 60–89% of IBD-associated cancers, and rather than being late events, they are frequently initiating mutations that may even precede the development of histologically observable dysplasia. Next-generation sequencing of IBD-associated cancers has revealed relatively high proportions of *MYC* amplifications and low rates of *KRAS* and *APC* mutations compared with sporadic cancers, and some actionable mutations, such as in *MLH1*, *RNF43*, and *RPL22*, were observed {783,1178,2739,3636}. A proportion (> 25% in one series) of IBD-associated cancers have high mutation rates that are associated mostly with defective mismatch repair and occasionally with defective DNA proofreading function of POLE {783,2739}.

Macroscopic appearance
There are no distinguishing features. Sampling of multiple areas is required to assess the presence of dysplasia, often resulting in many small endoscopic biopsies.

Histopathology
Dysplasia is classified according to either the Vienna {2886} or the Riddell {2712} system. In the Riddell system, which is popular in the USA, dysplasia is classified as negative, indefinite, low-grade, or high-grade.

The most common morphological subtypes of dysplasia in IBD include the intestinal (adenomatous) and serrated types. In general, and regardless of histological type, dysplasia is graded according to a combination of cytological and architectural alterations of the epithelium. In low-grade dysplasia (LGD), the crypts may be tubular and/or villous or serrated, and they demonstrate either no or only mild crypt budding and crowding. The dysplastic cells show nuclear enlargement, elongation, increased N:C ratios, hyperchromasia, stratification limited to the basal half of the cell cytoplasm, and either clumped chromatin or multiple small nucleoli. In serrated dysplasia, the dysplastic cells may show hypereosinophilic, mucin-depleted cytoplasm or microvesicular epithelium similar to that of sporadic sessile serrated lesions. Dysplastic epithelium normally involves both the crypt and the surface epithelium, but early cases may show only involvement of the crypts, which is termed crypt dysplasia. Other less common features of LGD include dystrophic goblet cells and endocrine and Paneth cell metaplasia.

In high-grade dysplasia (HGD), the cells show markedly enlarged, often pleomorphic, and hyperchromatic nuclei, with marked loss of cell polarity and nuclear stratification that involves the full thickness of the cell cytoplasm. Mitotic figures, both typical and atypical, are more frequent and often present in the upper portions of the crypts and surface epithelium. HGD is often

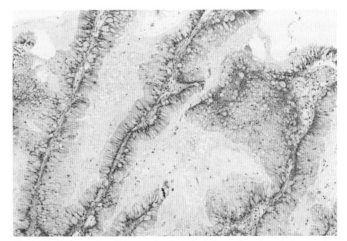

Fig. 6.21 Mucinous (gastric)-type dysplasia in inflammatory bowel disease, low grade.

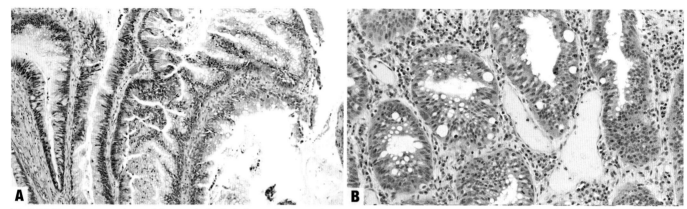

Fig. 6.22 Dysplasia, serrated type. **A** Low-grade dysplasia. Serrated crypts are lined by columnar and goblet cells with non-stratified hyperchromatic, crowded nuclei. **B** High-grade dysplasia. Serrated crypts are lined by columnar cells with eosinophilic cytoplasm and enlarged, haphazardly stratified nuclei.

accompanied by substantial architectural abnormalities, such as gland crowding, cribriforming, and marked budding and branching. Intraluminal necrosis may be present. There is no uniform agreement regarding the proportion of high-grade dysplastic crypts that are necessary to upgrade a biopsy specimen from low-grade to high-grade, but most authorities would categorize a biopsy specimen as high-grade if it had any high-grade focus.

Intramucosal carcinoma is defined by the presence of cells or glands that invade the lamina propria or into but not through the muscularis mucosae. Desmoplasia is typically absent when the carcinoma is limited to the mucosa, and its presence is virtually diagnostic of submucosal invasion.

Other less common types of dysplasia include a mucinous subtype, a subtype with eosinophilic cytoplasm and marked goblet cell depletion, and a "crypt cell" subtype comprising epithelial cells with atypical nuclei but near-normal cytoplasmic differentiation. Mucinous dysplasia often exhibits a tubulovillous pattern of growth, and it shows epithelium with small, hyperchromatic, basally oriented nuclei with minimal cytological atypia. Goblet cells are typically fewer in number, but the cytoplasm shows marked mucinous differentiation.

Patients with IBD may also develop hyperplastic polyp–like or sessile serrated lesion–like lesions without substantial nuclear atypia, but the natural history and risk of progression of these lesions is either not increased or unknown {2980,1659,2603}. Dysplastic serrated change shows more-substantial nuclear enlargement, hyperchromasia, and stratification, which typically reaches the surface of the epithelium. In many patients with dysplasia, mixed patterns of dysplasia are present. The most common is a mixture of intestinal and serrated dysplasia, ranging from hyperplastic change to high-grade serrated change. Rarely, traditional serrated adenoma–like lesions may also occur in IBD.

Cytology
Not clinically relevant

Diagnostic molecular pathology
Not clinically relevant

Essential and desirable diagnostic criteria
Essential: histological evidence of dysplasia in the setting of IBD.

Staging (TNM)
High-grade dysplasia is pTis.

Prognosis and prediction
The natural history and treatment of dysplasia varies according to the growth pattern {1769}. Endoscopically occult (flat, random, or non-targeted lesions) LGD has shown a 5-year rate of development to either HGD or carcinoma as high as 54% {659}. Higher rates of progression are noted if the dysplasia is found on initial colonoscopy (prevalent dysplasia) or is multifocal. Occult HGD has been associated with an even higher probability of cancer being detected at colectomy (40–67%) or progression to carcinoma, with 5-year predictive values of 40–90% {901,659,311}. Polypoid dysplasia, particularly if it is adenoma-like, has a very low rate of progression to carcinoma {863}. On long-term follow-up, the rate of progression to subsequent flat dysplasia is 0–5.1%, and to subsequent carcinoma 0–4.5%. In one long-term follow-up study of polypoid dysplasia, the risk of subsequent flat dysplasia or carcinoma was 2.9% after a mean of 82.1 months of follow-up {2409}. Similar rates of progression were noted for polypoid dysplasia in patients with Crohn disease in a recent study {2629}.

Colorectal adenocarcinoma

Nagtegaal ID
Arends MJ
Salto-Tellez M

Definition

Colorectal adenocarcinoma is a malignant epithelial tumour originating in the large bowel, showing glandular or mucinous differentiation.

ICD-O coding

8140/3 Adenocarcinoma NOS

ICD-11 coding

2B90.Y & XH74S1 Other specified malignant neoplasms of colon & Adenocarcinoma NOS

Related terminology

None

Subtype(s)

Serrated adenocarcinoma (8213/3); adenoma-like adenocarcinoma (8262/3); micropapillary adenocarcinoma (8265/3); mucinous adenocarcinoma (8480/3); poorly cohesive carcinoma (8490/3); signet-ring cell carcinoma (8490/3); medullary adenocarcinoma (8510/3); adenosquamous carcinoma (8560/3); carcinoma, undifferentiated, NOS (8020/3); carcinoma with sarcomatoid component (8033/3)

Localization

For practical purposes, colorectal carcinomas are divided into three groups by location: right-sided or proximal colon carcinomas (including those in the caecum, ascending colon, and transverse colon), left-sided colon carcinomas (located anywhere from the splenic flexure up to the sigmoid), and rectal carcinomas. Most colorectal cancers (CRCs) are left-sided or rectal {3126}. There has been a relative decrease in the incidence of left-sided CRC {649}, probably due to increased uptake of endoscopy.

Screening strategies, including faecal occult blood testing, are more sensitive for left-sided neoplasia {1192}. The molecular background of CRC also shows location-specific features (see *Pathogenesis*, below). Treatment is different, with a prominent role for neoadjuvant radiotherapy or radiochemotherapy for rectal carcinomas. Surgical complications are more often observed in the treatment of right-sided colon cancer {471}. Tumour location is also related to the outcome of metastatic CRC {689}, and it has an association with the success of systemic treatment {189,353}.

Clinical features

Common symptoms include persistent changes in bowel habits, anaemia and haematochezia, and abdominal pain. With the widespread introduction of population screening {1796}, the

Chapter 6

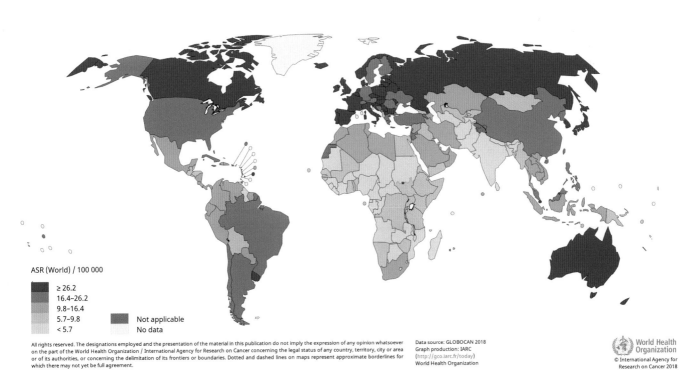

ASR (World) / 100 000

- ≥ 26.2
- 16.4–26.2
- 9.8–16.4
- 5.7–9.8
- < 5.7
- Not applicable
- No data

Data source: GLOBOCAN 2018
Graph production: IARC
(http://gco.iarc.fr/today)
World Health Organization

World Health Organization
© International Agency for Research on Cancer 2018

Fig. 6.23 Estimated age-standardized incidence rates (ASRs; World), per 100 000 person-years, of colorectal cancer in 2018.

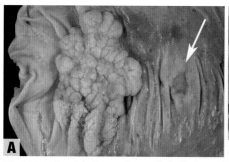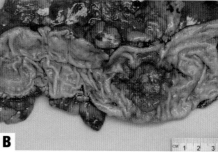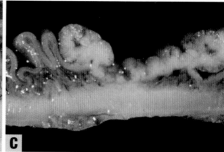

Fig. 6.24 Colorectal adenocarcinoma. **A** Small ulcerated invasive carcinoma (arrow) with a nearby protruding adenoma. **B** Note mucosal ulcer with rolled-up edges. **C** Cross-section of adenocarcinoma with extension into the submucosa.

clinical spectrum of CRC is changing, with increasing numbers of patients without symptoms. Depending on the accepted screening strategy, these patients' tumours are detected after selection by various types of faecal occult blood tests or during endoscopy {1796}.

Endoscopic evaluation allows visualization of CRC and precursor lesions on the mucosal surface of the large bowel. Therapeutic removal of early lesions can also be performed, by snare polypectomy, endoscopic mucosal resection, or submucosal dissection {979}. Advanced techniques, such as narrow-band imaging and magnifying chromoendoscopy, improve endoscopic detection and evaluation of CRC {216}.

Imaging can be applied for non-invasive detection of CRC with the use of CT colonography, but definite diagnosis is made on biopsy or resection. The main use of clinical imaging is for staging of CRC. Various techniques are applied. To determine invasion depth in early rectal cancers, endorectal ultrasonography is applied {3778}. For more-advanced lesions, MRI investigation is essential, in particular in the determination of the relation of the tumour with the mesorectal fascia {3752}. The evaluation of nodal status remains difficult {1766}. To identify distant metastases before extensive surgery is performed, CT or PET-CT can be used. Recently, the evaluation of tumour response (restaging) using imaging has become more important {3413,1999}.

Epidemiology

CRC, with an estimated 1 849 518 new cases worldwide in 2018, is the second most common cancer in women and the third most common cancer in men. The incidence varies widely,

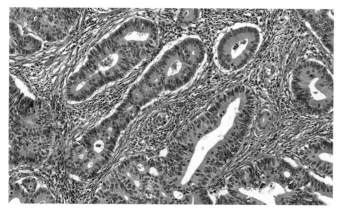

Fig. 6.25 Adenocarcinoma, low-grade.

with the highest rates seen in the highest-income countries {399}. In many low- and middle-income countries, the incidence of CRC is rapidly increasing, whereas stabilizing or decreasing rates have been observed in high-income, high-incidence countries {191}. Trends of increasing incidence in young adults have been reported recently in Australia, Canada, and the USA {3032,2546,3718}.

Etiology

A high incidence of CRC is consistently observed in populations with diets typical of high-income countries combined with a sedentary lifestyle. Established risk factors include consumption of processed and red meat {383}, consumption of alcohol {3473}, and excess body fat {1795}. The relation of smoking with CRC is controversial; some studies include smoking as a risk factor and others do not {1836}. Consumption of dietary fibre and dairy products {3473} and increased levels of physical activity {1742} decrease the risk, as do prolonged use of NSAIDS and hormone replacement therapy in women {1473,1094}. The molecular pathways underlying these epidemiological associations are poorly understood, probably because of complex interactions. Indeed, the effects of dietary interventions in CRC prevention seem minimal, and effective forms of chemoprevention are limited to NSAIDS {821}.

Genetic predisposition is an important risk factor for CRC, depending on the type of mutation. The risk can increase to 100% lifetime risk in patients with familial adenomatous polyposis. Table 6.06 (p. 187) provides an overview of hereditary cancer syndromes that involve CRC. Hereditary cancer syndromes are discussed in more detail in Chapter 14: *Genetic tumour syndromes of the digestive system* (p. 511).

Chronic bowel inflammation is an established risk factor for CRC. Inflammatory bowel diseases (Crohn disease and ulcerative colitis) are discussed in the section *Inflammatory bowel disease–associated dysplasia of the colorectum* (p. 174). Other rare but well-established risk factors are pelvic irradiation {2750}, cystic fibrosis {1136}, ureterosigmoidostomy {213}, and acromegaly {2746}.

Pathogenesis

Most CRCs develop via the conventional pathway through the classic adenoma–carcinoma sequence of pathogenesis, and the remainder evolve via either the hypermutant pathway or the ultramutant pathway. This involves transition from normal mucosal epithelial stem cells through adenomas to carcinomas, with stepwise accumulation of genetic and epigenetic

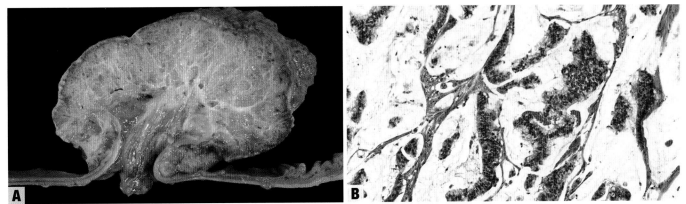

Fig. 6.26 Mucinous adenocarcinoma. **A** Note the cut surface with gelatinous appearance. **B** Malignant epithelial cells in clumps and layers in pools of extracellular mucin.

abnormalities in highly variable patterns in the evolving tumour cells. Cancers show underlying molecular changes associated with three main mechanisms of genetic instability: (1) chromosomal instability resulting in high levels of DNA somatic copy-number alterations (SCNAs), with DNA gains/amplifications and losses/deletions affecting a smaller group of genes {2611,178}; (2) microsatellite instability (MSI) with a high mutation rate (hypermutant) due to defective DNA mismatch repair affecting a large number of genes; or (3) defective proofreading polymerase with a very high mutation rate (ultramutant) affecting very large numbers of genes (mostly passenger mutations with few driver mutations) {474,2264}.

The most frequent and characteristic genetic changes in the conventional colorectal adenoma–carcinoma pathway include alterations to *APC, KRAS, TP53, SMAD4,* or *PIK3CA* (84%, chromosomal instability pathway); the mismatch repair genes *MLH1* and *MSH2* (13%, MSI hypermutant pathway); and *POLE* (3%, ultramutant pathway). *APC* alterations are mostly inactivating mutations, found in about 80% of both adenomas and carcinomas, which occur very early in the sequence and appear to initiate adenoma formation {178,1354}. These mutations usually lead to truncation of the APC protein, with reduced ability to direct degradation of β-catenin resulting in its accumulation and causing abnormal signalling through the WNT pathway {911,2216}. *KRAS* mutations, found in about 40% of both adenomas and cancers at specific sites (codons 12, 13, 61, and others), activate the KRAS oncoprotein by reducing or inactivating

its intrinsic GTPase enzymatic activity, thus locking the protein into its GTP-bound active state. This sends constitutive signals through the RAS-RAF-MEK-ERK (MAPK) proliferative signalling pathway, as can *BRAF* activating mutations {2264,2276}. Additionally, KRAS feeds into the PI3K apoptosis-suppressing pathway, which can also be activated by mutations in *PIK3CA* or *PTEN* {2275}. The *SMAD4* gene is usually inactivated by deletion (in ~60% cancers) of a large part of chromosome 18q or less often by mutation, reducing signalling through the TGF-β inhibitory pathway. The *TP53* tumour suppressor gene, which encodes p53, is sometimes called the guardian of the genome, because it responds to DNA damage and other stresses by either inducing cell-cycle arrest via p21, allowing an opportunity to repair small amounts of DNA damage, or inducing apoptotic cell death via BAX (and other proteins) when the DNA damage is more severe. Mutations that inactivate or subvert p53 function are found in about 60% of cancers, and this mutational event often maps to the late stage of adenoma–carcinoma transition in sporadic cancers, although it occurs earlier in inflammatory bowel disease–associated carcinogenesis, see also *Inflammatory bowel disease–associated dysplasia of the colorectum* (p. 174).

Serrated and other adenocarcinomas associated with defective mismatch repair account for about 13% of all CRCs and follow an alternative pathway in which the precursor lesions are serrated polyps (including hyperplastic polyps, sessile serrated lesions, traditional serrated adenomas, and mixed polyps)

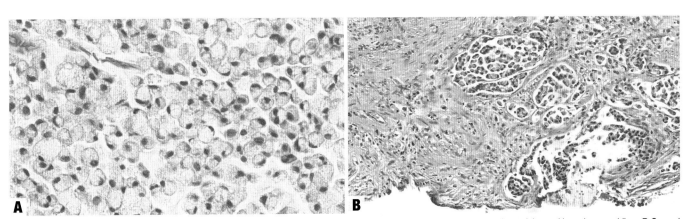

Fig. 6.27 Signet-ring cell carcinoma. **A** Note signet-ring cells with prominent intracytoplasmic mucin, displacing the nucleus to the periphery with nuclear moulding. **B** Serosal involvement.

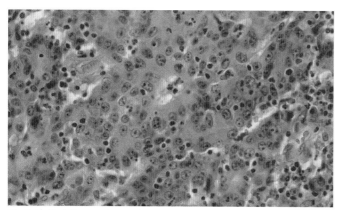

Fig. 6.28 Medullary carcinoma. Sheets of tumour cells and infiltration by lymphocytes.

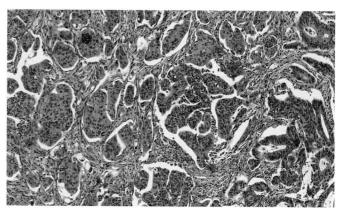

Fig. 6.30 Micropapillary carcinoma.

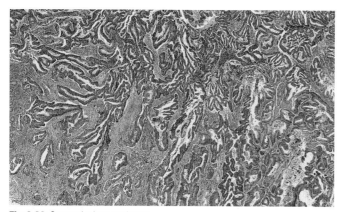

Fig. 6.29 Serrated adenocarcinoma.

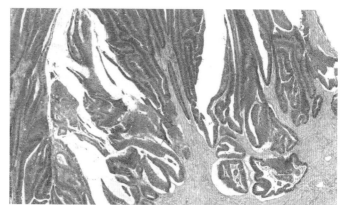

Fig. 6.31 Adenoma-like adenocarcinoma with a villous contour and a pushing infiltrative border configuration, due to the lack of desmoplastic reaction, which makes this tumour hard to identify on biopsy.

rather than conventional adenomas. Serrated polyps often have *BRAF* and (less often) *KRAS* activating mutations and the CpG island methylator phenotype, in which a range of susceptible genes develop epigenetic promoter hypermethylation that silences their expression, frequently including *MLH1*, leading to defective mismatch repair and MSI. About 3% of adenocarcinomas have mutations affecting the proofreading domain of POLE that confer very high mutation rates (ultramutant) {3654,1550}.

Macroscopic appearance
The appearances are variable, with endophytic and exophytic types and variable degrees of fibrosis. The usual type is an ulcer with rolled edges extending around the circumference of the colon.

Histopathology
The majority (90%) of all CRCs are adenocarcinomas. Their defining feature is invasion through the muscularis mucosae into the submucosa. Although most cases are diagnosed as adenocarcinoma NOS, several histopathological subtypes can be distinguished, with specific clinical and molecular characteristics.

Mucinous adenocarcinoma
A tumour is designated as mucinous adenocarcinoma if > 50% of the lesion is composed of pools of extracellular mucin that contain overt malignant epithelium as clumps, layers, or individual tumour cells including signet-ring cells. This is the most

common subtype, with a prevalence ranging from 5% to 20% {1324}. There is no prognostic difference compared with adenocarcinoma NOS {3464}, although there is a relatively poor response to systemic treatment in the metastatic setting {1323}. The proportion of cases with MSI is increased compared with adenocarcinoma NOS. The presence of MSI does not have independent prognostic value {1498,142}; therefore, grading should be based on glandular formation and epithelial maturation. Carcinomas with mucinous areas of < 50% are categorized as having a mucinous component.

Signet-ring cell carcinoma
A tumour is designated as signet-ring cell carcinoma if > 50% of the tumour cells have prominent intracytoplasmic mucin, typically with displacement and moulding of the nucleus. This subtype has a low prevalence rate, approximately 1% {1346}, and a predilection for the right colon. Tumours often present at advanced stages, but stage-corrected outcome is worse compared with adenocarcinoma NOS and mucinous carcinoma {1326}. Metastases develop rapidly and in multiple locations that are not typical for CRC {1325}. There is a high incidence of MSI, a strong association with Lynch syndrome {1499}, and possibly an enrichment of the MSI/PDL1 druggable phenotype {115}. Carcinomas with signet-ring cells in < 50% of the tumour are categorized as having a signet-ring cell component.

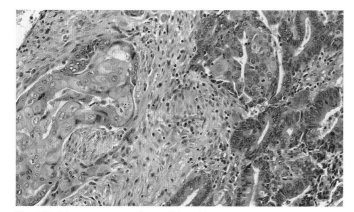

Fig. 6.32 Adenosquamous carcinoma of the colorectum.

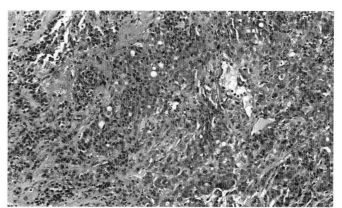

Fig. 6.33 Undifferentiated carcinoma.

Medullary carcinoma

This subtype is characterized by sheets of malignant cells with vesicular nuclei, prominent nucleoli, and abundant eosinophilic cytoplasm, exhibiting prominent infiltration by lymphocytes and neutrophilic granulocytes. Single-centre studies estimate its prevalence at 4% {1657,1789}. In cancer registries, this subtype is underreported {3296}. It frequently contains MSI, most frequently in combination with *BRAF* mutations {1657}, and it is associated with a good prognosis {1789}. Of note, this type of CRC shows an aberrant immunohistochemical pattern, with loss of CDX2 and CK20 {1237}. Neuroendocrine markers are negative on immunohistochemistry.

Serrated adenocarcinoma

This subtype is defined by morphological similarities with serrated polyps, with glandular serration that can be accompanied by mucinous areas. The tumour cells have a low N:C ratio. Approximately 10–15% of all CRCs can be classified as serrated adenocarcinoma {1012}.

Micropapillary adenocarcinoma

This subtype is characterized by small clusters of tumour cells within stromal spaces mimicking vascular channels; ≥ 5% of the tumour should present with this aspect for this diagnosis. Its incidence ranges from 5% to 20% in single-centre series {3462,1823,1193}. This subtype has a high risk of lymph node metastasis, and poor prognostic factors such as lymphatic invasion, extramural vascular invasion (EMVI), and perineural invasion are frequently present.

Adenoma-like adenocarcinoma

This subtype {1068}, previously described as "villous adenocarcinoma" {1955} and "invasive papillary adenocarcinoma" {2491}, is defined as an invasive adenocarcinoma in which ≥ 50% of the invasive areas have an adenoma-like aspect with villous structures, with a low-grade aspect. Minimal desmoplastic reaction is observed, and there is a pushing growth pattern. Its incidence ranges from 3% to 9% {1068,1955}. This subtype is characterized by difficulties in establishing a diagnosis of the invasive component on biopsies, a high *KRAS* mutation rate, and a favourable prognosis {1068}.

Adenosquamous carcinoma

This rare subtype has an incidence of < 0.1% {2071,456} and features of both adenocarcinoma and squamous cell carcinoma, similar to adenosquamous carcinomas seen elsewhere in the GI tract; see *Oesophageal adenosquamous and mucoepidermoid carcinomas* (p. 46) and *Gastric adenosquamous carcinoma* (p. 98).

Carcinomas with sarcomatoid components

A small subgroup of CRCs is characterized by partly undifferentiated histology and sarcomatoid aspects such as spindle cell components or rhabdoid features {626,2234,44}. In general, patients have a poor outcome {2234}. The tumours are typically large and show characteristic rhabdoid cells with abundant intracytoplasmic, eosinophilic rhabdoid bodies. The tumour cells are often dyscohesive and embedded in myxoid matrix. Pleomorphic giant or spindle cells, as well as areas of glandular differentiation, may also be seen. Loss of nuclear immunostaining for SMARCB1 (INI1), a core subunit of the SWI/SNF chromatin-remodelling complex, is characteristic {44}. These tumours appear to have loss/coactivation of multiple members of the SWI/SNF family of proteins, including SMARCA4, SMARCA2, and/or SMARCB1

Box 6.02 Essential and desirable diagnostic criteria for colorectal cancer

- Histological subtype
- Differentiation grade: Low/high
- Invasion depth: According to TNM, specify if invasion in other organs (pT4) or tumour perforation
- Presence of (lympho)vascular invasion: Intramural vascular invasion, extramural vascular invasion, lymphatic invasion
- Perineural growth: Present/absent
- Resection margin status (proximal, distal, circumferential): Positive, negative, distance in cm
- Diameter of the tumour
- Site/localization of the tumour
- Quality of the resection specimen
- Number of investigated lymph nodes
- Number of positive lymph nodes
- Presence of treatment response: Yes/no; if yes, partial or complete response
- Microsatellite status / presence of DNA mismatch repair proteins (MLH1, MSH2, MSH6, PMS2): Microsatellite-stable or -unstable, staining for mismatch repair proteins present or absent
- Tumour budding status
- Immune response
- Presence or absence of relevant mutations

Table 6.02 Histological prognostic factors in colorectal cancer: an overview of data derived from meta-analyses, depicted as hazard ratios (HRs) for overall survival

Risk factor	HR (95% CI) univariate	HR (95% CI) multivariate	Remarks	Reference
Subtypes				
Mucinous carcinoma	1.05 (1.02–1.08)		Compared with adenocarcinoma NOS	{3464}
Signet-ring cell carcinoma	1.49 (1.39–1.59)	2.66 (2.35–3.01)	Compared with adenocarcinoma NOS	{1323}
Medullary carcinoma	0.94 (0.80–1.00)		Compared with adenocarcinoma NOS	{2622}
Relevant histological features				
Perineural invasion	2.09 (1.68–2.61)	1.85 (1.63–2.12)	Compared with no perineural invasion	{1653}
Intramural vascular invasion	2.04 (1.39–2.99)	1.60 (1.15–2.24)	Compared with no intramural vascular invasion	{1654}
Extramural vascular invasion	3.6 (2.4–5.5)	1.72 (1.39–2.12)	Compared with no extramural vascular invasion	{1654}
Lymphatic invasion	2.15 (1.72–2.68)		In stage I/II colorectal cancer	{3725}
Tumour deposits	2.90 (2.20–3.92)	2.19 (1.72–2.77)	Compared with no tumour deposits	{2271}
Tumour budding	4.51 (2.55–7.99)[a]		Compared with no tumour budding	{2742A}
Treatment-related factors				
Circumferential margin	1.72 (1.28–2.27)		Compared with negative margins	{2272}
Tumour response	0.49 (0.28–0.85)		Partial response vs no response	{1847}
	0.44 (0.34–0.57)	0.54 (0.40–0.73)	Complete response vs other	{1990}

[a]Odds ratio instead of HR.

(indicating an association between SWI/SNF deficiency and rhabdoid phenotype), and some have ARID1A abnormalities.

Undifferentiated carcinoma

These carcinomas lack morphological, immunohistochemical, and molecular evidence of differentiation beyond that of an epithelial tumour. They differ from medullary carcinomas in their lack of pushing borders, syncytial growth pattern, and prominent lymphoplasmacytic infiltrates. They only infrequently show MSI.

Grading

Grading of CRC is based on gland formation: low-grade (formerly well- to moderately differentiated) and high-grade (formerly poorly differentiated) tumours. Grading is based on the least differentiated component. The invasive front, where formation of tumour budding and poorly differentiated clusters occurs as a sign of epithelial–mesenchymal transition {825}, should not be taken into account when grading the tumour, but should be reported separately.

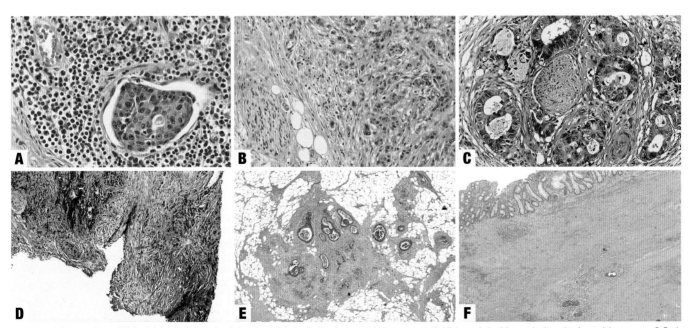

Fig. 6.34 Adenocarcinoma NOS. **A** Lymphatic invasion, in lymph vessels just below the muscularis mucosae. **B** High-grade budding at the invasive front of the tumour. **C** Perineural growth. **D** Involvement of the circumferential margin (black ink). **E** Tumour deposit. **F** Partial response to radiochemotherapy.

Table 6.03 Overview of the most commonly used systems for assessing tumour regression grade (TRG) {2036,1786}

Grade	Mandard	AJCC 2010	Rödel	MSKCC
TRG 0	–	No residual tumour cells	No regression	–
TRG 1	Absence of residual cancer, with fibrosis extending through the various layers of the oesophageal wall (complete regression)	Single cells or small groups	Fibrosis < 25% of tumour mass	100% response
TRG 2	Rare residual cancer cells scattered through the fibrosis	Residual cancer with desmoplastic response	Fibrosis 25–50% of tumour mass	86–99% response
TRG 3	An increase in the number of residual cancer cells, but fibrosis still predominates	Minimal evidence of tumour response	Fibrosis > 50% of tumour mass	< 86% response
TRG 4	Residual cancer outgrowing fibrosis	–	Complete regression	–
TRG 5	Absence of regressive changes	–	–	–

AJCC, American Joint Committee on Cancer; MSKCC, Memorial Sloan Kettering Cancer Center.

Important histological features
See Table 6.02.

Lymphatic invasion
Lymphatic invasion, i.e. the presence of single cells or groups of tumour cells in lymphatic channels (often defined as channels covered with endothelial cells devoid of erythrocytes) is a morphological risk factor for the presence of lymph node metastases in pT1 CRC. Additional immunohistochemistry can be helpful {1394}.

Intramural and extramural vascular invasion
Vascular invasion can be subclassified according to localization: within the bowel wall (intramural vascular invasion [IMVI]) versus outside the bowel wall (EMVI). IMVI is reported to have an incidence of 4–40% (12.5% overall reported incidence), and it is associated with poor outcome {1654}. The incidence of EMVI is higher than that of IMVI, but this feature is still considered to be underreported. The negative prognostic impact of EMVI is higher than that of IMVI {1654,550}. Features that are helpful in the recognition of EMVI are the orphan artery sign (a tumour nodule identified adjacent to an artery in a presumed vein) and the protruding tongue sign (a tongue of tumour protruding beyond the tumour border into a vein in the surrounding fat) {1617}. Elastin staining or immunohistochemistry is sometimes used to improve detection.

Perineural invasion
Growth along the nerve is called perineural invasion. Tumour cells should by definition surround at least one third of the nerve circumference {1904} and can be present in any of the three layers of the nerves (epineurium, perineurium, and endoneurium). The incidence is reported to be about 20%, with increased incidence in the rectum, in higher tumour stages, and in the presence of other risk factors (e.g. vascular and lymphatic invasion) {1653}. Perineural invasion is associated with local recurrence, distant recurrence, and decreased survival {1653}.

Tumour budding, poorly differentiated clusters, and growth pattern
Tumour budding is defined as single cells or clusters of as many as 4 tumour cells at the invasive margin of the tumour {1958}, which is determined on H&E staining in a hotspot at the invasive front using a three-tiered scoring system according to international consensus. The presence of high-grade budding is associated with poor outcome in various subgroups of CRC. Budding is considered to be the morphological manifestation of epithelial–mesenchymal transition {3786}. Poorly differentiated clusters are groups of ≥ 5 tumour cells, in the absence of glandular formation {3381}, and are an adverse prognostic feature {250}. Two types of growth patterns can be distinguished: infiltrative growth and pushing borders {1435}. Pushing borders are associated with improved outcome and lower stage.

Immune response
The relation of an immune response to outcome has been proven. Intratumoural lymphocytes {2772} and a Crohn-like reaction {2772} are associated with better outcome. Both features are associated with MSI {3075,1444}; however, the relation to outcome seems independent of MSI status. More recently, a standardized examination of the presence of lymphocytes at the invasive front of the tumour, using immunohistochemistry for CD3 and CD8, showed that this feature has significant prognostic power {2484}.

Resection margins and completeness of resection
The term "margin" refers to the areas of the resection or excision specimen that have been cut by the surgeon or endoscopist. Margins are not natural structures such as the serosal surface. Various margins can be defined: the proximal and distal margins are the easiest to distinguish. Those margins are rarely positive, but when the tumour is located close to these longitudinal margins, the risk of local recurrence is increased, particularly in rectal cancer when no radiotherapy is administered before surgery {2485}. The circumferential resection margin (considered positive if the distance between tumour and edge of resection is ≤ 1 mm) is more important, with a strong impact on local recurrence and overall survival {2272}. For caecal carcinomas, the circumferential or mesocolic margin is also important, but

Table 6.04 Predictive biomarkers in colorectal carcinoma

Biomarker	Type of abnormality	Predictive applicability	References
Established predictive biomarkers			
RAS genes	(DNA-based, tested primarily in tissues, increasing use in liquid biopsy) Mutation of codons 12, 13, 59, 61, 117, and 146 in the *KRAS* and *NRAS* genes	Mutant in 45–50% of all colorectal cancers. Establish predictive applicability 1. Anti-EGFR (HER1) therapy is ineffective in colorectal cancers with these mutations	{1072,2955,3596,1934, 3407,3570,3292,3257}
BRAF	(DNA-based, tested primarily in tissues, increasing use in liquid biopsy) Mutations in amino acid 600	Mutant in ~10% of colorectal cancers. Increasing/established predictive applicability 1. Potentially, *BRAF* mutations also identify colorectal cancer cases in which anti-EGFR therapy is ineffective 2. With microsatellite instability status (see below), it may predict response to chemotherapy	{946,175,2115,115, 1310,3292,3257}
Microsatellite instability	(DNA-based) Instability of microsatellites	Microsatellite instability in ~15% of colorectal cancers. Increasing predictive applicability 1. With *BRAF* status (see above), it may predict response to chemotherapy. Established predictive applicability 2. Predictive response to anti-PDL1 therapy	{818,1816,1815,2484}
Biomarkers partly established and/or under development			
Other cancer immune-related markers	DNA-based Tumour mutation burden Protein-based expression Immune score	Still to be determined for predictive purposes in colorectal cancer	
Gene expression signatures	RNA-based Gene expression	Restricted use. Predictive of recurrence after surgery	{3653,1554}
PIK3CA	DNA-based Mutations mainly in exons 9 and 20	Mutant in ~10% of cases. Restricted use. May identify colorectal cancer cases in which anti-EGFR therapy is ineffective. May predict successful adjuvant response to acetylsalicylic acid	{2849,2614,1897}
c-Met	Complex testing (DNA, RNA, and protein)		

less evidence is available {2922}. The strongest association with outcome is present when the margin is involved due to the primary tumour. Involvement due to positive lymph nodes, tumour deposits, vascular invasion, and perineural growth is less common and seems to have less impact on outcome {2272}. For a local excision specimen, the most important margin is the basal margin. Lateral resection margin positivity does not influence local recurrence rates {1838}.

In close correlation with the assessment of resection margins, the macroscopic evaluation of the completeness of the resection specimen and the achieved surgical plane of resection has been established as an important prognostic factor and as a quality indicator. The optimal planes of surgery are the mesorectal fascia {2274,2273} and the mesocolic plane {3552} for rectal and colonic tumours, respectively. Achievement of suboptimal planes of resection is associated with poor outcome.

Response to therapy
The application of neoadjuvant therapy, i.e. radiotherapy or radiochemotherapy for rectal carcinoma or systemic treatment for

CRC, interferes with the histopathology. A spectrum of tumour response can be observed, varying from complete pathological response to no detectable effects. Classification can be performed by assessment of downstaging (dependent on reliable pretreatment imaging) or evaluation of tumour regression grade (TRG). Various classification systems have been proposed, but all suffer from lack of reproducibility, although they have some features in common (see Table 6.03, p. 183) {3335}.

Cytology
Cytology is not clinically relevant, except in the metastatic setting, where FNA may be helpful.

Diagnostic molecular pathology
Two different approaches to the molecular pathological classification of CRC have been used: genomic (DNA-based) classification, supported by an integrated molecular analysis performed by The Cancer Genome Atlas (TCGA) network, and transcriptomic (RNA-based) profiling that characterizes CRC using RNA sequencing or array-based technologies {474,2264}.

Genomic classification

This approach classifies CRC into two main groups by mutation rate: hypermutated and non-hypermutated cancers, which match well with the MSI and chromosomal instability pathways and are consistent with previous DNA-based classification systems.

Hypermutated cases (~15% of CRCs) have a high frequency of mutations, and most show MSI due to defective DNA mismatch repair. This includes both sporadic hypermutated microsatellite-unstable cancers with *MLH1* promoter hypermethylation causing loss of MLH1 expression and inactivation of DNA mismatch repair (~13%). Almost all of these tumours have the CpG island methylator phenotype, with many other genes silenced by promoter hypermethylation. A small number of cancers show either inherited (Lynch syndrome) or somatic mismatch repair gene mutations. A further approximately 2–3% are ultramutated cancers, with extremely high mutation rates with a characteristic nucleotide base change spectrum (increased C→A transversions), resulting from the presence of a mutation that inactivates the proofreading function within the exonuclease domain of the DNA-replicating enzyme POLE, or rarely of POLD1 {409}. This results in failure to correct the misincorporation of nucleotides during DNA replication or repair by mutant POLE (or POLD1). Ultramutated and hypermutated cancers are usually combined into a single group with many more significantly recurrently mutated genes than the non-hypermutated CRCs, and these are shown in Table 6.05 (p. 186). Hypermutated microsatellite-unstable cancers have far fewer DNA SCNAs than do non-hypermutated CRCs, but they show the same pattern of affected chromosome arms and sub-arms {474}.

Non-hypermutated cases (~85% of CRCs) have a low frequency of mutations and are microsatellite-stable (MSS), but they have a high frequency of DNA SCNAs, often as chromosomal segment (arm and sub-arm) gains and losses, shown in Table 6.05 (p. 186). The genes that are significantly recurrently mutated in the non-hypermutated MSS CRC include *APC* (80%), *TP53* (60%), and *KRAS* (45%), among many others at lower frequencies, as shown in Table 6.05 (p. 186) {474}.

The most frequent alterations of signalling pathways by gene mutations, deletions, amplifications, and translocations are activation of the WNT, MAPK, and PI3K growth signalling pathways and inactivation of the TGF-β and p53 inhibitory pathways, which are relevant for targeted therapies {2264}. The WNT signalling pathway is activated in 93% of non-hypermutated and 97% of hypermutated cancers, involving biallelic inactivation of *APC* or activation of *CTNNB1* in > 80% of CRCs, together with changes to many other genes involved in regulation of the WNT pathway {474}.

Transcriptomic profiling

The Colorectal Cancer Subtyping Consortium (CRCSC) compiled RNA expression profiling data from multiple studies and produced a consensus identifying four main consensus molecular subtype (CMS) groups {1108}. Almost all hypermutated microsatellite-unstable cancers fell into the first category: CMS1 (MSI-immune, 14%). The remaining MSS cancers are subcategorized into three main groups: CMS2 (canonical, 37%), CMS3 (metabolic, 13%), and CMS4 (mesenchymal, 23%), with a residual unclassified group (mixed features, 13%) that may represent either a transition phenotype or intratumoural heterogeneity.

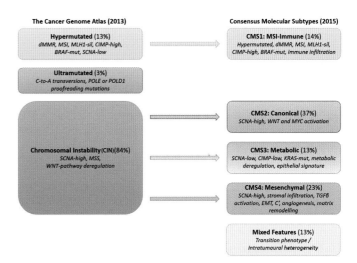

Fig. 6.35 Genomic and transcriptomic classifications of colorectal cancers. C', complement activation signature; CIMP, CpG island methylator phenotype; CMS, consensus molecular subtype; dMMR, defective mismatch repair; EMT, epithelial–mesenchymal transition; *MLH1*-sil, *MLH1* silencing by promoter hypermethylation; MSI, microsatellite instability; MSS, microsatellite stability; SCNA, somatic copy-number alteration.

CMS1 CRCs were hypermutated microsatellite-unstable due to *MLH1* silencing and accordingly CpG island methylator phenotype with frequent *BRAF* mutations, with a low number of SCNAs. This equates with the previously well-characterized sporadic microsatellite-unstable CRC subgroup. Gene expression profiling furthermore revealed evidence of strong immune activation in CMS1, consistent with pathological descriptions of prominent tumour-infiltrating CD8+ cytotoxic T lymphocytes, and this indicates potential responsiveness to immune checkpoint inhibitors {2264}. The CMS classification system is based on biological processes indicated by gene expression patterns and is suggested as a basis for future clinical stratification in trials and other studies with potential for subtype-based targeted interventions, although further studies are required to validate this {3187}.

An alternative system is the CRC intrinsic signature (CRIS), focused on cancer cell intrinsic expression signatures in order to avoid stromal-derived intratumoural heterogeneity {824}. This enabled concordant clustering of tumour samples regardless of region of origin, but it requires validation.

Essential and desirable diagnostic criteria

See Box 6.02 (p. 181).

Staging (TNM)

In staging, subdivision of T3 tumours and T1 tumours has been advocated for improved prognostication. Subdivision of T1 CRC has gained increased attention, with the increased case load observed after the introduction of population screening. After local resection of these tumours, the risk of lymph node metastasis can be estimated on the basis of various factors, including invasion depth (for sessile polyps the submucosal subdivision sm1–3 {1713}, for stalked polyps the Haggitt classification {1138}), in combination with differentiation grade, presence of lymphatic invasion, and tumour budding {373}. Alternatively, the submucosal invasion depth can be reported in mm {373}.

Nodal status depends on the number of positive lymph nodes in the region of the primary tumour: no positive lymph nodes

Table 6.05 Recurrently mutated genes and chromosome arm somatic copy-number alterations (SCNAs) in ultramutated and hypermutated versus non-hypermutated colorectal cancer (CRC)

	Ultramutated and hypermutated CRC	Non-hypermutated CRC
Significantly recurrently mutated genes[a]	*ACVR2A* (60%), *APC* (50%), *TGFBR2* (50%), *BRAF* (45%), *MSH3* (40%), *MSH6* (40%), *MYO1B* (30%), *TC-F7L2* (30%), *CASP8* (30%), *CDC27* (30%), *FZD3* (30%), *MIER3* (30%), *TCERG1* (30%), *MAP7* (25%), *PTPN12* (25%), and *TP53* (20%), as well as many others at lower frequencies	*APC* (80%), *TP53* (60%), *KRAS* (45%), *TTN* (30%), *PIK3CA* (20%), *FBXW7* (10%), *SMAD4* (10%), *NRAS* (10%), *TCF7L2* (10%), *AMER1* (also known as *FAM123B* and *WTX*; 7%), *SMAD2* (5%), *CTNNB1* (5%), as well as many others at lower frequencies
Chromosome arm SCNAs	Hypermutated CRCs have far fewer DNA SCNAs than do non-hypermutated CRCs, but there is no difference in the pattern of chromosome arms affected: Gains of 1q, 7p, 7q, 8p, 8q, 12q, 13q, 19q, 20p, 20q Deletions of 1p, 4q, 5q, 8p, 14q, 15q, 17p (includes *TP53*), 17q, 18p, 18q (includes *SMAD4*), 20p, 22q	

[a]The percentages in parentheses indicate the approximate proportion of the cancer group affected by each mutation (The Cancer Genome Atlas [TCGA] data) {474}.

(N0), 1–3 nodes (N1), or ≥ 4 nodes (N2). There has been a lot of discussion about the position of tumour deposits. In the current TNM classification (eighth edition) {408}, tumour deposits are only considered in the absence of nodal metastases and categorized as N1c, despite the evidence that their prognostic value is independent of nodal status {2271}. When only micro-metastases are present (no metastasis > 2 mm), this is indicated by the addition of "(mi)". Isolated tumour cells are single cells or small clusters of cells ≤ 0.2 mm in greatest extent; these are not considered lymph node metastases {408}.

The presence of distant metastases can be classified as M1a (metastases confined to one organ, without peritoneal metastases), M1b (metastases in more than one organ), and M1c (metastases to the peritoneum with or without other organs involved).

Prognosis and prediction

CRC is arguably the most studied cancer historically, resulting in very large numbers of potential prognostic and predictive biomarkers. Here, we aim to present the biomarkers routinely used as standard of care with clear-cut predictive value and those in which prognosis and prediction are intimately related, along with an indication of their level of acceptance in the diagnostic community. See also Table 6.04 (p. 184).

Established predictive biomarkers
RAS genes
RAS-encoded proteins are a family of small GTPase-related proteins involved in cell signal transduction {1072}. Mutations in RAS oncogenes are among the most common mutations in human cancers, and they are of biological significance in CRC. There are three RAS genes, two of which (*KRAS* and *NRAS*) have therapeutic significance. International guidelines {2955,3596} recommend the analysis of codons 12, 13, 59, 61,

117, and 146 in the *KRAS* and *NRAS* genes, because these codons generally correlate with resistance to monoclonal anti-bodies directed to the extracellular domain of EGFR (HER1) {1934,3407}. These antibodies (of which cetuximab and pani-tumumab are leading examples) prevent EGFR dimerization and subsequent downstream oncogenic signalling pathways. Almost 50% of CRCs harbour a clinically relevant RAS muta-tion and should not be treated with anti-EGFR antibody therapy. However, only 40–60% of RAS-wildtype cases show response to this therapy {3570}, suggesting a more complex biology in relation to this treatment option.

BRAF
BRAF is an oncogene of the family of RAF threonine kinases. *BRAF* is a super-biomarker relevant in the treatment and diagnosis of melanoma {946}, hairy cell leukaemia {175}, lung adenocarcinoma, and thyroid cancer {2115}. In CRC, *BRAF* is a biomarker of paramount importance. *BRAF* mutations in and around amino acid 600 (most frequently p.V600E) carry an adverse prognosis. Mutations of *BRAF* are of use for the exclu-sion of Lynch syndrome. *BRAF* mutations are overrepresented in some of the morphological subtypes {115}. In addition, *BRAF* may also have a predictive/therapeutic value: RAS and *BRAF* mutations are generally mutually exclusive, and although the evidence is less conclusive at present, due in part to the low prevalence of *BRAF* mutations in CRC, several studies have reported that patients with BRAF p.V600E mutations do not benefit from anti-EGFR therapy {1310}, and oncologists may use them in the therapeutic decision-making process.

Microsatellite instability
MSI results from the defective mismatch repair mechanism leading to predisposition to mutations. MSI drives one of the key mechanisms of oncogenesis in CRC, and it is one of the tests of reference in the diagnosis of Lynch syndrome. From a therapeutic decision-making standpoint, the presence of MSI is important in two main scenarios {818}. Firstly, in *BRAF*-wildtype cases, MSI confers a good prognosis, and regardless of *BRAF* status, MSI reduces the benefit of fluorouracil-based chemo-therapy. CRCs that are MSS, in the context of *BRAF* mutation, generally carry a poor prognosis. Secondly, the presence of MSI is important in the context of cancer immunotherapy. More recently, studies have reported significant responses of micro-satellite-unstable cancers (CRCs and others) to PDL1 inhibitors in patients who failed conventional therapy {1816,1815}. This test may serve in CRC as a surrogate for the tumour mutation bur-den test applicable in other cancer types.

Biomarkers partly established and/or under development
Cancer immunotherapy
The success of PD1/PDL1 inhibition in microsatellite-unstable CRC has been very encouraging, but it is limited by biology and disease stage to date. Important work is ongoing in the space of MSS CRCs and earlier disease presentation {357}, which makes this one of the most likely areas of development in the future for biomarker analysis in CRC. Pathologists have been at the forefront of the analysis of adaptive immunity in CRC and have validated the reproducibility of scoring systems in multicentre studies {2484}, but this represents today a disease classification and a prognostic tool

Table 6.06 Overview of hereditary cancer syndromes involving colorectal cancer (CRC)

Syndrome	Genes involved	Inheritance pattern	CRC risk
Lynch syndrome	Mismatch repair genes (*MLH1, MSH2, MSH6, PMS2*, others)	AD	10–50%[a]
Familial adenomatous polyposis	*APC*	AD	100%[b]
MUTYH-associated polyposis	*MUTYH*	AR	60–70%[b]
NTHL1-associated polyposis	*NTHL1*	AR	Unknown
Polymerase proofreading–associated polyposis	*POLD1, POLE*	AD	30–70%[c]
Constitutional mismatch repair deficiency syndrome	Mismatch repair genes (*MLH1, MSH2, MSH6, PMS2*)	AR	Unknown
Hereditary mixed polyposis syndrome	*GREM1*	AD	Unknown
MSH3-associated polyposis	*MSH3*	AR	Unknown
AXIN2-associated polyposis	*AXIN2*	AD	Unknown
Immune deficiency–associated polyposis	Various	Various	Unknown
Serrated polyposis	Unknown	Unknown	Unknown
Juvenile polyposis syndrome	*SMAD4* or *BMPR1A*	AD	68%[d]
Peutz–Jeghers syndrome	*STK11* (*LKB1*)	AD	39%[c]
Cowden syndrome	*PTEN*	AD	9%[b]
Li–Fraumeni syndrome	*TP53*	AD	Unknown

AD, autosomal dominant; AR, autosomal recessive.
[a]Risk at 75 years (varies by gene, age, and sex). [b]Lifetime risk. [c]Risk at 65–70 years. [d]Risk at 60 years.

rather than a predictive one. As such, it is more likely to complement our traditional staging procedures in the near future.

Other predictive biomarkers
The analysis of the transcriptome represents one of the most important classification systems in CRC. In addition, there are specific gene expression signatures that are able to predict recurrence after surgery. Both the Oncotype DX test {3653} and the ColDx test {1554} provide a score for recurrence in intermediate-stage CRC and are used in patient stratification. However, the central laboratory nature of these tests may diminish their applicability, particularly in universal health care systems.

PIK3CA, encoding the catalytic subunit of PI3K, is mutated in 10–20% of CRCs, mainly in exons 9 and 20. In RAS-wildtype CRC, *PIK3CA* mutations may be associated with a worse clinical outcome and with a negative prediction of response to targeted therapy by anti-EGFR monoclonal antibodies {2849,2614}. In addition, mutations in *PIK3CA* may predict successful adjuvant therapy with acetylsalicylic acid in CRC patients {1897}.

c-Met, a receptor tyrosine kinase, is frequently overexpressed in gastrointestinal tumours; in general, aberrant expression, activation, amplification, and mutation of c-Met has been reported in subgroups of patients with CRC, and *MET* copy-number gains or *MET* exon 14 skipping mutations may represent potential predictive biomarkers for c-Met inhibitors {392}.

Liquid biopsy, i.e. analysis of the patient's peripheral blood, has been used to diagnose metastatic CRC and to detect predictive markers of response. Among all the potential tests performed in blood (detecting circulating tumour cells, exosomes, or cell-free DNA), the detection of (K)RAS and BRAF mutations in the latter {3292,3257} is currently applicable in some centres and is likely to become widely acceptable in the near future.

Colorectal neuroendocrine neoplasms

Rindi G
Komminoth P
Scoazec JY
Shia J

Definition

Neuroendocrine neoplasms (NENs) of the colon and rectum are colorectal epithelial neoplasms with neuroendocrine differentiation, including well-differentiated neuroendocrine tumours (NETs), poorly differentiated neuroendocrine carcinomas (NECs), and mixed neuroendocrine–non-neuroendocrine neoplasms (MiNENs) – an umbrella category including mixed adenoneuroendocrine carcinoma (MANEC).

MiNENs are discussed in greater detail in the chapter on pancreatic tumours (see *Pancreatic MiNENs*, p. 370).

ICD-O coding

8240/3 Neuroendocrine tumour NOS
8246/3 Neuroendocrine carcinoma NOS
8154/3 Mixed neuroendocrine–non-neuroendocrine neoplasm (MiNEN)

ICD-11 coding

2B90.Y Other specified malignant neoplasms of colon
2B90.Y & XH9LV8 Other specified malignant neoplasms of colon & Neuroendocrine tumour, grade I
2B90.Y & XH0U20 Other specified malignant neoplasms of colon & Neuroendocrine carcinoma NOS
2B90.Y & XH9SY0 Other specified malignant neoplasms of colon & Small cell neuroendocrine carcinoma
2B90.Y & XH0NL5 Other specified malignant neoplasms of colon & Large cell neuroendocrine carcinoma
2B90.Y & XH6H10 Other specified malignant neoplasms of colon & Mixed adenoneuroendocrine carcinoma
2B90.Y & XH7NM1 Other specified malignant neoplasms of colon & Enterochromaffin cell carcinoid
2B90.Y & XH7LW9 Other specified malignant neoplasms of colon & L-cell tumour
2B90.Y & XH7152 Other specified malignant neoplasms of colon & Glucagon-like peptide-producing tumour
2B90.Y & XH9ZS8 Other specified malignant neoplasms of colon & Pancreatic peptide and pancreatic peptide-like peptide within terminal tyrosine amide-producing tumour

Related terminology

Acceptable: well-differentiated endocrine tumour; poorly differentiated endocrine carcinoma; mixed exocrine-endocrine carcinoma; mixed adenoneuroendocrine carcinoma.
Not recommended: carcinoid; well-differentiated endocrine carcinoma; composite carcinoid-adenocarcinoma.

Subtype(s)

Neuroendocrine tumour, grade 1 (8240/3); neuroendocrine tumour, grade 2 (8249/3); neuroendocrine tumour, grade 3 (8249/3); L-cell tumour (8152/3); glucagon-like peptide-producing tumour (8152/3); PP/PYY-producing tumour (8152/3); enterochromaffin-cell carcinoid (8241/3); serotonin-producing tumour (8241/3); large cell neuroendocrine carcinoma (8013/3); small cell neuroendocrine carcinoma (8041/3)

Localization

All NEN subtypes can be found anywhere in the colon and rectum, although NETs are more common in the rectum.

Clinical features

Most NETs are clinically silent or associated with nonspecific mass-related symptoms, bleeding, and pain {446,1454,3139}. There are cases with functioning serotonin-producing enterochromaffin cells (EC cells), as well as NET with classic carcinoid syndrome, often having liver metastases {2757}. NEC and MiNEN may present with widespread metastases {3073}.

Epidemiology

The observed incidence rates of rectal and colonic NENs in the USA are 1.2 and 0.2 new cases per 100 000 person-years,

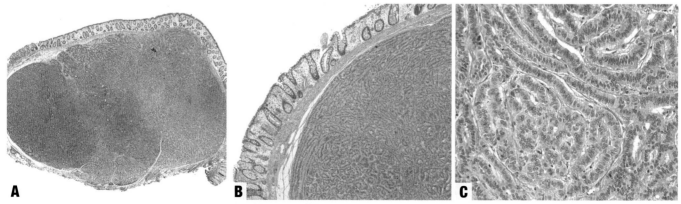

Fig. 6.36 Neuroendocrine tumour (NET), G2, L-cell type. **A** Mucosectomy specimen of rectal NET limited to the mucosa/submucosa. **B** NET of the rectum with typical trabecular pattern; higher-power view of panel A. **C** Trabeculae are composed of monomorphic tumour cells with mild to moderate atypia; higher-power view of panel B.

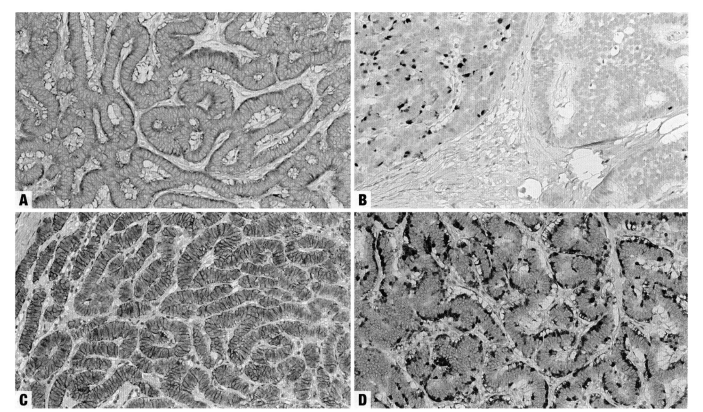

Fig. 6.37 Neuroendocrine tumour (NET), G2, L-cell type. **A** Synaptophysin immunoreactivity in rectal G2 NET. **B** Chromogranin A immunoreactivity in rectal G2 NET; note the limited cluster of positive cells (left part of the micrograph). **C** SSTR2A immunoreactivity; note the diffuse membrane expression. **D** PAP immunoreactivity; note the diffuse expression.

respectively {716}. Similar data have been reported worldwide, confirming the decade-long incremental trend observed for both NET and NEC. The prevalence is higher in Asian populations {1408,1860,1409}. Patients with NEN are often in the sixth or seventh decade of life. For rectal NEN the median age is 56 years; for colonic NEN, 65 years. There is a slight male predominance, especially among patients with NEC and MiNEN {3684,2164,2163}.

Etiology
The etiology is unknown, and little information is available about site-specific risk factors. A recent meta-analysis indicated increased risk associated with a family history of cancer, tobacco smoking, alcohol consumption, and increased body mass index, with the adjusted summary effect estimate of risk (odds ratio) ranging from 0.67 (increased body mass index) to 1.6 (alcohol consumption) {1861}.

Pathogenesis
Unknown

Macroscopic appearance
Colonic NETs are larger than their counterparts in the small intestine, appendix, and rectum, with a reported average size of 4.9 cm {302}. Rectal NETs, which are smaller, are usually detected as small submucosal polypoid nodules on endoscopy {3008}. More than half are < 1.0 cm in diameter, and only about 7% are > 2 cm {1668}. NECs of the colorectum are grossly similar to conventional adenocarcinomas.

Histopathology
NET

Serotonin-producing EC-cell NETs show the same histological, cytological, and immunohistochemical profile as jejunoileal EC-cell NETs. The solid-islet type (A structure) described by Soga and Tazawa in 1971 {3081} is usually observed. In addition, glandular (B structure) and trabecular (C structure) patterns may also be found. L-cell NETs are usually observed in the rectum and typically display the C structure. NET cells show bland features with mild to moderate atypia, abundant cytoplasm, and monomorphic nuclei with salt-and-pepper chromatin. Necrosis is usually absent; if present, it is inconspicuous and spotty, usually associating with more-solid structure and moderate to severe atypia. NETs are usually G1 or G2, although rare G3 NETs have been reported {2164,1207}.

NEC

NECs usually display an organoid structure with prevalent large trabeculae, rosette-like and palisading patterns, and solid nests with central necrosis, sometimes with single-cell necrosis and thick stroma. NEC cells display severe atypia, brisk mitotic activity (often with atypical mitoses), and small cell features (scant cytoplasm) or large/intermediate cell features (abundant cytoplasm and prominent nucleoli), thus fitting the definition of small cell NEC (SCNEC) or large cell NEC (LCNEC); see *Oesophageal neuroendocrine neoplasms* (p. 56) {2995}. Usually the solid pattern is observed in SCNEC and the organoid pattern in LCNEC. A minor non-neuroendocrine component

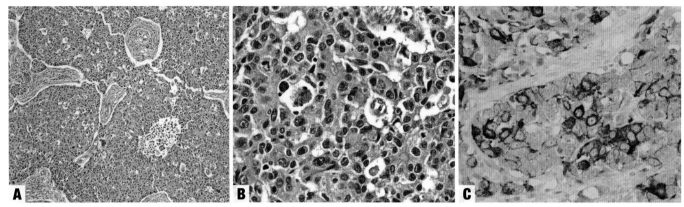

Fig. 6.38 Large cell neuroendocrine carcinoma (LCNEC). **A** LCNEC of the colon; note the solid structure with central necrosis. **B** At higher-power, the carcinoma cells show poor differentiation features with severe cytological atypia; note the cell size with relatively abundant cytoplasm and the prominent nucleoli. **C** Immunoreactivity for chromogranin A; note the diffuse but irregular staining in the cytoplasm of the large cells.

(either adenocarcinoma or squamous cell carcinoma) may be observed {2165}.

MiNEN

MiNENs are mostly made of a poorly differentiated NEC component, together with an adenocarcinoma component (colon and rectum). Exceedingly rare are MiNENs with a low-grade NET component. This tumour is usually found in a background of longstanding idiopathic inflammatory conditions {132,2315,1590}. Rarely, NETs are associated with adenomas {1331}.

Immunohistochemistry

EC-cell NETs are intensely and diffusely positive for chromogranin A and synaptophysin, as well as for serotonin. L-cell NETs are diffusely positive for synaptophysin and PYY, glicentin, and/

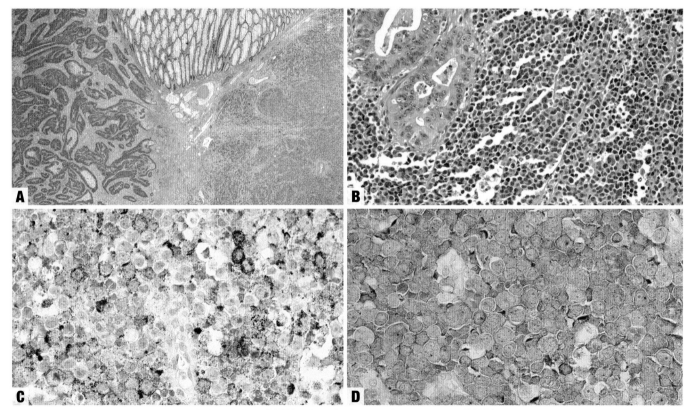

Fig. 6.39 Mixed neuroendocrine–non-neuroendocrine neoplasm (MiNEN) with small cell neuroendocrine carcinoma (SCNEC) and adenocarcinoma components. **A** Note the adenocarcinoma component on the left side and the SCNEC component on the right side, converging in the middle. **B** High-power view of a lymph node metastasis of the lesion shown in panel A; note the intimate admixture of the two components – the solid NEC component with abundant necrosis, small cells with severe atypia, scant cytoplasm, and inconspicuous nucleoli on the right side and the adenocarcinoma component with irregular glands and severe cytological atypia on the left side. **C** Chromogranin A immunoreactivity; note the faint but diffuse staining of the peripheral rim of the cytoplasm of small cells. **D** Immunoreactivity for synaptophysin; note the diffuse and intense staining of the cytoplasm of small cells.

or GLPs (GLP-1 and GLP-2), but often only focally positive for chromogranin A {940,912,2605}. Other peptide hormones and amines may also be observed, as well as CDX2 (EC-cell tumours only) and PAP (L-cell tumours only) {869,912}. Colorectal NETs are usually positive for SSTR2A {3699,1744,1682}.

Synaptophysin is intensely expressed in NEC, whereas chromogranin A may be scant or faint {1078,1485,2995}. In addition, neuron-specific enolase and CD56 (NCAM) are often positive. CDX2, TTF1, and at lesser extent SSTR2A may also be positive {1756,603,1682}.

Grading
Colorectal NENs are graded using the same system used for other gastroenteropancreatic NENs.

Cytology
Not clinically relevant

Diagnostic molecular pathology
Data are scant and limited by the difference in techniques used. Colorectal EC-cell NETs probably share the low genetic abnormality burden observed in EC-cell NETs of the small intestine {233,961}. No data are available for L-cell NETs.

NECs have a high burden of genetic abnormalities, usually including mutations in *TP53* and *RB1*. Other abnormalities in NECs include mutations in *APC*, *KRAS*, *FHIT* (3p), *DCC* and *SMAD4* (*DPC4*) (18q), *MEN1*, and *BRAF* {2597,986,2521,1682}. A few studies (mostly case reports) on MiNEN have shown MANEC having similar mutations to NEC, including mutations in *TP53*, *RB1*, *APC*, *KRAS*, *FOXP2*, *SMARCA4*, and *BCL9*. Some mutations are shared by the non-neuroendocrine counterpart {2877,3496}, but others are not {3435,3577,3376}.

Essential and desirable diagnostic criteria
NET
Essential: a uniform population of cells with round nuclei and finely stippled chromatin; architectural patterns include trabeculae, acini, nests, and ribbons; expression of synaptophysin and often chromogranin A.

NEC
Essential: a small cell carcinoma or large cell carcinoma pattern; sheets or trabeculae of poorly differentiated cells; a high mitotic count and Ki-67 proliferation index.

Staging (TNM)
The staging of colorectal NETs, which is presented in Chapter 1 (p. 20), follows the specific criteria defined in the eighth editions (2017) of the Union for International Cancer Control (UICC) TNM classification {408} and the American Joint Committee on Cancer (AJCC) cancer staging manual {127}. The staging of NEC and MiNEN follows the criteria for adenocarcinoma.

Prognosis and prediction
The prognosis of patients with NET largely depends on the grade and stage of the tumour, although tumour grade appears to play a more important role {716,1668,1736,3350,1599}. The median overall survival time of low-stage NET is excellent, with 24.6 years reported for rectum and about 21 years for colon. Similarly, low-grade NETs have an excellent median overall survival time of 30 years for rectum, but only about 12 years for colon {716}. Patients with colorectal G3 NET had poorer overall survival than those with NETs of all other digestive sites {2164,1207}. In one series, the median overall survival time observed in patients with colorectal G3 NET was approximately 12 months (compared with 22 months for NETs of other digestive sites) {2164}. NECs display an ominous outcome {2995,2963,663,2164}, directly related to the Ki-67 proliferation index. In one series, patients with NECs with a Ki-67 proliferation index < 55% had a median overall survival time of 25.4 months, whereas the other patients had a median survival time of 5.3 months {2164}. The prognosis of MiNEN with a NEC component depends on stage and the Ki-67 proliferation index of the NEC component. The median overall survival times of patients with colorectal MANEC and MANEC of all digestive sites were 12.2 months and 13.2 months, respectively {2163}.

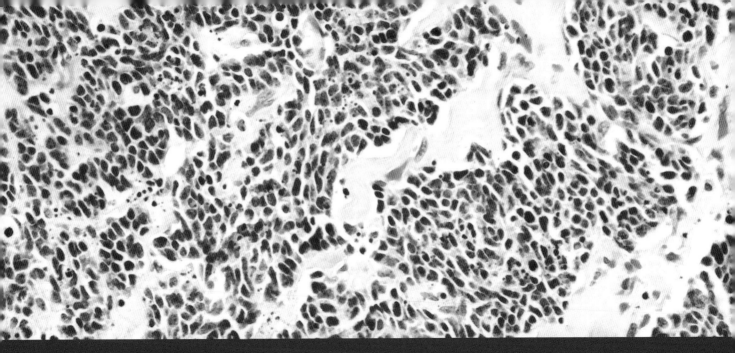

7

Tumours of the anal canal

Edited by: Goldblum JR, Klimstra DS, Lam AK

Benign epithelial tumours and precursors
   Inflammatory cloacogenic polyp
   Condyloma
   Squamous dysplasia (intraepithelial neoplasia)
Malignant epithelial tumours
   Squamous cell carcinoma
   Adenocarcinoma
   Neuroendocrine neoplasms

WHO classification of tumours of the anal canal

Benign epithelial tumours and precursors

8077/0	Squamous intraepithelial neoplasia, low grade
8077/2	Squamous intraepithelial neoplasia, high grade

Malignant epithelial tumours

8070/3	Squamous cell carcinoma NOS
8051/3	Verrucous squamous cell carcinoma
8140/3	Adenocarcinoma NOS
8240/3	Neuroendocrine tumour NOS
8240/3	Neuroendocrine tumour, grade 1
8249/3	Neuroendocrine tumour, grade 2
8249/3	Neuroendocrine tumour, grade 3
8246/3	Neuroendocrine carcinoma NOS
8013/3	Large cell neuroendocrine carcinoma
8041/3	Small cell neuroendocrine carcinoma
8154/3	Mixed neuroendocrine–non-neuroendocrine neoplasm (MiNEN)

These morphology codes are from the International Classification of Diseases for Oncology, third edition, second revision (ICD-O-3.2) {1378A}. Behaviour is coded /0 for benign tumours; /1 for unspecified, borderline, or uncertain behaviour; /2 for carcinoma in situ and grade III intraepithelial neoplasia; /3 for malignant tumours, primary site; and /6 for malignant tumours, metastatic site. Behaviour code /6 is not generally used by cancer registries.

This classification is modified from the previous WHO classification, taking into account changes in our understanding of these lesions.

TNM staging of tumours of the anal canal and perianal skin

Anal Canal and Perianal Skin

(ICD-O-3 C21, ICD-O-3 C44.5)

The anal canal extends from rectum to perianal skin (to the junction with hair-bearing skin). It is lined by the mucous membrane overlying the internal sphincter, including the transitional epithelium and dentate line. Tumours of anal margin and perianal skin defined as within 5 cm of the anal margin (ICD-O-3 C44.5) are now classified with carcinomas of the anal canal.

Rules for Classification

The classification applies only to carcinomas. There should be histological confirmation of the disease and division of cases by histological type.

The following are the procedures for assessing T, N, and M categories.

T categories	Physical examination, imaging, endoscopy, and/or surgical exploration
N categories	Physical examination, imaging, and/or surgical exploration
M categories	Physical examination, imaging, and/or surgical exploration

Regional Lymph Nodes

The regional lymph nodes are the perirectal, the internal iliac, external iliac, and the inguinal lymph nodes.

TNM Clinical Classification

T – Primary Tumour

TX   Primary tumour cannot be assessed
T0   No evidence of primary tumour
Tis Carcinoma in situ, Bowen disease, high-grade squamous intraepithelial lesion (HSIL), anal intraepithelial neoplasia II–III (AIN II–III)
T1   Tumour 2 cm or less in greatest dimension
T2   Tumour more than 2 cm but not more than 5 cm in greatest dimension
T3   Tumour more than 5 cm in greatest dimension
T4   Tumour of any size invades adjacent organ(s), e.g., vagina, urethra, bladder*

Note
* Direct invasion of the rectal wall, perianal skin, subcutaneous tissue, or the sphincter muscle(s) *alone* is not classified as T4.

N – Regional Lymph Nodes

NX   Regional lymph nodes cannot be assessed
N0   No regional lymph node metastasis
N1   Metastasis in regional lymph node(s)
  N1a   Metastases in inguinal, mesorectal, and/or internal iliac nodes
  N1b   Metastases in external iliac nodes
  N1c   Metastases in external iliac and in inguinal, mesorectal and/or internal iliac nodes

M – Distant Metastasis

M0   No distant metastasis
M1   Distant metastasis

pTNM Pathological Classification

The pT and pN categories correspond to the T and N categories.

pN0   Histological examination of a regional perirectal/pelvic lymphadenectomy specimen will ordinarily include 12 or more lymph nodes; histological examination of an inguinal lymphadenectomy specimen will ordinarily include 6 or more lymph nodes. If the lymph nodes are negative, but the number ordinarily examined is not met, classify as pN0.

pM – Distant Metastasis*

pM1   Distant metastasis microscopically confirmed

Note
* pM0 and pMX are not valid categories.

Stage

Stage 0	Tis	N0	M0
Stage I	T1	N0	M0
Stage IIA	T2	N0	M0
Stage IIB	T3	N0	M0
Stage IIIA	T1,T2	N1	M0
Stage IIIB	T4	N0	M0
Stage IIIC	T3,T4	N1	M0
Stage IV	Any T	Any N	M1

The information presented here has been excerpted from the 2017 *TNM classification of malignant tumours*, eighth edition (408,3385A). © 2017 UICC. A help desk for specific questions about the TNM classification is available at https://www.uicc.org/tnm-help-desk.

Chapter 7

Tumours of the anal canal: Introduction

Lam AK
Goldblum JR

Anatomy and histology

The anal canal begins distal to the rectum and ends at the anal verge (anal orifice, anus); it is completely extraperitoneal. The region beyond the anal verge, extending about 50 mm, is the perianal skin. The anal canal is 30–50 mm in length and is slightly longer in males. Internal and external smooth muscle sphincters form a complex encasing the canal. For surgeons and physiologists, the proximal border of the anal canal (anorectal junction) is the anorectal ring, which is a palpable structure on digital rectal examination at the level of the puborectalis muscle.

The dentate (pectinate) line is formed by the anal columns, which consist of a series of anal sinuses (draining anal glands). Two thirds to half of the anal canal is proximal to the dentate line (pectinate line). This portion is derived from hindgut (endodermal in origin), whereas the lower portion of the anal canal is from ectoderm. The dentate line is approximately 10–20 mm distal to the anorectal junction. It cannot be seen radiologically but can be identified on endoscopic examination, because the change of colour is obvious. The region from the dentate line to the anal verge is often labelled as the anatomical anal canal.

Histologically, the anal canal comprises three zones. The upper portion of the anal canal consists of colorectal-like columnar epithelium. The middle portion, above the dentate line, is covered by transitional epithelium, which is squamous metaplasia of the columnar epithelium. This portion of the anal canal is the anal transformation zone, which is susceptible to involvement by HPV. The lower portion of the anal canal is covered by non-keratinized stratified squamous epithelium devoid of epidermal appendages (hair follicles, apocrine glands, and sweat glands). Beyond the anal verge, the perianal skin is hair-bearing keratinizing squamous epithelium.

The ICD-O topographical coding for the anatomical sites covered in this chapter is presented in Box 7.01.

Clinical implications

The pathology of the anal region is different from that of the perianal region, and management of diseases in the regions differs. Clinically, if a lesion can be completely visualized with gentle traction on the buttocks, it is considered a perianal skin lesion, which is similar to skin lesions in other parts of the body.

Carcinomas located above the dentate line metastasize to the perirectal and internal iliac nodes, whereas carcinomas below the dentate line drain into the inguinal and femoral lymph nodes.

Box 7.01 ICD-O topographical coding for the anatomical sites covered in this chapter

C21 Anus and anal canal
    C21.0 Anus NOS
    C21.1 Anal canal
    C21.2 Cloacogenic zone
    C21.8 Overlapping lesion of the rectum, anus, and anal canal
C44 Skin
    C44.5 Perianal skin

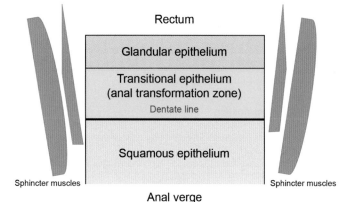

Fig. 7.01 Anatomy of the anal canal. The upper portion of the anal canal consists of colorectal-like columnar epithelium. The middle portion, above the dentate line, is covered by transitional epithelium, which is squamous metaplasia of the columnar epithelium. The lower portion of the anal canal is covered by non-keratinized stratified squamous epithelium devoid of epidermal appendages (hair follicles, apocrine glands, and sweat glands). Beyond the anal verge, the perianal skin is hair-bearing keratinizing squamous epithelium.

The treatment of perianal skin lesions depends on the exact nature of the lesion. Benign anal canal epithelial lesions are often removed endoscopically. Management of malignant epithelial lesions of the anal canal usually involves chemotherapy and radiotherapy, because these lesions are typically inoperable. Surgery such as abdominoperineal resection is reserved for those cancers if other treatments do not work or if the cancer recurs.

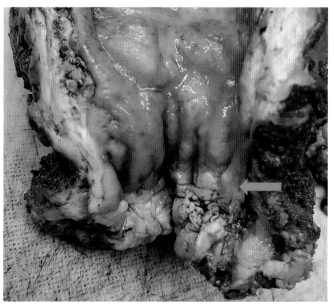

Fig. 7.02 Macroscopic appearance of the anal canal, showing the dentate line (arrow). Note the difference in colour of the mucosa above and below the line.

Classification

This chapter focuses on epithelial tumours and tumour-like lesions in the anal canal. Benign epithelial lesions most often present as polyps. The two main lesions are condyloma and inflammatory cloacogenic polyp, as well as their subtypes (see the corresponding sections). The other most common benign lesions that form tumour-like masses include haemorrhoids, fibroepithelial polyps, and ectopic tissue.

Haemorrhoids (piles) are the most common and well-known lesions in the area, often coexisting with other lesions. A tumour-like mass arises from abnormal dilation of the venous plexus because of elevated intra-abdominal pressure. Haemorrhoids may be external (distal to the dentate line and covered by squamous epithelium) or internal (proximal to the dentate line and covered by transitional or columnar epithelium).

Fibroepithelial polyp (skin tag, anal tag, hypertrophied anal papilla) is the second most common benign lesion in this region. It typically occurs on a background of chronic inflammation. The etiologies include haemorrhoids, mucosal prolapse, fissures, and Crohn disease. The polyp arises in the anal transformation zone and is covered by non-keratinizing stratified squamous epithelium or transitional epithelium. Areas of hyperkeratosis or parakeratosis could be seen reactive to trauma. The subepithelial stroma shows variable proliferation of vessels, smooth muscle, and chronic inflammation. The lesion is often clinically mistaken as a condyloma.

Ectopic gastric mucosa {593,3129} may present as an anal polyp. Patients are more often male and present with rectal bleeding, ulceration, and pain. Ectopic prostatic tissue of the anal canal has also been reported {3268}.

The most common malignant lesion in the anal canal is squamous cell carcinoma (and its subtypes), which is discussed in detail in the *Anal squamous cell carcinoma* section (p. 205). Adenocarcinoma is also common in the anal canal {3175}. Adenocarcinoma and its subtypes, as well as the related lesion Paget disease, are discussed in the *Anal adenocarcinoma* section (p. 208). The third most common malignant lesion is melanoma. Neuroendocrine tumour (NET), although rare, occurs in the anal canal and largely appears as neuroendocrine carcinoma (NEC; see *Anal neuroendocrine neoplasms*, p. 212).

Perianal tumours

Detailed descriptions of perianal epithelial lesions are outside the scope of this chapter. Common perianal carcinomas include basal cell carcinoma and squamous cell carcinoma.

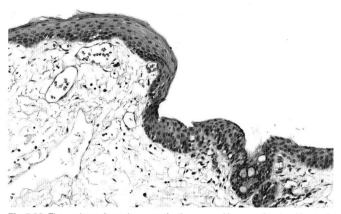

Fig. 7.03 The anal transformation zone. Anal mucosa with one end covered by stratified squamous epithelium and the other portion covered by transitional epithelium.

Developmental and acquired cysts may affect the perianal region, including anal duplication cyst, anal duct cyst, median raphe cyst, epidermoid cyst, mature cystic teratoma, and tailgut cyst {221,2813,179}. Many of these entities are more prevalent in childhood but may also affect adults.

Other non-neoplastic epithelial lesions in this region include endometriosis and ectopic breast tissue {548,944}. Infections (mycobacterial infection, condyloma latum, etc.) and granuloma (in Crohn disease) may form a tumour-like/polyploid lesion and should be detected using special stains and clinicopathological correlation.

Benign skin lesions in the perianal region include keratoacanthoma, hidradenitis suppurativa, and papillary hidradenoma. Keratoacanthoma is rare and should be differentiated from squamous cell carcinoma {1745}. Hidradenitis suppurativa (acne inversa) is an inflammatory lesion in the apocrine glands of the region {2588}. Papillary hidradenoma (hidradenoma papilliferum) is most often seen in the anogenital area and arises from anogenital mammary-like or apocrine adnexal glands {1679}. It occurs almost exclusively in middle-aged women, with highest incidence in the fifth and sixth decades of life {1938}. Papillary hidradenoma may be considered the cutaneous counterpart of intraductal papilloma of breast. The tumour is a well-circumscribed nodule with papillary architecture of ducts lined by double layers of epithelial cells with decapitation secretion.

Inflammatory cloacogenic polyp

Lam AK

Definition
Inflammatory cloacogenic polyp (ICP) is a non-neoplastic polyp that arises in the anal transitional zone and shows inflammation along with proliferation of glands and smooth muscle.

ICD-O coding
None

ICD-11 coding
DB71.0 Inflammatory anal polyp

Related terminology
Acceptable: cloacogenic polyp.

Subtype(s)
None

Localization
ICP is located in the anal transitional zone, but it may involve the lower rectum, often with origin from the anterior wall of the region.

Clinical features
The common clinical presentation of ICP includes rectal bleeding, constipation, swelling of the anus, and pruritus. ICP is often detected by endoscopic examination performed for other reasons. Haemorrhoids and diverticulosis may be seen in patients with ICP.

Epidemiology
ICP is uncommon and represents < 1% of lower GI tract polyps. It is predominantly reported in North American and European populations. There is no sex predilection. The polyp appears to have bimodal distribution, with peak occurrence in the second decade and the seventh decade of life {3731,2604,3534}, although it has also been reported in a 6-year-old girl {262} and an 85-year-old woman {2866}.

Etiology
ICP may be related to a low-fibre diet with a resultant increase in colonic intraluminal pressure.

Pathogenesis
The most accepted pathogenesis of ICP is the intraluminal pressure or abnormal pressure gradients leading to mucosal prolapse, hypoperfusion with ischaemic injury, necrosis, and regeneration.

Macroscopic appearance
ICP is usually small, ranging from 5 to 50 mm in greatest dimension (mean: ~20 mm) {2866}. It may be solitary or multiple. The surface of the polyp is often erythematous, oedematous, and eroded.

Histopathology
ICP is covered by stratified squamous epithelium, columnar epithelium, and transitional epithelium (intermediate between squamous and columnar epithelium). The epithelium shows hyperplastic changes with complex tubulovillous growth and goblet cell hypertrophy, with or without ulceration and regenerative nuclear atypia. There may be displacement of dilated (cystic) mucosal glands and pools of mucin in the lamina propria, resembling proctitis cystica profunda. Active chronic inflammation, granulation tissue, vascular ectasia, and oedema are often present. A classic feature is fibromuscular proliferation and obliteration of the lamina propria in a radial fashion. Reactive atypia in the ICP can be mistaken for dysplasia. p53 and Ki-67 immunohistochemistry may be useful in this distinction {2517}.

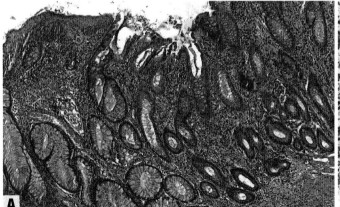 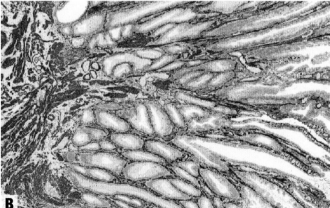

Fig. 7.04 Inflammatory cloacogenic polyp. **A** Inflammatory cloacogenic polyp is covered by stratified squamous epithelium and columnar epithelium. The epithelium shows hyperplastic changes with complex tubulovillous growth and goblet cell hypertrophy. **B** Desmin staining reveals the smooth muscle proliferation.

ICP is part of the spectrum of diseases with similar pathology and etiology referred to as mucosal prolapse syndrome, which includes solitary rectal ulcer syndrome, rectal prolapse, and proctitis cystica profunda.

Cytology
Not clinically relevant

Diagnostic molecular pathology
Not clinically relevant

Essential and desirable diagnostic criteria
Essential: epithelial hyperplasia without dysplasia; stromal inflammation; fibromuscular proliferation.

Staging (TNM)
Not clinically relevant

Prognosis and prediction
ICP does not recur after removal. Rare cases have been associated with squamous/columnar dysplasia {2866,1439,1162}.

Anal condyloma

Lam AK

Definition
Anal condyloma is a benign papillary squamous proliferation with a fibrovascular core, caused by HPV infection. Buschke–Lowenstein tumour (BLT) is a giant condyloma with features of deep growth and local destruction.

ICD-O coding
None

ICD-11 coding
1A95.0 Anal warts

Related terminology
Acceptable: wart; condyloma acuminatum.

Subtype(s)
None

Localization
Condyloma occurs in the anal canal, anal transformation zone, anal skin, and perianal region. BLT is large and often involves tissue both inside and outside the anal canal.

Clinical features
Patients with condyloma may be asymptomatic or could present with anal discomfort or pruritus. The lesion may be solitary or multiple and may present as a cauliflower-like mass. Patients with BLT present with a large pushing mass, with fistulas, abscesses, bleeding, and displacement of adjacent tissue. A anoscopy with biopsy is required for definitive diagnosis. Radio-logical examination (CT or MRI) is used to exclude malignant transformation.

Epidemiology
Condyloma is most common in young patients in the third dec-ade of life {2525}. The prevalence of anogenital condyloma is similar in men and women. Anal condyloma is more common in young men who have sex with men and HIV-positive individuals. In Australia, 4.5% of men who reported engaging in anorecep-tive sex had anal condyloma {2448}.

BLT (giant condyloma) may be seen in paediatric patients as young as 18 months of age {210}. Men are more commonly affected, with an M:F ratio of 2.7:1.

Etiology
The etiology of condyloma and BLT is linked to HPV infection, usually (in > 90% of cases) the low oncogenic risk subtypes HPV6 and HPV11. Risk factors for acquiring the virus include immunodeficient state (HIV infection, after organ and bone mar-row transplantation) and increased contacts (unprotected sex with multiple partners and anal intercourse) {1347}. The virus can also be transmitted via surface-to-surface contact without sexual intercourse {1864}.

Pathogenesis
HPV infection begins in the basal layer of stratified squamous epithelium, resulting in squamous proliferation of condyloma.

Macroscopic appearance
Condyloma appears as a warty tumour with an irregular sur-face. BLT is a giant condyloma, which may grow to 130 mm {3784}. It is a destructive lesion, with a propensity for infections and fistulations.

Histopathology
Microscopically, condyloma is characterized by hyperplastic papillary squamous epithelium with parakeratosis and a fibro-vascular core. The upper third of the squamous epithelium typically shows koilocytes. Coexisting squamous dysplasia or squamous cell carcinoma should be excluded. Condyloma without dysplasia is usually negative for p16 on immunohisto-chemistry {3035}. Strong, block-like p16 staining is often noted in dysplasia and carcinoma with high-risk HPV subtypes.

Large condyloma must be differentiated from verrucous carcinoma and BLT {3784}. Verrucous carcinoma invades the underlying stroma in the form of bulbous pegs with a pushing border. There is no koilocytosis or HPV in verrucous carcinoma {3784}. BLT resembles condyloma histologically but has deep local extension and displacement of surrounding tissues {1583}.

Squamous papilloma of anus is extremely rare {1028}. It may represent a form of burned-out condyloma with no HPV detected.

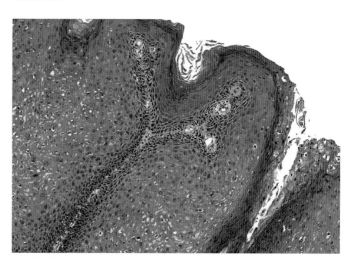

Fig. 7.05 Condyloma. Note the hyperplastic papillary squamous epithelium with para-keratosis and a fibrovascular core. The upper third of the squamous epithelium shows koilocytes.

Small condyloma must be distinguished from fibroepithelial polyp, which lacks papillary proliferation of squamous epithelium and does not show koilocytosis.

Cytology
Not clinically relevant

Diagnostic molecular pathology
Not clinically relevant

Essential and desirable diagnostic criteria
Essential: macroscopically, a warty lesion; histologically, epithelial hyperplasia with parakeratosis around fibrovascular cores (typically with koilocytes); no evidence of dysplasia.

Staging (TNM)
Not clinically relevant

Prognosis and prediction
Small condyloma can regress and be treated conservatively. Those located in the anal canal and distal end of the rectal ampulla require surgery {1864}. Large condyloma and BLT do not regress spontaneously and are prone to recurrence and malignant transformation. Recurrence of anal condyloma ranges from 4.6% to > 70%, depending on the treatment modality {2850}. The prevalence of high-grade dysplasia and carcinoma in patients with pre-existing anal condyloma is higher in HIV-positive patients {990}.

Chapter 7

Anal squamous dysplasia (intraepithelial neoplasia)

Graham RP

Definition
Anal squamous dysplasia (intraepithelial neoplasia [IEN]) consists of non-invasive cytological and architectural abnormalities of the squamous epithelium of the anal mucosa, associated with HPV infection.

ICD-O coding
8077/0 Squamous intraepithelial neoplasia, low grade
8077/2 Squamous intraepithelial neoplasia, high grade

ICD-11 coding
2E92.5 & XH3Y37 Benign neoplasm of anus or anal canal & Squamous intraepithelial dysplasia, low-grade
2E61.2 & XH9ND8 Carcinoma in situ of anal canal & Squamous intraepithelial dysplasia, high-grade

Related terminology
Acceptable: squamous intraepithelial lesion; anal intraepithelial neoplasia; anal squamous intraepithelial neoplasia.
Note: See also Table 7.01.

Subtype(s)
None

Localization
Anal squamous dysplasia (IEN) is localized in the anus.

Clinical features
Squamous dysplasia is often asymptomatic but may present as a mass lesion.

Epidemiology
Given the shared pathogenesis, the epidemiology of squamous dysplasia is similar to that of squamous cell carcinoma (SCC), which is described in *Anal squamous cell carcinoma* (p. 205).

Etiology
Squamous dysplasia of the anus is caused by HPV infection {711,3181}. Low-risk HPV genotypes mediate the development of low-risk lesions, whereas high-risk HPV genotypes, most commonly HPV16, cause high-risk lesions {3591,2544}.

Pathogenesis
HPV infection has two possible fates: transient productive infection, which gives rise to low-risk lesions, and proliferative oncogenic infection, which produces high-risk lesions {739,843}. Low-risk lesions do not progress to high-risk lesions in most instances. The risk of progression from a high-risk lesion to SCC is influenced by HPV genotype, immune status, and other factors {711,843,3591,348}.

Macroscopic appearance
Anal squamous dysplasia (IEN) presents as plaque-like lesions, occasionally presenting as masses in the anus.

Histopathology
Preinvasive lesions for anal SCC have been associated with confusion related to varying terminology being used by physicians from different fields and poor reproducibility of the intermediate category of dysplasia/IEN. The Lower Anogenital Squamous Terminology (LAST) standardization project proposed simple unified terminology for lesions across the anogenital tract. The terminology from the LAST project reflects the current understanding of HPV biology and facilitates clear communication across specialties. This terminology is now widely used in the USA {714}.

Low-grade squamous intraepithelial lesion (LSIL) includes what were previously classified as mild dysplasia, anal IEN I (AIN I), anal squamous intraepithelial lesion I, and condyloma acuminatum. Older IEN terms, including "condyloma acuminatum", may be included in parentheses {714}.

Table 7.01 The terminology applied to various anal and perianal dysplastic lesions

Description of lesion	Lower Anogenital Squamous Terminology (LAST) project	Anal squamous intraepithelial neoplasia (ASIN)	Anal intraepithelial neoplasia (AIN)
Condyloma acuminatum	LSIL (condyloma acuminatum)	Condyloma acuminatum	Condyloma acuminatum
Mild dysplasia	LSIL	ASIN-L	AIN I
Moderate dysplasia	HSIL	ASIN-H	AIN II
Severe dysplasia	HSIL	ASIN-H	AIN III
Carcinoma in situ	HSIL	ASIN-H	AIN III
Bowenoid papulosis	HSIL (bowenoid papulosis)	PSIN-H	n/a
Bowen disease	HSIL	PSIN-H	n/a

ASIN-H, high-grade anal squamous intraepithelial neoplasia; ASIN-L, low-grade anal squamous intraepithelial neoplasia; HSIL, high-grade squamous intraepithelial lesion; LSIL, low-grade squamous intraepithelial lesion; n/a, not applicable; PSIN-H, high-grade perianal squamous intraepithelial neoplasia.

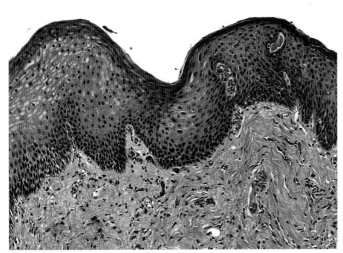

Fig. 7.06 Condyloma with low-grade squamous dysplasia. Note dysplasia of the squamous epithelium.

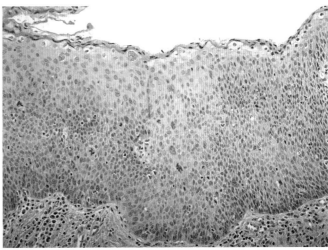

Fig. 7.08 High-grade squamous intraepithelial lesion (HSIL). HSIL (anal intraepithelial neoplasia III [AIN III]) shows full-thickness mucosal involvement by hyperchromatic cells with a high N:C ratio. Mitotic figures, including atypical forms, are seen in the upper two thirds of the mucosa.

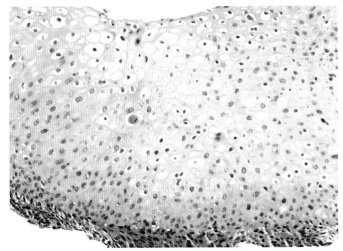

Fig. 7.07 Low-grade squamous intraepithelial lesion (LSIL). LSIL (anal intraepithelial neoplasia I [AIN I]) is characterized by koilocytosis with hyperchromatic raisinoid nuclei and perinuclear haloes. Dyskeratosis is noted. There are no atypical mitoses.

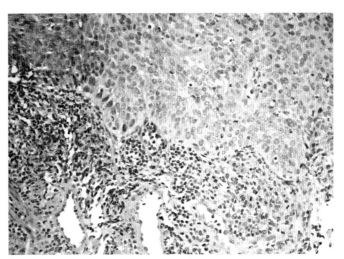

Fig. 7.09 Basaloid high-grade squamous intraepithelial lesion (HSIL). HSIL may show a basaloid morphology characterized by full-thickness involvement by immature-appearing hyperchromatic cells. Cases may show an admixture of basaloid and warty HSIL.

Histologically, LSIL shows cytological atypia and mitotic figures in the lower third of the epithelium only, and it is associated with koilocytotic atypia. Condyloma acuminatum, when included under LSIL, is a papillomatous exophytic growth with marked epithelial thickening, broad rete pegs, parakeratosis, and koilocytotic atypia. Immunohistochemistry may be confusing and is not recommended for the diagnosis of LSIL and reactive changes. Anal condylomas should be thoroughly sampled; infection with multiple HPV subtypes is not infrequent {2260,2654}, and both LSIL and high-grade squamous intraepithelial lesion (HSIL) may be seen in anal condylomas.

HSIL includes lesions that were previously classified as moderate dysplasia, severe dysplasia, carcinoma in situ, Bowen disease, and Bowenoid papulosis. It has been recognized that diagnosis using the three-tiered dysplasia terminology was associated with poor reproducibility {714}. Microscopically, HSIL shows involvement of two thirds or more of the squamous

epithelium by marked cytological atypia, mitotic figures in the upper two thirds of the epithelium, atypical mitotic figures, and loss of nuclear polarity. p16 immunohistochemistry is characteristically diffusely positive and can distinguish HSIL from reactive changes {714}.

The term "Bowen disease" refers to perineal and perianal plaques characterized by HSIL histological features with underlying chronic inflammation. The term is no longer encouraged, to avoid confusion. Bowenoid papulosis also shows the same histological features as HSIL and is located in the perianal skin. However, Bowenoid papulosis presents as papules and classically has a more indolent course, with reported regression {1364}. The term "Bowenoid papulosis" may be used in parentheses. It is reasonable to include this nomenclature if the clinical information is available, given the distinctive clinical presentation and propensity for regression of Bowenoid papulosis

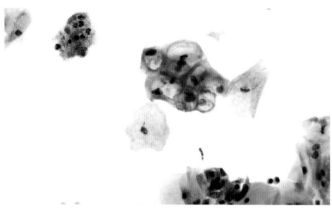

Fig. 7.10 Low-grade squamous intraepithelial lesion. Anal Papanicolaou staining showing nuclear enlargement, hyperchromasia, nuclear irregularity, and koilocytosis.

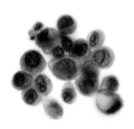

Fig. 7.11 High-grade squamous intraepithelial lesion (HSIL). Anal Papanicolaou staining shows cells with marked nuclear enlargement, irregularity, and dyskeratosis diagnostic of HSIL.

{714}. Histologically, Bowen disease and Bowenoid papulosis cannot be distinguished from HSIL involving the anus.

Cytology

For anal exfoliative cytology, the specimen swab should sample the entire length of the anal canal mucosa {2492}. Anal cytology should be reported as per the Bethesda system and adequacy criteria observed. A normal smear does not have abnormal squamous cells, by definition. Abnormal smears can be categorized as LSIL, HSIL, or atypical squamous cells of uncertain significance. This last category includes atypical cells that do not meet the criteria for LSIL or HSIL. LSIL typically shows koilocytotic atypia and > 3-fold nuclear enlargement in superficial squames. HSIL shows more severe nuclear atypia and involves more immature-appearing cells {276}. There has been some controversy regarding the cost-effectiveness of establishing routine cytology-based screening programmes for anal SCC, which has contributed to a lack of national screening programmes {2447,694,496}. However, several groups have recommended cytology sampling (anal Papanicolaou test) for patients at an increased risk of anal SCC, including patients with HIV, immunosuppressed patients who practise anoreceptive intercourse, and women with a diagnosis of HSIL or SCC of the gynaecological tract {694,835,999,2738}. The sensitivity and specificity of anal cytology for HSIL and SCC were 70% and 73%, respectively, in one large study {99}. There is modest correlation between biopsy results and cytology, indicating that cytology should be combined with other methods for screening {496,2951}.

Diagnostic molecular pathology

p16 staining and HPV subtyping by PCR can be helpful.

Essential and desirable diagnostic criteria

LSIL

Essential: cytological atypia and mitotic figures in the lower third of the anal squamous epithelium (associated with koilocytotic atypia), or papillomatous exophytic growth (condyloma) of the anal mucosa with marked epithelial thickening, broad rete pegs, parakeratosis, and koilocytotic atypia.

HSIL

Essential: involvement of at least two thirds of the anal squamous epithelium by marked cytological atypia; mitotic figures in the upper two thirds of the epithelium; atypical mitotic figures; loss of nuclear polarity.
Desirable: Diffuse p16 positivity.

Staging (TNM)

HSIL is staged as Tis.

Prognosis and prediction

Most cases of LSIL will regress and not progress further in immunocompetent hosts {714}. Consequently, LSIL is considered a preinvasive lesion rather than a precursor of SCC. HSIL may progress to (and is a precursor of) invasive SCC. HSIL has a 2-year recurrence risk of 53% in men who have sex with men {441}.

Anal squamous cell carcinoma

Graham RP

Definition
Anal squamous cell carcinoma (SCC) is a malignant epithelial tumour characterized by origin from the anal mucosa, keratin production, intercellular bridges, and frequent HPV infection.

ICD-O coding
8070/3 Squamous cell carcinoma NOS

ICD-11 coding
2C00.3 & XH0945 Squamous cell carcinoma of anus or anal canal & Squamous cell carcinoma

Related terminology
Acceptable: cloacogenic carcinoma; transitional carcinoma.

Subtype(s)
Verrucous squamous cell carcinoma (8051/3)

Localization
Anal SCC is localized in the anus.

Clinical features
Anal SCC generally presents with symptoms and signs related to the presence of a mass, such as discomfort, discharge, and haemorrhage. Clinical examination may detect a lump, indurated ulcer, friability, and or discolouration. In early disease, high-resolution anoscopy with acetic acid application to the anorectal mucosa improves lesion detection.

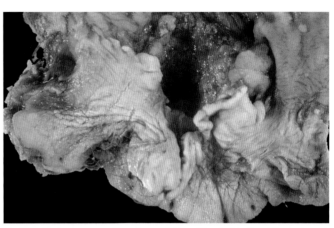

Fig. 7.12 Anal squamous cell carcinoma. Arising at the dentate line of the anal canal.

MRI {1441,2615} and endoanal ultrasound {2677} are used to assess local disease. MRI is also useful in assessing treatment response {1441,828,2615} after an appropriate interval {1051}. Regional lymph node assessment is enhanced by PET, but false positives may occur {2003,1290}.

Epidemiology
Most patients are diagnosed in the sixth decade of life or later {3005}. Cellular immune deficiency contributes to a younger presentation {3006,1943}.

The age-standardized incidence rate of invasive SCC ranges from 0.2 cases per 100 000 person-years in Asia to 1.7 cases

Table 7.02 Useful ancillary diagnostic markers for anal squamous cell carcinoma and its mimics

Tumour	Immunohistochemical markers					Other positive markers
	Pancytokeratin	CD45	S100	p40	Polyclonal CEA	
Anal squamous cell carcinoma	+	–	–	+	–	High-risk HPV in situ hybridization, p16
Basal cell carcinoma	+	–	–	+	–	Diffuse BerEP4
Neuroendocrine carcinoma (NEC)	+	–	–	–	Typically –	Chromogranin, synaptophysin, INSM1
Melanoma	Typically –	–	+	–	–	Melan-A, HMB45, SOX10
Extramammary Paget disease	+	–	–	–	+	GCDFP-15, GATA-3
Prostatic carcinoma	+	–	–	–	–	PSA, PSAP, NKX3-1
Colorectal carcinoma	+	–	–	–	+	CK20, CDX2, SATB2
Malignant lymphoma	–	+	–	–	–	PAX5 (often high-grade B-cell lymphoma)

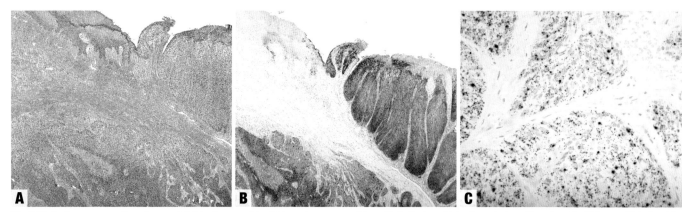

Fig. 7.13 Anal squamous cell carcinoma. **A** Arising from overlying high-grade squamous intraepithelial lesion with haphazard stromal invasion. **B** p16 immunohistochemistry is strongly and diffusely positive in the invasive carcinoma and overlying high-grade squamous intraepithelial lesion, characteristic of an HPV-positive carcinoma. **C** HPV E6/E7 mRNA in situ hybridization is positive, indicating transcriptionally active high-risk HPV in the tumour cells of the squamous cell carcinoma.

per 100 000 person-years in North America and northern Europe {3005,3566,1400,3079,384}. Rising incidence rates are believed to be related to evolving sexual behaviour and increased duration of HPV infection in HIV-positive patients {3006,1943,2411}. The incidence is higher in women and is unrelated to the prevalence of HIV, unlike in men {3005,3417,3079,384}.

Etiology

The etiological relationship between HPV and anal SCC is well established {711,2260,973}. HPV (most often HPV16) infection underlies 90% of cases {711,1103}. Multigenotype infection occurs {3591}. Additional risk factors include cellular immunodeficiency {3006,98}, anoreceptive intercourse {3353,646}, coinfection with other sexually transmitted infections {348,2099}, and cigarette smoking {646}. Longstanding perianal Crohn disease has been suggested as a potential risk factor for anal cancer {2779,2965}, but a large study revealed that only 2 of > 2900 such patients developed anal SCC {278}.

Pathogenesis

HPV infection is the main oncogenic driver, and its key oncoproteins are E6 and E7. E6 physically inactivates p53, facilitating survival of cells with genotoxic damage {1818}. E7 leads

to degradation and sequestering of RB1, allowing mutation-bearing cells to continue to proliferate {391}. Loss of RB1 function leads to overexpression of p16, which is used diagnostically {1956}. Additional factors such as immunosuppression {3006,98,3181,2544} are required for tumorigenesis, but the specific mechanisms/pathways by which they contribute to tumour development are unknown.

Macroscopic appearance

Thickening of the mucosa or a mass may be present, with or without ulceration.

Histopathology

Anal SCC is histologically heterogeneous and often composed of large eosinophilic cells characterized by keratinization. Alternatively, it may resemble urothelial carcinoma. Basaloid SCC refers to a pattern characterized by marked hyperchromasia, scant cytoplasm, and a peripheral palisade of tumour cells around the infiltrating trabeculae. This was previously called cloacogenic carcinoma. Rarely, basaloid tumour cell nests may be accompanied by hyalinization imparting an adenoid cystic-like appearance {1080,600}. Rarer still is a pattern composed of squamous cells with admixed mucin-containing cells. The descriptive term mucoepidermoid carcinoma is discouraged, to avoid clinical confusion {1080}. Recognition of these various histological patterns is useful to avoid misdiagnosis, but frequent admixture, subjectivity, lack of biological significance, and the predominance of biopsy-only sampling have contributed to the abandonment of histological subtyping for clinical purposes {918,1946}.

Verrucous carcinoma (VC) displays exophytic and endophytic growth of bulbous fronds of thickened epithelium with a pushing interface. VC lacks HPV cytopathic effect and severe cytological atypia. Mitoses are rare and basal. On small biopsies, the definitive diagnosis of VC is often impossible and may only be suggested based on clinical information. VC is locally destructive but does not metastasize. In some cases, areas of unequivocal conventional SCC are seen arising in VC. These cases can metastasize and should be diagnosed as conventional SCC. Thorough sampling is prudent before diagnosing VC. Giant condyloma of Buschke–Lowenstein was considered synonymous with VC. However, they are different entities; VC

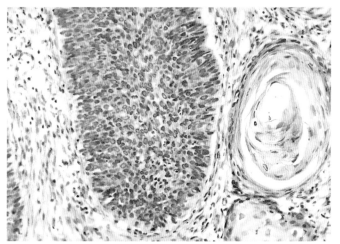

Fig. 7.14 Anal squamous cell carcinoma. The tumour shows a combination of basaloid features and keratinization.

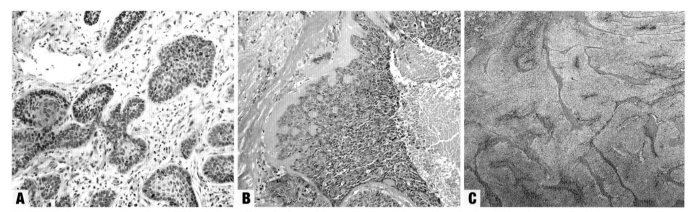

Fig. 7.15 Anal squamous cell carcinoma (SCC). **A** The neoplasm shows a peripheral palisade of darker-staining cells within the invasive trabecula; this imparts a basaloid appearance to the SCC. Focal keratinization is noted. **B** Hyaline material encircles and percolates into tumour trabecula, giving rise to an adenoid cystic–like appearance. This histological finding may be seen admixed with areas of conventional-looking SCC. **C** Anal SCC may display a morphological pattern reminiscent of urothelial carcinoma. In this field, overt squamous differentiation is inapparent, and the tumour cells have a transitional-like appearance.

is negative for HPV and giant condyloma is associated with low-risk HPV, viral cytopathic effect, and exophytic growth only {3784}.

Pseudoepitheliomatous squamous hyperplasia and basal cell carcinomas of the perianal skin may mimic SCC. Pseudoepitheliomatous hyperplasia shows limited cytological atypia and no invasion. An underlying granular cell tumour or syphilis may be identified. Retraction artefact, lack of atypical mitoses, and absence of an in situ component distinguish basal cell carcinoma from SCC {2552}. A broad range of neoplasms may mimic poorly differentiated SCC. Identification of an in situ component is frequently helpful in SCC diagnosis, but it should be interpreted cautiously, because mimics may involve the surface mucosa, including in a pagetoid manner.

Useful ancillary diagnostic markers for anal squamous cell carcinoma and its mimics are presented in Table 7.02 (p. 205).

Cytology

The cytology of SCC is described in the *Anal squamous dysplasia (intraepithelial neoplasia)* section (p. 202).

Diagnostic molecular pathology

Frequent mutations and genomic alterations in the PIK3CA/AKT/mTOR pathway, most commonly in *PIK3CA* {637,455}, have been identified. Overall, the tumour mutation burden is low {455}. HPV E6–mediated degradation inactivates p53, so *TP53* mutations are typically a feature of HPV-negative SCC {637}.

Essential and desirable diagnostic criteria

Essential: infiltrating squamous cell clusters and strands with malignant nuclei and eosinophilic cytoplasm; mitotic activity including atypical forms, intercellular bridges, and variable keratin production.

Note: See *Histopathology*, above, for other growth patterns of this histologically heterogeneous tumour.

Staging (TNM)

Anal SCC is staged according to the TNM system. Approximately 80% of patients present with the mass localized to the anal mucosa {2868}. Lymph from the anus drains towards the internal iliac and periaortic nodes or inguinal and femoral lymph nodes. Nodal metastases are detected in approximately 20% of patients {2868,1421}.

Prognosis and prediction

Pathological stage is the most important prognostic factor {1050}. The prognostic value of grade is confounded by stage, and morphological heterogeneity in anal SCC has rendered the value of grade on biopsies questionable {1050}. Tumour response by imaging correlates with outcome {1441,2003,2194}. HIV status does not alter disease-specific outcome, but HIV infection portends more treatment-related toxicity {1943,1248}. PDL1 expression by tumour cells has been identified in approximately half of anal SCC cases {3676}, and early data indicate encouraging responses to PD1 inhibition {2465}.

Anal adenocarcinoma

Shia J

Definition
Anal adenocarcinoma is an adenocarcinoma that arises in the glandular epithelium of the anal canal. Two subtypes exist: mucosal and extramucosal. The former arises in the luminal mucosa and is of intestinal type; the latter may be associated with anal gland, a pre-existing anal fistula, or other non-fistulating glandular structures of the anal canal (acquired or congenital malformations or embryological remnants) and may be of anal gland type, mucinous type, or intestinal type.

ICD-O coding
8140/3 Adenocarcinoma NOS

ICD-11 coding
2C00.0 Adenocarcinoma of anus or anal canal

Related terminology
Extramucosal anal canal adenocarcinoma
Acceptable: perianal adenocarcinoma.

Anal gland adenocarcinoma
Not recommended: anal duct adenocarcinoma.

Subtype(s)
None

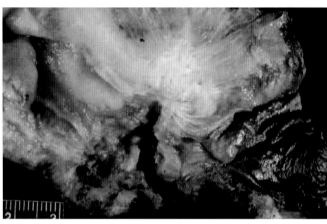

Fig. 7.16 Anal gland adenocarcinoma. A poorly defined infiltrative mass, intramurally and perianally located and closely approaching the inked radial margin.

Localization
Anal adenocarcinoma arises in the anal canal, including the perianal/ischiorectal region.

Clinical features
The mucosal type typically shares clinical features with distal rectal adenocarcinoma and anal squamous cell carcinoma. To date, our understanding of the characteristics of extramucosal-type

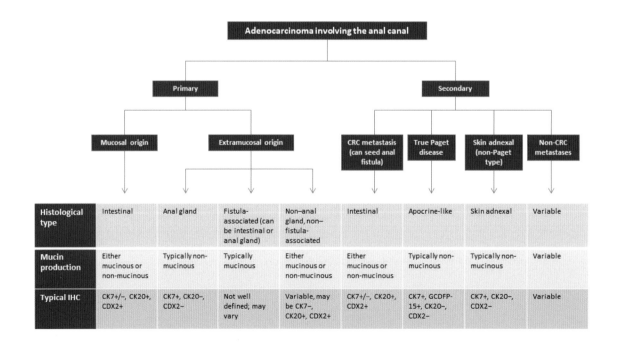

	Primary				Secondary			
	Mucosal origin	Extramucosal origin			CRC metastasis (can seed anal fistula)	True Paget disease	Skin adnexal (non-Paget type)	Non-CRC metastases
Histological type	Intestinal	Anal gland	Fistula-associated (can be intestinal or anal gland)	Non–anal gland, non–fistula-associated	Intestinal	Apocrine-like	Skin adnexal	Variable
Mucin production	Either mucinous or non-mucinous	Typically non-mucinous	Typically mucinous	Either mucinous or non-mucinous	Either mucinous or non-mucinous	Typically non-mucinous	Typically non-mucinous	Variable
Typical IHC	CK7+/–, CK20+, CDX2+	CK7+, CK20–, CDX2–	Not well defined; may vary	Variable, may be CK7–, CK20+, CDX2+	CK7+/–, CK20+, CDX2+	CK7+, GCDFP-15+, CK20–, CDX2–	CK7+, CK20–, CDX2–	Variable

Fig. 7.17 Classification scheme for adenocarcinomas involving the anal canal. CRC, colorectal carcinoma; IHC, immunohistochemistry.

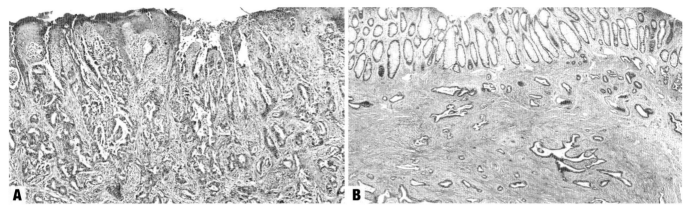

Fig. 7.18 Anal gland adenocarcinoma. **A** Note confluent anastomosing glands involving the wall and focally ulcerating the overlying squamous epithelium. **B** Elsewhere the tumour glands are less confluent and appear angulated.

tumours is from case studies. Reported cases of pathologically confirmed anal gland adenocarcinoma suggest a male predilection (M:F ratio: 1.7:1), with a mean age of 58 years. Patients typically present with pain, bleeding, or sensation of a mass {3741,7,1252,2124}. Most fistula-associated adenocarcinomas develop in the setting of Crohn disease {3298,2367,2416}, and in this setting there is a female predilection (M:F ratio: 0.7:1). The mean age at diagnosis is about 50 years (females younger than males). Fistula-associated adenocarcinomas unrelated to Crohn disease occur almost exclusively in men, with a mean patient age of 55 years {3668,2860,3037}. In most cases of fistula-associated carcinomas, the duration of the fistula before the diagnosis of carcinoma is characteristically ≥ 10 years. New-onset mucous discharge from the fistula is a common symptom. A high index of suspicion is key to the early detection of this malignancy.

Epidemiology

In 2018, 8580 new cases of anal cancer were projected to occur in the USA {3034}. It is estimated that adenocarcinomas account for as many as 10% of all anal cancers; most are mucosal.

Etiology

Risk factors include smoking, HIV infection, anoreceptive intercourse, anal Crohn disease, and chronic anal fistula {1859}. HPV infection has been implicated in a minor subset of anal canal adenocarcinomas {1692,1272,1219}, primarily in tumours arising from the anal transitional zone {1219}. The most commonly infecting genotype is HPV16, followed (distantly) by HPV18 {1219}.

Pathogenesis

Mucosal-type adenocarcinoma may share carcinogenesis pathways with other colorectal carcinomas. Fistula-associated carcinomas in the setting of Crohn disease are probably triggered by specific cytokines and transcriptional factors upregulated in an inflammatory microenvironment (see *Inflammatory bowel disease–associated dysplasia of the colorectum*, p. 174, and *Colorectal adenocarcinoma*, p. 177).

Macroscopic appearance

Anal adenocarcinomas may present as mucosal or submucosal lesions, sometimes associated with fistulas. Most are macroscopically indistinguishable from colorectal adenocarcinomas.

Histopathology

Mucosal-type anal adenocarcinomas arise within the luminal mucosa and typically have histopathological features indistinguishable from those of rectal adenocarcinoma.

Extramucosal-type anal canal adenocarcinomas, by definition, lack a luminal in situ component, although they may involve the surface mucosa by erosion, colonization, or pagetoid extension. On the basis of their relatedness to either an anal gland–like immunophenotype or anal fistula, these tumours are currently classified into three subtypes: anal gland adenocarcinoma; fistula-associated adenocarcinoma; and extramucosal anal canal adenocarcinoma, non–anal gland type and non–fistula-associated. Some fistula-associated carcinomas may have an anal gland–like immunophenotype.

Anal gland adenocarcinomas have their origin in the anal gland or duct. Grossly, they form firm, infiltrative masses, typically centred in the wall of the anorectal area, 2–5 cm in greatest dimension {1925,3592}. The histological spectrum of this subtype remains to be sharply defined. Typical cases exhibit haphazardly dispersed glands with cuboidal cells and scant mucin {1252}. Unusual subtypes may manifest tumour cell stratification, solid growth, or prominent mucin production. The tumour cells characteristically express CK7 and MUC5AC, and they do not express CK20 or CDX2 {1252,1728,2124}. CK5/6 and p63, markers constitutively positive in benign anal glands, are negative in anal gland carcinomas {1925,510,3741}. The main differential diagnoses include metastases from sites such as the gynaecological tract and breast.

Fistula-associated adenocarcinomas may be histogenetically related to anal gland epithelium {917,1961} or to transitional-type or rectal-type epithelium (via congenital or acquired mucosal duplication or malformations) {1961,1998,1478}. The majority of these tumours are mucinous, grossly and morphologically resembling ordinary colorectal-type mucinous adenocarcinoma. An adenoma or adenoma-like component may be seen {1998,1367}. Non-mucinous subtypes have been reported (as has squamous cell carcinoma) {3298,3698}. The available immunohistochemical studies support the presumed variability

Chapter 7

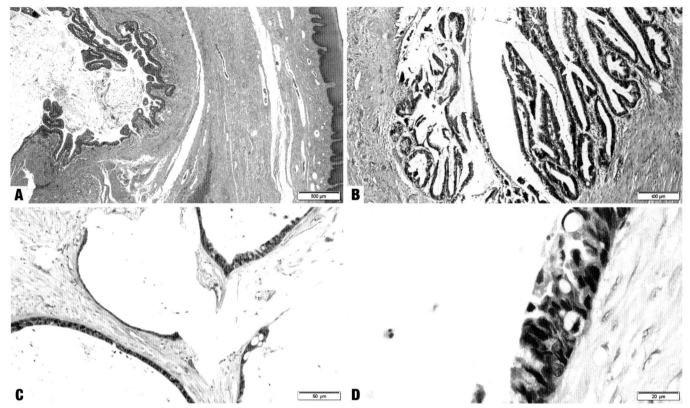

Fig. 7.19 Fistula-associated anal canal adenocarcinoma. **A** An example involving the wall of the lower anal canal. **B** Neoplastic glands are seen lining part of the fistula tract. Note the presence of inflammation and granulation tissue in upper left corner where the fistula tract is not lined by neoplastic glands. **C** Elsewhere, the tumour is composed predominantly of extracellular mucin. The neoplastic glands cling to the stroma and surround pools of mucin. Note that some of the tumour cells appear flattened, whereas others show more apparent stratification. **D** Higher-power view demonstrating a segment of neoplastic epithelium with nuclear stratification and intracellular mucin.

in histogenesis, with some cases showing an intestinal phenotype (positive for CK20 and MUC2) {1998,2367} and others exhibiting an anal gland–like mucin composition (no immunoreactivity to O-acetyl sialic acid groups) that is distinct from that of rectal epithelium {917,3597}. Diagnosis hinges on the presence

of a pre-existing, often longstanding fistula and the exclusion of subsequent involvement by a carcinoma from elsewhere, particularly the rectum or colon {3116}.

Extramucosal anal canal adenocarcinoma, non–anal gland type and non–fistula-associated, is a newly recognized group of tumours that may be histogenetically related to other non-fistulating intramural glandular structures (including acquired or congenital malformations or embryological remnants). A recent report described two such cases, both possessing an intestinal phenotype {1042}. Diagnosis requires the exclusion of a cutaneous primary or a metastasis.

All types of anal canal adenocarcinoma may show pagetoid spread to anal squamous mucosa or perianal skin, resulting in secondary anal Paget disease. Rarely, adenomas (without documented invasive disease) are also observed to give rise to secondary anal Paget disease {635}. The secondary Paget cells may be contiguous with the underlying neoplasm or manifest at sites distinctly away from it (with skip lesions). In some cases, the secondary anal Paget disease present months to years before or after the underlying adenocarcinoma becomes clinically detectable {2171}. It has been observed that Paget disease subsequent to rectal-type adenocarcinoma tends to express not only CK20 but also CK7 in both the Paget cells and the associated adenocarcinoma {1059}. Unlike secondary anal Paget disease, primary anal Paget disease is believed to originate in the perianal skin and to constitute an intraepithelial carcinoma with skin appendage differentiation. Typically presenting as erythematous eczematous plaque lesions, primary

Fig. 7.20 Extramucosal anal canal adenocarcinoma, non–fistula-associated. This example is not associated with a pre-existing anal fistula. The tumour shows an intestinal phenotype with nuclear stratification and intestinal-type mucin. By immunohistochemistry, it is negative for CK7 and positive for CK20 (not shown). This is currently classified as extramucosal anal canal adenocarcinoma, non–anal gland type and non–fistula-associated.

anal Paget disease can extend to the anal canal mucosa. It can also become invasive and involve the perianal or ischiorectal region, mimicking primary anal canal adenocarcinoma. Immunohistochemistry can facilitate the distinction: primary Paget disease cells typically coexpress CK7 and GCDFP-15, and they do not express CK20 or CDX2 {1059,2648}.

The main characteristics of the various primary and secondary anal canal adenocarcinomas are summarized in Fig. 7.17.

Cytology
Not clinically relevant

Diagnostic molecular pathology
The data are limited. One recent study observed rates of *KRAS* and *NRAS* mutation in anal canal adenocarcinoma to be 47% and 6%, respectively {1219}. Microsatellite instability was observed in only 1 of 48 intestinal-type tumours and 0 of 26 anal gland / transitional-type tumours {1219}.

Essential and desirable diagnostic criteria
See Fig. 7.17.

Staging (TNM)
Anal canal adenocarcinomas are staged according to the TNM classification for anal cancer. Carcinoma is defined by the presence of invasion and is staged on the basis of tumour size. pTis anal canal glandular neoplasia refers to high-grade glandular dysplasia.

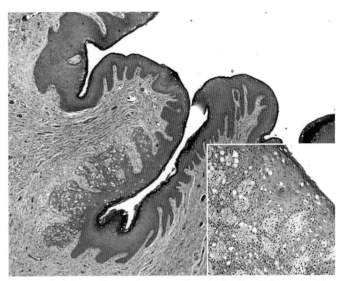

Fig. 7.21 Anal Paget disease. Low-power view showing Paget disease involving anal squamous mucosa in the form of skip lesions, with lesional areas separated by stretches of uninvolved epithelium. **Inset**: Large Paget cells with a signet-ring cell morphology. This is secondary anal Paget disease, associated metachronously with a mucosal-type anal canal adenocarcinoma.

Prognosis and prediction
The prognosis of anal canal adenocarcinoma has been shown to be worse than that of anal squamous cell carcinoma, and it is largely dependent on TNM staging {2256,586}.

Anal neuroendocrine neoplasms

Lam AK

Definition
Neuroendocrine neoplasms (NENs) of the anal canal are anal epithelial neoplasms with neuroendocrine differentiation.

ICD-O coding
8240/3 Neuroendocrine tumour NOS
8246/3 Neuroendocrine carcinoma NOS
8154/3 Mixed neuroendocrine–non-neuroendocrine neoplasm (MiNEN)

ICD-11 coding
2C00.2 Neuroendocrine neoplasm of anus or anal canal
2C00.2 & XH0U20 Neuroendocrine neoplasm of anus or anal canal & Neuroendocrine carcinoma NOS
2C00.2 & XH9SY0 Neuroendocrine neoplasm of anus or anal canal & Small cell neuroendocrine carcinoma
2C00.2 & XH0NL5 Neuroendocrine neoplasm of anus or anal canal & Large cell neuroendocrine carcinoma
2C00.2 & XH6H10 Neuroendocrine neoplasm of anus or anal canal & Mixed adenoneuroendocrine carcinoma

Related terminology
Acceptable: well-differentiated endocrine tumour/carcinoma; poorly differentiated endocrine carcinoma; mixed exocrine-endocrine carcinoma; mixed adenoneuroendocrine carcinoma.
Not recommended: carcinoid; composite carcinoid-adenocarcinoma.

Subtype(s)
Neuroendocrine tumour, grade 1 (8240/3); neuroendocrine tumour, grade 2 (8249/3); neuroendocrine tumour, grade 3 (8249/3); large cell neuroendocrine carcinoma (8013/3); small cell neuroendocrine carcinoma (8041/3)

Localization
NENs can occur in any portion of the anal canal.

Clinical features
Neuroendocrine carcinoma (NEC) appears to be slightly more common in women {639}. The median age of presentation of anal small cell NEC (SCNEC) is in the sixth decade of life {639}. Many NECs occur between the fifth and seventh decades of life. There are insufficient data in the literature on the sex and age distributions of anal canal neuroendocrine tumour (NET).

There have been no reports of patients with carcinoid syndrome. Patients with anal NENs could present with anal pain, discomfort, or bleeding {1560}. Obstruction of the anal canal by the tumour may cause constipation {1837}. A mass or ulcer may be apparent on endoscopic examination. These patients need radiological examination of the abdomen and pelvis to determine the extent of regional disease.

In cases of NET or large cell NEC (LCNEC) of the anal canal, 72.1% of patients had local disease at diagnosis. Anal SCNEC is often diagnosed at advanced stages, with 38.5% of patients having regional disease and 46.2% having distant disease. Liver, lung, and bone are common sites of distant metastases {3494}.

Epidemiology
NENs account for slightly more than 1% of all anal cancers {1622}. In the anal canal, LCNEC is far more common than NET {144}. SCNEC accounts for slightly more than one third of all NENs noted in the anal canal.

Etiology
The etiology of NENs of the anal canal is largely unknown. Anal canal SCNEC has been associated with HIV infection {2280,2050,100}. Similar to the association in squamous cell carcinoma (SCC), HPV could be an etiological factor for anal canal SCNEC {639,2430}.

Pathogenesis
Neuroendocrine cells are present in the basal layer of the anal transitional zone mucosa. The pathogenesis of the NENs is unknown.

Macroscopic appearance
Anal NETs often present as anal masses and may ulcerate.

Histopathology
Anal NETs are graded using the same system used for other gastroenteropancreatic NETs. They are often G1 or G2 {1128}. The tumour has a nesting or trabecular pattern, and the cells have granular cytoplasm {2769}. NEC has a diffuse architecture, and the cells show marked nuclear pleomorphism and brisk mitotic activity (a high Ki-67 proliferation index). Pagetoid spread to the anal epithelium has been reported in LCNEC {1115}. Anal SCNEC has small tumour cells with a high N:C ratio and nuclear moulding. There has been one reported case of melanoma coexisting with NEC {1366}. NENs of the anal canal are positive for neuroendocrine markers, chromogranin, and synaptophysin.

Mixed neuroendocrine–non-neuroendocrine neoplasms (MiNENs), which are rare in the anal canal, most often consist of NEC and adenocarcinoma {197,211}. MiNENs consisting of SCNEC and SCC can also occur. There has been a reported case of LCNEC coexisting with squamous intraepithelial neoplasia in an 80-year-old woman; both elements were positive for HPV18 {2430}.

Differential diagnosis

For NEC and MiNEN, differentiation from poorly differentiated / basaloid SCC, poorly differentiated adenocarcinoma, melanoma of the anal canal, and basal cell carcinoma of the peri-anal skin is important. Immunohistochemical markers (e.g. chromogranin and synaptophysin) could confirm the diagnosis of NEC or a NEC component in MiNEN {1255}. NEC is negative for p63 (positive in SCC and basal cell carcinoma), CK7 (positive in adenocarcinoma), CK20, and melanoma markers.

Merkel cell carcinoma occurs in the anal canal {2551,2446}. Similar to SCNEC, Merkel cell carcinoma expresses neuroendocrine markers. However, unlike SCNEC, classic polyomavirus-positive Merkel cell carcinoma shows perinuclear dot-like staining for CK20 and is negative for TTF1 {2543}.

Anal NEC may express TTF1 {1837}. Therefore, TTF1 cannot be used to differentiate anal NEC from metastatic NECs from other sites.

Cytology
Not clinically relevant

Diagnostic molecular pathology
Not clinically relevant

Essential and desirable diagnostic criteria
The essential and desirable diagnostic criteria for anal NENs are the same as those for NENs in other organs. The demonstration of neuroendocrine differentiation by immunohistochemistry is essential for the diagnosis of NEN. The subtypes are classified as described in the corresponding sections.

Staging (TNM)
NEC should be staged in the same way as other anal carcinomas.

Prognosis and prediction
In the anal canal, localized NET has a good prognosis, with a 10-year survival rate of 95% {1599}. In one series, survival time with extensive disease was only 25 months {1599}. NEC is reported to have a 5-year survival rate of 13% {309A}.

There is a lack of data on the predictive factors for anal NENs. In a study involving both anal and rectal NENs, large size, deep invasion, lymphovascular invasion, and an elevated mitotic count were predictive factors for aggressive biological behaviour {2998}.

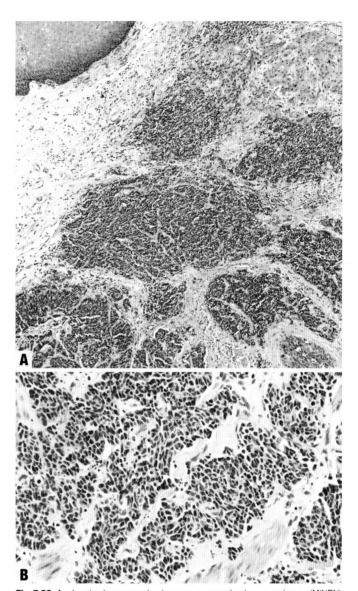

Fig. 7.22 Anal mixed neuroendocrine–non-neuroendocrine neoplasm (MiNEN) with small cell neuroendocrine carcinoma (SCNEC) and squamous cell carcinoma. **A** SCNEC is visible in the lower left; nests of tumour cells with a high N:C ratio are apparent; there is a separate area of squamous cell carcinoma in the upper right. **B** High-power view of the SCNEC component; note the small tumour cells with a high N:C ratio and nuclear moulding.

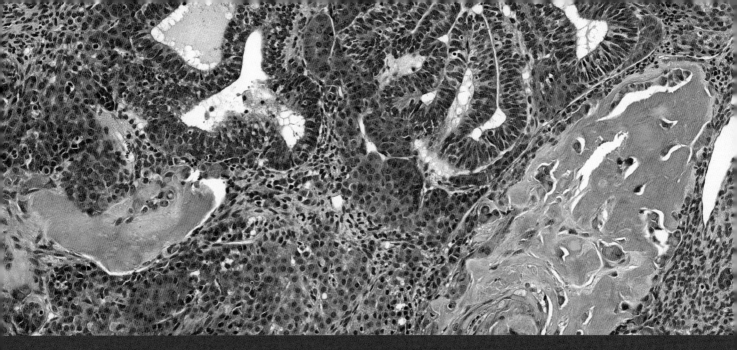

8

Tumours of the liver and intrahepatic bile ducts

Edited by: Paradis V, Fukayama M, Park YN, Schirmacher P

Benign hepatocellular tumours
   Focal nodular hyperplasia of the liver
   Hepatocellular adenoma
Malignant hepatocellular tumours and precursors
   Hepatocellular carcinoma
   Hepatoblastoma
Benign biliary tumours and precursors
   Bile duct adenoma
   Biliary adenofibroma
   Mucinous cystic neoplasm of the liver and biliary system
   Biliary intraepithelial neoplasia (see Chapter 9)
   Intraductal papillary neoplasm of the bile ducts (see Chapter 9)
Malignant biliary tumours
   Intrahepatic cholangiocarcinoma
Combined hepatocellular-cholangiocarcinoma and undifferentiated primary liver carcinoma
Hepatic neuroendocrine neoplasms

WHO classification of tumours of the liver and intrahepatic bile ducts

Benign hepatocellular tumours
8170/0   Hepatocellular adenoma
          HNF1A-inactivated hepatocellular adenoma
          Inflammatory hepatocellular adenoma
          B-catenin-activated hepatocellular adenoma
          B-catenin-activated inflammatory hepatocellular
          adenoma

Malignant hepatocellular tumours and precursors
8170/3   Hepatocellular carcinoma NOS
8171/3   Hepatocellular carcinoma, fibrolamellar
8172/3   Hepatocellular carcinoma, scirrhous
8174/3   Hepatocellular carcinoma, clear cell type
          Hepatocellular carcinoma, steatohepatitic
          Hepatocellular carcinoma, macrotrabecular
          massive
          Hepatocellular carcinoma, chromophobe
          Hepatocellular carcinoma, neutrophil-rich
          Hepatocellular carcinoma, lymphocyte-rich
8970/3   Hepatoblastoma NOS

Benign biliary tumours and precursors
8160/0   Bile duct adenoma
9013/0   Adenofibroma NOS
8148/0   Biliary intraepithelial neoplasia, low grade
8148/2   Biliary intraepithelial neoplasia, high grade
8503/0   Intraductal papillary neoplasm with low-grade
          intraepithelial neoplasia
8503/2   Intraductal papillary neoplasm with high-grade
          intraepithelial neoplasia
8503/3   Intraductal papillary neoplasm with associated invasive
          carcinoma
8470/0   Mucinous cystic neoplasm with low-grade
          intraepithelial neoplasia
8470/2   Mucinous cystic neoplasm with high-grade
          intraepithelial neoplasia
8470/3   Mucinous cystic neoplasm with associated invasive
          carcinoma

Malignant biliary tumours
8160/3   Cholangiocarcinoma
          Large duct intrahepatic cholangiocarcinoma
          Small duct intrahepatic cholangiocarcinoma
8020/3   Carcinoma, undifferentiated, NOS
8180/3   Combined hepatocellular carcinoma and
          cholangiocarcinoma
8240/3   Neuroendocrine tumour NOS
8240/3   Neuroendocrine tumour, grade 1
8249/3   Neuroendocrine tumour, grade 2
8249/3   Neuroendocrine tumour, grade 3
8246/3   Neuroendocrine carcinoma NOS
8013/3   Large cell neuroendocrine carcinoma
8041/3   Small cell neuroendocrine carcinoma
8154/3   Mixed neuroendocrine–non-neuroendocrine neoplasm
          (MiNEN)

These morphology codes are from the International Classification of Diseases for Oncology, third edition, second revision (ICD-O-3.2) {1378A}. Behaviour is coded /0 for benign tumours; /1 for unspecified, borderline, or uncertain behaviour; /2 for carcinoma in situ and grade III intraepithelial neoplasia; /3 for malignant tumours, primary site; and /6 for malignant tumours, metastatic site. Behaviour code /6 is not generally used by cancer registries.

This classification is modified from the previous WHO classification, taking into account changes in our understanding of these lesions.

TNM staging of tumours of the liver

Liver
(ICD-O-3 C22.0)

Rules for Classification
The classification applies to hepatocellular carcinoma.

Cholangio- (intrahepatic bile duct) carcinoma of the liver has a separate classification (see p. 218). There should be histological confirmation of the disease.

The following are the procedures for assessing T, N, and M categories.

T categories	Physical examination, imaging, and/or surgical exploration
N categories	Physical examination, imaging, and/or surgical exploration
M categories	Physical examination, imaging, and/or surgical exploration

Note
Although the presence of cirrhosis is an important prognostic factor it does not affect the TNM classification, being an independent prognostic variable.

Regional Lymph Nodes
The regional lymph nodes are the hilar, hepatic (along the proper hepatic artery), periportal (along the portal vein), inferior phrenic, and caval nodes.

TNM Clinical Classification
T – Primary Tumour
TX   Primary tumour cannot be assessed
T0   No evidence of primary tumour
T1a   Solitary tumour 2 cm or less in greatest dimension with or without vascular invasion
T1b   Solitary tumour more than 2 cm in greatest dimension without vascular invasion
T2   Solitary tumour with vascular invasion more than 2 cm dimension *or* multiple tumours, none more than 5 cm in greatest dimension
T3   Multiple tumours any more than 5 cm in greatest dimension
T4   Tumour(s) involving a major branch of the portal or hepatic vein or with direct invasion of adjacent organs (including the diaphragm), other than the gallbladder *or* with perforation of visceral peritoneum

N – Regional Lymph Nodes
NX   Regional lymph nodes cannot be assessed
N0   No regional lymph node metastasis
N1   Regional lymph node metastasis

M – Distant Metastasis
M0   No distant metastasis
M1   Distant metastasis

pTNM Pathological Classification
The pT and pN categories correspond to the T and N categories.

pN0   Histological examination of a regional lymphadenectomy specimen will ordinarily include 3 or more lymph nodes. If the lymph nodes are negative, but the number ordinarily examined is not met, classify as pN0.

pM – Distant Metastasis*
pM1   Distant metastasis microscopically confirmed

Note
* pM0 and pMX are not valid categories.

Stage – Liver

Stage IA	T1a	N0	M0
Stage IB	T1b	N0	M0
Stage II	T2	N0	M0
Stage IIIA	T3	N0	M0
Stage IIIB	T4	N0	M0
Stage IVA	Any T	N1	M0
Stage IVB	Any T	Any N	M1

TNM staging of tumours of the intrahepatic bile ducts

Intrahepatic Bile Ducts

(ICD-O-3 C22.1)

Rules for Classification

The staging system applies to intrahepatic cholangiocarcinoma, cholangiocellular carcinoma, and combined hepatocellular and cholangiocarcinoma (mixed hepatocellular/cholangiocellular carcinoma).

The following are the procedures for assessing T, N, and M categories.

T categories	Physical examination, imaging, and/or surgical exploration
N categories	Physical examination, imaging, and/or surgical exploration
M categories	Physical examination, imaging, and/or surgical exploration

Regional Lymph Nodes

For right-liver intrahepatic cholangiocarcinoma, the regional lymph nodes include the hilar (common bile duct, hepatic artery, portal vein, and cystic duct), periduodenal, and peripancreatic lymph nodes.

For left-liver intrahepatic cholangiocarcinoma, regional lymph nodes include hilar and gastrohepatic lymph nodes.

For intrahepatic cholangiocarcinoma, spread to the coeliac and/or periaortic and caval lymph nodes are distant metastases (M1).

TNM Clinical Classification

T – Primary Tumour

TX	Primary tumour cannot be assessed
T0	No evidence of primary tumour
Tis	Carcinoma in situ (intraductal tumour)
T1a	Solitary tumour 5 cm or less in greatest dimension without vascular invasion
T1b	Solitary tumour more than 5 cm in greatest dimension without vascular invasion
T2	Solitary tumour with intrahepatic vascular invasion *or* multiple tumours, with or without vascular invasion
T3	Tumour perforating the visceral peritoneum
T4	Tumour involving local extrahepatic structures by direct hepatic invasion

N – Regional Lymph Nodes

NX	Regional lymph nodes cannot be assessed
N0	No regional lymph node metastasis
N1	Regional lymph node metastasis

M – Distant Metastasis

M0	No distant metastasis
M1	Distant metastasis

pTNM Pathological Classification

The pT and pN categories correspond to the T and N categories.

pN0 Histological examination of a regional lymphadenectomy specimen will ordinarily include 6 or more lymph nodes. If the regional lymph nodes are negative, but the number ordinarily examined is not met, classify as pN0.

pM – Distant Metastasis*

pM1 Distant metastasis microscopically confirmed

Note
* pM0 and pMX are not valid categories.

Stage – Intrahepatic Bile Ducts

Stage	T	N	M
Stage 0	Tis	N0	M0
Stage I	T1	N0	M0
Stage IA	T1a	N0	M0
Stage IB	T1b	N0	M0
Stage II	T2	N0	M0
Stage IIIA	T3	N0	M0
Stage IIIB	T4	N0	M0
	Any T	N1	M0
Stage IV	Any T	Any N	M1

The information presented here has been excerpted from the 2017 *TNM classification of malignant tumours*, eighth edition {408,3385A}. © 2017 UICC.
A help desk for specific questions about the TNM classification is available at https://www.uicc.org/tnm-help-desk.

Tumours of the liver and intrahepatic bile ducts: Introduction

Schirmacher P
Fukayama M
Paradis V
Park YN

This chapter concerns neoplasms of the liver. The ICD-O topographical coding for the anatomical sites covered in this chapter is presented in Box 8.01. Due to the novel structure of the fifth edition, mesenchymal, germ cell, haematolymphoid neoplasia, and metastatic lesions are described in respective general chapters that cover these topics for all neoplasms of the digestive tract. The many tumour-forming non-neoplastic lesions of the liver are not specifically addressed, with the singular exception of focal nodular hyperplasia, for histological and imaging differential diagnostic relevance and quite recent demonstration of its reactive nature.

Many refinements of the fourth-edition classification have been made concerning liver tumours, supported by novel molecular findings. For example, a comprehensive picture of the molecular changes occurring in common hepatocellular carcinoma (HCC) has evolved from large-scale comprehensive molecular profiling studies. Meanwhile, several rarer HCC subtypes, which together may account for 20–30% of cases, have been defined by stable morphomolecular and clinical features, with fibrolamellar carcinoma and its diagnostic *DNAJB1-PRKACA* translocation being the paradigm. Intrahepatic cholangiocarcinoma (iCCA) is now better understood as being an entity combining two different subtypes: a large duct type, which resembles extrahepatic cholangiocarcinoma, and a small duct type, which shares etiological, pathogenetic, and imaging features with HCC. The two subtypes have very different etiologies, molecular alterations, growth patterns, and clinical characteristics, illustrating the conflict of anatomically and (histo)pathogenetically based classifications. It will be necessary to implement these findings into clinical research and study protocols. Also supported by molecular findings, the definition and distinction of combined hepatocellular-cholangiocarcinoma have become clearer. Cholangiolocarcinoma is no longer considered a subtype of combined hepatocellular-cholangiocarcinoma, but rather a subtype of small duct iCCA, putting all primary intrahepatic carcinomas with a ductal/tubular phenotype under the overarching category of iCCA. Nevertheless, primary liver cancer shows a spectrum of differentiation, making its strict typing arbitrary in some cases; the authors have addressed this aspect by emphasizing diagnostically relevant definitions, considering emerging genomic data, and aiming to simplify classification criteria to focus on morphologically recognizable distinctions.

Liver neoplasms provide several unusual aspects with clinical, diagnostic, and research impact. Not only is HCC one of the most frequent malignancies worldwide, it is the paradigm of cancer induced by infection and by metabolic and toxic agents linked to chronic necroinflammation. Although these findings have translated into primary and secondary preventive measures, as well as model systems of disease, the prognosis of clinically apparent HCC remains poor. iCCA stands out as a malignancy with a high percentage of cases showing translocations that may also represent future therapeutic targets.

Hepatocellular adenoma represents a beautiful example of consequent morphology-supervised molecular profiling leading to a now almost completely morphomolecularly subtyped neoplasia. This subtyping has gained high clinical relevance and has fuelled implementation of refined morphological criteria and molecular testing in routine diagnostics.

Box 8.01 ICD-O topographical coding for the anatomical sites covered in this chapter

C22 Liver and intrahepatic bile ducts
C22.0 Liver
C22.1 Intrahepatic bile duct

Focal nodular hyperplasia of the liver

Bioulac-Sage P
Kakar S
Nault JC

Definition

Focal nodular hyperplasia (FNH) of the liver is not a true neoplasm, but rather a mass-forming hyperplastic response of hepatocytes occurring as a result of localized vascular abnormalities.

ICD-O coding

None

ICD-11 coding

DB99.Y & XH0M86 Other diseases of liver & Focal nodular hyperplasia

Related terminology

None

Subtype(s)

None

Localization

FNH can appear anywhere in the liver.

Clinical features

In 80–90% of cases, FNH is discovered in young women, rarely in men or children. FNH is solitary in two thirds of cases {3524}. Most are asymptomatic, discovered as incidental findings. Exceptionally, large lesions can present with abdominal pain or compression of adjacent organs. Reports of haemorrhage or malignant transformation require further confirmation. FNH regression has been shown on serial imaging studies {2035,1725}.

The background liver is usually normal, but FNH can occur in association with vascular diseases (portal vein thrombosis or atresia, Budd–Chiari syndrome, hereditary haemorrhagic telangiectasia) and adjacent to mass lesions {3242,3526}.

FNH is associated with hepatic haemangioma in 20% of cases, and it can occasionally coexist with hepatocellular adenoma {1800,3007}.

In 90% of cases, an accurate diagnosis can be made by imaging, using contrast-enhanced ultrasonography or contrast-enhanced MRI (see Table 8.01) {448,1601,1092}. On contrast-enhanced ultrasonography, FNH shows a characteristic pattern of hypervascularity in the arterial phase, centrifugal filling, and stellate arteries producing a spoke-wheel sign. On MRI, the lesion is isointense or slightly hypointense on T1-weighted

Table 8.01 Typical features of focal nodular hyperplasia with various imaging modalities

Imaging modality	Main nodule	Central scar region
MRI		
T1-weighted	Isointense or slightly hypointense	Hypointense
Chemical shift sequences	No signal dropout	
T2-weighted	Isointense or slightly hyperintense	Hyperintense
Gadolinium-enhanced		
Arterial phase	Hyperintense homogeneous	Hypointense
Portal venous phase	Isointense or slightly hyperintense	Hypointense, isointense, or hyperintense
Delayed phase	Isointense	Hyperintense
Baseline greyscale ultrasonography	Slightly hypoechoic, isoechoic, or slightly hyperechoic	Slightly hyperechoic (inconstant)
Colour Doppler		
Vascularity	Hypervascular	
Arteries	Central feeding artery with a stellate or spoke-wheel pattern	Central stellate vasculature (inconstant); spoke-wheel aspect (inconstant)
Veins	Peripheral draining veins (inconstant)	
Contrast-enhanced ultrasonography		
Arterial phase	Hypervascular	Central scar not visualized
Filling pattern	Centrifugal and homogeneous, +/– spoke-wheel sign, +/– dendritic pattern	
Portal venous phase	Isoechoic or hyperechoic	Hypoechoic (inconstant)
Delayed phase	Isoechoic	Hypoechoic (inconstant)

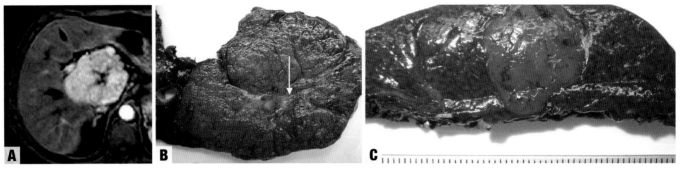

Fig. 8.01 Focal nodular hyperplasia. **A** MRI: fat-suppressed gadolinium-enhanced T1-weighted sequence (arterial phase). **B** Fresh specimen: note the multinodularity and central stellate scar (arrow). **C** Fresh specimen: small lesion without stellate scar; note the focal areas of congestion.

images and slightly hyperintense or isointense on T2. The central scar is typically hypointense on T1 and hyperintense on T2; during the arterial phase of gadolinium-enhanced imaging, FNH demonstrates intense homogeneous enhancement (except for the central scar) and returns to isointensity during the portal and delayed phase, whereas the central scar shows delayed enhancement. Biopsy is required in cases with atypical imaging features.

Epidemiology
FNH is the second most frequent benign liver nodule (after haemangioma), found in 0.8% of adult autopsies {3524}.

Etiology
There is no evidence of a relationship with oral contraceptive use {2076,1033}.

Pathogenesis
The pathogenesis of FNH is not fully established. The association with conditions having local or systemic vascular anomalies and the presence of unusually large vessels suggests that FNH is a nonspecific response to focally increased blood flow {3525}. A current hypothesis is that the primary lesion is outflow obstruction and the resulting congestive injury leads to parenchymal collapse and fibrosis, arteriovenous shunting, and loss of portal veins and ducts.

Clonal analysis using the HUMARA test has demonstrated the polyclonal nature of FNH {2512,334}. Studies showed that the mRNA expression of angiopoietin genes (*ANGPT1* and *ANGPT2*) involved in vessel maturation is altered, with an increased ANGPT1:ANGPT2 ratio compared with normal liver, cirrhosis, and other liver tumours {2510,2666}. The β-catenin pathway is activated without mutations in *CTNNB1* (encoding β-catenin) or *AXIN1* {2667}. This activation explains the expansion of glutamine synthetase (GS) staining in hepatocytes.

Macroscopic appearance
On cut section, classic FNH is a pale, firm, well-delineated, lobulated, and unencapsulated mass, from a few millimetres to > 10 cm. The lesion is composed of nodules 2–3 mm in size, separated by zones of fibrosis that give the lesion a multinodular appearance {2945}. The lesion characteristically has a central stellate fibrous scar with radiating extensions that partially surround nodules. Some cases of FNH may lack a central scar.

Histopathology
Nodules are composed of benign-looking hepatocytes arranged in plates no more than 2 cells in thickness. The central scar contains one or more large dystrophic vessels, accompanied by numerous small arterioles. The central fibrous region has radiating branches composed of portal tract–like structures that contain an artery unaccompanied by portal veins or ducts, often with a lymphocytic or mixed inflammatory infiltrate. At the interface of fibrous regions/nodules, a ductular reaction may be highlighted by CK7 and CK19 immunostaining, and there are often features of cholestasis, including feathery degeneration of

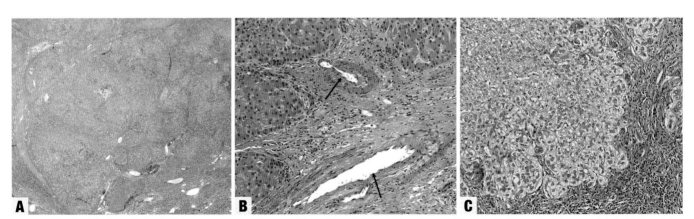

Fig. 8.02 Focal nodular hyperplasia. **A** Fibrous septa separate hepatocellular nodules of different sizes that resemble cirrhosis (Masson's trichrome staining). **B** The arteries in the central scar are variably thick-walled (arrows). **C** Focal nodular hyperplasia displaying cholestasis in periseptal hepatocytes (ballooned and clear), ductular reaction at the stromal–parenchymal interface, and septal inflammation.

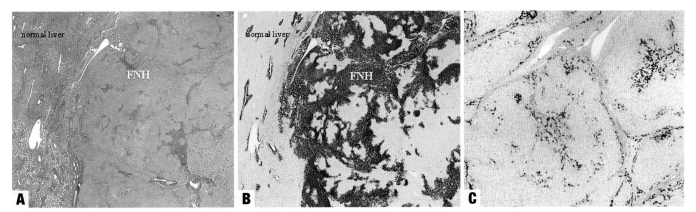

Fig. 8.03 Focal nodular hyperplasia (FNH). **A,B** Serial sections. General view (**A**). Immunolabelling for glutamine synthetase (GS) reveals a typical anastomosing map-like pattern of staining within the lesion, contrasting with the normal, perivenular pattern outside (**B**). **C** CK7 immunostaining highlights the prominent ductular reaction at the septal–parenchymal interface.

hepatocytes and Mallory–Denk bodies. The sinusoidal endothelium shows patchy to diffuse CD34 staining.

Immunohistochemistry for GS is useful for diagnosis, even on biopsies, showing broad, anastomosing areas of expression in hepatocytes adjacent to hepatic veins, leading to a characteristic map-like pattern {333,330}. However, the map-like pattern is not always discernible in needle biopsies, and strong staining of broad groups of hepatocytes without the anastomosing pattern can be observed, leading to difficulties in interpretation. Surgery may be required in rare instances when the diagnosis is not definitive on biopsy.

In some cases, one or more of the typical features (e.g. nodularity and ductular reaction) may not be present {2343}. Steatosis, steatohepatitis-like features, and large-cell change can occur {2343,1484,758}.

In some instances, especially in vascular diseases or around different kinds of neoplasms, regenerative nodules resembling FNH but without all the typical features can be present {187,2946}. Terms such as "FNH-like" have been used for such nodules {1901}.

Histological features such as fat, isolated arteries and sinusoidal dilatation are more common in hepatocellular adenoma, whereas nodularity, fibrous septa, and ductular reaction are more typical of FNH. However, there is histological overlap in 20–30% of cases, especially with inflammatory hepatocellular adenoma. Therefore, lesions previously characterized as telangiectatic FNH represent inflammatory hepatocellular adenoma {2509,334}.

Map-like GS staining plays a key role in this distinction. Absence of map-like GS staining and positivity for serum amyloid A and/or C-reactive protein are typical of inflammatory hepatocellular adenoma. However, patchy serum amyloid A or periseptal C-reactive protein staining can be seen in some FNH cases {1484}.

Hepatocellular carcinoma is distinguished from FNH by cytoarchitectural atypia and disruption of the reticulin framework. The periphery of FNH may show wider cell plates and focal loss of reticulin, which can mimic hepatocellular carcinoma, especially on needle biopsies. Map-like GS staining must not be erroneously interpreted as diffuse staining seen in β-catenin-mutated adenoma or hepatocellular carcinoma, especially in small biopsies.

On biopsy, cirrhosis is a differential diagnosis of FNH when the presence of a mass-forming lesion is unknown.

Cytology
Not clinically relevant

Diagnostic molecular pathology
Not clinically relevant

Essential and desirable diagnostic criteria
Essential: an unencapsulated nodule; nodular architecture; a central fibrous scar; dystrophic vessels; no features of malignancy.

Staging (TNM)
Not clinically relevant

Prognosis and prediction
There is no risk of malignant transformation.

Hepatocellular adenoma

Bioulac-Sage P
Kakar S
Nault JC

Definition
Hepatocellular adenoma (HCA) is a benign liver neoplasm composed of cells with hepatocellular differentiation.

ICD-O coding
8170/0 Hepatocellular adenoma

ICD-11 coding
2E92.7 & XH68V1 Benign neoplasm of liver or intrahepatic bile ducts & Liver cell adenoma

Related terminology
None

Subtype(s)
HNF1A-inactivated hepatocellular adenoma; inflammatory hepatocellular adenoma; β-catenin-activated hepatocellular adenoma; β-catenin-activated inflammatory hepatocellular adenoma

Localization
None

Clinical features
About 85% of HCAs occur in women of childbearing age; HCA is rare in children, men, and people aged > 65 years. HCAs can present with abdominal pain, palpable mass, or haemorrhage; however, most are incidentally discovered on imaging. HCAs can be single or multiple. When they are ≥ 10, the condition is known as adenomatosis {3472,608}. Clinically significant haemorrhage (20–25%) is mainly observed in tumours > 5 cm. Transformation to hepatocellular carcinoma (HCC) is uncommon (4–8%) and occurs mainly in men {2133,797,2944}; the risk varies with HCA subtype and is higher in some clinical settings (glycogenosis, anabolic steroid use, vascular diseases) {2948}.

Characteristic changes on imaging can be seen in some HCA subtypes (see Table 8.02) {396,1875A,1797}. However, histological evaluation remains the cornerstone for diagnosis of HCA.

Epidemiology
The incidence is 3–4 cases per 100 000 person-years in Europe and North America {2754}, possibly lower in Asia {1919}.

Etiology
Oral contraceptive use is a major risk factor, present in 80% of young women with HCA in North American and European countries. The risk increases with the duration of oral contraceptive usage. HCA can decrease in size after oral contraceptive cessation or after menopause. Men using anabolic steroids for body building are also at risk, as are patients taking anabolic steroids or androgens for aplastic anaemia {3455}.

Other risk factors include glycogenosis types 1 and 3, galactosaemia, tyrosinaemia, familial polyposis coli, polycystic ovary syndrome, and β-thalassaemia. The recent increase in HCA has been attributed to obesity and metabolic syndrome {2511,554,336}.

Pathogenesis
HCAs are clonal tumours. They are classified into several genotypic/phenotypic groups, which have important consequences for patient management {3789,335,331,2322,2324}. See *Diagnostic molecular pathology*, below.

Macroscopic appearance
HCAs are typically soft, poorly defined tumours that lack a fibrous capsule {2945}. Secondary changes such as necrosis, haemorrhage, and fibrosis can be present. The lesions range in size from microscopic to > 20 cm. Hundreds of minute subcapsular lesions may be visible in adenomatosis. The background liver is typically non-cirrhotic. Inflammatory HCA (IHCA) has been described in cirrhosis due to alcohol abuse and/or metabolic syndrome {462,2858}.

Histopathology
HCA, supplied by isolated arteries, is composed of benign cells with hepatocellular differentiation arranged in plates 1–2 cells thick and occasional pseudoglands. The cytoplasm can be normal, clear, or steatotic, or it can contain pigment such as bile or lipofuscin {2233}. Nuclear atypia is mild and may be related to ischaemic changes, but mitoses are unusual. Each molecular subtype has morphological hallmarks (see Table 8.02). *HNF1A*-inactivated HCAs (H-HCAs) often have lobulated contours and exhibit typically diffuse macrosteatosis/microsteatosis, ballooned and clear cells, and occasional pseudoglands. Microadenomas are often present in the background liver. Some atypical cases have no or only minor steatosis, rarely a myxoid stroma. IHCAs are typically characterized by sinusoidal dilatation, congestion, foci of inflammation, thick arteries, and more or less obvious ductular reaction leading to an aspect of pseudoportal tracts. Focal steatosis is not rare. Fibrotic bands and nodular organization due to remodelling can be misleading. β-catenin-activated HCA (b-HCA) can sometimes present some cytoarchitectural atypia, pseudoglands, and pigments (lipofuscins, bile). β-catenin-activated IHCAs (b-IHCAs) exhibit associated features of IHCA and b-HCA.

Table 8.02 summarizes the immunohistochemistry of HCA.

Features typical of focal nodular hyperplasia such as nodularity, fibrous septa, and ductular reaction can be seen in IHCA. Map-like glutamine synthetase (GS) staining in focal nodular hyperplasia and positive staining with inflammatory markers (serum amyloid A and C-reactive protein) in IHCA help in the diagnosis.

The presence of thick cell plates, frequent pseudoglands, small-cell change, mitoses, and loss/fragmentation of the reticulin network are typical of HCC. Immunohistochemistry for glypican-3 (GPC3) or HSP70 favours HCC, but is not helpful in most cases {2346}. Arterialized sinusoids (CD34+) are frequently seen in HCCs, but they can also be seen in benign lesions, including focal nodular hyperplasia and HCA.

Epithelioid angiomyolipoma can resemble HCA and can show diffuse GS staining {3664}. Demonstration of myomelanocytic differentiation by immunohistochemistry confirms the diagnosis of angiomyolipoma.

Table 8.02 Genotypic/phenotypic characteristics of the main hepatocellular adenoma (HCA) subtypes: *HNF1A*-inactivated HCA (H-HCA), inflammatory HCA (IHCA), β-catenin-activated HCA (b-HCA), and β-catenin-activated IHCA (b-IHCA)

Characteristics	HCA subtype		
	H-HCA	IHCA	b-HCA and b-IHCA[a]
Relative frequency	30–35%	35–40%	b-HCA: 10%; b-IHCA: 10–15%
Molecular findings	Biallelic inactivating mutations of *HNF1A*: • Somatic mutations: 90%; mainly in women • Germline mutations: 10% (MODY3) • *CYP1B1* mutations may predispose to H-HCA	IL-6/JAK/STAT activation due to mutations: *IL6ST* coding gp130 (60%); *FRK* (10%); *STAT3* (5%); *GNAS* (5%); *JAK1* (3%); unknown (20%)	*CTNNB1* activating mutations/deletions leading to different levels of β-catenin pathway activation: • Exon 3 (other than S45): high level • Exon 3 S45: moderate to weak level • Exon 7/8: weak level
MRI characteristics	Typical (massive fat component): • Diffuse and homogeneous signal dropout on T1-weighted images • Usually moderate arterial enhancement, not persistent during the delayed phase Atypical if no steatosis	Typical: • Hyperintense on T2, diffuse or predominant at the periphery (atoll sign) • Usually strong arterial enhancement, persistent in the delayed phase	No specific features
Clinical context	Females, childbearing Males (rare) MODY3 (both sexes; familial form) Solitary, multiple, adenomatosis	Females, childbearing Males (rare) Obesity, metabolic syndrome, alcohol Steatosis in background liver Solitary, multiple, adenomatosis	Females Males (more common than with other subtypes) Male hormones; metabolic diseases Solitary, rarely multiple
Histological features	Typical: lobulated contours, diffuse macrosteatosis/microsteatosis, ballooned, clear cells, a few pseudoglands Often: microadenomas in background liver Non-typical: no (or minor) steatosis; myxoid stroma	Typical: sinusoidal dilatation, congestion, foci of lymphocytic inflammation, thick arteries, ductular reaction, pseudoportal tracts Occasional: focal steatosis, fibrotic bands, nodular architecture (remodelling) Non-typical: lack of one or several features	Exon 3 mutation: often cytoarchitectural atypia, pseudoglands, pigments (lipofuscins, bile), focally decreased reticulin[b]
Immunomarkers (useful in practice)	Liver fatty-acid binding protein: absent in tumour (cytoplasmic staining in normal liver) GS: absent or positive around veins, or scattered patchy staining	C-reactive protein / serum amyloid A positivity: usually diffuse, with sharp demarcation from adjacent liver (adjacent liver can be focally or diffusely positive in some cases – haemorrhage, general inflammation, previous embolization, etc.) GS: absent or positive around veins, mainly at the periphery of nodule, or scattered patchy staining	GS overexpression[c], depending on the mutation types: • Exon 3 (other than S45): typically diffuse homogeneous staining (and often nuclear β-catenin) • Exon 3 S45: diffuse heterogeneous staining, starry-sky pattern (little or no nuclear β-catenin) • Exon 7/8: faint, with or without some perivascular staining (no nuclear β-catenin) In S45 and exon 7/8: often GS+ border and diffuse CD34 (except the border)
Risk of complications All subtypes: haemorrhage risk if > 5 cm	Low risk of HCC	Low risk of HCC	• Exon 3 mutation: high risk of HCC • Exon 7/8 mutation: no/low risk of HCC

GS, glutamine synthetase; HCC, hepatocellular carcinoma; MODY3, maturity-onset diabetes of the young type 3.
[a]Associated features of b-HCA and b-IHCA. [b]Also referred to as borderline lesion or atypical hepatocellular neoplasm (not sufficient for the diagnosis of HCC). [c]In non-tumoural liver, GS is restricted to a few rows of perivenular hepatocytes; the pattern of GS staining often correlates well with mutation type, but exceptions can occur.

Chapter 8

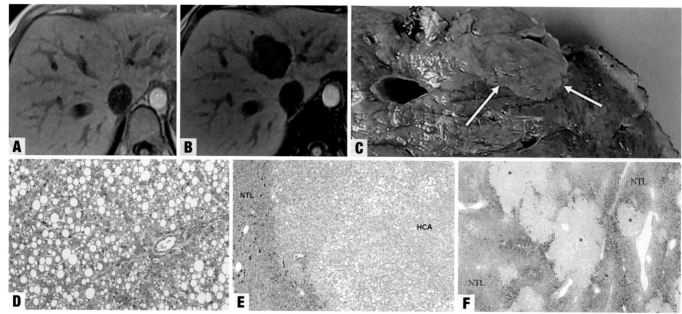

Fig. 8.04 *HNF1A*-inactivated hepatocellular adenoma (HCA). **A,B** MRI: homogeneous segment IV lesion displaying isointensity on T1-weighted image (**A**) and homogeneous signal dropout on opposed-phase T1-weighted image (**B**) due to high fat content. **C** Fresh specimen: yellowish tumour (arrows). **D** Benign, steatotic hepatocytes are intermingled with isolated thin-walled arteries. **E** Liver fatty-acid binding protein (LFABP) immunostaining: lack of LFABP in steatotic and non-steatotic tumoural hepatocytes (HCA), contrasting with normal expression of LFABP in non-tumoural liver (NTL). **F** LFABP immunostaining: numerous micronodules lacking LFABP (asterisks) are dispersed in the liver parenchyma (NTL).

Cytology

Not clinically relevant

Diagnostic molecular pathology

The molecular pathology (genotype/phenotype) of HCA is summarized in Table 8.02 (p. 225).

H-HCA accounts for 30–35% of all HCAs {350,217,1440}. *FABP1*, positively regulated by *HNF1A*, is a gene coding for liver fatty-acid binding protein, which is expressed in the cytoplasm of normal hepatocytes and is downregulated in H-HCA. Lack of liver fatty-acid binding protein expression by immunohistochemistry is a useful diagnostic marker for H-HCA.

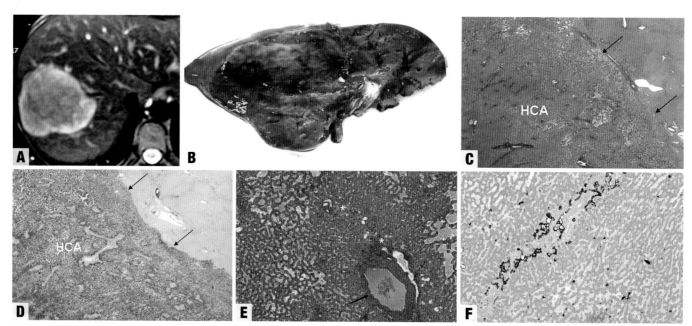

Fig. 8.05 Inflammatory hepatocellular adenoma (HCA). **A** Fat-suppressed T2-weighted MRI sequence: the tumour displays a high signal intensity, especially at the periphery (atoll sign). **B** Fresh specimen: poorly defined tumour with congestive areas. **C** The limits of the tumour (arrows) are poorly defined on H&E staining. **D** Amyloid A is strongly overexpressed by adenomatous hepatocytes, clearly demarcated from the non-tumoural liver (arrows). **E** Sinusoidal dilatation, inflammatory foci (asterisks) and thick-walled arteries (arrow) are the hallmarks of the tumour. **F** CK7 immunostaining highlights ductular reaction at the periphery of pseudoportal tracts.

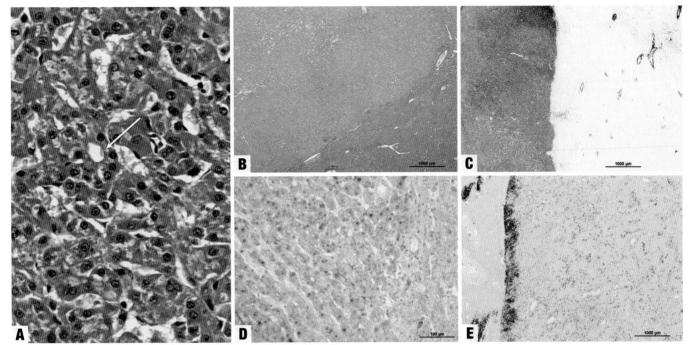

Fig. 8.06 β-catenin-activated hepatocellular adenoma (b-HCA). **A** b-HCA (exon 3) in a young boy treated with androgens for anaplastic anaemia: mild cytological atypia and rare pseudoglands (arrow). **B,C,D** β-catenin-activated inflammatory hepatocellular adenoma (b-IHCA). The tumour is well delimited from the non-tumoural liver, but unencapsulated (**B**); there is a strong and diffuse overexpression of glutamine synthetase (GS), contrasting with normal expression limited to a few centrilobular hepatocytes in non-tumoural liver (**C**); aberrant nuclear expression of β-catenin in numerous hepatocytes (**D**). This aspect (GS and β-catenin staining) is characteristic of *CTNNB1* mutation in exon 3 (non-S45). C-reactive protein staining was positive in the adenoma (not shown), leading to the diagnosis of b-IHCA exon 3. **E** b-HCA (exon 3 S45). GS expression is diffuse and heterogeneous (starry-sky pattern), with a strong GS border at the limit from the non-tumoural liver (left).

IHCA, which accounts for 35–40% of all HCAs, is characterized by recurrent somatic activating mutations in genes involved in the IL-6/JAK/STAT3 pathway {2665,2583}. IHCAs show increased expression of inflammation-associated proteins such as serum amyloid A and C-reactive protein at both the mRNA and protein levels. Serum C-reactive protein can be elevated, sometimes in association with fever and anaemia, which can regress after resection.

b-HCA accounts for 10% of all HCAs and b-IHCA for 10–15%. These subtypes show activation of the WNT signalling pathway, which results from mutation or deletion of *CTNNB1* (encoding β-catenin). Large deletions and most hotspot mutations in exon 3 lead to high levels of β-catenin activation, whereas exon 3 S45 and exon 7/8 mutations lead to moderate and weak activation of the pathway, respectively, leading to different GS patterns {2668,1143,335}. Nuclear β-catenin can be identified by immunohistochemistry, but the staining can be focal or even absent. Diffuse homogeneous GS staining is observed with mutations that lead to strong β-catenin activation, whereas more-modest activation (such as S45 mutation) tends to show a diffuse heterogeneous pattern (starry-sky pattern) {2668}. Most HCAs with mutations in exon 7/8 show weak patchy GS staining. In addition, b-HCA with exon 3 S45 and exon 7/8 mutations can show a strong peripheral border of GS staining; in these cases, CD34 is usually diffusely expressed in the tumour, except at the border. Therefore, GS is a good surrogate marker to identify different types of *CTNNB1* mutations; however, molecular analysis (on frozen or formalin-fixed, paraffin-embedded material) can be performed in cases with inconclusive GS pattern for evaluation of malignancy risk, which is high in cases with exon 3 mutations and low/absent in cases with exon 7/8 mutations.

The term "borderline lesion" has been used for b-HCA with focal cytoarchitectural atypias and/or reticulin abnormalities (but insufficient for definite diagnosis of HCC) {2583}. Other groups have proposed the term "atypical hepatocellular neoplasm" for all β-catenin-activated tumours (except those with exon 7/8 mutation), irrespective of cytoarchitectural atypia, in view of the high associated risk of HCC {888,1143}. Molecular and cytogenetic changes typical of HCC, such as *TERT* promoter mutations, are more common in b-HCA/b-IHCA with malignant transformation {888,2583}.

b-IHCAs have features of both IHCA and b-HCA, and they carry the same risk of malignant transformation as b-HCAs with exon 3 mutations.

An additional subtype, sonic hedgehog HCA (shHCA), has also been described. It accounts for 4% of HCAs and is characterized by activation of the sonic hedgehog pathway due to small somatic deletions of *INHBE* leading to the fusion of *INHBE* and *GLI1*. These cases may be identified by immunostaining for PTGDS {2324}. Overexpression of the enzyme ASS1 has also been reported in HCA (ASS1-positive HCA), including probably all shHCAs {1216}; both subtypes are reportedly associated with a high risk of haemorrhage, even for small nodules. Further studies are needed to further characterize these subtypes.

Unclassified HCAs, which account for 5–10% of all HCAs, lack well-defined pathological or genetic findings.

It is important to note that different HCA subtypes can occur in the same liver {2324}.

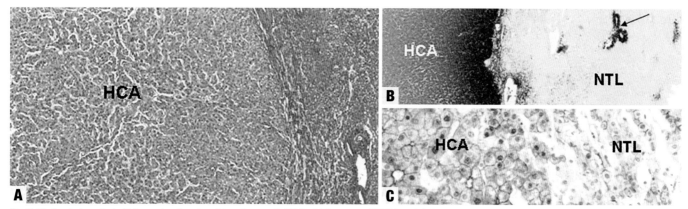

Fig. 8.07 β-catenin-activated inflammatory hepatocellular adenoma (b-IHCA). **A** The tumour (HCA) is well delimited from the non-tumoural liver, but unencapsulated. **B** There is a strong and diffuse overexpression of glutamine synthetase (GS), contrasting with normal expression limited to a few centrilobular hepatocytes (arrow) in non-tumoural liver (NTL). **C** Aberrant nuclear expression of β-catenin in numerous hepatocytes. This aspect (GS and β-catenin staining) is characteristic of *CTNNB1* mutation in exon 3 (non-S45). C-reactive protein staining was positive in the adenoma (not shown), leading to the diagnosis of b-IHCA exon 3.

Essential and desirable diagnostic criteria

Essential: a benign hepatocellular tumour; specific histological criteria according to subtype, with corresponding immunohisto-chemical surrogate markers; GS is a main marker in the clinical setting to identify b-HCA with risk of malignant transformation.

Staging (TNM)

Not clinically relevant

Prognosis and prediction

The management guidelines for HCA {884,2059} recommend biopsies mainly to assess the diagnosis of HCA, and surgical resection for tumours that are > 5 cm or irrespective of size if other high-risk features for malignant transformation are present, such as male sex, androgen-associated HCA, β-catenin activation, and borderline features for HCC {3326}. Ablative therapy can be used as an alternative to surgery. The treatment is similar for multiple tumours and is targeted towards nodule(s) with high-risk features. Because β-catenin activation can direct management, especially in small and multiple tumours, accurate assessment of GS staining is crucial for diagnosis. When GS results are equivocal, molecular/cytogenetic testing for *CTNNB1* mutation, *TERT* promoter mutations, and chromosomal gains (1, 7, and 8) can be helpful.

Hepatocellular carcinoma

Torbenson MS
Ng IOL
Park YN
Roncalli M
Sakamato M

Definition

Hepatocellular carcinoma (HCC) is a primary malignancy of the liver composed of epithelial cells showing hepatocellular differentiation.

ICD-O coding

8170/3 Hepatocellular carcinoma NOS

ICD-11 coding

2C12.02 Hepatocellular carcinoma of liver
XH4W48 Hepatocellular carcinoma NOS
XH4T58 Hepatocellular carcinoma, clear cell–type
XH9Q35 Hepatocellular carcinoma, fibrolamellar
XH5761 Hepatocellular carcinoma, scirrhous

Related terminology

None

Subtype(s)

Hepatocellular carcinoma, fibrolamellar (8171/3); hepatocellular carcinoma, scirrhous (8172/3); hepatocellular carcinoma, clear cell type (8174/3); hepatocellular carcinoma, steatohepatitic; hepatocellular carcinoma, macrotrabecular massive; hepatocellular carcinoma, chromophobe; hepatocellular carcinoma, neutrophil-rich; hepatocellular carcinoma, lymphocyte-rich

Localization

HCC can occur at any site within the liver.

Clinical features

Patients can present with clinical signs and symptoms related to the tumour or to underlying chronic liver disease. Symptoms include right upper quadrant abdominal pain, weight loss, and rapid deterioration in the setting of liver cirrhosis. Common clinical signs include hepatomegaly and splenomegaly, jaundice, and rapid increase of ascites. Symptomatic HCCs are invariably of advanced stage and have a poor prognosis. Serological biomarkers can support a clinical diagnosis of HCC or can be used to follow patients undergoing therapy, but they are less useful for screening purposes. Screening programmes are mostly based on imaging techniques and are important to detect HCC at an earlier, potentially curable stage.

Imaging is used to identify and stage HCC. The standard imaging techniques are contrast-enhanced ultrasonography, contrast-enhanced CT, and MRI. Typical vascular patterns on contrast-enhanced CT and/or MRI are enhancement on the arterial phase of imaging (wash-in) and hypointensity compared with the surrounding liver in the venous phase (washout). A particularly problematic area is accurately identifying HCC of < 2 cm diameter (small HCC) {2696}. Early HCCs (eHCCs; see below) usually appear isovascular or hypovascular, whereas

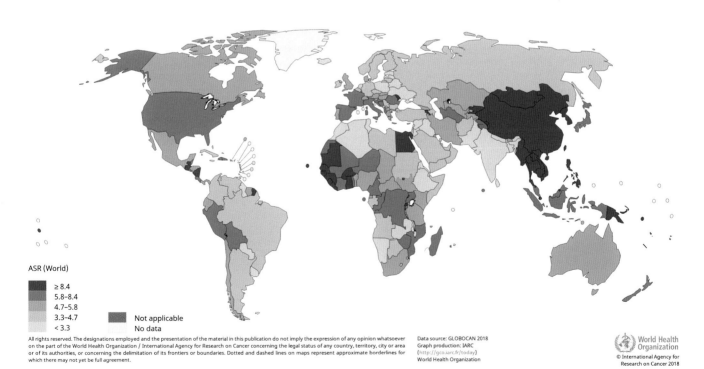

ASR (World)

- ≥ 8.4
- 5.8–8.4
- 4.7–5.8
- 3.3–4.7
- < 3.3
- Not applicable
- No data

Data source: GLOBOCAN 2018
Graph production: IARC
(http://gco.iarc.fr/today)
World Health Organization

World Health Organization
© International Agency for Research on Cancer 2018

Fig. 8.08 Estimated age-standardized incidence rates (ASRs; World), per 100 000 person-years, of liver cancer in 2018.

Table 8.03 Hepatocellular carcinoma (HCC) subtypes

Subtype	Relative frequency	Key clinical correlates	Prognosis[a]	Key histological features	Key molecular features
Steatohepatitic[b] {2835}	5–20%	Steatohepatitis may be in the background liver from metabolic syndrome or alcohol abuse	Similar	Tumour shows histological steato-hepatitis	IL-6/JAK/STAT activation; lower frequency of *CTNNB1*, *TERT*, and *TP53* mutations {461}
Clear cell {1888}	3–7%	None to date	Better	> 80% of tumour[c] shows clear cell morphology from glycogen accumulation; some steatosis is acceptable	None to date
Macrotrabecular massive {461}	5%	High serum AFP; poor prognosis	Worse	Macrotrabecular growth pattern in > 50% of tumour; vascular invasion common	*TP53* mutations and *FGF19* amplifications
Scirrhous {2086}	4%	Often mimics cholangiocarcinoma on imaging	Variable, no consensus in the literature	> 50% of tumour shows dense intratumoural fibrosis	*TSC1/2* mutations {461}; TGF-β signalling activation {2953}
Chromophobe {3600}	3%	None to date	Similar	Light, almost clear cytoplasm (chromophobe); mainly bland tumour nuclei, but focal areas of more striking nuclear atypia	Alternative lengthening of telomeres
Fibrolamellar carcinoma (synonym: fibrolamellar HCC) {1085}	1%	Young median age (25 years); no background liver disease	Similar to that of HCC in non-cirrhotic livers	Large eosinophilic tumour cells with prominent nucleoli; dense intratumoural fibrosis	Activation of PKA via a *DNAJB1-PRKACA* fusion gene
Neutrophil-rich {3327}	< 1%	Elevated white blood cell count, C-reactive protein, and IL-6	Worse	Numerous and diffuse neutrophils within tumour; can have sarcoma-toid areas	Tumour produces G-CSF
Lymphocyte-rich {3327}	< 1%	None to date	Better	On H&E staining, lymphocytes out-number tumour cells in most fields	None to date; not EBV-related

[a]As compared with the prognosis of conventional HCC. [b]In many cases, the background liver shows fatty liver disease; it is less clear whether this pattern represents a true subtype, because it is likely that the background liver and tumour are responding to the same systemic stimuli and the changes are not tumour-specific; in other cases, the steatohepatitis morphology is tumour-specific, being absent from the background liver. [c]The best percentage cut-off point has not been defined.

small progressed HCCs (pHCCs) mostly appear hypervascular on the arterial phase and hypovascular on the venous phase. Because of overlapping characteristics, imaging fails to reliably discriminate eHCCs from dysplastic nodules (DNs), particularly high-grade DNs.

Multifocal HCCs are common in cirrhotic livers. They may represent either independent HCCs arising simultaneously or intrahepatic metastases from a primary tumour {2432,2341}.

HCC can spread by lymphatic and haematogenous routes. Intrahepatic spread via the portal veins is the most common route, and the frequency increases with tumour size. HCC

Table 8.04 Molecular changes in multistep carcinogenesis {2323,2324,3170A,3385B,3331A}

	Low-grade dysplastic nodule	High-grade dysplastic nodule	Early hepatocellular carcinoma	Progressed hepatocellular carcinoma
Chromosomal alterations	0.5%	0.5%	3.4%	6.9%
TERT promoter mutation	6%	14–19%	43–61%	42–60%
TP53 mutation	–	–	–	12–48%
CTNNB1 mutation	–	–	0–21%	11–37%
Other gene mutations[a]	–	–	–	Variable[a]
DNA amplification[b]	–	–	–	22–47%
Methylation[c]	↑	↑	↑↑	↑↑↑
miR-375, let 7, miR-200f, miR-141, miR-429	↓	↑	↑	↑

[a]For example, mutations of *ARID2/1* (3–18%), *AXIN1* (5–15%), *TSC1/2* (3–8%), *NFE2L2* (3–6%), *RPS6KA3* (2–9%), *ATM* (2–6%), *KEAP1* (2–8%), *RB1* (3–8%), RAS family genes (2%). [b]For example, of *FGF19*, *CCND1*, *VEGFA*, *TERT*, *MYC*, *PTK2* (*FAK*). [c]APC, SOCS1, p16, COX-2, RASSF1A. ↑ ↓ as compared with surrounding non-tumorous liver.

invasion into the major bile ducts is found in about 5% of autopsy cases. Extrahepatic spread is common in advanced disease, including spread to the lungs, lymph nodes, bones, and adrenal glands.

Epidemiology

Primary liver cancer, of which HCC accounts for 75–85% of cases (the remainder are mostly intrahepatic cholangiocarcinoma and rare tumour types), is the sixth most common cancer and the fourth leading cause of cancer-related death worldwide, with an estimated 841 080 new cases and 781 631 deaths in 2018. Approximately three quarters of all new cases occur in low- and middle-income countries, with the highest incidence rates observed in Africa, China, and south-eastern Asia {399,920}.

Etiology

In the vast majority of patients (estimated to be > 90%), HCC can be related to a defined cause {1049}, being a chronic liver disease or exogenous exposure {2845}. The chronic liver diseases leading to HCC development are hepatitis B {3519}, hepatitis C {2643,1518}, steatohepatitis due to chronic alcohol abuse and non-alcoholic causes (e.g. metabolic syndrome) {2887,466}, and several inherited diseases affecting the liver (e.g. genetic haemochromatosis, glycogen storage diseases, and hereditary tyrosinaemia). In addition, the hepatocarcinogenic effect of numerous exogenous substances has been proven. On a global scale, exposure to fungal toxins (in particular aflatoxin B1) due to contamination of nutrients in tropical and subtropical regions is an important cause {633}. Rarely, HCC can arise from malignant transformation of hepatocellular adenoma (see *Hepatocellular adenoma*, p. 224) {2133}. The impact of the various HCC etiologies is related to their different prevalence and specific oncogenic potency. For example, the oncogenic potency is high for chronic hepatitis B and lower for alcoholic and non-alcoholic steatohepatitis.

Due to its causes, HCC is accompanied in most cases by substantial chronic liver disease and even cirrhosis (~80%) of the non-tumorous liver. Only in a minority of cases does HCC develop in a normal or near-normal liver {744}. Besides development from hepatocellular adenoma (rare) and exposure to hepatocarcinogenic substances, some correlation with metabolic syndrome / diabetes mellitus type 2 has been reported {2513,1843}.

For the various causes of HCC, hepatocarcinogenic mechanisms have been elaborated, which can be divided into etiology-specific and nonspecific mechanisms {1556,853}. The nonspecific mechanisms summarize the changes imposed by chronic liver disease, such as the sequence of hepatocellular death, regeneration, and stochastic acquisition of mutations, as well as oncogenic factors derived from the inflammatory milieu and effects due to fibrosis and vascular rearrangement. Specific oncogenic mechanisms have been shown for hepatitis B (transactivating viral factors, viral integration with constant cis- and trans-activation of oncogenic factors) {361} and aflatoxin (direct genotoxic effects leading to e.g. codon 249 mutation of *TP53*) {1311,403} and proposed for hepatitis C (oncogenic effects of core antigen and NS5A) {1783,815}.

Table 8.05 Summary of recurrent gene mutations in hepatocellular carcinoma (HCC) {2911,2873}

Driver genes	Frequency of mutations (%)			Pathways/role involved
	HBV	HCV	Non-viral	
TP53	10–65	24	16	DNA repair and surveillance; frequency varies by risk factors, with highest risk in areas of chronic aflatoxin B1 exposure
CTNNB1	15	30	39	WNT/β-catenin signalling pathway
AXIN1	12	13	6	
ARID1A	12	2	16	
ARID1B	0	4	2	Chromatin remodelling
ARID2	4	4	7	
NFE2L2	0	9	6	Oxidative stress
KEAP1	4	7	6	
RPS6KA3	4	9	6	Oncogenic MAPK signalling
KMT2A (MLL)	0	4	2	
KMT2C (MLL3)	8	0	3	Histone modification
KMT2D (MLL4)	4	4	2	
CDKN2A	0	4	2	DNA repair and surveillance
RB1	8	4	2	
TERT promoter	50	61	65	Most frequent mutation in HCC; also common in dysplastic nodules (6% in low-grade, 14–19% in high-grade)
HBV integration	65–100	n/a	n/a	
FGF19 amplification		5–10		Regulation of bile acid synthesis and hepatocyte proliferation via activation of its receptor FGFR4

n/a, not applicable

Pathogenesis

In most cases, HCC appears to follow an evolution starting from chronic liver disease providing the basis for premalignant lesions (dysplastic foci, DNs), which develop into highly differentiated, small/early HCC to progress into increasingly less differentiated HCC with intrahepatic and finally extrahepatic metastases. This development is accompanied by an increasing accumulation of clonal molecular alterations; the existence of clonal oncogenic mutations has already been shown for premalignant lesions. The type of molecular alteration shows some correlation with the underlying etiology {2958,2197}, which can be due to direct genotoxic mechanisms, as shown for aflatoxin exposure {1311,403}, or selection of complementary molecular driver mechanism. There is currently no evidence as to whether or to what extent the specific HCC subtypes outlined in Table 8.03 follow the outlined sequential tumour development.

The molecular features of high-grade DN are closer to those of HCC than those of low-grade DN, including telomere shortening, TERT activation, and inactivation of cell-cycle checkpoint

Chapter 8

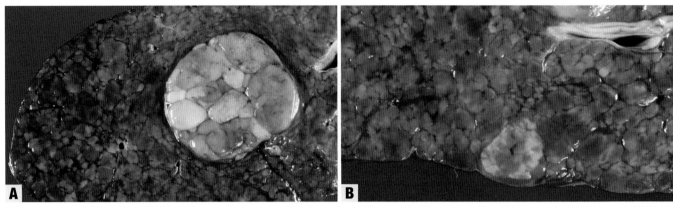

Fig. 8.09 Hepatocellular carcinoma (HCC). **A** Macroscopic photo of a soft yellow and tan HCC situated within a cirrhotic liver. **B** Macroscopic photo of an early HCC in the same patient.

regulators {1848}. There is a gradual increase in genetic changes from DN to eHCC to pHCC (see Table 8.04, p. 230) {2057}. *TERT* promoter mutations are an early event, seen in approximately 15% of high-grade DNs {2326,2323,3331A}.

Numerous large-scale genomic analyses have clarified the mutation landscape and identified key cell-signalling and metabolic pathways altered in tumorigenesis {478}. The molecular alterations in HCCs are quite variable {2911,478}, with the number of protein-altering mutations ranges from 5 to 121 per tumour {2325}. The diverse etiologies of HCC also influence their genetic profiles {1886}. Despite the many known mutations in HCC (see Table 8.05, p. 231), developing targeted therapy remains a challenge.

Macroscopic appearance

HCCs vary in colour from green to yellow to light tan, depending in part on their fat and bile content. The tumours often have a (pseudo)capsule composed of inflamed and fibrotic tissue, especially in HCC in cirrhotic livers. There are four main macroscopic patterns of HCC that are important for clinical staging purposes. First, there can be a single distinct nodule of HCC. Second, there can be a large dominant nodule of HCC with multiple smaller satellite nodules, usually present within 2 cm of the dominant nodule. Most satellite tumours in untreated HCC are located in close proximity to the dominant nodule and represent local spread of the HCC, usually through the portal venules. Third, there can be many small nodules of HCC (dozens to hundreds) that are approximately the same size and shape as cirrhotic nodules – a growth pattern called diffuse or

cirrhotomimetic. In these cases, the microscopic tumour burden is essentially always greater than that recognized by imaging or gross examination. Some of the small nodules can coalescence into a larger nodule and become more prominent by imaging and on gross examination. Fourth, there can be multiple distinct nodules of HCC that represent independent primaries. In these cases, the tumours are clearly separate from each other and do not fit a dominant tumour / satellite tumour pattern or a diffuse pattern. In some cases of independent primaries, the HCC can be seen to arise from a DN or as a nodule-in-nodule pattern with an outer nodule of well-differentiated HCC. Pedunculated HCCs protrude from the surface of the liver, but otherwise do not represent a unique macroscopic growth pattern and do not have distinct histological correlates {157}. In all cases, the size of the tumour and whether there is tumour rupture should be reported.

Histopathology

The tumour cells in HCC show hepatocytic differentiation by morphology and/or immunohistochemistry (see Table 8.06). The tumour shows loss of normal hepatic architecture, such as loss of portal tracts and reduction or loss of the normal reticulin framework. HCCs typically show increased arterialization, with aberrant arterioles in the parenchyma and sinusoidal capillarization. Cytological atypia varies from minimal to marked, and tumour cells commonly show increased proliferation.

HCCs have four principal histological growth patterns {2399}: trabecular, solid (synonym: compact), pseudoglandular (synonym; pseudoacinar), and macrotrabecular (composed mostly of trabeculae, being ≥ 10 cells thick). About 50% of resected

Table 8.06 Diagnostic tissue biomarkers for hepatocytic differentiation

Marker	Staining pattern	Approximate sensitivity (all HCC)[a]	Notes
Arginase-1 (ARG1)[b]	Cytoplasmic and nuclear	45–95%	Can occasionally be negative in well-differentiated cases; performs better than Hep Par-1 in poorly differentiated HCC
Hep Par-1[b]	Cytoplasmic	70–85%	Performs better than ARG1 in well-differentiated HCC
Polyclonal CEA	Canalicular	45–80%	Less useful given other, better stains
CD10	Canalicular	50–75%	Less useful given other, better stains
AFP	Cytoplasmic	30%	Frequently negative in well-differentiated HCC

HCC, hepatocellular carcinoma.
[a]The sensitivity of staining depends on tumour grade, the underlying liver disease, the presence or absence of cirrhosis, and the morphological subtype of HCC; for optimal specificity, all of these stains require careful correlation with morphology, with a final diagnosis requiring compatible H&E morphology. [b]Most commonly used in clinical practice.

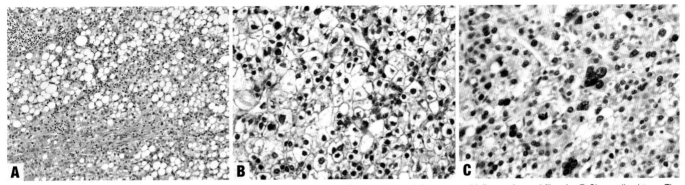

Fig. 8.10 Hepatocellular carcinoma. **A** Steatohepatitic subtype. The tumour cells contain fat and there is intratumoural inflammation and fibrosis. **B** Clear cell subtype. The abundant clear cytoplasm results from glycogen accumulation. **C** Chromophobe subtype. The tumour cells have a distinctive cytoplasm that can superficially resemble that of clear cell carcinoma. The nuclei are uniform in the background, with scattered single tumour cells and clusters of tumour cells with striking anaplasia.

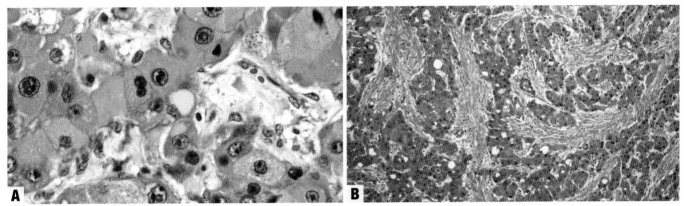

Fig. 8.11 Fibrolamellar carcinoma. **A** The tumour cells have abundant eosinophilic cytoplasm and prominent nucleoli. A pale body is also present. **B** There is abundant intratumoural lamellated fibrosis.

HCCs have mixed patterns, usually trabecular plus one or two others. The macrotrabecular pattern has been associated with a worse prognosis {1805}, but there are no other relevant clinical correlates for histological growth patterns. Histological growth patterns are important to recognize as part of the spectrum of HCC, but they do not need to be described in the pathology report. Any of the four growth patterns can be seen within the specific HCC subtypes.

Subsets of HCC show characteristic cellular changes, including bile production, lipofuscin deposits, glycogen accumulation leading to clear-cell change, and fatty change. The tumour cells can develop inclusions: hyaline bodies, Mallory–Denk bodies, or pale bodies. Pale bodies are common in fibrolamellar carcinoma but are not specific for it {3325}. Changes of the tumorous sinusoids include peliosis-like areas and small aggregates of macrophages.

Some HCCs have two or more distinct morphologies, which can include differences in architectural pattern, morphological subtype, and/or tumour grade. Most of these cases represent tumour progression, with a nodule of poorer differentiation arising within an existing HCC – a pattern called nodule-in-nodule growth.

As many as 35% of HCCs can be further subclassified into distinct subtypes (see Table 8.03, p. 230), representing distinct clinicopathological/molecular entities. All subtypes except fibrolamellar carcinoma have been described in cirrhotic and non-cirrhotic livers; fibrolamellar carcinoma occurs only in

Table 8.07 Nomenclature and features of small (≤ 2 cm) hepatocellular carcinoma (HCC)

Feature	Early HCC	Small progressed HCC
Gross margins	Indistinct	Distinct
Type of growth	Replacing	Expansive/infiltrative
Capsule	Absent	Common (> 50%)
Differentiation	Well differentiated	Well to moderately differentiated
Fatty change	Frequent (up to 40%)	Rare
Intratumoural portal tracts	Rare	Absent
Sinusoidal capillarization	Scattered/low density	Diffuse/high density
Stromal invasion	Focal/subtle	Obvious
Morphology	Non-tumoural liver mimic (low magnification), but increased cell density or cytological atypia deserves attention Little cellular and structural atypia (high magnification) requires careful distinction from HGDN	Increased cellular and structural atypia compared with early HCC Nodule-in-nodule pattern when arising within early HCC or HGDN

HGDN, high-grade dysplastic nodule.

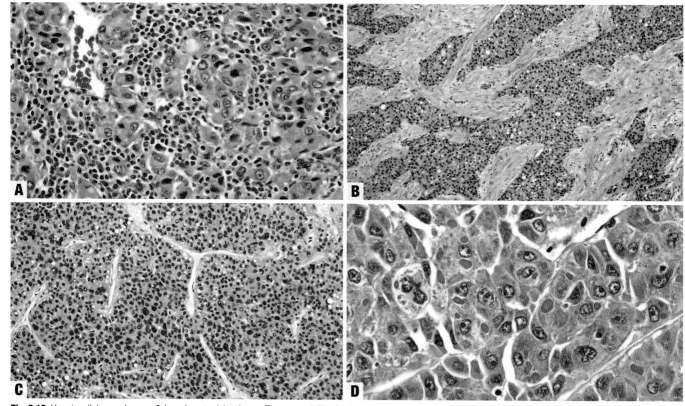

Fig. 8.12 Hepatocellular carcinoma. **A** Lymphocyte-rich subtype. The tumour-infiltrating lymphocytes outnumber the tumour cells. **B** Scirrhous subtype. There is dense intratumoural fibrosis. **C** Macrotrabecular growth pattern. The tumour trabeculae are > 10 cells in thickness. **D** Hyaline bodies; large eosinophilic cytoplasmic inclusions are present.

non-cirrhotic livers. In addition to the outlined standard morphological features, HCC includes several subtypes that represent distinct clinicopathological-molecular entities. These subtypes seem to have more-stable phenotypes. It has not been conclusively shown that they develop via the known premalignant lesions and follow a sequence of progressive changes.

eHCC and small pHCC
Small HCCs are defined as being ≤ 2 cm in diameter and are further divided into eHCC and small pHCC (see Table 8.07, p. 233). On gross examination, eHCC shows a vaguely nodular pattern with indistinct margins and no tumour capsule. On

microscopic examination, eHCCs are well differentiated and commonly show subtle stromal invasion but not vascular invasion {1379}. In contrast, small pHCCs show distinct margins on gross examination, frequently have a tumour capsule, and show expansive/infiltrative growth patterns by microscopy {1509}. Overall, small pHCCs are more likely to have histological features similar to those of larger HCCs.

There are differences in the vascular supply between eHCC and small pHCC. eHCCs may show a few portal tracts with portal veins and fewer unpaired (non-triadal) arteries, whereas pHCCs show no portal tracts and more unpaired arteries. Distinguishing between high-grade DN and eHCC is challenging,

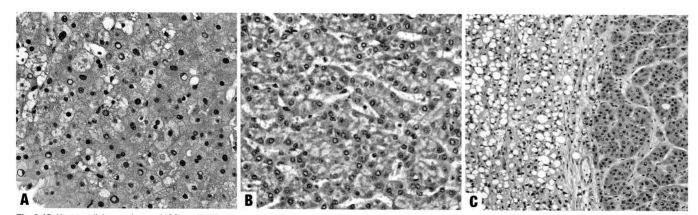

Fig. 8.13 Hepatocellular carcinoma (HCC), well-differentiated. **A** There is extensive reticulin loss, confirming HCC. **B** Minimal nuclear atypia, but abnormal lateralization of many of the hepatocyte nuclei and an increased N:C ratio. **C** Nodule-in-nodule pattern; well-differentiated steatohepatitic HCC (at left) with an inner nodule of moderately differentiated HCC (at right).

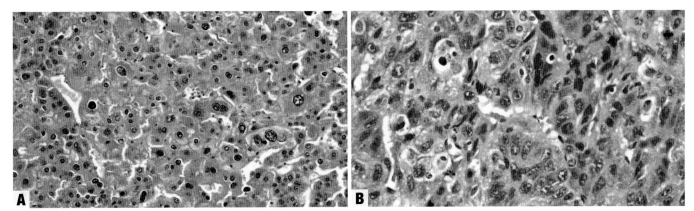

Fig. 8.14 Hepatocellular carcinoma. **A** Moderately differentiated. The tumour cells are clearly malignant but also show hepatic differentiation. **B** Poorly differentiated. The tumour shows marked nuclear atypia, prominent nucleoli, and an increased N:C ratio.

especially in biopsy material, but there are several useful discriminating features (see Table 8.09, p. 237). A nodule-in-nodule growth pattern essentially always indicates HCC. Stromal invasion is an objective and helpful feature for the diagnosis of HCC, and it can be defined by the lack of a CK7/CK19-positive ductular reaction around a nodule. In contrast, a ductular reaction is present around benign nodules {2533}. However, stromal invasion is often not detectable in biopsy specimens. Immunostaining can also be helpful, in particular the panel of HSP70, glypican-3 (GPC3), and glutamine synthetase (GS). Positivity for at least two of these markers strongly indicates HCC, with a near 100% specificity and 72% sensitivity {776}.

Histological grading

HCC tumour grade identifies the degree of differentiation based on H&E staining as compared with the morphology of a mature benign hepatocyte: well differentiated, moderately differentiated, and poorly differentiated. Undifferentiated carcinomas primary to the liver by definition have no compelling evidence for either hepatocellular or biliary differentiation, and they are not a grade of HCC (see *Combined hepatocellular-cholangiocarcinoma and undifferentiated primary liver carcinoma*, p. 260). Some HCCs can have more than one grade, in which case the worst grade (if in the minority) and the predominant grade can be reported. The worst grade tends to drive prognosis {1155}. Needle biopsy grade correlates well with the grade of the respective resection specimen {651}.

A rigorously defined, easy to use, reproducible, and broadly adopted HCC grading system remains to be developed. But even with the current heterogeneous approaches, tumour grade predicts patient survival and disease-free survival after resection with curative intent in cirrhotic livers {3777} and non-cirrhotic livers {1785}, as well as after liver transplantation {1477}. One example of a currently used grading system is the four-tiered modified Edmondson and Steiner system {2399}. Recent expert recommendations have favoured a three-tiered grading system {449}. A pragmatic grading approach (see Table 8.08) represents a synthesis of current published systems and experience.

Premalignant lesions

Premalignant lesions for HCC, found almost exclusively in cirrhotic livers, include dysplastic foci and DNs {1379}. Dysplastic foci are microscopic lesions, whereas DNs are most commonly identified (although not specified) by imaging that is performed in screening programmes for eHCC detection {885}, or in gross examination of resected or explanted specimens.

Dysplastic foci are < 1 mm in diameter and are incidental lesions discovered on histological examination of livers with advanced fibrosis. The foci are composed of groups of hepatocytes with cytological alterations and are further subclassified into large-cell change, small-cell change, and iron-free foci.

Small-cell change is defined as hepatocytes showing decreased cell volume, cytoplasmic basophilia, increased N:C ratio, mild nuclear pleomorphism, and hyperchromasia, giving the low-power impression of nuclear crowding / increased cell density. Hepatocytes with small-cell change have higher

Table 8.08 Proposed WHO grading system for hepatocellular carcinoma

Grade		Global assessment	Criteria
1	Well differentiated	Tumour cells resemble mature hepatocytes with minimal to mild atypia	Cytoplasm: ranges from abundant and eosinophilic to moderate and basophilic
		Hepatocellular adenoma or dysplastic nodule may have to be distinguished	Nuclei: minimal to mild nuclear atypia
2	Moderately differentiated	Clearly malignant on H&E staining, and morphology strongly suggests hepatocellular differentiation	Cytoplasm: ranges from abundant and eosinophilic to moderate and basophilic
			Nuclei: moderate nuclear atypia; occasional multinucleated tumour cells are acceptable
3	Poorly differentiated	Clearly malignant on H&E staining, but morphology is consistent with broad spectrum of poorly differentiated carcinomas	Cytoplasm: ranges from moderate to scant, usually basophilic
			Nuclei: marked nuclear pleomorphism, may include anaplastic giant cells

Notes: In grade 1, the diagnosis is often made only by loss of reticulin or by aberrant expression of immunostains such as glypican-3 (GPC3); cytology and morphology require distinction from hepatic adenoma in a non-cirrhotic liver and from a large regenerative nodule or dysplastic nodule in a cirrhotic liver. In grade 3, immunostaining is often necessary to confirm hepatocytic differentiation. Sarcomatoid and anaplastic morphology is classified as grade 3.

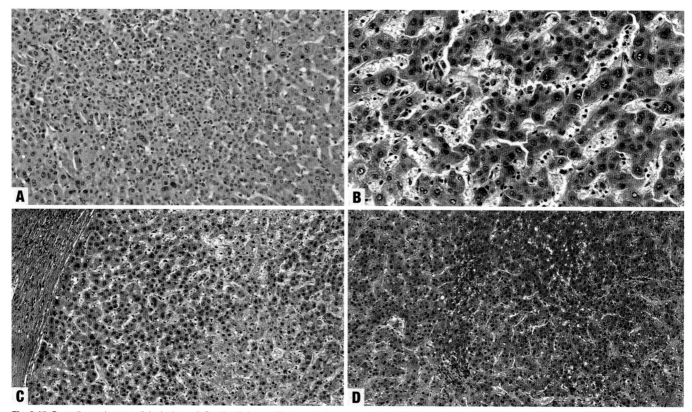

Fig. 8.15 Premalignant hepatocellular lesions. **A** Small-cell change. The hepatocytes in the centre of the image show small-cell change with increased N:C ratio; a few cells with large-cell change are also present. **B** Large-cell change. Scattered hepatocytes show nuclear hyperchromasia and multinucleation, but a normal N:C ratio is retained. **C** Low-grade dysplastic nodule. Patchy large-cell change is present. **D** High-grade dysplastic nodule. Small-cell change can be seen.

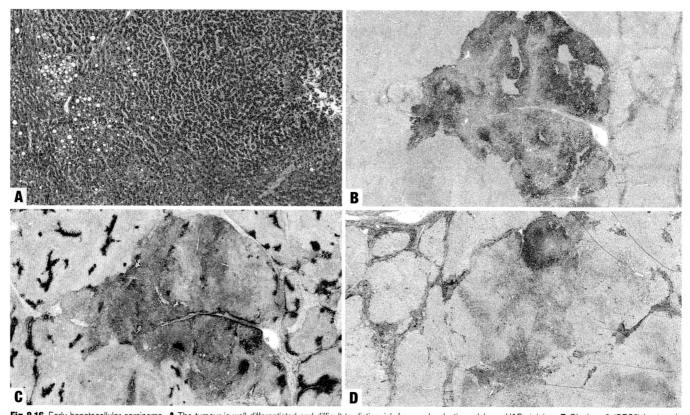

Fig. 8.16 Early hepatocellular carcinoma. **A** The tumour is well differentiated and difficult to distinguish from a dysplastic nodule on H&E staining. **B** Glypican-3 (GPC3) is strongly positive. **C** Glutamine synthetase (GS) staining is stronger and more diffuse in the early hepatocellular carcinoma than in the non-tumorous liver. **D** HSP70 is positive within the tumour.

Table 8.09 Histological features and diagnostic tools in dysplastic nodules and early hepatocellular carcinoma (HCC)

Histological features / diagnostic tools	LGDN	HGDN	Early HCC
Cytology			
Small-cell change	–	+	+
Large-cell change	±	±	–
Foci with clonal appearance	±	+	+
Growth patterns			
Increased cell density over surrounding liver parenchyma	< 1.3 times	1.3–2 times	> 2 times
Pseudoglandular/acinar changes	–	±	+
Architectural changes			
Portal tracts	Present	Present	Often absent
Reticulin framework[a]	Intact	Intact	Usually at least focal loss
Unpaired (non-triadal) arteries and sinusoidal capillarization (CD34)	±	±	+
Additional diagnostic tools			
Stromal invasion and loss of ductular reaction (CK7/CK19)[a]	–	–	±
Overexpression[a] (of ≥ 2 among HSP70[b], glypican-3 [GPC3][b], and GS[b]) {776,2919A}	–	–	+ (most)
Nodule-in-nodule growth[a]	–	–	±

–, absent; ±, may be present but not necessarily detectable in biopsy; +, present and usually detectable in biopsy; HGDN, high-grade dysplastic nodule; LGDN, low-grade dysplastic nodule.
[a]High discriminatory value; helpful immunohistochemical stain. [b]Recommended in international guidelines {885}.

proliferative activity than surrounding hepatocytes, chromosomal gains and losses, telomere shortening, and p21-checkpoint inactivation – together indicating the hepatocytes' premalignant nature {2600,2049}.

Large-cell change is defined as hepatocytes with both nuclear and cellular enlargement (therefore, a preserved N:C ratio), nuclear pleomorphism, frequent nuclear hyperchromasia, and often multinucleation. Large-cell change is a heterogeneous entity {2534}, and the evidence for its premalignant nature is less convincing, so far. It can be a risk indicator for HCC in chronic viral hepatitis B {1581}, but it can also result from cellular senescence in other settings {2318}.

Iron-free foci arise in the setting of iron storage disease and are precancerous lesions {765}.

There is no consensus on the need for reporting incidentally identified dysplastic foci in liver biopsy specimens, although reporting iron-free foci in iron storage disease and small-cell change in chronic viral hepatitis may have clinical value, indicating a higher risk for HCC development.

DNs are usually 5–15 mm in diameter and are detected either macroscopically or by imaging in cirrhotic livers, as single or multiple lesions. Their prevalence in cirrhotic livers ranges from 11% to 40% {529,372}. DNs are further classified as low-grade

or high-grade, depending on the degree of cytological and architectural atypia (see Table 8.09). The vascular remodelling of DNs leads to a progressive shift from a venous to an arterial blood supply. Portal tracts are commonly retained in DNs, but they may be reduced in number as newly formed unpaired lobular arteries gradually increase from low-grade DN to high-grade DN to HCC {2535}. Therefore, in the arterial phase of contrast-enhanced hepatic imaging, DNs are usually isovascular or hypovascular compared with the surrounding parenchyma.

The histological distinction between a low-grade DN and a large regenerative nodule (synonym: macroregenerative nodule) can be difficult. Reproducible and widely accepted histological criteria have not been developed, but the presence of unpaired arteries or cytological atypia greater than the background liver favours a DN.

Differential diagnosis

Histologically, HCC must be differentiated from other primary liver cancers (intrahepatic cholangiocarcinoma, combined hepatocellular-cholangiocarcinoma) and metastases of other malignant tumours (e.g. neuroendocrine tumours [NETs], urothelial and non-keratinizing squamous cell carcinoma, amelanotic melanoma), potentially supported by lineage-defining immunohistological criteria {3662,1500}. The differential diagnosis of highly differentiated HCC can be challenging, especially in biopsy; it must be distinguished from premalignant liver tumours (DN) and benign liver tumours (hepatocellular adenoma, focal

Multicentric tumours

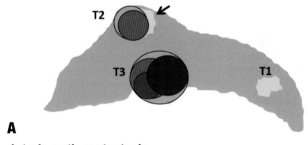

A

Intrahepatic metastasis

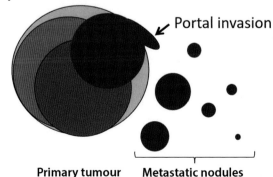

B

Fig. 8.17 Multicentric hepatocellular carcinoma (HCC). **A** Separate nodules of HCC can represent independent primaries. In cirrhotic livers, they can show a nodule-in-nodule pattern when arising within a high-grade dysplastic nodule. They are often in different Couinaud segments. **B** Separate nodules of HCC can also represent intrahepatic metastasis, usually by spread through the portal veins. This pattern typically shows a dominant nodule with smaller satellite nodules (typically < 5) closely approximated to the dominant nodule.

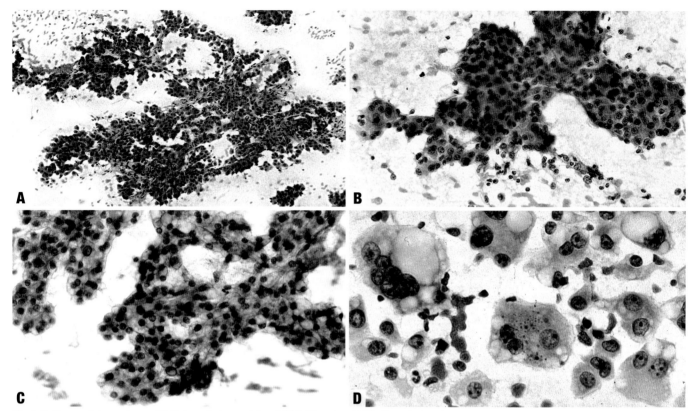

Fig. 8.18 Hepatocellular carcinoma (HCC), Papanicolaou staining. **A** Well-differentiated HCC. The cohesive clusters of malignant hepatocytes appear as slender arborizing cords. **B** Moderately differentiated HCC. The cohesive clusters of malignant hepatocytes with broad cords (> 5 cells thick) are wrapped by endothelium. Note the granular cytoplasm, increased N:C ratio, centrally located round nuclei with well-delineated nuclear membrane, granular chromatin, and distinct nucleolus. **C** HCC with trabecular arrangement and clear-cell change. **D** HCC with fatty change, bile, and giant cells. Dissociated malignant hepatocytes show pleomorphism and multinucleation.

nodular hyperplasia, regenerative nodule) with the help of histological criteria of malignancy {1674} and, if required, specific immunohistological algorithms (e.g. three-marker panel of GS, HSP70, and GPC3) {776}. In addition, some rare tumour entities primary to the liver, such as epithelioid angiomyolipoma or angiosarcoma, may pose a differential diagnostic challenge.

Cytology

On smears, findings that suggest hepatocytic differentiation include abundant eosinophilic granular cytoplasm, fatty change, and bile production. Findings that favour malignancy over a benign hepatic lesion include high cellularity, hyaline bodies, high N:C ratio, nuclear pleomorphism, multinucleated cells, naked nuclei, and mitotic figures. Architectural changes that suggest malignancy include pseudoacinar structures and thick trabeculae. The trabeculae can also demonstrate endothelial wrapping or transgressing vessels {3220,715}.

Diagnostic molecular pathology

The diagnosis of HCC is usually straightforward with the current tools of imaging and histology and does not require molecular confirmation. However, molecular analyses can aid in the diagnosis of difficult cases and in the identification of specific subtypes (see Table 8.03, p. 230), for example testing for the *DNAJB1-PRKACA* translocation to establish or confirm a diagnosis of fibrolamellar carcinoma {1086}.

There have been several proposed purely molecular HCC classifications {3790} and HCC classification systems using

combined histology and molecular findings {461}, but none of them have been incorporated into clinical care, because they do not provide additional relevant clinical information beyond that obtained by imaging and histology. Integrated morphological-molecular classifications of HCC are the most likely to be robust and clinically useful (see also Table 8.03, p. 230), but this has not yet been fully achieved.

Multikinase inhibitors have been established as first-line (sorafenib and lenvatinib) and second-line (regorafenib and cabozantinib) systemic treatment for HCC, but currently none of these use molecular testing to guide therapy. Other molecular markers, such as c-Met, NTRK gene fusions, and activated FGF19/FGFR4 axis, represent trial targets. Anti-PD1 immune checkpoint inhibitors (nivolumab and pembrolizumab) are currently approved for second-line treatment. Microsatellite instability is not relevant, being very rare in HCC.

Essential and desirable diagnostic criteria

Essential: hepatocellular differentiation as demonstrated by histology and potentially supported by respective immunohistological markers; proven malignancy using histological criteria in critical cases supported by respective immunohistological markers; absence of definite heterotypic, non-hepatocellular (e.g. cholangiocytic) differentiation (see also *Combined hepatocellular-cholangiocarcinoma and undifferentiated primary liver carcinoma*, p. 260).

Staging (TNM)

Staging of HCC follows the TNM classification {408}. Reflecting the peculiar situation of HCC in regard to the frequent coexistence of severe chronic liver disease and specific therapeutic options (e.g. transplantation), staging systems and decision algorithms partly based on clinical criteria have been developed and implemented internationally, including the Barcelona Clinic Liver Cancer (BCLC), Cancer of the Liver Italian Program (CLIP), Hong Kong Liver Cancer (HKLC), and Japan Integrated Staging (JIS) staging systems {1935,3285,3691A,1620}, to guide treatment decisions in HCC, as well as the (for example) Milan and University of California, San Francisco (UCSF) criteria for transplantation {2093,3682}.

Prognosis and prediction

DNs have a relative risk of developing HCC that ranges from 9% to 31%, mostly within 24–36 months, with the greatest risk found in high-grade DNs {372,1353}. However, a substantial proportion of DNs (20–50%) do not progress to HCC, and may even disappear during follow-up {372,2932}. Therefore, imaging-based surveillance and pathological evaluation by liver biopsy are crucial for patient management {885}.

The prognosis of patients with HCC is generally poor, particularly with advanced-stage HCC. Most studies report a 5-year survival rate of < 5% in symptomatic unresectable HCC patients. Long-term survival is likely only in patients with small, asymptomatic HCCs that can be treated by complete resection, by liver transplantation, or by adequate locoregional treatment

Box 8.02 Prognostic factors in hepatocellular carcinoma

Clinical/imaging features
- Serum AFP, des-γ carboxyprothrombin (DCP)
- Tumour size and number
- Invasion of major vessels on imaging
- Comorbidity; health condition

Morphological features
- Tumour grade
- Vascular invasion and intrahepatic metastasis
- Tumour stage
- Tumour subtype
- Presence or absence of liver cirrhosis
- Immunohistochemical expression of CK19

Molecular features
- *FGF19* amplification
- Gene expression profiling: proliferative vs non-proliferative subclasses

including percutaneous radiofrequency ablation or transarterial chemoembolization (TACE).

Clinical, morphological, and molecular factors are used to predict patient prognosis (see Box 8.02). As one example, HCCs have a worse prognosis when they demonstrate substantial CK19 immunostaining (> 5% of tumour cells), with higher recurrence rates and higher rates of lymph node metastasis {1579}. CK19-positive HCCs also have higher rates of resistance to locoregional therapy such as TACE and percutaneous radiofrequency ablation {2703,3358}.

Hepatoblastoma

Saxena R
Quaglia A

Definition
Hepatoblastoma is a malignant primary hepatic blastomatous tumour that recapitulates hepatic ontogenesis and consists of variable combinations of epithelial and mesenchymal elements.

ICD-O coding
8970/3 Hepatoblastoma NOS

ICD-11 coding
2C12.01 Hepatoblastoma

Related terminology
None

Subtype(s)
None

Localization
Hepatoblastoma occurs as a single mass in 80–85% of cases, involving the right lobe in 55–60% of cases, the left lobe in 15% of cases, and both lobes in the remaining cases. Multiple masses may occur in either or both liver lobes.

Clinical features
The majority (80–90%) of hepatoblastomas occur in patients aged between 6 months and 5 years, with a median age at onset of 18 months. The remaining cases occur in the prenatal and neonatal periods {1385}, in older children, and (rarely) in adults. There is a slight male predominance.

Hepatoblastoma may present as abdominal enlargement, discomfort, mass, or pain, accompanied by anorexia or weight loss. Jaundice is present in < 5% of patients. Serum AFP is markedly elevated in 90% of cases and is useful for monitoring chemotherapy-induced regression and recurrence of disease. Low or

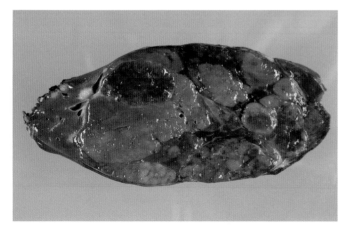

Fig. 8.19 Hepatoblastoma. A large (11 cm) example with a heterogeneous cut surface arising in a non-cirrhotic liver.

Box 8.03 International Pediatric Liver Tumors Consensus Classification of hepatoblastoma {1975}

Epithelial

Fetal
 -Fetal with low mitotic activity (well differentiated)
 -Fetal, mitotically active (crowded fetal)
 -Pleomorphic

Embryonal

Small cell undifferentiated
 -SMARCB1 (INI1)-negative
 -SMARCB1 (INI1)-positive

Cholangioblastic

Macrotrabecular

Mixed epithelial (any/all above)

Mixed epithelial and mesenchymal

Without teratoid features

With teratoid features

normal serum levels of AFP are associated with an aggressive course and the small cell undifferentiated (SCUD) subtype.

Hepatoblastomas appear as hyperechoic masses on ultrasonography and as hypoattenuated single or multiple well-delineated masses on CT. Areas of calcification and ossification may be seen.

Epidemiology
Hepatoblastoma is the most frequent malignant liver tumour in children, and it accounts for 1% of all paediatric malignances. The incidence, which is estimated to be 1–1.5 cases per million children, is uniform around the world. A rising incidence is observed in several countries, and appears to be related to the increasing cohort of low-birth-weight survivors {107}.

Etiology
Most cases of hepatoblastoma are sporadic, with no apparent underlying etiology. Hepatoblastoma is associated with familial adenomatous polyposis, Beckwith–Wiedemann syndrome, and trisomy 18 (Edwards syndrome). There is a strong association with low birth weight; the odds ratio increases with lower birth weights, and is highest for birth weights < 1000 g. Parenteral smoking, an established risk factor for low birth weight {3108}, is also a risk factor for hepatoblastoma {3102}.

Pathogenesis
Hepatoblastoma is postulated to arise from primary hepatoblasts or a highly proliferative undifferentiated multipotent hepatic progenitor cell with the capacity to differentiate along a variety of lineages. It is likely that the stage and microenvironmental milieu

Table 8.10 Molecular findings in hepatoblastoma

Gene or genetic pathway	Alteration	References
Microsatellite instability		{702}
TGFB1 (encoding TGF-β)	Upregulation	{27}
PPARA	Upregulation	{27}
Adipocytokine signalling	Upregulation	{27}
Extracellular matrix–receptor interaction	Upregulation	{27}
Apoptotic pathways	Downregulation	{27}
Upregulation of the WNT/β-catenin signalling pathway		{27}
CTNNB1	Mutation; deletions in exon 3 and exon 4	{702,1976,3259}
AXIN1	Mutations	{3259}
APC	Mutations (found in cases associated with familial adenomatous polyposis)	{1243,3667}
TP53	Mutations	{702}
Upregulation of cell-cycle pathways and loss of checkpoint control		
PLK1	Upregulation	{3638}
CDKN2A (encoding p16)	Promoter methylation	{3009}
CDKN1B (encoding p27/KIP1)	Loss of expression	{422}
DLK1, the Notch ligand	Upregulation	{1976,27}
Dysregulation of IGF signalling		{1091,3489,3321}
PLAG1	Overexpression	{3736}
11p15 gene cluster	Imprinting errors (found in cases associated with Beckwith–Wiedemann syndrome)	{668,1264}
Molecular markers with prognostic significance		
PLK1	Expression indicates poor prognosis	{3638}
RASSF1	Methylation indicates poor response to preoperative chemotherapy	{3165,1265,2825,1266}

at which the proliferating cells undergo mutations determine the differentiation pattern of the resulting tumour {291}.

Genetic abnormalities of the WNT/β-catenin signalling pathway are present in approximately 80% of hepatoblastomas; these abnormalities include long deletions in exon 3 of *CTNNB1*, as well as mutations in *CTNNB1*, the AXIN genes, and *APC*. Targets of WNT signalling, such as cyclin D1, survivin, and MYC, are overexpressed. Additionally, MYC enhances TERT expression, which further activates WNT signalling, setting up a vicious cycle {703}. A comprehensive list of molecular abnormalities in hepatoblastoma is presented in Table 8.10.

Gene expression profiling has identified two subclasses of hepatoblastoma, one of which is associated with greater genetic instability (gains of chromosomes 8q and 2p), overexpression of hepatic progenitor cell markers (AFP, CK19 [KRT19], EpCAM [TACSTD1]), and upregulated MYC signalling. These tumours correspond to a more aggressive clinicopathological phenotype with higher stage, greater propensity for invasion and metastasis, and less-differentiated histological patterns. This group corresponds to immature histological phenotypes such as embryonal and crowded fetal hepatoblastomas, whereas the group that lacks the above-mentioned genetic changes consists predominantly of the fetal (especially the pure fetal) phenotype {459}.

Macroscopic appearance

Hepatoblastomas appear as well-delineated single or multiple nodules with a nodular and bosselated appearance. An irregular, usually thin pseudocapsule formed by compressed liver may be present. The texture and colour of the cut surface depend on the tumour components and the presence or absence of necrosis and haemorrhage. Fetal hepatoblastomas display a tan-brown colour similar to that of normal liver. In the other patterns, the cut surface is often variegated, with soft or gelatinous brown to red areas. When osteoid is present, the tumour is typically gritty, and the cut surface exhibits multiple whitish and slightly transparent speckles, which may be clustered in a focal area.

Histopathology

Hepatoblastomas are classified by the International Pediatric Liver Tumors Consensus Classification as either epithelial or mixed epithelial and mesenchymal (see Box 8.03) {1975}. Epithelial hepatoblastoma may consist of fetal, embryonal, SCUD, cholangioblastic, and macrotrabecular patterns, occurring alone or in variable combinations.

The fetal pattern consists of thin trabeculae or nests of small to medium-sized cells resembling hepatocytes of the developing fetal liver. The cytoplasm is either clear or finely granular and eosinophilic, reflecting variable amounts of glycogen and

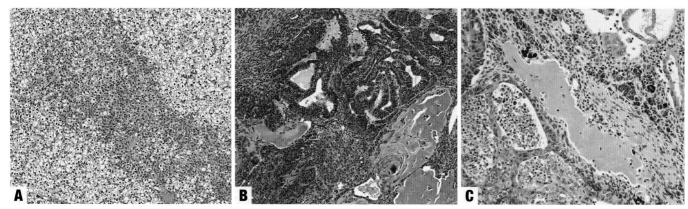

Fig. 8.20 Hepatoblastoma. **A** Epithelial hepatoblastoma, pure fetal. Showing light and dark areas; the light areas result from hepatoblasts that have a clear cytoplasm due to accumulation of glycogen and lipids, which are absent in the hepatoblasts forming the dark areas. **B** Mixed epithelial mesenchymal hepatoblastoma. Mixed hepatoblastoma with embryonal and fetal epithelial elements intermixed with mesenchymal elements that include fibrous, osteoid, and squamous components. **C** Mixed epithelial mesenchymal hepatoblastoma with teratoid features comprising embryonal and fetal epithelial elements intermixed with osteoid and melanin-containing neural components.

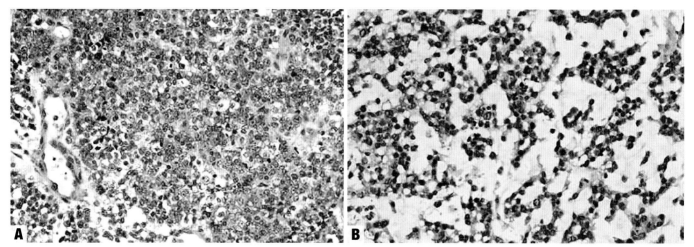

Fig. 8.21 Small cell undifferentiated hepatoblastoma. **A** Small immature cells with an increased N:C ratio form a diffuse growth pattern. **B** Clusters of small cells are embedded in a myxoid matrix (myxoid/mucoid subtype).

lipids, which impart a characteristic light and dark pattern at low magnification. The cells contain a small round nucleus with fine nuclear chromatin and an indistinct nucleolus. Foci of extramedullary haematopoiesis composed mainly of clusters of erythroid precursors are seen. The typical fetal pattern has low mitotic activity. This is referred to as well-differentiated fetal hepatoblastoma or fetal hepatoblastoma with low mitotic activity, to differentiate it from a subset of fetal hepatoblastomas that show considerable mitotic activity. The latter demonstrate larger, more pleomorphic nuclei and decreased cytoplasmic glycogen, creating a crowded, hypercellular appearance. This pattern is called crowded or mitotically active fetal hepatoblastoma. The fetal pattern may show pleomorphic nuclear features, especially after chemotherapy.

The embryonal pattern resembles the developing liver at 6–8 weeks of gestation. The cells are arranged as solid nests or glandular/acinar structures, with formation of pseudorosettes and papillary configurations. They have scant, dark granular cytoplasm devoid of visible glycogen and lipid droplets, and they contain enlarged nuclei with coarse chromatin, thus resembling blastemal cells found in other blastomatous tumours, such as nephroblastoma. Mitotic activity is more pronounced than

in the fetal areas, and extramedullary haematopoiesis is rarely present.

The SCUD pattern consists of solid sheets of dyscohesive small cells resembling the cells of neuroblastoma or other small blue cell tumours. Apoptosis, necrosis, and mitotic figures are abundant. Hepatoblastoma tissue showing the SCUD pattern can be either positive or negative for SMARCB1 (INI1). SMARCB1-negative SCUD tumours have features similar to those of rhabdoid tumours (advanced stage at diagnosis, chromosomal deletions or translocations of 22q11, and low serum AFP levels) and probably represent hepatic rhabdoid tumours {3342}. SMARCB1-positive SCUD tumours are associated with a better prognosis than SMARCB1-negative SCUD tumours.

The macrotrabecular pattern is characterized by the presence of thick trabeculae (5–12 cells thick), resembling the trabecular architecture of hepatocellular carcinoma. The trabeculae may be composed of fetal or embryonal hepatoblasts, pleomorphic cells, or cells that resemble those of hepatocellular carcinoma. The cholangioblastic pattern appears as small ducts that lie within or around hepatocellular components.

Neoplastic mesenchymal patterns (i.e. not tumour-induced stroma) in mixed hepatoblastoma most often comprise mature

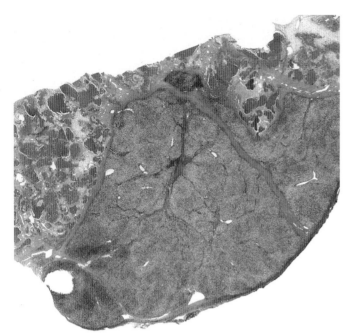

Fig. 8.22 Postchemotherapy resection showing fetal hepatoblastoma with abundant osteoid formation.

and immature fibrous tissue, osteoid or osteoid-like tissue, and hyaline cartilage. Osteoid is particularly more abundant after chemotherapy. A small percentage of mixed hepatoblastomas may display teratoid features, containing endodermal, neuro-ectodermal (melanin-producing cells, glial elements, neuronal cells), or complex mesenchymal tissues, such as striated muscle.

Immunohistochemistry

Immunohistochemistry is helpful for identifying residual neo-plastic tissue and demarcating its boundaries in surgical speci-mens after chemotherapy. Immunohistochemistry may assist in risk stratification and help to guide management {3171}. How-ever, there is no marker to differentiate hepatoblastoma from hepatocellular carcinoma.

Activation of the WNT/β-catenin signalling pathway explains the frequent nuclear and cytoplasmic expression of β-catenin in epithelial fetal (with the exception of the well-differentiated, low mitotic activity subtype) and mesenchymal components. Expression in other components is variable. Similarly, glutamine synthetase (GS), a downstream target of WNT signalling, is overexpressed, particularly in the fetal component.

AFP is expressed by the less-differentiated epithelial com-ponents, but interpretation may be challenging due to heavy background staining.

Hep Par-1, expressed by the fetal component, tends to be negative in more-immature epithelial components. Glypican-3 (GPC3) is expressed by epithelial fetal and embryonal compo-nents. The staining is usually finely granular in the low mitotic activity, well-differentiated component and coarser in other epi-thelial components. GPC3 may also be expressed by non-neo-plastic hepatocytes. Pancytokeratins are variably expressed by the epithelial components. CK7 and CK19 highlight cholan-gioblastic elements. SMARCB1 (INI1), which is usually positive

Note: PRETEXT groups the liver into four sections (previously referred to as sectors): the left lateral section (segments 2 and 3), the left medial section (segments 4a and 4b), the right anterior section (segments 5 and 8), and the right posterior section (segments 6 and 7).

Table 8.11 Prognostic factors by univariate analyses for hepatoblastoma {703}

Prognostic parameter	Good prognosis	Bad prognosis
Pretreatment extent of tumour	PRETEXT stage I, II	PRETEXT stage IV
		Multifocal disease
		Unresectable vascular involvement
		Extrahepatic tumour involvement
		Metastases at diagnosis
		Tumour rupture
Posttreatment extent of tumour		Poor response to chemotherapy
		Progressive disease on chemotherapy
		Positive surgical resection margins
		Surgically unresectable tumour
		Tumour relapse
Age	< 1 year	> 6 years
Serum AFP levels	Low (< 100 µg/L, 100–1000 µg/L)	Very high (> 1 million µg/L)
Histological subtype	Pure fetal with low mitotic activity (well-differentiated)	Small cell undifferentiated

PRETEXT, PRE-Treatment EXTent of tumor.

in all hepatoblastoma components, is helpful in identifying SMARCB1 (INI1)-negative SCUD tumours, which have a worse prognosis.

Table 8.12 Risk stratification backbones of the Children's Hepatic Tumors International Collaboration {2131}

Backbone	Criteria		
	PRETEXT group	Metastasis	AFP (μg/L)
1	I/II	No	> 100
2	III	No	> 100
3	IV	No	> 100
4	any (I, II, III, IV)	Yes	> 100
5	any (I, II, III, IV)	Yes or no	≤ 100

PRETEXT, PRE-Treatment EXTent of tumor.

Differential diagnosis

Rhabdoid tumour may resemble SCUD hepatoblastoma. Rhabdoid tumour consists of sheets of epithelioid cells with an eccentric nucleus and prominent PAS-positive intracytoplasmic inclusions. These tumours show loss of SMARCB1 (INI1) expression, corresponding to deletion or inactivation of *SMARCB1* on chromosome 22.

Well-differentiated hepatocellular carcinoma is differentiated from fetal hepatoblastoma by the presence of thickened trabeculae, higher N:C ratios, and the absence of light and dark areas

Cytology

Cytological diagnosis of hepatoblastoma relies on correlating cytological and immunohistochemical findings of immature hepatocellular cells with the presence of a hepatic mass in a young child with elevated serum AFP levels. High-grade elements and mesenchymal elements can be accurately identified on cytological smears. Necrosis, apoptosis, and mitotic figures are helpful clues to the diagnosis of embryonal and SCUD hepatoblastoma. These features are absent in fetal hepatoblastoma {3481}.

Diagnostic molecular pathology

Not clinically relevant

Essential and desirable diagnostic criteria

Essential: tumour cells recapitulating embryological stages of liver development; well-differentiated fetal hepatoblastoma: sheets of cells with light and dark areas, areas of haematopoiesis, low mitotic count; a mixture of patterns with epithelial and mesenchymal components including well-differentiated hepatoblasts, tubular structures, osteoid, cartilage, and squamous nests.

Staging

The PRETEXT (PRE-Treatment EXTent of tumor) system is the staging system adopted by the Pediatric Hepatic International Tumor Trial (PHITT) {3333}. The PRETEXT system has two components: the PRETEXT group and the annotation factors (see Box 8.04, p. 243). The PRETEXT group describes the extent of tumour within the liver, which is determined according to the number of contiguous sections that must be resected to completely excise the tumour. The annotation factors denote additional risk factors (vascular involvement, multifocality, rupture, extrahepatic extent of tumour, and metastases).

Prognosis and prediction

Univariate analyses have identified several prognostic factors that affect outcome in children with hepatoblastoma (see Table 8.11, p. 243) {703}. Five backbone groups have been identified (see Table 8.12) based on three traditional prognostic factors, namely, PRETEXT group, serum AFP level, and the presence of metastases at diagnosis. Further stratification was achieved by superimposing additional factors on these backbone groups, specifically, PRETEXT annotation factors, age at diagnosis (< 3 years, 3–7 years, and ≥ 8 years), and AFP levels (≤ 100 μg/L and 101–1000 μg/L). This has led to a refined system for risk stratification that also guides therapy {2131}.

Pure well-differentiated fetal hepatoblastoma with low mitotic activity has a favourable prognosis, and children with these tumours do not require chemotherapy if the tumour is completely resectable {2032}. In contrast, SCUD components impart an unfavourable prognosis, even when present only in small foci {1132}.

Bile duct adenoma

Tsui WM
Nakanuma Y

Definition

Bile duct adenoma (BDA) is a benign epithelial lesion composed of a proliferation of small, normal-looking bile ducts.

ICD-O coding

8160/0 Bile duct adenoma

ICD-11 coding

2E92.7 & XH6KR6 Benign neoplasm of liver or intrahepatic bile ducts & Bile duct adenoma

Related terminology

Acceptable: peribiliary gland hamartoma.

Subtype(s)

None

Localization

BDA is most commonly a solitary subcapsular nodule (90%), involving either liver lobe.

Clinical features

BDA is frequently an incidental finding at surgery or autopsy. It is mostly found in patients aged 20–70 years (range: 1.5–99 years; mean: 55 years), with no specific sex predilection.

Table 8.13 Differential diagnosis of solid-microcystic glandular lesions of the liver

Entity	Characteristics		
	Gross	**Histological**	**Immunohistochemical**
Von Meyenburg complex (bile duct microhamartoma)	Multiple discrete nodules, related to portal tracts, may contain bile; usually < 0.5 cm	Irregular or rounded ductal structures lined by flattened or cuboidal epithelium; lumina may contain proteinaceous fluid or bile concretions; dense fibrous stroma; usually portal or periportal	Expresses CK7 and CK19
Bile duct adenoma	Solitary subcapsular, whitish firm discrete nodule; usually < 2 cm	Small round tubules lined by cuboidal epithelium, may contain mucin; inflamed or hyalinized fibrous stroma; often contains pre-existing portal tracts	Expresses CK7, CK19, and often foregut antigens (MUC6, MUC5AC, TFF2, D10, 1F6)
Biliary adenofibroma	Circumscribed whitish solid-microcystic tumour; as large as 16 cm	Complex tubulocystic structures with complex branching; single-layered biliary epithelium of variable height, sometimes with mitotic activity; lumina may contain cellular debris or proteinaceous fluid; abundant fibroblastic stroma May be complicated by epithelial dysplasia	Expresses CK7, CK19, and occasionally CA19-9
Serous cystadenoma (microcystic adenoma)	Circumscribed, sponge-like tumour, with microcysts filled with clear watery fluid; any size	Multiple small cysts separated by thin fibrous septa, lined by a single layer of glycogen-rich clear cuboidal cells	Expresses CK7, CK19, and occasionally CA19-9 and B72.3
Cholangiocarcinoma	Variable appearances; any size: single firm nodule, multiple nodules, irregular periductal thickening, intraductal polypoid mass, diffuse growth, or any combination of the above	Haphazardly arranged tubules, acini, papillae, and solid nests; cuboidal or columnar cells with nuclear atypia; with or without mucin secretion; accompanying abundant sclerotic desmoplastic fibrous stroma Free extracellular mucin, perineural invasion, intrasinusoidal invasion between hepatocytic plates – features more common in primary than metastasis Predisposing conditions (e.g. hepatolithiasis) and precursor lesions (e.g. biliary intraepithelial neoplasia) may be present	CK7, CK19, and CEA: usually positive CK20: positive in 20% Ki-67 proliferation index: > 10% p53: often strong expression
Metastatic pancreatobiliary ductal adenocarcinoma	Single or multiple firm nodules of any size	Adenocarcinoma indistinguishable from cholangiocarcinoma either in morphology or by immunohistochemistry	
Metastatic colorectal adenocarcinoma	Single or multiple nodules of any size, often with central necrosis	Adenocarcinoma, often with garland pattern and central dirty necrosis	Positive for CK20, CDX2, MUC2, and CEA; negative for CK7
Metastatic adenocarcinoma from other sites	Single or multiple nodules of any size	Adenocarcinoma with variable appearance	Segregate according to CK7/CK20 pattern, then apply markers according to the suspected primary site

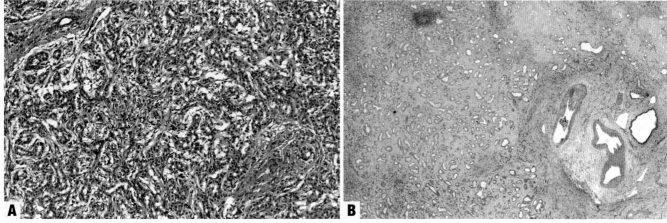

Fig. 8.23 Bile duct adenoma. **A** Postinjury pattern. Closely packed small ducts in scant fibrotic stroma enclosing some portal tracts. **B** Hamartomatous pattern. Mucin-secreting small ducts in collagenized stroma in vaguely lobular arrangement and in relation to a large bile duct.

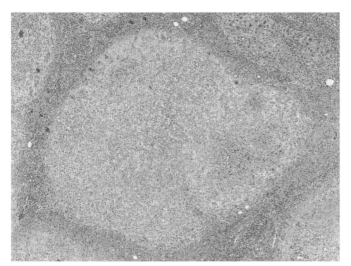

Fig. 8.24 Cirrhotic nodule transformed into a nodule of reactive ductules, representing a differential diagnosis to bile duct adenoma.

Epidemiology

The frequency of BDA was 0.6% in a large autopsy study {617} and 2.4% in a large resection cohort {66}.

Etiology

Unknown

Pathogenesis

The origin and pathogenesis of BDA are controversial. Early investigators proposed that BDA is a reactive process to a focal injury, possibly postinflammatory or traumatic {106}. A later study suggested that BDA is a peribiliary gland hamartoma {322}. More recently, *BRAF* p.V600E mutations were detected in a high proportion of cases (8 of 15 cases, 53%), some of which were multiple and associated with cholangiocarcinoma, suggesting that at least some BDAs are true neoplasms {2619,2620}.

Macroscopic appearance

BDA is usually a single, subcapsular, white, well-circumscribed but unencapsulated nodule. It is usually < 1 cm in size (range: 1–20 mm).

Histopathology

BDA is composed of a disordered collection of uniform small ducts in a connective tissue stroma without infiltrative or pushing margin. The ducts have no or little lumen and are formed by cuboidal cells that have regular nuclei, resembling ductules. The associated fibrous stroma shows varying degrees of chronic inflammation and collagenization. Portal tracts are often enclosed in the nodule. The cytokeratin immunophenotype of the ductal epithelium is similar to that of normal bile ducts, being positive for CK7 and CK19.

A portion of the lesions can express mucin and have more collagenized stroma. There is close association with large-calibre bile duct. BDA shows a secretory gland cell immunophenotype (foregut epithelial antigens D10 and 1F6 were positive) and mucous cell expression similar to those of peribiliary glands {322}. Further study has revealed that they also express other foregut antigens, such as MUC6, MUC5AC, and TFF2 {1328}.

Clear-cell and oncocytic changes have been described {89,177}, but their exact nature is uncertain and they should not be considered as part of the spectrum.

BDA's main clinical significance resides in its possible confusion with adenocarcinoma of pancreatobiliary differentiation, especially during intraoperative consultation.

Cholangiolocarcinoma and BDA both have innocent-looking small ductular structures, but these entities can be distinguished on the basis of tumour size, cytological and architectural patterns, and invasive features. Immunostaining for Ki-67, p53, EZH2, and p16 (p16INK4a) may be helpful {3355,2851}. The Ki-67 proliferation index is low in BDA (average: 2%, never > 10%), and strong p53 staining is not seen. EZH2 is expressed in carcinomas but not BDAs; p16 (p16INK4a) is expressed in BDAs but not carcinomas.

BDA should also be distinguished from other benign biliary conditions. Reactive ductular proliferation is usually not circumscribed or nodular in configuration. But in cirrhosis, ductular reaction can replace the hepatocytic nodule (parenchymal extinction in cirrhotic nodules) and form a nodular proliferation. Von Meyenburg complex and biliary adenofibroma are also mimics. Yet BDA does not show cystic changes and does not contain bile.

Cases reported to represent malignant transformation of BDA are questionable, because the cases exhibited atypical features, such as larger size {2587} and microcystic change {1179}. For more-detailed information about the differential diagnosis of solid-microcystic glandular lesions of the liver, see Table 8.13 (p. 245).

Cytology
Not clinically relevant

Diagnostic molecular pathology
Not clinically relevant

Essential and desirable diagnostic criteria
Essential: small nodular proliferation of benign small bile ducts with frequent inclusion of portal tracts; absence of infiltrative or pushing margin.
Desirable: may have fibrotic stroma with chronic inflammation; expression of CK7 and CK19.

Staging (TNM)
Not clinically relevant

Prognosis and prediction
Malignant transformation is not documented for classic BDA.

Biliary adenofibroma

Tsui WM
Nakanuma Y

Definition
Biliary adenofibroma (BAF) is a solid-microcystic epithelial neoplasm, comprising microcystic and tubuloacinar glandular structures lined by non–mucin-secreting biliary epithelium and supported by a fibroblastic stromal scaffolding.

ICD-O coding
9013/0 Adenofibroma NOS

ICD-11 coding
2E92.7 & XH91Y8 Benign neoplasm of liver or intrahepatic bile ducts & Adenofibroma NOS

Related terminology
None

Subtype(s)
None

Localization
Both lobes of the liver can be affected.

Clinical features
Abdominal pain is the presenting symptom in most patients. A few tumours are incidental findings.

Epidemiology
BAF is rare {3362,3447,1124,1496,186}. The mean age at presentation is 60 years (range: 37–83 years), with an M:F ratio of 0.5:1.

Etiology
Unknown

Pathogenesis
BAF is considered to be a primary epithelial neoplasm with a secondarily induced stroma {3447}. A close morphological resemblance to biliary microhamartoma (von Meyenburg complex) and a similar expression pattern of foregut epithelial antigens (D10-positive and 1F6-negative) have been noted, although there is no evidence of transformation of biliary microhamartoma to BAF. The immunophenotype is different from that of peribiliary glands, which makes them an unlikely source of this tumour {3447}.

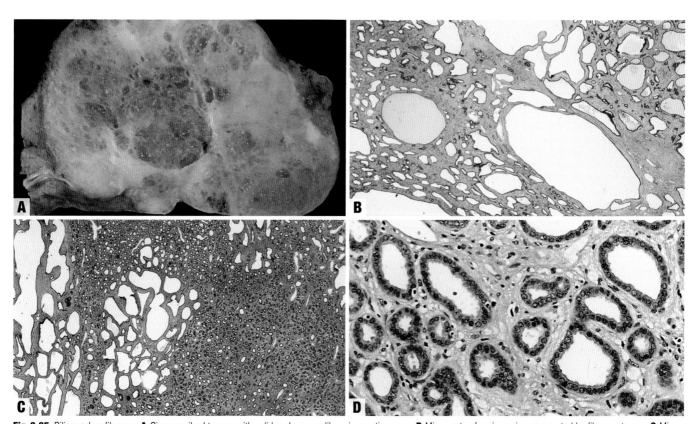

Fig. 8.25 Biliary adenofibroma. **A** Circumscribed tumour with solid and sponge-like microcystic areas. **B** Microcysts of various sizes separated by fibrous stroma. **C** Microcystic area merging with solid area of tubules and acini. **D** Lining epithelium of non–mucin-secreting cuboidal to low columnar biliary-type cells.

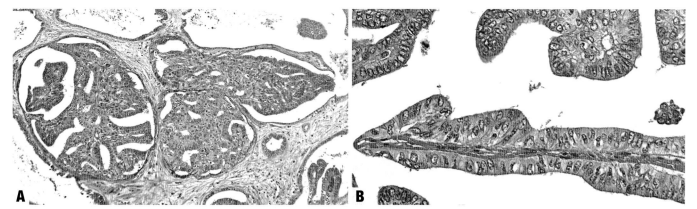

Fig. 8.26 Biliary adenofibroma with epithelial dysplasia. **A** Intracystic complex papillary proliferation and cribriform formation. **B** Lining epithelium displaying high-grade cellular dysplasia.

Multiplex PCR SNaPshot assay did not identify the presence of common cancer hotspot mutations in four BAFs {186}. By array comparative genomic hybridization, multiple clonal cytogenetic alternations were found, providing support for the neoplastic nature of BAF. The amplifications of *CCND1* and *ERBB2* suggest that BAF may have the ability to behave aggressively. A *CDKN2A* mutation was identified in one case with malignant transformation {3303}.

Macroscopic appearance
The tumour is typically solitary and 1.7–16 cm in diameter. It is unencapsulated, well circumscribed, and round to oval. On cut section, typically both solid and microcystic areas appear in varying proportions, with the latter often sponge-like in appearance. A few cases show some macrocysts > 1 cm in diameter.

Histopathology
BAF is composed of glandular structures shaped into acini, tubules, and cysts embedded in an abundant fibrotic stroma. The tubules are often dilated and branched and in places exhibit complex configurations. The cysts are of various sizes; some feature polypoid projections into their locules. The single layer of non–mucin-secreting epithelium is composed of cuboidal to low columnar cells, the portion lining the cysts being frequently flattened. The lining cells typically have amphophilic cytoplasm, bland round nuclei with inconspicuous nucleoli, and minimal contour irregularity. Apocrine snouts are notable in some cases. The background stroma is collagenous and contains bland spindle-shaped myofibroblasts. A patchy mononuclear inflammatory infiltrate can be present.

The biliary phenotype of the epithelial lining is reflected in its immunoreactivity with EMA, CK7, CK19, and CA19-9. The Ki-67 proliferation index is never > 10% in the epithelial component and is always < 1% in the stromal part.

A range of premalignant changes leading to invasive carcinoma is noted in half of the reported cases with epithelial dysplasia including elongated hyperchromatic nuclei and nuclear pseudostratification {186}, as well as architectural disturbance with intracystic complex papillary proliferation and cribriform formations {2345,3364}. The carcinoma arising is a conventional adenocarcinoma {3284,1052,3303}. A rare microcystic-cribriform carcinoma was observed in one case {1505}.

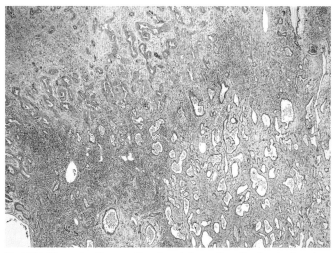

Fig. 8.27 Biliary adenofibroma with malignant change. Transition from benign microcystic areas to tubular adenocarcinoma with desmoplastic stroma.

Cytology
Not clinically relevant

Diagnostic molecular pathology
Not clinically relevant

Essential and desirable diagnostic criteria
Essential: solid-microcystic epithelial neoplasm; microcystic and tubuloacinar glandular structures lined by non–mucin-secreting biliary epithelium; supporting fibroblastic stroma.

Staging (TNM)
Not clinically relevant

Prognosis and prediction
BAF is a benign neoplasm with potential for malignant transformation, signified by the appearance of cellular and architectural atypia. Incomplete excision is followed by recurrence {186}.

Chapter 8

Mucinous cystic neoplasm of the liver and biliary system

Basturk O
Nakanuma Y
Aishima S
Esposito I

Klimstra DS
Komuta M
Zen Y

Definition

Mucinous cystic neoplasm (MCN) of the liver and biliary system is a cyst-forming epithelial neoplasm, typically showing no communication with the bile ducts, composed of cuboidal to columnar, variably mucin-producing epithelium, associated with ovarian-type subepithelial stroma. MCNs are categorized as MCN with either low/intermediate-grade dysplasia or high-grade dysplasia. Invasive carcinomas may occur in MCNs (MCN with associated invasive carcinoma).

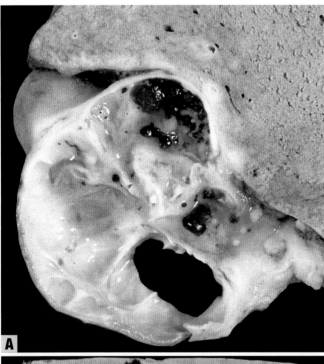

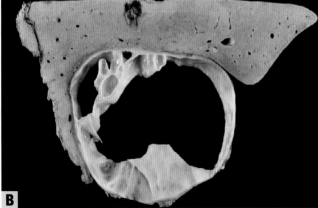

Fig. 8.28 Mucinous cystic neoplasm (MCN). **A** MCN of the gallbladder; a multilocular cystic lesion with mucinous and haemorrhagic content. **B** MCN of the liver; a gross photo showing multiloculated cystic tumour in the subcapsular region of the liver.

ICD-O coding

8470/0 Mucinous cystic neoplasm with low-grade intraepithelial neoplasia

8470/2 Mucinous cystic neoplasm with high-grade intraepithelial neoplasia

8470/3 Mucinous cystic neoplasm with associated invasive carcinoma

ICD-11 coding

2E92.6 & XH6NK7 Benign neoplasm of gallbladder, extrahepatic bile ducts or ampulla of Vater & Mucinous cystic neoplasm with low-grade intraepithelial neoplasia

2E61.Y & XH81P3 Carcinoma in situ of other specified digestive organs & Mucinous cystic tumour with high-grade dysplasia

2C15.1 Mucinous cystic neoplasm with associated invasive carcinoma of distal bile duct

2C18.1 Mucinous cystic neoplasm with associated invasive carcinoma of perihilar bile duct

2C17.1 Mucinous cystic neoplasm with associated invasive carcinoma of other or unspecified parts of biliary tract

Related terminology

Not recommended: hepatobiliary cystadenoma; cystadenocarcinoma.

Subtype(s)

None

Localization

MCNs occur principally in the liver {3748,2628,975}, particularly in the left hepatic lobe, and occasionally in the extrahepatic biliary system. Two cases were reported primary in the gallbladder {3164A,3750A}. MCNs are most often solitary.

Clinical features

MCNs nearly always cause symptoms at the time of presentation, typically abdominal pain and swelling. Serum levels of CA19-9 may be elevated, particularly if there is an associated invasive carcinoma. Cystic fluid CA19-9 and CEA levels are higher and help to distinguish MCN from non-neoplastic lesions {1821,1665}. Imaging shows a multilocular cystic mass with smaller cysts in the cyst wall. Irregular thickness of the wall, internal septation, and papillary projections are observed in malignant tumours {2812,1448}.

Epidemiology

MCNs are quite rare, with an incidence of 1 case per 20 000–100 000 person-years, and they constitute < 5% of liver cysts {3748,766,2812}. This neoplasm occurs almost exclusively in women {3748}. With the current requirement for ovarian-type stroma, it is likely that many cases previously reported in male patients as hepatobiliary cystadenoma or cystadenocarcinoma

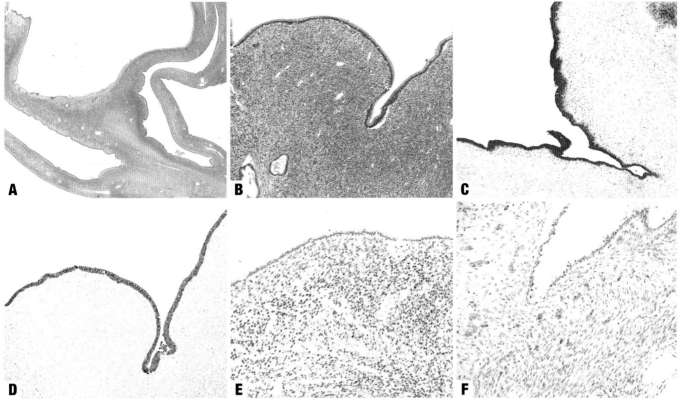

Fig. 8.29 Mucinous cystic neoplasm of the liver. **A** Multilocular cyst with compact cellular stroma and surrounding fibrous capsule. **B** The columnar lining epithelium is mucin-secreting and lies on an ovarian-like stroma. **C** Mucin is present in the supranuclear cytoplasm of the lining neoplastic cells (PAS after diastase digestion). **D** Lining epithelium is strongly positive for CK7. **E** Ovarian-like stroma is immunoreactive for ER. **F** Ovarian-like stroma is immunoreactive for α-inhibin.

{766} would now be classified as intraductal papillary neoplasm of the bile ducts. The mean age is 51 years (range: 28–76 years) {2628}. MCNs with associated invasive carcinoma tend to arise in older patients (mean age: 59 years) than do non-invasive MCNs (mean age: 45 years).

Etiology
The cause of MCN is unknown. The predominance in middle-aged to older patients suggests a hormonal influence {1821}.

Pathogenesis
Unknown

Macroscopic appearance
Grossly, MCNs are well-demarcated, multilocular cystic lesions, ranging from 5 to 29 cm in size (mean: 11 cm) {766,2628,975,85}. Most MCNs are separate from the biliary tree, but polypoid intraluminal extension into bile ducts can occur {88}. The inner surface is usually smooth or trabeculated, but rarely papillary projections can be seen. The cysts may contain mucinous, clear, or haemorrhagic fluid. An associated invasive carcinoma may appear as a solid area of greyish-white tumour.

Histopathology
Non-invasive MCNs are well delimited by a fibrous capsule. The inner surface of the cysts is lined by columnar, cuboidal, or flattened epithelial cells with pale eosinophilic to mucinous cytoplasm and basally oriented nuclei; polypoid or papillary projections may be present. Mucin can be demonstrated by

Table 8.14 Comparison of mucinous cystic neoplasm of the liver with other hepato-biliary cystic lesions

Lesion	Lining epithelium	Stroma	Papillary lesion	Communication with duct lumen
Mucinous cystic neoplasm	Mostly biliary	Ovarian-like stroma PR+, ER+	–/+++	Absent
Endometrial cyst	Endometrial	Endometrial stroma CD10+, PR+, ER+	–	Absent
Intraductal papillary neoplasm	Usually biliary, metaplastic	Fibrous	+++	Present
Bile duct cyst	Biliary	Fibrous	–	Absent
Peribiliary cyst	Biliary	Fibrous	–/+	Absent
Hepatic microcystic serous cystadenoma	Glycogen-rich cuboidal cells	Fibrous	–	Absent
Hepatic foregut cyst	Bronchial	Smooth muscle layer, fibrous	–	Absent

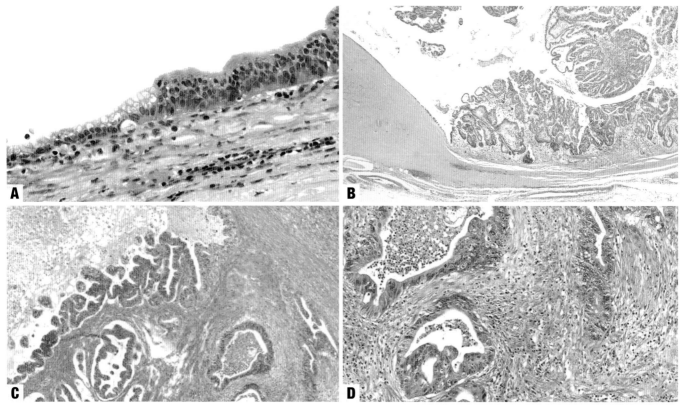

Fig. 8.30 Mucinous cystic neoplasm of the liver with high-grade intraepithelial neoplasia. **A** Transition from low-grade to high-grade dysplastic epithelium. **B** Complex papillary projections and crypt-like invaginations in the areas of high-grade neoplasia. **C** Invasion from high-grade dysplasia lining cyst wall; at higher magnification (**D**), invasive carcinoma in the cyst wall is apparent.

histochemical staining in some regions, but in 50% of cases much of the lining is composed of non-mucinous biliary-type epithelium, resembling the lining of non-neoplastic bile ducts {2628,3766}. The epithelial cells express CK7, CK8, CK18, CK19, EMA, CEA, and MUC5AC {2628}. Gastric and intestinal differentiation and squamous metaplasia may also occur. About half of the tumours contain scattered neuroendocrine cells {2628}.

Underlying the epithelium is the entity-defining ovarian-like hypercellular stroma, which in turn is surrounded by more collagenized fibrous tissue {2628,975}. The stromal cells may be focally luteinized, and hyalinization may occur in large MCNs or those in older patients. However, only half of all cases demonstrate diffuse ovarian-like stroma (present in > 75% of the cyst wall), whereas such stroma is focal in the remaining cases {2628}. Stromal inflammation and degenerative changes, such as haemorrhage, calcification, and necrosis, are common {2628}. The stromal cells are immunoreactive for ER, PR, and α-inhibin {2628,975,1314}.

The vast majority of hepatic and extrahepatic biliary MCNs have low/intermediate-grade dysplasia. Only rare cases display high-grade dysplasia, which is characterized by substantial architectural atypia as well as nuclear pleomorphism and numerous mitotic figures, or have an associated invasive

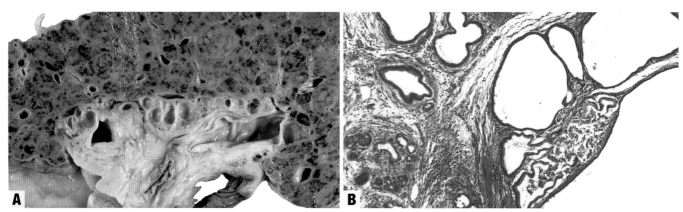

Fig. 8.31 Peribiliary cysts. **A** Large cysts in the connective tissue of the hilus; the background liver shows advanced cirrhosis. **B** Variably sized cysts are intermingled with peribiliary glands.

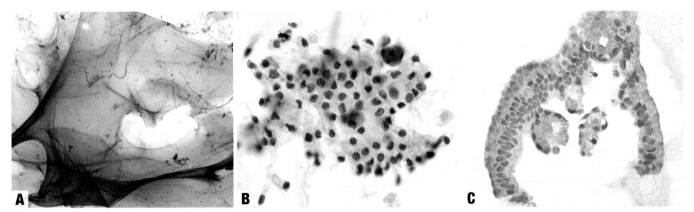

Fig. 8.32 Fine-needle aspirate of mucinous cystic neoplasm with low-grade dysplasia. **A** Mucinous background with some cellular debris and muciphages (Papanicolaou staining). **B** A sheet of columnar cells with bland nuclei in basal location (Papanicolaou staining). **C** Cell block material reveals a short strip of columnar cells with basally oriented nuclei and mucin-positive cytoplasm (mucicarmine).

carcinoma component, which typically occurs in large tumours with gross papillary projections {185,2628}. Associated invasive carcinomas, which are rare (occurring in 6% of cases), are adenocarcinomas with tubulopapillary or tubular growth patterns and a desmoplastic reaction {2628,975}. The invasive component may be focal, so these neoplasms must be extensively sampled {2628}.

Other diseases can mimic MCN clinically and pathologically (see Table 8.14, p. 251), but the presence of ovarian-like stroma is essential for the diagnosis of MCN, and its absence is mandatory for the diagnosis of other diseases {1314,3177}. Intrahepatic cystic carcinomas that communicate with bile ducts and do not contain ovarian-like stroma, previously reported as hepatobiliary cystadenocarcinomas {766}, are most likely to be intraductal papillary neoplasms with associated invasive carcinoma {2300}.

Cytology

FNA samples are characterized by aggregates of cuboidal to columnar epithelium with occasionally papillary arrangement. The background can be watery or composed of abundant thick mucin containing macrophages {3361}. The neoplastic cells show varying degrees of architectural and nuclear atypia. The ovarian-type stromal component is usually not seen {1941}, making it difficult to distinguish from intraductal papillary neoplasms with a cystic appearance on the basis of FNA.

Diagnostic molecular pathology

KRAS mutations are identified in 20% of MCNs, whereas *GNAS*, *RNF43*, and *PIK3CA* are wildtype in all cases {2628,975}. *KRAS* mutations are uncommon in cases with low-grade dysplasia (identified in 5%) but are found in most cases with high-grade dysplasia. *KRAS*-mutated MCNs more commonly have a multilocular cystic appearance and expression of EMA (MUC1), MUC2, and MUC5AC than *KRAS*-wildtype cases.

Essential and desirable diagnostic criteria

Essential: grossly visible multilocular cystic lesion, exclusively in female patients, with no communication to the bile duct system; cystic lesion with cuboidal and columnar neoplastic

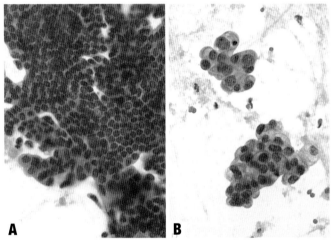

Fig. 8.33 Fine-needle aspirate of mucinous cystic neoplasm with high-grade dysplasia. **A** Sheets of moderately dysplastic epithelium with larger nuclei, nuclear crowding, and irregular nuclear membrane. **B** Clusters of highly atypical cells with enlarged, pleomorphic hyperchromatic nuclei and pale cytoplasm.

epithelia, at least partly positive for mucin staining and with variable atypia; ovarian-like, mesenchymal stroma, at least focally positive for ER and/or PR.

Staging (TNM)

Staging of MCN with associated adenocarcinoma follows the TNM classification for intrahepatic cholangiocarcinoma or carcinoma of the extrahepatic bile ducts {408}.

Prognosis and prediction

The prognosis for patients with a non-invasive biliary MCN is excellent if complete resection is possible {975,766}. The prognosis for patients with an invasive adenocarcinoma arising in association with MCN is much harder to predict. Recurrences are not uncommon after incomplete excision. It appears that invasive adenocarcinomas arising in association with biliary MCN have a better prognosis than conventional intrahepatic cholangiocarcinomas.

Intrahepatic cholangiocarcinoma

Nakanuma Y
Klimstra DS
Komuta M
Zen Y

Definition

Intrahepatic cholangiocarcinoma (iCCA) is a malignant intrahepatic epithelial neoplasm with biliary differentiation.

ICD-O coding

8160/3 Cholangiocarcinoma

ICD-11 coding

2C12.10 & XH7M15 Intrahepatic cholangiocarcinoma & Cholangiocarcinoma

Related terminology

Acceptable: intrahepatic bile duct carcinoma.
Not recommended: peripheral cholangiocarcinoma; cholangiocellular carcinoma; cholangiolocellular carcinoma.

Subtype(s)

iCCA has two main subtypes: large duct and small duct. Large duct iCCA arises in the large intrahepatic bile ducts near the hepatic hilus (proximal to the right and left hepatic ducts) and resembles perihilar and extrahepatic cholangiocarcinoma. Small duct iCCA preferentially occurs in the hepatic periphery (see Table 8.15) {71,65,1672}. Cholangiolocarcinoma and iCCA with ductal plate malformation–like pattern are subtypes of small duct iCCA. Rare subtypes described in perihilar and

Box 8.05 Subtypes of intrahepatic cholangiocarcinoma (iCCA)

Cholangiolocarcinoma (small duct type)
- Composed of ductular configuration (> 80%)
- Smaller cuboidal cells with round to oval nuclei with fine chromatin and scant cytoplasm
- Innocent-looking ductular tumour formations resembling reactive bile ductules
- Hyalinized fibrotic stroma
- Immunohistochemistry: CD56 (NCAM) and luminal expression of EMA

iCCA with ductal plate malformation pattern (small duct type)
- Tumour structures resembling ductal plate malformation, frequently with inspissated bile
- Benign-looking biliary neoplastic cells
- Fibrotic stroma
- Immunohistochemistry: CD56 (NCAM) and luminal expression of EMA

Other rare subtypes
- Adenosquamous and squamous carcinoma, mucinous carcinoma, signet-ring cell carcinoma, clear cell carcinoma, mucoepidermoid carcinoma, lymphoepithelioma-like carcinoma, sarcomatous iCCA

extrahepatic cholangiocarcinoma can also occur in large duct iCCA (see Box 8.05) {2947,2189,2298}.

Localization

iCCA arises in the liver peripheral/proximal to the left and right hepatic ducts. Large duct iCCA is preferentially located closer to the liver hilum and primarily spreads along the large portal

Table 8.15 Subclassification of intrahepatic cholangiocarcinoma (iCCA)

	Small duct type	Large duct type
Main location and gross features	Peripheral hepatic parenchyma MF pattern	Proximal to hepatic hilar regions PI pattern, PI + MF pattern
Risks	Non-biliary cirrhosis, chronic viral hepatitis	Primary sclerosing cholangitis, hepatolithiasis, liver fluke infection
Precursors	Unknown	Biliary intraepithelial neoplasia, intraductal papillary neoplasm
Histology	Small ductal components: tubular pattern with low columnar to cuboidal cells and desmoplastic reaction Ductular components: cuboidal epithelia showing ductular or cord-like pattern with slit-like lumen and desmoplastic reaction	Ductal or tubular pattern with columnar to cuboidal epithelium, with desmoplastic reaction
Mucin production	Non–mucin-secreting glands	Mucin-secreting glands
Perineural/lymphatic invasion	–/+	++
Origins of cells	Small bile ducts and bile ductules; hepatic progenitor cells?	Intrahepatic large bile ducts and peribiliary glands
Immune/molecular features		
Common markers	EMA (MUC1), CK7, CK19	EMA (MUC1), CK7, CK19
Characteristic features	CD56 (NCAM), C-reactive protein, N-cadherin, *IDH1/2* mutation	MUC5AC, MUC6, S100, TFF1, AGR2, MMP7, *KRAS* mutation
Similar to	Adenocarcinoma component of combined hepatocellular-cholangiocarcinoma	Perihilar cholangiocarcinoma
Synonyms	Peripheral small duct iCCA, peripheral iCCA	

MF, mass-forming; PI, periductal infiltrating.

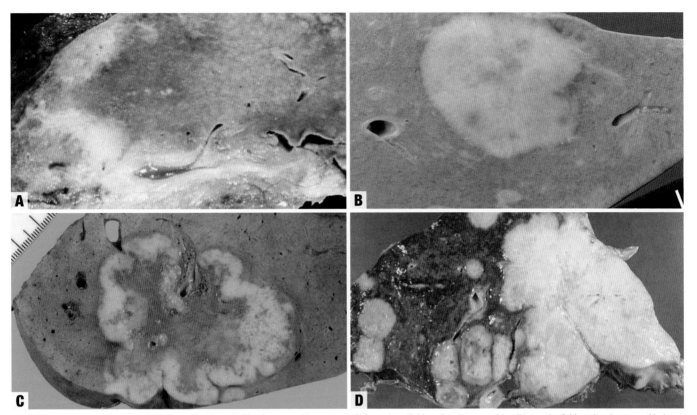

Fig. 8.34 Intrahepatic cholangiocarcinoma. **A** Periductal infiltrating type with some nodule formation. **B** Mass-forming type with solid growth. **C** Mass-forming type with dense central fibrosis. **D** Advanced stage.

tracts with a periductal infiltrating (PI) pattern. Small duct iCCA is mainly located in the peripheral parts of the liver and primarily shows a mass-forming (MF) pattern.

Clinical features

The average age at diagnosis is > 50 years, with a peak incidence between the fifth and seventh decades of life, and there is a slight male predominance. CA19-9 is typically elevated. General malaise, abdominal pain, and weight loss are frequent symptoms. Large duct iCCAs (PI pattern) with central bile duct obstruction may present with cholestasis or cholangitis. Small duct iCCA (MF pattern) often goes unnoticed until it reaches a relatively large size.

Epidemiology

iCCA is the second most common primary hepatic malignancy next to hepatocellular carcinoma and accounts for about 10–15% of primary liver cancers {3374}. The incidence of iCCA is increasing in many geographical areas {2815}. It is highest in south-eastern Asia (as many as 71.3 cases per 100 000 person-years), especially in Thailand (> 80 cases per 100 000 person-years), and lower in Europe (0.2–1.8 cases per 100 000 person-years). In the USA, the incidence increased from 0.92 cases per 100 000 person-years in 1995–2004 to 1.09 cases per 100 000 person-years in 2005–2014 {168}.

Etiology

Several risk factors for iCCA are well established and have a highly variable geographical prevalence. Small duct iCCA

exhibits the same risk factors as hepatocellular carcinoma, including viral hepatitis and non-biliary cirrhosis, whereas large duct iCCA shares the risk factors of extrahepatic and perihilar cholangiocarcinoma; it is associated with liver fluke infection, primary sclerosing cholangitis, and other more rare conditions (see Box 8.06) {1119,3186}. However, the exact etiology remains undefined in many iCCA cases.

Box 8.06 Risk factors for intrahepatic cholangiocarcinoma (iCCA)

Biliary tract inflammation and infection (large duct iCCA)
- Liver fluke infection
- Primary sclerosing cholangitis
- Hepatolithiasis

Biliary tract malformation
- Caroli disease
- Congenital hepatic fibrosis
- Bile duct cysts

Viral infection (small duct iCCA)
- Hepatitis virus (HBV and HCV) infection

Non-biliary cirrhosis (small duct iCCA)
- Alcoholic liver diseases
- Haemochromatosis
- Metabolic syndrome
- Diabetes and obesity

Chemical exposure
- Thorotrast
- Asbestos
- Occupational exposure to 1,2-dichloropropane and dichloromethane
- Smoking

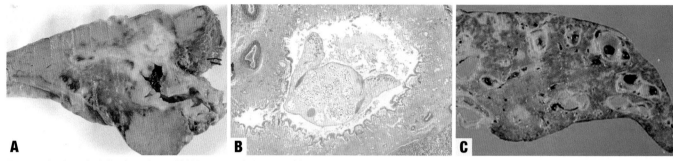

Fig. 8.35 Intrahepatic cholangiocarcinoma (iCCA). **A** Hepatolithiasis with iCCA. **B** Histology of the liver fluke *Opisthorchis viverrini* in an intrahepatic bile duct. **C** Caroli disease with congenital hepatic fibrosis associated with iCCA.

Pathogenesis

Large duct iCCA may evolve from two types of intraductal pre-malignant lesions: biliary intraepithelial neoplasia (BilIN; see also *Biliary intraepithelial neoplasia*, p. 273) and intraductal papillary neoplasm of the bile ducts (see also *Intraductal papillary neoplasm of the bile ducts*, p. 279) {65,2300,2301}. BilIN develops into PI carcinoma (PI type), which invades into the liver parenchyma, later on additionally adopting the morphological features of the MF type.

Liver progenitor cells have been discussed as cells of origin for small duct iCCA {2938,897}, but recent studies suggest that this entity may also derive from transformed and transdifferentiated hepatic progenitor cells and mature hepatocytes {1672,3028,2938}. No defined precursor lesion has been described for small duct iCCA; few cases were associated with a biliary adenofibroma {1505,321}.

Macroscopic appearance

Large duct iCCA grows along the bile duct wall as periductal nodular and sclerosing lesions proximal to the right or left hepatic ducts (PI type), developing strictures or obliterations of the affected large bile ducts and variably nodular parenchymal invasion. Small duct iCCAs primarily present as whitish or grey nodular mass lesions in the hepatic parenchyma (MF type) {65}. Both macroscopic patterns show a similar incidence among iCCAs {71,65}. At more advanced stages, iCCAs consist of variably sized, usually coalescent nodules.

Histopathology

iCCAs are almost exclusively adenocarcinomas. In most cases they show a ductal or tubular pattern with a variable-sized lumen, but a cord-like pattern with a slit-like lumen also occurs. Both patterns display a variable and frequently abundant fibrous stroma {2297,71}. A micropapillary component is occasionally admixed with the tubular pattern. The carcinoma cells are usually small or medium-sized, are cuboidal or columnar, and can be pleomorphic. The nuclei are smaller and the nucleoli are usually less prominent than in hepatocellular carcinoma. The majority of carcinoma cells have a pale, slightly eosinophilic or vacuolated cytoplasm; sometimes, the cytoplasm is clear and more abundant. Mucus secretion is common in large duct iCCA, whereas it is usually absent in small duct iCCA. iCCA frequently infiltrates into portal tracts, and it invades portal vessels (lymphatics and portal venules).

Large duct iCCA resembles the histology of perihilar and extrahepatic cholangiocarcinoma {2297,71}. It is an invasive tubular adenocarcinoma with desmoplastic reaction invading the portal connective tissue, the adjacent bile ducts, and the hepatic parenchyma. The large bile ducts from which it has arisen usually show sclerosis or obliteration by tumour tissue {2297,65}. Perineural and lymphatic invasion and lymph node metastasis are frequent.

BilIN is a microscopic precursor lesion of large duct iCCA (see also *Biliary intraepithelial neoplasia*, p. 273). It manifests as flat or micropapillary dysplastic lesions of the epithelium of

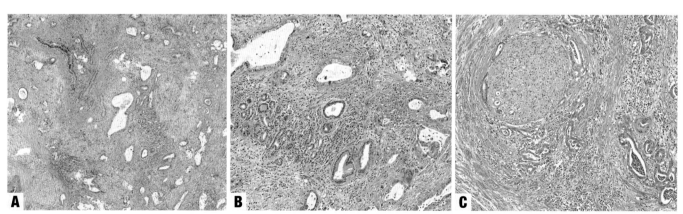

Fig. 8.36 Intrahepatic cholangiocarcinoma, large duct type. **A** Tubular adenocarcinoma with desmoplastic reaction is infiltrating into the portal tract adjacent to the branch of the left hepatic duct. **B** Invasive tubular adenocarcinoma is found in the portal tract; there are entrapped non-neoplastic peribiliary glands in cancerous tissue. **C** Invasion of the carcinoma into the portal tract and perineural invasion.

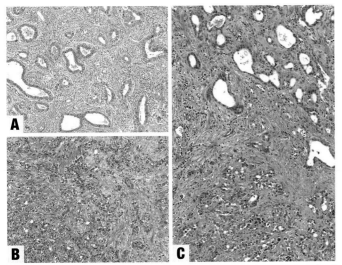

Fig. 8.37 Intrahepatic cholangiocarcinoma, small duct type. **A** Well-differentiated tubular adenocarcinoma. **B** Ductular component of cord-like structure with hyalinized fibrous stroma. **C** Mixture of small duct component (upper half) and ductular component (lower half) in the same case.

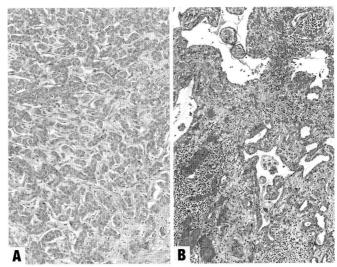

Fig. 8.38 Intrahepatic cholangiocarcinoma. **A** Cholangiolocarcinoma. **B** Intrahepatic cholangiocarcinoma with ductal plate malformation pattern.

the larger intrahepatic bile ducts {2297,2300,2301}. In contrast to reactive and hyperplastic alterations of the biliary epithelium, BilIN is characterized by a dysplastic epithelium with multilayered nuclei. It is subdivided into low-grade BilIN (low-grade dysplasia; including former BilIN-1 and BilIN-2) and high-grade BilIN (high-grade dysplasia; former BilIN-3) according to the extent of cellular and nuclear atypia (see Table 9.01, p. 273). In contrast to BilIN, intraductal papillary neoplasm of the bile ducts

is a macroscopic premalignant lesion that may also transform into large duct iCCA (see also *Intraductal papillary neoplasm of the bile ducts*, p. 279).

Small duct iCCA shows tubular formations with distinct lumina formed by cuboidal to low columnar tumour cells with scant cytoplasm or small tubular, cord-like, or spindle cell formations with a slit-like lumen {2297,65}. The components may be variably admixed {71,65}. Small duct iCCA exhibits replacement growth of the tumour cells in the hepatic lobules or regenerative

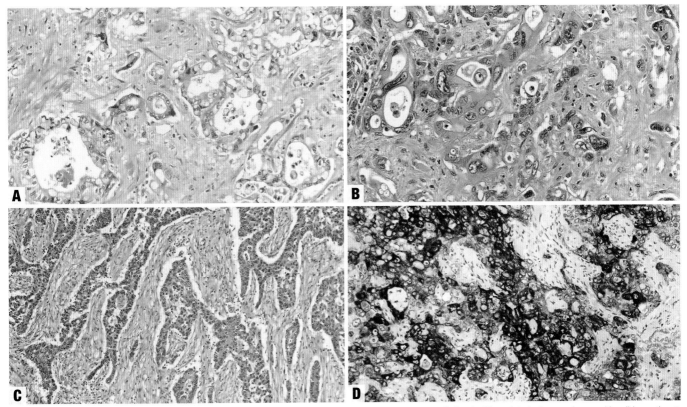

Fig. 8.39 Intrahepatic cholangiocarcinoma. **A** Poorly differentiated adenocarcinoma with pleomorphic pattern. **B** Poorly differentiated adenocarcinoma with solid growth pattern. **C** Adenocarcinoma with cord-like and solid pattern. **D** Poorly differentiated adenocarcinoma is positive for EMA.

nodules. Early-stage, small-sized iCCA may contain pre-existing portal tracts with preserved architecture and exhibit replacement growth features. Advanced small duct iCCA may show solid growth at the tumour periphery and extensively sclerotic and hypovascular central areas. The histopathological features of small duct iCCA subtypes (cholangiolocarcinoma and the subtype with ductal plate malformation pattern) are listed in Box 8.05 (p. 254).

iCCAs are graded as well-, moderately, or poorly differentiated adenocarcinoma according to their morphology.

iCCA must be distinguished from several benign biliary lesions and from metastatic adenocarcinoma, especially from pancreas, gallbladder, and extrahepatic bile ducts {1830,186,3355}.

Cytology

In bile and brush cytology of suspicious lesions including biliary strictures, epithelial cells with prominent nucleoli, thickening of the nuclear membrane, and increased chromatin are diagnostic for malignancy. The sensitivity of cytology is 9–24% and specificity 61–100%. In addition, supportive technologies, such as FISH, can be used for the evaluation of aneuploidy in cytology specimens {1615}. Percutaneous ultrasound-guided FNA is used for iCCA, especially in the MF type. In well-differentiated iCCAs, the sheets of cuboidal or columnar epithelial cells show crowding, piling up, and loss of nuclear polarity, as well as a honeycomb appearance with round to eccentric nuclei, fine chromatin, small to inconspicuous nucleoli, and ample lacy or vacuolated cytoplasm. Moderately and poorly differentiated iCCAs exhibit a greater degree of pleomorphism with dense cytoplasm and distinct cell borders.

Diagnostic molecular pathology

Recent studies of iCCAs disclosed many molecular alterations, such as mutations in KRAS, TP53, IDH1/2, ARID1A, BAP1, BRAF, and EGFR. Furthermore, mutations of genes involved in oncogenic pathways, such as PIK3CA and MET, and various gene fusions, especially involving FGFR2, have been described in iCCA {3787,549,3027}. Integrative analysis of expression and mutation pattern suggested two main molecular subtypes of iCCA: proliferation and inflammation subclasses showing clinicopathological correlations (see Box 8.07) {1081}.

Inflammation-related genetic/epigenetic alterations have been described in large duct iCCA. COX-2 is highly expressed in primary sclerosing cholangitis–associated cholangiocarcinoma {1395}. GNAS mutations were found in 9.2% of liver fluke–associated cholangiocarcinomas, but they were absent in hepatolithiasis-associated iCCA {2445}. KRAS mutation has been suggested as an early event of cholangiocarcinogenesis due to primary sclerosing cholangitis and hepatolithiasis {1899,1313}.

IDH1/2 and BRAF mutations and FGFR2 fusions occur only in small duct iCCA {71,2814}. In patients with iCCA, seropositivity for HBsAg was associated with TP53 mutations {3776}.

Essential and desirable diagnostic criteria

Essential: adenocarcinoma with biliary differentiation and variable desmoplastic reaction; absence of extrahepatic adenocarcinoma of comparable differentiation (especially adenocarcinoma of the pancreas, extrahepatic bile ducts, and gallbladder); in questionable cases compatible immunohistology (e.g. CK7, CK19, CA19-9) and absence of non-biliary lineage-defining markers.

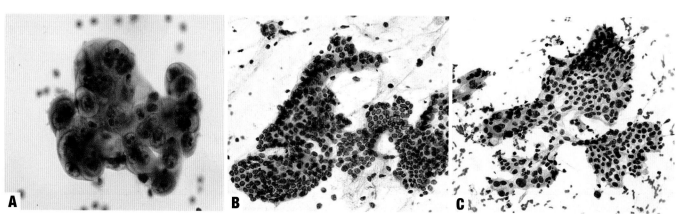

Fig. 8.40 Intrahepatic cholangiocarcinoma. **A** Exfoliative cytology; a cluster of malignant epithelial cells. **B** FNA; well-differentiated carcinoma. **C** Moderately differentiated carcinoma.

Staging (TNM)

Staging of iCCA follows the Union for International Cancer Control (UICC) TNM classification {408}.

Prognosis and prediction

iCCAs are aggressive carcinomas with high mortality and poor survival rates {65,405}. Resectability of iCCA indicates better prognosis. However, overall, few patients are candidates for surgical resection {3776,405}. Macroscopic vascular invasion, positive surgical margins, and advanced TNM stage are associated with a high recurrence rate and a poor prognosis {1456}. Small duct iCCA (MF pattern) has a higher 5-year postoperative survival rate than large duct iCCA (PI or PI+MF pattern) {1899}. At diagnosis, the large duct type typically has higher pT stages and more frequently shows perineural infiltration than the small duct type {71,65}. iCCA derived from intraductal papillary neoplasm of the bile ducts has a better postoperative prognosis than conventional iCCA {1963}. Small duct iCCA with cholangiolocarcinoma differentiation shows better overall survival and longer time to recurrence {2702}. In iCCA, expression of C-reactive protein is associated with a better prognosis, whereas expression of EMA (MUC1) indicates worse prognosis {3694,3028,1694,2081}. In cirrhotic patients, the clinical behaviour of iCCA is similar to that of hepatocellular carcinoma, whereas iCCAs in non-cirrhotic liver exhibit higher-risk pathological characteristics, a lower curative resection rate, and worse prognosis {3726}.

Combined hepatocellular-cholangiocarcinoma and undifferentiated primary liver carcinoma

Sempoux C
Kakar S
Kondo F
Schirmacher P

Definition

Combined hepatocellular-cholangiocarcinoma (cHCC-CCA) is a primary liver carcinoma (PLC) defined by the unequivocal presence of both hepatocytic and cholangiocytic differentiation within the same tumour; collision tumours are not part of this entity. Undifferentiated PLC lacks evidence of any differentiation beyond epithelial nature.

ICD-O coding

8020/3 Carcinoma, undifferentiated, NOS
8180/3 Combined hepatocellular carcinoma and cholangiocarcinoma

ICD-11 coding

2C12.00 Combined hepatocellular-cholangiocarcinoma
XH1YY4 Carcinoma, undifferentiated, NOS

Related terminology

cHCC-CCA
Acceptable: mixed hepatocellular-cholangiocarcinoma; mixed hepatobiliary carcinoma; hepatocholangiocarcinoma.

Subtype(s)

None

Localization

cHCC-CCA and undifferentiated PLC have an intrahepatic localization.

Clinical features

The age- and sex-specific incidence, variations in geographical distribution, and clinical features of cHCC-CCA (including the presence of underlying liver disease and cirrhosis) are similar to those of hepatocellular carcinoma (HCC) and intrahepatic cholangiocarcinoma (iCCA) {431}. Transarterial chemoembolization (TACE) of PLC has been associated with a higher frequency of cHCC-CCA {3743}. The imaging features overlap with those of HCC and iCCA, and they are often not specific {958,431}.

Epidemiology

cHCC-CCA is a rare tumour, accounting for 2–5% of PLCs {431}. Undifferentiated carcinoma is even more rare, with no definite incidence available.

Etiology

The etiologies established for HCC and iCCA apply to cHCC-CCA {431}. The etiologies for undifferentiated carcinoma are unclear.

Pathogenesis

The pathogenesis of cHCC-CCA is still debated. Plasticity or transdifferentiation of HCC, as demonstrated in several mouse models {1884} and supported by the occurrence of cHCC-CCA after TACE, has been proposed {3743}. Liver progenitor / stem cell origin has also been discussed {683}. The pathogenesis of undifferentiated carcinoma remains unclear.

Several molecular studies of cHCC-CCA have supported a common clonal origin of the HCC and iCCA components. The variability of the mutation spectrum in different studies probably reflects differences in collective composition. Some studies have shown a position of cHCC-CCA closer to iCCA than to HCC, while typical mutations of HCC (e.g. *CTNNB1*) and iCCA (e.g. *KRAS*, *IDH1*) have been found {530,977,1933,2856}. cHCC-CCAs enriched in cells with stem/progenitor morphology are frequently positive for SALL4, fetal-type growth factors, and stem cell signatures {2189}. Molecular data of undifferentiated carcinoma are limited.

Macroscopic appearance

cHCC-CCA and undifferentiated carcinoma show no specific macroscopic features. In cHCC-CCA, the macroscopic appearance depends on the major component, and detailed sampling of each of the heterogeneous macroscopic regions should be performed for microscopic examination.

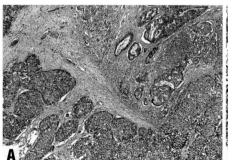 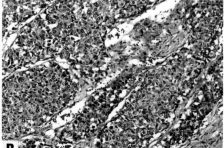 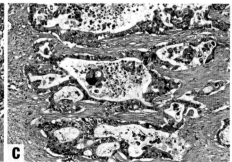

Fig. 8.41 Combined hepatocellular-cholangiocarcinoma. **A** Unequivocal cholangiocytic and hepatocytic areas of differentiation at low magnification. **B** Hepatocytic differentiation area. **C** Cholangiocytic differentiation area.

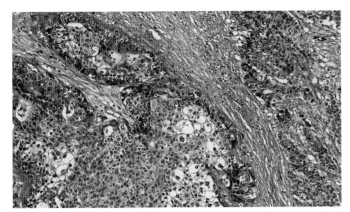

Fig. 8.42 Combined hepatocellular-cholangiocarcinoma, transitional zone. Small uniform tumour cells (so-called cancer stem cells) are located at the periphery of hepatocellular carcinoma trabeculae (at the left) or as small nests (at the right) in the transitional zone between cholangiocytic and hepatocytic differentiation components.

Fig. 8.43 Intermediate cell carcinoma. Monotonous tumour cells with scant cytoplasm showing intermediate morphological features between hepatocytes and cholangiocytes are arranged in strands in an abundant fibrous stroma.

Histopathology

In cHCC-CCA, the hepatocytic and cholangiocytic tumour areas may show all the architectural and cytological differentiation patterns described for HCC and iCCA, respectively. The two components are either close to each other or deeply intermingled, and the transition between them can be either poorly defined or sharp {431,2949}. There are no definite data at present to support the inclusion of minimum cut-off amounts of each component for the diagnosis of cHCC-CCA, and this diagnosis is made regardless of the percentage of each component, if they are unequivocal. The biphenotypic differentiation is based on the H&E morphology and can be confirmed by hepatocytic and cholangiocytic immunohistochemical markers. However, immunohistochemistry alone is not sufficient for a diagnosis of cHCC-CCA without supportive histomorphology. Distant metastases can show either cHCC-CCA features or an individual component of the original tumour {740}.

Small uniform tumour cells with scant cytoplasm and inconspicuous nucleoli (so-called cancer stem cells) can be identified in various proportions in the transitional zone between the two components, at the periphery of HCC trabeculae, or as

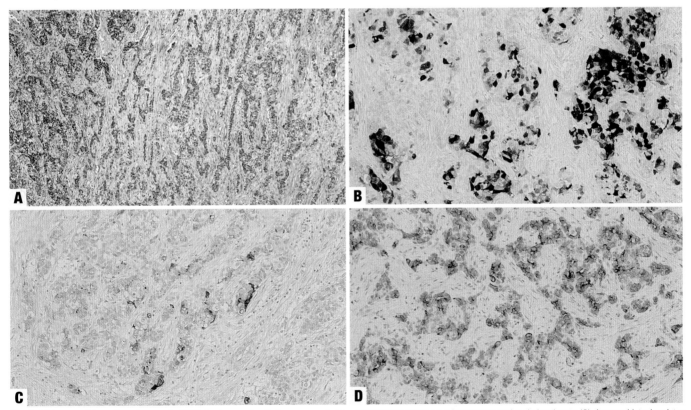

Fig. 8.44 Intermediate cell carcinoma. On H&E the tumoural cells have a morphology intermediate between a hepatocyte and a cholangiocyte (**A**). Immunohistochemistry demonstrates the biphenotypic nature of the tumour at the cellular level: the same cell expresses both hepatocytic markers, such as arginase-1 (ARG1) (**B**) and AFP (**C**), and cholangiocytic markers, such as CK19 (**D**).

small nests without specific location. Their presence and percentage can be mentioned in the pathology report but does not reflect the origin of the tumour {431}. A wide variety of immunohistochemical markers, such as CK19, EpCAM, CD56, KIT (CD117), and CD133, have been used to identify stem cell features. However, these markers are not specific for hepatic or cancer stem cells and can be present in both HCC and iCCA. In fact, CK19-positive HCC does not meet the diagnostic criteria for cHCC-CCA. Therefore, the use of the category "cHCC-CCA with stem cell features" is no longer recommended {431}. It should be emphasized that, so far, the established treatments for HCC and iCCA formally do not apply to cHCC-CCA. Therefore, the diagnosis of cHCC-CCA must be made carefully, to avoid preventing patients from benefiting from treatments specifically directed at HCC or iCCA.

Some PLCs show monotonous morphological features that are intermediate between those of hepatocytes and cholangiocytes at the cellular level, and these cases are therefore better called intermediate cell carcinoma of the liver {431,1582}. At lower magnification, the tumour is homogeneous. At higher magnification, the tumour cells are small with scant cytoplasm, and they are arranged in cords, strands, trabeculae, and occasional gland-like structures in an abundant fibrous stroma. The dual expression of hepatocytic and cholangiocytic markers in the tumour cells supports the intermediate hepatobiliary cell nature. This diagnosis should be reserved for PLCs in which intermediate features are present in the entire tumour {2855}. Focal presence of intermediate (hepatobiliary) tumour cells in a cHCC-CCA does not qualify for the diagnosis of intermediate cell carcinoma. There is no strong consensus as to whether intermediate cell carcinoma is a distinct entity or a histological pattern of cHCC-CCA, because of the limited data on molecular characteristics and clinical outcomes.

Cholangiolocarcinoma can be a component of cHCC-CCA if an HCC component is present. However, if cholangiolocarcinoma is present alone or admixed with conventional iCCA, it is now considered to be a subtype of iCCA. In addition, molecular profiling studies support the clustering of cholangiolocarcinoma as part of iCCA {2189}. The presence of a neuroendocrine component in HCC or iCCA is very rare, and such tumours belong to the group of mixed neuroendocrine–non-neuroendocrine neoplasms (MiNENs). Each component should be morphologically recognizable and confirmed by immunohistochemical markers {1758}. Carcinosarcoma is a very rare PLC showing both carcinomatous (HCC and CCA) and sarcomatous components. The sarcomatous component must lack any sign of epithelial differentiation on morphology, and is even better identified when there is morphological and/or immunohistochemical evidence of specific sarcoma differentiation {3327}.

Undifferentiated carcinoma lacks definitive morphological and immunohistochemical features of any differentiation beyond epithelial nature. There is no evidence of specific carcinoma differentiation, including HCC and CCA.

Cytology

Cytological diagnosis of these entities is at best limited. The cytology of cHCC-CCA is variable and reflects the cytomorphology of the respective components {3541}.

Diagnostic molecular pathology

Not clinically relevant

Essential and desirable diagnostic criteria

cHCC-CCA

Essential: a biphenotypic PLC showing unequivocal features of both hepatocytic and cholangiocytic differentiation based on H&E morphology; expression of immunohistochemical markers alone without histomorphological features is not sufficient for diagnosis.

Undifferentiated carcinoma

Essential: a PLC showing no specific differentiation, except for an epithelial nature based on H&E morphology and immunohistochemistry.

Staging (TNM)

According to the eighth edition (2017) of the Union for International Cancer Control (UICC) TNM classification {408}, the staging of cHCC-CCA is based on that of iCCA, and the staging of undifferentiated carcinoma is based on that of HCC.

Prognosis and prediction

cHCC-CCA has been associated with a worse prognosis than that of HCC after resection {3309,184}. Resectability is a positive prognostic factor. There are no established predictive markers concerning locoregional or systemic treatments. The prognosis of undifferentiated carcinoma is worse than that of HCC.

Hepatic neuroendocrine neoplasms

Klimstra DS

Definition
Neuroendocrine neoplasms (NENs) of the liver are hepatic epithelial neoplasms with morphological and immunohistochemical features of neuroendocrine differentiation, including well-differentiated neuroendocrine tumours (NETs) and poorly differentiated neuroendocrine carcinomas (NECs). Mixed neuroendocrine–non-neuroendocrine neoplasms (MiNENs) have a NEC component and a non-neuroendocrine component (either hepatocellular carcinoma or cholangiocarcinoma), each of which is morphologically and immunohistochemically recognizable as a discrete component and accounts for ≥ 30% of the neoplasm.

ICD-O coding
8240/3 Neuroendocrine tumour NOS
8246/3 Neuroendocrine carcinoma NOS
8154/3 Mixed neuroendocrine–non-neuroendocrine neoplasm (MiNEN)

ICD-11 coding
2C12.0Y & XH55D7 Other specified malignant neoplasm of liver & Neuroendocrine carcinoma, well-differentiated
2C12.0Y & XH9LV8 Other specified malignant neoplasm of liver & Neuroendocrine tumour, grade I
2C12.0Y & XH7F73 Other specified malignant neoplasm of liver & Neuroendocrine carcinoma, moderately differentiated
2C12.0Y & XH0U20 Other specified malignant neoplasm of liver & Neuroendocrine carcinoma NOS
2C12.0Y & XH9SY0 Other specified malignant neoplasm of liver & Small cell neuroendocrine carcinoma
2C12.0Y & XH0NL5 Other specified malignant neoplasm of liver & Large cell neuroendocrine carcinoma
2C12.0Y & XH6H10 Other specified malignant neoplasm of liver & Mixed adenoneuroendocrine carcinoma

Related terminology
Not recommended: carcinoid tumour of the liver; atypical carcinoid tumour of the liver.

Subtype(s)
Neuroendocrine tumour, grade 1 (8240/3); neuroendocrine tumour, grade 2 (8249/3); neuroendocrine tumour, grade 3 (8249/3); large cell neuroendocrine carcinoma (8013/3); small cell neuroendocrine carcinoma (8041/3)

Localization
Hepatic NENs can arise anywhere within the liver. Some NETs, NECs, and mixed cholangiocarcinoma-neuroendocrine carcinomas appear to arise from major bile ducts near the hilum, similar to extrahepatic bile duct primaries {1908}.

Clinical features
All types of hepatic NENs are very rare and are much less common than hepatic metastases of histologically similar neoplasms. NETs account for 0.4% of resected hepatic primaries, and NECs or MiNENs make up 0.5% {2382}. Therefore, the possibility that a NEN involving the liver is a metastasis must be rigorously excluded before the neoplasm can be accepted as a hepatic primary {919}. Reported cases of hepatic NENs have primarily occurred in adults (age range: 8–83 years; mean: 50 years), with a slight female predilection {1090,580}. Patients with NETs uncommonly experience carcinoid syndrome symptoms {2925,1411} and present with the effects of the mass lesion or incidentally {1090}; tumours near the hilum may cause jaundice. Cases presenting with Zollinger–Ellison syndrome and Cushing syndrome have been reported {2656,2964}.

Functional imaging of NETs may show positive labelling within the hepatic tumour, with negative results in extrahepatic sites.

Epidemiology
Few data are available, although most of the reported cases of hepatic NENs are from Asian populations.

Etiology
Occasional patients have a history of viral hepatitis, suggesting a role in etiology, although surveillance bias cannot be excluded {580,1916,1738}.

Pathogenesis
Hepatic NETs near the hilum may have originated from the major bile ducts rather than hepatocytes. Hepatic NECs may reflect aberrant differentiation of hepatocellular carcinoma or cholangiocarcinoma. Neuroendocrine differentiation is reported only rarely in conventional hepatic carcinomas and, despite early reports to the contrary, also appears to be uncommon in fibrolamellar hepatocellular carcinoma {3527}.

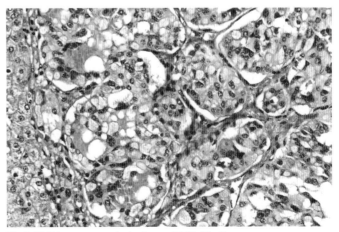

Fig. 8.45 Primary neuroendocrine tumour (NET) of the liver.

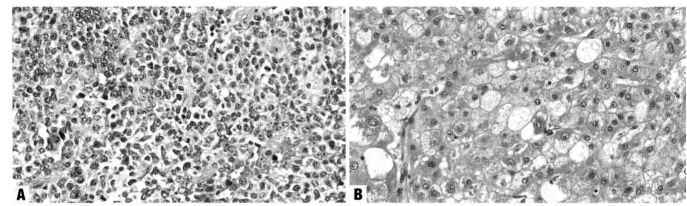

Fig. 8.46 Mixed hepatocellular-neuroendocrine neoplasm of the liver. **A** Large cell neuroendocrine carcinoma (LCNEC) component. **B** Hepatocellular carcinoma component of same case.

Macroscopic appearance

Hepatic NENs are typically solitary, circumscribed parenchymal masses, which average 6.5 cm {580}. NETs have a soft consistency and show little necrosis, whereas NECs and MiNENs may be grossly necrotic. MiNENs may have regions with gross features of hepatocellular carcinoma, or sclerotic foci reflecting the cholangiocarcinoma component.

Histopathology

NET: The histological features of hepatic NETs resemble those of well-differentiated NENs arising in the upper GI tract, pancreas, or rectum, with nests and cords of uniform polygonal cells with coarsely clumped chromatin. Focal necrosis can occur. The intense cytoplasmic granularity of midgut NETs is not typically found in hepatic primaries and would suggest a metastasis from an occult source. Hepatic NETs can be WHO grade G1 or G2 {3089}; G3 NETs have as yet not been reported in the liver. Strong and diffuse expression of synaptophysin and chromogranin A is typical {589}. The Ki-67 proliferation index is usually < 20% (mean: 7% {2382}).

NEC: Small cell carcinomas resemble their extrahepatic counterparts {3765,231,2977} and are typically encountered as a component of a mixed hepatocellular-neuroendocrine carcinoma. Necrosis and mitoses are abundant, and the Ki-67 proliferation index is very high (> 50%). Large cell NECs (LCNECs) are also typically mixed with non-NEC components. Both types express synaptophysin and, less frequently, chromogranin A.

MiNEN: Hepatic MiNENs appear to be more common than pure NECs. Most cases include a component of hepatocellular carcinoma {2438,620,2373,1738}, which may be the predominant component. The NEC and hepatocellular components can be intermingled or separate {2382}. Only a few cases of mixed cholangiocarcinoma-neuroendocrine carcinoma have been reported {3771,1517,1686}.

Cytology

The cytological features of hepatic NETs and NECs are indistinguishable from those of NENs arising elsewhere in the GI tract or pancreas. MiNENs may show evidence of the non-neuroendocrine component that, in the case of mixed hepatocellular-neuroendocrine carcinoma, may suggest a primary origin in the liver.

Diagnostic molecular pathology

Molecular studies on hepatic NENs have yet to be performed.

Essential and desirable diagnostic criteria

Essential: unequivocal evidence of neuroendocrine differentiation; NECs often mixed with other components; metastasis should be excluded.

Staging (TNM)

Hepatic NETs are staged using the Union for International Cancer Control (UICC) criteria for neoplasms of the intrahepatic bile ducts. There is no staging system specific for hepatic NECs or MiNENs.

Prognosis and prediction

Hepatic NETs are often amenable to surgical resection, and survival for many years without recurrence has been observed {1656,1784,2627}, although death from metastatic disease occurs in 18–47% of cases {919,1090,2989}, especially in G2 cases, sometimes after many years. In cases where extrahepatic disease appears within a relatively short interval after surgical resection, the hepatic lesion was a metastasis rather than a primary tumour {2914}. Both NECs and MiNENs are highly aggressive and rapidly lethal {2977,3765}. Given the markedly different proliferation rates of carcinomas and NETs, the Ki-67 proliferation index is a strong prognostic factor in all NENs {580}.

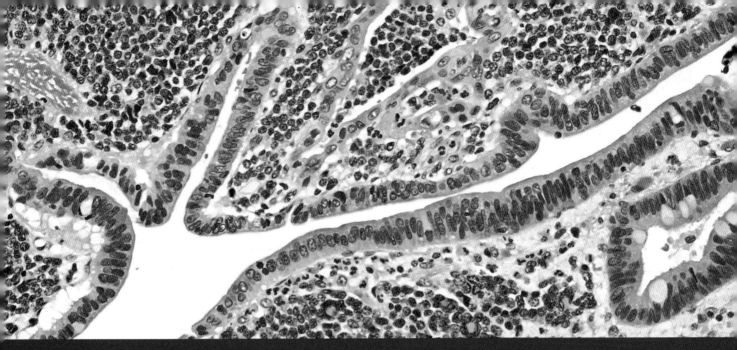

9

Tumours of the gallbladder and extrahepatic bile ducts

Edited by: Klimstra DS, Lam AK, Paradis V, Schirmacher P

Benign epithelial tumours and precursors
   Pyloric gland adenoma of the gallbladder
   Biliary intraepithelial neoplasia
   Intracholecystic papillary neoplasm
   Intraductal papillary neoplasm of the bile ducts
   Mucinous cystic neoplasm of the liver and biliary system (see Chapter 8)
Malignant epithelial tumours
   Carcinoma of the gallbladder
   Carcinoma of the extrahepatic bile ducts
   Neuroendocrine neoplasms of the gallbladder and bile ducts

WHO classification of tumours of the gallbladder and extrahepatic bile ducts

Benign epithelial tumours and precursors
8140/0   Adenoma NOS
8148/0   Biliary intraepithelial neoplasia, low grade
8148/2   Biliary intraepithelial neoplasia, high grade
8503/0   Intracystic papillary neoplasm with low-grade
         intraepithelial neoplasia
8503/2   Intracystic papillary neoplasm with high-grade
         intraepithelial neoplasia
8503/3   Intracystic papillary neoplasm with associated invasive
         carcinoma
8503/0   Intraductal papillary neoplasm with low-grade
         intraepithelial neoplasia
8503/2   Intraductal papillary neoplasm with high-grade
         intraepithelial neoplasia
8503/3   Intraductal papillary neoplasm with associated invasive
         carcinoma

Malignant epithelial tumours
8140/3   Adenocarcinoma NOS
8144/3   Adenocarcinoma, intestinal type
8310/3   Clear cell adenocarcinoma NOS
8470/3   Mucinous cystic neoplasm with associated invasive
           carcinoma
8480/3   Mucinous adenocarcinoma
8490/3   Poorly cohesive carcinoma
8503/3   Intracystic papillary neoplasm with associated
           invasive carcinoma
8070/3   Squamous cell carcinoma NOS
8020/3   Carcinoma, undifferentiated, NOS
8560/3   Adenosquamous carcinoma
8160/3   Cholangiocarcinoma
8240/3   Neuroendocrine tumour NOS
8240/3   Neuroendocrine tumour, grade 1
8249/3   Neuroendocrine tumour, grade 2
8249/3   Neuroendocrine tumour, grade 3
8246/3   Neuroendocrine carcinoma NOS
8013/3   Large cell neuroendocrine carcinoma
8041/3   Small cell neuroendocrine carcinoma
8154/3   Mixed neuroendocrine–non-neuroendocrine neoplasm
         (MiNEN)

These morphology codes are from the International Classification of Diseases for Oncology, third edition, second revision (ICD-O-3.2) {1378A}. Behaviour is coded /0 for benign tumours; /1 for unspecified, borderline, or uncertain behaviour; /2 for carcinoma in situ and grade III intraepithelial neoplasia; /3 for malignant tumours, primary site; and /6 for malignant tumours, metastatic site. Behaviour code /6 is not generally used by cancer registries.

This classification is modified from the previous WHO classification, taking into account changes in our understanding of these lesions.

TNM staging of tumours of the gallbladder

Gallbladder
(ICD-O-3 C23.9 and C24.0)

Rules for Classification
The classification applies only to carcinomas of gallbladder (C23.9) and cystic duct (C24.0). There should be histological confirmation of the disease.

The following are the procedures for assessing T, N, and M categories.

T categories	Physical examination, imaging, and/or surgical exploration
N categories	Physical examination, imaging, and/or surgical exploration
M categories	Physical examination, imaging, and/or surgical exploration

Regional Lymph Nodes
Regional lymph nodes are the hepatic hilus nodes (including nodes along the common bile duct, hepatic artery, portal vein, and cystic duct), coeliac, and superior mesenteric artery nodes.

TNM Clinical Classification
T – Primary Tumour

TX	Primary tumour cannot be assessed
T0	No evidence of primary tumour
Tis	Carcinoma in situ
T1	Tumour invades lamina propria or muscular layer
T1a	Tumour invades lamina propria
T1b	Tumour invades muscular layer
T2	Tumour invades perimuscular connective tissue; no extension beyond serosa or into liver
T2a	Tumour invades perimuscular connective tissue on the peritoneal side with no extension to the serosa
T2b	Tumour invades perimuscular connective tissue on the hepatic side with no extension into the liver
T3	Tumour perforates the serosa (visceral peritoneum) and/or directly invades the liver and/or one other adjacent organ or structure, such as stomach, duodenum, colon, pancreas, omentum, extrahepatic bile ducts
T4	Tumour invades main portal vein or hepatic artery or invades two or more extrahepatic organs or structures

N – Regional Lymph Nodes

NX	Regional lymph nodes cannot be assessed
N0	No regional lymph node metastasis
N1	Metastases to 1–3 regional nodes
N2	Metastasis to 4 or more regional nodes

M – Distant Metastasis

M0	No distant metastasis
M1	Distant metastasis

pTNM Pathological Classification
The pT and pN categories correspond to the T and N categories.

pN0 Histological examination of a regional lymphadenectomy specimen will ordinarily include 6 or more lymph nodes. If the regional lymph nodes are negative, but the number ordinarily examined is not met, classify as pN0.

pM – Distant Metastasis*
pM1 Distant metastasis microscopically confirmed

Note
* pM0 and pMX are not valid categories.

Stage – Gallbladder

Stage 0	Tis	N0	M0
Stage IA	T1a	N0	M0
Stage IB	T1b	N0	M0
Stage IIA	T2a	N0	M0
Stage IIB	T2b	N0	M0
Stage IIIA	T3	N0	M0
Stage IIIB	T1,T2,T3	N1	M0
Stage IVA	T4	N0,N1	M0
Stage IVB	Any T	N2	M0
	Any T	Any N	M1

The information presented here has been excerpted from the 2017 *TNM classification of malignant tumours*, eighth edition {408,3385A}. © 2017 UICC. A help desk for specific questions about the TNM classification is available at https://www.uicc.org/tnm-help-desk.

Chapter 9

TNM staging of tumours of the perihilar bile ducts

Perihilar Bile Ducts

(ICD-O-3 C24.0)

Rules for Classification

The classification applies to carcinomas of the extrahepatic bile ducts of perihilar localization (Klatskin tumour). Included are the right, left and the common hepatic ducts.

The following are the procedures for assessing T, N, and M categories.

T categories	Physical examination, imaging, and/or surgical exploration
N categories	Physical examination, imaging, and/or surgical exploration
M categories	Physical examination, imaging, and/or surgical exploration

Anatomical Sites and Subsites

Perihilar cholangiocarcinomas are tumours located in the extrahepatic biliary tree proximal to the origin of the cystic duct.

Regional Lymph Nodes

The regional nodes are the hilar and pericholedochal nodes in the hepatoduodenal ligament.

TNM Clinical Classification

T – Primary Tumour

TX	Primary tumour cannot be assessed
T0	No evidence of primary tumour
Tis	Carcinoma in situ
T1	Tumour confined to the bile duct, with extension up to the muscle layer or fibrous tissue
T2a	Tumour invades beyond the wall of the bile duct to surrounding adipose tissue
T2b	Tumour invades adjacent hepatic parenchyma
T3	Tumour invades unilateral branches of the portal vein or hepatic artery
T4	Tumour invades the main portal vein or its branches bilaterally; or the common hepatic artery; or unilateral second-order biliary radicals with contralateral portal vein or hepatic artery involvement

N – Regional Lymph Nodes

NX	Regional lymph nodes cannot be assessed
N0	No regional lymph node metastasis
N1	Metastases to 1–3 regional lymph nodes
N2	Metastases to 4 or more regional nodes

M – Distant Metastasis

M0	No distant metastasis
M1	Distant metastasis

pTNM Pathological Classification

The pT and pN categories correspond to the T and N categories.

pN0 Histological examination of a regional lymphadenectomy specimen will ordinarily include 15 more lymph nodes. If the regional lymph nodes are negative, but the number ordinarily examined is not met, classify as pN0.

pM – Distant Metastasis*

pM1 Distant metastasis microscopically confirmed

Note

* pM0 and pMX are not valid categories.

Stage – Perihilar Bile Ducts

Stage	T	N	M
Stage 0	Tis	N0	M0
Stage I	T1	N0	M0
Stage II	T2a,T2b	N0	M0
Stage IIIA	T3	N0	M0
Stage IIIB	T4	N0	M0
Stage IIIC	Any T	N1	M0
Stage IVA	Any T	N2	M0
Stage IVB	Any T	Any N	M1

TNM staging of tumours of the distal extrahepatic bile duct

Distal Extrahepatic Bile Duct
(ICD-O-3 C24.0)

Rules for Classification
The classification applies to carcinomas of the extrahepatic bile ducts distal to the insertion of the cystic duct. Cystic duct carcinoma is included under gallbladder.

The following are the procedures for assessing T, N, and M categories.

T categories	Physical examination, imaging, and/or surgical exploration
N categories	Physical examination, imaging, and/or surgical exploration
M categories	Physical examination, imaging, and/or surgical exploration

Regional Lymph Nodes
The regional lymph nodes are along the common bile duct, hepatic artery, back towards the coeliac trunk, posterior and anterior pancreaticoduodenal nodes, and nodes along the superior mesenteric artery.

TNM Clinical Classification
T – Primary Tumour

TX	Primary tumour cannot be assessed
T0	No evidence of primary tumour
Tis	Carcinoma in situ
T1	Tumour invades bile duct wall to a depth less than 5 mm
T2	Tumour invades bile duct wall to a depth of 5 mm up to 12 mm
T3	Tumour invades bile duct wall to a depth of more than 12 mm
T4	Tumour involves the coeliac axis, the superior mesenteric artery and/or the common hepatic artery

N – Regional Lymph Nodes

NX	Regional lymph nodes cannot be assessed
N0	No regional lymph node metastases
N1	Metastases to 1–3 regional nodes
N2	Metastasis to 4 or more regional nodes

M – Distant Metastasis

M0	No distant metastasis
M1	Distant metastasis

pTNM Pathological Classification
The pT and pN categories correspond to the T and N categories.

pN0　Histological examination of a regional lymphadenectomy specimen will ordinarily include 12 or more lymph nodes. If the regional lymph nodes are negative, but the number ordinarily examined is not met, classify as pN0.

pM – Distant Metastasis*
pM1　Distant metastasis microscopically confirmed

Note
* pM0 and pMX are not valid categories.

Stage – Distal Extrahepatic Bile Duct

Stage	T	N	M
Stage 0	Tis	N0	M0
Stage I	T1	N0	M0
Stage IIA	T1	N1	M0
	T2	N0	M0
Stage IIB	T2	N1	M0
	T3	N0,N1	M0
Stage IIIA	T1,T2,T3	N2	M0
Stage IIIB	T4	Any N	M0
Stage IV	Any T	Any N	M1

Chapter 9

Tumours of the gallbladder and extrahepatic bile ducts: Introduction

Paradis V
Klimstra DS

This chapter, covering tumours of the gallbladder and extrahepatic bile ducts (EHBDs), concerns epithelial tumours. The ICD-O topographical coding for the anatomical sites covered in this chapter is presented in Box 9.01.

Benign epithelial tumours and precursors include pyloric gland adenoma, biliary intraepithelial neoplasia, and intracholecystic and intraductal papillary neoplasms of the gallbladder, intrahepatic bile ducts, and EHBDs. Pyloric gland adenoma of the gallbladder, usually associated with cholelithiasis, plays a minor role in the pathogenesis of gallbladder carcinoma.

Tumours developed from the gallbladder and the EHBDs share a common pathogenetic mechanism, with a substantial role of chronic inflammation, commonly related to gallstones in the gallbladder or inflammatory conditions (e.g. sclerosing cholangitis) in the EHBDs, which promotes the development of precursor premalignant lesions: biliary intraepithelial neoplasia and intracholecystic papillary neoplasm (of the gallbladder) or intraductal papillary neoplasm (EHBDs) {1637}. All precursor lesions are now graded according to a two-tiered classification system, with the former low-grade and intermediate-grade dysplasia now classified as low-grade {267}, consistent with tumours in the pancreas and the tubular GI tract.

Carcinomas of the gallbladder and EHBDs display geographical variation, with high incidences of gallbladder carcinomas reported in Chile (among the indigenous Mapuche), India, and eastern Asia. EHBD carcinomas are much more frequent in Asian countries, especially the Republic of Korea.

Although adenocarcinoma is the most common type of biliary tract carcinoma, tumours may display a wide range of histological subtypes. Neuroendocrine tumours (NETs) are classified using the standardized system adopted in this volume for the entire GI tract and hepatopancreatobiliary system {2717}.

Carcinomas of the gallbladder and EHBDs are characterized by the accumulation of genetic abnormalities, with *TP53* mutations being the most common. In addition to common molecular alterations shared by gallbladder and EHBD carcinomas, some specific alterations have been described in EHBD carcinomas.

Box 9.01 ICD-O topographical coding for the anatomical sites covered in this chapter

C23 Gallbladder
  C23.9 Gallbladder
C24 Other and unspecified parts of the biliary tract
  C24.0 Extrahepatic bile duct NOS
  C24.1 Ampulla of Vater
  C24.2 Distal (extrahepatic) bile duct
  C24.3 Perihilar (or proximal) bile duct
  C24.4 Cystic duct
  C24.8 Overlapping lesion of the biliary tract
  C24.9 Biliary tract NOS

Pyloric gland adenoma of the gallbladder

Basturk O
Aishima S
Esposito I

Definition

Pyloric gland adenoma (PGA) of the gallbladder is a grossly visible non-invasive neoplasm of the gallbladder composed of uniform back-to-back mucinous glands arranged in a tubular configuration.

ICD-O coding

8140/0 Adenoma NOS

ICD-11 coding

2E92.6 Benign neoplasm of gallbladder, extrahepatic bile ducts or ampulla of Vater

Related terminology

Acceptable: intracholecystic papillary-tubular neoplasm, gastric pyloric, simple mucinous type {40}.

Subtype(s)

None

Localization

There is no preferential localization within the gallbladder.

Clinical features

PGAs are found in 0.2–0.5% of gallbladders removed for cholelithiasis or chronic cholecystitis {88}, and they account for about 10% of all grossly visible non-invasive neoplasms of the gallbladder {40}. They are more common in females, and most occur in adults {95,3583,83}.

PGAs are often < 2 cm and asymptomatic, and they are usually discovered incidentally. However, when they arise in the gallbladder neck, they may lead to gallbladder distension and right upper quadrant pain {40,88}.

Epidemiology

No conclusive epidemiological data are available.

Etiology

There are no well-established etiological factors for PGA. However, 50–65% of PGAs are associated with cholelithiasis {83}. Occasionally, they occur in association with Peutz–Jeghers syndrome {956} or familial adenomatous polyposis {88}.

Pathogenesis

There are few data on pathogenesis. PGAs do not harbour *TP53* or *CDKN2A* mutations, which are common in invasive carcinomas of the gallbladder {3583}. Several studies have found immunohistochemical expression of β-catenin and mutations of *CTNNB1* in 60% of PGAs {556,3665}, whereas mutations in *CTNNB1* are found in < 10% of the carcinomas {2657,556}. These data suggest that the molecular pathology of PGAs differs from that of invasive carcinomas, and that PGA plays only a minor role in gallbladder carcinogenesis {88}.

Macroscopic appearance

Some PGAs are sessile, whereas others are pedunculated {40}. The lesions are often readily detached from the mucosal surface and may be free-floating, mistaken as sludge in the lumen.

Histopathology

PGAs are composed of lobules of small, tightly packed, bland-looking pyloric-type or Brunner gland–like glands, some of which may be cystically dilated. The tumour cells reveal abundant apical mucinous cytoplasm, peripherally located nuclei, and a low N:C ratio. There is minimal or no intervening stroma {40,83,1733,2371}. Paneth cells and neuroendocrine cells are often present. The uninvolved gallbladder mucosa is mostly devoid of dysplasia or pyloric gland metaplasia {40,83,1733,2371}.

In the majority of the lesions, there is minimal cytological atypia, although the architecture is commonly complex. Foci of high-grade dysplasia may be seen in larger (> 1 cm) cases, which may occasionally even be associated with invasive carcinoma {82,83,40}.

The tumour cells are usually positive for CK7, and they diffusely and strongly express MUC6.

Pyloric gland metaplasia, when polypoid, can be confused with PGA; this appears to be the source of some controversy regarding the nature of these lesions in the literature {40}, because some major studies on adenomas have in fact predominantly involved subcentimetre foci of pyloric gland metaplasia {2728,2727,1407}. Unlike PGA, pyloric gland metaplasia is often

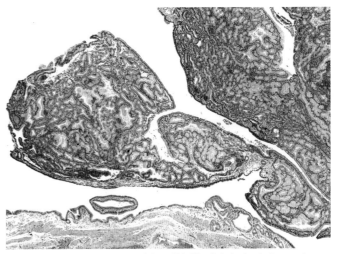

Fig. 9.01 Pyloric gland adenoma of the gallbladder. Pyloric gland adenoma is composed of tightly packed, evenly sized, small, bland-appearing pyloric-type glands and minimal intervening stroma.

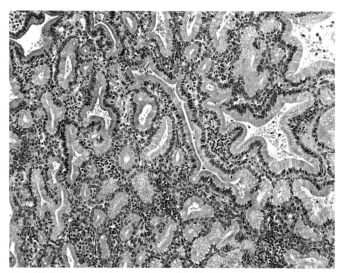

Fig. 9.02 Pyloric gland adenoma of the gallbladder. The cells have abundant apical mucinous cytoplasm, peripherally located nuclei, and a low N:C ratio.

microscopic and not well demarcated from the surrounding mucosa. Therefore, pyloric gland nodules < 0.5 cm arising in a background of pyloric gland metaplasia in the adjacent mucosa should not be designated as PGA {83}.

Cytology
PGAs are very rarely sampled by cytology.

Diagnostic molecular pathology
Not clinically relevant

Essential and desirable diagnostic criteria
Essential: non-invasive, benign glandular neoplasm of the gallbladder; usually composed of mucinous glands with pyloric
or Brunner gland features.

Staging (TNM)
PGAs with high-grade dysplasia are staged as pTis. If there is an associated invasive carcinoma, staging follows the protocol for carcinomas of the gallbladder {127}.

Prognosis and prediction
If invasive carcinoma is ruled out, PGAs are cured by chole-cystectomy, even when high-grade dysplasia is present. The potential for multifocal biliary neoplasm as found in intracholecystic papillary neoplasms is not thought to be substantial for PGAs. The prognosis for PGAs with associated invasive carcinoma probably depends on stage; however, the reported cases are too few to derive a conclusion {82,83,40}.

Biliary intraepithelial neoplasia

Basturk O
Aishima S
Esposito I

Definition

Biliary intraepithelial neoplasia (BilIN) consists of microscopic, non-invasive, flat or (micro)papillary lesions that are confined to the gallbladder lumen or bile ducts.

ICD-O coding

8148/0 Biliary intraepithelial neoplasia, low grade
8148/2 Biliary intraepithelial neoplasia, high grade

ICD-11 coding

2E92.6 & XH7BS0 Benign neoplasm of gallbladder, extrahepatic bile ducts or ampulla of Vater & Biliary intraepithelial neoplasia, low grade
2E61.Y & XH5U91 Carcinoma in situ of other specified digestive organs (or 2C18 Malignant neoplasms of perihilar bile duct) & Biliary intraepithelial neoplasia, high grade

Related terminology

BilIN
Acceptable: dysplasia (still the more widely used term for lesions in the gallbladder).

High-grade BilIN
Acceptable: carcinoma in situ (used parenthetically in some parts of the world).

Subtype(s)

None

Localization

Not applicable

Clinical features

Given its microscopic nature, BilIN is typically found incidentally in gallbladder and bile duct specimens resected for other reasons.

Epidemiology

In countries where gallbladder carcinoma is endemic, low-grade dysplasia is seen in as many as 15% of gallbladders with lithiasis, and high-grade dysplasia in 1–3.5% {547,2727,2725,1538,88}. These incidence rates were reported as < 5% and < 0.1%, respectively, in North America {2166}. The incidence of BilIN outside the setting of invasive adenocarcinoma is difficult to determine in the bile ducts because these are seldom biopsied unless there is a substantial pathology {2166}.

Etiology

In addition to lithiasis, BilIN is often encountered in the mucosa adjacent to invasive carcinoma and can be seen in patients with familial adenomatous polyposis, primary sclerosing cholangitis {1536,1878,1877}, choledochal cyst {1840}, and anomalous union of pancreatobiliary ducts {2378,2166}.

Pathogenesis

It has been suggested that chronic biliary inflammation may induce neoplastic change of biliary epithelium {64}.

KRAS mutations occur in approximately 40% of BilIN cases and are identified as an early molecular event during the progression of BilIN, whereas *TP53* mutation appears to be a late molecular event {2294,1313,2854}. Some evidence suggests that expression of autophagy-related proteins is also upregulated at an early stage {2854,1708}, and that p21, cyclin D1,

Table 9.01 Morphological features of biliary intraepithelial neoplasia (BilIN)

Features	Low-grade BilIN (BilIN-1/2)	High-grade BilIN (BilIN-3)
Histology	Flat pseudopapillary/micropapillary	Flat pseudopapillary/micropapillary
	Hyperchromatic nuclei	Hyperchromatic and irregular nuclei
	Increased N:C ratio	Pleomorphic, bizarre nuclei, increased N:C ratio
	Nuclear stratification	Complex nuclear stratification
	Preserved nuclear polarity	Loss of nuclear polarity
Biliary mucosa involvement	Relatively small foci or areas	Relatively extensive area
Involvement of peribiliary glands	Infrequent	Frequent
Ki-67 proliferation index	Mildly to moderately increased	Markedly increased
Immunostaining[a]		
S100	Mildly to moderately increased	Diffuse and strongly positive
p53	Usually negative	Frequently positive
p16	Relatively preserved	Decreased

[a]Overlaps in immunostaining results are wide, precluding their utility in individual cases (see text).

Chapter 9

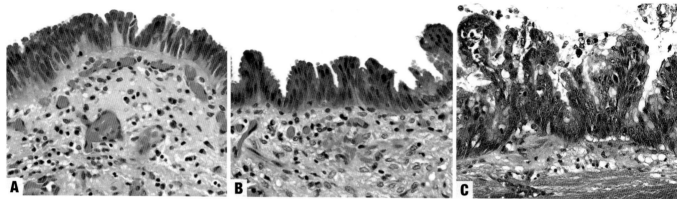

Fig. 9.03 Biliary intraepithelial neoplasia (BilIN). **A,B** Low-grade BilIN characterized by pseudostratification of nuclei (**A**) and focal papillary projections (**B**). The cells have an increased N:C ratio and nuclear hyperchromasia. **C** High-grade BilIN. There is complete loss of nuclear polarity and budding of cell clusters into the lumen. The nuclei are markedly pleomorphic.

SMAD4, and glucose transporters are also involved in the carcinogenesis of BilIN {2294,1708}.

Macroscopic appearance

BilIN lesions are usually not grossly visible but may be associated with subtle changes such as mucosal thickening.

Histopathology

BilIN consists of flat or (micro)papillary epithelial lesions that are graded, on the basis of the highest degree of cytoarchitectural atypia, as low-grade or high-grade {267}. This two-tiered classification replaces the former three-tiered classification (BilIN-1, BilIN-2, and BilIN-3) {3745}, with the former BilIN-1 and BilIN-2 categories now classified as low-grade and the former BilIN-3 now classified as high-grade (see Table 9.01, p. 273) {267}.

Low-grade BilIN is characterized by mild cytoarchitectural atypia, including a predominantly flat growth pattern, pseudostratification of nuclei, a high N:C ratio, hyperchromasia,

and prominent nucleoli. High-grade BilIN typically reveals more-complex patterns, such as micropapillae or tall papillae. Complete loss of polarity, marked nuclear atypia, and frequent mitoses are also identified. In the setting of hyalinizing cholecystitis, high-grade BilIN may have a denuded pattern, with only a few cells clinging to the stroma, akin to denuding carcinoma in situ seen in the urothelium {2549,2166}. High-grade BilIN in the gallbladder may arise from or extend into Rokitansky–Aschoff sinuses, a feature that should not be confused with invasion {94,2732}. Low-grade BilIN is of no clinical significance {2088,3023}. However, if high-grade BilIN is detected, thorough sampling is warranted.

Various cellular phenotypes, including biliary, intestinal, and gastric, are recognized {65,88,2166}. When BilIN is associated with an invasive carcinoma, the phenotype of BilIN does not necessarily correspond with that of the carcinoma.

The differential diagnosis with reactive epithelial atypia may be difficult. Reactive atypia often occurs at the deeper aspects

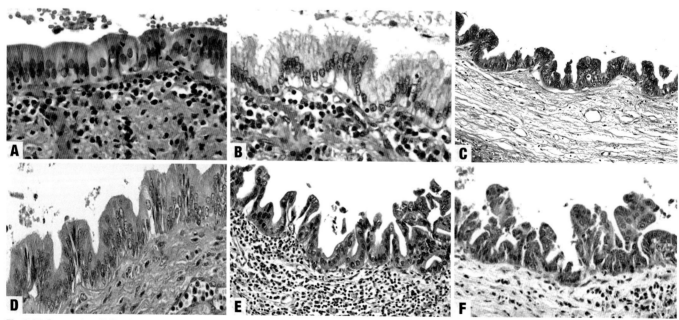

Fig. 9.04 Progression of biliary intraepithelial neoplasia (BilIN). **A** Normal biliary epithelium of a large intrahepatic bile duct. **B** Hyperplastic biliary epithelial cells of the intrahepatic large bile duct. **C,D** Low-grade BilIN. **E,F** High-grade BilIN.

of the epithelium and typically displays overlapping attenuated cells with overall basophilia, prominent intercellular clefts, and moulding of nuclei. The nuclei have relatively fine and diffuse chromatin, and the nucleoli are typically small or conspicuous. Mitotic activity may be brisk. Unlike in BilIN, reactive changes show a gradual transition. If present, overexpression of p53 favours BilIN {3582,2453,2863}. Similarly, MUC5AC expression appears to become more extensive with increasing degrees of BilIN {64,3749}. However, the overlaps are too wide for both stains, precluding their utility in individual cases. Recently, it has been suggested that S100 expression also increases during the multistep carcinogenesis process and may be used as an adjunct to distinguish high-grade BilIN from reactive atypia {63,2862,3762}.

Cytology

Isolated BilIN is not encountered in clinical cytology samples. However, if sampled, high-grade BilIN would be expected to show the classic features of adenocarcinoma {209,1134}. Cytology alone is insufficient to distinguish between preinvasive and invasive lesions.

Diagnostic molecular pathology

Not clinically relevant

Essential and desirable diagnostic criteria

Essential: microscopic non-invasive lesions with low-grade or high-grade epithelial dysplasia.

Staging (TNM)

High-grade BilIN is categorized as Tis (carcinoma in situ) {408}.

Prognosis and prediction

Early gallbladder cancer data suggest that most cases of high-grade BilIN in the gallbladder can be cured by cholecystectomy {2732,88}. However, a small proportion of patients experience recurrences and metastasis, usually several years after the diagnosis, indicating that there is a field effect in the biliary tree. Extensive disease, involvement of Rokitansky–Aschoff sinuses, and margin positivity may confer additional risk of recurrence {2292,2732,2166}.

Intracholecystic papillary neoplasm

Basturk O
Aishima S
Esposito I

Definition

Intracholecystic papillary neoplasm (ICPN) is a grossly visible, mass-forming, non-invasive epithelial neoplasm arising in the mucosa and projecting into the lumen of the gallbladder. If there is a component of invasive carcinoma, the lesion is called ICPN with associated invasive carcinoma.

ICD-O coding

8503/0 Intracystic papillary neoplasm with low-grade intraepithelial neoplasia
8503/2 Intracystic papillary neoplasm with high-grade intraepithelial neoplasia
8503/3 Intracystic papillary neoplasm with associated invasive carcinoma

ICD-11 coding

2E92.6 Benign neoplasm of gallbladder, extrahepatic bile ducts or ampulla of Vater
2E61.3 & XH6AH7 Carcinoma in situ of gallbladder, biliary tract or ampulla of Vater & Intraductal papillary neoplasm with high-grade intraepithelial neoplasia
2C13.0 & XH90W1 Adenocarcinoma of the gallbladder & Intraductal papillary neoplasm with associated invasive carcinoma

Related terminology

Not recommended: biliary adenoma; intestinal adenoma; papillary (villous) adenoma; tubulopapillary (tubulovillous) adenoma; non-invasive papillary neoplasm/carcinoma; intracystic papillary neoplasm; papillomatosis; papillary carcinoma.

Subtype(s)

None

Localization

Not applicable

Clinical features

ICPNs are twice as common in females as in males. Patient age ranges from 20 to 94 years (mean: 61 years) {40}. Almost half of all patients with ICPNs present with right upper outer quadrant pain. In the other half, the lesion is detected incidentally {2410}. Almost half of the cases are designated radiologically as gallbladder cancer {40}.

Epidemiology

ICPNs are found in 0.4% of cholecystectomies, and about 6% of gallbladder carcinomas arise in association with ICPN {40}.

Etiology

There are no known etiological factors. Unlike gallbladder carcinoma in general, ICPN has no known association with gallstones.

Pathogenesis

Unknown

Macroscopic appearance

ICPNs are characterized by granular, friable excrescences or by prominent exophytic growth. Granular lesions are usually broad-based, whereas others have stalks so thin that the lesions often detach from the surface and may be mistaken as sludge in the lumen {2166}. Approximately one third of ICPNs are multifocal. The median tumour size is 2.2 cm {40}.

Histopathology

Microscopically, the lesions reveal intraluminal growth of back-to-back epithelial units, typically in a predominantly papillary configuration. In some cases, tubulopapillary growth may be seen. Rarely, ICPNs extend into Rokitansky–Aschoff sinuses, a finding that should not be mistaken for invasive carcinoma. Adjacent mucosa often reveals flat dysplasia.

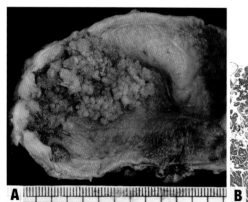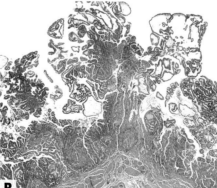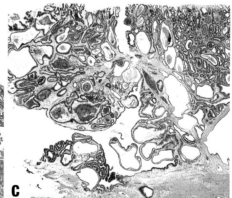

Fig. 9.05 Intracholecystic papillary neoplasm. **A** These are papillary or polypoid exophytic lesions distinct from adjacent gallbladder mucosa. **B,C** Intracholecystic papillary neoplasms reveal papillary (**B**) and/or tubular (**C**) growth patterns.

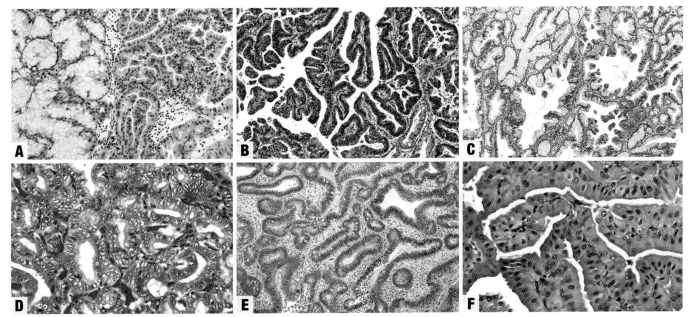

Fig. 9.06 Intracholecystic papillary neoplasm (ICPN). **A** Spectrum of dysplasia in ICPN. **B** Biliary morphology with nondescript cuboidal cells and extensive high-grade dysplasia. **C** Gastric morphology typically resembles gastric foveolar epithelium, with elongated interconnecting glands lined by tall columnar cells that have abundant pale mucin and diffuse MUC5AC expression. **D** A subset of ICPNs with gastric morphology is characterized by small, back-to-back, glandular units lined by uniform cuboidal cells without overt intracytoplasmic mucin, some with nuclear clearing and overlapping. MUC6 is consistently expressed in this pattern. **E** Intestinal morphology; a small percentage of ICPNs resemble intestinal adenomas, with overall basophilia and pseudostratified, cigar-shaped nuclei. **F** Rare ICPNs are oncocytic, showing features similar to those of intraductal oncocytic papillary neoplasms of the pancreas.

On the basis of the highest degree of cytoarchitectural atypia in the epithelium, ICPNs are classified as low-grade or high-grade. Low-grade ICPNs reveal only mild to moderate atypia. High-grade lesions are characterized by architectural complexity as well as loss of polarity and nuclear pleomorphism {2281,267}.

A variety of morphological patterns have been described, and various subtypes of ICPN have been proposed, such as tubular adenoma or papillary adenoma {88}. However, there is often substantial overlap of morphology and cellular differentiation between cases (making the specific definition of subtypes challenging) {40}, and there are no specific clinical implications to the subcategorization of subtypes; therefore, all neoplasms meeting the definition of ICPN are now classified together {40}. One related entity that can be separately defined is pyloric gland adenoma (see *Pyloric gland adenoma of the gallbladder*, p. 271).

Compared with their counterparts in the pancreas (intraductal papillary mucinous neoplasms), ICPNs more commonly display morphological heterogeneity and hybrid cell differentiation patterns, not only histologically but also immunohistochemically. Four morphological patterns are recognized, and the predominant pattern can be specified in the diagnosis:

Biliary morphology is the most common, with cuboidal cells showing clear to eosinophilic cytoplasm, enlarged nuclei, and prominent nucleoli. Biliary regions typically show CK7 and EMA (MUC1) expression {83,40}.

Gastric morphology is reflected in elongated glands lined by tall columnar cells with abundant pale cytoplasm and peripherally located nuclei (gastric foveolar type). Gastric regions are diffusely positive for MUC5AC, and some may also express MUC6 {83,40}. A distinctive pattern of gastric morphology seen in a subset of ICPNs is characterized by smaller tubular glands lined by relatively uniform cuboidal cells with a modest amount of cytoplasm, round nuclei, and visible nucleoli (gastric pyloric, non-mucinous type). Some of the glands are cystically dilated and contain acidophilic secretory material. Diffuse and strong MUC6 expression is uniform in this pattern {40}.

Intestinal morphology closely resembles that of colonic adenomas, with tall columnar cells showing pseudostratified cigar-shaped nuclei and basophilic cytoplasm. As expected, these regions are commonly positive for CK20, CDX2, and MUC2 {83,40}.

Oncocytic morphology is the least common in ICPNs, characterized by arborizing papillae lined by multiple layers of cells with abundant acidophilic granular cytoplasm and single prominent nucleoli {83,40}. Interestingly, oncocytic morphology in ICPNs does not correlate with the characteristic immunoprofile of intraductal oncocytic papillary neoplasms in the pancreas {268,265,270}; instead, there is diffuse positivity for EMA (MUC1) and no labelling with MUC6 {40}.

An associated invasive carcinoma is identified in about half of all ICPNs, particularly in lesions with predominantly biliary morphology or extensive high-grade dysplasia {1697,83,40}. The invasive component is often a tubular adenocarcinoma, although other types, such as mucinous, adenosquamous, or neuroendocrine carcinoma (NEC), have also been described {1251}. The carcinoma may be grossly inapparent and may also occur away from the main ICPN lesion. Therefore, thorough sampling and careful evaluation is warranted.

Cytology
Not clinically relevant

Diagnostic molecular pathology
Although *KRAS* mutations are common {3583,2490}, *TP53* mutation and *GNAS* mutation at codon 201 (which is seen in 50–70% of pancreatic intraductal neoplasms, particularly in the intestinal subtype {994,3617,2200,3231}) are rare in ICPNs {1313,2089}.

Essential and desirable diagnostic criteria
Essential: macroscopically, a mass-forming neoplasm arising in the gallbladder mucosa; microscopically, intraluminal growth of back-to-back epithelial units, in a papillary or tubulopapillary configuration.

Staging (TNM)
ICPNs with high-grade dysplasia are staged as pTis. The staging of ICPNs with associated invasive carcinoma follows that of gallbladder carcinoma.

Prognosis and prediction
ICPNs without an invasive carcinoma have a good prognosis after cholecystectomy. The 5-year survival rate for patients with non-invasive ICPNs is 78%, whereas patients with invasive carcinoma have a 5-year survival rate of 60% {40}. Even when only ICPNs with associated invasive carcinoma are considered, the overall outcome of ICPNs is incomparably better than that of conventional gallbladder carcinomas {40}. The fact that some patients with non-invasive ICPNs also die of biliary tract cancer, typically long after the diagnosis of ICPN, suggests that there is a field effect rendering the remainder of the biliary tract at risk of carcinoma; therefore, clinical follow-up is warranted after resection of ICPNs {40}.

Intraductal papillary neoplasm of the bile ducts

Nakanuma Y
Basturk O
Esposito I
Klimstra DS
Komuta M
Zen Y

Definition

Intraductal papillary neoplasm (IPN) of the liver and bile ducts is a grossly visible premalignant neoplasm with intraductal papillary or villous growth of biliary-type epithelium. If there is a component of invasive carcinoma, the lesion is designated IPN with associated invasive carcinoma.

ICD-O coding

8503/0 Intraductal papillary neoplasm with low-grade intraepithelial neoplasia
8503/2 Intraductal papillary neoplasm with high-grade intraepithelial neoplasia
8503/3 Intraductal papillary neoplasm with associated invasive carcinoma

ICD-11 coding

2E92.7 Benign neoplasm of liver or intrahepatic bile ducts

Related terminology

Acceptable: biliary papilloma and papillomatosis.
Not recommended: biliary adenoma; intestinal adenoma; papillary (villous) adenoma; tubulopapillary (tubulovillous) adenoma; non-invasive papillary neoplasm/carcinoma; papillary carcinoma; mucin-secreting biliary tumour.

Subtype(s)

None

Localization

The prevalent location of intraductal papillary neoplasm of the bile ducts (IPNB) is highly variable among studies (with ~80% of tumours located in the intrahepatic bile ducts in some studies and ~70% in the extrahepatic bile ducts in others) {2295}.

Table 9.02 Radiopathological correlation of intraductal papillary neoplasm of the bile ducts (IPNB)

Radiological pattern	Pathological characteristics
Intraductal mass and proximal ductal dilatation	Cast-like intraductal mass with upstream dilatation due to ductal obstruction by IPNB and absence of mucin
Intraductal mass and proximal and distal ductal dilatation	The most common and characteristic type Due to mass and excessive mucin secretion, the ducts containing mass and the proximal and distal bile ducts are markedly dilated
Cystic dilatation with mass	Unilocular or multilocular cystic lesions Mass on the internal surface of the cystic lesion or adjacent bile duct
Intraductal mass with macroinvasive lesion	In any of the above three types with grossly visible parenchymal invasion

Clinical features

The median patient age of IPNB is 50–70 years, with a male predominance. Symptoms include recurrent and intermittent abdominal pain and cholangitis (see Table 9.02) {1963,2524,1964,2740}.

Cholangiography usually shows filling defects in the biliary tract, due to polypoid tumours and/or mucin secretion, although the papillary tumour itself may be undetectable radiologically {1267,2999,1963}.

Epidemiology

IPNB occurs worldwide, but its incidence varies by geographical region {256,3692}. IPNs account for 10–38% of all bile duct tumours in eastern Asia but only 7–12% of all bile duct tumours in

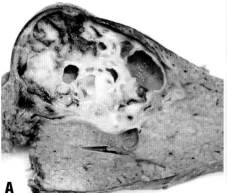
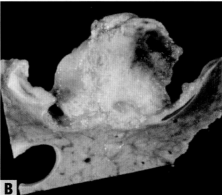
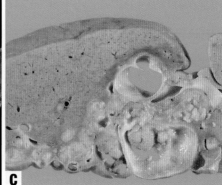

Fig. 9.07 Intraductal papillary neoplasm of the bile ducts. **A** Papillary tumours with multicystic dilatation of intrahepatic bile ducts. **B** Papillary tumour in a dilated bile duct. **C** Multiple papillary tumours in dilated bile ducts with parenchymal invasion.

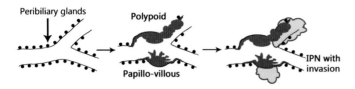

Fig. 9.08 Intraductal papillary neoplasm (IPN) of the bile ducts. Schematic representation of IPN presenting with polypoid and/or papillovillous growth (red) arising in the intrahepatic large bile duct and progressing to invasive carcinoma (IPN with invasion; orange).

North American and European countries {1964,2296,1711,2740}. Current reports are of sporadic cases without a tendency for familial aggregation.

Etiology

The etiology is unclear in most cases. Known risk factors are primary sclerosing cholangitis {1133}, hepatolithiasis, and liver fluke infection (clonorchiasis and opisthorchiasis) in eastern Asian countries {2524,2296,1489,3017}.

Pathogenesis

IPNB may progress from low-grade to high-grade dysplasia and then to invasive adenocarcinoma {1489,2300,2888}. The time lag between the development of IPNB in hepatolithiasis is 6–8 years, and high-grade dysplasia can take 1–2 years to develop into an invasive lesion {3507}.

The development of IPNB follows a sequential progression in association with the stepwise acquisition of molecular alterations affecting common oncogenic pathways, such as *KRAS* mutation, loss of p16, and *TP53* mutation {2888,12}. Overexpression of EZH2 may be associated with malignant behaviour {2853}. The expression of IMP3 and DNMT1 is significantly increased in invasive IPNB {2857}. In eastern Asia, *GNAS* mutations were detected in less than half of all cases of IPNB; all cases with *GNAS* mutations had intestinal differentiation with villous architecture and mucus hypersecretion {3348,2852,3349}.

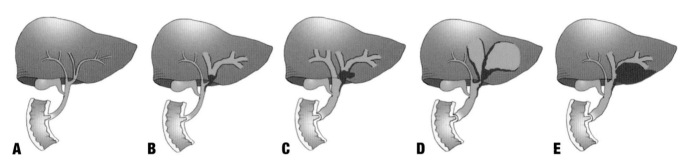

Fig. 9.09 Intraductal papillary neoplasm of the bile ducts (IPNB). Schematic representation of several pathoradiological patterns of IPNB (shown in red). **A** Normal hepatobiliary system. **B** Mass-forming IPNB with secondary dilatation of proximal bile ducts. **C** IPNB with proximal and distal bile duct dilatation due to excessive mucin hypersecretion. **D** Cystic dilatations of the proximal and distal bile ducts due to excessive mucin hypersecretion of the IPNB. **E** Cholangiocarcinoma derived from IPNB with marked invasion into the adjacent hepatic parenchyma (red).

Table 9.03 Characteristics of intraductal papillary neoplasms of the bile ducts based on similarities to their pancreatic counterparts, according to the Japan–Korea Cooperative Study Group {2295}

Characteristic	Type 1	Type 2
Preferential location	Intrahepatic bile ducts	Extrahepatic bile ducts
Gross features of ducts	Cystic, cylindrical dilatation	Cylindrical, fusiform dilatation
Excessive mucin	Frequent	Rare
Histology		
Lining epithelia	Regular, homogeneous Papillary > tubular	Irregular, complex Papillary > tubular; foci of cribriform and solid pattern
Fibrous core	Fine fibrovascular stroma	Fine vascular, focally fibrotic stroma
Subtype	Gastric, intestinal	Intestinal, pancreatobiliary
Grade	Mostly high grade, with foci of low/intermediate grade; infrequently low/intermediate grade	Always high grade, sometimes with foci of low/intermediate grade
Stromal invasion	Less common (< 50%) and minimal, occasionally nodular	Common (> 80%) and minimal, mild
Similarity to IPMN	Similar	Variably different
Aggressiveness	Less aggressive	More aggressive than type 1
Postoperative course	More favourable	Worse than type 1

IPMN, intraductal papillary mucinous neoplasm.

Mutations of *RNF43*, a tumour suppressor gene, were more frequent in the intestinal type of IPNB.

Macroscopic appearance

IPNB appears as a polypoid mass in dilated bile ducts that show cystic, cylindrical, or fusiform dilatation {1580,2740,2524}. The reported size of these dilated duct lumina is 4.1 ± 2.2 cm. The height of the intraluminal polypoid or papillary structures from their base is 5–20 mm. Some IPNBs appear as multiple contiguous papillary or polypoid lesions, whereas others are isolated papillary lesions, and multiple IPNBs may develop. IPNBs may present with mucus hypersecretion, more commonly in Asian patients than in European or North American patients {2999,2740}. IPNBs involving the peribiliary glands present as grossly visible cystic, papillary neoplastic lesions around the large bile ducts {2293,2299,2999}. If invasion into the periductal tissue is present, it is usually limited, but it can occasionally be nodular or mass-forming.

Histopathology

Papillary structures with fine fibrovascular cores covered by biliary epithelial cells are predominant, but tubular or glandular components may be admixed {2524,2300,2888}. The fibrous core of papillary structures may be widened by oedema or inflammatory cell infiltrations. At presentation, approximately 40–80% of IPNBs show minimal stromal invasive carcinoma, usually consisting of tubular adenocarcinoma and occasionally colloid carcinoma {2888,1489,2300}. Superficial spread may be found in the surrounding bile duct mucosa {2524,2300,2302}. On the basis of the highest degree of cytoarchitectural atypia in the epithelium, IPNBs are classified as low-grade or high-grade. Most IPNBs arising in the extrahepatic bile ducts show high-grade dysplasia {2295}.

Epithelia of IPNBs show intestinal, biliary, oncocytic, and gastric-type differentiation based on cytological appearance and immunophenotype {2300,3746,1589}. About half of all IPNBs contain two or more types of epithelia, so they are

Box 9.02 Differential diagnosis of intraductal papillary neoplasm of the bile ducts

Micropapillary biliary intraepithelial neoplasia (BilIN)
- Microscopically recognizable lesions in the intrahepatic large bile ducts
- < 3 mm in height
- Constantly intermixed with flat or pseudopapillary BilIN

Intraductal tubulopapillary neoplasm
- Cast-like lesion composed of densely packed neoplastic tubular glands in the duct
- Unequivocal architectural and cytological atypia (high grade)
- No mucinous content, negative for MUC5AC

Intraductal polypoid metastasis from extrahepatic organs
- Metastasis from colorectal carcinoma is common

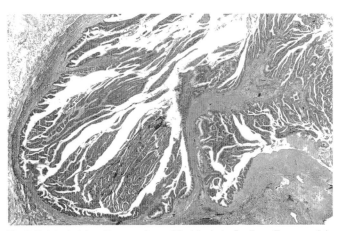

Fig. 9.11 Intraductal papillary neoplasm of the bile ducts. Papillary-villous growth in the cystically dilated bile duct.

classified according to the most prevalent morphological pattern. MUC5AC and MUC6 are frequently expressed by the gastric-type epithelium, and MUC2 by the intestinal type. EMA (MUC1) is frequently expressed by the pancreatobiliary-type epithelium and to a variable extent by the other epithelial types. Intestinal and gastric-type epithelia are most common in Asian

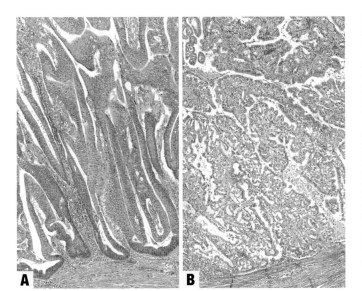

Fig. 9.10 Intraductal papillary neoplasm of the bile ducts. **A** Intestinal-type epithelium. **B** Gastric-type epithelium.

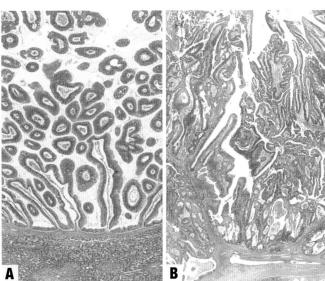

Fig. 9.12 Intraductal papillary neoplasm of the bile ducts with intestinal differentiation. **A** Regular and monotonous growth pattern (type 1). **B** Complex and heterogeneous growth pattern (type 2).

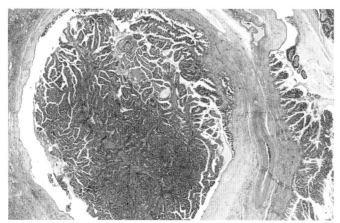

Fig. 9.13 Intraductal papillary neoplasm of the bile ducts (IPNB). Cystic subtype of IPNB closely mimicking high-grade mucinous cystic neoplasm (right side) but lacking the ovarian-like stroma. Note the IPNB in the adjacent dilated bile duct (left side).

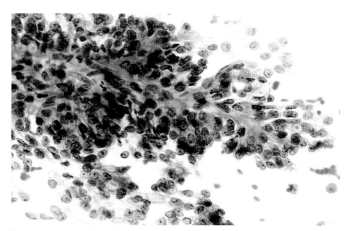

Fig. 9.14 Intraductal papillary neoplasm of the bile ducts. Cytology showing papillary neoplastic growth with fine stroma.

countries, whereas the pancreatobiliary subtype is most frequent in European and North American patients.

Recently, a different classification was proposed, dividing IPNBs into type 1 and type 2 categories on the basis of their similarity to their counterparts in the pancreas. Type 1 IPNBs are histologically similar to intraductal papillary mucinous neoplasm of the pancreas, whereas type 2 IPNBs differ from them to a variable extent. Type 1 is more frequent in the intrahepatic bile ducts, whereas type 2 is more common in the extrahepatic bile ducts. Invasive carcinoma is more frequent in type 2 than type 1 (see Table 9.03, p. 280) {2295,1251}.

Some IPNBs show a pattern called intraductal tubular neoplasm or intraductal tubulopapillary neoplasm of the bile ducts, which roughly corresponds to intraductal tubulopapillary neoplasm of the pancreas. The architecture is predominantly tubular, and mucin production is much less than in other IPNBs. In the pancreas there are good genomic and immunohistochemical data demonstrating that it is distinct from other intraductal neoplasms, but in the bile ducts these data do not yet exist {1537,2890}.

The differential diagnosis of IPNB is summarized in Box 9.02 (p. 281) {2301,2890,3656}.

Cytology

In FNA specimens, the hypercellular aspirates are composed of often broad, double-cell layered sheets of ductal columnar epithelium with distinctive, 3D, complex and branching papillary configurations with fibrovascular cores {3361,209,1134}. Dysplastic but not frankly malignant nuclear features are abundant in IPNB.

Diagnostic molecular pathology

Not clinically relevant

Essential and desirable diagnostic criteria

Essential: grossly visible papillary, villous, or polypoid lesion(s) predominantly growing in a bile duct lumen, variably dilated

due to obstruction by the neoplastic lesion and/or mucin secretion; cystic changes in continuity with adjacent bile duct lumen; fine fibrovascular cores lacking ovarian-like mesenchymal stroma covered by papillary, predominantly cuboidal or columnar, neoplastic epithelia showing variable atypia.

Staging (TNM)

The staging of cholangiocarcinoma derived from IPNB follows the TNM classification for intrahepatic cholangiocarcinoma {408}.

Prognosis and prediction

In IPNB with low-grade dysplasia, no tumour-related recurrence or death occurred after complete resection, whereas in cholangiocarcinoma derived from IPNB, the rates of tumour recurrence and overall survival were 47.0% and 68.8%, respectively, after 5 years {1963,1602,1964}. The prognosis of invasive carcinoma derived from IPNB has been consistently better than that of conventional intrahepatic and extrahepatic cholangiocarcinomas {2296,1489}. Both depth of invasion and percentage of the invasive carcinoma component correlate with survival. Invasive cholangiocarcinomas derived from IPNB with pancreatobiliary differentiation show higher histological grades, more lymph node metastases, more-frequent postoperative recurrences, and worse clinical outcome than invasive cholangiocarcinomas derived from IPNB with gastric and intestinal differentiation {1963,1602,2524}. EMA (MUC1)-expressing cholangiocarcinomas derived from IPNB show a shorter recurrence-free survival time than the EMA (MUC1) non-expressing group. In addition, colloid carcinomas derived from IPNB have a better prognosis than tubular adenocarcinomas {2999,1489}.

Carcinoma of the gallbladder

Roa JC
Adsay NV
Arola J
Tsui WM
Zen Y

Definition
Carcinoma of the gallbladder is a malignant epithelial neoplasm arising in the gallbladder from biliary epithelium.

ICD-O coding
8140/3 Adenocarcinoma NOS
8070/3 Squamous cell carcinoma NOS
8020/3 Carcinoma, undifferentiated, NOS

ICD-11 coding
2C13 Malignant neoplasms of the gallbladder

Related terminology
Not recommended: cholangiocarcinoma; gallbladder adeno-carcinoma.

Subtype(s)
Adenocarcinoma, intestinal type (8144/3); clear cell adenocarcinoma NOS (8310/3); mucinous cystic neoplasm with associated invasive carcinoma (8470/3); mucinous adenocarcinoma (8480/3); poorly cohesive carcinoma (8490/3); intracystic papillary neoplasm with associated invasive carcinoma (8503/3)

Localization
The most common site is the fundus (60%) followed by the body (30%) and neck (10%). Most tumours are flat, with extensive overlap into different sections of the gallbladder.

Clinical features
The signs and symptoms are nonspecific and indistinguishable from those produced by gallstones. Right upper quadrant pain is common. More than 50% of cases are diagnosed incidentally at a late stage. Ultrasound and CT are useful in a small fraction of cases involving non-flat tumours {2092}.

Epidemiology
Gallbladder cancers (GBCs) are the most common biliary tract carcinomas. The incidence of GBC varies geographically and ethnically. The highest incidence is reported in the indigenous Mapuche people of Chile, with an incidence among females of 27.3 cases per 100 000 person-years {315}. High incidences have also been found in parts of India, eastern Asia, and some central and eastern European countries {1337}. In Chile and India, GBC occurs predominantly in females with gallstones. In eastern Asia, it is almost as common in men, and the association with gallstones is much weaker, suggesting etiological differences in different regions.

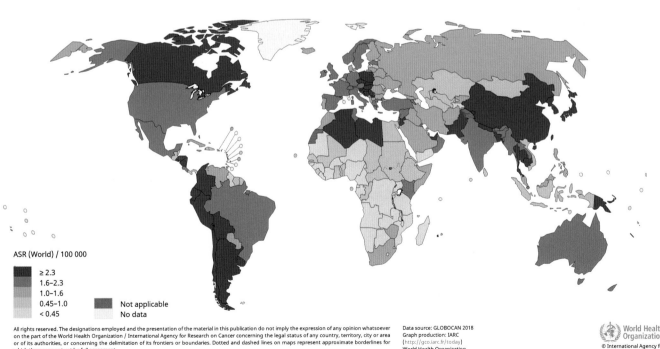

ASR (World) / 100 000

- ≥ 2.3
- 1.6–2.3
- 1.0–1.6
- 0.45–1.0
- < 0.45
- Not applicable
- No data

Data source: GLOBOCAN 2018
Graph production: IARC
(http://gco.iarc.fr/today)
World Health Organization

World Health Organization
© International Agency for Research on Cancer 2018

Fig. 9.15 Estimated age-standardized incidence rates (ASRs; World), per 100 000 person-years, of gallbladder carcinoma in 2018.

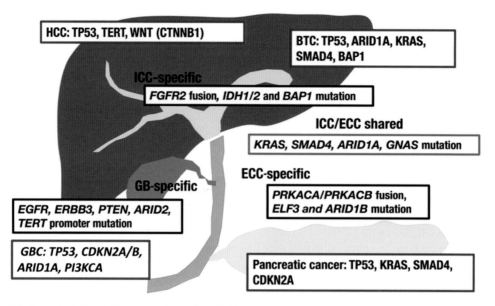

Fig. 9.16 Genomics of gallbladder and extrahepatic bile duct carcinoma. Specific driver genes across anatomical subtypes of biliary tract cancer (BTC) and comparison with core driver genes in hepatocellular carcinoma (HCC) and pancreatic cancer. ECC, extrahepatic cholangiocarcinoma; GB, gallbladder; GBC, gallbladder cancer; ICC, intrahepatic cholangiocarcinoma {3001}.

GBC is concentrated in certain racial and ethnic groups, and specific polymorphisms (SNPs) in the genes *DCC*, *CYP1A1*, *CYP17A1* (*P450C17*), *ERCC2*, *OGG1*, and *ABCG8* have been linked to a higher risk of GBC (odds ratio: 1.7–8.0). However, these correlations need validation in larger and independent cohorts {3791,2531,2530,540}.

Etiology

Among the established risk factors of GBC, gallstones are the most common; in some high-risk regions (e.g. Chile), they are found in > 80% of gallbladders harbouring carcinoma {2726}. However, the overall incidence of GBC in patients with chole-lithiasis is < 0.2% {1308}. The weight, volume, size, and length of the gallstones have been found to correlate with GBC incidence. The association of GBC with primary sclerosing cholangitis is attributable to inflammation. Aflatoxin B1, found in food not properly stored and conserved in rural areas, and *Salmonella typhi* have been implicated as triggers of the inflammatory cascade. Another established risk factor for GBC is pancreatobiliary maljunction, which is the supra-Oddi union of common bile duct with the main pancreatic duct. Rare cases have been

associated with familial cancer predisposition syndromes such as Lynch syndrome and familial adenomatous polyposis {645}.

Pathogenesis

Inflammation appears to be the main event in gallbladder carcinogenesis, including metabolic syndrome, in which the effects of growth factors, adipokines, and cytokines are believed to contribute to the risk {910}. It is believed that in these cases the carcinogenetic sequence involves inflammation, atrophy, metaplasia, dysplasia, and carcinoma, a process that may take decades. A distinct type of gallbladder injury called hyalinizing cholecystitis (also known as incomplete porcelain gallbladder) has also been identified with close association to GBC {2549}. It has been shown that selective mucosal calcification rather than the diffuse intramural calcification detected radiologically is the herald of the type of hyalinizing cholecystitis that has a substantial cancer risk {2549,3136}. Pancreatobiliary maljunction allows pancreatic enzymes to escape into the gallbladder and leads to a distinctive type of mucosal hyperplasia {2246}, followed by carcinogenesis that often undergoes a dysplasia–carcinoma sequence {2246}. In this disorder, a chemical phenomenon, not

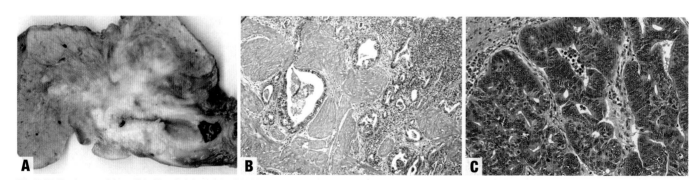

Fig. 9.17 Carcinoma of the gallbladder. **A** Advanced gallbladder cancer, gross appearance; note the scirrhous whitish thickening of the wall, absence of a polypoid mass protruding into the gallbladder lumen, and massive infiltration into the liver. Fragments of gallstones are present in the cystic duct and neck. **B** Well-differentiated adenocarcinoma infiltrating the gallbladder muscle layer, biliary type. **C** Adenocarcinoma of the gallbladder, intestinal type, resembling colonic adenocarcinoma.

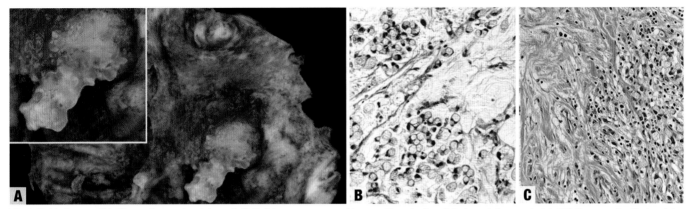

Fig. 9.18 Mucinous gallbladder carcinoma, signet-ring cell. **A** Nodular mucosa-covered tumour with protruding glistening gelatinous material. **B,C** Tumour cells with signet-ring morphology within the mucin pools and stroma.

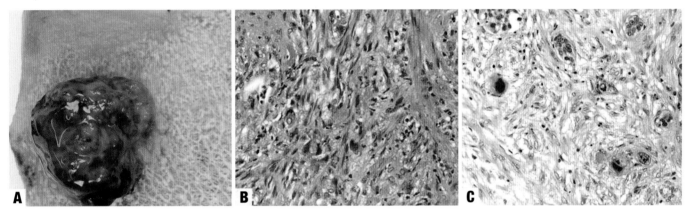

Fig. 9.19 Sarcomatoid gallbladder carcinoma. An example with a polypoid well-defined shape located in the fundus (**A**), exhibiting a spindle cell component (**B**); not infrequently, bizarre multinucleated giant tumour cells are noted (**C**).

necessarily inflammation, may be the culprit. Some carcinomas appear to arise in adenomyomas {2215}, but it remains to be determined whether these have a different etiopathogenesis or are dependent on the duration of chronic inflammation {878}.

Like other neoplasms, GBC is a product of the accumulation of multiple genetic alterations resulting from an interaction between a genetic predisposition and exposure to an environmental risk factor {340}. More than 50% of GBCs harbour *TP53* alterations {878}. Other more common mutations include alterations in *CDKN2A* or *CDKN2B* (19%), *ARID1A* (13%), *PIK3CA* (10%), and *CTNNB1* (10%). Amplifications of *ERBB2* (16%) have been reported {1462,1438}. Microsatellite instability and *CDKN2A* inactivation by promoter methylation have been reported in preinvasive and invasive lesions {2730}. The dysplasia–carcinoma sequence appears to go through different pathways, with paucity of mutations in *TP53* and *CDKN2A* and a higher frequency of mutations in *CTNNB1* (encoding β-catenin) {2890}. A higher *KRAS* mutation rate in lesions related to the pancreatobiliary maljunction but not in flat precursor lesions has been reported {3583,1811}.

Macroscopic appearance

Most GBCs (70%) arise in the fundus of the gallbladder. They are usually flat, firm, white, gritty, granular, and poorly defined tumours that typically grow diffusely. It is often difficult to distinguish carcinoma from chronic cholecystitis not only

preoperatively and in the operating room but also, as careful sampling studies from Chile elucidated, even with thorough macroscopic examination, which misses as many as 30% and 70% of advanced (pT2) and muscle-confined cases, respectively {2732}. GBCs arising from intracholecystic papillary neoplasms by definition have an exophytic component that can fill the lumen of the gallbladder {40}. Mucinous tumours have a more gelatinous appearance, and sarcomatoid and undifferentiated tumours might have a polypoid contour with fleshy appearance.

Histopathology

Adenocarcinoma is the most common subtype of GBC. The various patterns of adenocarcinoma are described below.

Biliary-type adenocarcinoma

Most ordinary GBCs belong to this group, which is also referred to as pancreatobiliary-type, because it is very similar in both morphology and behaviour to pancreatic ductal adenocarcinoma, being composed of widely separated tubular units lined by cuboidal to columnar cells embedded in a variably cellular or collagenized desmoplastic stroma. The cytoplasmic contents vary from case to case and between areas of a given case, and can range from more mucin-containing to foamy (also designated foamy gland adenocarcinoma) {41}, whereas some have more attenuated cytoplasm with a microcystic

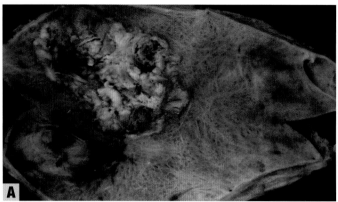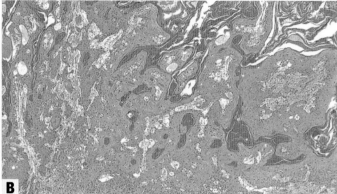

Fig. 9.20 Squamous cell carcinoma. An example with a broad-based polypoid mass located in the fundus. **A** The surface of the tumour is partially haemorrhagic. **B** Pure squamous cell carcinoma with extensive keratinization, including pearl formation and dyskeratotic cells.

glandular appearance. Some are exceedingly well differentiated to an extent that they can be difficult to distinguish from benign lesions. The vast majority of cases have the small tubular pattern, but some biliary adenocarcinomas exhibiting the large glandular pattern can have substantial papillary and cribriform areas. Poorly differentiated examples exhibit various patterns of growth, from single cells, cords, and nests to a sheet-like arrangement, often showing substantial pleomorphism and bizarre nuclei.

Micropapillary carcinoma as described in the lower pancreatobiliary tract or urothelium {1564,126} can also occur and raises concern for more aggressive dissemination potential. Of importance, ordinary biliary adenocarcinomas can be accompanied by any one of the other carcinoma types described below, but as long as the predominant pattern is the ordinary biliary type then the case is classified as such.

Some of the ordinary (biliary-type) adenocarcinomas display more cytoplasmic mucin with the nuclei compressed at the periphery, creating a picture reminiscent of gastric foveolar cells. Foamy gland adenocarcinomas have also been documented under this group by some authors. These adenocarcinomas have not been proven to be substantially different from ordinary biliary-type adenocarcinomas {87}.

Intestinal-type adenocarcinoma

Carcinomas with tubular configuration, more columnar cells, and elongated pseudostratified nuclei, resembling colonic adenocarcinomas, have been designated under the heading of "intestinal-type adenocarcinoma", but these appear to be very uncommon. In fact, if a carcinoma is displaying this morphology in the gallbladder, careful analysis is warranted to rule out involvement by a colonic adenocarcinoma. Distinctive features of colonic adenocarcinomas, including central necrosis, goblet cell–like intestinal mucin, and cellular basophilia, are uncommon in the gallbladder. An unusual subtype consisting of glands lined predominantly by goblet cells with variable amounts of Paneth and neuroendocrine cells has been described in this group {87}.

Mucinous adenocarcinoma

GBC shows some degree of stromal mucin deposition in approximately 7% of all cases, and a third fulfil the conventional criteria of > 50% of the tumour containing extracellular mucin.

These are similar to those arising in other anatomical sites, and some are mixed mucinous–signet-ring cell carcinomas. Pure colloid-type mucinous carcinoma is exceedingly uncommon in the gallbladder. Mucinous carcinomas are typically large and advanced at the time of diagnosis. They appear to exhibit more-aggressive behaviour than ordinary GBC, and unlike gastrointestinal mucinous carcinomas, they are microsatellite-stable {829}.

Clear cell carcinoma

Clear cell (hypernephroid) carcinoma is characterized by sheets of clear cells in an alveolar arrangement and separated by sinusoid vessels. Invariably, conventional patterns of ordinary adenocarcinoma growth are found somewhere in the tumour. It is an exceedingly uncommon type of carcinoma in the biliary tract {3442,92}. In fact, if it is a pure pattern, then the possibility of a metastatic clear cell renal carcinoma should be considered foremost.

Poorly cohesive carcinoma with or without signet-ring cells

These carcinomas are now defined as they are in the GI tract (in particular the stomach). They are characterized by individual cell (poorly cohesive cell) and cord-like patterns forming the diffuse infiltrative growth in which the cells dissect through the tissue planes, leaving the underlying structures such as the musculature intact, resulting in the linitis plastica pattern grossly {3365}. Plasmacytoid cells (as described in the urothelium) and signet-ring cells characterized by abundant mucin pushing the nucleus to the periphery and thus creating the signet-ring cell cytology occur in some cases but are not a requirement. As many as 8% of conventional biliary-type carcinomas in the gallbladder exhibit a focal component of this pattern. Tumours composed predominantly of this pattern occur rarely. They are more frequent in women and clinically show a behaviour more aggressive than that of ordinary GBC {3365}.

Adenosquamous carcinoma

Focal squamous differentiation is found in approximately 5% of gallbladder carcinomas {2731}. If squamous elements constitute a substantial part of the tumour (> 25%), the neoplasm is best classified as an adenosquamous carcinoma. Glandular and squamous components of the tumours have corresponding immunophenotypes. Additional sampling often reveals the adenocarcinoma component in a seemingly pure squamous cell carcinoma.

Squamous cell carcinoma

Bona fide examples of pure squamous cell carcinoma with squamous cell carcinoma in situ as well are exceedingly uncommon {2731}. They often show substantial keratinization. Like in the pancreas and breast, squamous differentiation appears to confer an even more aggressive behaviour on GBCs, with more-advanced presentation and worse prognosis {2731}.

Other differentiation patterns

Some carcinomas have an undifferentiated (non-glandular, nondescript) morphology. Some form patchy solid clusters of carcinoma cells without evidence of glandular differentiation. Various subtypes are recognized. Some form stroma-poor sheets of cells akin to medullary carcinomas of the GI tract, some also exhibiting the cytology of lymphoepithelioma-like carcinomas of the upper aerodigestive tract, although not yet with proven association with EBV {1114}.

Bona fide primary hepatoid carcinomas (as proven with the presence of high-grade dysplasia and/or a mixed ordinary adenocarcinoma component in the gallbladder, without pre-existing hepatocellular carcinoma) also occur and can show Hep Par-1 positivity, but they must be distinguished from hepatocellular carcinoma invading the gallbladder.

Sarcomatoid carcinoma with spindle cell morphology can also occur in the gallbladder. Sarcomatoid components may be subtle and fibroblast-like, but they are more commonly pleomorphic (including giant cells) or may show evidence of

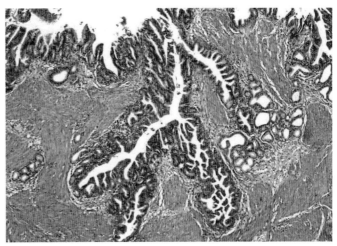

Fig. 9.22 Rokitansky–Aschoff involvement. Extension of a high-grade intraepithelial neoplasia into a Rokitansky–Aschoff sinus. Note the complexity of the micropapillary pattern.

heterologous differentiation (i.e. skeletal muscle, bone, and cartilage) {172,3184,2370}.

Differential diagnosis

Rokitansky–Aschoff sinuses and adenomyomatous changes can be difficult to distinguish from carcinomas that exhibit smaller, more densely packed glands with cellular atypia and often open round lumina or angulated contours sometimes oriented parallel to the mucosal surface, as well as carcinomas arising in hyalinizing cholecystitis {90}. Luschka ducts may have

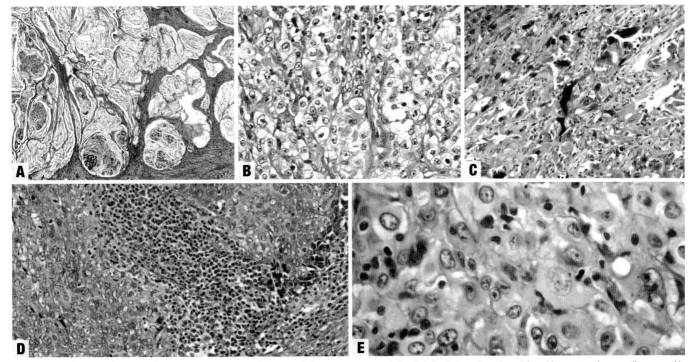

Fig. 9.21 Carcinoma of the gallbladder. **A** Colloid carcinoma with > 90% of the tumour composed of well-defined stromal mucin nodules with scant carcinoma cells encased in the mucin. **B** Clear cell carcinoma. Clear cell carcinoma change characterized by optically clear cytoplasm and distinct cell borders, mimicking renal cell carcinoma. **C** Undifferentiated carcinoma. Undifferentiated carcinomas exhibiting bizarre, pleomorphic tumour giant cells are occasionally identified. **D** Medullary carcinoma. The medullary pattern shows a syncytial growth; the cell borders are not distinct, with pushing borders and a predominantly lymphocytic infiltrate. **E** Hepatoid carcinoma. The hepatoid pattern is composed of polygonal cells with abundant eosinophilic cytoplasm; nuclei are centrally located and nuclei are usually prominent.

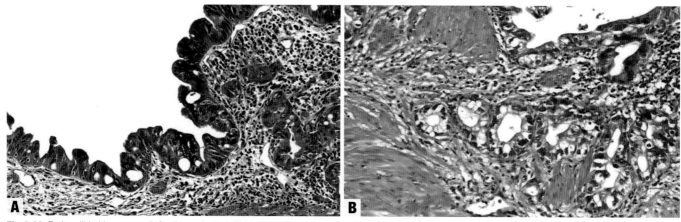

Fig. 9.23 Early gallbladder cancer. **A** Carcinoma in situ (pTis) in the surface, with conventional lamina propria infiltration (pT1a) underneath. **B** Well-differentiated adenocarcinoma focally infiltrating the muscle bundles (pT1b).

a proliferative atypical and pseudoinfiltrative appearance; however, this process is usually confined to the subhepatic area {3051}. No molecular or immunohistochemical markers are reliable to make these distinctions.

Cytology
Because many cases are undiagnosed before cholecystectomy and many of the unresectable overt carcinomas are diagnosable by radiology, FNA of the gallbladder is seldom used. However, in some parts of India where GBC is common, FNA is performed to confirm the diagnosis. These cases illustrate the corresponding cytology established in other sites of the pancreatobiliary tract {3635}.

Diagnostic molecular pathology
Early clinical data support the potential benefit of ERBB2 (HER2) immunohistochemistry to guide targeted therapy {2308A}. Clinical trial data are awaited. Microsatellite instability has been demonstrated and may have therapeutic implications in the future {3044}.

Essential and desirable diagnostic criteria
Essential: adenocarcinoma arising within the gallbladder showing invasion into at least the lamina propria; epithelia recapitulating other parts of the GI tract commonly occur; squamous or undifferentiated carcinoma occasionally occurs.
Desirable: may arise from intracholecystic papillary neoplasm; must exclude invasion from liver or metastases.

Staging (TNM)
The Union for International Cancer Control (UICC) TNM staging system for GBC has been extrapolated from the staging of other GI tract cancers, but only with limited data. Currently, the T1 category is divided into two subsets: T1a, invasion into lamina propria, and T1b, into tunica muscularis; however, studies have shown that reproducible classification of these minute invasions is not possible {2732}, with marked variations in the application of the criteria between different continents, similar to the controversy about intramucosal adenocarcinomas

of the GI tract. In high-risk regions where these cancers are seen much more commonly, a more practical approach with good prognostic correlation has been developed, categorizing Tis/T1a/T1b cancers into the category "early GBC (EGBC)". However, before a case can be classified as EGBC, total sampling of the specimen to rule out T2 (perimuscular invasion) is warranted, because small T2 foci are easy to miss otherwise {2729}. Of note, preliminary studies indicate that the amount/depth of perimuscular invasion may also be of importance, and cases that have only very minimal T2 invasion may have a prognosis closer to that of EGBC, if total sampling is performed to exclude deeper invasion {2729}.

Prognosis and prediction
If perimuscular invasion (T2) has been ruled out by total sampling of the gallbladder, muscle-confined (EGBC) cases may be curable in most instances {2729}. A small percentage of such cases that experience early progression are attributed to missed invasive carcinomas. There is also another small percentage that develop biliary tract cancers many years after the cholecystectomy despite being EGBC, and this group is attributed to the field effect rendering the biliary tract at risk. The extent of mucosal carcinoma, Rokitansky–Aschoff sinus involvement, and cystic duct margin status are suspected predictors of progression {2732,2729}.

Some T2 carcinomas that are very superficial/limited may also be successfully treated, but deeply invasive tumours are aggressive, with a 5-year overall survival rate ranging from 45% to 70%. These survival differences appear to be unrelated to pathological criteria and sampling, and reflect population or diagnosis/management differences.

Recently, only for T2 carcinomas, the demonstration of the location of the carcinoma as being serosal or hepatic surface oriented has been found to show differences in survival, and this parameter was therefore added to the TNM staging system as T2a and T2b {3020}. Whether the new T2a versus T2b (serosal vs hepatic localization of T2 cancer, respectively) is reproducible and will be a useful prognosticator remains to be seen {113,3020}.

Carcinoma of the extrahepatic bile ducts

Roa JC
Adsay NV
Arola J
Tsui WM
Zen Y

Definition

Carcinoma of the extrahepatic bile ducts (EHBDs) is a primary malignant epithelial neoplasm arising in the EHBDs.

ICD-O coding

8160/3 Cholangiocarcinoma
8070/3 Squamous cell carcinoma NOS
8560/3 Adenosquamous carcinoma
8020/3 Carcinoma, undifferentiated, NOS

ICD-11 coding

2C15.0 Adenocarcinoma of biliary tract, distal bile duct & XH7M15 Cholangiocarcinoma NOS

Related terminology

Acceptable: extrahepatic cholangiocarcinoma; bile duct cystadenocarcinoma.

Subtype(s)

None

Localization

The carcinomas arise in the extrahepatic hepatic ducts or common bile duct. Those arising in the hepatic ducts are referred to as perihilar.

Clinical features

Most patients with carcinoma of the EHBDs are in the sixth or seventh decade of life. Unlike in gallbladder carcinoma, there is no female predominance, presumably due to lack of association with gallstones.

Unlike those of the gallbladder, carcinomas of the EHBDs usually present relatively early with obstructive jaundice, which can rapidly progress or fluctuate. Jaundice usually appears while the neoplasm is relatively small, and it precedes widespread dissemination. Other symptoms include right upper quadrant pain, malaise, weight loss, pruritus, anorexia, nausea, and vomiting. If cholangitis develops, chills and fever appear.

Transhepatic cholangiograms and endoscopic retrograde cholangiopancreatography are essential for determining the exact localization of carcinomas of the EHBDs.

Early-stage biliary tract cancers are now detectable. The most useful imaging techniques are MRI and endoscopic retrograde cholangiopancreatography, EUS, and PET. Their role, after excluding metastatic disease, is to determine the T stage, which guides surgical management. Typically, the main imaging features are biliary duct obstruction (as evidenced by proximal ductal dilatation), periductal thickening, and enhancement {1215}.

Epidemiology

The incidence of EHBD carcinoma varies from 0.53 to 2 cases per 100 000 person-years worldwide, with higher frequency in Asian countries, in particular the Republic of Korea and Thailand {406}.

Etiology

Biliary conditions leading to chronic inflammation, such as primary sclerosing cholangitis (PSC), bile duct cysts, Caroli disease, and cholelithiasis, are known risk factors for carcinoma

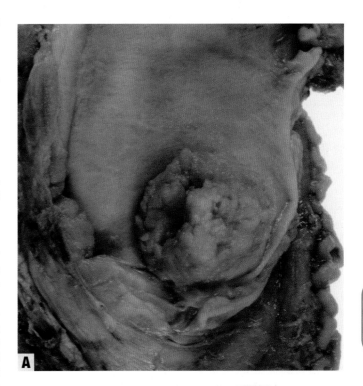

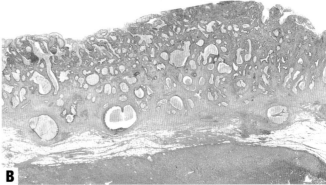

Fig. 9.24 Extrahepatic bile duct carcinoma. **A** Macroscopic photo of polypoid and papillary carcinoma involving the extrahepatic bile duct. **B** Low-power photomicrograph showing invasion to the level of the muscularis mucosae.

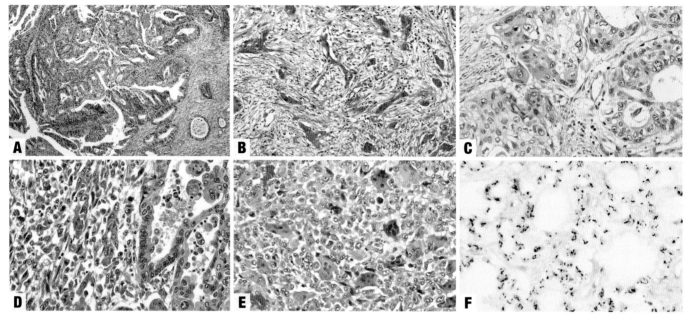

Fig. 9.25 Carcinoma of the extrahepatic bile ducts. **A** Moderately differentiated adenocarcinoma; cancer cells with intestinal-type features are arranged in a complex tubulopapillary architecture. **B** Poorly differentiated carcinoma with widely spaced epithelial nests and strands in a desmoplastic stroma. **C** Adenosquamous carcinoma. Both glandular differentiation and squamous differentiation are present. **D** Sarcomatous carcinoma. In addition to the adenocarcinoma component (right), sarcomatoid transformation with diffuse proliferation of spindle-shaped tumour cells is seen (left). **E** Undifferentiated carcinoma with osteoclast-like giant cells. Many giant cells are present against the background of diffusely arranged polygonal cancer cells. Adenocarcinoma components were also present elsewhere. **F** Extrahepatic bile duct carcinoma. *MDM2* amplification; dual-colour in situ hybridization reveals many clustered signals for *MDM2*. Dark-brown dots represent *MDM2* and red signals indicate a chromosome 12 control.

of the EHBDs {3373}. The risk of cholangiocarcinoma among patients with PSC seems to be higher among male patients and patients with inflammatory activity in bile duct cytology. Certain bile microbiota may also be associated with development of biliary neoplasia {390,389,2567}. Inflammatory bowel disease as a risk factor for cholangiocarcinoma is related to coexisting PSC. In south-eastern Asia, endemic parasites (in particular *Opisthorchis viverrini* and *Clonorchis sinensis*) are the main etiological factor for extrahepatic cholangiocarcinoma (eCCA) {3770}. Recently discovered risk factors for eCCA from large US cohort data included various metabolic conditions, type 1 diabetes, chronic pancreatitis, and gout. Smoking is also a risk factor for eCCA {2577}. Occupational exposure to 1,2-dichloropropane is a plausible risk factor for cholangiocarcinoma {1717}.

Pathogenesis

Two types of precursor lesions are thought to precede the development and progression of EHBD carcinoma: biliary intraepithelial neoplasia and intraductal papillary neoplasm of the bile ducts {1637}. Biliary intraepithelial neoplasia and intraductal papillary neoplasm of the extrahepatic and intrahepatic biliary tree share similar morphological and immunophenotypical features (see the above sections).

Genetic features vary widely among cases of extrahepatic biliary malignancy. *TP53* is mutated in about 50% of cases {2283}, typically in the late stage of the carcinogenetic process. *KRAS* mutations, considered to be an early event, are observed in 20–30% of eCCAs. *MDM2* amplification occurs in 12% of perihilar cholangiocarcinomas {1595}, but this genetic event appears to be exceptional in distal cholangiocarcinomas {1595}.

Intrahepatic and eCCAs share some alterations in several genes (*TP53*, *KRAS*, *SMAD4*, *ARID1A*, *GNAS*). EHBD cancer–specific alterations are *PRKACA/PRKACB* fusion, *ELF3* mutation, and *ARID1B* mutation (see Fig. 9.16, p. 284) {3001,3528}.

Macroscopic appearance

Macroscopically, EHBD carcinomas can present as sclerosing, nodular, or papillary types. The sclerosing type is most common and causes annular constrictive thickening of the bile ducts. Often the gross boundaries of the carcinoma are difficult to determine with certainty.

Histopathology

Most of the carcinomas are pancreatobiliary-type adenocarcinomas, characterized by widely spaced, well-formed irregular glands and small cell clusters associated with a sclerotic desmoplastic stroma, often with perineural infiltration and lymphovascular invasion. Other histological patterns of adenocarcinoma include intestinal-type, foveolar-type, mucinous, signet-ring cell, clear cell, pyloric gland {84}, hepatoid {3521}, and invasive micropapillary {3716}. Rare types of EHBD carcinoma include squamous cell, adenosquamous, sarcomatoid, and undifferentiated carcinomas.

Adenocarcinoma should be distinguished from reactive periductal glands. Involvement by pancreatic ductal adenocarcinoma is indistinguishable by histological features and immunophenotypes.

Cytology

Because histological sampling from EHBDs is often not possible, brush cytology is usually the primary sampling method for EHBD carcinoma. Where available, cholangioscopy biopsies also have moderate sensitivity for biliary neoplasia {2327}. In a PSC cohort meta-analysis, the sensitivity of brush cytology was only 43%, but the specificity was 97% {3340}. Adequate sampling is mandatory. Features suggestive of malignancy include irregularities of nuclear contour, increased N:C ratio, nuclear pleomorphism and overlapping coarse or pale chromatin, prominent nucleoli, 3D cell clusters, polarity disorders, and high mitotic activity. Another helpful feature is the existence of two distinguishable populations of cells: one benign and the other clearly neoplastic {3704,352}. Coexisting inflammatory activity with regenerative and inflammatory atypia found in the brush cytology of patients with PSC makes diagnosis of neoplasia more difficult. The distinction of invasive rather than in situ growth cannot be made from the brush cytology. The diagnostic value of cytology can be improved using immunohistochemical and molecular techniques, for example demonstration of *TP53* and *KRAS* mutations. Ploidy analysis using FISH, DNA flow cytometry, or digital image analysis can improve the sensitivity for detecting malignancy {1923,1065,390}.

Diagnostic molecular pathology
Molecular investigation is not required for diagnosis.

Essential and desirable diagnostic criteria
Essential: presence of an adenocarcinoma or more rarely a squamous carcinoma within the EHBDs or cystic duct; adjacent high-grade dysplasia may be present; multiple histological patterns may be present.

Staging (TNM)
Carcinoma of the EHBDs is staged according to the Union for International Cancer Control (UICC) TNM classification of tumours of the perihilar bile duct or distal EHBD, depending on the location of the tumour.

Prognosis and prediction
The stage of disease at presentation is the most important determination of prognosis {954,1269,838}. Resectability is another critical factor associated with outcome, with the 5-year overall survival rate estimated to be 20–30% for resectable

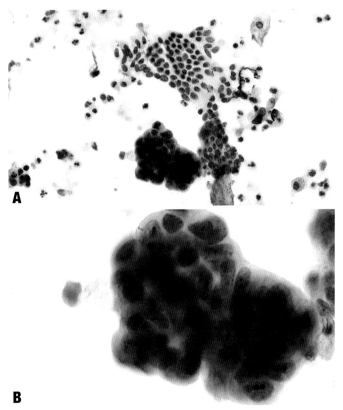

Fig. 9.26 Biliary epithelium suspicious for neoplasia/dysplasia. **A** Both normal epithelium and neoplastic epithelium are present. **B** Higher power shows a cluster of neoplastic cells with pleomorphic nuclei, prominent nucleoli, and a mitosis.

EHBD cancers, whereas it declines to almost 0% for unresectable cases {759,3717,3020}. Patients with papillary cholangiocarcinoma have a better prognosis than those with non-papillary cancer {976}. Other microscopic factors associated with poor prognosis include poor differentiation, vascular invasion, and perineural infiltration {2729}.

Neuroendocrine neoplasms of the gallbladder and bile ducts

Adsay NV
La Rosa S

Definition

Neuroendocrine neoplasms (NENs) of the gallbladder and bile ducts are biliary tract epithelial neoplasms with neuroendocrine differentiation, including well-differentiated neuroendocrine tumours (NETs) and poorly differentiated neuroendocrine carcinomas (NECs).

ICD-O coding

8240/3 Neuroendocrine tumour NOS
8246/3 Neuroendocrine carcinoma NOS
8154/3 Mixed neuroendocrine–non-neuroendocrine neoplasm (MiNEN)

ICD-11 coding

2C14.2 & XH55D7 Neuroendocrine neoplasms of cystic duct & Neuroendocrine carcinoma, well-differentiated
2C14.2 & XH9LV8 Neuroendocrine neoplasms of cystic duct & Neuroendocrine tumour, grade I
2C14.2 & XH7F73 Neuroendocrine neoplasms of cystic duct & Neuroendocrine carcinoma, moderately differentiated
2C14.2 & XH0U20 Neuroendocrine neoplasms of cystic duct & Neuroendocrine carcinoma NOS
2C14.2 & XH9SY0 Neuroendocrine neoplasms of cystic duct & Small cell neuroendocrine carcinoma
2C14.2 & XH0NL5 Neuroendocrine neoplasms of cystic duct & Large cell neuroendocrine carcinoma
2C14.2 & XH6H10 Neuroendocrine neoplasms of cystic duct & Mixed adenoneuroendocrine carcinoma

Related terminology

NET
Not recommended: carcinoid; well-differentiated endocrine tumour/carcinoma.

NEC
Acceptable: poorly differentiated endocrine carcinoma; high-grade neuroendocrine carcinoma; small cell endocrine carcinoma; large cell endocrine carcinoma.

Subtype(s)

Neuroendocrine tumour, grade 1 (8240/3); neuroendocrine tumour, grade 2 (8249/3); neuroendocrine tumour, grade 3 (8249/3); large cell neuroendocrine carcinoma (8013/3); small cell neuroendocrine carcinoma (8041/3)

Localization

NENs are more common in the gallbladder than in the bile ducts. In the gallbladder, NECs seem to substantially outnumber NETs {2689,574,1503,3634}. Both NETs and NECs can involve any portion of the gallbladder (fundus, body, or neck).

Extrahepatic bile duct (EHBD) NENs may arise throughout, but are more common in the distal common bile duct {850,2616}, with a predilection for junctional/transitional areas of EHBD {1577,1286,3101}.

Clinical features

Gallbladder NETs are usually detected incidentally after cholecystectomy or because of nonspecific abdominal symptoms. EHBD NETs can produce bile duct obstruction {2798}. Rare cases produce gastrin, leading to Zollinger–Ellison syndrome {2060,2616}.

The primary clinical symptom of NEC is abdominal pain. Other findings include abdominal distension or mass, jaundice, weight loss, and ascites {2368,1503,3634}. Cushing syndrome {3111} or other paraneoplastic syndromes such as sensory neuropathy {3390} and hyponatraemia {2832} may be seen occasionally.

Epidemiology

NETs of the gallbladder and bile ducts are extremely rare, estimated to account for 0.2% and 0.01%, respectively, of all NETs {2187,3634}. NETs are slightly more common in females and in the early to mid-seventh decade of life {81}. NECs account for 4% of all malignant gallbladder neoplasms {2689}. NECs also show female predominance and present at an average age in the early to mid-seventh decade of life (age range: 26–93 years) {2689,81,1503,574}.

Etiology

The cause of NENs of the gallbladder and bile ducts is unknown. Some NETs are associated with von Hippel–Lindau syndrome (VHL) and multiple endocrine neoplasia type 1. Gallbladder NEC etiology seems to be closer to that of adenocarcinomas and is therefore frequently associated with gallstones {2689} and to a lesser extent pancreatobiliary maljunction {2247,2084}.

Pathogenesis

Some gallbladder and EHBD NETs may be associated with VHL {2266,3064} and multiple endocrine neoplasia type 1 {2616}. Microsatellite instability has been identified in occasional small cell NECs (SCNECs) of the gallbladder {1885}.

Few studies have addressed genetic alterations in NENs of the gallbladder and EHBDs {1908,1885}. Mutations of *TP53*, *KRAS*, and *SMAD4* appear not to play a substantial role in the pathogenesis of NETs {2010}. Accumulation of p53 and inactivation of the RB1/p16 pathway have been found in most NECs of the gallbladder {2689,2537}. Expression of SMAD4 protein is usually retained, and *KRAS* mutations are rare {2011,2537}. Somatic alterations in *ERBB4*, *HRAS*, *NRG1*, *HMCN1*, and *CDH10*; fusions (*NCAM2-SGCZ* and *BTG3-CCDC40*); and genome-wide copy-number variations and microsatellite instability have also been identified in SCNECs of the gallbladder {1885}.

Macroscopic appearance

NETs are usually small (generally < 2 cm), greyish-white or yellow submucosal nodules {88,850,2436,933}. Tumours are pedunculated {1497,2436} or polypoid, mimicking papillary bile duct neoplasms {1321,3314}. Multifocality has been rarely reported {2480}.

Histopathology

Tumours appear nodular {2368}, often have a substantial polypoid component {1594,1726,3652}, and tend to be associated with an intraepithelial papillary neoplasm {40,2689,2247}. These neoplasms can be quite large and may extensively involve the duct system and invade the liver and adjacent tissues {2011,1569}.

NET tumour cells are arranged in nests, trabeculae, and occasionally tubules {3088}; they have uniform round to oval nuclei, inconspicuous nucleoli, and a fair amount of cytoplasm on cytology {3634}.

Tumour cells are immunoreactive for synaptophysin {2010}, chromogranin A {147,3045}, and keratins {3064}, as well as hormones to a variable degree {147,2010,2060,1676}. Clear cell NETs of the gallbladder are characterized by foamy non-glycogenated, non-mucinous cytoplasm. Some clear cell NETs are associated with VHL {1676,3064,3314}. NENs associated with VHL may be positive for inhibin, unlike sporadic cases {1676,3314}.

NECs encompass small cell and large cell subtypes as defined in the lungs {2689,1503,1726,2011}. Small cell carcinomas are composed of moulded round or fusiform cells with hyperchromatic nuclei and inconspicuous nucleoli, arranged in sheets, nests, cords, and festoons {2689,3634}. Rosette-like structures and tubules are occasionally present. Large cell NEC (LCNEC) displays organoid growth with rosette formation and is composed of large, monotonous or pleomorphic cells with vesicular nuclei, prominent nucleoli, and variable amounts of cytoplasm {1487,2506,3634}. NECs show a characteristically high proliferation index, with brisk mitotic activity and single-cell and confluent necrosis {2689,1503}. Occasionally, tumour giant cells are observed {88,2689,2011}. NEC shows diffuse positivity for epithelial markers (AE1/AE3) and variable positivity for neuroendocrine markers (synaptophysin staining is often diffuse and strong, and chromogranin A staining is often patchy) {2689}. Overexpression of p53 and loss of RB1 are common findings {2537}. TTF1 staining may be seen, particularly in SCNEC. Loss of ATRX or DAXX is uncommon {2689}.

More than a third of NECs are accompanied by an adenocarcinoma component (mixed neuroendocrine–non-neuroendocrine neoplasm [MiNEN]) {1514,1503,3634}. The presence and extent of the NEC component should be acknowledged, because this component is the primary driver of behaviour and clinical management {1514,1503}.

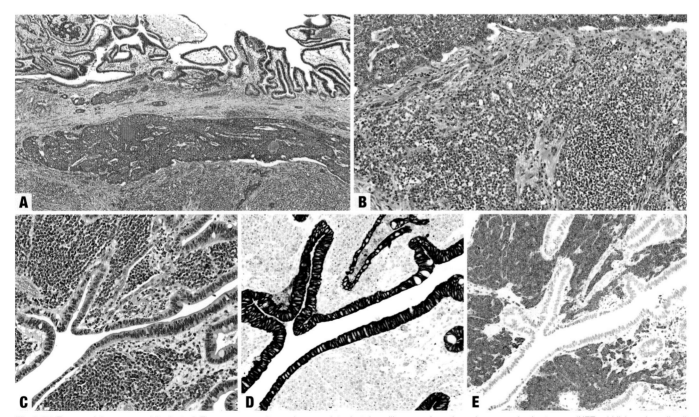

Fig. 9.27 Tumour of the common bile duct. **A** Three components can be seen: intraductal papillary neoplasm (upper), neuroendocrine tumour (NET; middle), and small cell neuroendocrine carcinoma (SCNEC; lower). **B** At higher magnification. **C,D,E** The small cell carcinoma component is seen in the cores of the papillae; it is positive for CAM5.2 in a dot pattern (**D**) and synaptophysin (**E**).

Cytology

NENs of the gallbladder and bile ducts are seldom aspirated, because of the inaccessibility of these sites and the rarity of these tumours. Their cytological characteristics are similar to those in other organs {3634}. In NECs, moulding, smudge cells, and high cellular turnover (due to mitotic activity, necrosis, and apoptosis) are common.

Diagnostic molecular pathology

Not clinically relevant

Essential and desirable diagnostic criteria

The diagnostic criteria are similar to those of NETs and NECs elsewhere in the GI tract.

Staging (TNM)

NENs of the gallbladder and bile ducts are generally staged like other gallbladder carcinomas.

Prognosis and prediction

The data on prognosis of NETs of the gallbladder and bile ducts is highly limited because of the rarity of these tumours; however, their prognosis seems to be similar to that of NETs in the GI tract. Metastases and locally invasive progression can occur {147,2106,148}. The risk of malignant behaviour largely depends on tumour size {88}. NETs > 2 cm often extend into the liver and/or metastasize {850}. Approximately one third of patients with bile duct NETs exhibit metastases at diagnosis {850}. Aggressive surgical therapy offers the only chance for cure and should be considered whenever possible {1125,1413,2188}. In one study analysing a national database, the 10-year survival rates were 36% for gallbladder NETs and 80% for EHBD NETs {81}.

NECs have a poor prognosis {1487,1503}. More than half of all patients have disseminated disease at diagnosis {2689,1503,974}. SCNEC appears to be highly responsive to cisplatinum-based chemotherapy as well as radiotherapy, and survival times of > 1 year have been reported by some, using regimens similar to those for small cell carcinoma of lung {974}. The median survival time is < 1 year {1503}, and the 5-year and 10-year survival rates are 20% and 0%, respectively {2689,513,1503,81}.

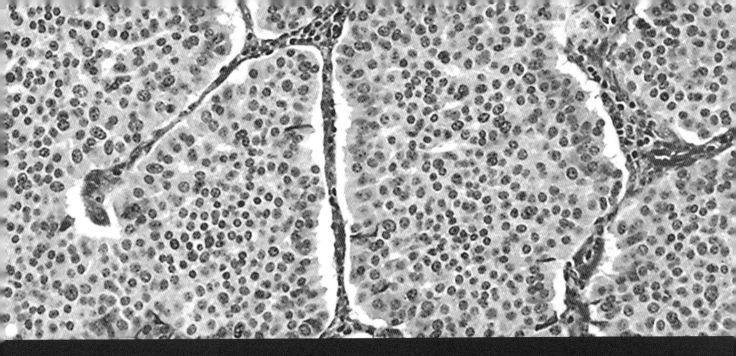

10

Tumours of the pancreas

Edited by: Gill AJ, Klimstra DS, Lam AK, Washington MK

Benign epithelial tumours and precursors
    Acinar cystic transformation
    Serous neoplasms
    Intraepithelial neoplasia
    Intraductal papillary mucinous neoplasm
    Intraductal oncocytic papillary neoplasm
    Intraductal tubulopapillary neoplasm
    Mucinous cystic neoplasm
Malignant epithelial tumours
    Ductal adenocarcinoma
    Acinar cell carcinoma
    Pancreatoblastoma
    Solid pseudopapillary neoplasm

Neuroendocrine neoplasms
    Non-functioning neuroendocrine tumours
    Functioning neuroendocrine tumours
        Insulinoma
        Gastrinoma
        VIPoma
        Glucagonoma
        Somatostatinoma
        ACTH-producing neuroendocrine tumour
        Serotonin-producing neuroendocrine tumour
    Neuroendocrine carcinoma
    MiNENs

WHO classification of tumours of the pancreas

Benign epithelial tumours and precursors

8441/0	Serous cystadenoma NOS
	Macrocystic (oligocystic) serous cystadenoma
	Solid serous adenoma
	Von Hippel–Lindau syndrome–associated serous cystic neoplasm
	Mixed serous-neuroendocrine neoplasm
8441/3	Serous cystadenocarcinoma NOS
8148/0	Glandular intraepithelial neoplasia, low grade
8148/2	Glandular intraepithelial neoplasia, high grade
8453/0	Intraductal papillary mucinous neoplasm with low-grade dysplasia
8453/2	Intraductal papillary mucinous neoplasm with high-grade dysplasia
8453/3	Intraductal papillary mucinous neoplasm with associated invasive carcinoma
8455/2*	Intraductal oncocytic papillary neoplasm NOS
8455/3*	Intraductal oncocytic papillary neoplasm with associated invasive carcinoma
8503/2	Intraductal tubulopapillary neoplasm
8503/3	Intraductal papillary neoplasm with associated invasive carcinoma
8470/0	Mucinous cystic neoplasm with low-grade dysplasia
8470/2	Mucinous cystic neoplasm with high-grade dysplasia
8470/3	Mucinous cystic neoplasm with associated invasive carcinoma

Malignant epithelial tumours

8500/3	Duct adenocarcinoma NOS
8480/3	Colloid carcinoma
8490/3	Poorly cohesive carcinoma
8490/3	Signet-ring cell carcinoma
8510/3	Medullary carcinoma NOS
8560/3	Adenosquamous carcinoma
8576/3	Hepatoid carcinoma
8014/3	Large cell carcinoma with rhabdoid phenotype
8020/3	Carcinoma, undifferentiated, NOS
8035/3	Undifferentiated carcinoma with osteoclast-like giant cells
8550/3	Acinar cell carcinoma
8551/3	Acinar cell cystadenocarcinoma
8154/3	Mixed acinar-neuroendocrine carcinoma
8154/3	Mixed acinar-endocrine-ductal carcinoma
8552/3	Mixed acinar-ductal carcinoma
8971/3	Pancreatoblastoma
8452/3	Solid pseudopapillary neoplasm of the pancreas
	Solid pseudopapillary neoplasm with high-grade carcinoma

Pancreatic neuroendocrine neoplasms

8150/0	Pancreatic neuroendocrine microadenoma
8240/3	Neuroendocrine tumour NOS
8240/3	Neuroendocrine tumour, grade 1
8249/3	Neuroendocrine tumour, grade 2
8249/3	Neuroendocrine tumour, grade 3
8150/3	Pancreatic neuroendocrine tumour, non-functioning
	Oncocytic neuroendocrine tumour, non-functioning pancreatic
	Pleomorphic neuroendocrine tumour, non-functioning pancreatic
	Clear cell neuroendocrine tumour, non-functioning pancreatic
	Cystic neuroendocrine tumour, non-functioning pancreatic

Functioning pancreatic neuroendocrine tumours

8151/3*	Insulinoma
8153/3*	Gastrinoma
8155/3*	VIPoma
8152/3*	Glucagonoma
8156/3*	Somatostatinoma
8158/3	ACTH-producing tumour
8241/3	Enterochromaffin-cell carcinoid
8241/3	Serotonin-producing tumour
8246/3	Neuroendocrine carcinoma NOS
8013/3	Large cell neuroendocrine carcinoma
8041/3	Small cell neuroendocrine carcinoma
8154/3	Mixed neuroendocrine–non-neuroendocrine neoplasm (MiNEN)
8154/3	Mixed acinar-endocrine carcinoma
8154/3	Mixed acinar-neuroendocrine carcinoma
8154/3	Mixed acinar-endocrine-ductal carcinoma

These morphology codes are from the International Classification of Diseases for Oncology, third edition, second revision (ICD-O-3.2) {1378A}. Behaviour is coded /0 for benign tumours; /1 for unspecified, borderline, or uncertain behaviour; /2 for carcinoma in situ and grade III intraepithelial neoplasia; /3 for malignant tumours, primary site; and /6 for malignant tumours, metastatic site. Behaviour code /6 is not generally used by cancer registries.

This classification is modified from the previous WHO classification, taking into account changes in our understanding of these lesions.

* Codes marked with an asterisk were approved by the IARC/WHO Committee for ICD-O at its meeting in April 2019.

TNM staging of carcinomas of the pancreas

Pancreas
(ICD-O-3 C25)

Rules for Classification
The classification applies to carcinomas of the exocrine pancreas and/or high-grade neuroendocrine carcinomas. Well-differentiated neuroendocrine tumours of the pancreas are classified as shown on p. 20. There should be histological or cytological confirmation of the disease.

The following are the procedures for assessing T, N, and M categories.

T categories	Physical examination, imaging, and/or surgical exploration
N categories	Physical examination, imaging, and/or surgical exploration
M categories	Physical examination, imaging, and/or surgical exploration

Anatomical Subsites
C25.0 Head of pancreas[a]
C25.1 Body of pancreas[b]
C25.2 Tail of pancreas[c]
C25.3 Pancreatic duct

Notes
[a] Tumours of the head of the pancreas are those arising to the right of the left border of the superior mesenteric vein. The uncinate process is considered as part of the head.
[b] Tumours of the body are those arising between the left border of the superior mesenteric vein and left border of the aorta.
[c] Tumours of the tail are those arising between the left border of the aorta and the hilum of the spleen.

Regional Lymph Nodes
The regional lymph nodes for tumours in the head and neck of the pancreas are the lymph nodes along the common bile duct, common hepatic artery, portal vein, pyloric, infrapyloric, subpyloric, proximal mesenteric, coeliac, posterior, and anterior pancreaticoduodenal vessels, and along the superior mesenteric vein and right lateral wall of the superior mesenteric artery.

The regional lymph nodes for tumours in body and tail are the lymph nodes along the common hepatic artery, coeliac axis, splenic artery, and splenic hilum, as well as retroperitoneal nodes and lateral aortic nodes.

TNM Clinical Classification
T – Primary Tumour
TX   Primary tumour cannot be assessed
T0   No evidence of primary tumour
Tis   Carcinoma in situ*
T1   Tumour 2 cm or less in greatest dimension
   T1a   Tumour 0.5 cm or less in greatest dimension
   T1b   Tumour greater than 0.5 cm and no more than 1 cm in greatest dimension
   T1c   Tumour greater than 1 cm but no more than 2 cm in greatest dimension
T2   Tumour more than 2 cm but no more than 4 cm in greatest dimension
T3   Tumour more than 4 cm in greatest dimension
T4   Tumour involves coeliac axis, superior mesenteric artery and/or common hepatic artery

Note
* Tis also includes the 'PanIN-III' classification.

N – Regional Lymph Nodes
NX   Regional lymph nodes cannot be assessed
N0   No regional lymph node metastasis
N1   Metastases in 1 to 3 regional lymph node(s)
N2   Metastases in 4 or more regional lymph nodes

M – Distant Metastasis
M0   No distant metastasis
M1   Distant metastasis

pTNM Pathological Classification
The pT and pN categories correspond to the T and N categories.

pN0   Histological examination of a regional lymphadenectomy specimen will ordinarily include 12 or more lymph nodes. If the lymph nodes are negative, but the number ordinarily examined is not met, classify as pN0.

pM – Distant Metastasis*
pM1   Distant metastasis microscopically confirmed

Note
* pM0 and pMX are not valid categories.

Stage – Pancreas

Stage	T	N	M
Stage 0	Tis	N0	M0
Stage IA	T1	N0	M0
Stage IB	T2	N0	M0
Stage IIA	T3	N0	M0
Stage IIB	T1,T2,T3	N1	M0
Stage III	T1,T2,T3	N2	M0
	T4	Any N	M0
Stage IV	Any T	Any N	M1

Note: Neuroendocrine tumours (NETs) of the pancreas are staged using the NET-specific TNM staging system, which is presented in Chapter 1 (p. 20).

The information presented here has been excerpted from the 2017 *TNM classification of malignant tumours*, eighth edition {408,3385A}. © 2017 UICC.
A help desk for specific questions about the TNM classification is available at https://www.uicc.org/tnm-help-desk.

Chapter 10

Tumours of the pancreas: Introduction

Klimstra DS
Gill AJ
Washington MK

The ICD-O topographical coding for the anatomical sites covered in this chapter is presented in Box 10.01. The classification of pancreatic neoplasms is based on the lines of cellular differentiation (ductal, acinar, neuroendocrine, or other) that they display, as well as on their gross configuration (solid, cystic, or intraductal). Most epithelial neoplasms of the pancreas have one or more readily definable lines of differentiation that recapitulate normal adult epithelial cell types in the gland {1631}. Ductal differentiation is reflected in the formation of glandular or true papillary structures by the neoplasm, often accompanied by the production of mucin, which can be visualized on routinely stained slides, with histochemical stains for mucins, or using immunohistochemistry for glycoproteins such as CA19-9, CEA, and mucins – in particular EMA (MUC1), MUC2, MUC5AC, and MUC6 {1302}. Mucin production is absent in some ductal-type neoplasms, such as serous neoplasms, intraductal tubulopapillary neoplasms, and undifferentiated carcinomas, which are known to be of ductal type based on their common co-occurrence with elements of typical ductal adenocarcinoma. Acinar differentiation is defined by the production of pancreatic exocrine enzymes by the neoplastic cells, which can be demonstrated using immunohistochemical staining for trypsin, chymotrypsin, lipase, and BCL10 {1634,1748}. Neuroendocrine differentiation is demonstrated by immunolabelling for the general neuroendocrine markers, chromogranin A and synaptophysin {1630}. The only well-characterized epithelial neoplasm of the pancreas for which one or more lines of differentiation cannot be demonstrated is solid pseudopapillary neoplasm, which remains a neoplasm of uncertain histogenesis {468}. Mesenchymal and haematolymphoid neoplasms are classified using the same criteria as in other anatomical sites. Both are rare as primary pancreatic neoplasms.

Nearly 90% of adult pancreatic neoplasms are invasive ductal adenocarcinomas or related subtypes thereof {943}, to the extent that the term "pancreatic cancer" is used colloquially as a synonym for ductal adenocarcinoma. Cystic and intraductal neoplasms make up 4–5%, pancreatic neuroendocrine tumours (PanNETs) are 3–4%, and acinar cell carcinoma and other uncommon entities account for the remaining 2–3%. The increased use of cross-sectional imaging has resulted in greater detection of cystic and intraductal neoplasms, as well as small PanNETs. Intraductal papillary mucinous neoplasms (IPMNs) now constitute 60% of cyst-forming neoplasms of the pancreas and are commonly detected incidentally, raising the issue of the preoperative features that should indicate surgical intervention {3119}. Intraductal neoplasms cause cystic change due to the dilatation of the involved ducts, but cysts are characteristic of solid pseudopapillary neoplasm {34}. Other cyst-forming neoplasms include the true cystic neoplasms, such as serous cystic neoplasms and mucinous cystic neoplasms, as well as those with degenerative cystic changes, which can

C25 Pancreas
  C25.0 Head of the pancreas
  C25.1 Body of the pancreas
  C25.2 Tail of the pancreas
  C25.3 Pancreatic duct
  C25.4 Islets of Langerhans
  C25.7 Other specified parts of the pancreas
  C25.8 Overlapping lesion of the pancreas
  C25.9 Pancreas NOS

occur in any typically solid neoplasm, such as invasive ductal adenocarcinoma or PanNET.

Pancreatic neoplasms are rare in childhood, and the relative frequencies of the various entities differ from those in adults {3024,2258}. Ductal adenocarcinomas and intraductal neoplasms are extremely rare in childhood. The most frequent neoplasms in the first decade of life are pancreatoblastomas, acinar cell carcinomas, and PanNETs. In the second decade, solid pseudopapillary neoplasms, PanNETs, and acinar cell carcinomas are most prevalent.

The recent enhanced availability of genomic sequencing has substantially increased the volume of data related to pancreatic tumour genetics. The genetic basis of ductal adenocarcinoma was established more than a decade ago {1481}, and the importance of germline mutations in its pathogenesis is becoming increasingly clear {1954}. Recent work has demonstrated that numerous less common mutations also play an important role, some of which may be targetable therapeutically {1480,1942,606}. Molecular subcategories are also emerging based on genomic and transcriptomic analysis {224,2390}. For pancreatic neoplasms other than ductal adenocarcinoma, genomic analysis has helped validate existing morphological classifications, demonstrating mutation profiles different from those of ductal adenocarcinoma and sometimes revealing novel genomic alterations highly characteristic of an entity (e.g. MEN1, DAXX, and ATRX mutations in PanNETs {1463} or GNAS and RNF43 mutations in IPMNs {120}). Sequencing of intraductal neoplasms with oncocytic morphology has revealed abnormalities entirely distinct from those of other IPMNs, allowing separation of intraductal oncocytic papillary neoplasm from the other subtypes of IPMN {270}. Intraductal tubulopapillary neoplasms also have distinctive genetic alterations {264}. These and other genomic studies have further informed the WHO classification presented in this volume.

Precursors to invasive ductal adenocarcinoma include microscopic foci of pancreatic intraepithelial neoplasia, which in low-grade form commonly occur in a substantial proportion of adults, as well as the increasingly detected macroscopic precursor neoplasms, IPMNs, intraductal oncocytic papillary neoplasms, intraductal tubulopapillary neoplasms, and mucinous cystic neoplasms. All of these precursors are now classified into two tiers of dysplasia, on the basis of the highest grade of dysplasia detected, rather than the three-tiered system used in the previous edition of the WHO classification {267}. The high-grade category is intended to reflect only the most dysplastic third of the morphological spectrum of dysplasia, such that PanIN-2 or intermediate-grade dysplasia in the prior classification is now included with low-grade in the new one. When invasive carcinoma is present in association with a macroscopic precursor lesion, it should be diagnosed separately and graded and staged using the parameters for invasive carcinomas (e.g. IPMN with associated invasive colloid carcinoma).

An important change in the fifth edition of the WHO Classification of Tumours regards neuroendocrine neoplasms (NENs), following the WHO uniform classification framework for NENs published in 2018 (see *Classification of neuroendocrine neoplasms of the digestive system*, p. 16) {2717}. This framework sharply separates well-differentiated neoplasms (neuroendocrine tumours [NETs]) from poorly differentiated neoplasms (neuroendocrine carcinomas [NECs]) and further acknowledges that NETs can be separated into low, intermediate, and high grades based on the parameters proposed for gastroenteropancreatic NENs by the European Neuroendocrine Tumor Society (ENETS) {2719} and adopted in the fourth edition of the WHO Classification of Tumours. The recognition that PanNETs can be high-grade {272} was incorporated into the fourth-edition *WHO classification of tumours of endocrine organs* in 2017, which served as the basis for the recent uniform classification proposal {2717}. Included for the first time in this fifth-edition volume are detailed sections on each functioning and nonfunctioning PanNET subtype. Also relevant to the classification of pancreatic NENs (PanNENs) is the novel concept of mixed neuroendocrine–non-neuroendocrine neoplasms (MiNENs), which was also first advanced for pancreatic neoplasms in the fourth-edition *WHO classification of tumours of endocrine organs*, replacing the prior term "mixed adenoneuroendocrine carcinoma (MANEC)". MiNEN is a conceptual category rather than a specific diagnosis, and in the pancreas, it encompasses a range of neoplasms with mixed differentiation, such as mixed ductal-neuroendocrine carcinoma and some mixed acinar-neuroendocrine carcinomas.

The only other emerging new entity in the pancreas is sclerosing epithelioid mesenchymal tumour, which is covered in Chapter 12: *Mesenchymal tumours of the digestive system* (p. 433). The subtypes of ductal adenocarcinoma now include invasive micropapillary carcinoma, which (like in other anatomical locations) has a particularly aggressive clinical course. Other subtypes remain as classified in the fourth edition.

Acinar cystic transformation of the pancreas

Singhi AD
Adsay NV
Hiraoka N
Terris B

Definition
Acinar cystic transformation of the pancreas is a non-neoplastic cystic lesion lined by benign-appearing acinar and ductal epithelium.

ICD-O coding
None

ICD-11 coding
DC30.0 Cyst of pancreas

Related terminology
Acceptable: acinar cell cystadenoma.

Subtype(s)
None

Localization
These lesions can occur throughout the pancreas, but they are more common in the pancreatic head; some diffusely involve the entire gland {3734,1566,3061,3509}.

Clinical features
Fewer than 50 cases have been described, with a mean age at presentation of 43 years (range: 9–83 years) and a female predominance of 3:1 {3734,97,569,685,1651,2102,3588,1566, 3061,3509,3759}. Cases are divided into two categories: clinically recognized macroscopic lesions and incidental microscopic findings. Patients with macroscopic lesions may present with abdominal pain, dyspepsia, and/or a palpable mass, but a substantial proportion are asymptomatic {1566,3061,3509,3759}. Incidental cases are only detected upon pathological review of pancreata removed for other indications.

Epidemiology
Unknown

Etiology
The etiology is unknown, but some cases may occur because of obstruction {3759}.

Pathogenesis
Recent evidence suggests that this lesion represents a non-neoplastic dilatation of the acinar and ductal epithelium {3061,307}. Chromosomal gains, but not losses, were reported for one case by array comparative genomic hybridization and suggest a possible neoplastic process {1566}. However, a subsequent study found a random X-chromosome inactivation pattern for 5 cases, which would support these lesions as non-neoplastic {3061}. Unlike in pancreatic ductal adenocarcinoma and its cystic precursor neoplasms, alterations in *KRAS*, *GNAS*, *RNF43*, *TP53*, *CDKN2A*, and *SMAD4* have not been reported in these lesions {3058}.

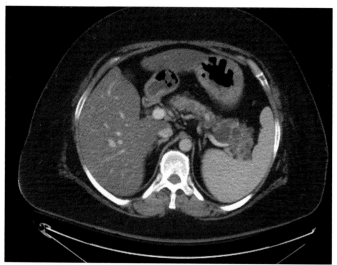

Fig. 10.01 Acinar cystic transformation. CT of an acinar cystic transformation involving the pancreatic tail.

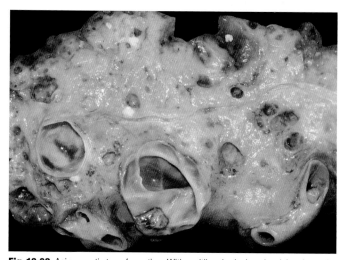

Fig. 10.02 Acinar cystic transformation. With multilocular lesions involving the entire length of the pancreas.

Macroscopic appearance
Clinically recognized lesions measure 1.5–19.7 cm (mean: 5.8 cm) in diameter and form multilocular or unilocular cystic masses {3588,1566,3061,3509}. Multicentricity is common and may diffusely involve the entire gland. The cyst wall is typically thin, smooth and translucent, and filled with clear watery fluid. Incidentally detected cases are usually < 1.0 cm and unilocular, and they may not be apparent grossly. Communication with the main pancreatic duct is rare.

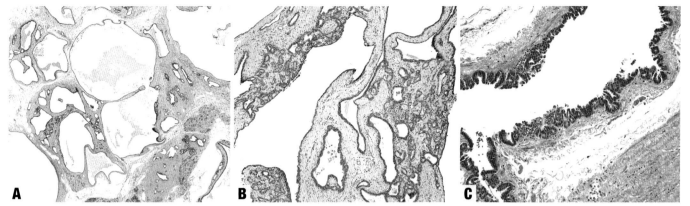

Fig. 10.03 Acinar cystic transformation. **A** Multilocular acinar cystic transformation consists of variably sized cysts with incomplete septa that appear as broad papillary projections and are surrounded by fibrotic and atrophic pancreatic parenchyma. **B** Multilocular acinar cystic transformation is characterized by dilated and interconnecting clusters of acinar epithelium that open into larger cysts lined by epithelium with separate regions of acinar and ductal differentiation. **C** Unilocular acinar cystic transformation is characterized by 1–2 cell layers of acinar epithelium with little intervening ductal epithelium and an underlying hyalinized wall.

Histopathology

Microscopically, multilocular lesions are characterized by innumerable cysts of varying sizes. The cysts are composed of dilated and interconnecting clusters of pancreatic acini that surround and open into larger cysts. Residual pancreatic elements are often present between the larger cysts. The cysts are lined by epithelium with pale or granular apical cytoplasm and basally oriented nuclei. No substantial nuclear atypia or mitotic activity has been reported. The epithelium exhibits separate regions of either pancreatic acinar or ductal differentiation. In some areas, the cysts form large fusiform locules with incomplete septa and club-like pseudopapillae. In contrast, unilocular lesions are lined by 1–2 cell layers of epithelium with acinar differentiation and little intervening ductal differentiation. The cyst lumina may contain inspissated eosinophilic enzymatic secretions, and the surrounding pancreatic parenchyma is typically fibrotic and atrophic. Incidental microscopic cases usually consist of a single cyst lined by cells with predominantly acinar differentiation, and they are often found in the setting of pancreatic ductal obstruction. Immunohistochemistry is usually necessary to confirm that the cyst-lining epithelium exhibits distinct regions of acinar and ductal differentiation, and to exclude other cystic pancreatic lesions within the differential diagnosis.

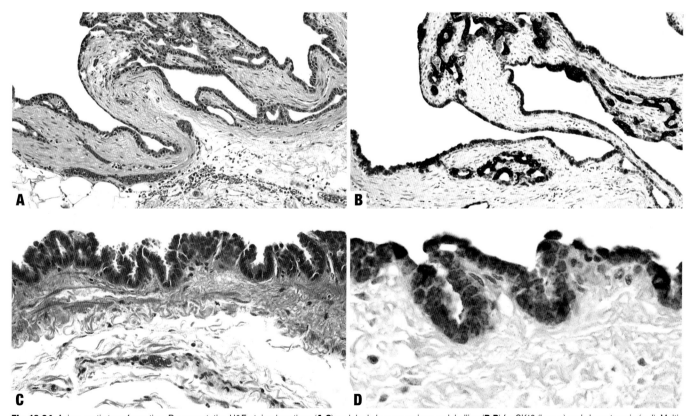

Fig. 10.04 Acinar cystic transformation. Representative H&E-stained sections (**A,C**) and dual chromogen immunolabelling (**B,D**) for CK19 (brown) and chymotrypsin (red). Multilocular lesions coalesce with regions of ductal epithelium (brown) among long stretches of acinar epithelium (red).

Acinar cystic transformation can be confused with serous cystadenomas, squamoid cysts of the pancreatic ducts, intraductal papillary mucinous neoplasms, and mucinous cystic neoplasms. Recognition of both acinar and ductal differentiation with supporting immunohistochemical stains, such as trypsin, chymotrypsin, BCL10, and CK19, can aid in establishing the correct diagnosis. Acinar cystic transformation lacks the glycogen-rich epithelium of serous cystadenomas, the squamous differentiation of squamoid cysts, the prominent mucinous epithelium of intraductal papillary mucinous neoplasms and mucinous cystic neoplasms, and the underlying ovarian-type stroma of mucinous cystic neoplasms.

Cytology
Because the lesional epithelium is indistinguishable from normal acinar and ductal cells, FNA specimens are often interpreted as non-diagnostic or benign {3700,3041,573}.

Diagnostic molecular pathology
Not clinically relevant

Essential and desirable diagnostic criteria
Essential: a benign unilocular or multilocular cystic lesion; evidence of both ductal and acinar differentiation.

Staging (TNM)
Not clinically relevant

Prognosis and prediction
All cases reported to date have been clinically benign, and there is no evidence of recurrence, malignant transformation, or association with acinar cell carcinoma {3734,3588,3061,3509}.

Serous neoplasms of the pancreas

Singhi AD
Adsay NV
Hiraoka N
Terris B

Definition

Serous cystadenoma of the pancreas is a benign epithelial neoplasm composed of uniform cuboidal, glycogen-rich cells that often form cysts containing serous fluid. The diagnosis of malignancy in pancreatic serous neoplasms is restricted to cases with unequivocal distant metastasis beyond the pancreatic/peripancreatic bed.

ICD-O coding

8441/0 Serous cystadenoma NOS
8441/3 Serous cystadenocarcinoma NOS

ICD-11 coding

2E92.8 & XH8TJ0 Benign neoplasm of pancreas & Serous cystadenoma NOS
2C10.Y & XH7A08 Other specified malignant neoplasms of pancreas & Serous cystadenocarcinoma NOS

Related terminology

Serous cystadenoma
Acceptable: microcystic adenoma; glycogen-rich adenoma; oligocystic ill-demarcated adenoma.

Subtype(s)

Macrocystic (oligocystic) serous cystadenoma; solid serous adenoma; von Hippel–Lindau syndrome–associated serous cystic neoplasm; mixed serous-neuroendocrine neoplasm

Localization

Serous cystadenomas can occur anywhere in the pancreas, but they arise most frequently (50–75%) in the pancreatic body or tail and are generally solitary {1562,1608,1419,2686}. Unless associated with germline alterations in *VHL*, these neoplasms rarely involve the full length of the pancreas or are multifocal {567,2973,1360}. Serous cystadenocarcinomas often arise in the body and/or tail of the pancreas.

Clinical features

Serous cystadenoma
The mean age at presentation is 58 years (range: 18–91 years), with a female predominance of 3:1 {3710,1419,1608,2686}. Patients may exhibit symptoms related to local mass effect, such as nonspecific abdominal and back pain, a palpable mass, nausea and vomiting, diabetes, and weight loss {656,1002,3710,1419}. Jaundice caused by obstruction of the distal common bile duct is unusual, even in association with neoplasms within the pancreatic head. However, 60% of patients are asymptomatic at clinical presentation {980,1608,1419}.

Most serous cystadenomas are discovered incidentally by abdominal imaging. A classic CT finding is a well-circumscribed and multilocular cystic/microcystic mass {623,632}. Approximately 30% of cases demonstrate a central scar with a sunburst

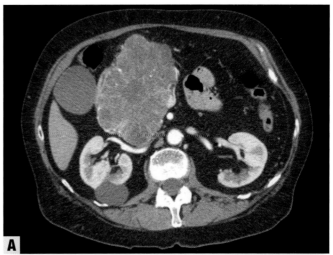
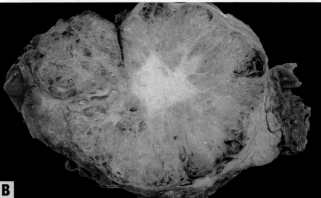

Fig. 10.05 Serous cystadenoma. **A** CT of a microcystic serous cystadenoma in the pancreatic head; note the presence of a central scar. **B** Gross appearance of a microcystic serous cystadenoma; note the central stellate scar and sponge-like appearance.

calcification pattern. On MRI, serous cystadenomas are usually hyperintense on T2-weighted images and hypointense on T1-weighted images {3772,623,1502}. Occasionally, debris (especially haemorrhage) in the cyst alters this signal intensity pattern. The septa of the neoplasm are well depicted on T2-weighted images, but the central scar is not. EUS reveals an echogenic mass with numerous cysts, which produce a characteristic honeycomb pattern {1608}. The sensitivity of EUS can be increased by using it in conjunction with needle-based confocal laser endomicroscopy, but this technique is limited to larger cysts {2310,1705}. There is no visible communication between the cyst and the pancreatic ductal system, but upstream ductal dilatation has been documented in 11% of cases {1419}. Despite the typical radiographical appearance of most cases, the probability of a misdiagnosis based on preoperative imaging is high {1562,1608}. Serum tumour markers are generally within normal limits.

Serous cystadenocarcinoma

Serous cystadenocarcinomas have been reported to account for as many as 1–3% of serous neoplasms in some series. However, when strict criteria requiring the presence of true distant metastases are used, < 20 cases have been reported {3612, 1397,870,1691,3715,1002,1121,3152,962,238,3780,2763,395, 1608,3532,1027,1330,1419,3418}, and true malignancy may occur in as few as 0.2% of serous neoplasms {1419}. These patients are 52–86 years of age, and two thirds are women. The signs and symptoms associated with serous cystadenocarcinomas are difficult to ascertain within the literature, but they include abdominal pain, gastrointestinal bleeding, jaundice, weight loss, diarrhoea, and a palpable mass {3612,1397,870, 1691,3715,1002,1121,3152,962,238,3780,2763,395,1608,3532, 1027,1330,1419,3418}. Radiological imaging typically reveals a large cystic mass. Serum CEA and CA19-9 levels are usually normal or slightly elevated.

Epidemiology

Serous cystadenomas account for 1–2% of all pancreatic neoplasms and 10–16% of surgically resected cystic lesions {1689,1608,3404,3058}.

Etiology

There are no known etiological factors, although some cases are associated with germline alterations in *VHL*. As many as 90% of patients with von Hippel–Lindau syndrome (VHL) develop serous cystadenomas {1154,2195,3495,567}.

Pathogenesis

The pathogenesis remains largely unknown, but a centroacinar origin with abnormal regulation of the VHL/HIF pathway, similar to the origin of other glycogen-rich neoplasms, has been proposed {114,3660,3295}.

VHL is considered the main tumour suppressor gene responsible for the formation of both familial and sporadic serous cystadenomas. Somatic mutations in *VHL* (located on chromosome 3p25.3) and loss of heterozygosity of 3p occur in 50% and 90% of cases, respectively {3495,22927,3118}. Allelic loss of chromosome 10q has also been reported in 50% of serous cystadenomas {2207}.

Macroscopic appearance

Microcystic serous cystadenomas account for 45% of cases. They are usually well-circumscribed, slightly bosselated, rounded lesions, 1–25 cm in diameter {657,1002,1689,2686}. On cross-section, they are sponge-like and composed of numerous tiny cysts (> 0.1–1.0 cm in diameter). The cysts at the periphery are often larger than those near the centre of the tumour. A central scar is often present and may be calcified. Macrocystic (oligocystic) subtypes tend to be poorly demarcated, and a central scar is usually absent {1689,1691,1875,2686}. They are composed of 1 (unilocular) to < 10 (multilocular) large cysts of 1–3 cm in diameter and can grossly mimic mucinous cystic neoplasms and intraductal papillary mucinous neoplasms. Solid serous adenomas are well-circumscribed neoplasms with a solid gross appearance (similar to that of well-differentiated neuroendocrine tumours [NETs]), usually 2–4 cm in diameter {2839,1992,519}. They show complete absence of cystic change. Diffuse serous cystadenomas replace the entire pancreas with innumerable cysts and are closely associated with VHL {50}.

Histopathology
Serous cystadenoma

Microcystic serous cystadenoma: Microscopically, the cysts are lined by a single layer of cuboidal to flat epithelial cells with clear cytoplasm, well-defined cytoplasmic borders, and a small round nucleus with dense homogeneous chromatin and an inconspicuous nucleolus. Owing to the presence of abundant intracytoplasmic glycogen, PAS staining is positive but PASD staining is negative. Nuclear atypia and mitoses are typically absent, but symplastic changes may occur {2686}. Blunt papillary projections, tufting, and micropapillae may be found focally {2686}, but well-formed or complex papillae are unusual. Satellite nodules are found in as many as a third of cases {2686}. The epithelium is immunoreactive for inhibin, GLUT1, and MUC6. Underlying the epithelium is an interweaving network of capillaries. The central scar consists of hyalinized stroma with few clusters of tiny cysts.

Macrocystic (oligocystic) serous cystadenoma: The cyst lining is microscopically identical to that of the microcystic type.

Solid serous adenoma: This tumour type is composed of small back-to-back acini with no or minute central lumina and cytological features that are otherwise typical of a serous cystadenoma.

VHL-associated serous cystic neoplasm: Approximately 35–90% of patients with VHL develop multiple microcystic and macrocystic serous cystadenomas {1154,2973,567,1360}. Microscopically, these cysts are virtually indistinguishable from those occurring sporadically. The lesions vary from single, minute cystic dilatations of the centroacinar lumen to involvement of the entire gland – known as diffuse serous cystadenoma {50}.

Mixed serous-neuroendocrine neoplasm: In rare cases, serous cystadenomas are associated with pancreatic neuroendocrine neoplasms (PanNENs). The neuroendocrine proliferation can be independent or intermingled with the cysts {344,3071}. Such an association is highly suggestive of VHL: 10–17% of patients with VHL are reported to have neuroendocrine neoplasms (NENs), and 70% have neuroendocrine microadenomatosis {1154,2623,567,1360}. However, in a few cases, no genetic syndrome is identified. It is unclear whether these rare cases represent true mixed neoplasms with both exocrine and endocrine differentiation, or whether they are coincidental collision tumours.

Serous cystadenocarcinoma

Malignant behaviour of serous neoplasms has been reported (serous cystadenocarcinoma), but it is extraordinarily rare, and the diagnosis of malignancy in pancreatic serous neoplasms is restricted to cases with unequivocal distant metastasis beyond the pancreatic/peripancreatic bed.

Although atypical and potentially a sign of aggressive behaviour, vascular, perineural, and adjacent organ and lymph node involvement by direct spread is insufficient for the diagnosis of serous cystadenocarcinoma, which requires metastasis (almost always to the liver) {1419}. These exceptional neoplasms are grossly and microscopically similar to microcystic serous cystadenomas, but they tend to be larger, with a mean diameter of 10 cm. A subset of benign serous neoplasms show cytological atypia or are locally aggressive, with lymphovascular and

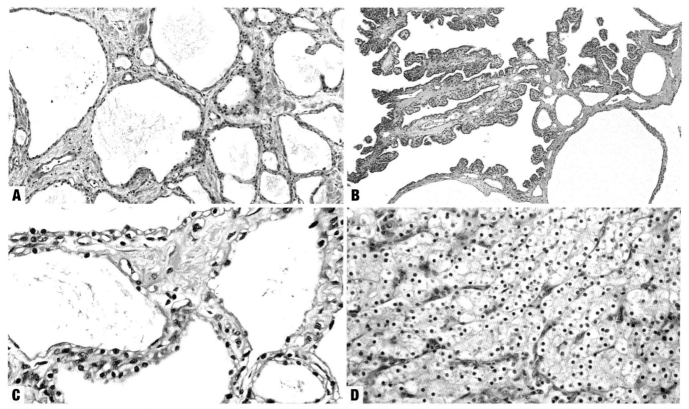

Fig. 10.06 Serous cystadenoma. Microcystic serous cystadenoma consists of numerous tiny cysts lined by a flattened layer of epithelium (**A**), with rare microscopic papillae that project into the cyst lumen (**B**); the cysts contain proteinaceous fluid and are lined by cuboidal epithelium with clear cytoplasm and uniform, round nuclei (**C**). **D** Solid serous adenoma is composed of cells morphologically indistinguishable from those of microcystic and macrocystic serous cystadenomas, but in the absence of cyst formation.

perineural invasion, as well as direct invasion into the spleen, stomach, and lymph nodes, and these tumours may be at higher risk of metastasis and subsequent classification as serous cystadenocarcinoma. Of note, some serous neoplasms reported as being cytologically malignant have not behaved aggressively {1121,3780}, and overt cytological features of malignancy have not been reported in truly malignant (metastatic) cases.

Cytology
FNA specimens are usually paucicellular {294,1911}. Smears predominantly show proteinaceous debris and blood with few (if any) epithelial cells. When seen, the neoplastic epithelium forms small monolayered fragments of cuboidal-type cells with round, uniform nuclei and scant to moderate, often clear cytoplasm. If sufficient material is present, ancillary studies for glycogen, inhibin, and MUC6 are useful. Biochemical and molecular fluid analyses are also helpful in establishing a diagnosis {1479,3118,3058}.

Diagnostic molecular pathology
Serous cystadenoma: Genomic alterations in *VHL* can be detected in preoperative pancreatic cyst fluid and used clinically for diagnostic purposes {1479,3058}. Alterations in *KRAS*, *GNAS*, *CDKN2A*, and *SMAD4* have not been reported in serous cystadenomas, unlike in pancreatic ductal adenocarcinoma and its cystic precursor neoplasms {22927}.
Serous cystadenocarcinoma: Limited molecular data are available due to the paucity of reported cases. However, one

case of carcinoma ex microcystic adenoma was wildtype for *KRAS* {3780}.

Essential and desirable diagnostic criteria
Essential: usually a cystic lesion; low, cuboidal, bland glycogenated epithelium.

Staging (TNM)
Serous cystadenocarcinomas are staged as carcinomas of the exocrine pancreas.

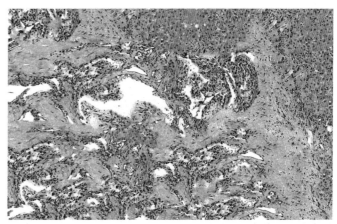

Fig. 10.07 Serous cystadenocarcinoma metastatic to the liver. Note the bland cytological features that are indistinguishable from those of an ordinary serous cystadenoma.

Prognosis and prediction

The prognosis for patients with a serous cystadenoma is excellent {1608,1419,2686}. A minority exhibit growth on follow-up, and the reported annual median growth rate is 0.4–0.6 cm, which is dependent on cyst size {3354,1419}. Considering the indolent behaviour and the potentially substantial postoperative morbidity and mortality, conservative management has been proposed when serous cystadenomas are small and asymptomatic and show typical radiological and cyst fluid characteristics {1853,886}. Surgical resection is almost always curative. Although not technically classified as malignant, serous cystadenomas with locally aggressive features, such as direct extension into adjacent structures, can rarely recur or even metastasize (and are then classified as serous cystadenocarcinoma). Therefore, postoperative follow-up may be warranted in atypical cases.

For serous cystadenocarcinoma, the most common site of metastasis is the liver {2686}. However, it is important to consider the possibility of multifocality and synchronous disease when evaluating these cases, because primary hepatic serous cystadenomas occur even in the absence of pancreatic tumours {2686}. Regardless, these neoplasms are slow-growing and characterized by an indolent behaviour. In fact, only one death has been attributed to extrapancreatic dissemination {962}, and long-term survival in the presence of liver lesions interpreted as metastasis is usual {1419,2686}. Surgical resection may be helpful for symptomatic disease.

Pancreatic intraepithelial neoplasia

Basturk O   Hong SM
Esposito I   Klöppel G
Fukushima N Maitra A
Furukawa T   Zamboni G

Definition
Pancreatic intraepithelial neoplasia (PanIN) is a microscopic, non-invasive, flat or micropapillary, epithelial neoplasm confined to the pancreatic ducts.

ICD-O coding
8148/0 Glandular intraepithelial neoplasia, low grade
8148/2 Glandular intraepithelial neoplasia, high grade

ICD-11 coding
2E92.8 & XH6AF9 Benign neoplasm of pancreas & Glandular intraepithelial neoplasia, low grade
2E61.Y & XH28N7 Carcinoma in situ of other specified digestive organs & Glandular intraepithelial neoplasia, high grade

Related terminology
PanIN
Not recommended: mucinous metaplasia; papillary hyperplasia; atypical hyperplasia; ductal dysplasia.

High-grade PanIN
Acceptable: carcinoma in situ (used parenthetically in some parts of the world).

Note: The current two-tiered grading system for PanIN recently replaced the former three-tiered grading scheme (PanIN-1, PanIN-2, PanIN-3) {1301}; neoplasms belonging to the former PanIN-1 and PanIN-2 categories are now categorized as low-grade PanIN, and those belonging to the former PanIN-3 category are now categorized as high-grade PanIN {267}.

Subtype(s)
None

Localization
PanIN is more common in the head of the pancreas {1695,1303}.

Clinical features
Given their microscopic nature, PanIN lesions are asymptomatic, generally cannot be detected on preoperative imaging studies, and are typically found incidentally in pancreatic specimens resected for other reasons. However, in patients with a familial predisposition to pancreatic ductal adenocarcinoma (PDAC), PanIN lesions, especially high-grade lesions, associated with lobulocentric atrophy, are more frequently observed and tend to be multifocal {2987,428}. It may be possible to detect lobulocentric atrophy on imaging studies such as EUS, suggesting a potential screening tool for identification of individuals at higher risk of invasive neoplasia {480}.

Epidemiology
Low-grade PanIN is a common incidental finding in the general population {133,1678} and can be found in more than half of all individuals aged > 50 years with thorough examination of the pancreas {1305}. In contrast, high-grade PanIN is seldom seen in pancreata without PDACs {133,2082}.

Etiology
Like PDAC, PanIN has been suggested to be associated with advanced age, obesity, pancreatic fatty infiltration, and diabetes mellitus {1695,1303,2913,2669,2082}. Also, PanIN lesions are more numerous and of a higher grade in the pancreata from patients with a familial predisposition to PDAC {2987}.

Pathogenesis
Multiple clinicopathological studies suggest that high-grade PanIN is the main precursor of PDAC {133,1695,698,397,2098}. Molecular studies have supported this hypothesis by showing that PanIN lesions share critical genetic abnormalities with adjacent PDAC, and histological progression of PanIN parallels the accumulation of molecular abnormalities {3563,914,1285,1284}. The evolution of invasive carcinoma from the first genetic change appears to occur over decades, and the relatively common occurrence of low-grade PanIN lesions, most of which never progress to PDAC, suggests that this phase of carcinogenesis lasts many years.

The histological progression of PanIN to invasive carcinoma is mirrored by genetic progression, manifesting as either an increasing frequency of molecular aberrations overall, or a trend towards a higher degree of clonality for any individual molecular aberration in high-grade PanIN than in low-grade PanIN {2009}. For example, > 90% of PanIN lesions of all grades harbour *KRAS* mutations; however, the mutant allele frequency (a measure of clonality) is substantially higher in high-grade PanIN {1510}. Although the precise sequence of alterations is not well defined, certain genetic abnormalities, such as telomere shortening and activating mutations of the *KRAS* oncogene, are early changes, observed even in low-grade PanIN, and probably contribute to disease initiation. In contrast, widespread clonal copy-number alterations, as well as biallelic inactivation of *CDKN2A* (*P16*), are observed in high-grade PanIN, suggesting an association between these late changes and disease progression {1187,1284}. In contrast to what had been previously reported, recent studies have shown that mutations of *TP53* are rare, if not absent, and there are no mutations or homozygous deletions of *SMAD4* in isolated high-grade PanIN lesions, indicating that inactivation of these two genes predominantly occurs in bona fide invasive carcinomas {1284,1187}. Also, some evidence suggests a pathway to invasive carcinoma via chromothripsis-like events (chromosomal shattering with chaotic reassembly), which causes sudden, catastrophic

Chapter 10

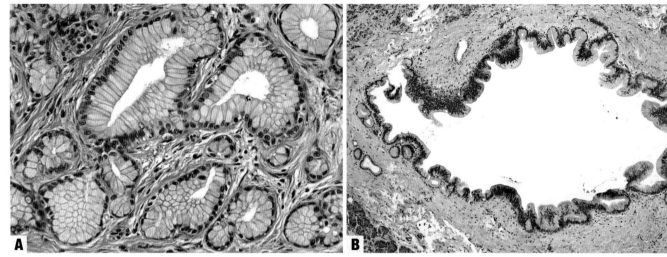

Fig. 10.08 Pancreatic intraepithelial neoplasia. Low-grade pancreatic intraepithelial neoplasia with simple, columnar, mucin-filled, perfectly polarized cells (**A**) or mild folding of the epithelium and pseudostratification of nuclei (**B**).

accumulation of molecular alterations to drive PanIN to invasive carcinoma {2664,2390,1187}.

The molecular features of PanIN lesions differ from those of intraductal papillary mucinous neoplasms (IPMNs), the next most common precursor lesion of PDAC. Specifically, certain genetic alterations that are common in IPMNs, such as activating mutations of *GNAS* and inactivating mutations of *RNF43*, are rare in PanIN lesions {22927,3617,1284,3231}.

Macroscopic appearance

PanIN lesions are usually not grossly visible but may be associated with changes such as lobulocentric atrophy and duct stricture in the immediately adjacent pancreatic parenchyma {764,428,2985,2986}.

Histopathology

Microscopically, PanIN lesions are composed of cuboidal to columnar cells producing varying amounts of mucin {1301,1306}. PanIN lesions are graded on the basis of the highest degree

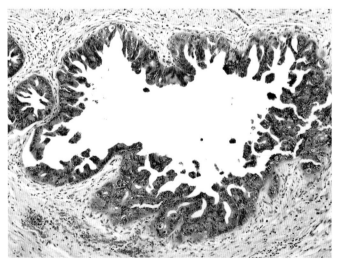

Fig. 10.09 Pancreatic intraepithelial neoplasia. High-grade pancreatic intraepithelial neoplasia with predominantly micropapillary architecture. Note the loss of polarity and the enlarged, irregular nuclei with prominent nucleoli.

of cytoarchitectural atypia as low-grade or high-grade. Low-grade PanIN lesions are flat or papillary, with basally located or pseudostratified nuclei and mild to moderate cytological atypia. Marked architectural alterations (cribriforming, micropapillae, and budding of epithelial cell clusters into the duct lumen) are absent. Mitoses are infrequent. High-grade PanIN lesions are typically micropapillary or papillary, with marked loss of polarity, irregular nuclear stratification, budding of cell clusters into the lumen, severe cytological atypia, and mitoses. Uncommonly there can be cribriform architecture. Occasionally intraluminal necrosis may be observed {1306,267}.

The immunohistochemical labelling pattern of PanIN parallels that of PDAC. None of the lesions express MUC2 {2008}, but most express EMA (MUC1), MUC4, and MUC5AC {36,2008}. MUC6 expression is limited to the low-grade lesions that have pyloric gland features {268}. Alterations in other glycoproteins include cytoplasmic expression of CEA and aberrant expression of B72.3, both of which are more common in high-grade PanIN. An increasing Ki-67 proliferation index has been shown with increasing grades of PanIN {1626}. Recent studies have shown that aberrant expression of p53 is rare and SMAD4 immunolabelling is retained in high-grade PanIN lesions {1284}.

Oncocytic and intestinal subtypes of PanIN have been described, but genetic analysis to confirm their neoplastic nature has yet to be performed {96}.

The differential diagnosis with IPMNs may be difficult. Size is the main feature used to distinguish these lesions: PanIN lesions are usually < 0.5 cm, whereas IPMNs are usually > 1.0 cm in diameter {1306,267,42}. The direction of differentiation of the neoplastic cells is also important. The epithelial cells in almost all PanIN lesions have gastric differentiation, whereas those in IPMNs can have various differentiation {28,37,993,268}; lesions with intestinal or oncocytic differentiation most likely represent IPMNs or intraductal oncocytic papillary neoplasms. The term "incipient IPMN" or "incipient intraductal oncocytic papillary neoplasm" can be applied to lesions 0.5–1.0 cm in diameter with long finger-like papillae, intestinal or oncocytic differentiation, or a *GNAS* mutation {267,42,2090}.

Intraductal spread of invasive carcinoma (ductal cancerization or colonization), which is seen in as many as 70% of surgically resected PDACs, can sometimes be impossible to distinguish from high-grade PanIN {3251}. If present, continuity of the intraductal lesion with invasive carcinoma in the adjacent stroma and abrupt transition from morphologically normal epithelium to markedly atypical epithelium within the same duct are helpful in recognizing intraductal spread {267}. Loss of SMAD4 (DPC4) expression also favours intraductal spread {1284,3705}.

A pattern of vascular invasion by PDAC may also histologically mimic PanIN. The presence of a subtle circumferential layer of smooth muscle fibres indicates vascular invasion {234,1268}.

Cytology
Because these are microscopic lesions and are not detectable preoperatively, PanIN is rarely encountered in clinical cytology samples.

Diagnostic molecular pathology
Not clinically relevant

Essential and desirable diagnostic criteria
Essential: microscopic foci of low-grade or high-grade epithelial dysplasia within ducts; absence of invasion.

Staging (TNM)
High-grade PanIN is categorized as Tis (carcinoma in situ).

Prognosis and prediction
Low-grade PanIN is very common and of no proven clinical significance. In contrast, high-grade PanIN, especially in isolation, may have clinical significance and may serve as a surrogate marker for invasive carcinoma elsewhere in the organ {133,397,42,267}. Therefore, in the absence of an established invasive carcinoma, if high-grade PanIN is present at a margin, additional surgery may be justifiable {2098,42,267}. However, once invasive carcinoma is present, it is highly unlikely that the clinical course will be affected by the presence of any grade of PanIN, even at the margin {267}.

Pancreatic intraductal papillary mucinous neoplasm

Basturk O
Esposito I
Fukushima N
Furukawa T
Hong SM
Klöppel G
Maitra A
Zamboni G

Definition

Intraductal papillary mucinous neoplasm (IPMN) of the pancreas is a grossly visible (typically > 5 mm) intraductal epithelial neoplasm of mucin-producing cells, arising in the main pancreatic duct and/or its branches.

ICD-O coding

8453/0 Intraductal papillary mucinous neoplasm with low-grade dysplasia

8453/2 Intraductal papillary mucinous neoplasm with high-grade dysplasia

8453/3 Intraductal papillary mucinous neoplasm with associated invasive carcinoma

ICD-11 coding

2E92.8 & XH8MD2 Benign neoplasm of pancreas & Intraductal papillary-mucinous tumour with low-grade dysplasia

2E61.Y & XH3MB3 Carcinoma in situ of other specified digestive organs & Intraductal papillary mucinous neoplasm with high-grade dysplasia

Related terminology

High-grade IPMN

Acceptable: carcinoma in situ (used parenthetically in some parts of the world).

Note: The current two-tiered grading system for IPMN recently replaced the former three-tiered grading scheme; neoplasms belonging to the former categories of "IPMN with low-grade dysplasia (LGD)" and "IPMN with intermediate-grade dysplasia" {1301,1306} are now categorized as low-grade IPMN. Those belonging to the former category of "IPMN with high-grade dysplasia (HGD)" are now categorized as high-grade IPMN {267}.

Subtype(s)

Gastric-type intraductal papillary mucinous neoplasm; intestinal-type intraductal papillary mucinous neoplasm; pancreatobiliary-type intraductal papillary mucinous neoplasm.

Oncocytic-type intraductal papillary mucinous neoplasm is now recognized as a distinct entity {28,270,2048,265}. The designations "main duct-type intraductal papillary mucinous neoplasm", "branch duct-type intraductal papillary mucinous neoplasm", and "mixed duct-type intraductal papillary mucinous neoplasm" are imaging terms used by clinicians (see *Clinical features*, below) rather than pathological subtypes.

Localization

IPMNs can occur anywhere in the main pancreatic duct and/or its branches; however, most are located in the head of the pancreas {212,1663,266}. Multicentricity is observed in as many as 40% of cases {35,3241,1939,3091,2560,1423}.

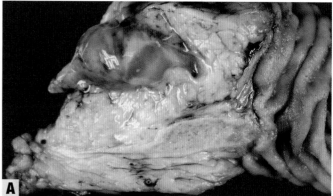

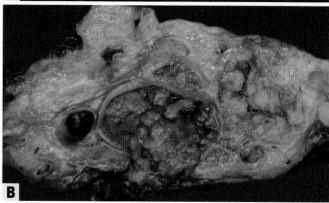

Fig. 10.10 Intraductal papillary mucinous neoplasm (IPMN). **A** Main duct-type IPMN; the duct is diffusely dilated and often filled with sticky mucin. **B** IPMN involving both the main and secondary pancreatic ducts; markedly dilated pancreatic ducts are filled with friable papillary formations.

Clinical features

IPMNs are fairly common, particularly in elderly people. In consecutive CT scans, the prevalence was reported as 1.7%, rising to 6.7% in people in their eighth decade of life {563}. Patients with IPMNs with associated invasive carcinoma are 3–5 years older than those without an associated invasive carcinoma, suggesting that progression occurs over a period of years {1689,3091}. Clinical symptoms include epigastric pain, chronic pancreatitis, weight loss, diabetes mellitus, and jaundice {3338,1649,3687,2837,3091}. Branch duct-type IPMNs are often detected incidentally {3240}.

By imaging, three distinct types of IPMN can be discerned {1663,3239,3240,42}. Main duct-type IPMNs are characterized by primary involvement of the main pancreatic duct with segmental or diffuse dilatation. Branch duct-type IPMNs typically involve the smaller, secondary ducts without affecting the main pancreatic duct {2837,3170,3238,3239}. Mixed duct-type IPMN is a combination of the other two types {3239,3240,42,1640}. Mural nodules and/or irregularities in the duct contours may correspond to HGD or invasive carcinoma {995,1667}.

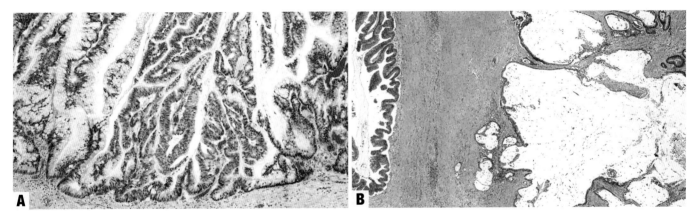

Fig. 10.14 Intestinal-type intraductal papillary mucinous neoplasm. **A** With high-grade dysplasia. There is more complex architecture and the nuclei are stratified, hyperchromatic, and pleomorphic. **B** With associated invasive colloid carcinoma (right).

pattern of mucins, as well as CDX2 (a marker of intestinal differentiation), is useful for distinguishing the morphological subtypes, although overlaps in expression patterns commonly occur (see Table 10.01) {36,37,993,268}.

The differential diagnoses of IPMNs include other pancreatic intraductal neoplasms, mucinous cystic neoplasms (MCNs), and retention cysts. PanIN is a microscopic non-invasive, flat or papillary epithelial neoplasm arising in the pancreatic ducts, usually < 5 mm in diameter {1306}. The epithelial cells in almost all PanIN lesions have gastric foveolar differentiation. In contrast, IPMNs are > 5 mm in diameter and can have varying differentiation {1306,267,42}. Therefore, although small gastric-type IPMNs are difficult to distinguish from large PanIN lesions, lesions with intestinal differentiation are most likely IPMNs {267,42}. Intraductal oncocytic papillary neoplasms are characteristically complex, with florid proliferation of monotonous cells that have intensely eosinophilic granular cytoplasm, round enlarged nuclei with a prominent nucleolus, and intraepithelial lumina {28}. The term "incipient IPMN" or "incipient intraductal oncocytic papillary neoplasm" can be applied to lesions 0.5–1.0 cm in diameter with long finger-like papillae, intestinal or oncocytic differentiation, or a *GNAS* mutation {267,42,2090}. Intraductal tubulopapillary neoplasms may be difficult to distinguish from pancreatobiliary-type IPMNs {3643}. Predominantly tubular architecture, diffuse HGD, minimal intracellular mucin, and lack of MUC5AC expression favour intraductal tubulopapillary neoplasm {263,1640,2687,2755}. Unlike IPMNs, MCNs typically occur in women, are almost always located in the tail or body of the pancreas, and do not communicate with the duct system. Also, MCNs contain cellular ovarian-type stroma that expresses hormone receptors by immunohistochemistry {1424}.

Retention cysts (dilatation of the pancreatic ducts due to an obstructive process) are usually unilocular and lined by a flat single layer of ductal epithelium without nuclear atypia. When these are involved by PanIN, they may mimic IPMNs. The location of the lesions (commonly in the periphery of a mass lesion) and lack of florid papillae may help differentiate these from true IPMNs {1651,42,1699}. Of note, in the absence of a visible obstructive process, > 1 cm mucinous cysts that do not have characteristic features of IPMNs or MCNs are classified as simple mucinous cysts {267,42,1699}.

Cytology

FNA specimens range from hypocellular to hypercellular, with isolated single cells or loosely cohesive groups of mucin-producing columnar cells. Papillary structures or sheets may also be seen. There is abundant, thick, viscid mucus in the background in nearly all cases {2595,3134,245,2134}.

Because the ovarian-type stroma is often not sampled, IPMN may not be distinguished from MCN on FNA {2670}. In such cases, the nonspecific diagnosis of mucinous neoplastic cyst is preferred, with a comment indicating that the differential diagnosis includes both types of cystic lesions {42}. Once a cyst is determined to be a mucinous neoplastic cyst, it is important to determine the grade of cytological atypia (low-grade vs high-grade), but it may be impossible to distinguish HGD (carcinoma in situ) from invasive carcinoma {2687,42,267}.

Table 10.01 Immunohistochemical profile of intraductal papillary mucinous neoplasm (IPMN), intraductal oncocytic papillary neoplasm (IOPN), and intraductal tubulopapillary neoplasm (ITPN)

	CK7/CK8/CK18/CK19	CK20	EMA (MUC1)	MUC2	MUC5AC	MUC6	CDX2
IPMN							
Gastric	+	–	–	–	+	–/+	–
Pancreatobiliary	+	–	+	–	+	+	–
Intestinal	+	+	–	+	+	–	+
IOPN	+	+ in goblet cells	+	+ in goblet cells	+	+	+ in goblet cells
ITPN	+	–	+	–	–	+	–

Diagnostic molecular pathology

Not clinically relevant

Essential and desirable diagnostic criteria

Essential: a grossly visible epithelial lesion within the pancreatic ductal system, with papillary formation; may have gastric-type, intestinal-type, or pancreatobiliary-type epithelium; associated invasive carcinoma must be excluded.

Staging (TNM)

High-grade IPMNs are categorized as Tis (carcinoma in situ), and staging of IPMNs with an invasive carcinoma is based on the size of the invasive carcinoma, following the protocol for PDAC {2822,42,110,269}. For IPMNs previously staged as early invasion (≤ 2 cm, pT1), the Union for International Cancer Control (UICC) recently created the substages of pT1a (≤ 0.5 cm), pT1b (> 0.5 to < 1 cm), and pT1c (≥ 1 cm).

Prognosis and prediction

The classification of IPMNs as main duct-type versus branch duct-type is of utmost importance during the preoperative management of patients with an IPMN, because main duct-type IPMNs are associated with a higher risk of HGD and invasive carcinoma {2837,2741,3185,690}. However, once the neoplasm is resected, this classification is superseded by the absence or presence of an associated invasive carcinoma {3238,3239,42}.

IPMNs without an invasive carcinoma are often curable; the 5-year survival rates for patients with resected low-grade IPMNs and high-grade IPMNs were reported as 100% and 85–95%, respectively {2007,566,992}. Although some of the mortality in the latter group represents deaths from other causes and the presence of residual neoplasm at a margin, these data suggest that metachronous multifocal disease remains a substantial risk for these patients, and careful clinical follow-up is warranted after the resection {3558}.

The prognosis for IPMNs with invasive carcinoma is significantly worse; the 5-year survival rate was reported to be between 36% and 90%, depending on the histological type and size (stage) of the invasive carcinoma {3558,3011,566,2172}. IPMNs with a colloid type of invasion have a better prognosis than do those with a tubular type of invasion {37}. Those with invasion of < 5 mm have an excellent prognosis {2311}, whereas the prognosis for IPMNs with an advanced-stage invasion is as poor as for conventional PDACs {2311,2902}. The phenotype of the neoplastic cells also has predictive value for clinical outcome {992,2172}.

Pancreatic intraductal oncocytic papillary neoplasm

Basturk O
Esposito I
Fukushima N
Furukawa T
Hong SM
Klöppel G
Maitra A
Zamboni G

Definition

Intraductal oncocytic papillary neoplasm (IOPN) of the pancreas is a grossly cystic epithelial neoplasm composed of exophytic nodular projections lined by oncocytic glandular epithelium, which grows within dilated pancreatic ducts. If there is a component of invasive carcinoma, the lesions are designated IOPN with associated invasive carcinoma.

ICD-O coding

8455/2 Intraductal oncocytic papillary neoplasm NOS
8455/3 Intraductal oncocytic papillary neoplasm with associated invasive carcinoma

ICD-11 coding

2E92.8 & XH8MD2 Benign neoplasm of pancreas & Intraductal papillary-mucinous tumour with low-grade dysplasia

Related terminology

Acceptable: oncocytic subtype of intraductal papillary mucinous neoplasm.

Subtype(s)

None

Localization

Approximately 70% of IOPNs occur in the head of the pancreas and involve the main duct; 10% diffusely involve the gland {28,2048,706}.

Clinical features

IOPNs account for 4.5% of all intraductal neoplasms of the pancreas {706} and are more common in females. Patient age ranges from 36 to 87 years (mean: 59 years) {3520}. IOPNs either are incidentally discovered {706} or present with symptoms attributed to chronic pancreatitis and/or to the mass effect of the neoplasm, such as jaundice {28,2048}. Endoscopic biopsy or cytology may provide histological confirmation {3712,706,2690}.

Epidemiology

Unknown

Etiology

Unknown

Pathogenesis

There are few data on pathogenesis. IOPNs typically lack the alterations reported to be related to ductal adenocarcinoma and intraductal papillary mucinous neoplasm, such as mutations in *KRAS*, *GNAS*, and *RNF43* {3622,265,2196,22927,3118}. In contrast, genes including *ARHGAP26*, *ASXL1*, *EPHA8*, and *ERBB4* are recurrently mutated in some IOPNs, but there are no entity-defining genomic alterations present in most cases {270}.

Macroscopic appearance

Grossly, IOPNs typically form large (average size: 5.5 cm), tan-brown, friable papillary projections or solid nodules within cystically dilated pancreatic ducts, with little intraductal mucin accumulation {28,3487}. Occasionally, the connection of the cysts to the ductal system may not be apparent grossly.

Histopathology

Microscopically, the tumours form complex and arborizing papillae with delicate fibrovascular cores. Sometimes the intraductal

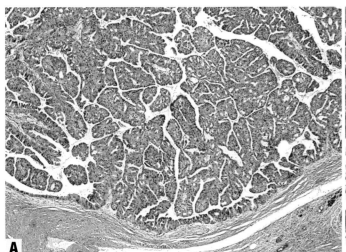
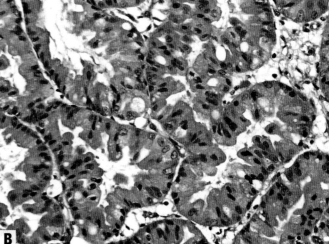

Fig. 10.15 Intraductal oncocytic papillary neoplasm. **A** These neoplasms are characterized by complex arborizing papillae with delicate fibrovascular cores. **B** The cells have distinctive oncocytic cytoplasm and nuclei with single, prominent nucleoli. Intracellular lumina are also seen.

Chapter 10

growth may be difficult to recognize, but at least focal involvement of the ductal system can be demonstrated {28,35,3520}. The papillae are lined by 2–5 layers of cuboidal to columnar cells with mitochondrion-rich eosinophilic granular cytoplasm that contains a large, round nucleus with a prominent nucleolus. These cells form cribriformed structures, with mucin-containing intraepithelial lumina. Interspersed goblet cells are also common. In some cases, the epithelium of adjacent papillae may fuse, producing a solid growth pattern. An intense stromal and intraepithelial infiltration by neutrophilic granulocytes may also be seen. Based on both the architectural complexity and the degree of nuclear atypia, essentially all IOPNs have high-grade dysplasia.

Associated invasive carcinoma occurs in about 30% of IOPNs and is usually limited in extent {28,2048,3520}. The invasive component is mostly composed of small infiltrating tubules or solid nests composed of oncocytic cells. In rare cases, the invasive component has abundant stromal mucin accumulation {28,3520}.

Immunohistochemically, IOPNs diffusely label for EMA (MUC1) and MUC6, whereas MUC2 and MUC5AC expression is largely restricted to goblet cells {1983,3280,268,265}. In addition, there is consistent immunolabelling with Hep Par-1; however, in situ hybridization for albumin, a more specific test for hepatocellular differentiation, is negative {265}.

IOPNs should be distinguished from intraductal papillary mucinous neoplasms, especially the pancreatobiliary subtype. The complex cribriform architecture of the papillae that are composed of intensely eosinophilic (oncocytic) cells is the hallmark of IOPNs {28,1640}. IOPNs with a predominantly solid growth pattern may resemble acinar cell carcinoma or pancreatic neuroendocrine neoplasm (PanNEN). Immunohistochemistry is helpful in these distinctions.

Cytology
The unique cytological features of IOPN include sheets or papillary groups of oncocytic cells with abundant granular cytoplasm, as well as well-defined cell borders, large central nuclei, prominent eccentric nucleoli, and intercellular punched-out spaces. IOPNs produce far less intracellular mucin and have less extracellular colloid-like mucin – features typically reported in intraductal papillary mucinous neoplasms {3301,1226,2205,2690}.

IOPNs qualify as exhibiting high-grade atypia by virtue of their architectural and cellular complexity {2134,2591,2690}. However, the high-grade atypia observed in these tumours does not necessarily signify the presence of invasive carcinoma {2048,3520}.

The cellularity and complex architecture of IOPNs, combined with the paucity of mucin, may lead to their misdiagnosis as ductal adenocarcinoma on cytological samples {2690}.

Diagnostic molecular pathology
Not clinically relevant

Essential and desirable diagnostic criteria
Essential: a complex arborizing papillary neoplasm with oncocytic epithelial features; location within a cystically dilated duct; examine carefully for an associated invasive carcinoma.

Staging (TNM)
Staging of IOPNs with associated invasive carcinoma is based on the size of the invasive component and follows the protocol for ductal adenocarcinoma {2822,42,110}. For IOPNs previously staged as early invasion (≤ 2 cm, pT1), the Union for International Cancer Control (UICC) recently introduced the substages pT1a (≤ 0.5 cm), pT1b (> 0.5 to < 1 cm), and pT1c (≥ 1 cm).

Prognosis and prediction
Although IOPNs are associated with invasive carcinoma in about 30% of cases, patients' 5-year disease-specific survival rate approaches 100% {3520}. Local recurrences, which are seen in as many as 45% of cases and may occur > 10 years after the initial resection, can often be successfully treated with additional resection {28,2048,3520}.

Pancreatic intraductal tubulopapillary neoplasm

Basturk O   Hong SM
Esposito I   Klöppel G
Fukushima N   Maitra A
Furukawa T   Zamboni G

Definition

Intraductal tubulopapillary neoplasm (ITPN) of the pancreas is an intraductal, predominantly tubule-forming, epithelial neoplasm with high-grade dysplasia and ductal differentiation without overt production of mucin. Invasive carcinoma may occur, and these cases are designated ITPN with associated invasive carcinoma.

ICD-O coding

8503/2 Intraductal tubulopapillary neoplasm
8503/3 Intraductal papillary neoplasm with associated invasive carcinoma

ICD-11 coding

2E61.Y & XH64S7 Carcinoma in situ of other specified digestive organs & Intraductal tubular-papillary neoplasm, high grade
2C10.0 & XH90W1 Adenocarcinoma of pancreas & Intraductal papillary neoplasm with associated invasive carcinoma

Related terminology

Not recommended: intraductal tubular carcinoma.

Subtype(s)

None

Localization

About half of all ITPNs occur in the head of the pancreas and a third involve the gland diffusely {263}.

Clinical features

ITPNs account for < 1% of all pancreatic exocrine neoplasms and 3% of intraductal neoplasms of the pancreas {3643}. ITPNs are slightly more common in females. Patient age ranges from 25 to 84 years (mean: 55 years) {263}. Patients present with non-specific symptoms including abdominal pain, vomiting, weight loss, steatorrhoea, and diabetes mellitus. Obstructive jaundice is uncommon. Some ITPNs are detected incidentally {263}.

Epidemiology

Unknown

Etiology

Unknown

Pathogenesis

There are few data on pathogenesis. The genetic features of ITPNs differ from those of ductal adenocarcinomas and other intraductal neoplasms of the pancreas. Most of the reported alterations related to ductal adenocarcinoma and intraductal papillary mucinous neoplasm (IPMN), including *KRAS* mutations, are absent in ITPNs {3643,3641,3642,120}. However, certain chromatin remodelling genes (*KMT2A* [*MLL1*], *KMT2B*

[*MLL2*], KMT2C [*MLL3*], *BAP1*) and PI3K pathway genes (*PIK3CA*, *PTEN*) can be mutated. A subset of cases harbour *FGFR2* fusions {264}, which might be targetable.

Macroscopic appearance

ITPNs form solid, fleshy to rubbery, nodular masses within dilated pancreatic ducts {879,1244,3160,3643}, but the intraductal growth may be difficult to recognize. Cyst formation is often less evident than in IPMNs. Mucinous secretions are not present. The average ITPN is 4.5 cm in diameter (range: 0.5–15.0 cm).

Histopathology

Microscopically, ITPNs form nodules of back-to-back tubular glands, resulting in large cribriform structures {263,3208,3643}. The intraductal location of at least some of the nodules is evidenced by continuity of the neoplastic epithelium with non-neoplastic ductal epithelium. However, most intraductal tumour nodules obliterate the ductal lumen, appearing as sharply circumscribed nests surrounded by fibrotic stroma. Although most ITPNs are predominantly tubular, papillae may be seen {3643}. ITPNs are architecturally complex and typically have high-grade dysplasia. The tumour cells are predominantly cuboidal, with modest amounts of eosinophilic to amphophilic and rarely clear cytoplasm {57,263}. In some cases, intraluminal secretions may be seen. However, intracellular mucin is typically not detectable or is minimal {1743,3643}. The nuclei are

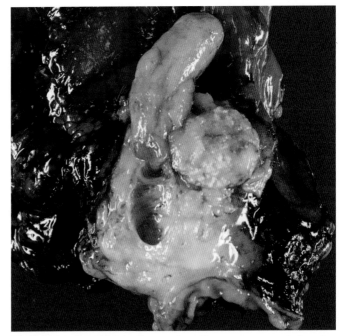

Fig. 10.16 Intraductal tubulopapillary neoplasm. Gross appearance; note the polypoid component within the dilated main pancreatic duct.

Chapter 10

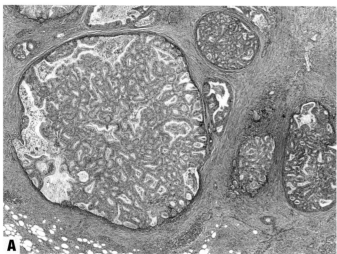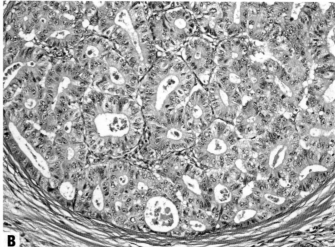

Fig. 10.17 Intraductal tubulopapillary neoplasm. **A** Intraductal tubulopapillary neoplasm is composed of multiple smooth-contoured, cellular nodules that exhibit a predominantly tubular architecture. **B** The tubules are typically well formed, with recognizable lumina of various sizes. The tumour cells contain minimal cytoplasm, and nuclei are atypical.

round to oval and atypical but uniform. Mitotic figures are often readily identifiable {3643}. Most cases show foci of necrosis within the nodules, often with a comedo-like pattern.

ITPNs typically have a relatively homogeneous appearance, and there are no transitions to areas with less-marked cyto-architectural atypia or to IPMNs or pancreatic intraepithelial neoplasia {3208,3209,3643}. Invasive carcinoma is found in association with 70% of cases, and the invasive component is usually limited in extent {263,3160,3643}. Because many of the individual neoplastic nodules lack a peripheral rim of non-neoplastic ductal epithelium, it is often difficult to determine whether invasive carcinoma is present, and even for cases with established invasive carcinoma, it may be challenging to determine its extent. Individual cells or small, angulated non-mucinous glands extending away from the periphery of the nodules into surrounding desmoplastic stroma represent invasive carcinoma. Therefore, careful sampling and evaluation is warranted.

The neoplastic cells are consistently positive for pancy-tokeratins and commonly label for CK7 and CK19. Labelling for acinar markers and neuroendocrine markers is negative. Most commonly, EMA (MUC1) and MUC6 are expressed, but MUC2 is consistently negative, and MUC5AC, a marker of all types of IPMNs, is almost never expressed in ITPNs {2249,717,263}.

Pancreatobiliary-type IPMNs can be difficult to distinguish from ITPNs. A mucinous nature in parallel with MUC5AC expression, as well as the presence of a spectrum of dysplasia, favours pancreatobiliary-type IPMN {263,1640,2687,2755}.

ITPN is also difficult to distinguish from acinar cell carcinomas, which may show intraductal growth {273}. Unlike ITPNs, acinar cell carcinomas often show apical acidophilic granules and occasionally display intraluminal crystals (enzymatic concretions). Immunohistochemical labelling for markers of pancreatic exocrine enzymes, such as trypsin, is essential in this differential diagnosis {1748}.

Cytology

Although there have been no systematic analyses, case reports describe highly cellular, relatively cohesive clusters with cribriform and tubular patterns and tumour cells without intracytoplasmic mucin in cytological smears of ITPNs {202,989,1106,3207,2869}.

Diagnostic molecular pathology

Not clinically relevant

Essential and desirable diagnostic criteria

Essential: nodules of back-to-back tubular glands, resulting in large cribriformed structures; expression of cytokeratins; lack of MUC5AC expression.

Staging (TNM)

Staging of ITPNs with associated invasive carcinoma is based on the size of the invasive component and follows the protocol for ductal adenocarcinoma {2822,42,110}. For ITPNs previously staged as early invasion (≤ 2 cm, pT1), the Union for International Cancer Control (UICC) recently introduced the substages pT1a (≤ 0.5 cm), pT1b (> 0.5 to < 1 cm), and pT1c (≥ 1 cm). ITPNs without an associated invasive carcinoma are staged as Tis.

Prognosis and prediction

Despite the difficulties of determining the extent of invasive carcinoma in many cases, the overall outcome of ITPNs seems to be significantly better than that of ductal adenocarcinoma {263,3160,3208,3643}. Even when only the ITPNs with invasive carcinoma are considered, the 5-year survival rate is 71% {263}.

Pancreatic mucinous cystic neoplasm

Basturk O
Esposito I
Fukushima N
Furukawa T
Hong SM
Klöppel G
Maitra A
Zamboni G

Definition

Mucinous cystic neoplasm (MCN) of the pancreas is a cyst-forming and mucin-producing epithelial neoplasm associated with distinctive ovarian-type subepithelial stroma. If there is an invasive carcinoma component, the lesion is designated MCN with associated invasive carcinoma.

ICD-O coding

8470/0 Mucinous cystic neoplasm with low-grade dysplasia
8470/2 Mucinous cystic neoplasm with high-grade dysplasia
8470/3 Mucinous cystic neoplasm with associated invasive carcinoma

ICD-11 coding

2E92.8 & XH6H73 Benign neoplasm of pancreas & Mucinous cystadenoma NOS
2E92.8 & XH6NK7 Benign neoplasm of pancreas & Mucinous cystic neoplasm with low-grade intraepithelial neoplasia
2E61.Y & XH81P3 Carcinoma in situ of other specified digestive organs & Mucinous cystic tumour with high-grade dysplasia
2C10.0 & XH1K19 Adenocarcinoma of pancreas & Mucinous cystic tumour with associated invasive carcinoma

Related terminology

MCN
Acceptable: mucinous cystadenoma.

MCN with associated invasive carcinoma
Acceptable: mucinous cystadenocarcinoma.

High-grade MCN
Acceptable: carcinoma in situ (used parenthetically in some parts of the world).

Subtype(s)

None

Localization

The majority (> 98%) of MCNs occur in the body or tail of the pancreas {3733,3302,3655,1424}.

Clinical features

MCNs account for about 8% of resected cystic lesions of the pancreas {1689,563}. The vast majority of MCNs (> 98%) occur in women, and the average age at diagnosis is 48 years (range: 14–95 years) {3733,3302,3655,1424}. Patients with an invasive carcinoma component are 5–10 years older than patients with a non-invasive MCN, suggesting that progression occurs over a period of years {1689}.

Small tumours (< 3 cm) are usually found incidentally. Larger tumours may produce symptoms due to compression of adjacent structures, often accompanied by a palpable abdominal

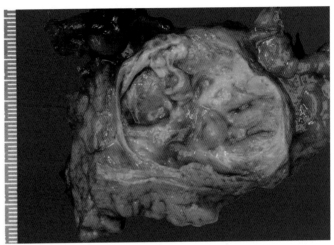

Fig. 10.18 Mucinous cystic neoplasm. Macroscopically, mucinous cystic neoplasms are typically single unilocular or multilocular cysts containing thick mucin or haemorrhagic material.

mass. Imaging studies reveal a large well-defined cystic lesion with thick-walled loculations without connection to the pancreatic ducts {266,1689,3655}. Features suggestive of an associated invasive carcinoma include large tumour size (> 5 cm), irregular thickening of the cyst wall, intracystic mural nodules, and elevated serum CA19-9 level (> 37 kU/L) {3655,1424}. Preoperative cyst fluid CEA levels {1240,2223,2277} and molecular analysis {2360,2594,1014} may also supplement other findings in assessing the risk of carcinoma in MCNs.

Epidemiology

There are no known geographical variations in the occurrence of MCNs.

Etiology

Unknown

Pathogenesis

Pancreatic MCNs share many clinicopathological features with their counterparts in the hepatobiliary tree, ovary, and other organs {3022,3733}. It is conceivable that ectopic ovarian stroma incorporated during embryogenesis in the pancreas and other organs may become activated in the setting of a hormonal imbalance, releasing hormones and growth factors and causing nearby ductal epithelium to proliferate and form cystic neoplasms {3733,1415}. This hypothesis cannot account for MCNs in males. Another possibility is that the ovarian-type stroma represents persistent fetal periductal mesenchyme, which may respond and proliferate in response to hormonal stimulation {1304}.

The epithelial component of MCNs harbours activating mutations in codon 12 of *KRAS* in 50–66% of cases, as well as

Chapter 10

loss-of-function alterations in *RNF43* {3617,22927,3118}. Mutations of *TP53* are rare. Because *TP53* mutations are often associated with aggressiveness {1511}, it is possible that the MCNs with mutations in *TP53* are the ones most likely to progress to high-grade dysplasia or invasive carcinoma {3616,3118}.

Macroscopic appearance

MCN typically presents as a cystic mass with a fibrous wall of variable thickness, occasionally containing calcifications. MCNs range from 2 to 35 cm in greatest dimension (mean: 6 cm), but MCNs with invasive carcinoma are considerably larger (mean: 9 cm) {1424}. The unilocular or multilocular cysts contain thick mucin and/or haemorrhagic, necrotic material. The internal surface may be smooth; however, higher-grade MCNs often have nodules or papillary projections {3655,1424}.

Histopathology

Histologically, the cysts of MCNs are lined by epithelium and have underlying ovarian-type stroma. The epithelium is predominantly columnar, with mucin-producing cells; however, cuboidal cells lacking mucin, similar to non-neoplastic ductal cells, can occur as well {91,3766}. On the basis of the highest degree of cytoarchitectural atypia in the epithelium, MCNs are categorized as low-grade or high-grade. The current two-tiered grading system for MCN recently replaced the former three-tiered grading scheme; neoplasms belonging to the former categories of "MCN with low-grade dysplasia" and "MCN with intermediate-grade dysplasia" {1301,1306} are now categorized as low-grade MCN, and those belonging to the former category of "MCN with high-grade dysplasia" are now categorized as high-grade MCN {267}.

Low-grade MCNs are characterized by mild to moderate atypia and may or may not reveal papillary projections and mitoses. High-grade MCNs display severe atypia, with the formation of papillae with irregular branching and budding, nuclear stratification with loss of polarity, pleomorphism, and prominent nucleoli; mitoses are numerous.

The distinctive ovarian-type stroma consists of densely packed spindle-shaped cells with round or elongated nuclei and sparse cytoplasm, and its presence is required for the diagnosis {3238,2166,1304}. It can be particularly useful when the epithelial lining is extensively denuded. The stroma frequently displays clusters of epithelioid cells with round to oval nuclei and abundant clear or eosinophilic cytoplasm, resembling luteinized cells {3733}. In large MCNs or in those occurring in postmenopausal patients, the stroma may become hypocellular and hyalinized. Similarly, the amount of stroma may be decreased around areas of high-grade dysplasia and invasive carcinoma {1424}.

About 15% of MCNs have an associated invasive carcinoma component {2848,3655,1097,1424}, which typically occurs in large (> 5 cm) tumours with gross papillary nodules {3733,439,3282}. The invasive component is usually tubular-type adenocarcinoma, but other subtypes have been described, including adenosquamous carcinoma and undifferentiated carcinoma with osteoclast-like giant cells; colloid carcinoma does not occur in MCNs {3409,39,101,349}. The invasive component can be focal. Therefore, thorough (if not complete) sampling is warranted {1424}.

The neoplastic epithelial cells are immunoreactive with CK7, CK8, CK18, CK19, EMA, CEA, and MUC5AC {982,2959}. Whereas non-invasive MCNs express SMAD4 protein but not EMA (MUC1), invasive carcinomas in MCNs may lose the expression of SMAD4 and express EMA (MUC1) {1977,1349}. The ovarian-type stroma expresses SMA, MSA, desmin, PR (60–90%), and ER (30%) {983,3733}. Luteinized cells stain for tyrosine hydroxylase, calretinin, and α-inhibin {3733,1393}.

The differential diagnosis with intraductal papillary mucinous neoplasms can be relatively straightforward for main duct-type intraductal papillary mucinous neoplasms, but may be difficult for branch duct-type intraductal papillary mucinous neoplasms. Two features distinguish these entities: MCNs do not grow within the pancreatic duct system, and they contain (by definition) ovarian-type stroma. Differentiating a pseudocyst from an MCN may be a problem, because some MCNs can have substantial degenerative changes, including almost entirely denuded epithelium. Extensive sampling is needed to identify the diagnostic features of MCN, the mucin-producing epithelial lining, or the ovarian-type stroma {2166,1304}.

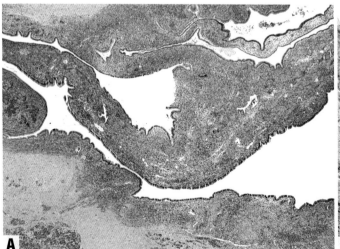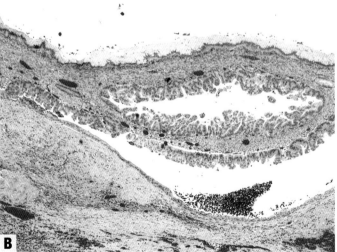

Fig. 10.19 Mucinous cystic neoplasm. **A** At low power, mucinous cystic neoplasm is surrounded by a fibrous capsule. The cysts are lined by mucinous epithelium, and the stroma of the septa is of hypercellular ovarian type. **B** Mucinous cystic neoplasm with both low-grade (top) and high-grade (centre) dysplasia.

Cytology

Aspirates contain varying amounts of thick mucin and often only few epithelial cells. The neoplastic cells form sheets and small clusters and the cytoplasm contains mucin. The degree of dysplasia in cytological samples often underrepresents that observed histologically when the lesion is resected. The ovarian-type stroma is often not present in aspirates. In such cases, only the nonspecific diagnosis of mucinous neoplastic cyst can be made {42}.

Diagnostic molecular pathology

Not clinically relevant

Essential and desirable diagnostic criteria

Essential: a grossly visible, multilocular cystic lesion, almost exclusively in female patients, with no communication to the ductal system; a cystic lesion with cuboidal and columnar neoplastic epithelia, staining at least partly positive for mucin, with variable atypia; ovarian-like, mesenchymal stroma, at least focally positive for ER and/or PR.

Staging (TNM)

High-grade MCNs are categorized as Tis (carcinoma in situ). Staging of MCNs with associated invasive carcinoma is based on the size of the invasive component and follows the protocol for pancreatic ductal adenocarcinoma {2822,42,110,269}. For MCNs previously designated as having early invasion (≤ 2 cm, pT1), the Union for International Cancer Control (UICC) recently introduced the substages pT1a (≤ 0.5 cm), pT1b (> 0.5 to < 1 cm), and pT1c (≥ 1 cm).

Prognosis and prediction

If invasive carcinoma is ruled out by thorough sampling of the neoplasm, the prognosis of non-invasive MCNs is excellent, with a 5-year survival rate of 100% {3561,3733,2672,691,3655,227}. However, invasive carcinomas arising in MCNs have an aggressive clinical course, with 3-year and 5-year survival rates of 44% and 26%, respectively. Also, the prognosis in these patients depends on the size (T stage) of the invasive component, nodal and distant metastasis, and resectability {3733,1424}. Earlier data suggesting that invasive carcinomas limited to the septa of the cysts were unlikely to metastasize {3733} conflict with a recent report of metastases from microscopic, cyst-limited (pT1a) carcinomas {1424}.

Pancreatic ductal adenocarcinoma

Hruban RH
Adsay NV
Esposito I
Fukushima N
Furukawa T
Klöppel G
Maitra A
Notohara K
Offerhaus GJA
Ohike N
Pitman MB
Zamboni G

Definition

Pancreatic ductal adenocarcinoma (PDAC) is an invasive pancreatic epithelial neoplasm with glandular (ductal) differentiation, usually demonstrating luminal and/or intracellular mucin production, without a substantial component of any other histological type.

ICD-O coding

8500/3 Duct adenocarcinoma NOS

ICD-11 coding

2C10.0 Adenocarcinoma of pancreas

Related terminology

Ductal adenocarcinoma
Acceptable: duct cell adenocarcinoma; infiltrating duct carcinoma; tubular adenocarcinoma.

Adenosquamous carcinoma
None

Colloid carcinoma
Acceptable: mucinous non-cystic carcinoma.

Undifferentiated carcinoma, anaplastic type
Acceptable: giant cell carcinoma; anaplastic carcinoma; pleomorphic large cell carcinoma.

Undifferentiated carcinoma, sarcomatoid type
Acceptable: spindle cell carcinoma; sarcomatoid carcinoma.

Undifferentiated carcinoma with osteoclast-like giant cells
Acceptable: osteoclastic giant cell carcinoma.

Subtype(s)

Colloid carcinoma (8480/3); poorly cohesive carcinoma (8490/3); signet-ring cell carcinoma (8490/3); medullary carcinoma NOS (8510/3); adenosquamous carcinoma (8560/3); hepatoid carcinoma (8576/3); large cell carcinoma with rhabdoid phenotype (8014/3); carcinoma, undifferentiated, NOS (8020/3); undifferentiated carcinoma with osteoclast-like giant cells (8035/3)

Localization

Two thirds of ductal adenocarcinomas arise in the head of the pancreas, and the remainder in the body or tail of the gland {1304}. The vast majority of ductal adenocarcinomas are solitary, but multifocal disease can occur {1304,2803}. Very rarely, ectopic pancreatic tissue can give rise to pancreatic intraepithelial neoplasia (PanIN) lesions and even to an invasive carcinoma {1062,3260,1488,3754}.

Clinical features

Clinical features include decreased appetite and indigestion, changes in bowel habits, fatigue, back pain, unexplained weight loss, and jaundice {3505}. New-onset diabetes (type 3c) may be the first manifestation of pancreatic cancer {1175,2975}. Depression may be a presenting symptom {3589}. Symptoms of advanced disease are related to liver metastasis and/or invasion of adjacent organs (e.g. the duodenum) or of the peritoneal cavity (ascites). Patients occasionally present with migratory thrombophlebitis {1706} and rarely with acute pancreatitis {1887}.

Multidetector CT with dual-phase or multiphase dynamic contrast using early arterial, pancreatic, and late venous phases is one of the best imaging modalities for the pancreas and the surrounding vasculature {3589}. PDAC usually appears as an irregular solid hypodense mass with abrupt cut-off and upstream dilatation of the pancreatic duct. The double-duct sign (dilatation of both the biliary and the pancreatic ducts) is virtually pathognomonic of carcinoma of the head of the pancreas. MRI may be more sensitive than CT for the detection and evaluation of liver metastases {2232}, and magnetic resonance cholangiopancreatography provides excellent resolution of the duct system. EUS allows high-resolution imaging of the pancreas and surrounding lymph nodes and vessels; it also allows tissue sampling, which remains the gold standard for diagnosis. PET may have diagnostic value, especially in cases with enlarged lymph nodes or of persisting masses after therapy {2520}. The serum markers CA19-9 and CEA are not useful, by themselves, for screening of asymptomatic individuals but can be used to monitor established disease {2606}.

Epidemiology

The epidemiological study of PDAC is complicated by substantial geographical and temporal variations in the sensitivity and specificity of clinical diagnosis and in the proportion of cases that are histologically verified. Differences in access to health care (e.g. across different social classes or age groups) can affect the reported incidence and mortality rates.

Worldwide, 458 918 new cases of PDAC were estimated in 2018, with an age-adjusted incidence rate among both sexes of 6.2 cases per 100 000 person-years in higher-income countries and 1.5 cases per 100 000 person-years in lower-income countries {399}. The highest rates have been recorded among black people in the USA (about 17 cases per 100 000 person-years among men and 14 cases per 100 000 person-years among women {3183}) and in indigenous populations in Oceania. The lowest rates (< 2 cases per 100 000 person-years among men and 1 case per 100 000 person-years among women), which may be partially attributable to underdiagnosis, have been recorded in India, northern and central Africa, and south-eastern Asia. Most patients are diagnosed at an age of 55–85 years (median age at diagnosis in the USA: 70 years). Globally, the M:F ratio is 1.1:1. Because of the very poor survival, mortality

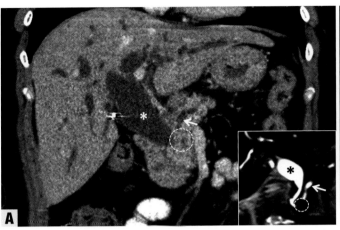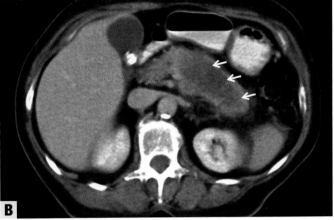

Fig. 10.20 Pancreatic cancer. **A** Coronal CT of a pancreatic head ductal adenocarcinoma showing the characteristic double duct sign. The arrow indicates the dilated pancreatic duct, and the asterisk the dilated bile duct; the dotted circle indicates the slightly hypodense neoplasm. **Inset**: The same case shown on MRI / magnetic resonance cholangiopancreatography. **B** Ductal adenocarcinoma of the pancreatic body-tail presenting as a large hypodense mass on CT.

rates are similar to incidence rates, with a mortality-to-incidence ratio of 0.94 {399,923}.

An apparent increase in incidence and mortality has occurred since the 1970s, in particular in high-income countries, where this increase can be partially attributed to diagnostic improvements. Although some data suggest a levelling off of incidence and mortality rates over the past 10 years {3183}, recent reports indicate a steady increase of incidence rates in Europe and North America, probably as a result of ageing populations and increasing risk factors {1075,922,3593,374}. It has been predicted that by 2030, pancreatic cancer will become the second leading cause of cancer-related death in the USA {2641}.

Urban populations have higher rates than rural populations, but this may again reflect differences in quality of diagnosis. Migrant studies suggest that first-generation migrants from low-risk to high-risk areas experience, after 15 or 20 years, rates that are higher than those of the country of emigration, suggesting an important role of environmental exposures occurring late in life {135}.

Etiology

The best-known risk factor for pancreatic cancer is tobacco smoking. The risk in smokers is 2–3 times that in non-smokers, and a dose–response relationship and a favourable effect of quitting smoking have been shown in many populations {1382,1973,3499}. The proportion of cases of pancreatic cancer attributable to tobacco smoking has been estimated to be 20–30% in men and 10% in women {1352}. Passive (secondhand) smoking and the use of smokeless tobacco products have also been linked to pancreatic cancer risk {354,241}.

Nutritional and dietary factors have been suggested to be related to pancreatic cancer, including obesity, low physical activity, high intake of (saturated) fats, and low intake of vegetables and fruits {3144,1021,905,1461,1693}.

A positive association between alcohol consumption and pancreatic cancer has been reported in some (but not all) studies that have addressed this question. The current evidence is consistent with a possible weak effect of heavy alcohol consumption {1022,1123}.

Several medical conditions are associated with subsequent risk of pancreatic cancer, most notably diabetes mellitus

and chronic pancreatitis {3633,236}. A history of pancreatitis increases the risk 2-fold to 10-fold, and the risk is particularly high in individuals with hereditary pancreatitis {236,1952,2644}. An increased risk has also been shown in several studies of patients with diabetes mellitus; the relative risk is likely to fall in the range 1.5–2 {1915,376}. Although studies are conflicting, gastrectomy patients may have an increased risk of pancreatic cancer {2414,375,1067}. Some of the features of the descriptive epidemiology of pancreatic cancer (i.e. a high incidence among Black people in the USA but a low incidence in Africa, and a higher risk among men and urban residents) can be explained by differences in smoking habits, diabetes, and obesity {190,1985}.

Genome-wide association studies have linked variants in the *ABO* locus to pancreatic cancer susceptibility; individuals with type O blood were found to have a lower risk than those with type A or B {3590}. For further details on genetic predisposition, see *Familial pancreatic cancer* (p. 539).

Pathogenesis

The mechanisms by which several of the causes described in the etiology subsection lead to neoplastic progression are well defined. For example, cigarette smoking is one of the leading causes of pancreatic cancer. Cigarette smoke contains carcinogens that damage DNA such as 4-(methylnitrosamino)-1-(3-pyridyl)-1-butanone (NNK) and benzo[a]pyrene (BaP), and as discussed below, DNA mutations are known to drive the formation of pancreatic cancer {1307,342}. Longstanding chronic pancreatitis is also a risk factor for pancreatic cancer, and repeated episodes of inflammation, injury, and repair drive neoplasia {1194}.

Pancreatic cancer is essentially a genetic disease, caused by inherited (germline) and somatic mutations. The inherited mutations are described in the *Familial pancreatic cancer* section (p. 539). The main somatic genetic drivers of pancreatic cancer were discovered in the late 1980s and the 1990s {1141,460,3072,255}. The exomes of pancreatic cancer were first sequenced in 2008 {1481}. Several large publicly funded next-generation sequencing efforts, such as the International Cancer Genome Consortium (ICGC) and The Cancer Genome Atlas (TCGA), have further defined the comprehensive

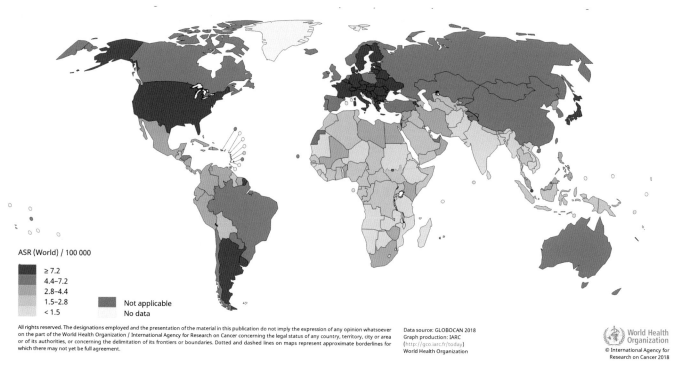

Data source: GLOBOCAN 2018
Graph production: IARC
(http://gco.iarc.fr/today)
World Health Organization

World Health Organization
© International Agency for Research on Cancer 2018

Fig. 10.21 Estimated age-standardized incidence rates (ASRs; World), per 100 000 person-years, of pancreatic cancer in 2018.

ASR (World) / 100 000

≥ 7.2
4.4–7.2
2.8–4.4
1.5–2.8
< 1.5
Not applicable
No data

molecular landscapes of pancreatic cancer {224,327,477,2192}. These studies have identified four "mountains" (i.e. the most common recurrent abnormalities in the pancreatic cancer genome): oncogenic mutations of *KRAS* (chromosome 12p), as well as loss-of-function mutations and/or deletions of the tumour suppressor genes *TP53* (chromosome 17p), *SMAD4* (*DPC4*) (chromosome 18q), and *CDKN2A* (*P16*) (chromosome 9p).

Oncogenic point mutations of *KRAS* on codon 12, 13, or 61 are found in > 90% of pancreatic cancers. The resulting constitutive activation of the RAS signalling pathway has a profound impact on cell-autonomous growth and survival, as well as paracrine effects on the tumour microenvironment that enable cancer cells to escape the immune system {3538,1623,3492,433}. As described in the chapter on PanIN lesions, *KRAS* mutations are one of the earliest genetic alterations in the multistep progression of pancreatic cancer, and animal models have validated its seminal role in pancreatic cancer initiation and maintenance {1235,1236,3703,653}. The *CDKN2A* (*P16*) tumour suppressor gene is inactivated in 40% of pancreatic carcinomas by homozygous deletion, in 40% by loss of one allele coupled with an intragenic mutation in the other, and in an additional 15% by hypermethylation of the *CDKN2A* (*P16*) promoter {460,2912}. The *TP53* gene is inactivated in 75% of pancreatic carcinomas by loss of one allele coupled with an intragenic mutation in the second allele {255,2674}. The *SMAD4* (*DPC4*) tumour suppressor gene is inactivated in 55% of pancreatic carcinomas {1141}: in 35% by homozygous deletion and in 20% by loss of one allele coupled with an intragenic mutation in the second allele.

In addition to these four mountains, a large number of genomic "hills" are altered at a lower prevalence in pancreatic cancer, and the individual genes can be grouped into several core pathways that are hallmarks of cancers. For example, mutations of genes involved in DNA repair (most commonly *BRCA2*

mutations, but also other somatic mutations such as *PALB2*, *ATM*, *CHEK2*, and *RAD51* mutations) can be found in as many as 15–20% of pancreatic cancers {3500,661,1954}. Pancreatic cancers with defects in DNA repair represent a unique subset that can be targeted with platinum drugs (e.g. cisplatin) or with a new class of agents known as poly (ADP-ribose) polymerase (PARP) inhibitors {2817}. Similarly, defects in epigenetic drivers that regulate chromatin accessibility, and therefore gene expression, are found in almost 40% of pancreatic cancers, including abnormalities of the COMPASS-like complex (*KMT2C* [*MLL3*], *KDM6A*) and the DNA-binding helicase multiprotein complex known as the SWI/SNF complex – *ARID1A*, *PBRM1*, *SMARCA4* (*BRG1*) {224,477}. Defects in these chromatin regulators cause widespread transcriptional deregulation in pancreatic cancer that promotes tumour growth and metastases {143,2770}. Identifying therapeutic agents that can target pancreatic cancers with these driver mutations remains an area of active investigation.

Macroscopic appearance

Ductal adenocarcinomas are firm and poorly defined yellowish-white masses, usually without haemorrhagic necrosis but occasionally with microcystic or macrocystic areas. Most resected carcinomas of the pancreas head (60%) are 2–4 cm (mean: 3.5 cm) {2891,1203}, whereas carcinomas of the body/tail are usually somewhat larger. Cancers < 2 cm are rare (12%) {2891,1203}. Carcinomas in the pancreatic head typically lead to stenosis and proximal dilatation of the common bile duct and/or the main pancreatic duct (double duct sign on imaging), and this in turn causes fibrosclerotic atrophy of the upstream non-neoplastic pancreatic tissue (obstructive chronic pancreatitis). Moreover, most pancreatic carcinomas infiltrate surrounding structures, including the ampulla of Vater, the duodenal wall, peripancreatic and retroperitoneal tissues, and the superior mesenteric vessels {710}. Carcinomas in the pancreatic body or tail typically do not involve the common bile duct, but may infiltrate the stomach wall, left side of the colon, spleen, and left adrenal gland {3702}.

Histopathology
Histopathological appearance
Most ductal adenocarcinomas are well to moderately differentiated and form duct-like glandular structures, which haphazardly infiltrate the pancreatic parenchyma and elicit a strong desmoplastic stromal response {1304}. In well-differentiated carcinomas, the duct-like structures, which may be difficult to recognize as neoplastic glands, occur side by side with glands showing features more diagnostic of adenocarcinoma, including ducts with angular contours, branching, ruptured glands, and/or a multilayered papillary epithelium with cribriform patterns. Most characteristic are ruptured glands that are partly lined by cellular stroma, into which mucin is leaking. The lumina of these glands may contain cellular debris and some neutrophils. Rarely, the histology of the carcinoma is dominated by a large duct pattern {1688,2893}. In moderately differentiated adenocarcinomas, the intratumoural heterogeneity is more conspicuous, with abundant glands forming cribriform, papillary, micropapillary, and/or gyriform patterns {1552,2893}. Foci of smaller and more irregular glands and some individual pleomorphic cells are often found at the tumour margins. Common to both well-differentiated and moderately differentiated carcinomas is a desmoplastic stroma that encompasses the neoplastic glands, sometimes in a ductocentric pattern. The stroma is hypovascular and composed of collagen fibres, which are often interspersed with fibroblasts, myofibroblasts, scattered lymphocytes, and macrophages.

The neoplastic cells are columnar to cuboidal and produce mucins that stain with Alcian blue and the PAS stain. The cytoplasm of the neoplastic cells is eosinophilic but sometimes foamy or even clear. The nuclei are round to ovoid with little pleomorphism. Occasionally there are bigger nuclei, 3–4 times the size of non-neoplastic nuclei. The nucleoli are often distinct, and the mitotic count is moderate.

Neoplastic glands can infiltrate the peripancreatic fatty tissue (following interlobular septa) and infiltrate pre-existing structures such as nerves, vessels, and ducts {2393}. Some neoplastic glands may lie individually within fatty tissue (naked ducts) or invade the duodenum and the ampulla up to the mucosa. Perineural invasion is common and occurs within and particularly outside the pancreas, where nerves are abundant {2267,1548}. Perineural invasion is a highly tumour-specific finding; non-neoplastic glandular inclusion in a nerve is exceedingly rare. Lymphatic invasion is found in the peripancreatic tissue and is associated with lymph node metastasis. When adenocarcinoma invades veins, it may replace the vascular endothelium and can even mimic PanIN {1268}. Carcinomas may invade back into non-neoplastic ducts, a process called cancerization of the ducts {1344A}. This change is usually accompanied by ductocentric desmoplasia, and it can be indistinguishable from high-grade PanIN (see *Pancreatic intraepithelial neoplasia*, p. 307). Perineural invasion, venous invasion, and cancerization of the ducts are all pathways by which the invasive carcinoma can reach far beyond the main neoplastic mass {1644}.The

infiltrating neoplastic glands may be intimately associated with non-neoplastic islets or single islet cells {2424}. A gland in an islet is not specific for cancer, and only in exceptional cases do the endocrine cells constitute a truly neoplastic component of the ductal carcinoma. In cases of severe duct obstruction by the carcinoma, there is marked upstream duct dilatation and almost complete fibrotic atrophy of the upstream parenchyma, often with intense non-neoplastic clustering (aggregation) of the remaining islets.

Poorly differentiated ductal adenocarcinomas are heterogeneous, and they are composed of solid or cribriform cell sheets and individual pleomorphic cells embedded in loosely arranged stroma {2893}. Foci of necrosis and haemorrhage may occur. The pleomorphic neoplastic cells (occasionally with squamoid or spindle cell differentiation) are not well polarized, produce little or no mucin, and have many mitoses. The neoplastic tissue destroys the parenchyma and may infiltrate widely into the peripancreatic tissue. Intraductal tumour extension is seen less often than in better-differentiated carcinomas, whereas perineural, lymphatic, and blood vessel invasion are equally prevalent.

Morphological patterns of ductal adenocarcinoma
Carcinomas of ductal lineage with distinct prognostic or molecular features are discussed in detail below, under the subheading *Histological subtypes*. There are also morphological patterns of conventional ductal adenocarcinomas that are not considered among the above entities because they do not alter prognosis and they do not appear to have distinct biological behaviour or clinical symptomatology to warrant classification as a specific subtype.

Perhaps the most important histological pattern of ductal adenocarcinoma that one should be aware of is the large duct pattern, which is characterized by neoplastic ducts measuring > 0.5 mm and sometimes having a deceptively bland-looking morphology {1688}. This pattern can mimic the branching of an intraductal papillary mucinous neoplasm (IPMN), until one recognizes that the glands are haphazardly arranged and the neoplastic cells are markedly dysplastic. Ductal adenocarcinoma

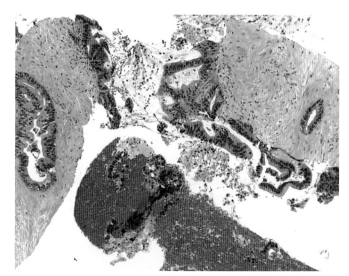

Fig. 10.22 Adenocarcinoma. Next-generation needle biopsy; ultrathin needles acquire small core tissue fragments, which may demonstrate invasive growth in desmoplastic stroma (cell block).

with a foamy gland pattern is also important to recognize {41}. The neoplastic cells of foamy gland adenocarcinoma have a lacy-looking microvesicular cytoplasm, basally located hyperchromatic (and often raisinoid) nuclei reminiscent of gastric foveolar epithelium, and a brush border–like apical condensation zone at the luminal side of the neoplastic cells. These cells look deceptively bland, particularly on frozen sections or small biopsies {41}. A clear cell subtype that resembles metastatic renal carcinoma has also been described {1981}. Some PDACs exhibit a substantially vacuolated pattern {830}.

Finally, a cystic papillary pattern, which may be related to the large duct pattern, has been reported, and this should not be mistaken for IPMN, because it has the histological features of and behaves similarly to a poorly differentiated ductal adenocarcinoma {1552}.

Immunohistochemistry

To date, there is no immunohistochemical marker that unequivocally distinguishes ductal adenocarcinoma from extrapancreatic mucin-producing adenocarcinomas, notably bile duct and gastric carcinomas. CK7, CK8, CK18, and CK19 are consistently expressed {1304}. Other markers that are usually positive are CEA, CA19-9, CA125, B72.3, DUPAN-2, EMA (MUC1), and MUC5AC (but not MUC2) {2269}. However, some of these markers also label the apical cell membranes of normal duct cells, particularly in chronic pancreatitis. Ductal adenocarcinomas are usually negative for vimentin and (with rare exceptions) neuroendocrine markers (synaptophysin, chromogranin A) or acinar markers (trypsin, BCL10) {1752}. Nuclear expression of

SMAD4 (DPC4) and p16 (CDKN2A) is lost in 55% and 75% of the carcinomas, respectively. p53 expression is altered in 75–80% of the cancers with either nuclear overexpression or no expression (null pattern) {2893,1304}. Other markers whose overexpression has been reported in PDACs include EGF and its receptor ERBB2 (c-erbB-2, HER2), TGF-α and TGF-β, PDGFA and PDGFB, VEGF and its receptors, metallothionein, CD44v6, claudin-4, claudin-18, ANXA8, disintegrin and metalloproteinase domain–containing protein 9 (ADAM9), K homology domain containing protein overexpressed in cancer (KOC), S100A4, S100A6, and S100P {1104,805,484,3681,2431,3065, 1524,1173}.

Grading

The grading of ductal adenocarcinoma is based on combined assessment of the degree of glandular differentiation, mucin production, mitotic activity, and nuclear features {1979,31}. If there is intratumoural heterogeneity (i.e. variation in the degree of differentiation and mitotic activity), the higher grade is assigned. This rule also applies if only a minor component (< 50% of the tumour) is of higher grade. Using this system, there is a correlation between grade and survival, and grade is an independent prognostic variable {1979,31}.

Differential diagnosis

Ductal adenocarcinoma must be distinguished from advanced chronic pancreatitis and other primary neoplasms of the pancreas {1636}. The most relevant criteria for the differential diagnosis are listed in Table 10.02 (p. 327) and Table 10.03 (p. 330).

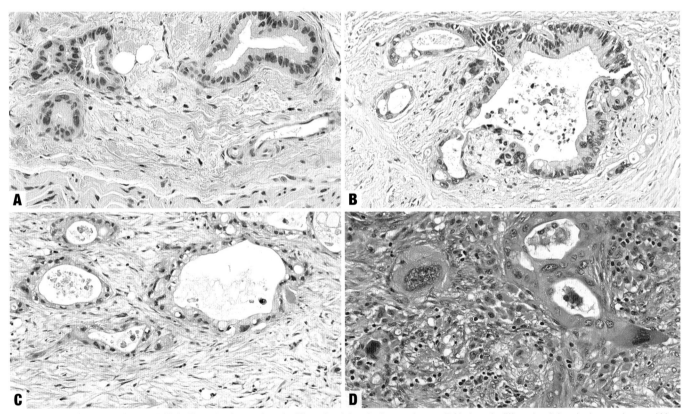

Fig. 10.23 Ductal adenocarcinoma. **A** Well-differentiated to moderately differentiated ductal adenocarcinoma. **B** Moderately differentiated ductal adenocarcinoma within a desmoplastic stroma. **C** Moderately differentiated adenocarcinoma. **D** Poorly differentiated ductal adenocarcinoma with giant cells.

Histological subtypes
Adenosquamous carcinoma and squamous cell carcinoma

Squamous differentiation is uncommon in pancreatic carcinomas and usually occurs in association with conventional ductal adenocarcinoma. True squamous cell carcinomas show exclusively squamous differentiation, with no evidence of gland formation or mucin production. The squamous component arbitrarily should account for ≥ 30% of the neoplasm in order for it to qualify as adenosquamous. Such cases account for only 1–4% of exocrine pancreatic malignancies {367,1312,1997}. Pure squamous cell carcinoma of the pancreas is extremely rare, and a metastasis from another site (e.g. lung) should be excluded if a neoplasm has purely squamous differentiation. Sampling often reveals glandular differentiation or histochemical evidence of mucin production in a pancreatic carcinoma with predominantly squamous differentiation. Macroscopically, most adenosquamous carcinomas are infiltrative, yellowish-white to grey, firm masses {2768}. Central necrosis and cystic degeneration are common. Some adenosquamous carcinomas are deceptively demarcated (radiologically detected as ring-enhancing {1370}), accentuating the differential diagnosis with a metastasis from another site. Histologically, the adenocarcinoma component forms glandular structures, often with intracellular or luminal mucin. Squamous differentiation is characterized by solid clusters or sheets of polygonal cells with distinct cellular borders, prominent intercellular junctions, dense eosinophilic cytoplasm, and varying degrees of keratinization. As expected, the squamous component often expresses p63 {412}, p40, and low-molecular-weight cytokeratins {2051,899}. Almost all cases harbour KRAS mutations at codon 12 {367}, and they also show

highly enriched *TP53* mutations, along with 3p loss {899} and mutations in the RNA surveillance gene *UPF1* {1927}. Immunohistochemically, they show loss of p16 (CDKN2A) protein expression, loss of SMAD4 (DPC4) protein, and strong nuclear p53 immunoreactivity, which is similar to the molecular signature found in PDACs {412,1526}. Emerging evidence suggests that adenosquamous carcinomas belong to the basal-like genomic subtype of pancreatic carcinoma {224}. Adenosquamous carcinomas appear to have a worse prognosis than pure ductal adenocarcinomas even when resected, with a median survival time

Table 10.02 Histological criteria for the differential diagnosis of ductal adenocarcinoma versus chronic pancreatitis {1636}

	Ductal adenocarcinoma	Chronic pancreatitis
Ductal features		
Distribution	Irregular, haphazard	Organized, lobular
Location	Perineural, intravascular, extrapancreatic (naked ducts in fat tissue)	Intrapancreatic
Contours	Rupture	Intact ducts
Contents	Neutrophils, necrotic debris	Calculi, secretory plugs
Cytological features		
Nucleus	Pleomorphic Mitosis Prominent nucleoli	Uniform, round-oval No mitosis No or small nucleoli
Nuclear polarity	Commonly lost	Retained

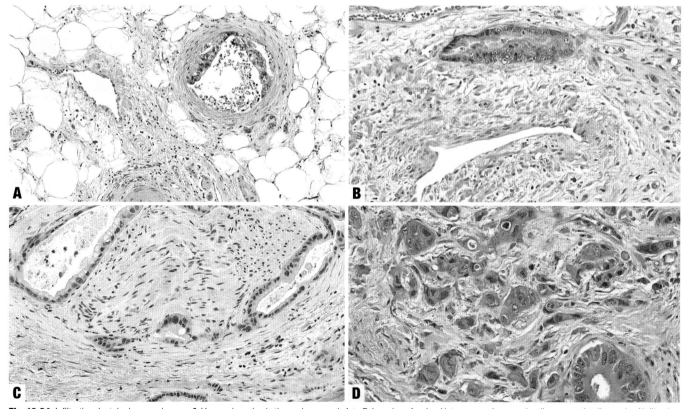

Fig. 10.24 Infiltrating ductal adenocarcinoma. **A** Venous invasion in the peripancreatic fat. **B** Invasion of a gland into a muscular vessel wall supports the diagnosis of infiltrating ductal adenocarcinoma. **C** Perineural invasion supports the diagnosis of infiltrating ductal adenocarcinoma. **D** Poorly differentiated ductal adenocarcinoma.

of about 9 months {1526,2433,3493,1670,1369,388}. The presence of any squamous component in the neoplasm appears to portend a worse prognosis {3493}.

Colloid carcinoma

Colloid carcinomas are adenocarcinomas in which ≥ 80% of the neoplastic epithelium is suspended in extracellular mucin pools. The tumours tend to be large and well demarcated, and most arise in association with intestinal-type IPMNs {39,2930}. The epithelium within the mucin is arranged in strips (either free-floating or attached to the surrounding fibrous stroma), as well as in clusters, in glands, and as individual cells. Some floating cells may be of the signet-ring type. The neoplastic cells of colloid carcinoma show intestinal differentiation; there is strong expression of CDX2 and MUC2, which are not substantially expressed in conventional ductal adenocarcinoma. In patients with IPMN, neoplastic cells floating in pools of stromal mucin and perineural invasion help distinguish a colloid carcinoma component from stromal mucin spillage {39,2230,2682}.

Colloid carcinomas have a substantially better prognosis than conventional ductal adenocarcinomas {39,2612,3231}, with a 5-year survival rate > 55% {38}.

Hepatoid carcinoma

Hepatoid carcinoma of the pancreas is an extremely rare malignant epithelial neoplasm {1327,2501,3261,3677,3437}. It is defined as a carcinoma in which ≥ 50% of the neoplasm displays histological and immunohistochemical evidence of hepatocellular differentiation. Hepatoid carcinomas are composed of large polygonal cells with abundant eosinophilic cytoplasm. An associated component of ductal adenocarcinoma may be present, and some hepatoid carcinomas are probably related to acinar cell carcinomas, which can express hepatocellular markers and produce AFP {640,200}. Many other tumour types can have hepatocyte-like morphology; therefore, this diagnosis should be used very stringently. AFP is not specific for hepatocellular differentiation and can also be observed in pancreatoblastomas and acinar, neuroendocrine, and ductal neoplasms without hepatoid morphological features {640,1542}. The expression of hepatocyte-specific antigen (Hep Par-1) can be seen in non-hepatoid neoplasms including intraductal oncocytic papillary neoplasm. A canalicular pattern of labelling with antibodies to polyclonal CEA and CD10 can be helpful but is not entirely specific either {701,1150}. FISH for albumin and immunohistochemistry for arginase are more-reliable markers of hepatocellular differentiation {200}. A pancreatic metastasis from an occult hepatocellular carcinoma must be excluded before establishing the diagnosis of a hepatoid carcinoma primary in the pancreas. Data on the prognosis of hepatoid carcinomas are minimal.

Medullary carcinoma

These are poorly differentiated carcinomas with limited gland formation, a pushing border, and syncytial growth, frequently with abundant tumour-infiltrating lymphocytes. Medullary carcinoma is composed of sheets and nests of poorly differentiated epithelial cells that largely lack gland formation. The periphery is circumscribed, pushing rather than infiltrating the surrounding fibrous stroma. Intercellular borders are indistinct, producing a syncytial growth pattern, and tumour-associated inflammatory infiltrates are typical, both within the stroma and admixed with the neoplastic cells (tumour-infiltrating lymphocytes) {1055,3562,2306}. Medullary carcinomas express keratin, and immunohistochemistry may demonstrate the loss of expression of one or more DNA mismatch repair proteins {239,1673,2306,3562}. Medullary carcinomas are more common in the ampulla and duodenum and are exceedingly uncommon in the pancreas; therefore, before this diagnosis can be rendered, origin in the adjacent GI tract must be excluded. Medullary carcinomas may arise sporadically or in the setting of Lynch syndrome {239,3649,3562}. They are often microsatellite-unstable {3562} and wildtype for the KRAS gene {463,1055,1213,1233,3157,3649}. Some poorly differentiated carcinomas with EBV infection of the neoplastic cells {3562} histologically resemble medullary carcinoma. Despite poor differentiation, the prognosis for patients with medullary carcinomas may be somewhat better than for those with conventional ductal adenocarcinomas {2306,3562,3649}. Based on the presence of microsatellite instability, medullary carcinomas may be responsive to treatment with immunotherapy {1816}.

Invasive micropapillary carcinoma

Invasive micropapillary carcinoma is an adenocarcinoma in which ≥ 50% of the neoplasm consists of small solid nests of cells suspended within stromal lacunae. A micropapillary pattern, as originally described in the breast and later in the urothelium, can also be seen in the pancreas, more commonly as a focal finding, which occurs in < 5% of pancreatobiliary-type adenocarcinomas {1564}. However, in some cases, it can be the predominant pattern, warranting a diagnosis of invasive micropapillary carcinoma {1618,1129}. Micropapillary carcinomas are often associated with prominent intra-epithelial neutrophilia. Micropapillary carcinomas behave more aggressively.

Signet-ring cell (poorly cohesive cell) carcinoma

The extremely rare pancreatic signet-ring cell carcinoma shows infiltration of individual poorly cohesive cells or of cords or sheets {889,3334,3275,2636}. At least 80% of the neoplasm consists of individually arrayed, poorly cohesive cells, often with intracellular mucin vacuoles peripherally displacing the nuclei. A variable amount of extracellular mucin is usually present. A carcinoma with this morphology in the pancreas should be presumed to be metastatic (from the stomach or breast in particular) before it can be classified as primary.

Undifferentiated carcinoma

Undifferentiated carcinoma is a malignant epithelial neoplasm in which a substantial component of the neoplasm does not show a definitive direction of differentiation. Typically, these neoplasms have a more diffuse sheet-like growth pattern without overt glandular differentiation in this component {3151}. Unlike ductal adenocarcinomas, undifferentiated carcinomas are poorly cohesive and hypercellular, and they often have only scant stroma {3351}. Immunohistochemically, most of these carcinomas express vimentin and usually also keratin but not E-cadherin {1271,2482,3580}. The prognosis is extremely poor, with an average survival time of just 5 months {1271,2482,3351}. Three morphological patterns of this subtype have been recognized.

Anaplastic undifferentiated carcinomas are composed of pleomorphic mononuclear cells admixed with bizarre-appearing

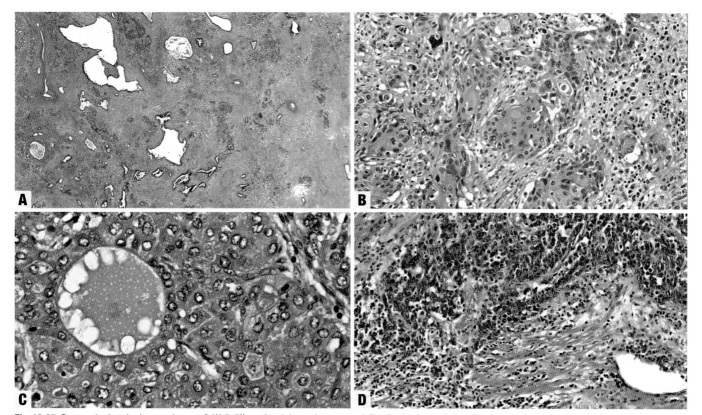

Fig. 10.25 Pancreatic ductal adenocarcinoma. **A** Well-differentiated, large duct pattern infiltrating haphazardly into fibrotic, atrophic pancreatic stroma. **B** Adenosquamous subtype. **C** Hepatoid subtype. **D** Medullary or lymphoepithelial subtype.

giant cells with eosinophilic cytoplasm. At least 80% of the neoplasm consists of solid sheets of cells lacking gland formation and showing markedly pleomorphic nuclei. The cells are non-cohesive, and a neutrophilic inflammatory infiltrate may be prominent, with emperipolesis of neutrophils within the cytoplasm of the neoplastic cells. Keratin expression is typically present.

Sarcomatoid undifferentiated carcinomas have cells with spindle cell morphology, which may contain heterologous elements including bone and cartilage. At least 80% of the neoplasm displays spindle cell features, with or without heterologous differentiation. Very rare examples of sarcomatoid undifferentiated carcinomas with rhabdoid cells have been described in the pancreas {2841}. They are characterized by diffuse sheets of rhabdoid cells, often with some degree of non-cohesiveness and a myxoid matrix. They can have pleomorphic giant cells, spindle cell areas, and tubular components. Immunohistochemically, loss of nuclear expression of SMARC1 (INI1), which is a core subunit of the SWI/SNF chromatin-remodelling complex, is characteristic {2426}, but this can also be found in carcinomas with more-conventional morphological features.

Carcinosarcomas have a biphasic pattern, containing both sarcomatoid elements (with or without heterologous elements) and components with obvious epithelial morphology, which can be conventional ductal adenocarcinoma. Each component should arbitrarily constitute 30% of the neoplasm to qualify as carcinosarcoma. Each component is immunophenotypically similar to its pure counterpart.

Undifferentiated carcinoma with osteoclast-like giant cells
The mean age of patients with an undifferentiated carcinoma with osteoclast-like giant cells is 62 years, but there is a wide range (32–93 years) {2380,2248,2688}. This distinctive neoplasm occurs mostly in the pancreas but rarely also in the bile ducts and other organs. It contains three cell types: non-neoplastic osteoclast-like multinucleated giant cells, a mononuclear histiocytic component, and the neoplastic mononuclear cell component. The multinucleated cells express histiocytic markers and lack epithelial differentiation, and they are often found in areas adjacent to haemorrhage or necrosis {2248,2688}. These cells are believed to be attracted by the tumour via mechanisms yet to be discovered. The mononuclear histiocytic component may be inconspicuous by routine histology but is abundantly demonstrated by immunohistochemistry for histiocytic markers. The neoplastic cells vary from spindle-shaped to epithelioid and can be very large and pleomorphic. They are usually non-cohesive and may be found within the cytoplasm of the osteoclast-like giant cells. These cells can show keratin positivity, but not inevitably. They have a high Ki-67 proliferation index and mutations in *KRAS* and *TP53*, which along with the commonly associated presence of a conventional ductal adenocarcinoma or adenocarcinoma precursor component provides evidence of the relationship of undifferentiated carcinomas with osteoclast-like giant cells to ductal adenocarcinomas {2823,1271,1959, 2198,3555,308,3283}. The clinical behaviour of this tumour type appears to be unpredictable, but many behave unexpectedly well and in fact a substantial proportion of patients are alive after many years {2248,2688}. Grading this tumour on the basis

Table 10.03 Differential diagnosis of the most common pancreatic tumours, on the basis of histological and immunohistological features

Diagnosis	Histology	CK7, CK19	CK8, CK18	EMA (MUC1)	MUC2	Tryp.	Syn.	CG	CEA	AFP	Nuclear β-catenin
Ductal adenocarcinoma	Infiltrative	+	+	+	–	–	–	–	+	–	–
Intraductal papillary mucinous neoplasm	Intraductal	+	+	+[a]	+[b]	–	–	–	+	–	–
Mucinous cystic neoplasm	Extraductal, ovarian stroma	+	+	+	–	–	–	–	+	–	–
Serous cystic neoplasm	Microcystic	+	+	–	–	–	–	–	–	–	–
Acinar cell carcinoma	Solid	+/–	+	–	–	+	+[c]	+[c]	–	+[d]	+[d]
Pancreatoblastoma	Solid	+	+	–	–	+	+[c]	+[c]	–	+[d]	+[d]
Solid pseudopapillary neoplasm	Loosely cohesive, pseudocystic	–	+[d]	–	–	–	+[e]	–	–	–	+
Neuroendocrine neoplasms (NENs)	Solid	+/–	+	–	–	–	+	+	–	–	–

CG, chromogranin; Syn., synaptophysin; Tryp., trypsin.
[a]In pancreatobiliary-type. [b]In intestinal-type. [c]Focal and in ~40% of cases. [d]Occasionally. [e]Focal and faint.

of the predominance of the neoplastic cell component may have prognostic value.

Other neoplasms
Additionally, rare neoplasms of uncertain clinical significance have been reported. Among these, carcinomas of probable ductal phenotype include oncocytic carcinoma {2507}; non-mucinous, glycogen-poor cystadenocarcinoma {971}; choriocarcinoma {3732}; clear cell carcinoma {1508,1593,1947,1981,3269}; and ciliated cell adenocarcinoma {2217}. Although most of these neoplasms are reported to have a distinctive histological appearance, their clinical and biological significance is not well defined, and they are therefore not considered separate subtypes at this time. Some have been reclassified immunohistochemically as other specific types of pancreatic carcinoma, and others are regarded as patterns of growth rather than distinct subtypes.

Cytology
Cytology diagnostic of adenocarcinoma is most often obtained by FNA (typically EUS-guided FNA) {1019}. Ultrathin needles, which allow for the acquisition of tissue fragments for formalin-fixed, paraffin-embedded cytohistology, have improved diagnostic yield and accuracy of EUS-guided FNA {235}. Pancreatobiliary duct brushing techniques have also improved {3379}, but brushing cytology is inferior to EUS-guided FNA for the diagnosis of malignancy {3542}. Ancillary tests of bile duct brushing specimens, such as FISH {249} and next-generation sequencing {819}, may add value to cytology for the detection of malignancy.

Ductal adenocarcinomas are distinguished from other solid neoplasms of the pancreas on the basis of both smear pattern and cytomorphology. The smear pattern of adenocarcinomas is one of scattered cellular glandular clusters admixed with single cells, in contrast to the diffuse, uniform solid cellular smear pattern produced by the monotonous tumour cells of parenchyma-rich, stroma-poor neoplasms such as acinar cell carcinomas and neuroendocrine tumours (NETs) {533}.

Moderately-poorly differentiated adenocarcinomas are recognized by overt features of malignancy. Nuclei are enlarged and hyperchromatic and display irregular nuclear membranes; the cytoplasm ranges from scant and non-mucinous to abundant and mucinous {533,2593}. Subtypes such as adenosquamous carcinoma, undifferentiated carcinoma, and undifferentiated carcinoma with osteoclast-type giant cells can also be recognized by unique cytological features that recapitulate the histology {1808,2640}.

Well-differentiated adenocarcinomas are more challenging, because the aspirated ductal cells can be difficult to distinguish from atypical but reactive glandular cells in pancreatitis {762,1704}, as well as from gastrointestinal contamination from the EUS-guided biopsy procedure {2328}. Cytological criteria for well-differentiated adenocarcinoma include irregular spacing of cells in a cohesive group, anisonucleosis of 4:1 in a single group, parachromatin clearing, irregular nuclear membranes, and finely vacuolated lacy-looking cytoplasm {533,2593}.

Diagnostic molecular pathology
The consequential loss of the SMAD4 (DPC4) protein is relatively cancer-specific and thus serves as a diagnostic aid in the histopathological evaluation of pancreatic biopsies {3564}.

While next-generation DNA sequencing has definitively established the genomic landscape of pancreatic cancer, transcriptomic profiling has defined discrete subtypes of pancreatic cancer characterized by distinct gene signatures, therapeutic responsiveness, and natural history {477,224}. Specifically, pancreatic cancers can be dichotomized into the basal-like subtype (also known as the squamous or quasimesenchymal subtype) and the classic subtype, based on expression patterns in the epithelium. Along the same lines, two subtypes (normal and activated) have been suggested based on expression pattern restricted to the stroma. The basal-like epithelial signature and activated stromal signature each tend to be independently associated with more-aggressive disease, reduced response to cytotoxic therapies, and worse survival outcomes than the classic epithelial or normal stromal subtypes of cancer {2192,208}. Certain genomic alterations (e.g. chromatin driver mutations) are more frequently associated with the aggressive basal-like cancers {143}, and this subtype also demonstrates a particularly immune-suppressive milieu that favours tumour progression {479}. Not surprisingly, each of the two main epithelial subtypes is associated with distinct transcription factor profiles and epigenetic alterations that underlie the defining gene signatures {1944}, and their elucidation provides an opportunity for therapeutic targeting of subtype-specific dependencies in pancreatic cancer.

Essential and desirable diagnostic criteria
Essential: malignant glands of varying degrees of differentiation haphazardly infiltrating pancreatic and peripancreatic tissue.
Desirable: perineural and vascular invasion; recognition of one of the specific subtypes of pancreatic carcinoma.

Staging (TNM)
Ductal adenocarcinomas spread early to the retroperitoneal tissues, the various local peripancreatic and more-distal lymph node groups (depending on the location of the primary tumour {1619}), and the liver. Lung, bone, and adrenal metastases are mostly seen in advanced tumour stages {3631}; cerebral metastases are uncommon. For accurate staging of resected pancreatic carcinomas, the use of protocols that describe standardized processing and sampling of tumour tissue is recommended {3460,32,1304,472}. Because involvement of the retroperitoneal resection margin is one of the factors determining survival, careful sampling and examination of this area has also been recommended {2889,880}.

Ductal adenocarcinoma is pathologically staged according to the eighth edition (2017) of the Union for International Cancer Control (UICC) TNM classification {408}, in which the T category is based on tumour size and independent of any extrapancreatic tumour extension. Node-positive disease has been subdivided into N1 and N2, based on the number of positive lymph nodes. A slightly modified classification is proposed by the Japan Pancreas Society {1388}.

Neoadjuvant chemoradiation or chemotherapy is increasingly used as a treatment option in addition to surgical resection. Several scoring systems have been reported for evaluation of the extent of residual carcinoma in posttherapy resection specimens. Correlation of the extent of residual carcinoma with survival reveals that patients with < 5% viable residual tumour have much better disease-free and overall survival than those with > 5% viable residual tumour {570,3763,472}.

Prognosis and prediction
Ductal adenocarcinoma is fatal in almost all cases. The mean survival time of untreated patients is 3–5 months, and the mean survival time after surgical resection is 10–20 months {658,2335,1714,2085}. Only 10–20% of patients have surgically resectable carcinomas at the time of diagnosis {658,660,2952,3112}. The overall 5-year survival rate is 8% {1443,3331}, whereas that of patients treated by surgical resection is 15–25% {1914}.

Resectability is the most important determinant of prognosis. However, 70–90% of surgically resected carcinomas recur within 2 years after surgery {3411,261}, most commonly locally in the bed of the pancreas and more distantly in the liver. The peritoneal cavity or lymph nodes are also common sites of recurrence {3411,261}. Neoadjuvant and adjuvant chemotherapy with combinations that include gemcitabine or fluorouracil prolong survival time only slightly {2334,2336,2412}.

Stage is the most important prognosticator. Survival time is longer in patients with carcinomas confined to the pancreas and < 30 mm in greatest dimension than in patients with carcinomas that extend beyond the gland and are > 30 mm in size {3092,1220,3013,1914}. As reflected in the most recent staging system, size is more important than extension beyond the pancreas {110,2046}.

Patients with no evidence of residual tumour after resection (R0) have the most favourable prognosis of those who are treated surgically {1220,2335,3578}. Lymph node metastases substantially worsen prognosis {3092,2903,1291,1914}. Lymph

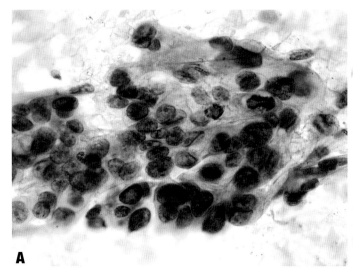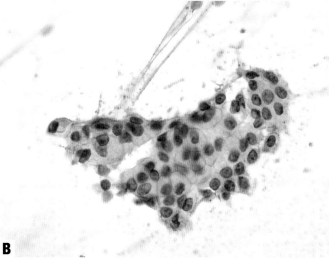

A **B**

Fig. 10.26 Pancreatic ductal adenocarcinoma. **A** High-grade adenocarcinoma. Cytology; moderately-poorly differentiated adenocarcinoma demonstrates enlarged, hyperchromatic, crowded, and disordered nuclei (direct smear, Papanicolaou staining). **B** Well-differentiated adenocarcinoma displays nuclei with irregular spacing, anisonucleosis of 4:1, parachromatin clearing, irregular nuclear membranes, and finely vacuolated, lacy-looking cytoplasm (direct smear, Papanicolaou staining). This may be difficult to differentiate from the reactive cells of pancreatitis.

node status is a factor not only determining short-term survival (< 5 years) after surgical resection but also predicting long-term survival (≥ 5 years) {2903}. The lymph node ratio (the ratio of the number of nodes harbouring a metastasis to the total number of nodes examined) is an important predictor of survival after surgery {2554}. It is suggested that at least 12 lymph nodes must be examined for proper staging of node-negative resections {2916,3322,1210,1322,3038}. Carcinomas of the body or tail of the pancreas tend to present at a more advanced stage than those of the head {3012}.

Histological features are not as strong prognosticators as stage. Tumour grade, mitotic count, and severity of cellular atypia have been correlated with postoperative survival {1979}. Major vessel involvement {2304}, vessel invasion, perineural invasion, and resection margin status are also prognostic indicators {2303,2478,2178,3430,3150}. Other reported prognosticators include CA19-9 {932,305,3169,3375}, obesity {947,2108,1532}, race {604,1563}, site of metastases (with lung-only being favourable) {3523,579}, and *SMAD4* gene status of the cancer {343,3579,2893}.

A postresection nomogram has been developed to predict survival of a patient with pancreatic cancer, accounting for various variables in addition to stage {3469}.

Pancreatic acinar cell carcinoma

La Rosa S
Klimstra DS
Wood LD

Definition

Acinar cell carcinoma of the pancreas is a malignant pancreatic epithelial neoplasm showing acinar cell differentiation.

ICD-O coding

8550/3 Acinar cell carcinoma

ICD-11 coding

2C10.0 & XH3PG9 Adenocarcinoma of pancreas & Acinar cell carcinoma

Related terminology

None

Subtype(s)

Acinar cell cystadenocarcinoma (8551/3); mixed acinar-neuroendocrine carcinoma (8154/3); mixed acinar-endocrine-ductal carcinoma (8154/3); mixed acinar-ductal carcinoma (8552/3)

Localization

Acinar cell carcinomas may arise in any portion of the pancreas, but they are most frequent in the head, followed by the tail and the body {1748,1628}.

Clinical features

Presenting symptoms are usually related to tumour growth and/or metastatic spread and include weight loss, abdominal pain, vomiting, and nausea. Jaundice can be present but is rare. Patients with extensive metastatic disease may show symptoms due to lipase hypersecretion, which include subcutaneous fat necrosis and polyarthralgia {1629,1748,1628,1757}. Rare patients, especially when young, can show increased blood levels of AFP {640,2045}.

Epidemiology

Acinar cell carcinomas account for about 1–2% of pancreatic neoplasms in adults and about 15% in children {1628}. The average age of adult patients is approximately 60 years (range: 20–88 years). Males are more commonly affected, with an M:F ratio of 2.1:1 {1748,1628,1257}.

Etiology

Although most acinar cell carcinomas are sporadic, rare cases diagnosed in the context of Lynch syndrome, Carney complex, or familial adenomatous polyposis have been documented {1017,1748,1522,1931,2931}.

Pathogenesis

Little is known about the pathogenesis. Although some cytogenetic similarities between acinar cell carcinomas and ductal adenocarcinomas have been observed, the cytogenetic profile is globally different between the two entities. Acinar cell carcinomas show a mutation signature associated with tobacco use and defective DNA repair {1490}. Acinar cell carcinomas show chromosomal instability characterized by high degrees of allelic loss and gains. The regions more frequently involved by losses included 1p, 3p, 5q, 6q, 8p, 9p, 11, 17p, and 18q, whereas the gained regions were mainly 1q, 7, 8q, 12, 17q, and 20q {1464,1270,3264,306}. Interestingly, a hierarchical clustering of comparative genomic hybridization findings did not find differences between pure acinar cell carcinomas, cystic acinar cell carcinomas, and mixed acinar-neuroendocrine carcinomas, indicating that these subtypes have the same cytogenetic background {306}. *MYC* alterations, including gene amplification and/or chromosome 8 polysomy, have been described in a subset of acinar cell carcinomas and in all mixed acinar-neuroendocrine carcinomas investigated, but they were not associated with a different prognostic signature {306,1750}. Loss of 18q has been correlated with loss or substantial reduction of

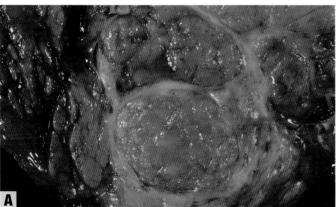
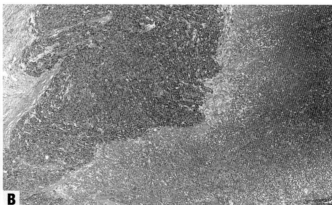

Fig. 10.27 Acinar cell carcinoma. **A** The cut surface shows a well-circumscribed, encapsulated, solid tumour with a homogeneous pink surface. **B** At low power, acinar cell carcinoma appears as a highly cellular tumour with scant fibrous stroma showing a lobular pattern of growth and necrosis.

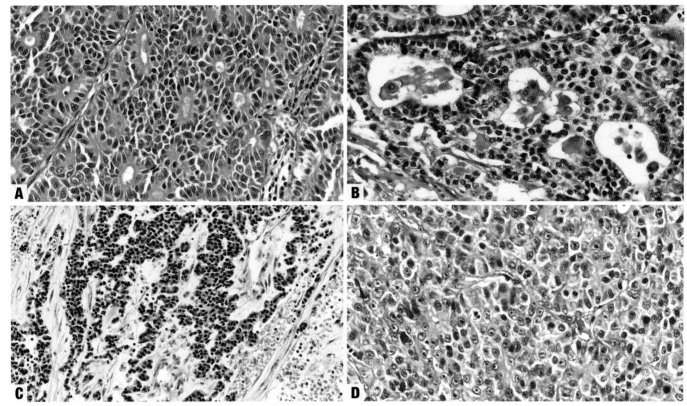

Fig. 10.28 Acinar cell carcinoma. **A** The acinar pattern is characterized by structures resembling normal acini, with small lumina and cells distributed in a monolayer with basally located nuclei. **B** The glandular pattern is characterized by acinar structures with dilated lumina and stratified nuclei. **C** The trabecular pattern is characterized by ribbons of cells strongly resembling those of pancreatic neuroendocrine tumours (PanNETs). **D** The solid pattern is characterized by large sheets of cells without lumina.

the protein DCC and has been considered an early step in the development of acinar cell carcinoma {306}. Acinar cell carcinomas show low levels of hypermethylation, and no tumours characterized by concerted hypermethylation at multiple loci have been identified. However, some genes, including *RASSF1* and *APC*, are frequently methylated {987}.

Macroscopic appearance
Acinar cell carcinomas are generally well circumscribed, at least partially encapsulated, solid, and large (average diameter: 8–10 cm). They have a homogeneous pink to tan cut surface and are fleshy or even friable in consistency. Haemorrhage and necrosis are not infrequent {1629,1748,1628}. Acinar cell carcinomas exclusively characterized by variable-sized cysts are defined as acinar cell cystadenocarcinomas {655}.

Histopathology
Histologically, acinar cell carcinomas are highly cellular, with scant fibrous stroma showing a lobular pattern of growth and frequent necrosis. The cells have moderate amounts of granular eosinophilic cytoplasm containing zymogen granules, which are PASD-positive. Nuclei are generally uniform and a single prominent nucleolus is characteristic. The mitotic count is variable but generally high {1748}. Acinar cell carcinomas may have different architectural features. The acinar pattern is characterized by structures resembling normal acini, sometimes with minute lumina. Cells are distributed in a monolayer, with basally located nuclei. The glandular pattern is characterized by acinar structures with dilated lumina. The trabecular pattern is characterized

by ribbons of cells strongly resembling those of pancreatic neuroendocrine tumours (PanNETs). The solid pattern is characterized by large sheets of cells without lumina that can also resemble the appearance of PanNETs. The most frequent patterns are acinar and solid, although a mixture is frequently found within an individual acinar cell carcinoma. In addition, uncommon subtypes including oncocytic, spindle, clear, and pleomorphic cell types have been described {1748,1757}. Intraductal growth and papillary features are also described {273}. The lack of squamoid nests is helpful for the differential diagnosis with pancreatoblastoma (see *Pancreatoblastoma*, p. 337), a pancreatic neoplasm showing predominantly acinar differentiation.

Immunohistochemistry plays a key diagnostic role in demonstrating acinar cell differentiation, but antibodies commonly used in routine practice (trypsin, chymotrypsin, lipase, amylase) show different sensitivity {1748,1752}. The monoclonal antibody directed against the COOH-terminal portion of the BCL10 protein (clone 331.3), which recognizes the COOH-terminal portion of pancreatic carboxyl ester lipase, is highly specific and sensitive in detecting acinar differentiation {1752}. Amylase is rarely expressed, and lipase antibodies show low sensitivity. Trypsin, chymotrypsin, and BCL10 antibodies are the most sensitive. Simultaneous use of two of them allows the detection of nearly 100% of acinar cell carcinomas {1752,1748}. Acinar cell carcinomas may also express CK7 and CK19 and are positive for PDX1. Nuclear expression of β-catenin is found in about 10% of cases {1748}. Markers typically expressed in hepatocellular carcinoma, including AFP, Hep Par-1, glypican-3 (GPC3), and albumin mRNA (by in situ hybridization), can be found in acinar

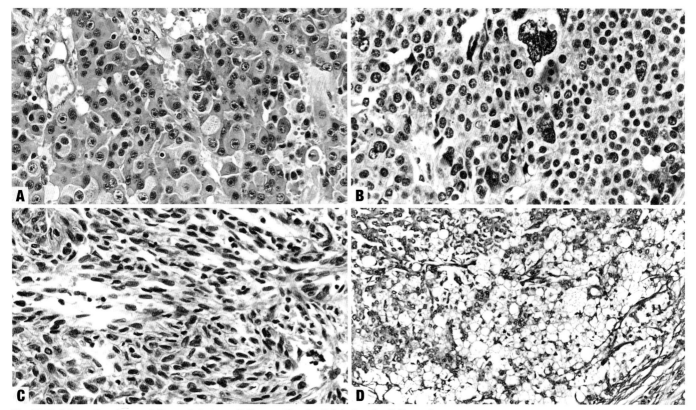

Fig. 10.29 Acinar cell carcinoma. **A** Oncocytic features. **B** Pleomorphic cells. **C** Spindle cells. **D** Clear cells.

cell carcinomas {200}. Scattered neuroendocrine cells positive for chromogranin A and/or synaptophysin can be observed.

Mixed acinar carcinomas

Pancreatic carcinomas with mixed differentiation are rare, and in many, the primary component demonstrates acinar differentiation. Mixed carcinomas are defined as having > 30% of each line of differentiation. The most common is mixed acinar-neuroendocrine carcinoma, which is defined on the basis of the immunohistochemical finding of coexpression of acinar and neuroendocrine markers {1632}. Most cases have an intimate mixture of the two cell types, although rare cases with morphologically distinct acinar and neuroendocrine components exist and fit the definition of a mixed neuroendocrine–non-neuroendocrine neoplasm (MiNEN; see *Pancreatic MiNENs*, p. 370). Mixed acinar-neuroendocrine carcinomas are best regarded as a subtype of acinar cell carcinoma, because they share its clinical behaviour and genomic features {616}. Importantly, the possibility of a mixed acinar-neuroendocrine carcinoma should be considered for a pancreatic neoplasm expressing neuroendocrine markers when the morphological features are not perfectly typical of a well-differentiated neuroendocrine tumour (NET).

Mixed acinar-ductal carcinomas

Mixed acinar-ductal carcinomas have one of two different patterns {3133}. Some exhibit extensive intracellular or extracellular mucin accumulation in association with acinar elements. There may be nests of acinar cells floating in colloid-like pools of mucin, or the neoplastic elements may have a combination of typical acinar elements mixed with nests of columnar or signet-ring cells with cytoplasmic mucin. Mucin staining (with mucicarmine or Alcian blue) is positive, as is immunohistochemical labelling for trypsin and chymotrypsin. Other mixed acinar-ductal carcinomas have an individual gland pattern of infiltration with an associated desmoplastic stromal response (reminiscent of infiltrating ductal adenocarcinoma), but nonetheless show substantial acinar differentiation by immunohistochemistry. Rare mixed acinar-neuroendocrine-ductal carcinomas show mixed morphology, with acinar patterns, cells with neuroendocrine differentiation, and areas simulating infiltrating ductal adenocarcinoma, with immunohistochemical staining supporting the three lines of differentiation {3133,3212,136}. One of the reported cases arose in association with high-grade pancreatic intraepithelial neoplasia {1304}. Data are limited but suggest aggressive behaviour for mixed acinar-ductal and mixed acinar-neuroendocrine-ductal carcinomas {2424}.

Cytology

Aspirate smears are moderately cellular with a generally clean background, although cytoplasmic granules and naked nuclei can be observed. Neoplastic cells are arranged in irregularly shaped groups, small glandular structures, or large sheets, although they can also be isolated. Tumour cells are polygonal with abundant finely granular cytoplasm and uniform nuclei. The chromatin is coarsely clumped, with one or two evident nucleoli.

Diagnostic molecular pathology

The most common molecular alterations found in ductal adenocarcinomas (*KRAS*, *SMAD4*, and *CDKN2A*), cystic neoplasms (*GNAS* and *RNF43*), and PanNETs (*MEN1*, *DAXX*, and *ATRX*) are largely absent in acinar cell carcinomas {1628,1757}. There is no genetic alteration that can be considered the hallmark

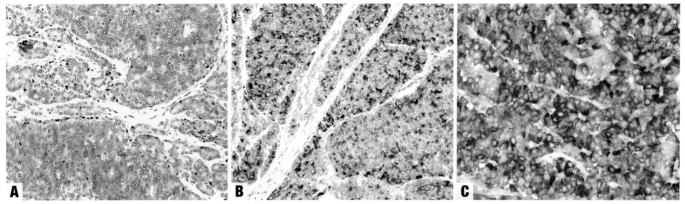

Fig. 10.30 Acinar cell carcinoma, immunohistochemical staining. **A** For trypsin. **B** For chymotrypsin. **C** For BCL10; this staining pattern confirms acinar differentiation.

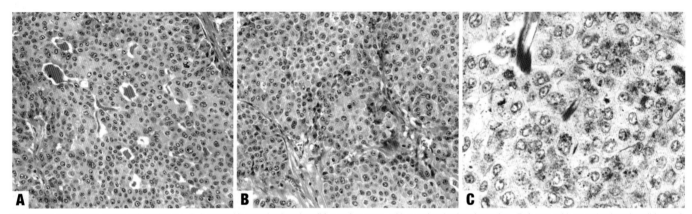

Fig. 10.31 Pancreatic acinar cell carcinoma. **A** A case with a predominantly solid growth pattern, with very focal acinar formation. **B** A case with a predominantly solid growth pattern. **C** A case with a predominantly solid growth pattern, with very focal acinar formation. The tumour cells show cytoplasmic granular staining for diastase-PAS.

present in the majority of acinar cell carcinomas, but recent next-generation sequencing–based technologies have identified SMAD4 and CDKN2A or CDKN2B mutations in a minority of cases, and the tumour suppressor genes ID3, ARID1A, APC, and CDKN2A are frequently affected in acinar cell carcinomas {616,1464,1490}. Alterations in the APC/β-catenin pathway have been well documented and include mutations of both APC and CTNNB1, which have been found in 8% and 7% of cases, respectively. However, the most frequent alterations of the APC gene are gene loss and promoter hypermethylation, identified in 48% and 56% of cases, respectively {987}. TP53 mutation and/or gene loss has been identified in 12–24% of acinar cell carcinomas {616,1464,1749,767}. The concomitant presence of both TP53 mutations and gene loss has been found to correlate with a worse prognosis {1749}. BRAF mutations are very rare {1464}, but about 23% of acinar cell carcinomas harbour rearrangements involving BRAF and RAF1, and the most prevalent fusions are SND1-BRAF and HERPUD1-BRAF {616,3516}. Although acinar cell carcinoma is an unusual tumour found in the context of Lynch syndrome {1522,1953}, microsatellite instability (MSI) has been identified in 8–14% of acinar cell carcinomas {1931,1757}. Considering the promise of immunotherapy in other microsatellite-unstable neoplasms, MSI-targeted therapy may represent a new therapeutic approach for microsatellite-unstable acinar cell carcinomas that needs to be explored.

Essential and desirable diagnostic criteria

Essential: a lobular pattern of growth, with high cellularity; cells with moderate amounts of granular eosinophilic cytoplasm and uniform nuclei with single prominent nucleoli; scant to absent fibrous stroma; moderate to abundant necrosis; immunohistochemical evidence of acinar cell markers.

Staging (TNM)

The Union for International Cancer Control (UICC) staging system for acinar cell carcinoma is the same as that used for pancreatic carcinoma.

Prognosis and prediction

The survival of patients with acinar cell carcinoma is poor, with a median survival time of about 19 months and a 5-year survival rate of 25%. Although the prognostic meaning of several morphological features, immunohistochemical markers, and molecular abnormalities has been investigated in recent years, only stage has proven to be an independent prognostic factor in multivariate analysis {1748}.

SND1-BRAF–transformed cells are sensitive to treatment with MEK inhibitors, suggesting a new therapeutic approach to acinar cell carcinomas {616}.

Pancreatoblastoma

Ohike N
La Rosa S

Definition
Pancreatoblastoma is a malignant epithelial neoplasm of the pancreas showing predominantly acinar differentiation with squamoid nests.

ICD-O coding
8971/3 Pancreatoblastoma

ICD-11 coding
2C10.Y & XH27L5 Other specified malignant neoplasms of pancreas & Pancreatoblastoma

Related terminology
None

Subtype(s)
None

Localization
Pancreatoblastoma has no preferential location within the pancreas.

Clinical features
The presenting features of pancreatoblastoma are nonspecific, and many cases are discovered incidentally. Common symptoms include abdominal pain, weight loss, nausea, and diarrhoea. Jaundice is uncommon. An abdominal mass is often palpable, especially in children. Isolated case reports have described patients with Cushing syndrome as a result of the inappropriate secretion of ACTH by the tumour {2632,1627,2542}. Serum AFP, which can be used to monitor the effectiveness of therapy, is elevated in two thirds of children, with levels often in excess of 1000 µg/L {834}, but it is not consistently elevated in adults {2647}. CEA may be elevated in children.

Epidemiology
Although pancreatoblastoma is a rare neoplasm, with approximately 200 cases reported, it is one of the most frequent pancreatic neoplasms in childhood, accounting for approximately 25% of pancreatic neoplasms occurring in the first decade of life (median age: ~4–5 years) {3024,2259}. Approximately 40 cases have been reported in patients of between 18 and 78 years of age {2396}. No sex predominance is seen.

Etiology
The precise etiology is unknown. Although most cases are sporadic, there are associations with genetic syndromes (Beckwith–Wiedemann syndrome and familial adenomatous polyposis) and with the corresponding genetic mutations.

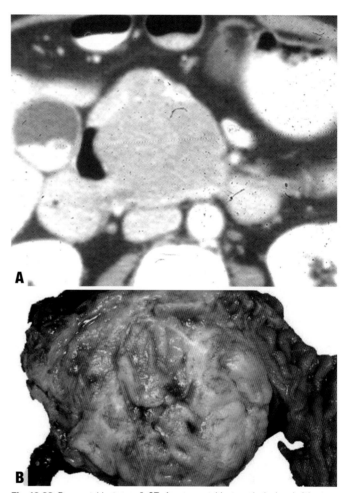

Fig. 10.32 Pancreatoblastoma. **A** CT of a pancreatoblastoma in the head of the pancreas. **B** The cut section of the neoplasm reveals the lobulated surface.

Pathogenesis
Unknown

Macroscopic appearance
Pancreatoblastomas are usually large at presentation, ranging from 1.5 to 20 cm in size (mean: 10 cm) {2425}. Most are solitary, at least partially well-circumscribed or encapsulated, solid masses. Sectioning reveals tan to whitish-yellow soft lobules separated by fibrous stromal bands. Some may contain cystic spaces due to haemorrhagic necrosis and cystic degeneration, which appear as a heterogeneous or multiloculated mass on radiological imaging. Congenital cases in association with Beckwith–Wiedemann syndrome may be predominantly cystic {813}. Biliary and pancreatic ductal dilatation may be present.

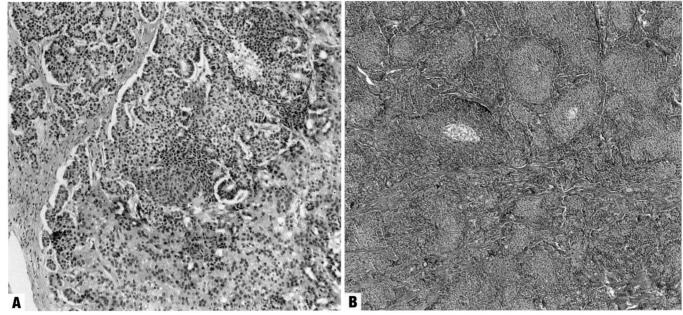

Fig. 10.33 Pancreatoblastoma. **A** A geographical low-power appearance. **B** A lymphoid follicle low-power appearance.

Histopathology

Histologically, the tumours are composed of highly cellular lobules separated by fibrous bands, producing a geographical or lymphoid-follicle, multiphasic low-power appearance. The neoplastic cells within the lobules usually show an organoid arrangement of acinar, solid, or trabecular formations akin to acinar cell carcinomas. They are polarized around small lumina and have nuclei with a single prominent nucleolus. Nuclear atypia is generally modest. The acinar differentiation is supported in the form of PASD-positive cytoplasmic granules, as well as by immunohistochemical labelling for pancreatic enzymes (trypsin, chymotrypsin, and lipase) and BCL10 (clone 331.1).

The squamoid nests are considered a defining component of pancreatoblastoma and are critical for establishing the diagnosis {281,1273}. They are composed of distinctive cells with eosinophilic to clear cytoplasm in formations varying from islands of epithelioid cells to whorled nests of spindle cells with a squamous appearance, and they may demonstrate overt keratinization. Their nuclei are larger and more oval-shaped than those of the surrounding cells. They lack cellular atypia, prominent nucleoli, and mitoses. Occasionally, nuclear clearing

due to the intranuclear accumulation of biotin may be seen {3245}. Squamoid nests are also positive for EMA. It is important to keep in mind that the density and distribution of the squamoid nests varies by region as well as by neoplasm, and that it may be difficult to detect the squamoid nests in small samples. In addition to the acinar component and squamous nests, a neuroendocrine component is detected with the help of specific immunohistochemical stains (chromogranin A, synaptophysin). Glandular spaces lined by mucin-containing cells and a more primitive round cell component are focally present.

The stroma of pancreatoblastomas is often hypercellular, in some instances achieving a neoplastic appearance. Rarely, heterologous stromal elements, including neoplastic bone and cartilage, have been reported. Pancreatoblastomas in adults have similar histological features to those in children; however, the stromal bands may be less abundant and less cellular. An abnormal (nuclear and cytoplasmic) immunolabelling pattern for β-catenin and the overexpression of its target gene *CCND1* are seen in most cases, in some cases being patchy or limited to the squamoid nests. Immunohistochemical positivity for AFP is detectable, especially in cases with elevated serum

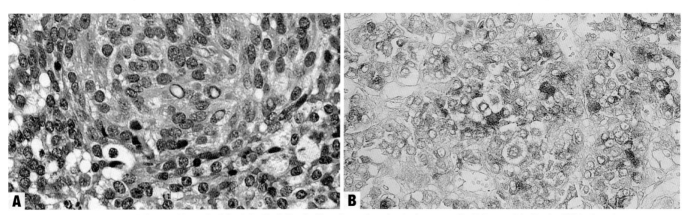

Fig. 10.34 Pancreatoblastoma. **A** Squamoid nest-like island of epithelioid cells. Note the nuclear clearing in some cells. **B** Immunolabelling for AFP in the acinar component.

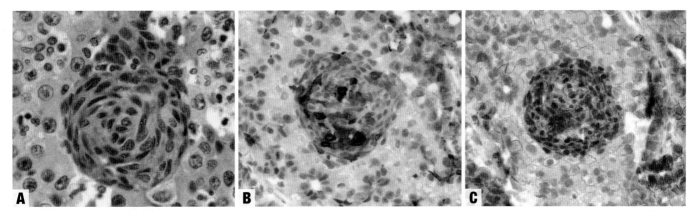

Fig. 10.35 Pancreatoblastoma. **A** Squamoid area showing whorled nest of spindled cells. **B** Immunolabelling for EMA limited to the squamoid nest. **C** Immunolabelling for β-catenin limited to the squamoid nest.

AFP. Ultrastructural studies show the heterogeneity of cellular differentiation in the tumour by demonstrating zymogen (size: 400–800 nm), neuroendocrine granules (size: 125–250 nm), and mucinous granules (size: 500–900 nm). The cells of the squamoid nests contain numerous desmosomes but only focally well-developed desmosome-tonofilament complexes.

Cytology

FNA specimens show a loosely cohesive and/or clustered cellular pattern. Most of the neoplastic cells are polygonal with round to oval nuclei; one or more small nucleoli; and a granular, amphophilic, or eosinophilic cytoplasm. These nuclear features are similar to those of acinar cell carcinoma. The squamoid nests are usually more difficult to appreciate and may be detected in the cell block preparations. Optically clear nuclei may be recognized in some of the neoplastic cells forming the squamoid nests.

Diagnostic molecular pathology

Loss of heterozygosity of the short arm of chromosome 11p {19,1557} is commonly identified. The locus is also affected in children with Beckwith–Wiedemann syndrome, where the maternal allele is typically lost. The loss of 11p also occurs in > 80% of sporadic pancreatoblastomas. Alterations in the APC/β-catenin pathway have been reported in 50–80% of pancreatoblastomas {19,3247}. These alterations most often involve mutation of *CTNNB1* (encoding β-catenin), which results in the abnormal nuclear accumulation of the β-catenin protein. *APC* gene abnormalities are reported in pancreatoblastomas arising in patients with and without familial adenomatous polyposis {19,3647}. *KRAS* mutations and the accumulation of p53 protein, typically found in ductal adenocarcinoma of the pancreas, are not identified. Loss of SMAD4 expression is infrequent.

Essential and desirable diagnostic criteria

Essential: multiple lines of differentiation, including acinar, endocrine, and sometimes ductal differentiation; squamoid nests.

Staging (TNM)

The TNM classification of pancreatoblastomas follows the criteria for classifying ductal adenocarcinoma (see *Pancreatic ductal adenocarcinoma*, p. 322).

Prognosis and prediction

Pancreatoblastomas are indolent and curable tumours, but they exhibit a malignant behaviour with local invasion, recurrence, and occasionally distant metastasis. They can invade adjacent structures such as the spleen, colon, duodenum, portal vein, and common bile duct. Metastases are present in 17–35% of patients at the time of the diagnosis, and some patients develop metastases later in the course of their disease {774}. The liver is the most common site of metastasis, followed by lymph nodes and lung. Surgical resection of the tumour is the mainstay of therapy, with or without a variable combination of radiotherapy and chemotherapy.

The overall survival rate of patients with pancreatoblastoma is approximately 50%. The postoperative prognosis in patients with localized surgically resectable disease is favourable, with a 5-year survival rate of 65%, whereas patients with non-resectable disease do not usually survive beyond 5 years {774}. After complete resection, 18% of patients with pancreatoblastoma develop local recurrence after a median of 20 months, and 26% develop metachronous metastases {774}. Factors associated with a worse prognosis include metastasis and non-resectable disease {774}. The outcome in children may be more favourable than that in adults. One of the reasons appears to be that children often present with non-metastatic and well-encapsulated neoplasms. Although no standardized treatment protocol has been defined, chemotherapy and radiotherapy may have a role in the treatment of recurrent, residual, unresectable, and metastatic disease. Neoadjuvant chemotherapy (cisplatin-based regimens are commonly used) may allow for complete surgical resection of previously unresectable pancreatoblastoma. Stage and response to treatment are predictors of the outcome.

Solid pseudopapillary neoplasm of the pancreas

Klöppel G
Basturk O
Klimstra DS
Lam AK
Notohara K

Definition

Solid pseudopapillary neoplasm (SPN) of the pancreas is a low-grade malignant pancreatic tumour composed of poorly cohesive epithelial cells forming solid and pseudopapillary structures that lack a specific line of pancreatic epithelial differentiation.

ICD-O coding

8452/3 Solid pseudopapillary neoplasm of the pancreas

ICD-11 coding

2C10.Y & XH3FD4 Other specified malignant neoplasms of pancreas & Solid pseudopapillary tumour

Related terminology

Acceptable: solid-pseudopapillary tumour; solid-cystic tumour; papillary-cystic tumour; solid and papillary epithelial neoplasm; Frantz tumour {964}.

Subtype(s)

Solid pseudopapillary neoplasm with high-grade carcinoma (8452/3)

Localization

SPNs have a slight preference for the tail region {2005,2100}. Extrapancreatic SPNs have been reported in retropancreatic tissue, ovary, and testis {1645,1671,3279,2135,1304}.

Clinical features

They occur predominantly (90%) in adolescent girls and young women (mean age: 28 years; range: 7–79 years), are rare in men (mean age: 35 years; range: 25–72 years) {1646,3279}, and account for 30% of all pancreatic neoplasms in patients aged < 40 years {1980}.

SPNs are often found incidentally by imaging or present with abdominal discomfort and pain {1304}. Intratumoural haemorrhage after abdominal trauma can produce acute abdomen. All known tumour markers are normal, and the neoplasms are not associated with a functional endocrine syndrome. The diagnosis is established by imaging (ultrasonography, CT, MRI), which reveals a well-demarcated, variably solid and pseudocystic mass, occasionally with calcifications.

Epidemiology

SPNs are rare, accounting for 0.9–2.7% of all exocrine pancreatic neoplasms and only 5% of cystic neoplasms {1689,1304}. There is no apparent ethnic predilection.

Etiology

Rare cases have been reported in the setting of familial adenomatous polyposis {2802,1377}.

Pathogenesis

The striking sex and age distribution suggests a role for hormonal factors, but no association with endocrine disturbances has been noted to date. The somatic mutation of *CTNNB1* (encoding β-catenin), which most likely occurs early in life, results in a protein that has lost its function as an adhesion molecule at the cell membrane and might be a cause of the tumour cell discohesion that is typical of SPNs. Because SPNs identical to those in the pancreas have also been described in the ovary and testis {1671,3047,2135}, it is possible that the cells giving rise to SPNs occur in the genital ridges and may be translocated into pancreatic parenchyma during embryogenesis {1690}.

The mutation leads to a β-catenin protein that escapes intracytoplasmic phosphorylation and forms complexes with the

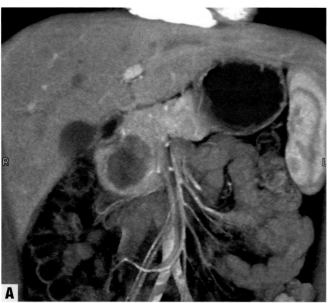

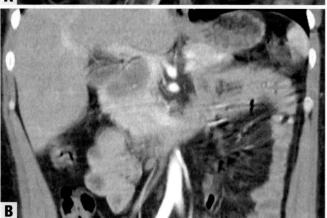

Fig. 10.36 Solid pseudopapillary neoplasm. **A** Coronal CT revealing a solid pseudopapillary neoplasm in the head of the pancreas. **B** Coronal CT demonstrating a solid pseudopapillary neoplasm in the head of the pancreas.

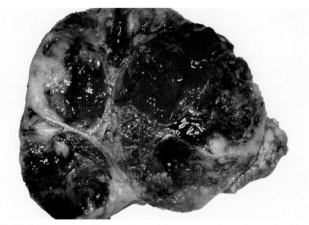

Fig. 10.37 Solid pseudopapillary neoplasm of the pancreas. A neoplasm with a lobulated, fleshy surface showing marked haemorrhage and degenerative changes.

T-cell transcription factor / lymphoid enhancer-binding factor in the nucleus, as indicated by nuclear expression of β-catenin. The complex activates the transcription of oncogenes such as *MYC* and *CCND1* and activates the WNT/β-catenin signalling pathway. Although this activation increases proliferation in other neoplasms, in SPNs the signalling cascade seems to be interrupted by an as yet unexplained overexpression of p21 and p27 {3310}, resulting in a very low proliferation rate. Gene expression studies have revealed an expression profile that is distinct from that of either ductal adenocarcinoma or neuroendocrine neoplasm (NEN), and have demonstrated the involvement of the WNT/β-catenin and Notch signalling pathways {207,3279}.

Macroscopic appearance

SPNs are solitary, round, well-demarcated, and large tumours (average size: 8–10 cm; range: 0.5–25.0 cm), usually with some small solid areas, large areas of haemorrhagic necrosis, and large pseudocystic spaces {3095,1304}. Small tumours tend to be more solid. The wall of the neoplasm may contain calcifications. Rarely, the tumour extends into the duodenal wall or other adjacent structures {2892}.

Histopathology

Solid and pseudopapillary structures are combined with haemorrhage and pseudocystic changes in various proportions {3095,1304}. The solid tumour component, which may mimic a NEN, is composed of poorly cohesive monomorphic cells that cling to hyalinized or myxoid fibrovascular cords. Pseudopapillae are formed when the neoplastic cells detach from the fibrovascular stalks. Cholesterol crystals surrounded by foreign body giant cells, foamy histiocytes, and calcifications or even ossifications may occur. The tumour is generally well demarcated, but it may focally infiltrate the surrounding pancreatic tissue, entrapping acinar cells and islets. Vascular and perineural invasion is rare. The neoplastic cells are eosinophilic or vacuolated, often containing small PASD-positive hyaline globules. At the ultrastructural level, these globules correspond to zymogen-like α1-antitrypsin granules, whose contents may disintegrate, forming multilamellated vesicles and lipid droplets

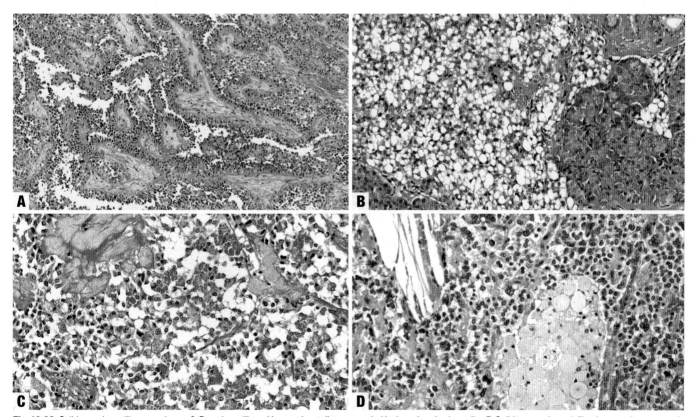

Fig. 10.38 Solid pseudopapillary neoplasm. **A** Pseudopapillae with vascular stalks surrounded by loosely cohesive cells. **B** Solid tumour tissue infiltrating exocrine pancreatic parenchyma and composed of cells with clear cytoplasm. **C** An example showing aggregates of hyaline globules between loosely cohesive tumour cells. **D** An example with cholesterol crystals next to a group of foamy histiocytes.

Chapter 10

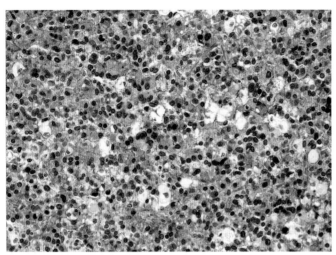

Fig. 10.39 Solid pseudopapillary neoplasm. An example with nuclear and cytoplasmic β-catenin labelling.

{3095}. Glycogen is not prominent and mucin is absent. The round to oval nuclei are often grooved or indented and have finely dispersed chromatin without a prominent nucleolus. Bizarre nuclei may occasionally occur. Mitoses are uncommon. Metastases have largely the same morphological appearance as the primary tumour, but the cells may be more pleomorphic and show more mitoses {2892}.

SPNs with foci of high-grade malignant transformation are considered a histological subtype. These SPNs, which are clinically extremely aggressive, are characterized by diffuse sheets of cells with increased nuclear atypia, as well as abundant mitoses. One case has been reported to contain a focus of sarcomatoid (spindle cell) carcinoma {3252}.

SPNs always show nuclear/cytoplasmic expression of β-catenin and often also E-cadherin {1690,3246,10,3310,601,2344}. The tumour cells also express cyclin D1, vimentin, PR, CD10, CD99 (dot-like), CD56, claudin-5, claudin-7, and α1-antitrypsin. Cytokeratins are detected in 30–70% of cases, depending on the method of antigen retrieval used. As many as 50% of SPNs express KIT (CD117) but show no *KIT* mutation {483}. Synaptophysin and neuron-specific enolase may be focally positive. The tumours are usually negative for chromogranin A and are consistently negative for trypsin and CEA {2344,708}.

Solid SPNs may mimic well-differentiated NENs or acinar cell carcinomas. In these cases, the diagnosis is established by nuclear expression of β-catenin and absent labelling for chromogranin A, trypsin, and/or BCL10.

Cytology

FNA specimens typically contain numerous discohesive small and monomorphic neoplastic cells clinging to thin branching vessels. Naked nuclei are also present. The cytoplasm of the cells is eosinophilic or foamy and may contain hyaline globules. The nuclei have indented or grooved membranes and may be stripped of cytoplasm. The background often contains haemorrhagic debris, foamy histiocytes, and multinucleated giant cells {3095,1304}.

Diagnostic molecular pathology

Somatic activating mutation in exon 3 of *CTNNB1* is the only genetic alteration known in SPNs {3246,10,22927}.

Essential and desirable diagnostic criteria

Essential: a neoplasm occurring in a patient of the characteristic age group and sex; solid, papillary, and cystic structures; positive nuclear and cytoplasmic staining for β-catenin.
Desirable: cholesterol crystals with granulomatous reaction; PAS-positive hyaline globules.

Staging (TNM)

Rarely, these neoplasms may directly infiltrate the duodenum, stomach, spleen, or portal vein. In 5–15% of patients, metastases may occur (even years after the resection of the primary) in the peritoneum and liver. Lymph nodes and skin are exceptionally rare sites of metastatic disease {3095}. The staging follows that of other carcinomas of the exocrine pancreas {3095,127,1304}.

Prognosis and prediction

The long-term prognosis is generally excellent for localized, metastatic, and recurrent disease, with long disease-free periods after complete surgical resection {2673,2047}. Only a few patients have died of a metastasizing SPN, mostly patients whose tumours harboured an undifferentiated component {2673}.

Metastatic behaviour cannot be predicted by perineural invasion, angioinvasion, and/or deep infiltration of surrounding structures. Consequently, all SPNs are currently classified as low-grade malignant neoplasms. However, it has been suggested that older patients do worse than younger patients, that patients with tumours with an aneuploid DNA content do worse than those with diploid tumours, and that an elevated mitotic count and certain nuclear features of the tumours (e.g. mean nuclear diameter and size) are associated with the presence of metastases {2369,3252}.

Pancreatic neuroendocrine neoplasms: Introduction

Klöppel G
Adsay NV
Couvelard A
Hruban RH
Kasajima A
Klimstra DS
La Rosa S

Perren A
Rindi G
Sasano H
Scarpa A
Shi C
Singhi AD

Like other neuroendocrine neoplasms (NENs), pancreatic NENs (PanNENs) express synaptophysin and usually chromogranin A. They include malignant well-differentiated NENs, called neuroendocrine tumours (NETs), and poorly differentiated NENs, designated neuroendocrine carcinomas (NECs).

Clinical features

Pancreatic NETs (PanNETs) are generally slow-growing, with overall survival rates of 33% at 5 years, 17% at 10 years, and 10% at 20 years {963}. Surgical resection markedly improves survival rates (see *Non-functioning pancreatic neuroendocrine tumours*, p. 347). In contrast, patients with fast-growing pancreatic NECs (PanNECs) rarely survive 1 year {271}.

PanNETs are divided into functioning and non-functioning neoplasms. Tumours associated with clinical syndromes caused by abnormal secretion of hormones by the tumours are considered functioning (syndromic) PanNETs and include insulinomas, gastrinomas, glucagonomas, and VIPomas, along with other less common tumours producing serotonin, ACTH, GHRH, PTHrP, and CCK.

Non-functioning (non-syndromic) tumours are not associated with a clinical hormone hypersecretion syndrome, but they may secrete peptide hormones and biogenic substances, such as PP, somatostatin, and chromogranins, which either are secreted at levels insufficient to cause symptoms or by themselves do not give rise to a clinical syndrome. Non-functioning tumours are incidentally discovered or become clinically apparent because of their large size, invasion of adjacent organs, or metastasis. Tumours with a diameter of < 5 mm (the minimum size for detection by imaging) are typically non-functioning and are designated neuroendocrine microadenomas. In the past, functioning PanNETs accounted for 60–85% of all PanNENs, with insulinomas being the most frequent type (accounting for as many as 70% of cases), followed by gastrinomas, glucagonomas, VIPomas, and other functioning PanNETs (e.g. PanNETs producing serotonin, ACTH, GHRH {1010}, PTHrP {1507}, and CCK {2678}). Recent data show that non-functioning PanNETs outnumber functioning NETs and account for > 60% of all PanNENs {895,894}.

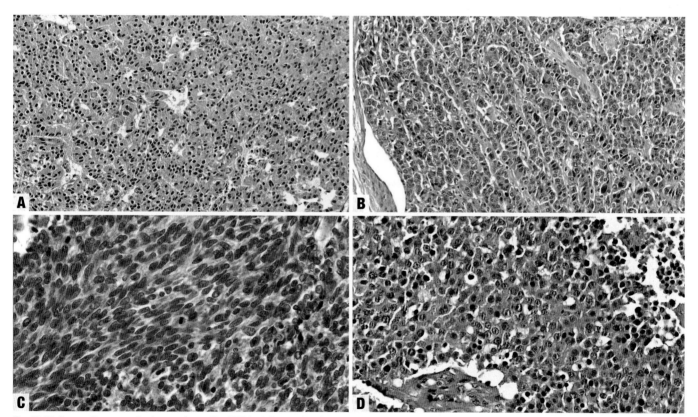

Fig. 10.40 Pancreatic neuroendocrine neoplasms (PanNENs). **A** Neuroendocrine tumour (NET), G1. A well-differentiated PanNEN with solid and trabecular pattern and monomorphous cytoplasm-rich cells. **B** NET, G2, with trabecular pattern, showing a well-differentiated to intermediately differentiated histology. **C** Neuroendocrine carcinoma (NEC) with poorly differentiated histology, small cell type. **D** NEC with poorly differentiated histology, large cell type.

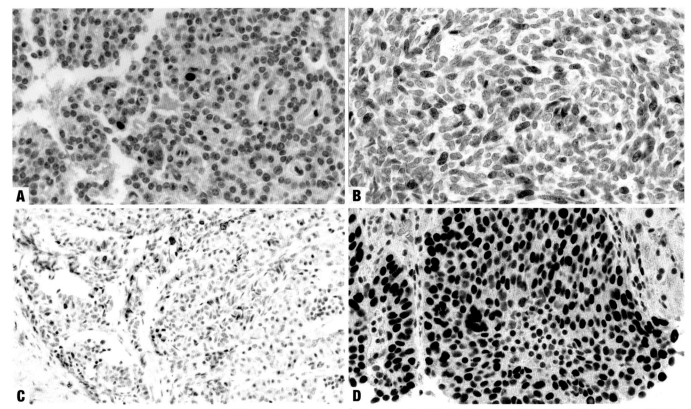

Fig. 10.41 Pancreatic neuroendocrine neoplasms (PanNENs). **A** Pancreatic neuroendocrine tumour (PanNET). Ki-67 immunostaining of a well-differentiated PanNEN. The Ki-67 proliferation index was < 3%, qualifying the tumour as G1. **B** Pancreatic neuroendocrine carcinoma (PanNEC). Ki-67 immunostaining of a poorly differentiated PanNEN, small cell type, with a Ki-67 proliferation index > 50%. **C** PanNET with wildtype *TP53* status, showing a low (< 20% of tumour cells) and weak nuclear p53 expression. **D** PanNEC with *TP53* mutation, showing a high and strong nuclear p53 expression.

Epidemiology

The relative prevalence of NENs among the pancreatic tumours is 2–5%, and their estimated incidence is < 1 case per 100 000 person-years {963,1145}. Autopsy studies that take into account tumours measuring ≤ 5 mm give a higher prevalence {1607} (see *Non-functioning pancreatic neuroendocrine tumours*, p. 347). PanNENs show no substantial sex difference and occur over a wide age range, with the highest incidence found in patients aged 30–60 years. The incidence of well-differentiated PanNENs has steadily increased over the past 40 years, for both low-grade and high-grade neoplasms {963,387,1860}, probably as a result of advances in imaging. Risk factors include family history of cancer, smoking, alcohol consumption, obesity, and diabetes {1861}.

Updated WHO classification

The 2010 WHO classification {379} effectively stratified groups predictive of patient survival, but in the years since its publication, some PanNENs with the histological features of PanNET have been reported to have a Ki-67 proliferation index > 20%. This is particularly common in liver metastases developing during the course of the disease. According to the 2010 WHO criteria, these histologically bland but mitotically active tumours would be classified as PanNEC. Although these tumours appear to have a somewhat worse prognosis than G2 PanNET, their behaviour is less aggressive than that of PanNECs {272,1207}. They show the features associated with PanNETs (i.e. hormone expression and association with hormonal as well as genetic

syndromes) and they usually lack the genetic abnormalities found in the histologically high-grade PanNENs (i.e. changes in expression and mutation of *TP53* and *RB1*) {271,3632,1681}. Furthermore, patients with PanNECs as defined by the 2010 WHO classification whose neoplasms had a Ki-67 proliferation index < 55% had a lower response rate but better survival than patients with neoplasms that had a Ki-67 proliferation index > 55% when treated with first-line platinum-based chemotherapy as used for the treatment of poorly differentiated NENs {3103}. Therefore, a novel tumour category, called G3 PanNET, was included in the 2017 WHO classification {1936}. These tumours retain a well-differentiated histological pattern and have a Ki-67 proliferation index > 20% and usually < 55% (see Table 1.01, p. 16).

Primary G3 PanNETs almost always have intact *TP53* and *RB1*. Only occasionally, there may be a G3 PanNET that develops a *TP53* mutation during its metastatic progression {1681}. No upper limit has been defined for the mitotic count or the Ki-67 proliferation index of G3 PanNET, but the lower limits, respectively, are > 20 mitoses/2 mm² and > 20%, by definition. G3 PanNETs may contain lower-grade components, or they may be found as metastases in patients with a prior G1 or G2 PanNET. The Ki-67 proliferation index of PanNECs is by definition > 20%.

PanNECs have a poorly differentiated histology (of either small cell or large cell type), often show p53 nuclear accumulation, lack RB1 expression, lack insulin gene enhancer protein ISL1 expression, and retain expression of DAXX and ATRX {3632,45}. Genetically, PanNECs may show similarities to ductal adenocarcinomas, because PanNECs frequently harbour *KRAS* mutations that characterize ductal adenocarcinomas {3632,1681,1231}. They may also express ductal lineage markers such as EMA (MUC1) and CEA {1681}.

Studies in large patient cohorts have shown that the subgroups of patients with G1 or G2 tumours have a significantly higher risk of progression when 5% is used as the Ki-67 proliferation index cut-off point instead of 3% {2563,2716,2879,2716A}. However, the evidence of differences in clinical management based on this higher cut-off point is insufficient to justify changing it at this time.

The terminology used for mixed neoplasms was changed in the 2017 WHO classification of NETs of the pancreas from "mixed adenoneuroendocrine carcinoma (MANEC)" to "mixed neuroendocrine–non-neuroendocrine neoplasm (MiNEN)". There are two reasons for this change. First, the complex neoplasms that are usually poorly differentiated in both components may occasionally be well differentiated, and second, they may contain a non-neuroendocrine component other than adenocarcinoma. The term "neuroendocrine" is the only one maintained from the previous terminology, because the neuroendocrine part is the constant component of these mixed tumours.

The category of hyperplastic and preneoplastic lesions included in the 2010 WHO classification was abolished in the 2017 WHO classification of NETs of the pancreas, because PanNEN precursor changes have not been clearly identified in association with sporadic neoplasms. They are described in the settings of multiple endocrine neoplasia type 1, von Hippel–Lindau syndrome (VHL) {3110}, and glucagon cell hyperplasia and neoplasia {881,3066,1638}.

Definition of PanNET

PanNET is a well-differentiated NEN of low, intermediate, or high grade, composed of cells with minimal to moderate atypia, displaying organoid patterns, lacking necrosis, and expressing general markers of neuroendocrine differentiation (diffuse/intense synaptophysin and usually also chromogranin A staining) and hormones (usually intense but not necessarily diffuse), either orthotopic or ectopic to the pancreas. On the basis of their proliferative activity, PanNETs are graded as G1 (< 2 mitoses/2 mm^2 and a Ki-67 proliferation index < 3%), G2 (2–20 mitoses/2 mm^2 or a Ki-67 proliferation index of 3–20%), or G3 (> 20 mitoses/2 mm^2 or a Ki-67 proliferation index > 20%) (see Table 1.01, p. 16). In cases with an associated hormonal

syndrome, PanNETs are categorized as insulinoma, glucagonoma, somatostatinoma, gastrinoma, VIPoma, serotonin-producing tumour (with or without carcinoid syndrome), ACTH-producing tumour, etc.

Definition of PanNEC

PanNEC is a poorly differentiated high-grade NEN, composed of highly atypical small cells or intermediate to large cells expressing the markers of neuroendocrine differentiation (diffuse/faint synaptophysin staining as well as faint/focal chromogranin A staining) and rarely hormones. The carcinoma lacks expression of acinar cell markers such as trypsin or carboxyl ester hydrolase (detected by BCL10). Based on their proliferative activity (> 20 mitoses/2 mm^2 or a Ki-67 proliferation index > 20%), PanNECs are considered high-grade neoplasms (see Table 1.01, p. 16).

Definition of MiNEN

MiNEN is a mixed neoplasm with a neuroendocrine component combined with a non-neuroendocrine component (typically ductal adenocarcinoma or acinar cell carcinoma). Both components are usually high-grade (G3), but occasionally one or both components may be G1 or G2. Therefore, when the components are morphologically distinguishable, each component should be graded on the respective grading system. Of particular importance is the grading of the neuroendocrine component, because it seems that the Ki-67 proliferation index of this component drives the prognosis of the MiNEN {2163}. For a tumour to qualify as MiNEN, each component should account for ≥ 30% of the tumour cell population. Non-neuroendocrine carcinomas with scattered neuroendocrine cells by immunohistochemistry do not fulfil this criterion; the presence of focal (< 30%) neuroendocrine differentiation can be mentioned but does not affect the diagnostic categorization. MiNEN is a conceptual category rather than a discrete entity; individual diagnoses indicating the specific cellular components should be applied (i.e. mixed acinar-neuroendocrine carcinoma, mixed ductal-neuroendocrine carcinoma, etc.) (see *Pancreatic MiNENs*, p. 370, and Box 1.01, p. 19).

Reporting of PanNENs

PanNENs could be NET or NEC based on histology and immunohistochemistry. PanNETs are graded as G1, G2, or G3. Endocrine function assessment should be provided upon clinical

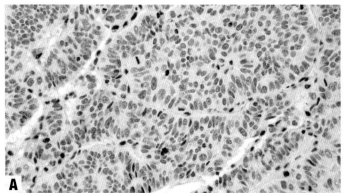
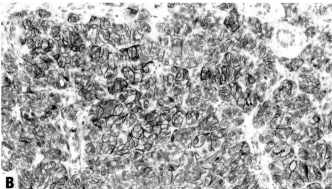

Fig. 10.42 Pancreatic neuroendocrine neoplasms (PanNENs). **A** Pancreatic neuroendocrine carcinoma (PanNEC) with *RB1* mutation and loss of nuclear RB1 expression. **B** Pancreatic neuroendocrine tumour (PanNET) with complete membranous expression of SSTR2A.

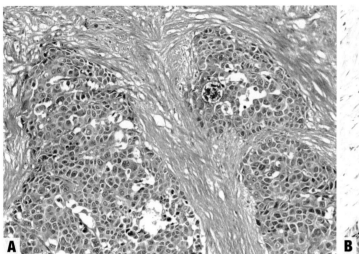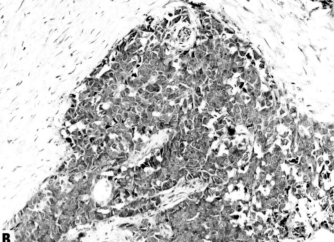

Fig. 10.43 Pancreatic mixed neuroendocrine–non-neuroendocrine neoplasm (MiNEN). **A** MiNEN with an adenocarcinoma component of numerous small glandular structures admixed with the neuroendocrine component (PASD). **B** Synaptophysin staining of the neuroendocrine component of the same tumour.

request. See the sections that follow for the tumour-type–specific requirements.

Genetic syndromes

In 10–20% of cases, PanNETs are associated with genetically determined hereditary syndromes such as multiple endocrine neoplasia type 1, VHL, neurofibromatosis type 1, tuberous sclerosis, glucagon cell hyperplasia and neoplasia {881,3066,2392}, and familial insulinomatosis {1350}. Germline mutations in DNA repair genes (*MUTYH*, *CHEK2*, and *BRCA2*) have been described in patients with apparently sporadic PanNETs {2878}. PanNECs do not show these associations {881}.

Molecular genetics

The *MEN1* gene is somatically inactivated in about 40% of PanNETs. This gene codes for menin, a tumour suppressor protein with diverse functions. In addition, approximately 40% of PanNETs showed mutation in either *DAXX* or *ATRX*. The function of DAXX and ATRX proteins is to maintain chromatin remodelling at telomeric and pericentromeric regions. *DAXX* and *ATRX* mutations are strongly associated with the alternative lengthening of telomeres pathway for telomere maintenance, as well as with chromosomal instability. About 15% of PanNETs have alterations in mTOR pathway genes such as *TSC2* and *PTEN*. This mTOR pathway is important because it is a potential therapeutic target. There are also PanNETs with *HIF1A* and *VHL* alterations {881,3066,2878,811,1463,2555,2897,2988}.

Germline alterations affecting *MEN1*, *VHL*, *NF1*, *GCGR*, and *MAFA* are found in PanNETs associated with multiple endocrine neoplasia type 1, VHL, neurofibromatosis type 1, glucagon cell hyperplasia and neoplasia, and insulinomatosis, respectively {1350}. Some of these PanNETs have distinctive morphologies. Mutations in *VHL* result in dysregulation of the HIF pathway, and PanNETs that arise in patients with VHL often have clear cell morphology {1250}. Mutations in *GCGR* alter glucagon receptor signalling and lead to glucagon cell hyperplasia and subsequent neoplasia, but the mechanism through which these alterations occur is not yet clear {3066}. Missense mutations of the *MAFA* gene in familial insulinomatosis cause the development of familial multifocal trabecular insulin-producing PanNETs {1350}.

In PanNECs, only somatic genetic alterations have been reported. These include mutations of cell-cycle regulatory genes, such as *TP53*, *RB1*, and *CDKN2A*, whereas chromatin remodelling genes such as *MEN1*, *ATRX*, and *DAXX* are not involved {3632,1681}. In addition, PanNECs may show *KRAS* mutations identical to those that occur in conventional ductal adenocarcinomas {3632,1681,1231}.

Staging (TNM)

PanNEN staging, which is presented in Chapter 1 (p. 20), follows the eighth editions (2017) of the Union for International Cancer Control (UICC) TNM classification {408} and the American Joint Committee on Cancer (AJCC) cancer staging manual {127,636}, which rely on macroscopic assessment of site, tumour size, and metastases. This approach largely corresponds to that of the European Neuroendocrine Tumor Society (ENETS) classification {2716,2716A}.

Prognosis and prediction

The criteria that predict the risk of tumour progression of PanNEN are summarized in the TNM staging table (p. 20). The listed criteria have a high probability and statistical significance (in particular Ki-67 proliferation index {2563,2716,2716A}) for predicting the behaviour of a given PanNEN {2896}. However, predicting the outcome of a PanNEN often requires long clinical follow-up, particularly for PanNETs, because metastasis may occur many years after resection of the primary.

Prognostic immunohistochemical markers other than Ki-67 (e.g. CK19, KIT, CD99, CD44, and p27) have been reported {2896,761} (see also *Non-functioning pancreatic neuroendocrine tumours*, p. 347), but these have not been validated in a large cohort. Recent genetic studies in PanNETs showed that patients with *DAXX* or *ATRX* mutations had a worse clinical outcome than those with wildtype *DAXX* and *ATRX*. This was particularly obvious in patients with G2 PanNET {2878,2527,3436,1586,3057}. Furthermore, primary PanNETs with loss of trimethylation of histone H3 lysine 36 (H3K36me3), ARID1A expression, and/or *CDKN2A* deletion have been reported to have a poorer prognosis {2771}, but further investigations are required to confirm the clinical relevance of these genetic abnormalities.

Non-functioning pancreatic neuroendocrine tumours

Klöppel G
Hruban RH
Klimstra DS
Rindi G
Scarpa A

Definition

Non-functioning (non-syndromic) pancreatic neuroendocrine tumours (NF-PanNETs) are well-differentiated epithelial pancreatic neuroendocrine neoplasms (PanNENs) that measure ≥ 0.5 cm, without a distinct hormonal syndrome. Microadenomas are NF-PanNETs measuring < 0.5 cm. Microadenomatosis is the multifocal occurrence of microadenomas.

ICD-O coding

8150/0 Pancreatic neuroendocrine microadenoma
8240/3 Neuroendocrine tumour NOS
8150/3 Pancreatic neuroendocrine tumour, non-functioning

ICD-11 coding

2C10.1 & XH3709 Neuroendocrine neoplasms of pancreas & Pancreatic endocrine tumour, non-functioning

Related terminology

Acceptable: non-functioning pancreatic endocrine tumour; islet cell tumour.
Not recommended: low-grade endocrine carcinoma of the pancreas (has potential to be confused with poorly differentiated pancreatic neuroendocrine carcinoma).

Subtype(s)

Neuroendocrine tumour, grade 1 (8240/3); neuroendocrine tumour, grade 2 (8249/3); neuroendocrine tumour, grade 3 (8249/3); oncocytic neuroendocrine tumour, non-functioning pancreatic; pleomorphic neuroendocrine tumour, non-functioning pancreatic; clear cell neuroendocrine tumour, non-functioning pancreatic; cystic neuroendocrine tumour, non-functioning pancreatic

Localization

Two thirds of surgically resected NF-PanNETs occur in the head of the pancreas {3457}.

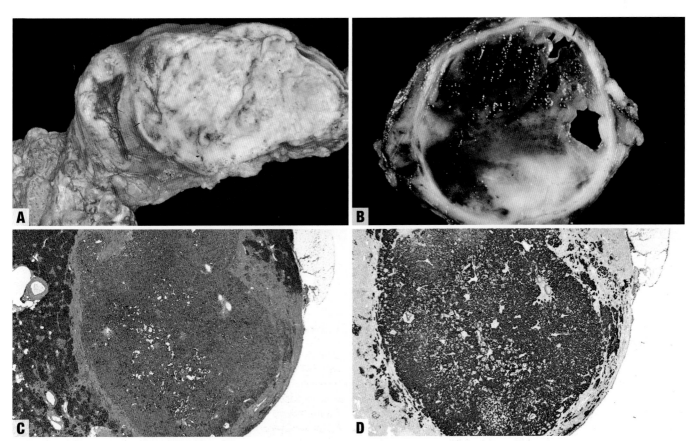

Fig. 10.44 Non-functioning neuroendocrine tumour (NET). **A** Large, well-demarcated, solid, and lobulated tumour in the pancreatic body, with a pinkish-tan to white cut surface lacking necrosis. **B** Tumour with central unilocular cyst surrounded by a small rim of neoplastic tissue. **C** Neuroendocrine microadenoma. The tumour is well circumscribed and has a trabecular architecture. **D** Immunostaining for glucagon.

Chapter 10

Clinical features

The patient age at which sporadic NF-PanNETs are clinically detected ranges widely (12–79 years), with a mean age of 50–55 years {3024,934,2879,1151,2716,3457,2716A}. Both sexes are equally affected, with an M:F ratio of 1:1.15. Many NF-PanNETs are detected incidentally, particularly if they are small or localized in the tail of the gland. The remaining NF-PanNETs present with symptoms due to local or metastatic tumour spread {1716}. As many as half of patients present with metastatic disease {3684,2716,2716A}. The clinical diagnosis is supported by elevated serum levels of chromogranin A or neuron-specific enolase, EUS, CT, MRI, and somatostatin receptor scintigraphy (octreoscan and 68Ga-DOTATOC PET) {895}. 68Ga-DOTATOC PET specifically locates and stages NF-PanNETs and their metastases {1716,2718}.

Metastases occur both to regional lymph nodes and to the liver. Distant metastases usually occur late in the course of the disease and are mainly found in lung and bone {1716,3457}.

Epidemiology

The prevalence of clinically diagnosed sporadic NF-PanNET is much lower (0.2–2 cases per million person-years) than that of microadenomas detected in postmortem examinations. The prevalence of microadenomas ranges from 1% to 10%, depending on the amount of pancreatic tissue examined {1607}. The prevalence of clinically detected NF-PanNETs {1145} seems to have steadily increased over the past 40 years {1807,716}, most likely because of improved imaging. There is also an increase in the relative prevalence of NF-PanNETs. Two to three decades ago, they were reported to constitute only a third of all Pan-NETs {423,1643}, but now they account for as many as 70–80% {934,2879,2716,2716A}. In multiple endocrine neoplasia type 1, 30–75% of patients have clinical evidence of a PanNET, and there is pancreatic involvement in nearly 100% of patients with multiple endocrine neoplasia type 1 at autopsy {2013}. In these patients, a high percentage of individual tumours are non-functioning {1111,156}, but the majority of multiple endocrine neoplasia type 1 patients with pancreatic involvement also have at least one functioning PanNET {1648,1813}. In von Hippel–Lindau syndrome (VHL), PanNETs are observed in 11–17% of patients {345,1154,2710}, and all are non-functioning {345,2623}. This also holds true for glucagon cell hyperplasia and neoplasia {3066}.

Etiology

Familial NF-PanNETs are found in several hereditary syndromes (see *Pancreatic neuroendocrine neoplasms: Introduction*, p. 343).

Pathogenesis

The pathogenesis of NF-PanNETs is largely unknown, and precursors in both the ducts and the islets have been suggested. During disease progression, accumulation of additional genomic alterations accompanies the grade progression that may occur.

Macroscopic appearance

NF-PanNETs in the head of the gland may narrow the common bile duct and infiltrate the duodenum; tumours in the tail of the gland extend into peripancreatic soft tissues and spleen. Tumour thrombi within large veins may be found.

Because of their small size (< 5 mm), microadenomas are barely visible grossly. The average greatest dimension of NF-PanNETs ranges from 2 to 5 cm, and most tumours are well circumscribed {1716}. Large tumours are often lobulated, with a heterogeneous and nodular-infiltrative appearance. The consistency of NF-PanNETs varies from soft and fleshy to hard and fibrous, and the colour varies from reddish-tan to brownish-yellow. Necrosis is uncommon. Cystic change may occur, usually with a unilocular cyst filled with serous fluid surrounded by a rim of neoplastic tissue {1680,3052,1909}.

Histopathology

NF-PanNETs have well-differentiated organoid growth patterns that do not differ from those of most types of functioning Pan-NETs {2988,699}. The spectrum includes solid-nesting and solid-paraganglioma-like growth patterns, trabecular and gyriform patterns, and a glandular pattern. Intratumoural heterogeneity is rare in small tumours and relatively common in larger neoplasms {1643,1642}. Necrosis is uncommon. The stroma is richly vascular, but otherwise varies considerably, from simple, fine, capillary-sized vessels between neoplastic cell nests to broad areas of dense, hyalinized collagen. Some tumours exhibit stromal calcifications (sometimes including psammoma bodies).

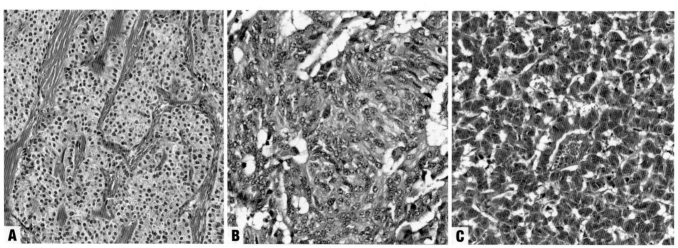

Fig. 10.45 Non-functioning neuroendocrine tumour (NET). **A** Solid nested pattern. **B** Solid paraganglioma-like pattern. **C** Reticulated trabecular pattern.

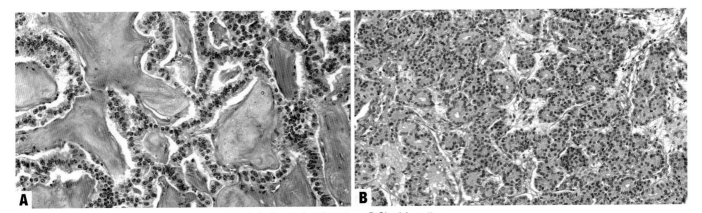

Fig. 10.46 Non-functioning neuroendocrine tumour (NET). **A** Gyriform trabecular pattern. **B** Glandular pattern.

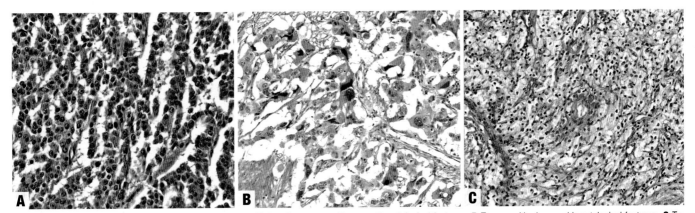

Fig. 10.47 Non-functioning neuroendocrine tumour (NET). **A** Trabecular tumour with oncocytic cytological features. **B** Tumour with pleomorphic cytological features. **C** Tumour with clear cell features.

Most of the neoplastic cells are cuboidal and eosinophilic, with finely granular cytoplasm. The nuclei are round to oval, with minimal atypia and coarsely clumped (salt-and-pepper) chromatin. They are centrally located or polarized, particularly in trabecular tumours. Uncommon are eccentric nuclei associated with a rhabdoid cell appearance {2568}, enlarged nuclei, irregular nuclear membranes {3740}, and prominent nucleoli. Mitoses are generally sparse; in most cases there are < 5 mitoses/2 mm^2 and almost always < 20 mitoses/2 mm^2. Some NF-PanNETs contain small non-neoplastic ductules and islets intermingled with the neoplastic cells {3419,1520}.

A number of NF-PanNETs have distinctive cytological features. Oncocytic NF-PanNETs are composed of cells with voluminous intensely eosinophilic cytoplasm due to abundant mitochondria {3485,514,3166}. The nuclei are often enlarged and frequently contain prominent nucleoli. Pleomorphic NF-PanNETs are characterized by marked nuclear pleomorphism, but these pleomorphic nuclei have no adverse prognostic significance, because they are associated with a normal N:C ratio and no increased proliferation rate {3740}. Clear cell NF-PanNETs have innumerable lipid vacuoles in the cytoplasm, scalloping the nucleus . Such tumours have been reported particularly in patients with VHL {1250,3048}.

The ultrastructure of NF-PanNETs is characterized by variable numbers of membrane-bound electron-dense neurosecretory granules, either non-polarized within the cytoplasm or oriented near the basal surfaces facing the capillaries. The granule

morphology is often nonspecific. The characteristic granule types of α or β cells sometimes found in functioning PanNETs are absent.

Immunohistochemistry
NF-PanNETs express synaptophysin (usually diffuse and strong) and chromogranin A (usually more focal and apical). They also express neuron-specific enolase, CD56, and CD57, which are not specific for neuroendocrine differentiation {3378,2988,1209}. Many NF-PanNETs, although clinically non-functioning, immunolabel for peptide hormones in highly variable proportions of the tumour cells. About 40% of the tumours are multihormonal {1520}. The hormones most often expressed are glucagon, PP, and somatostatin {1520,1254}. Rarely, the entire tumour fails to label for any hormone. In some tumours, in which one hormone predominates, distinctive histological patterns may occur. Glucagon-positive NF-PanNETs frequently demonstrate cystic changes, trabecular pattern, or reticular pattern {1680}. Somatostatin-positive NF-PanNETs may show paraganglioma-like pattern and/or glandular structures with psammoma bodies {1009}. Serotonin-positive NF-PanNETs often display small cell nests and tubules embedded in dense stromal sclerosis, and they frequently arise adjacent to the main duct, causing duct obstruction and dilatation (see *Serotonin-producing neuroendocrine tumour*, p. 365) {1555,2097}. Microadenomas are more likely to show diffuse expression of a single peptide, most often glucagon, followed by PP {156}.

Table 10.04 Differential diagnostic considerations for pancreatic neuroendocrine carcinomas (PanNECs)

Diagnosis	Architecture	Cytomorphology	Immunophenotype
PanNEC {272,3632,271}	Infiltrative; necrotic	Small cell or large cell cytology; diffuse or nested pattern; > 20 mitoses/2 mm²; desmoplastic stroma; may have an adenocarcinoma component	Chromogranin, synaptophysin (weak or +); p53 (+); RB1 (lost); DAXX, ATRX (retained); Ki-67 (usually > 50%)
Acinar cell carcinoma {3601,1752}	Solid and acinar patterns	Granular eosinophilic cytoplasm; prominent nucleoli	Trypsin, chymotrypsin, lipase, BCL10 (+); chromogranin, synaptophysin (focal)
Pancreatoblastoma {3601,1752}	Solid and acinar patterns; lobulated	Acinar cytomorphology; squamoid nests; hypercellular stromal bands	Trypsin, chymotrypsin, lipase, BCL10 (+); chromogranin, synaptophysin (focal)
Solid pseudopapillary neoplasm {1633,3279,3248}	Solid and cystic with degenerative changes	Loosely cohesive cells; pseudopapillae; cytoplasmic vacuoles; hyaline globules; foamy histiocytes; nuclear grooves	Vimentin, CD10, CD56, α1-antitrypsin, β-catenin (+); keratin, synaptophysin (focal); trypsin, chymotrypsin, chromogranin (−)
Ductal adenocarcinoma	Solid; infiltrative	Individual mucin-producing glands; desmoplastic stroma; substantial mitotic activity	CK7, CEA, EMA (MUC1), chromogranin, synaptophysin (− or focally +)

NF-PanNETs express the transcription factor insulin gene enhancer protein ISL1, which may be useful to support pancreatic origin for a metastatic neuroendocrine tumour (NET) of unknown primary {45,1084}. Less useful for determining the site of origin are PDX1, PAX8, and CDX2 {1767,72,1221}. Immunolabelling for DAXX and ATRX reveals loss of expression in 45% of NF-PanNETs {2053,1463,3544}. There is generally no overexpression of p53 or loss of expression of RB1 or SMAD4 {3632,2988}. Among the various somatostatin receptors, SSTR2A is often strongly expressed in a membranous pattern, and its expression correlates with molecular imaging {3483}. Occasionally, NF-PanNETs immunolabel for CEA and CA19-9 {1506,3678} or have scattered trypsin-positive cells {1506}. PanNETs associated with VHL typically express HIF1A and CAIX, as do associated foci of islet cell hyperplasia not identifiable on routinely stained sections in these patients {670,2623}.

Grading
See *Pancreatic neuroendocrine neoplasms: Introduction* (p. 343).

Differential diagnosis
The main differential diagnosis includes pancreatic neuroendocrine carcinoma (PanNEC), acinar cell carcinoma, solid pseudopapillary neoplasm, pancreatoblastoma, and ductal adenocarcinoma (for diagnostic criteria, see Table 10.04).

Metastasis from renal cell carcinoma may resemble a clear cell PanNET, particularly in patients with VHL, whereas metastases from hepatocellular carcinoma or adrenal cortical carcinoma may resemble oncocytic PanNETs {3485,1250}.

Microadenomas can be distinguished from enlarged islets by immunohistochemical staining for islet peptides, because microadenomas lose the normal proportions and non-random distribution of peptide cell types that characterize islets {156}.

Cytology
FNA specimens from PanNETs are usually highly cellular with a clean background. The neoplastic cells are found in loosely cohesive clusters and individually. A plasmacytoid configuration is characteristic. The nuclei are uniform and round to oval, and they contain coarsely granular chromatin. Mitotic figures are usually not identified. Grading of NF-PanNETs in cytological specimens can underestimate the true grade because of limited material {3478,902,3042}.

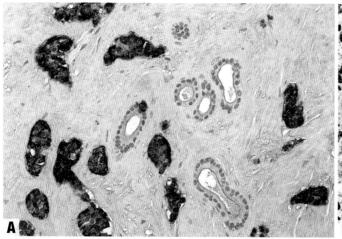
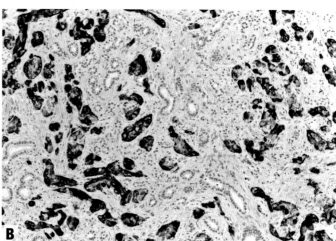

Fig. 10.48 Non-functioning neuroendocrine tumour (NET). **A** Entrapped non-neoplastic ducts between glucagon-positive tumour cells. **B** Tumour with serotonin-positive cells embedded in sclerotic stroma.

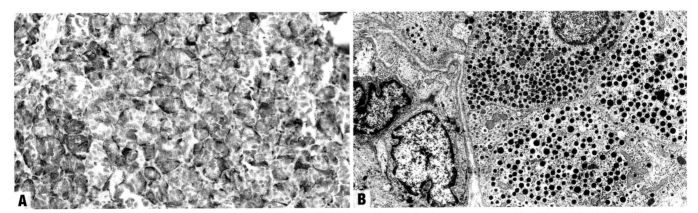

Fig. 10.49 Non-functioning neuroendocrine tumour (NET). **A** Tumour with somatostatin-positive cells forming a paraganglioma-like pattern. **B** Ultrastructure of tumour cells with membrane-bound hormone containing granules.

Diagnostic molecular pathology
The genetic features of NF-PanNETs are similar to those described for PanNETs in general (see *Pancreatic neuroendocrine neoplasms: Introduction*, p. 343). The most frequent recurring genetic features are inactivation of the genes *MEN1*, *DAXX* or *ATRX*, *SETD2*, *PTEN*, and *TSC1/2*; hyperactivation of the PI3K/mTOR pathway; and alternative lengthening of telomeres {1463}.

Essential and desirable diagnostic criteria
Essential: usually well circumscribed; regular cytological features, with salt-and-pepper nuclei and a nested organoid growth pattern; positive staining for neuroendocrine markers.
Desirable: positive staining for a variety of hormone products may be seen; other histological patterns may be seen.

Staging (TNM)
The staging of NF-PanNETs, like that of all PanNENs, follows the eighth editions (2017) of the Union for International Cancer Control (UICC) TNM classification {408} and the American Joint Committee on Cancer (AJCC) cancer staging manual {127,636}, which rely on macroscopic assessment of site, tumour size, and metastases. This approach largely corresponds to that of the European Neuroendocrine Tumor Society (ENETS) classification {2716,2716A}. The staging of well-differentiated PanNENs is presented in Chapter 1 (p. 20).

Prognosis and prediction
Microadenomas are considered to be benign, and it is unknown whether all or only a subset of these tumours may progress to clinically relevant PanNETs.

Table 10.05 Prognostic factors for non-functioning pancreatic neuroendocrine tumours (PanNETs)

Factor	Method of assessment	In routine use?	References
Tumour size	Gross evaluation	Yes	{1716,1111,2896}
Invasiveness (vascular invasion, extrapancreatic invasion)	Microscopic evaluation	Yes	{1716,2896}
Necrosis	Microscopic evaluation	No	{1254}
Stage	Microscopic evaluation; clinical/radiographical evaluation	Yes	{2716,2716A}
Grade	Microscopic evaluation and immunohistochemistry	Yes	{2896,934,2879,2716,2716A}
Mitotic count	Microscopic evaluation	Yes	{2896,934,2879,2716,2716A}
Ki-67 proliferation index	Immunohistochemistry	Yes	{2896,934,2879,3675,2716,1643A,2716A}
PTEN loss	Immunohistochemistry	No	{881A}
PR loss	Immunohistochemistry	No	{881A}
Aneuploidy	Flow cytometry	No	{802A}
CK19 expression	Immunohistochemistry	No	{2896,3754A}
KIT (also known as CD117 and c-KIT) expression	Immunohistochemistry	No	{3754A}
Loss of heterozygosity at 1p, 3p, 6q, 17p, 22q, and X	Comparative genomic hybridization	No	{246,2597A}
DAXX/ATRX	Immunohistochemistry; FISH	No	{2053,3057}

Approximately 55–75% of all other NF-PanNETs behave in a malignant manner, with extrapancreatic spread, metastasis, or recurrence {3457,2716,2716A}. After surgical resection, the 5-year survival rate of NF-PanNETs is reportedly 65–86%, and the 10-year survival rate is 45–68% {2716,1151,934,1254}. Most patients with metastatic PanNETs survive for several years. The median survival time after recurrence is 2.3 years {1151}. The 5-year survival rate of patients with metastatic PanNETs is 59%, and the 10-year survival rate is 36% {1561}.

A number of factors have been shown to predict the prognosis of PanNETs. The most important histological factor predictive of outcome is proliferative rate, based on mitotic count and Ki-67 proliferation index {1026} (see *Pancreatic neuroendocrine neoplasms: Introduction*, p. 343). Abundant data demonstrate the prognostic stratification of G1 and G2 NF-PanNETs, both in the setting of a resected primary tumour and for metastatic disease. In biopsies of metastases, the Ki-67 proliferation index may be difficult to assess accurately because of the limited tissue available or tumour heterogeneity regarding highest proliferative activity {3675}. Both G1 and G2 PanNETs are prognostically separated from PanNECs {2164}. This is also true for the G3 PanNET group (see also *Pancreatic neuroendocrine neoplasms: Introduction*, p. 343), which is somewhat more aggressive than G2 PanNET but not as rapidly progressive as PanNEC {2716A}. The 5-year survival rate for G3 PanNETs is 29%, for G2 PanNETs 62%, and for PanNECs 16% {272}.

Another predictor of outcome is tumour size. Tumours < 2 cm uncommonly demonstrate clinical aggressiveness, whereas tumours > 3 cm have a higher risk of metastasis {1716,1111}. Small (< 2.0 cm), low-grade NF-PanNETs have very indolent biology. Therefore, it has been suggested that asymptomatic cases may be closely monitored radiographically rather than resected {895}. The likelihood of metastasis also increases with extent of invasive growth (especially vascular invasion), necrosis, and the status of regional lymph nodes {2896}.

Immunolabelling for a peptide in the absence of a clinical syndrome has no prognostic relevance. The histological patterns of NF-PanNETs are not prognostically distinctive in general. Cystic PanNETs frequently lack adverse prognostic factors and often present at a lower stage {1680,1909}. Oncocytic NF-PanNETs appear to be aggressive {3485}. Other immunohistochemical and molecular factors reported as prognostic are listed in Table 10.05 (p. 351).

Insulinoma

Perren A
Couvelard A
Singhi AD

Definition
Insulinoma is a functioning neuroendocrine neoplasm (NEN) composed of insulin-producing cells, with uncontrolled secretion of insulin causing a hypoglycaemic syndrome.

ICD-O coding
8151/3 Insulinoma

ICD-11 coding
2C10.1 & XH3UK0 Neuroendocrine neoplasms of pancreas & Insulinoma, malignant

Related terminology
None

Subtype(s)
None

Localization
The vast majority of insulinomas are found in the pancreas, where they are evenly distributed {2110}. Extrapancreatic insulinomas, which are extremely rare, have been described in the duodenal wall, the ileum, the jejunum, and the hilum of the spleen {25,1666,2562,2970,1755}.

Clinical features
Insulinomas are the most common functioning pancreatic NENs (PanNENs) and account for about 4–20% of resected PanNENs {3683,1408}. The peak incidence is in the sixth decade of life, but individuals of any age can be affected {2110}. Insulinomas are rare in children and young adults (1% in patients aged < 30 years) {2110}. Women seem to be slightly more affected than men. About 10% of insulinomas develop metastases, which occur more frequently in men {2956,2359}. Multiple insulinomas are seen in about 10% of the patients, most often in the

setting of multiple endocrine neoplasia type 1, but also rarely in the setting of insulinomatosis {150}.

Hyperinsulinaemic hypoglycaemia leads to autonomic and neuroglycopenic symptoms. The adrenergic symptoms include palpitations and tremor. The cholinergic symptoms include sweating, hunger, and/or paraesthesia. The neuroglycopenic symptoms comprise severe weakness and a wide variety of psychiatric and neurological manifestations. Other common signs and symptoms include confusion, agitation, slow reaction pattern, blurred vision, seizures, transient loss of consciousness, and hypoglycaemic coma {1089}. The diagnosis is based on the hypoglycaemic symptoms, low plasma glucose levels (< 2.2 mmol/L [< 40 mg/dL]), and symptom relief after glucose administration (the Whipple triad). The best diagnostic test is prolonged fasting (48–72 hours) with measurement of blood glucose, serum insulin, C-peptide, and proinsulin {2957}.

The tumours are usually detected by CT, MRI, EUS, and or 68Ga-DOTATOC/TATE PET {1641,3180,871}. Recently, radiolabelled GLP analogue scintigraphy has been introduced as a sensitive method to localize small insulinomas {630}. Malignant insulinomas can change hormone production and clinical syndrome during the course of the disease.

Epidemiology
Insulinomas have an estimated incidence of 0.4 cases per 100 000 person-years {2956}.

Etiology
There are no known etiological factors for sporadic solitary insulinomas. There may be an association with diabetes {1144}. Families with germline mutations in MEN1 develop insulinomas among other pancreatic neuroendocrine tumours (PanNETs) and endocrine tumours. Familial insulinomatosis has recently been attributed to a MAFA germline mutation {1350}.

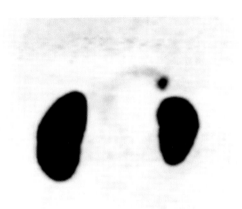

Fig. 10.50 Insulinoma. 68Ga-DOTA-exendin-4 whole-body PET highlighting insulinoma and kidneys via GLP receptor binding.

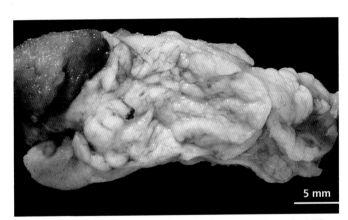

5 mm

Fig. 10.51 Insulinoma. Resection specimen showing a well-circumscribed 1.5 cm tumour.

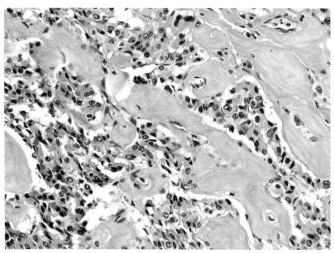

Fig. 10.52 Insulinoma. Typical insulinoma morphology with predominantly trabecular growth. Note stromal amyloid deposition.

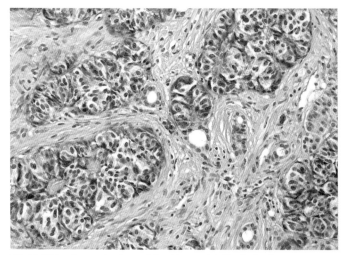

Fig. 10.53 Insulinoma showing peripheral immunolabelling for insulin.

Pathogenesis

Unknown

Macroscopic appearance

Insulinomas are usually small, solitary, and well-demarcated PanNETs with greyish-white to yellowish-tan, sometimes haemorrhagic cut surfaces. About 80% of insulinomas are smaller (1–2 cm in diameter) than other functioning PanNETs, making diagnosis difficult. Insulinomas that metastasize are typically > 2 cm, with a mean diameter of 3 cm.

Histopathology

The growth pattern of insulinomas is mainly trabecular or solid. Some insulinomas show a tubuloacinar growth pattern with psammoma bodies, as is seen in somatostatin-producing Pan-NET. Non-neoplastic ducts may be entrapped, and intense hyalinized sclerosis may be present. Stromal deposits of islet amyloid polypeptide (IAPP; also called amylin) are specific for insulinomas but occur in only about 5% of cases.

The demonstration of insulin is not mandatory for the diagnosis of insulinoma in the setting of a solitary PanNET. However, if multiple PanNETs are present, it is important to stain for insulin to identify the insulinoma, because the largest Pan-NET is not always responsible for the clinical syndrome {156}. Insulin staining is required for the diagnosis of insulinomatosis {150}. About half of insulinomas include scattered non–insulin-staining cells positive for glucagon, PP, somatostatin, and/or other hormones. This is particularly the case in malignant insulinomas.

Cytology

The cytological features are identical to those of other PanNETs.

Diagnostic molecular pathology

Insulinomas share most mutational events with other PanNETs (e.g. mutations in *MEN1*, *DAXX*, *ATRX*, *PTEN*, and *TSC2*). Nevertheless, insulinomas cluster at the RNA level as an independent PanNET group {2809}. A recurrent p.T372R mutation in *YY1* has been reported in 30% of sporadic insulinomas {488,1902} but is absent in other PanNETs.

Essential and desirable diagnostic criteria

Essential: clinical diagnosis (see *Clinical features*, above); neuroendocrine tumour (NET) histology.

Staging (TNM)

The staging of insulinomas, like that of all PanNENs, follows the eighth editions (2017) of the Union for International Cancer Control (UICC) TNM classification {408} and the American Joint Committee on Cancer (AJCC) cancer staging manual {127,636}, which rely on macroscopic assessment of site, tumour size, and metastases. This approach largely corresponds to that of the European Neuroendocrine Tumor Society (ENETS) classification {2716}. The staging of well-differentiated PanNENs is presented in Chapter 1 (p. 20).

Prognosis and prediction

Like for other PanNETs, the most important prognostic markers are stage and grade of the tumours {1641}. Insulinomas > 2 cm {3517} and with loss of DAXX and/or ATRX {2053,2771,2878} have an increased risk of metastasis.

Gastrinoma

Kasajima A
Couvelard A

Definition
Gastrinoma of the pancreas is a functioning well-differentiated pancreatic neuroendocrine neoplasm (PanNEN) composed of gastrin-producing cells (G cells), with uncontrolled gastrin secretion causing Zollinger–Ellison syndrome (ZES).

ICD-O coding
8153/3 Gastrinoma

ICD-11 coding
2C10.1 & XH0GY2 Neuroendocrine neoplasms of pancreas & Gastrinoma, malignant

Related terminology
None

Subtype(s)
None

Localization
Gastrinomas have no preferential localization in the pancreas {641,1446,1698}. In the duodenum, where gastrinomas are much more common {1639}, especially in patients with multiple endocrine neoplasia type 1 (MEN1), they occur mainly in the proximal part {153,1639}. Extrapancreatic and extraduodenal gastrinomas have been reported in the stomach, liver, and lymph node {1446}. The diagnosis of primary lymph node gastrinoma requires careful exclusion of metastatic disease from occult duodenal gastrinoma {151}.

Clinical features
The typical clinical features of ZES are duodenal ulcer and/or gastro-oesophageal reflux disease {750}. These symptoms are caused by marked gastric acid hypersecretion associated with inappropriately elevated fasting serum gastrin. ZES may also lead to fundic enterochromaffin-like–cell (ECL cell) hyperplasia, and in the setting of MEN1 to fundic neuroendocrine tumours (NETs) of type 2.

Epidemiology
Gastrinomas account for 4–8% of all pancreatic NETs (PanNETs) {153,1408}. ZES is the second most common hormonal syndrome associated with functioning PanNETs {2096,1408}. Patients with sporadic pancreatic gastrinomas are usually younger than those with non-functioning PanNETs, often in their fifth or sixth decade of life, with no sex predilection {1446,2716}. Patients with MEN1-associated gastrinomas are usually a decade younger {1037,1446}.

Etiology
There are no known etiological factors specific to sporadic pancreatic gastrinomas. Approximately 25% of all gastrinomas are associated with MEN1, but almost all of them arise in the duodenum {895}. Gastrinomas associated with neurofibromatosis (neurofibromatosis type 1 or 2) {1845,2072} or tuberous sclerosis {2917} are extremely rare.

Pathogenesis
The pathogenesis of pancreatic gastrinoma is unknown. Multicentric preneoplastic gastrin-cell proliferation has only been identified in association with MEN1-related duodenal gastrinomas {155}.

Sporadic gastrinomas may harbour somatic *MEN1* mutations, which are identified in 33% of cases {3782}. *MEN1* mutations lead to abnormal menin that interacts with FOXN3 (CHES1). This may lead to the aggressive behaviour of the tumours noted in patients with MEN1 {259}.

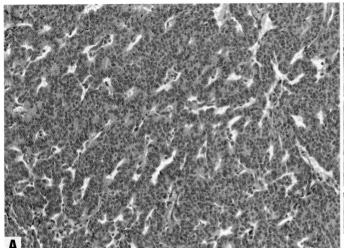
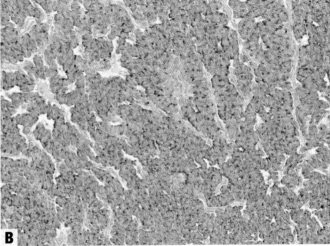

Fig. 10.54 Pancreatic gastrinoma. **A** Tumour cells display trabeculae with mild to moderate cellular atypia. **B** Tumour cells stain positively for gastrin.

Macroscopic appearance

Pancreatic gastrinomas are generally large (mean: 3.8 cm; only 6% < 1 cm), but their macroscopic appearance does not otherwise differ from that of the other PanNETs.

Histopathology

Gastrinomas often display trabecular or glandular structures. The margin of the tumour can be expansive or focally infiltrative. The stroma is normally delicate and may only be prominent in large tumours. The tumour cells express synaptophysin, chromogranin A, SSTR2, and gastrin (often focal). Other hormones that may be expressed include insulin, glucagon, PP, and somatostatin. Rarely, a switch in hormone hypersecretion from gastrin to another hormone, with consequent change in the associated clinical syndrome, has been reported {728,2045}.

Cytology

The cytology is the same as that of other PanNETs.

Diagnostic molecular pathology

Not clinically relevant

Essential and desirable diagnostic criteria

Essential: clinical syndrome; NET histology.

Staging (TNM)

The staging of gastrinomas, like that of all PanNENs, follows the eighth editions (2017) of the Union for International Cancer Control (UICC) TNM classification {408} and the American Joint Committee on Cancer (AJCC) cancer staging manual {127,636}, which rely on macroscopic assessment of site, tumour size, and metastases. This approach largely corresponds to that of the European Neuroendocrine Tumor Society (ENETS) classification {2716}. The staging of well-differentiated PanNENs is presented in Chapter 1 (p. 20).

Prognosis and prediction

Ki-67 proliferation index and mitotic counts of the tumour determine the grading of pancreatic gastrinoma. TNM staging is the most important prognostic factor (see *Pancreatic neuroendocrine neoplasms: Introduction*, p. 343). Approximately 60% of patients with pancreatic gastrinoma show lymph node metastases {748,260}. Liver metastasis occurs more frequently in patients with pancreatic gastrinoma than in those with duodenal gastrinoma, leading to a lower overall survival in the former {3084,260}.

VIPoma

Shi C
Kasajima A
La Rosa S

Definition
VIPoma is a functioning well-differentiated neuroendocrine neoplasm (NEN) composed of tumour cells with uncontrolled secretion of VIP, causing the syndrome of watery diarrhoea, hypokalaemia, and achlorhydria (WDHA syndrome, also called Verner–Morrison syndrome). A minority of VIPomas (typically occurring in children) are neurogenic tumours arising in the sympathetic paraganglia and adrenal glands.

ICD-O coding
8155/3 VIPoma

ICD-11 coding
2C10.1 & XH8LS0 Neuroendocrine neoplasms of pancreas & VIPoma, malignant

Related terminology
Not recommended: diarrhoeagenic tumour of the pancreas; islet cell tumour with watery diarrhoea.

Subtype(s)
None

Localization
Approximately 75–90% of VIPomas are located in the pancreas, and 10–25% outside the pancreas {3085,895}. Within the pancreas, the most common tumour location is the tail, with 70% in the body or tail and 30% in the head {3074,1030,3085}. Most of the extrapancreatic VIPomas belong to the group of neurogenic neoplasms occurring in the adrenal glands, retroperitoneum, and mediastinum, such as phaeochromocytoma, ganglioneuroma, and ganglioneuroblastoma {1702,3085}.

Clinical features
The key clinical features of WDHA syndrome are large-volume secretory diarrhoea (usually > 1 L of stool per day) that persists with fasting, hypokalaemia, hypochlorhydria/achlorhydria, and acidosis. Other common clinical presentations are weight loss, hypercalcaemia, glucose intolerance, and flushing {3085,3074,1702}. The diagnosis is confirmed by demonstrating high plasma VIP levels, usually > 80 pmol/L for the full syndrome. CT, MRI, EUS, MRI, octreoscan, and 68Ga-DOTATATE PET-CT can be used to detect primary and metastatic VIPomas {3074,1716}. The radiographical appearance is similar to that of other pancreatic neuroendocrine tumours (PanNETs).

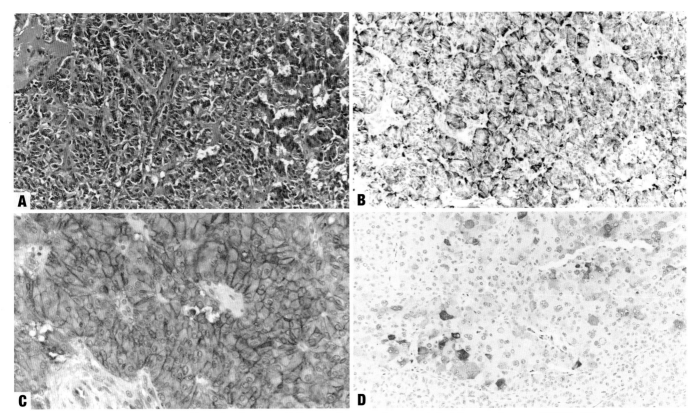

Fig. 10.55 VIPoma. **A** Tumour cells arranged in a trabecular pattern. **B** Tumour cells express chromogranin A. **C** Tumour cells express SSTR2A. **D** Tumour cells express VIP (scattered).

Chapter 10

Epidemiology

Pancreatic VIPoma is very rare, accounting for only 0.6–1.5% of all pancreatic NENs (PanNENs) {2096,1408} and approximately 2–6% of functioning tumours {1408,1558}. The incidence is 0.05–0.2 cases per 1 million person-years {895}.

Etiology

There are no known etiological factors. Approximately 10% of pancreatic VIPomas are seen in patients with multiple endocrine neoplasia type 1 {3085,3074}.

Pathogenesis

Pancreatic VIPomas originate from non-β islet cells of the pancreas that produce VIP {3468}. These tumours can produce excessive amounts of VIP, which causes intestinal secretion by activating G protein–coupled receptors on the intestinal epithelial cells, leading to watery diarrhoea and consequently dehydration and electrolyte imbalance {2733,890}.

Somatic mutations in *MEN1* are found in some sporadic pancreatic VIPomas. However, *VHL*, *PTEN*, or *SMAD4* (*DPC4*) mutations have also been found {246,257}. Chromosomal gains/losses in pancreatic VIPoma, detected by comparative genomic hybridization, are frequently aberrations of 11q, Xq, and Y {3109}. Allelic losses of 3p and 6q in the tumours, found by loss-of-heterozygosity analysis, may be involved in tumour progression {246,247}.

Macroscopic appearance

Pancreatic VIPomas are usually solitary, well circumscribed, and large (mean size: 4.5–5.3 cm) {3096,1030,3085}.

Histopathology

The histopathology of pancreatic VIPomas resembles that of other well-differentiated PanNETs. The tumour cells are arranged in a solid, trabecular, or tubuloacinar pattern {3096}. Mitoses are generally rare (< 2 mitoses/mm^2), even in tumours with metastases {3085,2096}. Most cases are either G1 or G2 {2096}. Lymphovascular and perineural invasion is common {3085}. Tumour cells express synaptophysin, chromogranin A, cytokeratin AE1/AE3, CK8/18, CK19, PDX1, and SSTR2A. In some cases, low-molecular-weight cytokeratin is expressed as perinuclear dots. In most pancreatic VIPomas, VIP-immunoreactive cells are scattered. In addition, PP is frequently expressed in tumour cells {3096}.

Cytology

The tumour cells generally have modest amounts of eosinophilic cytoplasm and bland nuclei without prominent nucleoli. Like other PanNETs, VIPomas can display focal or extensive oncocytic or clear-cell changes {3096}.

Diagnostic molecular pathology

Not clinically relevant.

Essential and desirable diagnostic criteria

Essential: clinical syndrome; neuroendocrine tumour (NET) histology.

Staging (TNM)

The staging of pancreatic VIPomas, like that of all PanNENs, follows the eighth editions (2017) of the Union for International Cancer Control (UICC) TNM classification {408} and the American Joint Committee on Cancer (AJCC) cancer staging manual {127,636}, which rely on macroscopic assessment of site, tumour size, and metastases. This approach largely corresponds to that of the European Neuroendocrine Tumor Society (ENETS) classification {2716}. The staging of well-differentiated PanNENs is presented in Chapter 1 (p. 20).

Prognosis and prediction

Tumour grade (determined by Ki-67 proliferation index and mitotic count) and tumour stage are the two main prognostic factors. Approximately 50–80% of cases present with distant metastases at diagnosis, mostly in the liver {3085,1702,3074}. Postoperative 5-year survival rates are 60% and 94%, respectively, for patients with and without metastasis {3085}.

Glucagonoma

Couvelard A
Klöppel G
Shi C

Definition
Glucagonoma is a well-differentiated functioning pancreatic neuroendocrine tumour (PanNET) composed of cells producing glucagon and preproglucagon-derived peptide, with uncontrolled glucagon secretion, causing glucagonoma syndrome. Glucagon cell hyperplasia and neoplasia (GCHN) is found in patients with inherited mutations in *GCGR* leading to hyperplasia and neoplasia of the islet glucagon cells.

ICD-O coding
8152/3 Glucagonoma

ICD-11 coding
2C10.1 & XH87C1 Neuroendocrine neoplasms of pancreas & Glucagonoma, malignant

Related terminology
Glucagonoma
None

GCHN
Acceptable: glucagon cell adenomatosis; Mahvash disease.

Subtype(s)
None

Localization
Glucagonoma predominantly involves the tail of the pancreas {3098}. GCHN affects the pancreas diffusely.

Clinical features
Diagnosis of the tumour depends on elevated glucagon levels and the typical triad of glucagonoma syndrome: skin rash (necrolytic migratory erythema), diabetes mellitus, and weight loss. The necrolytic migratory erythema is usually located in the groin and migrates to the limbs, buttocks, and peritoneum. Angular stomatitis, cheilitis, or atrophic glossitis is present in approximately 40% of patients. Other features are amino acid deficiency, normochromic normocytic anaemia, and widespread venous thrombosis with pulmonary embolism in late-stage disease. The average time from symptom onset to diagnosis is 31.4 months {3098}. Metastatic disease at initial diagnosis is common, most commonly affecting the liver, followed by lymph nodes, mesentery/peritoneum, bone, lung, and spleen {3098}.

Elevated glucagon levels without glucagonoma syndrome may be found in patients with GCHN. In these patients, upper abdominal discomfort usually leads to the detection of multiple pancreatic tumours by CT, MRI, ultrasound, octreoscan, and/or 68Ga-DOTATATE PET-CT {2767}.

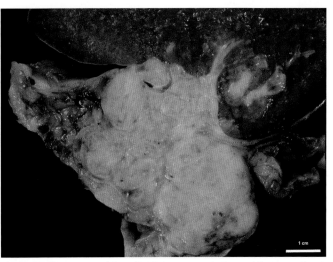

Fig. 10.56 Glucagonoma. A large (6 cm) glucagonoma in the caudal pancreas, invading the spleen.

Epidemiology
Glucagonoma accounts for 1–2% of all PanNETs and is the fourth most common functioning PanNET, after insulinoma, gastrinoma, and VIPoma {3683,1446}. Its incidence is approximatively 1 case per 20 million person-years. The average patient age at diagnosis is 52.5 years, and the reported M:F ratio is 0.8:1 {3082}.

GCHN is an extremely rare autosomal recessive disease, with only about 10 cases reported to date. Males and females are equally affected. Patient age ranges from 25 to 68 years.

Etiology
Unknown

Pathogenesis
Excessive glucagon produced by the tumour acts on the liver and increases both amino acid oxidation and gluconeogenesis from amino acid substrates, consequently causing glucagonoma syndrome.

GCHN results from *GCGR* gene mutations that probably lead to deficient receptor expression. Lack of glucagon signalling in the liver probably causes a disturbance in a presumed feedback mechanism between the liver and the glucagon cells, which in turn leads to glucagon cell hyperplasia and elevated glucagon levels.

Macroscopic appearance
Glucagonomas are usually solitary, well-demarcated tumours, varying in size from 3 to 7 cm {3551,3098}. Rarely, they are cystic {427,1680}. They occasionally infiltrate the pancreatic tissue or the spleen.

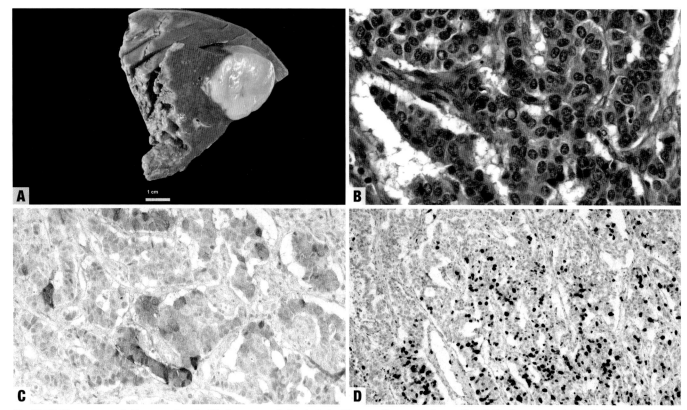

Fig. 10.57 Glucagonoma. **A** Liver resection of a G3 glucagonoma that metastasized 3 years after pancreatic resection. **B** The liver metastasis is well differentiated on HES staining. **C** The liver metastasis is well differentiated, with focal positive immunostaining for glucagon. **D** Ki-67 expression is heterogeneous, with areas of high staining; the Ki-67 proliferation index was calculated at 52%.

In GCHN, the pancreas may be diffusely involved, with multiple whitish-yellow nodules ranging in size from a few millimetres to 8 cm.

Histopathology

Glucagonomas are well-differentiated PanNETs with densely packed trabecular formations and a scant stromal reaction. Mitotic figures are rare. No poorly differentiated glucagonomas have been described, but glucagonomas may progress to G3 PanNETs. The tumour cells express synaptophysin, chromogranin A, glucagon, and often PP {3551}.

In GCHN, the pancreatic tissue shows normal-sized and hypertrophic islets (with glucagon cell hyperplasia) randomly distributed between glucagon cell microadenomas, and in some cases a single macrotumour. Calcification is often noted. All express glucagon {3066,3773}. Metastatic disease is rare {3066}.

Cytology

The cytology is the same as that of other PanNETs.

Diagnostic molecular pathology

Rarely, glucagonoma occurs in multiple endocrine neoplasia type 1 {1446,3082}. FOXA2, which plays a crucial role in islet development, is reported to be deregulated in multiple endocrine neoplasia type 1–associated glucagonomas {362}. In addition, a biallelic inactivation of *DAXX* was reported in a sporadic glucagonoma {3228}. In GCHN, about 50% of the examined patients showed germline mutations of *GCGR*, located on chromosome 17q25.3 {3066,3773}.

Essential and desirable diagnostic criteria

Essential: clinical diagnosis (see *Clinical features*, above); neuroendocrine tumour (NET) histology.

Staging (TNM)

The staging of glucagonomas, like that of all pancreatic neuroendocrine neoplasms (PanNENs), follows the eighth editions (2017) of the Union for International Cancer Control (UICC) TNM classification {408} and the American Joint Committee on Cancer (AJCC) cancer staging manual {127,636}, which rely on macroscopic assessment of site, tumour size, and metastases. This approach largely corresponds to that of the European Neuroendocrine Tumor Society (ENETS) classification {2716}. The staging of well-differentiated PanNENs is presented in Chapter 1 (p. 20).

Prognosis and prediction

The prognosis depends on grade and stage {3683,1587}. In a recent series, Ki-67 proliferation index was not found to be of prognostic relevance {1611}. Recent data show that 70% of patients survive 5 years, with a mean survival time of > 6 years {855,3551}. In another retrospective study, the average survival time was 32.1 months {3098}. Death is usually related to tumour growth rather than tumour-related functional complications {3551,1611}.

Somatostatinoma

Singhi AD
Adsay NV
Sasano H

Definition

Somatostatinoma is a functionally active, well-differentiated pancreatic neuroendocrine tumour (PanNET) that is associated with clinical manifestations of inappropriate somatostatin secretion (somatostatinoma syndrome). Tumours that demonstrate D-cell differentiation based on immunohistochemical labelling with somatostatin but lack symptoms of somatostatinoma syndrome, such as those observed within the ampulla and duodenum, should be designated as somatostatin-producing well-differentiated neuroendocrine tumours (NETs) and not considered somatostatinomas.

ICD-O coding

8156/3 Somatostatinoma

ICD-11 coding

2C10.1 & XH9Z82 Neuroendocrine neoplasms of pancreas & Somatostatinoma, malignant

Related terminology

None

Subtype(s)

None

Localization

Somatostatinomas can arise throughout the pancreas, but approximately two thirds arise within the pancreatic head {1790, 1677,3083,145,2214,487,2337}.

Clinical features

The clinical findings indicative of excess somatostatin secretion are not as dramatic or distinctive as the features of other functioning PanNETs {1790,1677,3083,145,2214,487,2337}.

The classic triad of somatostatinoma syndrome comprises diabetes / glucose intolerance, cholelithiasis, and diarrhoea/ steatorrhoea. Many patients with somatostatinomas also have gastric hypochlorhydria due to decreased gastric secretion. Somatostatinoma syndrome can be confirmed by a fasting plasma somatostatin level > 18.33 pmol/L (> 30 pg/mL). However, many of the symptoms are nonspecific and often not present at clinical presentation {1677}. Therefore, the initial diagnosis of a PanNET is usually based on imaging studies, such as CT, MRI, and EUS. Adjunct tests include somatostatin receptor scintigraphy (octreoscan) and functional PET tracers: 18F-DOPA, 11C-5-HTP, 68Ga-DOTATOC, and 68Ga-DOTA-TATE {1701}.

Epidemiology

Somatostatinomas are rare neoplasms, with an incidence of 1 case per 40 million person-years, and they account for < 1% of functioning PanNETs {2337}. The mean patient age at diagnosis is 55 years (range: 30–74 years), and it occurs more commonly in females {3083,3479}.

Etiology

The etiology and pathogenesis of pancreatic somatostatinoma are unknown. Ampullary and duodenal somatostatinomas are often associated with a history of neurofibromatosis type 1, but pancreatic somatostatinomas are rarely found in neurofibromatosis {2044}. Patients with other predisposing genetic syndromes for PanNETs, such as multiple endocrine neoplasia type 1 and von Hippel–Lindau syndrome, infrequently develop somatostatinomas {3083,1974,2020,1154}.

Pathogenesis

Unknown

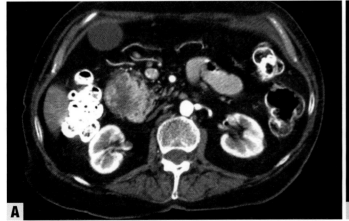
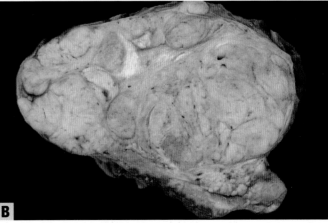

Fig. 10.58 Somatostatinoma. **A** CT of a large somatostatinoma in the pancreatic head. **B** Gross appearance of a large somatostatinoma with yellow to tan parenchyma and multinodular growth pattern.

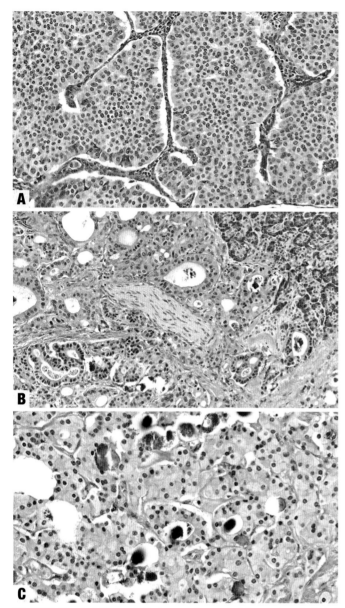

Fig. 10.59 Somatostatinoma. **A** Most pancreatic somatostatinomas have the typical appearance of other pancreatic neuroendocrine tumours (PanNETs), with trabecular, solid, and/or acinar architecture. **B,C** A subset of somatostatinomas exhibit histological features similar to those of their ampullary/duodenal analogues, with tubular and glandular architecture (**B**) and intraglandular psammomatous calcifications (**C**).

Macroscopic appearance

Pancreatic somatostatinomas are grossly indistinguishable from other PanNETs. These neoplasms are solitary, well circumscribed, and large (average diameter: 5–6 cm) {3083,3751}. On cross-section, pancreatic somatostatinomas are unencapsulated and composed of yellow to tan parenchyma. They are usually multinodular and demonstrate invasive growth into adjacent structures, such as the duodenum and spleen. Because

ampullary and duodenal somatostatinomas are considerably more common than pancreatic somatostatinomas, careful inspection of the central location of the tumour and correlation with the microscopic findings are critical.

Histopathology

A subset of pancreatic somatostatinomas exhibit histological features similar to those of ampullary/duodenal somatostatinomas, with a tubular and glandular architectural pattern and intraglandular psammomatous calcifications. However, the majority have the typical appearance of other PanNETs. The neoplastic cells are cuboidal to round, with eosinophilic cytoplasm and uniform nuclei. They are often characterized by a trabecular, solid, and/or acinar architecture. Vascular invasion and perineural invasion are frequent, but extensive necrosis is typically absent. A systematic analysis of mitotic count and Ki-67 proliferation index has not been documented for pancreatic somatostatinomas, but most cases are G2.

The tumour shows diffuse positivity for synaptophysin and somatostatin and less consistently positive or absent chromogranin A. It may also show scattered positivity for PP, calcitonin, gastrin, ACTH, glucagon, and insulin.

Cytology

The cytology is similar to that of other PanNETs {784}.

Diagnostic molecular pathology

The molecular pathology of sporadic pancreatic somatostatinomas is not well studied. There are no known genetic differences when compared with non-functioning PanNETs.

Essential and desirable diagnostic criteria

Essential: clinical diagnosis (see *Clinical features*, above) – fasting plasma somatostatin level > 18.33 pmol/L (> 30 pg/mL); NET histology.

Staging (TNM)

The staging of pancreatic somatostatinomas, like that of all pancreatic neuroendocrine neoplasms (PanNENs), follows the eighth editions (2017) of the Union for International Cancer Control (UICC) TNM classification {408} and the American Joint Committee on Cancer (AJCC) cancer staging manual {127,636}, which rely on macroscopic assessment of site, tumour size, and metastases. This approach largely corresponds to that of the European Neuroendocrine Tumor Society (ENETS) classification {2716}. The staging of well-differentiated PanNENs is presented in Chapter 1 (p. 20).

Prognosis and prediction

There is insufficient survival data for patients with pancreatic somatostatinomas. However, the 5-year overall survival rate ranges from 60–100% in patients with localized disease to 15–60% in patients with distant metastases. Large tumour size (> 3 cm) and lymph node involvement are poor prognostic markers {3083}.

ACTH-producing neuroendocrine tumour

La Rosa S
Rindi G

Definition
ACTH-producing neuroendocrine tumour (NET) is a functioning well-differentiated NET producing ACTH, resulting in Cushing syndrome.

ICD-O coding
8158/3 ACTH-producing tumour

ICD-11 coding
2C10.1 & XH7AG8 Neuroendocrine neoplasms of pancreas & ACTH-producing tumour

Related terminology
Acceptable: ectopic ACTH-producing pancreatic neuroendocrine tumour.

Subtype(s)
None

Localization
There is no site predilection.

Clinical features
The clinical symptoms encompass all manifestations of Cushing syndrome, which include weight gain, central obesity, moon face, violaceous striae, hypertension, insulin resistance, glucose hypersensitivity, overt diabetes mellitus, severe hypokalaemia, life-threatening infections, psychiatric disorders, cutaneous hyperpigmentation, osteoporosis, and fractures {1189}. Approximately 40% of patients have Zollinger–Ellison syndrome and 5% have insulinoma syndrome. These signs and symptoms may rarely be synchronous with Cushing syndrome, but they are usually metachronous, most frequently occurring before Cushing syndrome becomes overt {2045}.

Epidemiology
ACTH-producing pancreatic NETs (PanNETs) are rare and occur most frequently in young or middle-aged females (M:F ratio: 0.5:1), with about two thirds of patients being < 50 years old. They can also occur in children. No population-based information is available.

Etiology
The etiology is unknown. A few rare cases have been related to genetically transmitted syndromes, including multiple endocrine neoplasia type 1 {3178} and von Hippel–Lindau syndrome {2045}.

Pathogenesis
Unknown

Macroscopic appearance
Macroscopically, the tumour is well circumscribed and unencapsulated, with a mean diameter of 4.8 cm (range: 2.5–15 cm). The cut surface is grey to pink and usually homogeneous {2045}.

Histopathology
The neoplasms are composed of relatively uniform cuboidal cells with centrally located nuclei and eosinophilic or amphophilic granular cytoplasm, arranged in nests, trabeculae, pseudoglands, or solid sheets. Lymphovascular invasion and perineural invasion are frequently observed, whereas necrosis is unusual. No morphological feature may distinguish ACTH-producing PanNETs from other PanNETs. Most cases are of low grade, usually G2 {2045}. By immunohistochemistry, all ACTH-producing PanNETs are positive for synaptophysin and chromogranin A, as well as for ACTH and/or ACTH-related peptide hormones, including POMC, melanotropin (MSH), β-endorphin, and met-enkephalin {2442}. The expression of other diverse peptide hormones is not a rare event. All tumours associated with Zollinger–Ellison syndrome are positive for gastrin, whereas tumours associated with insulinoma syndrome are positive for insulin and/or insulin-related peptides. ACTH-producing PanNETs may be immunoreactive for KIT (CD117) and galectin 3, the clinical significance of which is unclear {2045}. ACTH-secreting PanNETs show weak expression of SSTR2A, possibly due to the downregulation of somatostatin receptors by high levels of glucocorticoids {531,731,640}. Rarely, PanNETs associated with ectopic Cushing syndrome are negative for ACTH but positive for CRH {2532}. In some PanNETs associated with Cushing syndrome, ACTH expression has been reported in recurrences or metastatic deposits, even though the primary lesion was ACTH-negative {2532,2634}.

Cytology
Not clinically relevant

Diagnostic molecular pathology
Not clinically relevant

Essential and desirable diagnostic criteria
Essential: clinical syndrome; NET histology.

Staging (TNM)
The staging of ACTH-producing PanNETs, like that of all pancreatic neuroendocrine neoplasm (PanNENs), follows the eighth editions (2017) of the Union for International Cancer Control (UICC) TNM classification {408} and the American Joint Committee on Cancer (AJCC) cancer staging manual {127,636}, which rely on macroscopic assessment of site, tumour size, and metastases. This approach largely corresponds to that of the European Neuroendocrine Tumor Society (ENETS)

Chapter 10

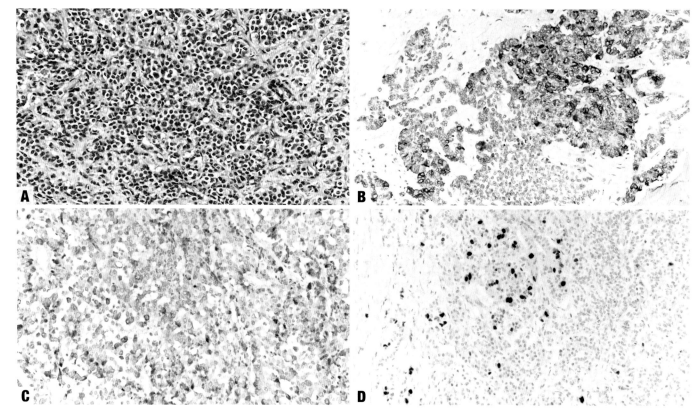

Fig. 10.60 ACTH-producing pancreatic neuroendocrine tumour (PanNET). **A** ACTH-producing PanNET showing a trabecular and nested pattern of growth. **B** Tumour cells are positive for ACTH. **C** Tumour cells are also positive for β-endorphin. **D** Most ACTH-producing PanNETs are G2, showing a Ki-67 proliferation index > 3%.

classification {2716,2716A}. The staging of well-differentiated PanNENs is presented in Chapter 1 (p. 20).

Prognosis and prediction
The prognosis depends on the grading and staging of the tumour. About 80% of patients present with metastases at the time of diagnosis or develop distant metastases during follow-up. The liver is the most frequent metastasis site, followed by lung, bones, and pelvic organs (e.g. ovaries). ACTH-producing

PanNETs are aggressive, with a median overall survival time of 30 months and a 5-year overall survival rate of 35% {2045}. Patients with both Cushing syndrome and Zollinger–Ellison syndrome appear to have poorer survival than those with Cushing syndrome only {103,2045}. In contrast, those with insulinoma syndrome or with the detection of other peptide hormones do not {2045}. Treatment usually entails surgery when feasible and multimodal therapy. Cases positive for SSTR2A may respond to somatostatin-analogue therapy {796}.

Serotonin-producing neuroendocrine tumour

Hruban RH
Sasano H
Shi C

Definition

Serotonin-producing neuroendocrine tumour (NET) is a well-differentiated pancreatic neuroendocrine neoplasm (PanNEN) composed of cells that express serotonin, which in some cases produces carcinoid syndrome, usually after metastasizing to the liver.

ICD-O coding

8241/3 Serotonin-producing tumour

ICD-11 coding

2C10.1 & XH7NM1 Neuroendocrine neoplasms of pancreas & Enterochromaffin cell carcinoid (includes serotonin-producing carcinoid)

Related terminology

Not recommended: pancreatic carcinoid.

Subtype(s)

None

Localization

There is no site predilection within the pancreas; however, ductocentric examples of non-syndromic serotonin-producing neoplasms have been reported {1751,2097}.

Clinical features

Carcinoid syndrome is usually present only when there are liver metastases, but rare cases with carcinoid syndrome without liver metastasis have been reported {3738}. Most patients with functioning tumours present with atypical carcinoid syndrome, with abdominal pain being the most common symptom (66%), followed by diarrhoea (52%), weight loss (45%), and flushing (34%) {2091}. Only one case with cardiac valve disease has been reported in the literature {1029}. The diagnosis is confirmed by demonstrating high urinary 5-HIAA excretion.

Epidemiology

Pancreatic serotonin-producing tumours are extremely rare, and those responsible for carcinoid syndrome are even rarer {3086}. Serotonin-immunoreactive tumours account for 0.58–4.1% of all pancreatic NETs (PanNETs) {1751,1587,2097,3356}. Only slightly more than 50 well-documented functioning neoplasms have been reported {1751}. They are more common in females than males. The mean ages of patients with functioning and non-functioning tumours, respectively, are 41 years and 56 years {1751}.

Etiology

There are no known etiological factors. No association with genetic syndromes has been documented.

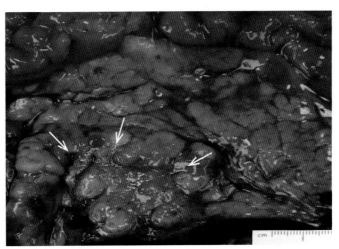

Fig. 10.61 Serotonin-producing pancreatic neuroendocrine tumour (PanNET). Gross photograph showing a well-circumscribed mass, measuring 5 cm, in the pancreatic head (arrows).

Pathogenesis

Unknown

Macroscopic appearance

Most are large (1–6 cm {1751,3086}) and do not have distinctive gross features. Functioning tumours are usually larger than non-functioning tumours (mean diameters: 5.2 cm vs 4.2 cm) {1751}. There have been reports of rare small non-syndromic serotonin-producing tumours centred on the main pancreatic duct that cause dilation of the upstream duct system, mimicking an intraductal papillary mucinous neoplasm {1543,3506}.

Histopathology

Most serotonin-producing tumours are well differentiated, G1 or G2 with rare mitosis; very exceptional cases of poorly differentiated neoplasms have been reported {1751}. However, vascular, perineural, and adjacent organ/structural invasion is frequent, with rare tumour necrosis. Serotonin-producing PanNETs usually do not resemble their intestinal counterparts. The neoplastic cells are frequently arranged in a trabecular pattern and less frequently in solid nests, with variable amounts of stroma {1751,2097}. The stroma is prominent in ductocentric tumours {2097}. Phenotypically and ultrastructurally, neoplastic cells resemble gastric-type and not intestinal-type enterochromaffin cells (EC cells): unlike their intestinal counterparts, they rarely express substance P, aFGF, VMAT1, and CDX2, but they usually express serotonin and VMAT2 {1751}. SSTR2A is usually detectable by immunohistochemistry {1751}.

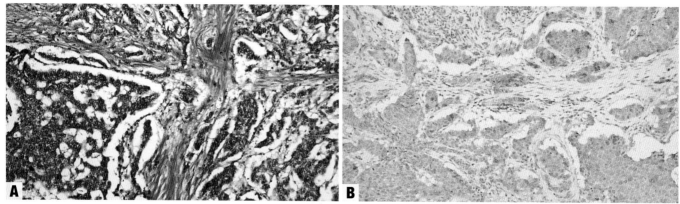

Fig. 10.62 Serotonin-producing pancreatic neuroendocrine tumour (PanNET). **A** NET histology in a sclerotic background. Many cases are even more sclerotic than this example. **B** Immunolabelling of the same case for serotonin.

Cytology

The cytology is not different from that of typical PanNET. The neoplastic cells contain finely granular cytoplasm and monomorphic round nuclei.

Diagnostic molecular pathology

The only genetic alterations described to date are monosomy and rearrangements of chromosome 18 {1751}.

Essential and desirable diagnostic criteria

Essential: clinical syndrome; NET histology.

Staging (TNM)

The staging of serotonin-producing NETs, like that of all PanNENs, follows the eighth editions (2017) of the Union for International Cancer Control (UICC) TNM classification {408} and the American Joint Committee on Cancer (AJCC) cancer staging manual {127,636}, which rely on macroscopic assessment of site, tumour size, and metastases. This approach largely corresponds to that of the European Neuroendocrine Tumor Society (ENETS) classification {2716}. The staging of well-differentiated PanNENs is presented in Chapter 1 (p. 20).

Prognosis and prediction

Serotonin-producing tumours do not differ substantially from non-functioning PanNENs in terms of size, Ki-67 proliferation index, or distant metastases {2097}. Functioning tumours are associated with a poorer prognosis than non-functioning ones, because they are almost always metastatic {1751}.

Pancreatic neuroendocrine carcinoma

Adsay NV
Perren A
Singhi AD

Definition
Pancreatic neuroendocrine carcinoma (PanNEC) is a high-grade malignant epithelial neoplasm with neuroendocrine differentiation.

ICD-O coding
8246/3 Neuroendocrine carcinoma NOS

ICD-11 coding
2C10.1 & XH0U20 Neuroendocrine neoplasms of pancreas & Neuroendocrine carcinoma NOS
2C10.1 & XH9SY0 Neuroendocrine neoplasms of pancreas & Small cell neuroendocrine carcinoma
2C10.1 & XH0NL5 Neuroendocrine neoplasms of pancreas & Large cell neuroendocrine carcinoma

Related terminology
Acceptable: high-grade (poorly differentiated) neuroendocrine carcinoma {271,272,3104}; small cell carcinoma; small cell undifferentiated carcinoma {1207,3632,2684}.

Subtype(s)
Large cell neuroendocrine carcinoma (8013/3); small cell neuroendocrine carcinoma (8041/3)

Localization
PanNECs show a mild predilection for occurring in the head of the pancreas, with a 2:1 ratio {271}.

Clinical features
The presentation of PanNECs is similar to that of pancreatic ductal adenocarcinomas (PDACs) {1616,271,272,1207}, including back pain, jaundice, and/or nonspecific abdominal symptoms {1862,3104}. Serum hormone activity is very unusual {677}, and increased serum chromogranin does not seem to be a feature. Calcitonin may be elevated in some patients {3377}. Serum CA19-9 levels may also be high. The vast majority (> 90%) of patients present with metastasis at the time of diagnosis. Somatostatin receptor scintigraphy is often negative due to lack of expression of SSTR2 and SSTR5, and this may be a helpful criterion to distinguish PanNECs from well-differentiated pancreatic neuroendocrine tumours (PanNETs) clinically.

Epidemiology
PanNECs are rare, accounting for < 1% of all pancreatic tumours and no more than 2–3% of PanNETs {2700,272,1146,2354}. They seem to be slightly more common in males. They mostly occur in patients aged 50–60 years {271,272,1207,3104}, but they can occur in younger patients as well.

Etiology
Similar to their counterparts in other organs, PanNECs show an association with cigarette smoking {598}, although this requires further confirmation.

Pathogenesis
Syndromes that are associated with well-differentiated neuroendocrine tumours (NETs), such as multiple endocrine neoplasia type 1 and von Hippel–Lindau syndrome, do not seem to be involved in PanNECs. A case with BRCA1 mutation was noted in a study of 44 PanNECs {271}, a frequency similar to that seen in PDACs.

Specific genetic alterations common in well-differentiated NETs (alterations in MEN1, ATRX, DAXX) or PDAC (alterations in KRAS, SMAD4) {3632} are not features of PanNEC {277,2558}. Instead, PanNECs seem to be characterized by the presence of mutations of TP53 and inactivation of the RB1/p16 pathway determined by either mutations in RB1 or loss of expression of p16 {3632,1047}. The role of epigenetic and microRNA expression modifications {1116,2748} or increased CDK4 or CDK6 {3254} identified in NETs has yet to be determined for PanNECs.

Macroscopic appearance
PanNECs present as relatively large (mean size: 4 cm; largest reported size: 18 cm), solid, compact tumours that are typically more fleshy than ordinary PDACs. They tend to be whitish-grey or tan-red to yellowish, and they often exhibit vague nodularity {271}. They tend to appear more demarcated than PDACs. Haemorrhage is common, and necrosis is often visible.

Histopathology
Histologically, PanNECs are defined similarly to their counterparts in other organs, particularly their pulmonary counterparts {271,2684,272,3153}. Poorly differentiated NECs of small cell type are characterized by diffuse sheets of cells with scant cytoplasm, round or elongated nuclei (some with moulding), and finely granular chromatin with inconspicuous nucleoli. The large cell subtype, which is more common (60%) {271,272}, shows a nesting/trabecular pattern, with relatively uniform round to polygonal cells having amphophilic cytoplasm, large nuclei, vesicular chromatin, and in some cases prominent nucleoli. Necrosis with peritheliomatous preservation of cells can be seen {271}. Mitoses are easily identified, typically multiple in each high-power field. The Ki-67 proliferation index is by definition > 20%, in the vast majority of cases > 50%, and commonly > 60–80% {271,272,3104}.

Neuroendocrine carcinomas (NECs) can be associated with other (non-neuroendocrine) carcinoma types, in particular ductal adenocarcinoma or acinar cell carcinoma. When each component accounts for ≥ 30% of the tumour area, the term "mixed neuroendocrine–non-neuroendocrine carcinoma (MiNEC)" is applicable; however, in reporting such cases, it is advisable to emphasize the NEC component, because these mixed cases behave very similarly to pure NECs {271}.

NEC is defined by morphology {271,272,3153,2684}, but it is important to establish the neuroendocrine differentiation in these poorly differentiated malignant neoplasms. Synaptophysin is the most sensitive marker. However, other neoplasms (including acinar and solid pseudopapillary neoplasms) can also express synaptophysin. Chromogranin is a highly specific marker, but its sensitivity is relatively low, and its expression can be especially faint in small cell carcinomas where the cytoplasm is less abundant and contains fewer granules {2984}. CD56 by itself is not conclusive, due to its low specificity. Moreover, the expression of all these markers is often focal in distribution {271}; conversely, focal/scattered neuroendocrine differentiation is not uncommon in some non-neuroendocrine neoplasms. In rare cases, small cell PanNEC may be diagnosed in the absence of synaptophysin/chromogranin staining {271}.

Acinar cell carcinomas are often mistaken for NECs due to their characteristically monotonous appearance, high-grade nature, and common expression of neuroendocrine markers (at least focally). In one study {271}, 15% of cases originally classified as NEC proved to be acinar carcinomas on further analysis (see *Pancreatic acinar cell carcinoma*, p. 333).

NEC should be differentiated from lymphoma and melanoma by negative lymphoid and melanoma markers. Metastatic carcinoma to the pancreas should be excluded and requires clinical correlation {29}. Immunohistochemical analysis may

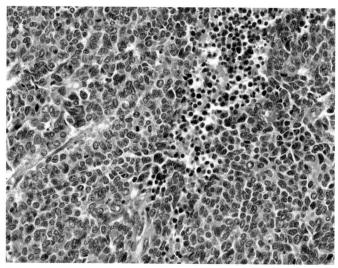

Fig. 10.64 Pancreatic neuroendocrine carcinoma (PanNEC; poorly differentiated neuroendocrine neoplasm [NEN]), small cell type. The cells have high-grade cytology, with minimal cytoplasm and a high N:C ratio. Mitotic activity is brisk, and necrosis is readily evident.

not be helpful in this regard, given the ubiquitous expression of otherwise organ-specific transcription factors, such as TTF1, CDX2, and insulin gene enhancer protein ISL1 or PDX1, which are commonly seen in small cell carcinomas of any location {3471,45}. Loss of SMAD4 may be of some value but requires

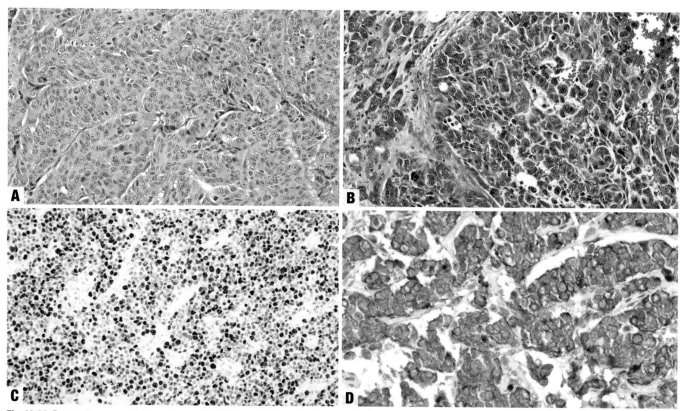

Fig. 10.63 Pancreatic neuroendocrine carcinoma (PanNEC; poorly differentiated neuroendocrine neoplasm [NEN]), large cell type. **A** Diffuse growth of relatively monotonous cells with a nested/organoid pattern compartmentalized by delicate vasculature, indicating neuroendocrine differentiation, which was confirmed by synaptophysin staining. Cytological atypia and prominent mitotic activity indicate the high-grade (poorly differentiated) nature of this carcinoma. **B** Large nuclei with prominent nucleoli and moderate cytoplasm. **C** Ki-67 immunostaining shows diffuse nuclear labelling, with a Ki-67 proliferation index > 80%. **D** Synaptophysin staining shows diffuse labelling with focal, punctate positivity in rare cells.

further investigation. Similarly, immunohistochemical staining is also helpful in small blue cell tumours of young adulthood, which can occur in the pancreas and mimic NEC {2236,339}.

The Ki-67 proliferation index is typically very high in NECs (commonly > 60–80%). In a tumour with a low Ki-67 proliferation index (< 40%), other possibilities must be considered more carefully {272}.

Cytology

The cytological characteristics of small cell and large cell Pan-NECs are similar to those of NECs in other organs {2681,2906}. Often, the high-grade malignant nature of the process is readily evident, with necrotic material and mitotic figures easily identified. The carcinomas should be differentiated from other malignancies, including lymphomas, melanomas, and other carcinomas. Their distinction from well-differentiated NETs can be challenging; immunohistochemical studies on cell blocks may be helpful {3042}. Proliferation index analysis may also serve as an adjunct {984}.

Diagnostic molecular pathology

Not clinically relevant

Essential and desirable diagnostic criteria

Essential: a poorly differentiated neoplasm of small or large cells, with vague neuroendocrine features; usually weak expression of neuroendocrine markers; mitotic count of > 20 mitoses/2 mm² and Ki-67 proliferation index > 20%.
Desirable: Ki-67 proliferation index > 50%.

Staging (TNM)

The pathological staging of PanNECs is based on the eighth edition (2017) of the Union for International Cancer Control (UICC) TNM classification {408} for carcinomas of the exocrine pancreas, rather than the staging for better-differentiated NETs (PanNETs).

Prognosis and prediction

PanNECs are highly aggressive malignant neoplasms {271,2906,272}. Metastasis is present in the vast majority of patients at the time of diagnosis {1207,1862,3104}. Even in resected cases and with platinum-based therapy, the median survival time is very short (< 1 year), and < 25% of patients survive beyond 2 years. The survival of patients with large cell PanNECs seems to be only very slightly better than for the small cell subtype. In addition, PanNECs with other carcinoma components (such as ductal adenocarcinoma) appear to behave aggressively, emphasizing the importance of recognition of the PanNEC component in such cases.

In terms of molecular targets for therapy, the current literature suggests that PanNECs may not be good candidates for somatostatin-receptor analogues, whereas there is emerging evidence that, similar to NECs of other sites, pancreatic primaries may warrant platinum-based therapy instead {3104,272}. One potential target that may be worth further investigation is the mTOR pathway {3104,1013,3004}, and some efficacy of the mTOR inhibitor everolimus has been shown {528,358,2177}.

Pancreatic MiNENs

La Rosa S
Klimstra DS

Definition
Pancreatic mixed neuroendocrine–non-neuroendocrine neoplasms (MiNENs) are neoplasms composed of morphologically recognizable neuroendocrine and non-neuroendocrine components, each constituting ≥ 30% of the tumour volume. Poorly differentiated neuroendocrine components should display immunoreactivity for specific neuroendocrine markers (synaptophysin or chromogranin). MiNENs include a range of specific diagnostic entities in the pancreas.

ICD-O coding
8154/3 Mixed neuroendocrine–non-neuroendocrine neoplasm (MiNEN)

ICD-11 coding
2C10.1 & XH6H10 Neuroendocrine neoplasms of pancreas & Mixed adenoneuroendocrine carcinoma

Related terminology
Acceptable: mixed adenoneuroendocrine carcinoma.

Subtype(s)
Mixed acinar-endocrine carcinoma (8154/3); mixed acinar-neuroendocrine carcinoma (8154/3); mixed acinar-endocrine-ductal carcinoma (8154/3)

Localization
Pancreatic MiNENs can arise anywhere in the pancreas, although mixed ductal-neuroendocrine carcinomas are more frequently located in the pancreatic head.

Clinical features
The symptoms are usually nonspecific and related to tumour growth and/or metastatic dissemination. One patient with mixed ductal-neuroendocrine carcinoma presenting with Zollinger–Ellison syndrome has been reported {3270}.

Epidemiology
Mixed ductal-neuroendocrine carcinomas account for about 0.5–2% of all ductal adenocarcinomas {1650,2422}. About 18% of poorly differentiated neuroendocrine carcinomas (NECs) have components of adenocarcinoma {271}. There is no sex predilection. The average patient age at presentation is 68 years (range: 21–84 years).

Mixed acinar-neuroendocrine carcinomas are rare and account for 15–20% of all acinar cell carcinomas {1632,1748}. Both carcinomas have a similar age distribution. However, a male predominance is noted only in acinar cell carcinoma and not the mixed carcinomas {1632,1748,2424}. Mixed acinar-neuroendocrine carcinomas rarely display morphologically distinguishable acinar and neuroendocrine components {1632}.

Etiology
Unknown

Pathogenesis
Limited molecular investigations have been performed, but the available evidence points to clonal selection within cells capable of giving rise to cells with glandular or neuroendocrine differentiation. These tumours may therefore represent a subtype of adenocarcinoma, but their unique characteristics warrant separate classification at present. Collision tumours may also occur and can theoretically result in similar appearances.

For mixed ductal-neuroendocrine carcinoma, no definitive molecular data are yet available, and no association with genetic syndromes has been documented. The genetic alterations in these tumours may be extrapolated from information about ordinary ductal carcinomas and neuroendocrine neoplasms

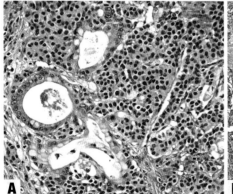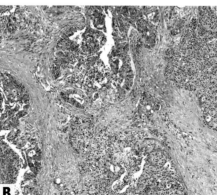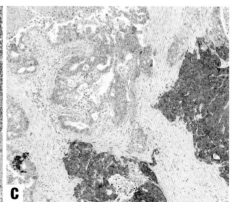

Fig. 10.65 Mixed ductal-neuroendocrine carcinoma. **A** The ductal component (left) is intimately admixed with the neuroendocrine component (right). **B** PAS staining shows tumour tissue composed of a ductal adenocarcinoma component and neuroendocrine carcinoma (NEC) of the large cell type. **C** In the same tumour tissue, immunostaining for synaptophysin reveals the neuroendocrine component.

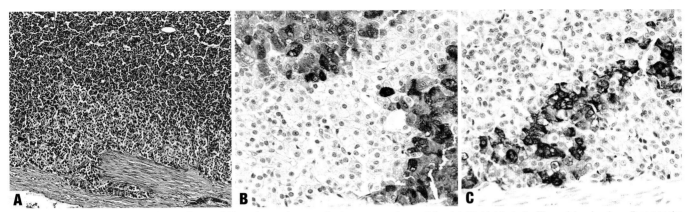

Fig. 10.66 Mixed acinar-neuroendocrine carcinoma. **A** The acinar and neuroendocrine components are distinguishable histologically. The peripheral region adjacent to the fibrous pseudocapsule is composed of a band of neuroendocrine cells, whereas the central portion is acinar. **B** The acinar component is positive for trypsin. **C** The neuroendocrine component is positive for chromogranin.

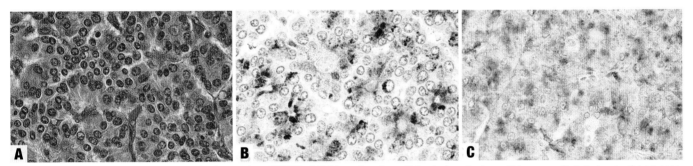

Fig. 10.67 Mixed neuroendocrine–non-neuroendocrine neoplasm (MiNEN). **A** Solid growth pattern with focal acinar structures. **B** Immunopositivity for trypsin. **C** Immunopositivity for synaptophysin.

(NENs) and include a variety of somatic mutations involving *KRAS*, *CDKN2A* (*P16*), *TP53*, and *SMAD4* (*DPC4*) for the ductal adenocarcinoma component and *TP53* and *RB1* for the NEC component. Data from gastrointestinal mixed adenoneuroendocrine carcinomas (MANECs) suggest a monoclonal origin of the two components. However, this has not been tested in pancreatic mixed ductal-neuroendocrine carcinoma.

For mixed acinar-neuroendocrine carcinoma, no association with genetic syndromes has been documented. The tumours seem to share the genetic changes of acinar cell carcinomas, including APC/β-catenin pathway alterations and *BRAF* fusions {987,616}. Mutations found in pancreatic neuroendocrine tumours (PanNETs), such as *DAXX*, *ATRX*, and *MEN1* mutations, are not typically observed. *MYC* amplification may be a mechanism involved in the neuroendocrine differentiation of acinar cell carcinomas {1750}.

Macroscopic appearance

Mixed ductal-neuroendocrine carcinomas are solid tumours measuring 2–10 cm in diameter. Mixed acinar-neuroendocrine carcinomas are large (4–8 cm) nodular neoplasms with a fleshy, focally necrotic cut surface.

Histopathology

In some mixed ductal-neuroendocrine carcinomas, the two components are intermingled and characterized by neoplastic ductal and neuroendocrine cells forming glandular, cribriform, solid, and/or trabecular structures. In other cases, the two

components are distinct and consist of a ductal adenocarcinoma usually combined with a NEC. In very rare cases, the neuroendocrine component is well differentiated, although it is possible that such cases in fact represent collision tumours, in which the two components are not clonally related. The ductal adenocarcinoma component is positive for CEA, EMA (MUC1), and/or MUC2, and the neuroendocrine component is positive for synaptophysin and chromogranin A. Mixed ductal-neuroendocrine carcinomas must be distinguished from ductal adenocarcinomas with entrapped islets, which can be intimately attached to well-differentiated neoplastic glands. Conversely, mixed ductal-neuroendocrine carcinomas must be distinguished from PanNETs with entrapped ductules, which are biologically similar to other PanNETs.

Most mixed acinar-neuroendocrine carcinomas resemble pure acinar cell carcinomas, with the neuroendocrine differentiation only demonstrated using immunohistochemistry. Such cases do not fit the definition of MiNEN and are discussed in the *Pancreatic acinar cell carcinoma* section (p. 333). A few mixed acinar-neuroendocrine carcinomas show histologically separate acinar and neuroendocrine components, which form closely connected sheets and nests. In such cases, the neuroendocrine component can be graded. Immunohistochemistry for acinar and neuroendocrine cell markers demonstrates distinct compartments in the tumour tissue. Carcinomas with only scattered neuroendocrine cells (< 30% of the tumour cells) do not qualify as mixed carcinomas and should be diagnosed as acinar cell carcinoma with a neuroendocrine component.

Cytology

Not clinically relevant

Diagnostic molecular pathology

Diagnostic molecular pathology is not yet required for diagnosis. However, molecular investigation may be helpful in distinguishing the components of these tumours in small biopsies.

Essential and desirable diagnostic criteria

Essential: a mixed tumour composed of at least two components; ≥ 30% of the neoplasm should be composed of each type; the neuroendocrine component must be substantiated by immunohistochemistry.

Desirable: usually composed of carcinomas but occasionally includes a well-differentiated neuroendocrine tumour (NET).

Staging (TNM)

Pancreatic MiNENs are staged using the Union for International Cancer Control (UICC) or American Joint Committee on Cancer (AJCC) staging system for pancreatic carcinoma.

Prognosis and prediction

Mixed ductal-neuroendocrine carcinomas usually metastasize to lymph nodes and liver. Resectability of the carcinoma is the most important prognostic factor. Patients rarely survive > 3 years. The 2-year and 5-year survival rates are 25% and 0%, respectively. However, the few prognostic data available seem to suggest that mixed ductal-neuroendocrine carcinomas have a slightly longer median survival time than pure NECs (20 months vs 12 months) {271}.

After surgery, patients with mixed acinar-neuroendocrine carcinomas show the same 5-year survival rate (30–50%) as patients with pure acinar cell carcinomas.

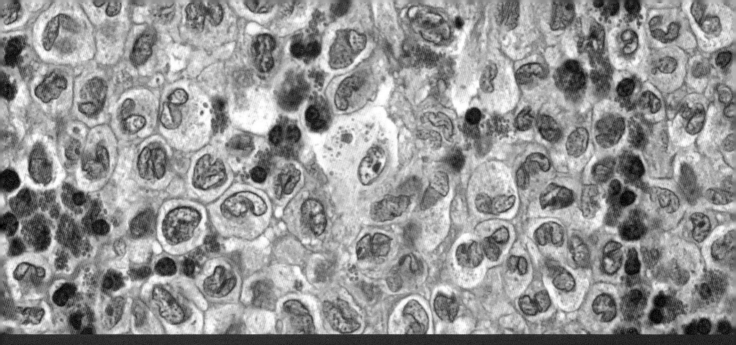

11

Haematolymphoid tumours of the digestive system

Edited by: Chan JKC, Fukayama M

Site-specific haematolymphoid tumours
  MALT lymphoma
  Duodenal-type follicular lymphoma
  Enteropathy-associated T-cell lymphoma
  Monomorphic epitheliotropic intestinal T-cell
    lymphoma
  Intestinal T-cell lymphoma NOS
  Indolent T-cell lymphoproliferative disorder of the
    GI tract
  Hepatosplenic T-cell lymphoma
  EBV+ inflammatory follicular dendritic cell
    sarcoma

Haematolymphoid tumours occurring with some
    frequency in the digestive system
  Diffuse large B-cell lymphoma
  Follicular lymphoma
  Mantle cell lymphoma
  Burkitt lymphoma
  Plasmablastic lymphoma
  Posttransplant lymphoproliferative disorders
  Extranodal NK/T-cell lymphoma
  Systemic mastocytosis
  Langerhans cell histiocytosis
  Follicular dendritic cell sarcoma
  Histiocytic sarcoma

WHO classification of haematolymphoid tumours of the digestive system

Site-specific haematolymphoid tumours

9699/3	MALT lymphoma
9764/3	Immunoproliferative small intestinal disease
9695/3	Follicular lymphoma, duodenal type
9717/3	Enteropathy-associated T-cell lymphoma
9717/3	Monomorphic epitheliotropic intestinal T-cell lymphoma
9717/3	Intestinal T-cell lymphoma
9702/1	Indolent T-cell lymphoproliferative disorder of the gastrointestinal tract
9716/3	Hepatosplenic T-cell lymphoma
9758/3	Follicular dendritic cell sarcoma

Haematolymphoid tumours occurring with some frequency in the digestive system

9680/3	Diffuse large B-cell lymphoma NOS
9690/3	Follicular lymphoma NOS
9695/3	Follicular lymphoma, grade 1
9691/3	Follicular lymphoma, grade 2
9698/3	Follicular lymphoma, grade 3A
9698/3	Follicular lymphoma, grade 3B
9673/3	Mantle cell lymphoma
	Conventional mantle cell lymphoma
	Leukaemic non-nodal mantle cell lymphoma
9687/3	Burkitt lymphoma NOS
	Endemic Burkitt lymphoma
	Sporadic Burkitt lymphoma
	Immunodeficiency-associated Burkitt lymphoma
9735/3	Plasmablastic lymphoma
9971/1	Posttransplant lymphoproliferative disorder NOS
	Non-destructive posttransplant lymphoproliferative disorder
	Polymorphic posttransplant lymphoproliferative disorder
	Monomorphic posttransplant lymphoproliferative disorder
	Classic Hodgkin lymphoma posttransplant lymphoproliferative disorder
	Mucocutaneous ulcer posttransplant lymphoproliferative disorder
9719/3	Extranodal NK/T-cell lymphoma, nasal type
9740/3	Mast cell sarcoma
9741/1	Indolent systemic mastocytosis
9741/3	Aggressive systemic mastocytosis
9741/3	Systemic mastocytosis with associated haematological clonal non-mast cell disorder
9742/3	Mast cell leukaemia
9751/1	Langerhans cell histiocytosis NOS
9751/3	Langerhans cell histiocytosis, disseminated
9758/3	Follicular dendritic cell sarcoma
9755/3	Histiocytic sarcoma

These morphology codes are from the International Classification of Diseases for Oncology, third edition, second revision (ICD-O-3.2) {1378A}. Behaviour is coded /0 for benign tumours; /1 for unspecified, borderline, or uncertain behaviour; /2 for carcinoma in situ and grade III intraepithelial neoplasia; /3 for malignant tumours, primary site; and /6 for malignant tumours, metastatic site. Behaviour code /6 is not generally used by cancer registries.

This classification is modified from the previous WHO classification, taking into account changes in our understanding of these lesions.

Haematolymphoid tumours of the digestive system: Introduction

Chan JKC
Fukayama M

Various types of haematolymphoid tumours, in particular lymphomas, occur in the digestive system with variable frequencies, either as primary disease or as part of systemic involvement. Primary lymphoma of the digestive system, if strictly defined, refers to an extranodal lymphoma arising in a specific site of the digestive system, with the bulk of disease localized to the site, with or without regional lymph node involvement. However, less stringent inclusion criteria are commonly used, allowing for contiguous involvement of other organs and for distant nodal disease, provided that the extranodal tumour is the presenting site and constitutes the predominant disease. Therefore, results reported in different studies are not necessarily comparable, due to the use of different inclusion criteria.

Although the frequencies and spectrum of haematolymphoid tumours differ in the various anatomical sites of the digestive system, the same haematolymphoid tumour type can occur in different anatomical sites. To avoid repetition, all gastrointestinal haematolymphoid tumours are covered in this chapter. Details are also available in the 2017 *WHO classification of tumours* *of haematopoietic and lymphoid tissues* (revised fourth edition) {3189}.

Lymphoid neoplasms (but not the histiocytic/dendritic cell neoplasms) are staged according to the Lugano classification, which has been adopted by the eighth edition of the Union for International Cancer Control (UICC) TNM classification {596}.

Gastrointestinal (GI) tract

The GI tract is the most common site for occurrence of extranodal lymphomas, accounting for 30–40% of all extranodal lymphomas {968,2466,2467}. The most commonly involved site is the stomach (50–60%), followed by the small intestine (30%) and large intestine (10%); in the Middle East, a higher percentage of lymphomas occur in the small intestine {696,1664,1398, 1895,704}. The various types of primary lymphomas of the GI tract are listed in Table 11.01. Histiocytic/dendritic cell tumours {763,1277,1239,1258}, myeloid sarcoma, and mastocytosis {2237,1829} can also occur in the GI tract.

Table 11.01 Primary haematolymphoid neoplasms of the digestive tract

Neoplasm	Most common sites of involvement in the digestive tract
B-cell lymphomas	
Diffuse large B-cell lymphoma	Stomach, ileocaecal region
Extranodal marginal zone lymphoma, including immunoproliferative small intestinal disease	Stomach, small intestine
Follicular lymphoma	Small intestine, large intestine
Duodenal-type follicular lymphoma	Duodenum
Mantle cell lymphoma	Any site of the GI tract
Burkitt lymphoma	Ileocaecal region, stomach, small intestine
Plasmablastic lymphoma	Anorectum, other parts of the GI tract
Posttransplant lymphoproliferative disorder	Any site of the GI tract
T-cell and NK-cell lymphomas	
Enteropathy-associated T-cell lymphoma	Small intestine
Monomorphic epitheliotropic intestinal T-cell lymphoma	Small intestine
Intestinal T-cell lymphoma NOS	Large intestine, small intestine
Indolent T-cell lymphoproliferative disorder of the GI tract	Small intestine, large intestine
Extranodal NK/T-cell lymphoma, nasal-type	Small intestine, large intestine
Others	
EBV+ inflammatory follicular dendritic cell sarcoma	Liver
Systemic mastocytosis	GI tract, liver
Langerhans cell histiocytosis	GI tract, liver
Follicular dendritic cell sarcoma	GI tract, pancreas, liver
Histiocytic sarcoma	GI tract

Primary lymphomas of the oesophagus are rare, accounting for 0.2% of extranodal lymphomas and < 1% of all oesophageal tumours {968,1120}. Involvement of the oesophagus by lymphoma from elsewhere is more common, including direct extension from adjacent structures such as the mediastinum and stomach, or spread from distant sites. The most frequent types of primary oesophageal lymphomas are diffuse large B-cell lymphoma (DLBCL) and extranodal marginal zone lymphoma.

In the stomach, DLBCL and extranodal marginal zone lymphoma account for the majority of cases.

In the small intestine, the ileum and ileocaecal region are the most commonly affected. DLBCL is the most common type of lymphoma, and the frequencies of other types of lymphomas vary depending on series and ethnic background.

In the large intestine, the most common type of lymphoma is DLBCL (> 50%), followed by extranodal marginal zone lymphoma, follicular lymphoma, mantle cell lymphoma, and Burkitt lymphoma. The incidence of large intestinal lymphoma has increased over the years, attributable to acquired or iatrogenic immunodeficiency {1127}.

Liver

Although the liver is frequently involved in advanced-stage lymphoma of any type, primary lymphoma of the liver is very rare, accounting for only 0.4% of extranodal lymphomas {968,851}.

Primary hepatic lymphoma shows a strong association with viral infection and immunological disorders {159,386,2833}, such as chronic hepatitis (HBV, HCV) {274,413,2444}, immunodeficiency (HIV, posttransplant and iatrogenic immunosuppression) {274,1924,2314}, and autoimmune disease (e.g. Felty syndrome, systemic lupus erythematosus, autoimmune cytopenia, and primary biliary cirrhosis) {832,1572}.

The most common types of primary hepatic lymphomas are DLBCL and extranodal marginal zone lymphoma. Hepatosplenic T-cell lymphoma typically involves the liver as part of systemic disease.

The liver is a characteristic primary site for the occurrence of EBV-positive inflammatory follicular dendritic cell sarcoma, previously known as inflammatory pseudotumour-like follicular/fibroblastic dendritic cell sarcoma {602}. Histiocytic sarcoma and myeloid sarcoma can uncommonly affect the liver {602, 1159,1707,2389}. Systemic mastocytosis commonly shows liver involvement.

Pancreas, gallbladder, and extrahepatic bile ducts

Primary lymphomas of the pancreas, gallbladder, and extrahepatic bile ducts are very rare. The most common types are DLBCL and extranodal marginal zone lymphoma {2176}.

Dendritic cell sarcoma has rarely been reported in the pancreas {1896,2981}. Myeloid sarcoma may rarely affect the pancreatobiliary tract {2389}.

Extranodal marginal zone lymphoma of mucosa-associated lymphoid tissue (MALT lymphoma) involving the digestive tract

Nakamura S
Delabie J

Definition

Extranodal marginal zone lymphoma of mucosa-associated lymphoid tissue (MALT lymphoma) involving the digestive tract is an extranodal low-grade B-cell lymphoma arising in mucosal or glandular tissues, recapitulating the cytoarchitectural features of mucosa-associated lymphoid tissue (MALT). It is composed of small lymphoid cells, often including marginal zone cells.

ICD-O coding

9699/3 Extranodal marginal zone lymphoma of mucosa-associated lymphoid tissue (MALT lymphoma)

ICD-11 coding

2A85.1 Extranodal marginal zone B-cell lymphoma of mucosa-associated lymphoid tissue of stomach
2A85.3 Extranodal marginal zone B-cell lymphoma, primary site excluding stomach or skin

Related terminology

None

Subtype(s)

Immunoproliferative small intestinal disease (9764/3)

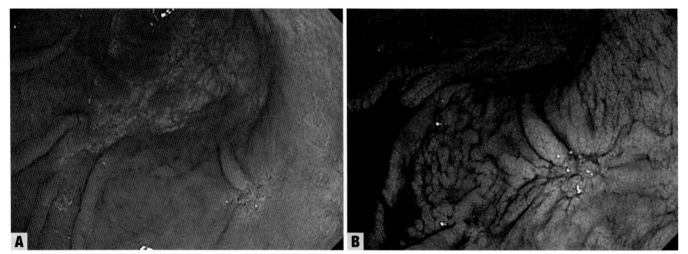

Fig. 11.01 Gastric extranodal marginal zone lymphoma of mucosa-associated lymphoid tissue (MALT lymphoma) with *Helicobacter pylori* infection without t(11;18)/*BIRC3-MALT1*. **A** The tumour regressed after *H. pylori* eradication. Endoscopy reveals a superficially depressed lesion. **B** The spraying of indigo carmine highlights the depressed lesion.

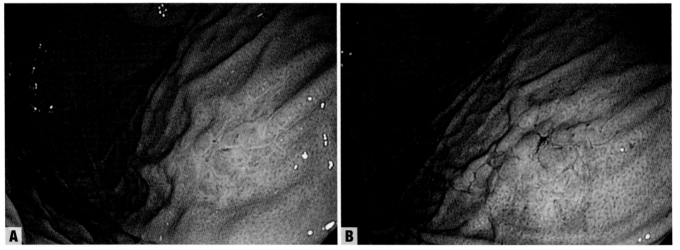

Fig. 11.02 Gastric extranodal marginal zone lymphoma of mucosa-associated lymphoid tissue (MALT lymphoma) with t(11;18)/*BIRC3-MALT1* and without *Helicobacter pylori* infection. **A** Endoscopy reveals a superficial lesion with small nodules mimicking cobblestones. **B** The spraying of indigo carmine highlights the cobblestone lesion.

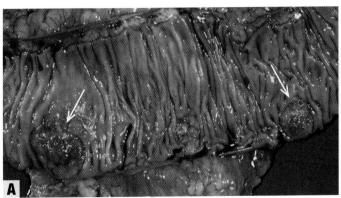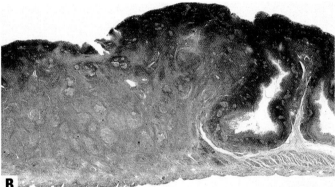

Fig. 11.03 Colonic extranodal marginal zone lymphoma of mucosa-associated lymphoid tissue (MALT lymphoma) with t(11;18)/*BIRC3-MALT1*. **A** Multiple lesions are evident (arrows). **B** The lymphomatous infiltrate extends into the muscularis propria.

Localization

Primary MALT lymphoma may occur at any site in the digestive system, including the GI tract, liver, and pancreatobiliary tract {666,3788}. Immunoproliferative small intestinal disease (IPSID), also called α-heavy chain disease (αHCD), involves the GI tract (mainly the small intestine) and mesenteric lymph nodes.

Clinical features

Patients with MALT lymphoma present with site-related or non-specific symptoms, although some can be asymptomatic {666, 3788}. Endoscopically, MALT lymphoma of the GI tract appears as superficial spreading and mass-forming lesions {2285}. It is often multifocal within the involved organ.

Epidemiology

MALT lymphoma accounts for 7–8% of all B-cell lymphomas {3286}, 30–60% of primary gastric lymphomas, and 2–28% of primary intestinal lymphomas {795,2633,957,2909}. IPSID/αHCD predominantly occurs in young adults, with a geographical restriction to the Middle East, Africa, and eastern Asia. Primary MALT lymphomas of oesophagus {2221,1987}, liver {3147,801}, biliary tract {2039,1262}, and pancreas {3289} are very rare.

Most patients are adults, with a median age in the sixth decade of life. Men and women are about equally affected {3286, 1559,3788}.

Etiology

The best-studied association involves *Helicobacter pylori* and gastric MALT lymphoma, with the bacterium present in as many as 90% of cases {3609,3291,931}. The proliferation of lymphoma cells in *H. pylori*–infected patients depends on the presence of T cells specifically activated by *H. pylori* antigens {1344}. The importance of this stimulation in vivo has been clearly demonstrated by the induction of remission in MALT lymphomas with *H. pylori* eradication {3608}. Recent studies suggest that the incidence of gastric MALT lymphoma is decreasing and that only 32% of cases are now associated with *H. pylori*, as a result of effective therapy {1960,2950}. A similar role has been suggested for *Campylobacter* infection in IPSID/αHCD {3291}.

There are variations in the role of chronic inflammation and type of recurrent genetic alterations in the various anatomical sites (see Table 11.02).

Table 11.02 Summary of the main characteristics of extranodal marginal zone lymphoma of mucosa-associated lymphoid tissue (MALT lymphoma) of the digestive tract

Primary site	% of EMZL	Infection, autoimmunity, and other characteristics	Genetic alterations
Oesophagus		Unknown	Not reported
Stomach	70%	*Helicobacter pylori* (85%) and *H. heilmannii* (< 1%)	t(11;18)(q21;q21)/*BIRC3-MALT1* (6–26%), t(14;18)(q32;q21)/IGH-*MALT1* (1–5%), t(3;14)(p14;q32)/IGH-*FOXP1* (0–3%), t(1;14)(p22;q32)/IGH-*BCL10* (0–2%), trisomy 3 (11%), trisomy 18 (6%), and *TNFAIP3* inactivation (5%)
Intestinal tract	2%	*Campylobacter jejuni* (50%)	t(11;18)(q21;q21)/*BIRC3-MALT1* (12–56%), t(1;14)(p22;q32)/IGH-*BCL10* (0–13%), trisomy 3 (75%), and trisomy 18 (25%)
Liver	10%	HCV (23%), HBV (16%), hepatitis of other causes (10%), *H. pylori* (13%), autoimmune hepatitis / primary biliary cirrhosis / Sjögren syndrome (12%), ascariasis (4%), and synchronous malignant tumours (11%)	t(14;18)(q32;q21)/IGH-*MALT1* (0–67%), t(3;14)(p14;q32)/IGH-*FOXP1*, trisomy 3, and trisomy 18
Gallbladder and extrahepatic bile duct	14%	Gallstones	t(11;18)(q21;q21)/*BIRC3-MALT1*
Pancreas		Unknown	Not reported

EMZL, extranodal marginal zone lymphoma.
Data summarized according to Streubel et al. {3146}, Remstein et al. {2694}, and Schreuder et al. {2909}.

Pathogenesis

Four translocations are specifically associated with MALT lymphomas: t(11;18)(q21;q21), t(1;14)(p22;q32), t(14;18)(q32;q21), and t(3;14)(p14;q32). They result in the production of a chimeric protein (BIRC3-MALT1) or in transcriptional deregulation of BCL10, MALT1, and FOXP1, respectively {68,3149,814,314}. Trisomy of chromosome 3 or 18 is frequent in MALT lymphomas but is nonspecific. The frequencies of the translocations or trisomies vary markedly with the primary site of disease. The chromosomal translocations all converge on the activation of the same oncogenic pathway associated with NF-κB {900}. The t(11;18)(q21;q21)/BIRC3-MALT1 translocation, which occurs in 6–26% of gastric MALT lymphomas, is significantly associated with H. pylori negativity and nuclear BCL10 expression, and it can identify cases that will not respond to H. pylori eradication {2290, 1930,2291,2288}. This translocation is also found in 12–56% of intestinal MALT lymphomas {3148}, sometimes together with gastric and multifocal intestinal involvement. The translocation is rarely seen in colorectal MALT lymphoma. The t(11;18)(q21;q21)/BIRC3-MALT1 translocation is associated with a low risk of additional genetic damage and hence transformation into diffuse large B-cell lymphoma (DLBCL). The t(14;18)/IGH-MALT1 translocation is often detected in hepatic MALT lymphoma {3147}. The translocations t(1;14)/BCL10-MALT1 and t(3;14)/IGH-FOXP1 are infrequently found. The latter is associated with an increased risk of transformation to DLBCL. Extra copies of MALT1 and FOXP1, often suggestive of partial and complete trisomies 18 and 3, are detected in 25% and 17% of gastric cases, respectively. The presence of extra copies of MALT1 is significantly associated with progression or relapse of lymphoma, and is an adverse prognostic factor for event-free survival {2289}.

Macroscopic appearance

Thickening of the mucosa may be mild or macroscopically obvious. Mass-forming lesions {2285} may occur. MALT lymphoma is often multifocal within the involved organ.

Histopathology

MALT lymphomas variably recapitulate the cytoarchitectural features of Peyer patches, the prototypical normal MALT. Tumours arising at any anatomical site share similar histopathological characteristics, despite site-specific differences in etiology and molecular cytogenetic abnormalities (see Table 11.02, p. 379).

MALT lymphoma is composed of small B cells that most typically include marginal zone cells (small to intermediate-sized cells with pale cytoplasm and a slightly irregular nucleus, also called centrocyte-like cells), monocytoid cells, and small lymphocytes, as well as scattered immunoblasts and centroblast-like cells {666}. Plasma cell differentiation is occasionally observed in MALT lymphomas of the GI tract, but it is a constant feature of IPSID. Dutcher bodies, immunoglobulin inclusions (crystals or globules), and amyloid can be present.

The lymphoma cells infiltrate around reactive lymphoid follicles in a marginal zone pattern. They also extend to the

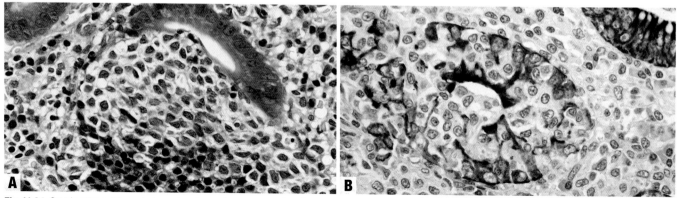

Fig. 11.04 Gastric extranodal marginal zone lymphoma of mucosa-associated lymphoid tissue (MALT lymphoma). **A** Lymphoepithelial lesions consisting of centrocyte-like cells infiltrating and expanding glandular epithelium. **B** Immunostaining for keratin highlights lymphoepithelial lesions.

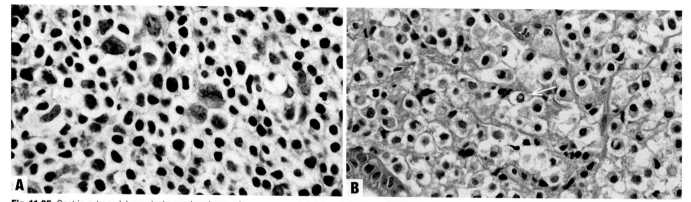

Fig. 11.05 Gastric extranodal marginal zone lymphoma of mucosa-associated lymphoid tissue (MALT lymphoma) with *Helicobacter pylori* infection without t(11;18)/*BIRC3-MALT1*; variation in appearance of centrocyte-like cells. **A** Clear cell subtype. **B** Prominent plasma cell differentiation and Dutcher bodies (arrow).

interfollicular regions. The neoplastic cells can erode, colonize, and eventually overrun the reactive follicles (a process called follicular colonization). Lymphoma cells typically infiltrate the epithelium, forming lymphoepithelial lesions, which are defined as aggregates of ≥ 3 marginal zone cells with destruction of the glandular epithelium, often together with eosinophilic degeneration of epithelial cells {2503}. Lymphoepithelial lesions are usually less prominent in non-gastric sites.

Scattered large cells resembling centroblasts or immunoblasts are usually present, but are in the minority. When solid or sheet-like proliferations of transformed cells are present, the tumour should be diagnosed as DLBCL, with the presence of concurrent MALT lymphoma noted. The term "high-grade MALT lymphoma" should not be used, and the term "MALT lymphoma" should not be applied to a DLBCL even if it has arisen in a MALT site or is associated with lymphoepithelial lesions.

The immunophenotype of lymphoma cells in MALT lymphoma is similar to that of marginal zone B cells: CD20+, CD79a+, BCL2+, BCL6−, CD5−, CD10−, CD23−, CD43+/−, CD11c+/− (weak), and typically expressing IgM (less often IgA or IgG and rarely IgD). There is no specific marker for MALT lymphoma, with IRTA1 and MNDA1 being possible markers for marginal

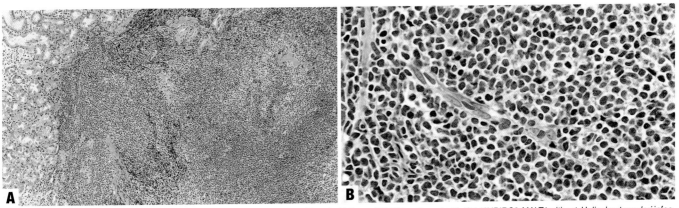

Fig. 11.06 Gastric extranodal marginal zone lymphoma of mucosa-associated lymphoid tissue (MALT lymphoma) with t(11;18)/*BIRC3-MALT1* without *Helicobacter pylori* infection. **A** The diffuse lymphomatous infiltrate extends into the submucosa. **B** A relatively monotonous proliferation of centrocyte-like cells with few scattered large cells.

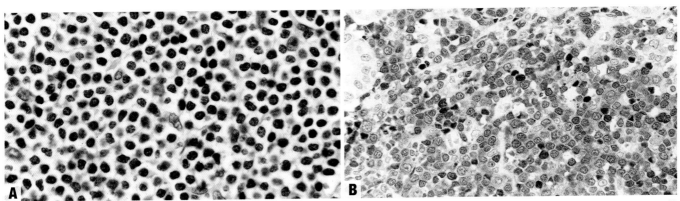

Fig. 11.07 Colonic extranodal marginal zone lymphoma of mucosa-associated lymphoid tissue (MALT lymphoma) with t(11;18)/*BIRC3-MALT1*. **A** A relatively monotonous proliferation of centrocyte-like cells with scattered large cells. **B** Immunostaining for BCL10 highlights the tumour cells.

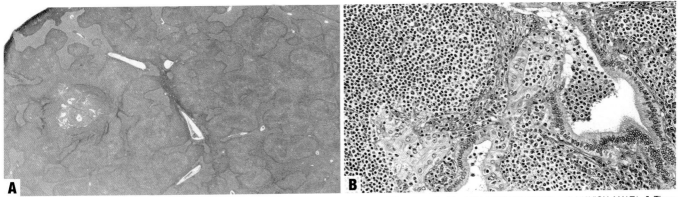

Fig. 11.08 Hepatic extranodal marginal zone lymphoma of mucosa-associated lymphoid tissue (MALT lymphoma) without t(11;18)/*BIRC3-MALT1* or t(14;18)/IGH-*MALT1*. **A** There is a dense lymphoid infiltrate with portal and parenchymal involvement. **B** A monotonous proliferation of centrocyte-like cells, forming a lymphoepithelial lesion with bile duct epithelium.

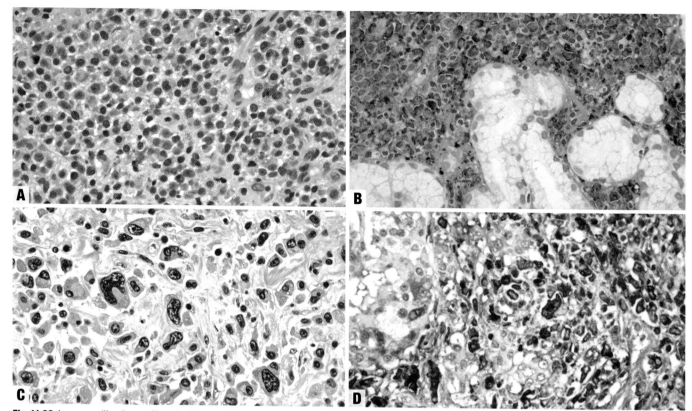

Fig. 11.09 Immunoproliferative small intestinal disease. **A** It is characterized by a dense lymphoplasmacytic infiltrate. **B** Immunostaining for IgA highlights tumour cells. **C** Transformation to diffuse large B-cell lymphoma with plasmacytic differentiation. **D** Immunostaining for IgA highlights tumour cells.

zone lymphomas {896,1513,2127}. Negative staining for cyclin D1/SOX11 and CD10/BCL6 is useful for distinguishing MALT lymphoma from mantle cell lymphoma and follicular lymphoma, respectively. Coexpression of CD5, CD23, and LEF1 distinguishes chronic lymphocytic leukaemia from MALT lymphoma, although occasional expression of CD5 or CD23 may be seen in MALT lymphoma. Immunostaining with antikeratin antibodies may aid in the identification of lymphoepithelial lesions.

IPSID/αHCD

IPSID/αHCD is a subtype of gastrointestinal MALT lymphoma with secretion of defective immunoglobulin α-heavy chain {665,75,1386,325}. IPSID is a MALT lymphoma with marked plasma cell differentiation {1386,75,325}.

Early stages manifest as a dense lymphoplasmacytic infiltrate confined to the mucosa and/or submucosa. Villous blunting or atrophy of the small intestine may be seen. Advanced stages are characterized by histological transformation to DLBCL, usually also with plasmacytic differentiation. Immunohistochemical studies demonstrate the production of α-heavy chain without light chain. This peculiar feature is due to the deletion of most of the IGHV (VH) and all of the CH1 domains, but with intact C-terminal regions resulting in expression of a truncated heavy chain, which is unable to assemble with light chains.

Cytology
Not clinically relevant

Diagnostic molecular pathology
Not clinically relevant

Essential and desirable diagnostic criteria
Essential: involvement of extranodal site; diffuse to perifollicular infiltrate of centrocyte-like cells and small lymphoid cells, often with scattered large lymphoid cells; monocytoid cells and plasma cells may or may not be present; positivity for B-lineage markers; immunohistochemical exclusion of mantle cell lymphoma (CD5, cyclin D1) and follicular lymphoma (CD10, BCL6).
Desirable: presence of lymphoepithelial lesions.

Staging (TNM)
Lymphoid neoplasms are staged according to the Lugano classification, which has been adopted by the eighth edition of the Union for International Cancer Control (UICC) TNM classification {596}.

Prognosis and prediction
MALT lymphomas have an indolent clinical course and are slow to disseminate {2635}. *H. pylori* eradication results in complete remission in 60–100% of gastric MALT lymphoma patients {2288,2287}. Early-stage IPSID/αHCD also responds to antibiotics. The t(11;18)/*BIRC3-MALT1* translocation confers resistance to *H. pylori* eradication therapy. MALT lymphomas are sensitive to radiotherapy, and local treatment can be followed by prolonged disease-free intervals. Involvement of multiple extranodal sites and even bone marrow involvement do not appear to confer an adverse prognosis {3290,3291}.

Duodenal-type follicular lymphoma

Yoshino T
Chott A

Definition

Duodenal-type follicular lymphoma (DTFL) is a neoplasm of follicular B lymphocytes showing follicular architecture with highly characteristic clinical and biological features, including presentation most commonly in the second portion of the duodenum, low histological grade, indolent clinical course, and excellent outcome.

ICD-O coding

9695/3 Follicular lymphoma, duodenal type

ICD-11 coding

2A80.0 Follicular lymphoma grade 1
2A80.1 Follicular lymphoma grade 2
XA9780 Duodenum

Related terminology

Acceptable: primary intestinal follicular lymphoma.

Subtype(s)

None

Localization

DTFL is usually detected endoscopically in the second portion of the duodenum. There is commonly simultaneous involvement of the jejunum or ileum {3216}.

Clinical features

Most DTFLs are detected incidentally; some patients may present with abdominal pain and/or discomfort {2056}.

Epidemiology

Two comprehensive studies, one performed in Europe and the other in Japan, reported median patient ages of 65 and 59 years, respectively, and both studies reported a 1:1 M:F ratio. The disease may affect younger individuals, with about 10% in their fourth decade of life in the European study. DTFL accounts for about 4% of all gastrointestinal lymphoma cases. One case of DTFL is diagnosed in 3000–7000 gastroduodenoscopies {2894,3216}.

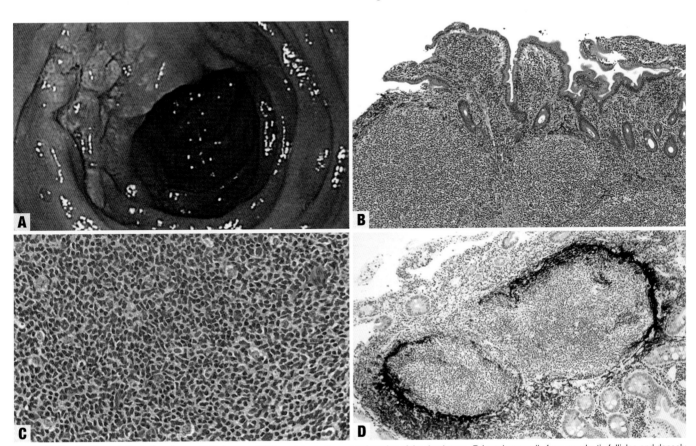

Fig. 11.10 Duodenal-type follicular lymphoma. **A** Endoscopy. White nodules in the second portion of the duodenum. **B** Lymphoma cells form neoplastic follicles and densely infiltrate the lamina propria of the villi. **C** Uniform lymphoma cells without tingible-body macrophages. **D** CD21+ follicular dendritic cells located at the periphery of follicles.

Etiology

Unknown

Pathogenesis

DTFL harbours the same t(14;18)(q32;q21) as nodal follicular lymphoma. Studies on immunoglobulin heavy variable (IGHV [VH]) gene rearrangements, comparative genomic hybridization studies, and comparative gene expression profiling have revealed similarities of gene and protein expression profiles with both extranodal marginal zone lymphoma of mucosa-associated lymphoid tissue (MALT lymphoma) and other subtypes of follicular lymphoma. Ongoing hypermutations and selective usage of IGHV (VH) gene segments suggest an underlying antigen-driven mechanism {3218}. An inflammatory background may be produced by the overexpression of the pro-inflammatory chemokine CCL20 and its receptor CCR6 {3219}. The propensity to remain localized to the mucosa may relate to the site in which the relevant antigen is first encountered and to the expression of characteristic homing receptors {296}. DTFL might arise from a bone marrow–derived t(14;18) precursor that has already experienced antigen challenge and germinal-centre transit before settling in the specific mucosal environment in the memory B-cell stage. Although some genomic alterations are shared with nodal follicular lymphoma, the selection pressure to malignant pathways appears to be limited {2034}.

Macroscopic appearance

Not clinically relevant

Histopathology

The neoplastic follicles are located in the mucosa/submucosa and often result in a polypoid architecture. They are non-polarized and largely composed of centrocytes, constituting grade 1–2 disease according to the grading system for nodal follicular lymphoma. Tingible-body macrophages and mantle zones are lacking. Usually sheets of small lymphoid cells with dark round nuclei, which belong to the neoplastic population, are present in the lamina propria outside the follicles {2894}.

The immunophenotype is similar to that of nodal follicular lymphoma. The neoplastic cells are usually CD20+, CD10+, BCL6+, and BCL2+, and the proliferation rate is usually low {3218}. Follicular dendritic cells, identified by CD21, are lacking in the central area of the neoplastic germinal centres, but redistributed to the periphery as a condensed rim of enhanced staining {3217}.

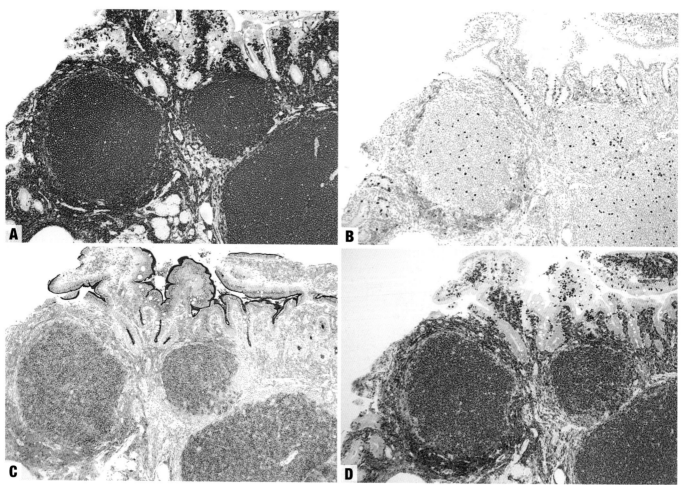

Fig. 11.11 Duodenal-type follicular lymphoma. **A** CD20 highlights the neoplastic follicles as well as neoplastic cells in the lamina propria. **B** Very low Ki-67 proliferation index. **C** Lymphoma cells positive for CD10. **D** Lymphoma cells strongly positive for BCL2.

Cytology

Not clinically relevant

Diagnostic molecular pathology

Not clinically relevant

Essential and desirable diagnostic criteria

Essential: lymphoma confined to mucosa and/or submucosa of small bowel, most commonly duodenum; neoplastic follicles predominated by centrocytes; lamina propria also infiltrated; immunophenotype: CD20+, CD10+, BCL2+.

Staging (TNM)

Most patients have disease limited to the mucosa/submucosa, without lymph node involvement. Lymphoid neoplasms are staged according to the Lugano classification, which has been adopted by the eighth edition of the Union for International Cancer Control (UICC) TNM classification {596}.

Prognosis and prediction

The prognosis is excellent. There is low risk of progression to nodal disease, and large cell transformation occurs rarely {2894,3216,3262}. Given the indolent clinical course, a watch-and-wait approach is reasonable for most patients {2894,3263}.

Enteropathy-associated T-cell lymphoma

Bhagat G
Chott A

Definition

Enteropathy-associated T-cell lymphoma (EATL) is an intestinal T-cell lymphoma derived from intraepithelial lymphocytes (IELs), which occurs in individuals with coeliac disease.

ICD-O coding

9717/3 Enteropathy-associated T-cell lymphoma

ICD-11 coding

2A90.7 Enteropathy-associated T-cell lymphoma
XA6452 Small intestine
XA9780 Duodenum
XA8UM1 Jejunum
XA0QT6 Ileum
XA2520 Overlapping lesion of small intestine

Related terminology

Acceptable: enteropathy-type intestinal T-cell lymphoma; enteropathy-associated T-cell lymphoma, type I.

Subtype(s)

None

Localization

The jejunum is most often involved, but other segments of the small bowel, and less commonly the stomach and colon, may be affected. As many as a third of EATLs evolving from refractory coeliac disease (RCD) type 2 (RCD2; see below) may arise at extraintestinal locations {2025}. Dissemination to extragastrointestinal sites occurs most frequently to abdominal lymph nodes, but other organs, including bone marrow, lung, or liver, may show evidence of disease in 10–20% of cases {842,2025,746}.

Although some series have described low-stage disease in the majority of patients at presentation using the Lugano staging system, recent studies using more-sensitive imaging modalities report stage IV disease in almost 50% of cases {2025}.

Clinical features

Abdominal pain, diarrhoea, and weight loss are common symptoms and signs. Almost half of all patients present with an acute abdominal emergency due to small bowel perforation or obstruction. Many patients are known to have adult-onset coeliac disease, but not infrequently, coeliac disease is diagnosed only at the time of EATL diagnosis. Occasionally, adult coeliac disease patients become unresponsive to a gluten-free diet before the development of EATL, a condition referred to as RCD. Such patients usually present with anorexia and severe malnutrition. B symptoms other than weight loss are present in a third of cases, and elevated LDH or hypercalcaemia is detected in a subset of patients {3036,3420,746,2025}.

Refractory coeliac disease

Approximately 0.3–1% of individuals with adult-onset coeliac disease have persistent villous atrophy and fail to improve clinically or develop recurrent malabsorptive symptoms and signs despite being on a strict gluten-free diet for > 12 months. Upon exclusion of other gastrointestinal disorders and coeliac disease–related malignancies, these patients are diagnosed as having RCD {78,1368,1957}. Two subtypes of RCD are recognized based on the absence (type 1; RCD1) or presence (type 2; RCD2) of abnormal IELs {720}.
RCD1: The IELs are of TCRαβ+ lineage and express surface CD3 and CD8 (i.e. a normal immunophenotype). TRB or TRG rearrangement analysis shows no clonal rearrangements.

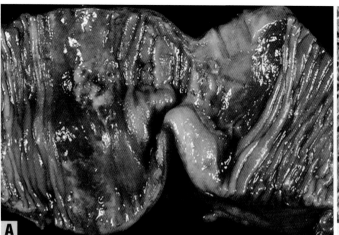
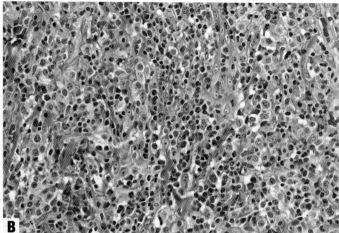

Fig. 11.12 Enteropathy-associated T-cell lymphoma. **A** In a small intestinal resection specimen, circumferential induration and ulceration of the jejunum are seen adjacent to a stricture. **B** With a prominent inflammatory cell infiltrate. Clusters of large monomorphic neoplastic cells admixed with numerous histiocytes and eosinophils and a few small lymphocytes (note the rich vascularity).

Mucosal histopathological changes are the same as in uncomplicated coeliac disease. RCD1 is the more common subtype and it generally has a benign course with a low risk of EATL development {2024,78,1368,2778}.

RCD2: The IELs usually express cytoplasmic CD3 but lack surface CD3, CD8, and T-cell receptor expression. Flow cytometry is the best modality to detect IEL phenotype, and a cut-off point of > 20% abnormal cells has been proposed to discriminate between RCD2 and RCD1 {3458}. For immunohistochemistry, a threshold of > 50% CD8– (of all CD3ε+) IELs has been recommended for classification as RCD2, although this threshold might not be stringent enough {3434,2027}. Clonal TRB or TRG gene rearrangements can be demonstrated in the majority of cases. However, one must be aware that about 25% of cases lack clonal TR gene rearrangements, and a minority of uncomplicated coeliac disease or RCD1 cases may show clonal TRB/TRG rearrangements {3198,1343}. Villous atrophy is usually severe. The abnormal IELs lack substantial cytological atypia, and they may disseminate along the entire GI tract (or to extragastrointestinal sites), with frequent infiltration of the lamina propria {3465,3459}. Mucosal ulcers are observed in some cases (ulcerative jejunitis). Recent molecular and phenotypic investigations of RCD2 have suggested an origin of at least a proportion of, if not all, cases from innate (T/NK precursor) IELs that show variable commitment to a T-cell lineage {3198,2898, 883}. In contrast to RCD1, RCD2 is considered a low-grade lymphoma of IELs or EATL in situ, and it has a high propensity to transform to EATL (30–52% within ~5 years), with a 5-year survival rate of about 50% {2024,78,1368,2778}.

Epidemiology

EATL constitutes < 5% of all gastrointestinal lymphomas {746}. It usually occurs in adults aged > 50 years, with a slight male predominance. All patients have the genetic background of coeliac disease. Therefore, EATL is more common in regions with a high seroprevalence of coeliac disease, particularly Europe and the USA {1387}.

Etiology

EATL is strongly associated with coeliac disease. Evidence for an association between coeliac disease and EATL comes from the following: identical HLA-DQ2 haplotypes of coeliac disease and EATL patients, the demonstration of gluten sensitivity in EATL patients, and the protective effect of a gluten-free diet {1300,2404,1260}. Homozygosity for HLA-DQ2 alleles, observed in 53–56% of EATL patients (compared with 21% in

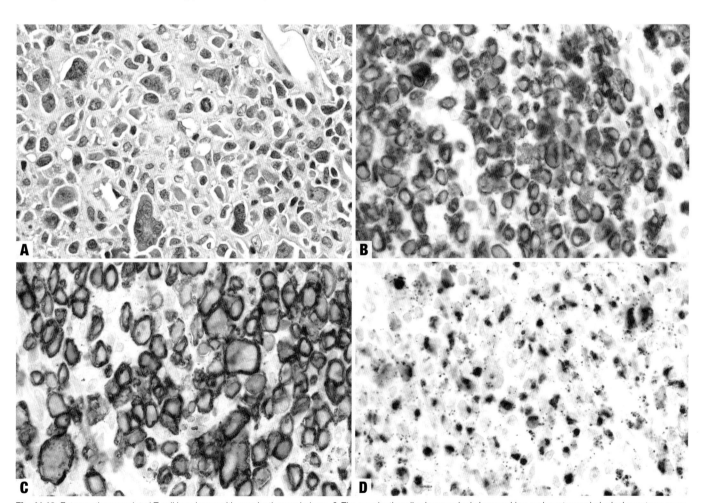

Fig. 11.13 Enteropathy-associated T-cell lymphoma with anaplastic morphology. **A** The neoplastic cells show marked pleomorphism and a cytomorphological spectrum, ranging from medium to large to bizarre-appearing binucleated and multinucleated cells. Some of the neoplastic cells resemble Reed–Sternberg cells. The neoplastic cells show expression of CD3 (**B**), CD7 (not shown), CD30 (**C**), and granzyme B (**D**), but they do not express TCRβ (βF1) (not shown).

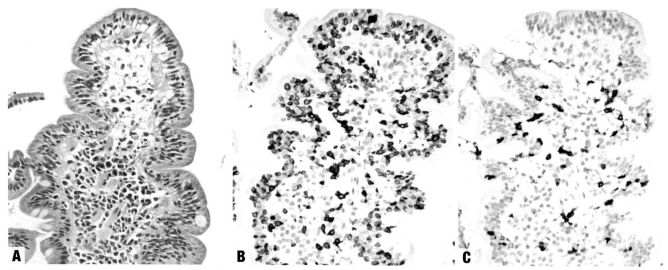

Fig. 11.14 Refractory coeliac disease type 2. **A** The villus tip shows increased intraepithelial lymphocytes, which are small in size and lack cytological atypia. The intraepithelial lymphocytes show uniform, intense CD7 expression (not shown) and cytoplasmic CD3 expression (no surface CD3 expression was detected by flow cytometry) (**B**), and they lack CD8 expression (**C**).

uncomplicated coeliac disease) and older age, both connoting increased exposure to gluten (gliadin peptides), are risk factors for the development of EATL {77,2025}.

Pathogenesis

EATL can occur de novo or can progress in a stepwise manner, with an intermediate phase of RCD2, in approximately 50% of cases {2025,721}. In active coeliac disease, gliadin peptide–mediated enterocyte damage leads to IL-15 production by enterocytes and lamina propria macrophages, promoting the development of cytotoxic IELs by activating the perforin/granzyme system. In addition, IL-15 induces NK-activating receptors (e.g. NKG2D, NKp46) on IELs and the non-classic MHC class I ligands (MIC-A and HLA-E) on epithelial cells, resulting in epithelial destruction {2122,883,2898}. Protracted inflammation due to sustained IL-15 expression and production of other cytokines (e.g. IL-21, TNF-α) by gliadin-responsive CD4+ T cells in the lamina propria is thought to contribute to DNA damage, acquisition of genomic alterations, and inhibition of IEL apoptosis, fostering clonal expansion of IELs and progression to EATL {883,2026,3198,1685}. This pathogenetic sequence has been proposed for RCD2-derived EATLs, but the disease-initiating factors for de novo EATL are unknown.

Most cases show clonal TRB or TRG rearrangements. Comparative genomic hybridization studies have reported segmental amplifications of chromosome 9q31.3-qter or deletions at 16q12.1 in > 80% of EATLs, as well as gains at 1q and 5q34-q35.2 {749}. These changes are not specific for EATL; they are also detected in monomorphic epitheliotropic intestinal T-cell lymphoma. Whole-exome sequencing has shown the JAK/STAT pathway to be the most frequently mutated pathway in EATLs, with *JAK1*, *STAT3*, *STAT5B*, and *SOCS1* being commonly involved. Recurrent *JAK1* and *STAT3* mutations have also been observed in RCD2, suggesting early acquisition of these genetic alterations in lymphomagenesis {883}. Interestingly, EATLs and monomorphic epitheliotropic intestinal T-cell

lymphomas have highly overlapping genetic alterations, implying shared mechanisms of disease pathogenesis {2191}.

Macroscopic appearance

The intestinal tumour is often multifocal, with circumferentially oriented ulcers, ulcerated nodules, plaques, and strictures. The mesentery and mesenteric lymph nodes may be involved.

Histopathology

The majority of EATLs are composed of pleomorphic medium and large cells, and some exhibit anaplastic morphology. The tumours may have a pronounced inflammatory background consisting of histiocytes, eosinophils, small lymphocytes, and plasma cells, which can obscure the tumour cells. Intraepithelial spread may be striking. Mucosa adjacent to the tumour usually shows villous atrophy, crypt hyperplasia, and intraepithelial lymphocytosis – histopathological features of coeliac disease. Importantly, these coeliac disease–associated alterations are variable: more pronounced in the upper jejunum and less in the distal small intestinal segments {1387}.

The immunophenotype of the neoplastic cells is usually CD3+, CD5–, CD7+, CD4–, CD8–, CD56– and CD103+; cytotoxic markers (TIA1, granzyme B, perforin) are commonly expressed. A proportion of de novo EATLs may be CD8+, and rare cases express TCRγδ {2025,3433}. Lymphomas with large cell morphology are often CD30+ and at times EMA+, but ALK1 is not expressed {628,2025}. EATLs frequently lack surface and cytoplasmic T-cell receptor expression {3312}. Demonstration of a substantial number of EBV-infected tumour cells precludes the diagnosis of EATL.

Cytology

Not clinically relevant

Diagnostic molecular pathology

Not clinically relevant

Essential and desirable diagnostic criteria

Essential: intestine infiltrated by pleomorphic medium-sized to large lymphoid cells, which may even be anaplastic; accompanied by a variable inflammatory background often including many eosinophils and histiocytes; uninvolved intestinal mucosa shows features of coeliac disease (villous atrophy, crypt hyperplasia, intraepithelial lymphocytosis); T-cell lineage, often with CD4– CD8– phenotype and expression of cytotoxic markers; CD30 can be positive.

Staging (TNM)

Lymphoid neoplasms are staged according to the Lugano classification, which has been adopted by the eighth edition of the Union for International Cancer Control (UICC) TNM classification {596}.

Prognosis and prediction

The prognosis of EATL is very poor because of the frequent multifocal nature of the disease, high rate of intestinal (or extraintestinal) recurrence, and poor nutritional condition of patients, especially those with preceding RCD2. Prognostic factors are not well established for EATL. Recently, an EATL prognostic index (EPI) was introduced, which reportedly performs better than the International Prognostic Index (IPI) and another prognostic model for T-cell lymphomas (the prognostic index for peripheral T-cell lymphoma [PIT]) {729}. The median overall survival time is < 10 months. Better outcomes have been reported for patients receiving multiagent chemotherapy and autologous stem cell transplantation {3036}.

Chapter 11

Monomorphic epitheliotropic intestinal T-cell lymphoma

Tan SY
de Leval L

Definition

Monomorphic epitheliotropic intestinal T-cell lymphoma (MEITL) is a primary intestinal T-cell lymphoma derived from intraepithelial T lymphocytes, characterized by monomorphic cytomorphology and epitheliotropism, typically lacking coeliac disease association.

ICD-O coding

9717/3 Monomorphic epitheliotropic intestinal T-cell lymphoma

ICD-11 coding

2A90.C Peripheral T-cell lymphoma NOS
XA6452 Small intestine
XA9780 Duodenum
XA8UM1 Jejunum
XA0QT6 Ileum
XA2520 Overlapping lesion of small intestine

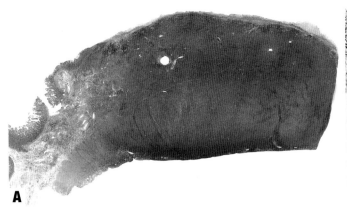
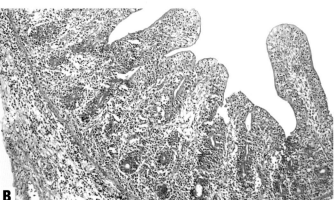

Fig. 11.15 Monomorphic epitheliotropic intestinal T-cell lymphoma. **A** The lymphoma shows transmural infiltration of the small bowel wall, with ulceration but no necrosis. **B** The mucosa adjacent to the tumour shows expanded and distorted intestinal villi containing epitheliotropic lymphoma cells.

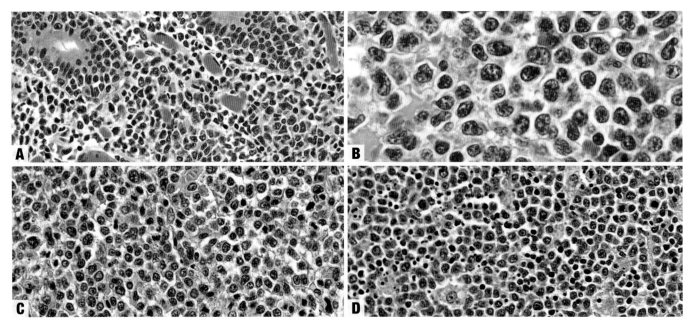

Fig. 11.16 Monomorphic epitheliotropic intestinal T-cell lymphoma. **A** The epitheliotropic lymphoma cells in the peripheral zone are cytologically atypical, featuring medium-sized lymphoid cells with irregular nuclear contours, moderate nuclear pleomorphism, more open chromatin, and distinct nucleoli. **B** Neoplastic lymphocytes are medium-sized, showing regular, round to slightly irregular nuclei with slightly open chromatin and inconspicuous nucleoli. There are few admixed inflammatory cells. **C** In this case, the lymphomatous population is somewhat pleomorphic morphologically, with occasional larger cells. **D** This case has a high-grade appearance, with frequent apoptotic bodies and macrophages, imparting a starry-sky pattern.

Related terminology

Acceptable: type II enteropathy-associated T-cell lymphoma.

Subtype(s)

None

Localization

Most cases present as ulcerative masses in the small intestine or (less commonly) in the colon, duodenum, or stomach, and a small subset of patients may present with multifocal gastrointestinal lesions {3235,3352,1391}. In addition to mesenteric lymph nodes, the disease may also disseminate to the lung, liver, and brain.

Clinical features

Most patients present with abdominal pain, gastrointestinal bleeding, obstruction or perforation, diarrhoea, and weight loss {3235,3352,544}. A history of malabsorption or coeliac disease is generally absent.

Epidemiology

MEITL has a worldwide distribution. It accounts for many primary intestinal T-cell lymphomas in Asia {544,1011,3173}. It occurs predominantly in adults, with a median patient age in the sixth decade of life and an M:F ratio of about 2:1 {3235}.

Etiology

Unknown

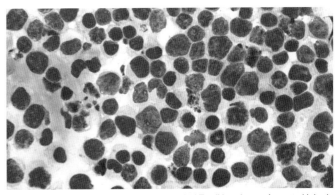

Fig. 11.18 Monomorphic epitheliotropic intestinal T-cell lymphoma. A case with brain and cerebrospinal fluid involvement showing neoplastic lymphocytes with occasional prominent nucleoli in the cerebrospinal fluid (Diff-Quik).

Pathogenesis

There is clonal rearrangement of the TR genes. Apart from gains of *MYC* {3235,2437}, also reported are gains at 9q34.3 {3320, 1661}, 1q32.3, 4p15.1, 5q34, 7q34, 8p11.23, 9q22.31, 9q33.2, and 12p13.31, as well as losses of 7p14.1 and 16q12.1 {3320, 2279}. Unlike in type I enteropathy-associated T-cell lymphoma, gains at 1q32.2-q41 and 5q34-q35.5 are uncommon {2279}.

Activating mutations of *STAT5B* are noted in cases of both γδ and αβ derivation {2279,1747}. Mutations of *JAK3* and *GNAI2* may be seen {2279}. *SETD2* is frequently silenced through nonsense mutations, frameshift insertions, and deletions {2735, 2191}. EBV is usually negative {3235,544}.

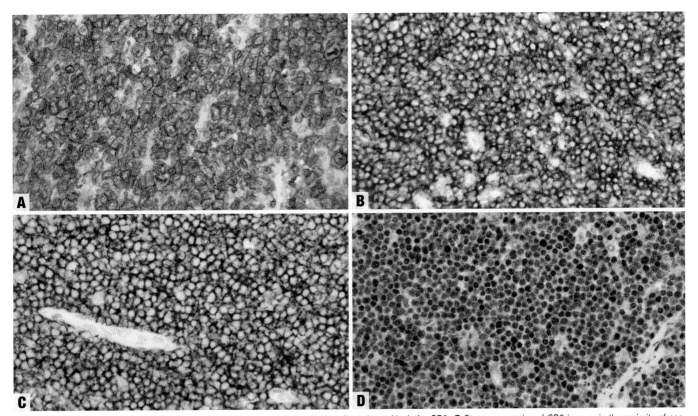

Fig. 11.17 Monomorphic epitheliotropic intestinal T-cell lymphoma. **A** Neoplastic cells stain positively for CD3. **B** Strong expression of CD8 is seen in the majority of cases. **C** This example shows strong staining for CD56, but some cases display weak to negative expression. **D** Nuclear staining for MATK is seen in many cases of monomorphic epitheliotropic intestinal T-cell lymphoma.

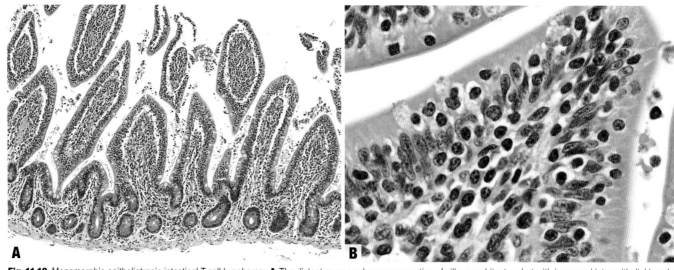

Fig. 11.19 Monomorphic epitheliotropic intestinal T-cell lymphoma. **A** The distant mucosa shows preservation of villous architecture but with increased intraepithelial lymphocytes. **B** Intraepithelial lymphocytes have a bland cytological appearance, with round nuclei, condensed chromatin, and inconspicuous nucleoli.

Macroscopic appearance
Not clinically relevant

Histopathology
The tumour is often ulcerated, with transmural invasion. Neoplastic cells are monotonous, small to medium-sized cells with round nuclei, dispersed chromatin, and ample clear cytoplasm. Occasionally neoplastic cells may appear high-grade with a starry-sky appearance or feature greater pleomorphism or more open chromatin. Areas of necrosis and an inflammatory background are uncommon. In the peripheral zone, the tumour invades the adjacent mucosa, which features distorted, broadly expanded villi containing epitheliotropic lymphoma cells. The distant intestinal mucosa features normal architecture and often shows an increase of morphologically bland intraepithelial lymphocytes which may mimic coeliac disease and lymphocytic colitis {3235,544,1391}.

The usual immunophenotype is CD2+, CD3+, CD4–, CD5–, CD7+, CD8+, CD56+ {3235,544}. Expression of TCRγ or TCRβ may be seen {3235,206,3569}, although a minority is T-cell receptor–silent, and rarely both T-cell receptors are expressed {3235,544}. One study reported a high incidence of CD8a homodimers {3235}. The cytotoxic marker TIA1 is expressed in most cases, whereas expression of granzyme B and perforin is less consistent {3320}. Extensive nuclear expression of MATK is noted {3236}, and aberrant expression of CD20 is reported

in 20% of cases {3235}. The intraepithelial lymphocytes in the distant zone express CD3, CD8, and TIA1, but they can be positive or negative for CD56 {3235,1391,544} and may represent precursor lesions of MEITL.

Cytology
Not clinically relevant

Diagnostic molecular pathology
Not clinically relevant

Essential and desirable diagnostic criteria
Essential: intestine densely infiltrated by monotonous medium-sized T-lineage lymphoid cells, typically lacking necrosis; epithelial invasion commonly present; most common immunophenotype: CD3+, CD5–, CD4–, CD8+, CD56+, cytotoxic marker +.

Staging (TNM)
Lymphoid neoplasms are staged according to the Lugano classification, which has been adopted by the eighth edition of the Union for International Cancer Control (UICC) TNM classification {596}.

Prognosis and prediction
The clinical outcome for MEITL is poor, with a median survival time of 7 months {3235}.

Intestinal T-cell lymphoma NOS

Bhagat G
Tan SY

Definition

Intestinal T-cell lymphoma (ITCL) NOS is an aggressive GI tract T-cell lymphoma that lacks the clinical and pathological features of enteropathy-associated T-cell lymphoma (EATL), monomorphic epitheliotropic ITCL (MEITL), anaplastic large cell lymphoma, or extranodal NK/T-cell lymphoma.

ICD-O coding

9717/3 Intestinal T-cell lymphoma

ICD-11 coding

2A90.C Peripheral T-cell lymphoma NOS
XA6452 Small intestine
XA9780 Duodenum
XA8UM1 Jejunum
XA0QT6 Ileum
XA2520 Overlapping lesion of small intestine

Related terminology

None

Subtype(s)

None

Localization

ITCL-NOS can occur in or be confined to a particular gastrointestinal organ or involve multiple sites; dissemination to regional lymph nodes and extragastrointestinal sites is not uncommon {206,1541}. The colon and small intestine are the more commonly involved organs {206}. Limited data suggest that multicentric disease is less common in ITCL-NOS than in MEITL {3173}.

Clinical features

The symptoms and signs of ITCL-NOS depend on the type and extent of organ involvement. The clinical presentation of patients with intestinal disease is similar to those with EATL and MEITL, although malabsorption is infrequent. Epigastric pain and haematemesis are common in individuals with primary gastric lymphomas {3173,1541}. Approximately 50% of patients present with stage III/IV disease {3173,1596}.

Epidemiology

The geographical distribution of ITCL-NOS is wide, but a higher frequency has been reported in Asia, where it is one of the more common subtypes of ITCL {2529}. The mean patient age is similar to or slightly lower than that of MEITL, and males are more commonly affected {3173,2529}.

Etiology

The etiology of ITCL-NOS is unknown, but it is probably multifactorial, given the disease heterogeneity. Occasional cases have been reported in individuals with inflammatory gastrointestinal disorders (inflammatory bowel disease and autoimmune

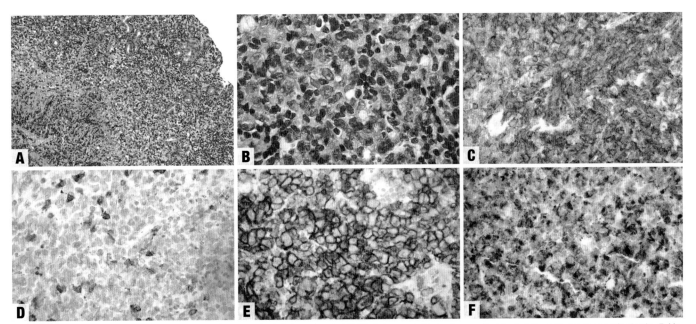

Fig. 11.20 Intestinal T-cell lymphoma NOS involving the stomach. **A** A dense lymphoid infiltrate is seen in the lamina propria, interdigitating between the gastric glands. **B** Medium-sized to large pleomorphic lymphocytes are seen, which have dispersed chromatin and prominent nucleoli. The neoplastic cells are diffusely positive for CD4 (**C**), lack CD8 expression (**D**), and display strong CD30 expression (**E**). **F** The neoplastic cells are also positive for granzyme B, indicating a cytotoxic phenotype.

Chapter 11

enteropathy) {206,2028,638}. If the patient is immunosuppressed or has received immunosuppressive or immunomodulatory therapy, the lymphoma is better classified as an immunosuppression-related or immunomodulatory therapy–related lymphoproliferative disorder {222}.

Pathogenesis
The types and frequencies of chromosome alterations in ITCL-NOS are unknown, but JAK/STAT and MAPK pathway mutations, similar to those found in EATL and MEITL, have been identified in the few cases evaluated {2352}.

Macroscopic appearance
ITCL-NOS more commonly has an ulcerated plaque-like appearance, and protruding luminal masses can be seen in some cases {3173}.

Histopathology
The lymphoma cells vary in size from medium to large and often show pleomorphism. Epithelial infiltration is only present in a minority of cases (~20%) {3173,1541}. CD4+ and CD4–/CD8– are the more frequent phenotypes. The majority express βF1 (TCRαβ), and a subset of tumours can be T-cell receptor–silent {1541,3173,206}. A high proportion of tumours express the cytotoxic granule protein TIA1, whereas granzyme B and CD30 expression is variable, and a minority of tumours (10%) are EBV-positive {1541,3173,206}.

Cytology
Not clinically relevant

Diagnostic molecular pathology
Not clinically relevant

Essential and desirable diagnostic criteria
Essential: primary T-cell lymphoma of the GI tract not conforming to EATL, MEITL, anaplastic large cell lymphoma, or extranodal NK/T-cell lymphoma; infiltration by medium-sized to large lymphoma cells; expression of T-lineage markers, and often CD4+ or CD4– CD8–.

Staging (TNM)
Lymphoid neoplasms are staged according to the Lugano classification, which has been adopted by the eighth edition of the Union for International Cancer Control (UICC) TNM classification {596}.

Prognosis and prediction
ITCL-NOS patients have a poor prognosis, although some studies report better median (35 months) and overall survival times than EATL and MEITL patients {1596,3173}. High stage and large cell morphology have been associated with worse 5-year survival rates {1541,1596}.

Indolent T-cell lymphoproliferative disorder of the GI tract

Jaffe ES
Chan WC

Definition
Indolent T-cell lymphoproliferative disorder of the GI tract is an indolent clonal T-cell lymphoproliferative disorder comprising non-epitheliotropic mature small lymphoid cells that infiltrate the lamina propria, most commonly in the small intestine and colon.

ICD-O coding
9702/1 Indolent T-cell lymphoproliferative disorder of the gastrointestinal tract

ICD-11 coding
2B2Y & XH2LK2 Other specified mature T-cell or NK-cell neoplasms & Lymphoproliferative disorder NOS

Related terminology
None

Subtype(s)
None

Localization
Most patients present with disease affecting the small bowel or colon {2571,2653}. However, all sites in the GI tract can be involved, including the oral cavity and oesophagus {844}. Disease spares bone marrow and peripheral blood.

Clinical features
Presenting symptoms include abdominal pain, diarrhoea, vomiting, dyspepsia, and weight loss {2571,495}. Peripheral lymphadenopathy is not present, but a subset of patients exhibit mesenteric lymphadenopathy {2052}.

Epidemiology
The disease presents in adulthood, more frequently in men than women, and rarely in children.

Etiology
Unknown

Pathogenesis
Cases show clonal rearrangement of TR genes, either TRG or TRB {2571,2052}. Activating mutations of *STAT3* are not found. However, cases expressing CD4 show a high incidence of recurrent *STAT3-JAK2* fusions, with t(9;17)(p24.1;q21.2) identified by cytogenetics {2974}. Most fusion-positive cases express STAT5 but not STAT3. In situ hybridization for EBV-encoded small RNA (EBER) is negative in all cases studied.

Macroscopic appearance
The mucosa of affected sites in the GI tract is thickened, with prominent folds or nodularity. In some tumours, the infiltrate produces intestinal polyps resembling lymphomatous polyposis {1238,1403}.

Histopathology
The lamina propria is expanded by a dense, non-destructive lymphoid infiltrate {2571}. Infiltration of the muscularis mucosae and submucosa may be seen focally. Epitheliotropism is usually absent. The infiltrate is composed of small, round,

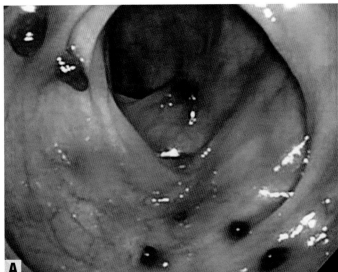 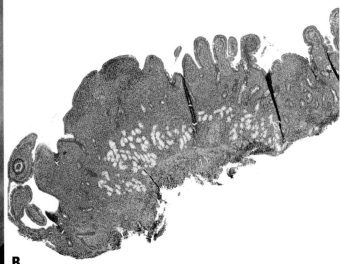

Fig. 11.21 Indolent T-cell lymphoproliferative disorder of the GI tract. **A** Colon. Small polypoid lesions are hyperaemic. **B** Duodenal biopsy. Infiltrate fills the lamina propria and focally extends beyond the muscularis mucosae. However, glands are largely intact.

Chapter 11

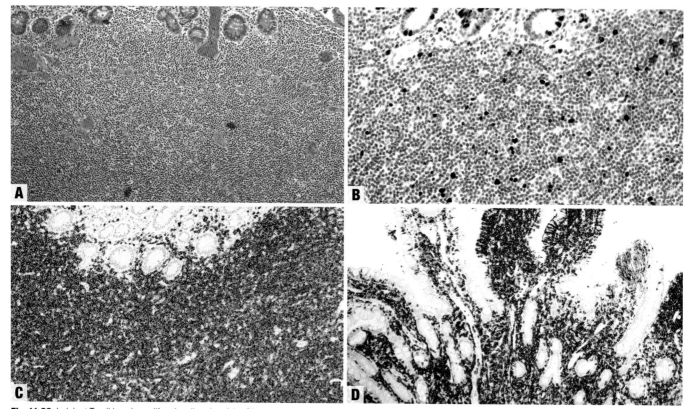

Fig. 11.22 Indolent T-cell lymphoproliferative disorder of the GI tract. **A** Ileum. The lamina propria is diffusely infiltrated by small lymphoid cells. **B** Ileum. The proliferative rate is extremely low (Ki-67 staining). **C** Ileum. Lymphocytes are positive for CD3. **D** Duodenal biopsy. Glands are largely intact, but some epitheliotropism is seen (CD8 staining).

mature-appearing lymphocytes. Admixed inflammatory cells are rare, but epithelioid granulomas may be focally present, causing resemblance to Crohn disease {2571,495,2052}. The cells have a mature T-cell phenotype, positive for CD3. Most reported tumours have been positive for CD8 {2571}, and others express CD4 {495,2052}. The CD8+ tumours express TIA1, but granzyme B is generally negative. Other mature T-cell markers are expressed. All reported cases expressed TCRαβ and are negative for TCRγδ. CD56 is negative. CD103 has been reported in some cases. The proliferation rate is extremely low, with a Ki-67 proliferation index < 10% in all cases studied. Phenotypic aberrancy may be an indication of progression in recurrent lesions.

Cytology
Not clinically relevant

Diagnostic molecular pathology
Not clinically relevant

Essential and desirable diagnostic criteria
Essential: a non-destructive, non-epitheliotropic small lymphoid cell infiltrate confined to the gastrointestinal mucosa and/ or submucosa; immunophenotype: T-lineage, with TCRαβ expression; low proliferative fraction (Ki-67 proliferation index < 10%).

Staging (TNM)
Lymphoid neoplasms are staged according to the Lugano classification, which has been adopted by the eighth edition of the Union for International Cancer Control (UICC) TNM classification {596}.

Prognosis and prediction
Multiple sites in the GI tract are involved, with a chronic relapsing clinical course. A subset of patients are at risk for disease progression and more-widespread disease, usually after many years. Response to conventional chemotherapy is poor, but patients have prolonged survival with persistent disease. The presence of an aberrant T-cell phenotype in a small subset may indicate the potential for more-aggressive clinical behaviour. Additionally, cases expressing CD4 rather than CD8 appear to be at higher risk for progression, although data are limited {2571,2052,2974}.

Hepatosplenic T-cell lymphoma

Gaulard P
Jaffe ES

Definition

Hepatosplenic T-cell lymphoma (HSTL) is an aggressive extra-nodal lymphoma characterized by a proliferation of cytotoxic T cells, usually γδ T cells, with a hepatosplenic presentation and no lymphadenopathy.

ICD-O coding

9716/3 Hepatosplenic T-cell lymphoma

ICD-11 coding

2A90.8 Hepatosplenic T-cell lymphoma

Related terminology

None

Subtype(s)

None

Localization

The spleen and liver are involved, whereas lymph nodes are usually not involved. Bone marrow is consistently affected {3453,288,206}.

Clinical features

HSTL typically presents with hepatosplenomegaly and systemic symptoms. Patients usually manifest marked thrombocytopenia, often with anaemia and leukopenia. Peripheral blood involvement, which is uncommon at presentation, may occur late in the clinical course {288,667,206,3453}.

Epidemiology

HSTL is a rare form of lymphoma, reported in North America, Europe, and Asia {3497,736}. Peak incidence occurs in adolescents and young adults, with a male predominance {288,667, 206}.

Etiology

As many as 20% of HSTLs arise in the setting of chronic immune suppression, most commonly long-term immunosuppressive therapy for solid-organ transplantation or prolonged antigenic stimulation {3615,288,3454}. A number of cases have been reported in patients, especially children, with immune disorders (including Crohn disease, rheumatoid arthritis, and psoriasis) treated with azathioprine or mercaptopurine, often in combination with TNF inhibitors {1994,3159,743,3630}.

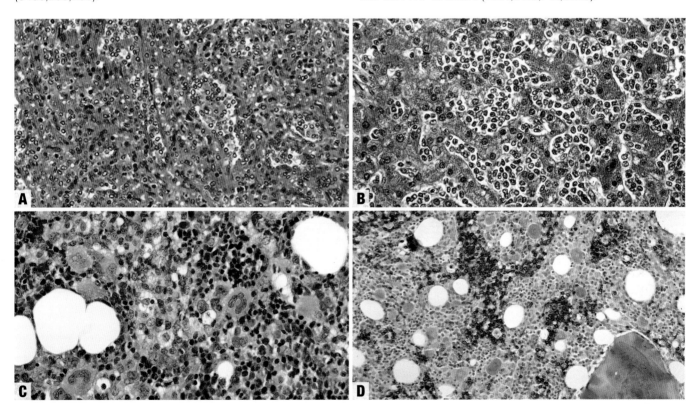

Fig. 11.23 Hepatosplenic T-cell lymphoma. **A** Cords and sinusoids of the spleen are infiltrated by a monotonous population of neoplastic lymphoid cells with medium-sized nuclei and a moderate rim of pale cytoplasm. **B** The neoplastic cells diffusely infiltrate the hepatic sinusoids. **C** The bone marrow is usually hypercellular, with neoplastic cells infiltrating sinusoids. **D** Neoplastic cells in the bone marrow are highlighted with immunohistochemistry for CD3.

Chapter 11

Pathogenesis

HSTL shows clonally rearranged TRG genes. Cases of γδ origin show a biallelic rearrangement of TRD genes. TRB genes are rearranged in αβ cases; however, unproductive rearrangements of TRB genes have been reported in some γδ cases {1018}. Isochromosome 7q is present in most cases {3586}. The common gained region mapped at 7q22 is associated with increased expression of several genes, including the multidrug resistance gene *ABCB1* {939}. Trisomy 8 may also be present. In situ hybridization for EBV is generally negative. Gene expression profiling studies have shown that HSTL exhibits a distinctive signature unifying γδ and αβ cases {3339}. Mutations in the chromatin-modifying gene *SETD2* have been reported in 62% of cases; mutations in *STAT5B* (found in 40% of cases), and more rarely in *STAT3*, indicate substantial enrichment of genes encoding the JAK/STAT pathway {2353,2105,3339}.

Macroscopic appearance

The liver and spleen show diffuse enlargement without an identifiable mass lesion.

Histopathology

The neoplastic cells of HSTL are typically monotonous, with medium-sized nuclei, small inconspicuous nucleoli, and a rim of pale cytoplasm. Some degree of pleomorphism may occasionally be seen {206}. The neoplastic cells involve the cords and sinuses of the splenic red pulp, with atrophy of the white pulp. The liver shows a predominantly sinusoidal infiltration. Neoplastic cells are nearly always present in the bone marrow, with a predominantly intrasinusoidal distribution. This may be difficult to identify without the aid of immunohistochemistry or flow cytometry. Cytological atypia with large-cell or blastic changes may be seen, especially with disease progression {3453,288, 206}.

The neoplastic cells are CD3+, CD5−, CD4−, CD8−/+, CD56+/−, and usually TCRγδ+ and TCRαβ− {667,288}. A minority of tumours are of TCRαβ type {1995,206}. The cells express TIA1 but are usually negative for granzyme B and perforin. Therefore, the cells appear to be mature, non-activated cytotoxic T cells with phenotypic aberrancy.

Cytology

Not clinically relevant

Diagnostic molecular pathology

Not clinically relevant

Essential and desirable diagnostic criteria

Essential: uniform medium-sized lymphoid cells with indistinct nucleoli; sinusoidal localization in liver, spleen, and bone marrow; cytotoxic T-cell phenotype, with TIA1 expression.
Desirable: usual expression of TCRγδ, but sometimes TCRαβ; EBV-negative.

Staging (TNM)

Lymphoid neoplasms are staged according to the Lugano classification, which has been adopted by the eighth edition of the Union for International Cancer Control (UICC) TNM classification {596}.

Prognosis and prediction

The course is aggressive. Patients may initially respond to chemotherapy, but relapses are the rule. The median survival time is < 2 years {893}. Platinum-cytarabine {288} and pentostatin have been shown to be active agents. Early use of high-dose therapy followed by allogeneic haematopoietic stem cell transplantation may improve survival {3498,3250}.

EBV+ inflammatory follicular dendritic cell sarcoma of the digestive tract

Cheuk W
Li XQ

Definition
EBV-positive inflammatory follicular dendritic cell (FDC) sarcoma is a neoplasm of spindled FDCs with a rich lymphoplasmacytic infiltrate and a consistent association with EBV.

ICD-O coding
9758/3 Follicular dendritic cell sarcoma

ICD-11 coding
2B31.Y Other specified histiocytic or dendritic cell neoplasms
XA5DY0 Liver
XA7FU9 Spleen
XA9607 Gastrointestinal tract

Related terminology
Not recommended: inflammatory pseudotumour-like follicular/fibroblastic dendritic cell sarcoma; inflammatory pseudotumour-like follicular dendritic cell tumour; follicular dendritic cell sarcoma of the inflammatory pseudotumour-like subtype; EBV-positive inflammatory pseudotumour.

Subtype(s)
None

Localization
It most frequently involves the liver or spleen and rarely the GI tract in the form of polypoid lesions {2495,1066}.

Clinical features
Patients are asymptomatic or present with abdominal discomfort, sometimes accompanied by constitutional symptoms such as malaise, weight loss, or low-grade fever. Laboratory investigations may reveal anaemia, elevated C-reactive protein, hypoalbuminaemia, hypergammaglobulinaemia, raised CA125, and (occasionally) peripheral eosinophilia {585,1891}.

Epidemiology
It occurs predominantly in young to middle-aged adults (mean age: 54.5 years), with a female predominance {1020}. A predilection for Asians is possible, given that the vast majority of cases have been reported in China, the Republic of Korea, and Japan.

Etiology
The neoplastic cells are consistently associated with clonal EBV genome {1876,2942}. It has been postulated that the tumour may arise from a common EBV-infected mesenchymal cell that differentiates along the follicular or fibroblastic dendritic cell pathway {3405}. This tumour is not associated with IgG4-related disease.

Pathogenesis
Monoclonal EBV genome with a 30 bp deletion or point mutations in exon 3 of the *LMP-1* gene has been reported {583,2942, 2979,1274}. EBV is currently assumed to be the causative agent.

Macroscopic appearance
Tumours occurring in the liver or spleen are well circumscribed and unencapsulated, consisting of fleshy tan tissue with large areas of haemorrhage and/or necrosis. Tumours involving the intestines occur as mucosal polyps with or without involvement of the muscularis.

Histopathology
The neoplastic spindled cells with poorly defined borders are inconspicuous or form loose whorled fascicles in the background

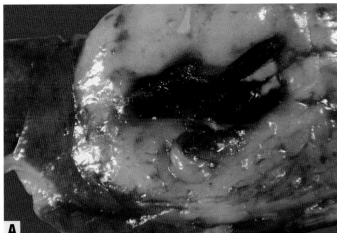
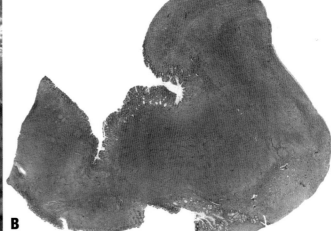

Fig. 11.24 EBV+ inflammatory follicular dendritic cell sarcoma. **A** Macroscopically, this tumour in the liver is well circumscribed and shows a fleshy cut surface with haemorrhage at the centre. **B** This histological image shows a tumour of the colon centred in the submucosa, presenting as a polyp.

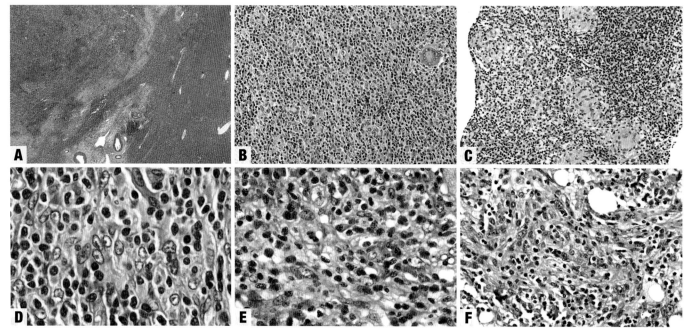

Fig. 11.25 EBV+ inflammatory follicular dendritic cell sarcoma. **A** The tumour exhibits a pushing invasive growth in the liver parenchyma. **B** The spindly tumour cells are accompanied by numerous lymphocytes and plasma cells as well as some eosinophils. A multinucleated giant cell is present. **C** Multiple small non-caseating granulomas can occur. **D** The scattered neoplastic spindled cells have oval nuclei, fine chromatin, distinct nucleoli, and eosinophilic cytoplasm with poorly defined cell borders. **E** Large numbers of lymphocytes, plasma cells, and eosinophils overshadow the scattered neoplastic cells with oval nuclei and fine chromatin. **F** Focally, the neoplastic cells form loose, whorled fascicles and have large pleomorphic nuclei.

of a prominent lymphoplasmacytic infiltrate. The nuclei show vesicular chromatin and small distinct nucleoli. Nuclear atypia is highly variable, but at least some cells with overt atypia such as enlarged, irregularly folded or hyperchromatic nuclei are always found. Some tumour cells may even resemble Reed–Sternberg cells {2942}. Necrosis and haemorrhage are often present and can be associated with histiocytic or granulomatous inflammation. In some cases, the tumour shows massive infiltration of eosinophils or numerous epithelioid granulomas {1891}. The blood vessels frequently show fibrinoid deposits in the vessel walls, a finding frequently seen in EBV-associated neoplasms.

The neoplastic cells are often positive for FDC markers, but the staining can be focal, and application of a large panel of FDC markers, such as CD21, CD35, CD23, CXCL13, D2-40, CNA.42, and clusterin, may be required. Some cases may be negative for FDC markers but express actin, raising the possibility of fibroblastic reticular cell differentiation. EBV LMP1 protein expression is found in 70% of cases.

Cytology

Cytological preparations reveal hypercellular samples with dual populations of neoplastic spindled cells and inflammatory cells.

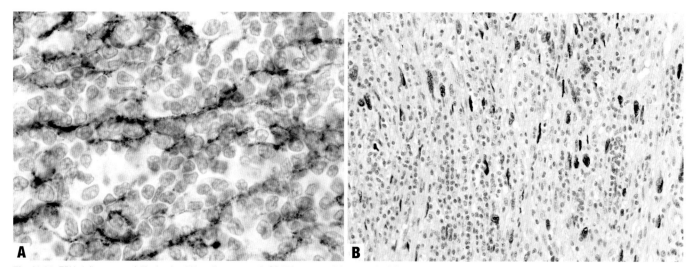

Fig. 11.26 EBV+ inflammatory follicular dendritic cell sarcoma. **A** CD35 immunostaining reveals delicate cytoplasmic processes of the tumour cells. **B** In situ hybridization for EBV-encoded small RNA (EBER) highlights tumour cells with uniform slender nuclei as well as cells with overt nuclear pleomorphism.

Tumour cells appear as syncytial groups, whorls, fascicles, or single cells with variable nuclear atypia and prominent nucleoli. Multilobated and multinucleated forms can be seen {1087}.

Diagnostic molecular pathology
In situ hybridization for EBV-encoded small RNA (EBER) is the most sensitive marker to highlight the neoplastic cells. The positively stained tumour cells typically encompass slender bland-looking nuclei as well as large pleomorphic nuclei.

Essential and desirable diagnostic criteria
Essential: atypical spindle cell proliferation accompanied by abundant lymphocytes and plasma cells; spindle cells have indistinct cell borders, vesicular chromatin, and distinct nucleoli; EBV positivity; positivity of neoplastic cells for FDC markers.

Staging (TNM)
Not clinically relevant

Prognosis and prediction
The tumour is indolent. Rare porta hepatis lymph node involvement has been reported {602}. Tumours occurring in the liver have a worse prognosis than those occurring in the spleen. Based on several series on liver tumours, the recurrence rate is 26% and the tumour mortality rate is 6% {1891,585,1020}.

Diffuse large B-cell lymphoma

Chan WC
Lai J
Nakamura S
Rosenwald A

Definition

Diffuse large B-cell lymphoma (DLBCL) is a diffuse neoplastic proliferation of large B lymphocytes lacking features of other defined types of large B-cell lymphoma.

ICD-O coding

9680/3 Diffuse large B-cell lymphoma NOS

ICD-11 coding

2A81.Z Diffuse large B-cell lymphoma NOS
XA7MC7 Stomach
XA0QT6 Ileum
XA6J68 Caecum

Related terminology

None

Subtype(s)

None

Localization

DLBCL can involve practically any part of the digestive tract but most commonly involves the stomach and ileocaecal region.

Clinical features

Patients with gastrointestinal lymphoma present with abdominal pain or discomfort or symptoms/signs related to bleeding, obstruction, or perforation. Regional nodes may be involved, but when widespread systemic disease is present, it is difficult to be sure that the patient has primary gastrointestinal lymphoma. B symptoms may be present.

Patients with liver lymphoma present with abdominal pain or mass, sometimes accompanied by constitutional symptoms {413,2387,2462}.

Epidemiology

The GI tract is the most frequent site of involvement in extra-nodal lymphomas, accounting for 30–40% of all cases {968, 2466}. DLBCL is the most common type of lymphoma, and it accounts for 55–69% of lymphomas occurring in various sites in the GI tract {1664}. In the GI tract, this lymphoma type occurs predominantly in middle-aged to elderly patients, with a median age in the seventh decade of life. There is a slight male predilection {1664}.

Etiology

Patients with immunodeficiency are more prone to develop DLBCL, and the tumour may be EBV-positive, in which case the classification should change to EBV-positive DLBCL NOS.

Pathogenesis

The mutation landscape of DLBCL is fairly well defined, although the studies are not specifically focused on gastrointestinal tumours. The profiles of germinal-centre B-cell (GCB)

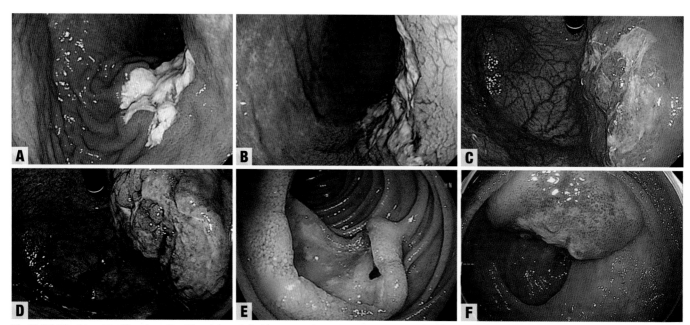

Fig. 11.27 Primary gastric diffuse large B-cell lymphoma. **A** Endoscopy reveals an ulcerative lesion, which is highlighted by the spraying of indigo carmine (**B**). **C** Endoscopy reveals a large tumorous lesion, with the image enhanced by the spraying of indigo carmine (**D**). **E** Endoscopy reveals an ulcerative lesion in the jejunum. **F** Endoscopy reveals a polypoid lesion in the rectum.

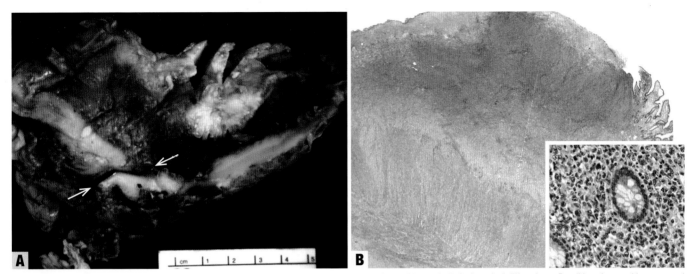

Fig. 11.28 Diffuse large B-cell lymphoma. **A** Sigmoid colon with a large tumour mass that perforated (arrows). **B** An intestinal diffuse large B-cell lymphoma with transmural infiltration of large lymphoma cells and surface ulceration.

and activated B-cell (ABC) DLBCL overlap, but a number of mutations are preferentially associated with each subtype {2671,2541}. DLBCLs can also be divided into genetic subgroups based on their mutations, with different biological and prognostic significance {2899,564}. *BCL2*, *BCL6*, and *MYC* translocations are relatively frequent, and double-hit (*MYC* with either *BCL2* or *BCL6*) and triple-hit cases are now classified as high-grade B-cell lymphoma with *MYC* and *BCL2* and/or *BCL6* rearrangements {3189}.

BCL6 rearrangement is present in about 25% of DLBCL cases, more commonly in ABC DLBCL {1383}. *BCL2* rearrangement occurs almost exclusively in GCB DLBCL and is associated

with BCL2 expression {1384}. BCL2 is frequently expressed in ABC DLBCL but is unrelated to *BCL2* translocation {1384}. Mutations of epigenetic modifiers, NF-κB pathway regulators, the B-cell receptor signalling pathway, the PI3K/AKT/mTOR pathway, immunosurveillance factors, differentiation (*BCL6*, *PRDM1*), and *TP53* are common {2541,2671}.

Macroscopic appearance

Gastrointestinal DLBCL often takes the form of a solitary infiltrative fleshy tumour mass with ulceration of the mucosa. It usually shows transmural infiltration {1188,799}.

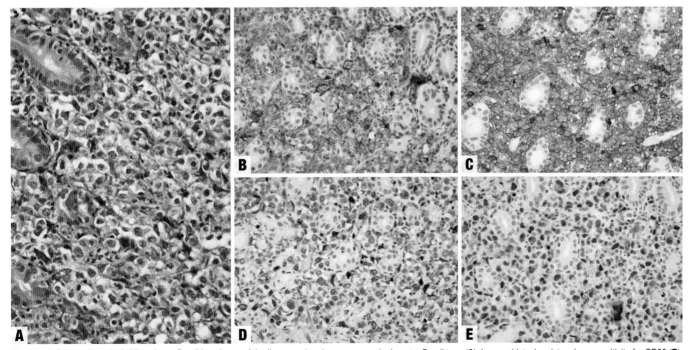

Fig. 11.29 Primary intestinal diffuse large B-cell lymphoma of the ileocaecal region, non–germinal-centre B-cell type (**A**). Immunohistochemistry shows positivity for CD20 (**B**), PDL1 (**C**), BCL2 (**D**), and IRF4 (MUM1) (**E**).

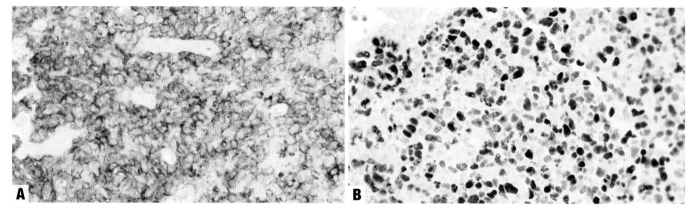

Fig. 11.30 Diffuse large B-cell lymphoma, germinal-centre B-cell type. Strong expression of CD10 (**A**) and BCL6 (**B**).

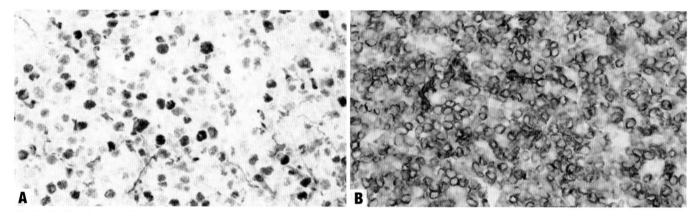

Fig. 11.31 Diffuse large B-cell lymphoma. A double expressor of MYC (**A**) and BCL2 (**B**).

DLBCL of the liver usually takes the form of a large solitary fleshy mass or multiple masses. Rarely, it shows diffuse liver involvement resulting in hepatomegaly {2920,413,3783,2429,2462}.

Histopathology

The morphology is similar to that of nodal disease showing sheets of large cells with high proliferation (Ki-67 proliferation index generally > 40%). Most of the tumour cells may resemble centroblasts or immunoblasts and rarely may be anaplastic.

The lymphoma cells should express one or more B-cell markers (CD19, CD20, CD79a, PAX5, or surface/cytoplasmic immunoglobulin). If there is suspicion of a follicular component,

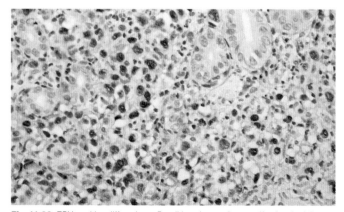

Fig. 11.32 EBV-positive diffuse large B-cell lymphoma. A case affecting the jejunum, showing EBV infection by in situ hybridization for EBV-encoded small RNA (EBER).

immunostaining for follicular dendritic cell markers is helpful. A component of extranodal marginal zone lymphoma of mucosa-associated lymphoid tissue (MALT lymphoma) may also be detected in some DLBCLs and should be noted. GCB DLBCLs are more often positive for CD10, GCET1, and LMO2, whereas the ABC type is generally strongly positive for IRF4 (MUM1) and FOXP1. Strong BCL6 positivity with weak or negative IRF4 staining favours a GCB subtype. mRNA profiling {2921} has been reported to have higher accuracy and reproducibility in cell-of-origin subtyping of DLBCL. Strong MYC and BCL2 expression (double expressor) has been found to be associated with a worse prognosis in some studies {1474,2570}. The presence of EBV may not be suggested morphologically or clinically, and requires in situ hybridization for EBV-encoded small RNA (EBER) {1396}.

Cytology

Not clinically relevant

Diagnostic molecular pathology

Not clinically relevant

Essential and desirable diagnostic criteria

Essential: diffuse infiltrate of atypical large lymphoid cells; immunoreactivity for B-lineage markers; lack of immunoreactivity for EBV.

Staging (TNM)

Lymphoid neoplasms are staged according to the Lugano classification, which has been adopted by the eighth edition of the Union for International Cancer Control (UICC) TNM classification {596}. Because of the special anatomical location of DLBCL, several attempts have been made to include important information unique to the site of involvement utilizing some modifications of the TNM system {2802A}.

Prognosis and prediction

Primary extranodal DLBCLs generally have a tendency to localize in their anatomical sites and are prognostically more favourable than nodal equivalents. The International Prognostic Index (IPI) is a robust prognosticator. The ABC DLBCL subtype has worse prognosis than the GCB subtype. Stromal signatures may have prognostic power independent of the subtype distinction {1855}. Many other markers have been reported to be predictive of survival (although the findings are not consistent). These include *MYC* translocation {3626}, CD5 expression {2180}, CD30 expression (excluding EBV-positive cases) {1317}, LMO2 expression {2320}, and double MYC/ BCL2 expressor status. *TP53* mutation {3627} and *CDKN2A* deletion, particularly in combination with trisomy 3 {1856}, are associated with poorer survival. There are some biomarkers that may predict response to targeted therapy such as BTK inhibition {3571}.

Follicular lymphoma

Ott G
Yoshino T

Definition
Follicular lymphoma (FL) is a malignant lymphoid neoplasm of follicular-centre B cells, typically showing follicular architecture.

ICD-O coding
9690/3 Follicular lymphoma NOS

ICD-11 coding
2A80.0 Follicular lymphoma grade 1
2A80.1 Follicular lymphoma grade 2
2A80.2 Follicular lymphoma grade 3
2A80.Z Follicular lymphoma, unspecified

Related terminology
None

Subtype(s)
Follicular lymphoma, grade 1 (9695/3); follicular lymphoma, grade 2 (9691/3); follicular lymphoma, grade 3A (9698/3); follicular lymphoma, grade 3B (9698/3)

Localization
Primary digestive tract FL occurs most often in the small and large intestines, whereas its occurrence in the stomach, liver {1064}, pancreas, and biliary ducts {2039} is rare. By definition, it is set apart from duodenal-type FL {2894,3216,3214}.

Clinical features
The clinical features depend on the localization of the tumour. Lymphomas in the small or large intestine may cause abdominal discomfort, intestinal obstruction, or intestinal bleeding if ulcerated, whereas FL of the biliary tract may cause jaundice. However, many localized digestive tract FLs are incidentally detected.

Epidemiology
Primary FLs of the GI tract are rare and constitute < 4% of primary GI tract lymphomas. However, the GI tract is the most commonly involved site in which primary extranodal FLs are diagnosed {1417}. The tumours are rare in the liver and pancreatobiliary system. Primary GI tract FLs are usually diagnosed in middle-aged patients, with a mean patient age of 50 years.

Etiology
Unknown

Pathogenesis
The findings of ongoing hypermutations and selective usage of IGHV (VH) gene segments suggest an underlying antigen-driven pathogenesis {3218}. The expression of characteristic homing factors points to the importance of local factors in the maintenance of localized disease {296}.

Genetic analyses have shown ongoing somatic hypermutations in most cases {3217}. The FL hallmark translocation t(14;18), which results in fusion of *BCL2* and IGH genes, is detected in about 90% of gastrointestinal FLs, a frequency very similar to that in nodal FL.

Macroscopic appearance
Not clinically relevant

Histopathology
Unlike duodenal-type FL, primary FL in the hollow gut usually presents with transmural infiltration of the organ wall. Multiple polyps in the small or large intestine (lymphomatous polyposis) may also be seen. The diagnosis requires recognition of at least partly follicular proliferation of centroblasts and centrocytes, and most cases are indistinguishable from their nodal counterparts.

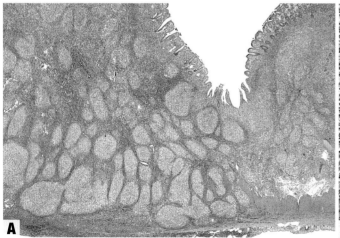
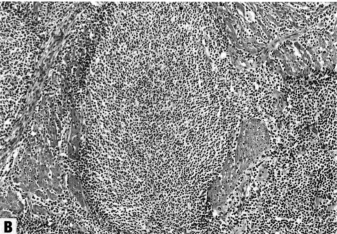

Fig. 11.33 Primary intestinal follicular lymphoma. **A** The small bowel shows transmural replacement by closely packed abnormal lymphoid follicles. **B** The lymphoid follicles are neoplastic, as evidenced by the lack of mantle, lack of tingible-body macrophages, predominance of centrocytes, and lack of polarity.

They grow in atypical follicular structures that usually lack the zonation phenomenon and starry-sky pattern characteristic of reactive follicles, and the follicles are often crowded. Most cases are of grade 1 or 2. Sclerosis may be present.

The immunohistochemical profile is similar to that of FL in general. The FL cells express the B-cell–associated markers CD19, CD20, and/or PAX5 and are positive for CD10, BCL6, and BCL2; rare cases may be CD5-positive. FLs arising primarily in the GI tract, especially the stomach and colorectum, often downregulate CD10 and BCL6 expression {2427}. Unlike in duodenal-type FL, follicular dendritic cell meshworks are well preserved and similar to those of typical nodal FLs {3218}.

Cytology
Not clinically relevant

Diagnostic molecular pathology
The FL hallmark translocation t(14;18), which results in fusion of BCL2 and IGH genes, is detected in about 90% of cases and may be helpful in the diagnosis of problematic cases.

Essential and desirable diagnostic criteria
Essential: lymphoid proliferation with cytological features of follicular-centre cells (centrocytes and centroblasts); at least focal atypical follicle formation (crowding, lack of polarization, lack of tingible-body macrophages); B-lineage neoplasm with expression of follicular-centre cell markers (CD10, BCL6); follicles BCL2-positive.

Staging (TNM)
A diagnosis of FL in the stomach, small intestine, colorectum, or hepatobiliary system primarily warrants the exclusion of systemic disease. Most cases are localized, but regional lymph node involvement is not rare. Lymphomatous polyposis is a special type of spread that may occur throughout the hollow gut. Lymphoid neoplasms are staged according to the Lugano classification, which has been adopted by the eighth edition of the Union for International Cancer Control (UICC) TNM classification {596}.

Prognosis and prediction
Histological transformation of gastrointestinal FL is extremely rare (as compared with nodal FL), and only few cases have been reported so far {3263}.

Mantle cell lymphoma

Campo E
Seto M

Definition
Mantle cell lymphoma (MCL) is a mature B-cell neoplasm usually composed of monomorphic small to medium-sized lymphoid cells with irregular nuclear contours that commonly express CD5 and in > 95% of tumours carry the t(11;14)(q13;q32) translocation leading to cyclin D1 overexpression.

ICD-O coding
9673/3 Mantle cell lymphoma

ICD-11 coding
2A85.5 Mantle cell lymphoma

Related terminology
None

Subtype(s)
Conventional mantle cell lymphoma; leukaemic non-nodal mantle cell lymphoma

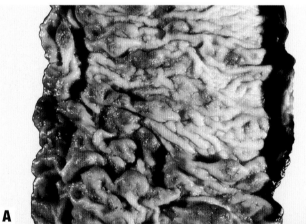

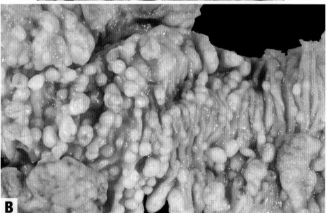

Fig. 11.34 Mantle cell lymphoma involving the colon (multiple lymphomatous polyposis). **A,B** Closer view showing numerous small polypoid mucosal lesions.

Localization
Lymph nodes are the most commonly involved site in conventional MCL (cMCL), although extranodal involvement is frequent. Subclinical tumour cell infiltration of the GI tract is common in patients with MCL {2828,2749}. Superficial ulcers, large tumour masses, and diffuse thickening of the gastrointestinal mucosa may be seen {959}. Presentation as multiple intestinal polyps (multiple lymphomatous polyposis) is distinctive, although not specific for MCL {1718,2238}. Circulating cells in leukaemic non-nodal MCL (nnMCL) may reversibly infiltrate extranodal inflammatory sites (e.g. *Helicobacter pylori*–associated gastritis) {876}.

Clinical features
Most patients present with stage III/IV disease with lymphadenopathy and bone marrow involvement. Extranodal involvement usually occurs in association with lymphadenopathy. nnMCL presents as isolated bone marrow and blood involvement, sometimes accompanied by splenomegaly; nodal dissemination may occur with clinical progression.

Epidemiology
MCL accounts for 3–10% of all lymphoid neoplasms. It is more common in males than females (> 2:1), with a median patient age of about 60 years.

Etiology
Unknown

Pathogenesis
The t(11;14)(q13;q32) translocation between an IGH gene and *CCND1* is present in > 95% of cases of MCL, and this is considered the primary genetic event. The translocation results in deregulated overexpression of *CCND1* mRNA and the cyclin D1 protein. The cases of MCL lacking *CCND1* translocation show *CCND2* (~75%) or *CCND3* translocations, usually with an IG partner, often either IGK or IGL {3191}.

cMCL shows complex karyotypes, particularly in blastoid/pleomorphic subtypes. nnMCL shows few genetic alterations other than t(11;14). Frequently mutated genes in cMCL include *ATM* (40–75%), *KMT2D* (14–18%), and *NOTCH1* or *NOTCH2* (5–12%) {2617}. *CDKN2A* deletions/mutations (20–25%) in cMCL and *TP53* mutations (15–35%) in both cMCL and nnMCL are associated with high proliferation and aggressive behaviour {875}.

Macroscopic appearance
There may be subclinical tumour cell infiltration of the GI tract or superficial ulcers, large tumour masses, and diffuse thickening of the gastrointestinal mucosa. Presentation as multiple intestinal polyps (multiple lymphomatous polyposis) is distinctive but not specific.

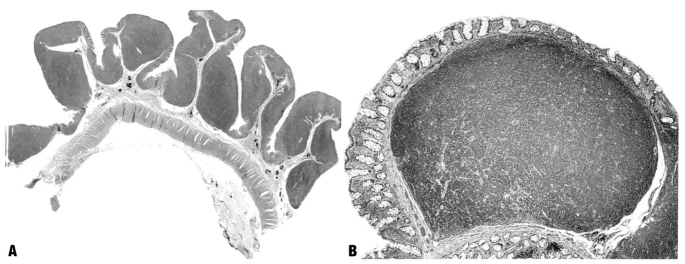

Fig. 11.35 Mantle cell lymphoma involving the colon. **A** Polypoid lesions involving the lamina propria and submucosa. **B** Predominantly infiltrating the submucosa, causing a polypoid lesion.

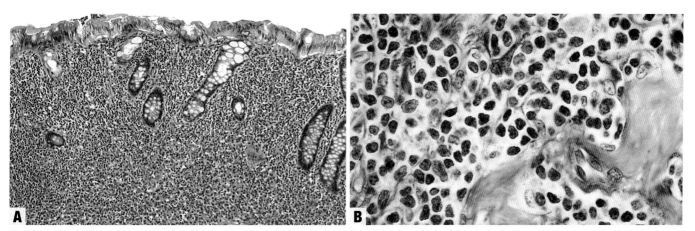

Fig. 11.36 Mantle cell lymphoma of the colon. **A** Low power. **B** High power demonstrating a homogeneous population of cells that resemble centrocytes (PAS staining).

Histopathology

Classic MCL is a monomorphic proliferation of small-intermediate lymphoid cells with scant cytoplasm and irregular nuclei that have dispersed chromatin and inconspicuous nucleoli. The tumour may show a mantle zone and a nodular or diffuse growth pattern. Tumour cells may have a spectrum of cytological subtypes. The small cell subtype is more common in nnMCL and shows round nuclei mimicking chronic lymphocytic leukaemia, but without nucleolated cells. The blastoid subtype is characterized by intermediate-sized cells with round nuclei and finely dispersed chromatin, mimicking lymphoblasts, and numerous mitoses. The pleomorphic subtype shows large irregular nuclei with nucleoli.

Mantle cell neoplasia in situ is characterized by the presence of cyclin D1–positive cells restricted to the mantle zone of otherwise reactive follicles. When mantle cell neoplasia in situ is found incidentally, progression to overt MCL is uncommon {1531}.

MCL cells express mature B-cell markers (CD20, CD79a), CD5, and CD43. CD10/BCL6 and CD23 are usually negative. Nuclear cyclin D1 is expressed in > 95% of MCLs, including those that are CD5-negative. SOX11 is expressed in cMCL but is negative in nnMCL. LEF1 is negative but may be expressed

in the blastoid and pleomorphic subtypes. CD200 is negative in cMCL, but it is expressed in 40–90% of nnMCL cases {2617}. The subset of cyclin D1–negative MCL shows the same morphology, phenotype, and clinical features as cyclin D1–positive cases, including SOX11 expression {2831}.

Cytology

Not clinically relevant

Diagnostic molecular pathology

The t(11;14)(q13;q32) translocation between an IGH gene and *CCND1* is present in > 95% of cases of MCL, and it is a desirable diagnostic criterion if other features are absent.

Essential and desirable diagnostic criteria

Essential: diffuse, nodular to mantle zone proliferation of small to medium-sized cells with irregular nuclear contours, dispersed chromatin, and inconspicuous nucleoli – blastoid and pleomorphic subtypes will show different cytological features; B-cell neoplasm with expression of CD5 and cyclin D1; SOX11 often positive.

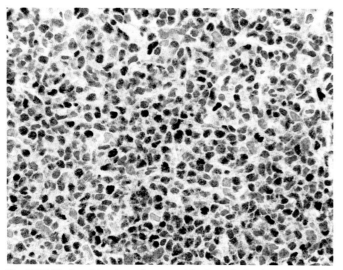

Fig. 11.37 Mantle cell lymphoma. Immunostaining for cyclin D1 shows nuclear positivity.

Desirable: morphological features suggestive of MCL and CD5-positive but cyclin D1–negative: diagnosis to be confirmed by SOX11 positivity and/or *CCND2/3* translocations.

Staging (TNM)

Lymphoid neoplasms are staged according to the Lugano classification, which has been adopted by the eighth edition of the Union for International Cancer Control (UICC) TNM classification {596}.

Prognosis and prediction

Proliferative activity is the most important independent prognostic parameter in MCL {1288}. The Ki-67 proliferation index adds value to the Mantle Cell Lymphoma International Prognostic Index (MIPI) {1287}. Genomic complexity confers poor outcome {644}.

Burkitt lymphoma

Leoncini L
Siebert R

Definition

Burkitt lymphoma (BL) is a highly aggressive B-cell lymphoma characterized by frequent presentation in extranodal sites or as an acute leukaemia, with high proliferative activity and usually *MYC* gene translocation to an IG locus.

ICD-O coding

9687/3 Burkitt lymphoma NOS

ICD-11 coding

2A85.6 Burkitt lymphoma, including Burkitt leukaemia

Related terminology

Acceptable: Burkitt cell leukaemia (9826/3).

Not recommended: Burkitt tumour; malignant lymphoma, undifferentiated, Burkitt type; malignant lymphoma, small non-cleaved, Burkitt type.

Subtype(s)

Endemic Burkitt lymphoma; sporadic Burkitt lymphoma; immunodeficiency-associated Burkitt lymphoma

Localization

In the GI tract, the most frequent site of involvement is the ileocaecal region, followed by the stomach, small intestine, and ascending colon.

Clinical features

Patients often present with bulky disease and high tumour burden due to the short doubling time of the tumour. Specific clinical manifestations at presentation vary according to the epidemiological subtype and the site of involvement. The most frequent presentation of the sporadic subtype is abdominal involvement. In gastrointestinal BL, the most common symptoms are vomiting, abdominal pain, constipation, weight loss, and progressive anaemia. Fatal haemorrhage, jejunal intussusception, and jaundice (with pancreatic localization) may also occur.

Epidemiology

Endemic BL occurs in equatorial Africa and in Papua New Guinea, with a distribution that overlaps with regions endemic for malaria. In these areas, BL is the most common childhood malignancy, with an incidence peak among children aged 4–7 years and an M:F ratio of 2:1 {447,3610}.

Sporadic BL is seen throughout the world, mainly in children and young adults {2095}. The incidence is low, with sporadic BL accounting for only 1–2% of all lymphomas in western Europe and the USA. In these parts of the world, BL accounts for approximately 30–50% of all childhood lymphomas. The median age of adult patients is 30 years, but an incidence peak has also been reported in elderly patients {2095}. The M:F ratio is 2:1 to 3:1.

Immunodeficiency-associated BL is more common in the setting of HIV infection than in other forms of inborn or acquired immunodeficiency. In HIV-infected patients, BL appears early in the evolution of the disease, when CD4+ T-cell counts are still high {1996,2655}.

Etiology

A number of infectious agents (e.g. EBV, *Plasmodium falciparum*, and HIV), environmental factors, and genetic predispositions (e.g. germline mutations in *ATM*, *BLM*, or *SH2D1A*) are known etiological cofactors.

Pathogenesis

In endemic BL, the EBV genome is present in > 95% of cases. There is also a strong epidemiological link with holoendemic malaria. Therefore, EBV and *P. falciparum* are considered to be associated with endemic BL {741,1475}. Recent data have provided new insight into how these two human pathogens interact to cause the disease, supporting the emerging concepts of polymicrobial disease pathogenesis {592,2201,2418,2645, 2734}. The polymicrobial nature of endemic BL is further supported by the status of B-cell receptor, which carries the signs of antigen selection due to chronic antigen stimulation {121,2579}.

In sporadic BL, EBV can be detected in as many as 20–30% of cases {2000}; however, more-sensitive tools are able to identify EBV infection in a higher percentage of cases {2244}. The proportion of EBV-positive sporadic BL cases appears to be much higher in adults than in children {2864}.

In immunodeficiency-associated BL, EBV is identified in 25–40% of cases {1153,2745}.

The variation in EBV association among the different forms of BL and among different countries makes it difficult to determine the role of the virus in BL pathogenesis. EBV may affect host cell homeostasis in various ways by encoding its own genes and microRNAs and by interfering with cellular microRNA expression {123,1551,1865,2580,3463}. However, recent studies have shown that the mutation and viral landscape of BL is more complex than previously reported. In fact, a distinct latency pattern of EBV involving the expression of LMP2A along with that of lytic genes has been demonstrated (non-canonical latency programme) {195,3311}. Nonetheless, expression of the latency pattern in BL is heterogeneous, not only from case to case, but also within a given case from cell to cell, suggesting that the tumour is under selective pressure and needs alternative mechanisms to survive and proliferate. The inverse correlation between the EBV viral load and the number of somatic mutations suggests that these mutations may substitute for the virus in maintaining the neoplastic phenotype {1044,2}.

The molecular hallmark of BL is the translocation of *MYC* at band 8q24 to the IGH locus on chromosome 14q32, t(8;14) (q24;q32), or less commonly to the IGK light chain locus on 2p12 [t(2;8)] or the IGL light chain locus on 22q11 [t(8;22)].

Chapter 11

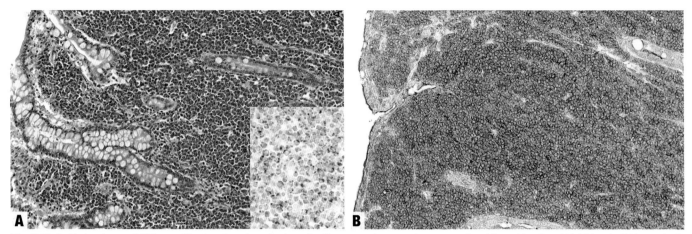

Fig. 11.38 Burkitt lymphoma. **A** Diffuse proliferation of regular, cohesive cells with a starry-sky pattern is present; adipophilin staining (**inset**) highlights the lipid vacuoles in paraffin sections. **B** The neoplastic cells are CD10-positive.

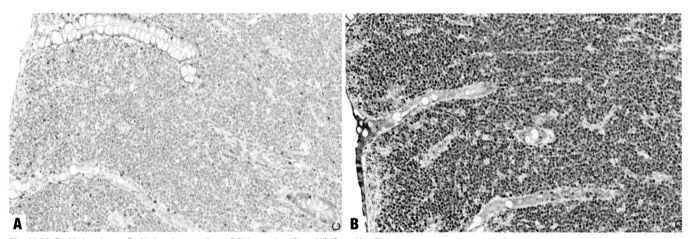

Fig. 11.39 Burkitt lymphoma. Burkitt lymphoma cells are BCL2-negative (**A**) and MYC-positive (**B**).

Most breakpoints originate from class switching or aberrant somatic hypermutation mediated by the activity of the mutagenic enzyme activation-induced cytidine deaminase. Additional chromosomal abnormalities may also occur in BL, including gains of 1q, 7, and 12 and losses of 6q, 13q32-q34, and 17p. Approximately 10% of classic BL cases lack an identifiable *MYC* rearrangement {1168,1335,1865}. However, none of the techniques currently used to detect genetic changes can unambiguously rule out all *MYC* translocations. The expression of *MYC* mRNA and MYC protein in these cases suggests that alternative mechanisms deregulating *MYC* also exist {2451, 2905}. In these cases, strict clinical, morphological, and phenotypic criteria should be used to exclude lymphomas that mimic BL. At least some of these cases represent the new provisional entity Burkitt-like lymphoma with 11q aberrations {2830}.

Next-generation sequencing analysis has revealed the importance of the B-cell receptor signalling pathway in the pathogenesis of BL. Mutations of the transcription factor *TCF3* (*E2A*) or its negative regulator *ID3* have been reported in about 70% of sporadic BL cases. These mutations activate B-cell receptor signalling, which sustains BL cell survival by engaging the PI3K pathway {1950,2711,2900,2840}. Mutations of *MYC*, *CCND3*, *TP53*, *RHOA*, *SMARCA4*, and *ARID1A* are other recurrent mutations, found in 5–40% of BL cases {1044}. The numbers of mutations

overall and mutations in *TCF3* or *ID3* are lower in endemic BL than in sporadic BL {2}.

Macroscopic appearance

Soft, tan, fleshy tumours with haemorrhage and necrosis infiltrate the bowel and/or involved organs.

Histopathology

BL is characterized by a diffuse monotonous infiltrate of medium-sized lymphoid cells. The cells appear to be cohesive but often exhibit squared-off borders of retracted cytoplasm. The nuclei are round with finely clumped chromatin, and they contain multiple basophilic medium-sized paracentrally located nucleoli. The cytoplasm is deeply basophilic and usually contains lipid vacuoles, which are better seen in imprint preparations or FNA specimens. The characteristic lipid vacuoles can also be demonstrated by immunostaining for adipophilin {124}. The tumour has an extremely high proliferation rate, with many mitotic figures, as well as a high rate of spontaneous cell death (apoptosis). A starry-sky pattern is usually present, as a result of the presence of numerous tingible-body macrophages.

The tumour cells typically express moderate to strong membrane IgM with light chain restriction, B-cell antigens (CD19, CD20, CD22, CD79a, and PAX5) and germinal-centre markers

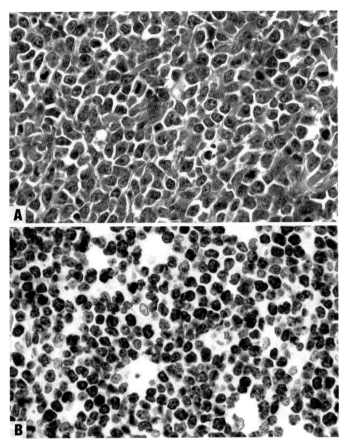

Fig. 11.40 Burkitt lymphoma. **A** This example shows slightly greater nuclear irregularity. **B** Immunohistochemistry shows strong and homogeneous positivity for Ki-67 by MIB1 antibody staining.

(CD10 and BCL6). CD38, CD77, and CD43 are also frequently positive {252,1768,2312}. Almost all BLs show strong expression of MYC protein in the majority of neoplastic cells {122}. The proliferation rate is very high, with nearly 100% of the cells positive for Ki-67. The neoplastic cells are usually negative for CD5, CD23, CD138, and BCL2. However, BCL2 expression in a variable number of cells may be observed. This immunophenotype

may be more variable in sporadic BL in older patients and at extranodal sites {252}. TdT is negative, allowing differential diagnosis from pre-B acute lymphoblastic leukaemia with *MYC* translocation {2312,788}.

Cytology

In cytology or touch imprint preparations, the nuclei are round with fine chromatin, multiple nucleoli, and mitotic figures. The cytoplasm is basophilic and contains numerous lipid vacuoles.

Diagnostic molecular pathology

The presence of translocations involving *MYC* can provide helpful diagnostic information in cases of doubt, but it is rarely required for diagnosis. These translocations are usually of band 8q24 to the IGH locus on chromosome 14q32, t(8;14)(q24;q32), or less commonly to the IGK light chain locus on 2p12 [t(2;8)] or the IGL light chain locus on 22q11 [t(8;22)]. Approximately 10% of classic BL cases lack an identifiable *MYC* rearrangement {1168,1335,1865}.

Gene and microRNA expression profiling can define molecular signatures that are characteristic of BL and different from those of other lymphomas, such as diffuse large B-cell lymphoma {722,1335}. Slight differences in the expression profiles have been identified between the endemic BL and sporadic BL subtypes {2579,1857}.

Essential and desirable diagnostic criteria

Classic features

Essential: diffuse monotonous infiltrate of medium-sized lymphoid cells with squared-off contours, round nuclei with finely clumped chromatin, multiple nucleoli, and basophilic cytoplasm; numerous mitotic figures and apoptotic bodies; immunophenotype: B-lineage marker–positive, CD10-positive, BCL2-negative, MYC protein expression in > 80% of neoplastic cells, near 100% Ki-67 proliferation index.

Cases with deviations from the above-listed features

Essential: when morphology or immunophenotype is atypical and/or MYC protein expression is present in < 80% of neoplastic cells, additional testing is required to confirm a diagnosis

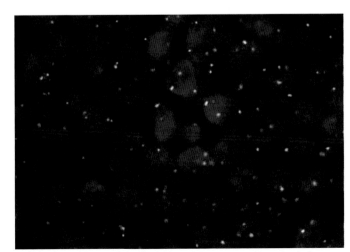

Fig. 11.41 Burkitt lymphoma. Break-apart FISH probes for *MYC* show one allele with colocalization of both probes (red and green) and one allele with separation of the probes.

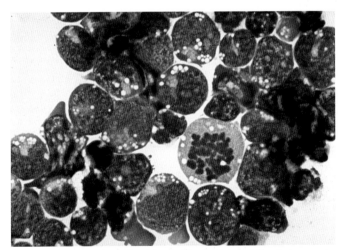

Fig. 11.42 Burkitt lymphoma. Touch imprint. The deeply basophilic cytoplasm can be appreciated, as can abundant lipid vacuoles in the cytoplasm.

of BL: FISH analysis for *MYC*, *BCL2*, *BCL6* rearrangements, and 11q abnormality to exclude high-grade B-cell lymphoma with *MYC* and *BCL2* and/or *BCL6* rearrangements, high-grade B-cell lymphoma NOS, and Burkitt-like lymphoma with 11q abnormality.

Staging (TNM)
Paediatric BL is staged according to the system of Murphy et al. {2253}. A revised International Pediatric Non-Hodgkin Lymphoma Staging System (IPNHLSS) has recently been proposed {2758}.

Prognosis and prediction
BL is a highly aggressive but potentially curable tumour; intensive chemotherapy can result in long-term overall survival in 70–90% of patients, with children doing better than adults. Adverse prognostic factors include advanced-stage disease, bone marrow and CNS involvement, unresected tumour > 10 cm in diameter, and high serum LDH levels {2162,527,438}. The overall survival rate in endemic BL has improved from no more than 10–20% to almost 70% as a result of the introduction of the International Network for Cancer Treatment and Research (INCTR) protocol INCTR 03-06 in African institutions {2342}.

Plasmablastic lymphoma

Campo E
Montes-Moreno S

Definition
Plasmablastic lymphoma (PBL) is an aggressive lymphoma composed of large B cells with plasmablastic and immunoblastic morphology, exhibiting a terminal B-cell differentiation phenotype with downregulation of mature B-cell markers and expression of plasma cell–associated antigens.

ICD-O coding
9735/3 Plasmablastic lymphoma

ICD-11 coding
2A81.2 Plasmablastic lymphoma

Related terminology
None

Subtype(s)
None

Localization
PBL usually involves extranodal locations such as the nasal/oral cavity (~50%), digestive system (~20%), bone and soft tissues (~15%), and skin (~5%). PBL can affect any portion of the GI tract, with predilection for the anorectal area, stomach, and intestines. The liver and gallbladder can rarely be involved {525, 1940,1799,2203,2202}.

Clinical features
PBL presents as a local mass, but disseminated stage III/IV disease is present at diagnosis in 75% of HIV-positive patients, 50% of posttransplant patients, and 25% of patients without apparent immunodeficiency {525}. Uncommonly, large B-cell lymphomas with plasmablastic characteristics may transform from previous follicular lymphoma, chronic lymphocytic leukaemia, and other small B-cell lymphomas {2064,2497,2468}.

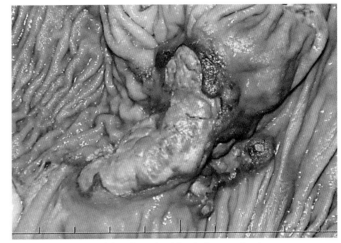

Fig. 11.44 Plasmablastic lymphoma involving the ileocaecal region.

Epidemiology
PBL is more common in males than females (3:1) and accounts for approximately 1% of all large B-cell lymphomas and 2% of HIV-related lymphomas {525,2631}. Most cases are associated with immunodeficiency due to HIV infection (31–62%) or immunosuppressive therapy for bone marrow or solid organ transplantation or autoimmune diseases (3–7%). PBL may also occur in apparently immunocompetent patients (27–55%), who are usually older (mean age: 59 years; range: 45–92 years) than HIV-positive patients, with presumptive immunosenescence {525,1940,1799,2203,2225}. Rarely, PBL can occur in children.

Etiology
Immune deficiency is a predisposing factor in a substantial fraction of patients.

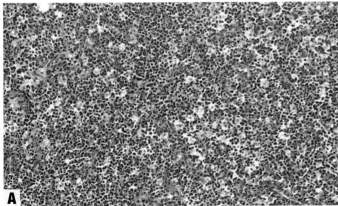

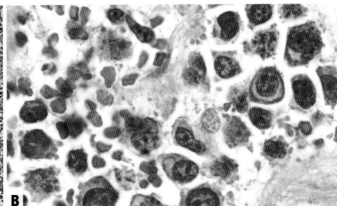

Fig. 11.43 Plasmablastic lymphoma. **A** The tumour has a prominent starry-sky pattern. **B** Neoplastic cells are atypical immunoblasts and plasmablasts with vesicular nuclei, prominent nucleoli, and basophilic cytoplasm with a paranuclear pale-staining Golgi zone.

Chapter 11

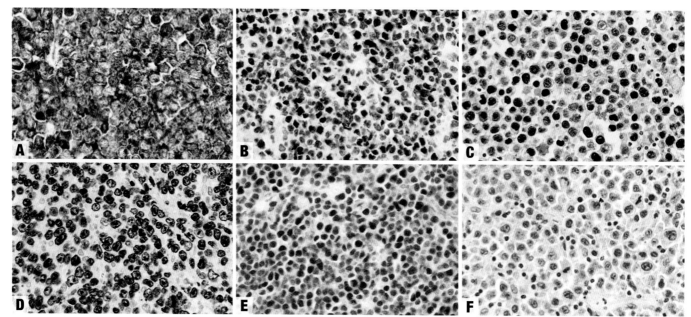

Fig. 11.45 Plasmablastic lymphoma. **A** The cells are positive for CD138. **B** The cells are positive for IRF4 (MUM1). **C** In situ hybridization for EBV-encoded small RNA (EBER) is frequently positive. **D** The Ki-67 proliferation index is usually > 90%. **E** MYC protein is overexpressed. **F** The lymphoma cells are negative for B-cell markers, such as CD20.

Pathogenesis

IGHV genes are clonally rearranged and may be either mutated or unmutated {998}. *MYC* translocations, usually with IG genes, are more frequent in HIV-positive patients (80%) than HIV-negative patients (40–60%). *MYC* gains/amplifications are uncommon {2225,3401}. Karyotypes are usually complex. Combined *MYC* and *BCL2* or *BCL6* translocations have only been seen in cases transformed from previous follicular lymphoma {355, 3199,3401,2468}. *PRDM1*/Blimp1 mutations have been found in 45% of tumours {2203}; Blimp1 is the master regulator of plasma cell differentiation. Gene expression profiling has demonstrated downregulation of B-cell receptor signalling genes and upregulation of *MYC* and genes involved in plasma cell differentiation {563A}.

Macroscopic appearance

Not clinically relevant

Histopathology

PBL is characterized by a diffuse infiltration of large atypical immunoblasts and plasmablasts. Lymphoplasmacytoid and plasma cells may constitute a minor component in some cases. A prominent starry-sky pattern and abundant mitotic figures are common. Necrosis and granulomatous reaction may be seen.

The tumour cells are virtually CD20-negative and have reduced/absent expression of PAX5 and CD45. CD79a is positive in 40% of cases. IRF4 (MUM1) is constantly positive. Plasma cell markers (CD138, CD38, VS38c, Blimp1, and XBP1) are found in the majority of cases {525,2203,2202,2225}. Light chain restriction can usually be demonstrated. MYC protein is overexpressed in the vast majority of cases, irrespective of the presence or absence of *MYC* translocation. The Ki-67 proliferation index is usually > 90% {1940,2203}. PDL1 overexpression

and loss or aberrant expression of MHC class II have been demonstrated in a variable number of cases {1799,2895}. CD10, CD56, and CD30 are positive in 20–30% of cases. BCL6 is usually negative. EBV-encoded small RNA (EBER) is more frequently positive in HIV-infected patients (82%) than in other individuals (40–60%). EBV LMP1 is usually negative. ALK protein and HHV8 are negative {525}.

Cytology

Not clinically relevant

Diagnostic molecular pathology

Not clinically relevant

Essential and desirable diagnostic criteria

Essential: lymphoma with immunoblastic or plasmablastic morphology; immunophenotypic features of terminal B-cell differentiation (loss of conventional B-cell markers, especially CD20 and PAX5, and expression of plasma cell markers); lack of ALK expression; HHV8-negative.

Staging (TNM)

Lymphoid neoplasms are staged according to the Lugano classification, which has been adopted by the eighth edition of the Union for International Cancer Control (UICC) TNM classification {596}.

Prognosis and prediction

The prognosis is poor (median overall survival time: 9–15 months). HIV-negative status is associated with worse overall survival {525,2225}. *MYC* translocation has been associated with adverse outcome in both HIV-positive and HIV-negative patients {2225,526}.

Posttransplant lymphoproliferative disorders

Chadburn A
Ferry JA

Definition

Posttransplant lymphoproliferative disorders (PTLDs) are characterized by abnormal, heterogeneous lymphoid proliferations (usually of B-cell origin and usually EBV-positive) that occur in the setting of iatrogenic immunosuppression to prevent rejection of transplanted solid organs or haematopoietic stem cells.

ICD-O coding

9971/1 Posttransplant lymphoproliferative disorder NOS

ICD-11 coding

2B32.0 Posttransplant lymphoproliferative disorder, early lesion
2B32.1 Reactive plasmacytic hyperplasia
2B32.2 Posttransplant lymphoproliferative disorder, infectious mononucleosis-like
2B32.3 Polymorphic posttransplant lymphoproliferative disorder
2B32.Y Other specified immunodeficiency-associated lymphoproliferative disorders

Related terminology

None

Subtype(s)

Non-destructive PTLD; polymorphic PTLD; monomorphic PTLD; classic Hodgkin lymphoma PTLD; mucocutaneous ulcer PTLD

Localization

PTLDs arise in nodal and extranodal sites. The GI tract is the most common extranodal site (10–30% of cases); other frequent extranodal sites include liver, lung, CNS, and allograft

Table 11.03 Risk factors for posttransplant lymphoproliferative disorders (PTLDs)

Factor	Increased risk
EBV status	EBV-seronegative recipient, especially with EBV-seropositive donor
Cytomegalovirus status	Lack of prior cytomegalovirus exposure (in some studies)
Type of transplant	Intestinal, multivisceral (~20%) > heart/lung > liver > kidney, haematopoietic stem cell, pancreas (~1%)
Type of immunosuppression	More intense, T-cell depleting
	Treatment for rejection
	Longer duration of immunosuppression
Sex	Male
Age	Early-onset PTLD: childhood and old age
	Late-onset PTLD: older age

References: {773,3192,2228,781,2838}.

{3785,773,960}. More than 20% of liver and > 70% of intestinal transplant PTLDs occur in the allograft {1414}.

Clinical features

Symptoms are often nonspecific (fever, mass, pain, graft dysfunction) or reflect the site(s) involved. Gastrointestinal PTLD patients present with abdominal pain, diarrhoea, gastrointestinal bleeding, obstruction, perforation, and/or intussusception {486,1373,3205,772}. On endoscopy, gastrointestinal PTLD lesions are usually raised, rubbery, and erythematous, with central ulceration {1373}.

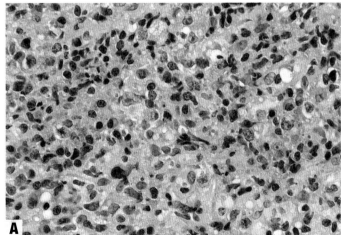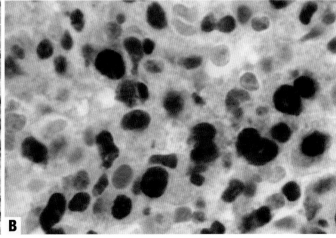

Fig. 11.46 Polymorphic posttransplant lymphoproliferative disorder (PTLD). **A** Polymorphic PTLDs destroy the underlying architecture of the tissue and are composed of a heterogeneous mixture of cells, including lymphocytes, plasma cells, immunoblasts, and Reed–Sternberg–like cells. **B** These lesions are almost always positive for EBV, as demonstrated by in situ hybridization for EBV-encoded small RNA (EBER).

Table 11.04 Clinicopathological features of the five categories of posttransplant lymphoproliferative disorders (PTLDs)

Type of PTLD	Onset	Sites	Architecture	Composition	Immunophenotype	EBV	Clonality (IGH, TR)	Cytogenetic and oncogene abnormalities
Non-destructive PTLD[a] 1. Plasmacytic hyperplasia 2. Infectious mononucleosis 3. Florid follicular hyperplasia	Usually early onset after transplantation	Mass lesions in tonsils, adenoids, lymph nodes; gastrointestinal involvement is rare	Intact or distorted, not obliterated	1. Small lymphocytes, plasma cells, occasional immunoblasts 2. Similar to that of infectious mononucleosis in the general population 3. Floridly hyperplastic follicles with centrocytes and centroblasts	Polyclonal B cells and T cells	+, almost always	Polyclonal or very small clonal B-cell populations; polyclonal, occasionally oligoclonal or clonal T cells	Cytogenetic changes: uncommon
P-PTLD	Tends to occur earlier after transplantation than M-PTLD	Lymph nodes, GI tract, liver, bone marrow, other extranodal sites	Obliterated; criteria for a specific type of lymphoma are not fulfilled	Small lymphocytes, plasma cells, medium-sized lymphoid cells, immunoblasts, +/− Reed–Sternberg–like cells, +/− necrosis	Polyclonal B cells +/− clonal B cells, admixed T cells	+, almost always	Clonal B cells, polyclonal T cells	BCL6 mutation in some; mutations of other genes (rare); fewer cytogenetic abnormalities than M-PTLD
M-PTLD 1. B-lineage: DLBCL, Burkitt and Burkitt-like lymphoma, MZL 2. T/NK-cell lymphomas: PTCL-NOS, HSTL, others 3. Plasma cell neoplasms	Early and late onset	Lymph nodes, GI tract, liver, bone marrow, other extranodal sites; MZL involves skin and soft tissue	Obliterated; criteria for a specific type of lymphoma are fulfilled	As for the same type of lymphoma in the general population	As for the same type of lymphoma in the general population EBV+ DLBCL M-PTLDs have non-GCB phenotype; EBV− DLBCL M-PTLDs may have GCB phenotype	+ (especially early-onset B-PTLD and MZL) or − (many late-onset B-PTLDs and most T-PTLDs)	B-PTLDs have clonal B cells and may have clonal or oligoclonal T cells; T-PTLDs have clonal T cells	B-lineage M-PTLD: BCL6 mutation (common); abnormal karyotypes, often complex (common) EBV+ DLBCL M-PTLD: TP53 mutation (infrequent); 9q24 gains (common) EBV− DLBCL M-PTLD: TP53 usually mutated; gains of 3/3q and loss of 6q23 (common) Burkitt lymphoma: MYC rearranged Burkitt-like lymphoma: 11q abnormalities
CHL-PTLD	Late onset	Lymph nodes > extranodal sites	Obliterated; criteria for CHL are fulfilled	As for CHL in the general population; the mixed cellularity subtype is most common	As for CHL in the general population; neoplastic cells may be CD20+	+	Typically polyclonal B and T cells	Complex abnormal karyotype reported, but limited data
Mucocutaneous ulcer PTLD	Late onset more common; early onset in some cases	Oral cavity, GI tract	Discrete ulcer	Polymorphic infiltrate of lymphoid cells of a range of sizes, including immunoblasts and/or Reed–Sternberg–like cells, with histiocytes, plasma cells, and eosinophils; band of small T cells at base of lesion	Large cells are B-antigen + with non-GCB phenotype, CD30+, CD15+/−	+	Clonal or polyclonal B cells; oligoclonal T cells may be present	n/a

B-PTLD, B-lineage PTLD; CHL, classic Hodgkin lymphoma; CHL-PTLD, classic Hodgkin lymphoma PTLD; DLBCL, diffuse large B-cell lymphoma; GCB, germinal-centre B-cell; HSTL, hepatosplenic T-cell lymphoma; M-PTLD, monomorphic PTLD; MZL, marginal zone lymphoma; n/a, not available; P-PTLD, polymorphic PTLD; PTCL-NOS, peripheral T-cell lymphoma NOS; T-PTLD, T-lineage PTLD.
[a]Formerly called early lesions.
References: {3192,1174,3297,929,928,684,3399,1655,536,538,1176}.

Epidemiology

The risk for PTLD varies based on several factors (see Table 11.03, p. 417), the most important of which is recipient EBV seronegativity at transplantation {771,773,3540,2573}. PTLDs occurring within 1 year of transplantation are more likely EBV-positive and relatively more often non-destructive or polymorphic lesions, whereas the incidence of EBV-negative and monomorphic PTLD (M-PTLD) is higher with longer times after transplantation {772,2573,542,1414}. In recent years, the number of M-PTLDs and the time from transplantation to PTLD have

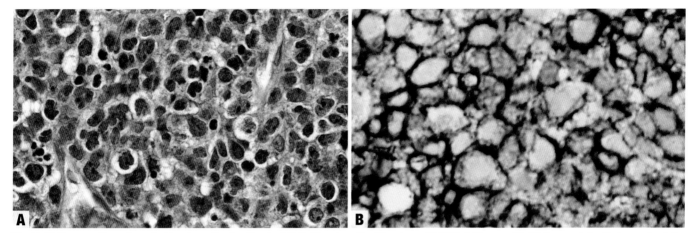

Fig. 11.47 Monomorphic posttransplant lymphoproliferative disorder (PTLD) diffuse large B-cell lymphoma (DLBCL). **A** Monomorphic PTLDs are subclassified according to the 2017 *WHO classification of tumours of haematopoietic and lymphoid tissues* (revised fourth edition). **B** These lesions, like this CD20+ monomorphic PTLD DLBCL, are frequently EBV-negative (immunoperoxidase).

increased {3345}. Most PTLDs related to haematopoietic stem cell transplantation are of donor origin, whereas most PTLDs related to solid organ transplantation are of recipient origin {1609}.

Etiology
EBV-positive PTLDs (60–80%) arise as a result of impaired immunity due to therapeutic immunosuppression, resulting in reactivation of a latent EBV infection or a poor response to a new EBV infection. The etiology of EBV-negative PTLDs is unknown {772,2575,1504}.

Pathogenesis
PTLD pathogenesis is multifactorial. In EBV-positive PTLDs, latent EBV plays a crucial role, encoding for gene products involved in disease development, including a number that are transforming {1031,1455}. For example, EBV-encoded LMP1 activates several pathways (i.e. NF-κB, MAPK, and JAK/ STAT) important in the transformation of B cells, expression of cytokines and antiapoptotic proteins, and suppression of the EBV lytic cycle. Furthermore, T-cell function is hampered not only by immunosuppression, but also by EBV-induced expression of PDL1, IL-6, and IL-10 and by EBV-encoded microRNAs {2065,2575,773,2226}. The pathogenesis of EBV-negative PTLDs is probably similar to that of immunocompetent lymphomas, because they exhibit genomic alterations seen in diffuse large B-cell lymphomas {928,2224,2226}.

Macroscopic appearance
The macroscopic appearance is similar to that of non–immunosuppression-related lymphomas.

Histopathology
PTLDs are classified as non-destructive PTLD, polymorphic PTLD, monomorphic PTLD, classic Hodgkin lymphoma, or mucocutaneous ulcer. They are morphologically heterogeneous, depending on the subtype (see Table 11.04) {3192,1655, 54,1174}.

Except for EBV-positive marginal zone lymphoma, low-grade lymphomas are not considered PTLDs {3192,1174,54,1039}.

Cytology
Not clinically relevant

Diagnostic molecular pathology
Polymorphic PTLDs (P-PTLDs) and M-PTLDs are composed of monoclonal T cells or B cells, a subset of which contain genetic alterations (see Table 11.04) {3192,1655}. Some patients with multiple PTLDs have different clones in separate lesions {2037, 541}. Gene expression profiling shows different upregulated genes in EBV-positive (i.e. in innate immunity, tolerance) and EBV-negative (i.e. in B-cell development) M-PTLDs, consistent with differences in pathogenesis {2224,688}.

Essential and desirable diagnostic criteria
Table 11.04 lists the diagnostic criteria for each PTLD type {3192}.

Staging (TNM)
Most patients (~60%) present with Ann Arbor stage III–IV disease {3785,3130,1652,1719}. Lymphoid neoplasms are staged according to the Lugano classification, which has been adopted by the eighth edition of the Union for International Cancer Control (UICC) TNM classification {596}.

Prognosis and prediction
The survival rate has been poor (30–60%) {1719,1414,3130}, but recent data suggest improving outcomes {1703}. In general, non-destructive PTLDs regress after immunosuppression reduction {2332,1504}, whereas EBV-negative M-PTLDs often require multiagent chemotherapy, immunotherapy, and/or adoptive T-cell therapy {857,1504,804,3337}. Poor prognostic factors include late onset, M-PTLD, CNS involvement, thoracic organ transplantation, elevated LDH, and disseminated disease {1652,3337,458,2663}.

Chapter 11

Extranodal NK/T-cell lymphoma

Ko YH
Li GD
Takeuchi K

Definition

Extranodal NK/T-cell lymphoma (ENKTL) is a neoplasm of NK cells or cytotoxic T cells characterized by extranodal occurrence, frequent presence of angioinvasion, and association with EBV infection.

ICD-O coding

9719/3 Extranodal NK/T-cell lymphoma, nasal type

ICD-11 coding

2A90.6 Extranodal NK/T-cell lymphoma, nasal type

Related terminology

Not recommended: angiocentric T-cell lymphoma; malignant midline reticulosis; polymorphic reticulosis; lethal midline granuloma; angiocentric immunoproliferative lesion.

Subtype(s)

None

Localization

The GI tract is the third most common site of involvement, after the nasal cavity and the skin. ENKTL, nasal-type (ENKTL-NT), occurs predominantly in the small and large intestines rather than in the stomach. The liver may be involved in disseminated ENKTL-NT {1660,1597,1458}.

Clinical features

Patients present with fever, abdominal pain, GI tract bleeding, or (less commonly) bowel perforation. Endoscopically, ENKTL-NT is characterized by single or multiple ulcerative tumours or diffuse irregular ulcers.

Epidemiology

ENKTL-NT is uncommon in Europe and North America but is more prevalent in eastern Asian countries and among indigenous peoples of Central and South America. In China, ENKTL-NT accounts for 8.3% of all GI tract lymphomas {1662, 1966,3497,3174,1801,786}. The patients are younger than those with other types of mature T-cell lymphomas (median age: 35–45 years), with a male predominance {1597,1458}.

Etiology

Genetic predisposition to EBV infection contributes to an individual's susceptibility to ENKTL-NT. A recent genome-wide association study suggests that a common genetic variation at HLA-DPB1 is a strong contributor to the disease {1894}.

Pathogenesis

EBV plays an important role in tumour pathogenesis, but the precise mechanism of action is unknown. EBV induces extensive DNA methylation and genomic instability in the host cell. During expansion of EBV-infected T cells or NK cells, additional genetic, environmental, or microenvironmental triggers contribute to the development of ENKTL-NT {578,1196}.

Clonal TR gene rearrangements are detected in some cases and reflect the T-cell subset. Recurrent mutations have been reported for genes such as *DDX3X*, *BCOR*, *STAT3*, *STAT5B*, *JAK1*, and *JAK3* {1683,1457,1747,1839,794}, which affect gene expression, cell-cycle progression, apoptosis, and immune evasion by EBV-infected cells.

Macroscopic appearance

The GI tract shows tumour infiltration with mass formation, often accompanied by necrosis, ulceration, and/or perforation.

Histopathology

Lymphoma cells infiltrate diffusely and frequently show an angiocentric and angiodestructive pattern. Coagulative necrosis and admixed apoptotic bodies are usually present. The cells tend to be medium in size and have irregular nuclei with pale to clear cytoplasm, but they can be small or large. ENKTL-NT

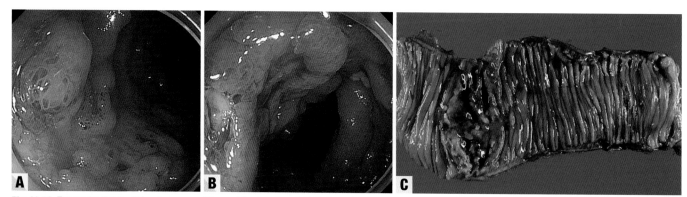

Fig. 11.48 Extranodal NK/T-cell lymphoma, nasal-type, of the intestine. **A,B** Endoscopic views of multifocal polypoid submucosal disease. **C** The small intestinal mucosa shows focal ulceration and necrosis.

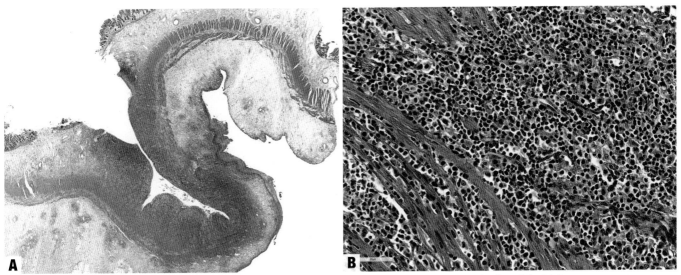

Fig. 11.49 Extranodal NK/T-cell lymphoma. **A** Low power showing transmural involvement with ulceration. **B** High power showing cellular detail.

is typically positive for CD2, cytoplasmic CD3, CD56, cytotoxic molecules (TIA1, granzyme B, and perforin), and EBV-encoded small RNA (EBER). ENKTL-NT is variably positive for CD7 but not for surface CD3, CD4, CD5, CD8, CD16, or CD57. Cases positive for surface CD3, CD5, CD8, and/or T-cell receptor constitute a T-cell subset of ENKTL-NT.

The differential diagnosis includes lymphomatoid gastropathy / NK-cell enteropathy, which is a rare benign NK-cell proliferative process that presents as one to several mucosal surface lesions (~1 cm in diameter) in the stomach and/or intestines {3452,3222,2042,3244,3651,3277,1392,3215,

1402}. Most cases reported from Japan are localized in the stomach {3222,3244,3651,3277,1392,3215,1402}, but intestinal cases have been recognized {3452,2042}. Individual lesions spontaneously regress in a few months, but some patients may develop new lesions for years.

The biopsy shows superficial infiltration of atypical cells that destroy the gastric or intestinal glands, mimicking lymphoepithelial lesions in extranodal marginal zone lymphoma. The cells are medium to large in size and usually have eosinophilic granules in the cytoplasm. The immunophenotype is the same as that of ENKTL-NT, except for consistent negativity for EBER.

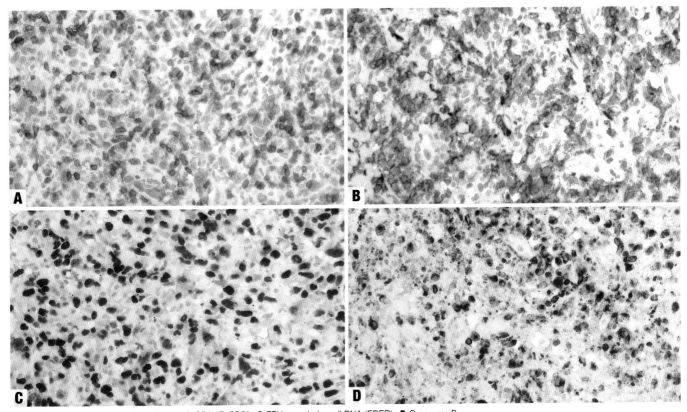

Fig. 11.50 Extranodal NK/T-cell lymphoma. **A** CD3. **B** CD56. **C** EBV-encoded small RNA (EBER). **D** Granzyme B.

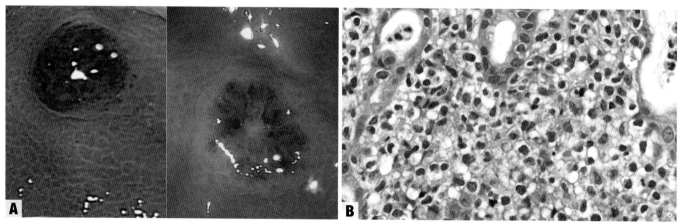

Fig. 11.51 Lymphomatoid gastropathy / NK-cell enteropathy. **A** Endoscopic findings. The mucosal superficial lesions show various appearances, including blood blister–like (**left**) and flat elevations with a shallow depression (**right**). **B** The gastric mucosa shows infiltration by atypical medium-sized cells with irregular nuclei and pale cytoplasm. Some cells contain brightly eosinophilic granules.

Cytology

Not clinically relevant

Diagnostic molecular pathology

Not clinically relevant

Essential and desirable diagnostic criteria

Essential: destructive infiltrate of lymphoma cells; neoplastic cells are either NK or T cells with expression of cytotoxic proteins; EBV positivity.

Desirable: angiocentric growth and necrosis; CD56 is expressed in the vast majority of cases, but can be negative.

Staging (TNM)

Lymphoid neoplasms are staged according to the Lugano classification, which has been adopted by the eighth edition of the Union for International Cancer Control (UICC) TNM classification {596}.

Prognosis and prediction

ENKTL-NT involving the GI tract has a dismal prognosis despite chemotherapy and surgery. The median overall survival time is 2.8–7.8 months. Poor prognostic factors include high International Prognostic Index (IPI), high NK/T-cell lymphoma prognostic index, bowel perforation, and high viral load in peripheral blood {1597,1458}.

Systemic mastocytosis

Horny H-P
Pileri SA
Valent P

Definition
Systemic mastocytosis is a neoplasm characterized by proliferation of clonally mutated (typically *KIT*-mutant) mast cells in various organs/tissues.

ICD-O coding
9740/3 Mast cell sarcoma
9741/1 Indolent systemic mastocytosis
9741/3 Aggressive systemic mastocytosis
9741/3 Systemic mastocytosis with associated haematological clonal non-mast cell disorder
9742/3 Mast cell leukaemia

ICD-11 coding
2A21.00 Mast cell leukaemia
2A21.2 Mast cell sarcoma
2A21.0Z Systemic mastocytosis, unspecified
2A21.0Y Other specified systemic mastocytosis

Related terminology
Not recommended: systemic mast cell disease.

Subtype(s)
None

Localization
Systemic mastocytosis may affect mucosal layers of all parts of the digestive tract: oesophagus, stomach, and small and large intestines. Involvement of the liver in patients with systemic mastocytosis has also been reported, but histologically confirmed infiltration of the pancreas or the bile tract has not been described.

Clinical features
There is a wide range of abdominal symptoms, including abdominal discomfort, constipation, cramping, diarrhoea, and diffuse pain. In patients with advanced systemic mastocytosis, these symptoms are frequently associated with progressive weight loss and/or hypoalbuminaemia. These patients may also present with ascites, abdominal lymphadenopathy, and hepatosplenomegaly. In addition, rapidly increasing serum tryptase levels and elevated liver enzymes (including alkaline phosphatase) may be seen in advanced systemic mastocytosis. There are many review articles and case reports that focus on gastrointestinal manifestations of systemic mastocytosis, including its differential diagnoses {3760,1447,128,1828}.

Most systemic mastocytosis patients with digestive tract involvement have indolent systemic mastocytosis. In these cases, the symptoms are usually mild to moderate and can be kept under control using histamine receptor H_2 blockers. Systemic mastocytosis with predominant digestive tract involvement does occur, but isolated involvement of the digestive tract seems to be extremely uncommon, and infiltration of the bone marrow, although sometimes to a very low degree, is found in almost all patients.

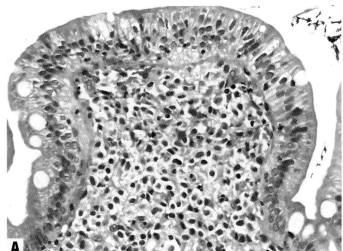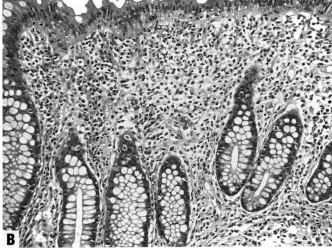

Fig. 11.52 Systemic mastocytosis involving the digestive tract. **A** Systemic mastocytosis involving the GI tract mucosa shows compact infiltration with broadening of a duodenal villus by a mixed infiltrate mainly consisting of medium-sized cells with ample pale cytoplasm, intermingled with loosely scattered eosinophils. Note the intact surface epithelium. Diagnosis of mastocytosis is highly likely but should be confirmed with appropriate immunostains. **B** Colonic mucosa with slightly distorted crypts (without dysplastic features) and a mixed infiltrate mainly affecting the upper parts of the mucosa. The infiltrate mainly consists of medium-sized cells with pale cytoplasm and inconspicuous nuclei. Loosely distributed eosinophils can also be seen. Diagnosis of mastocytosis is highly likely but must be confirmed with appropriate immunostains.

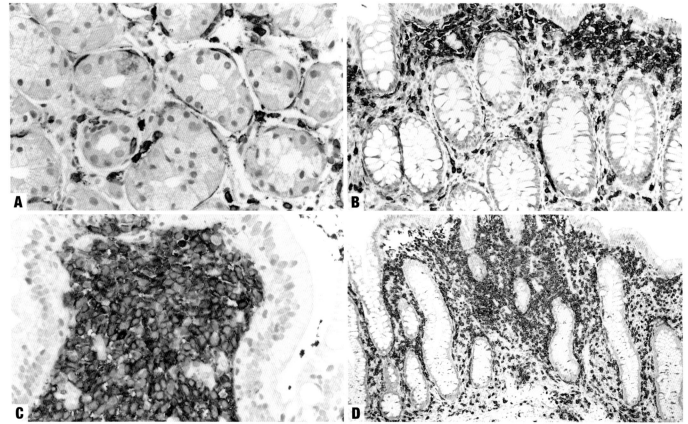

Fig. 11.53 Systemic mastocytosis involving the GI tract mucosa. **A** Immunostaining of the stomach mucosa (corpus/fundus) with anti-CD117 (KIT) reveals a substantial increase of at least 20% spindly mast cells either loosely scattered throughout or forming small (subdiagnostic) groups. Note that compact (diagnostic) mast cell infiltrates are missing. **B** Immunostaining with anti-CD117 (KIT) reveals a band-like subepithelial mast cell infiltrate. Note that mast cells in the deeper layers of the mucosa do not form compact or micronodular infiltrates. **C** In the same case shown in Fig. 11.52A, immunostaining with an antibody against CD117 (KIT) reveals a compact mast cell infiltrate in an intravillous position. **D** In the same case shown in Fig. 11.52B, immunostaining with an antibody against CD117 (KIT) reveals diffuse and partially packed infiltration of the colonic mucosa by atypical mast cells.

Epidemiology

Systemic mastocytosis is generally diagnosed after the second decade of life, and reported M:F ratios range from 1:1 to 0.67:1 {1279}.

Etiology

Unknown

Pathogenesis

In all systemic mastocytosis subtypes, clinical symptoms result from an inappropriate release of mast cell–derived mediators, including histamine, prostaglandin D2, leukotrienes, and/or cytokines. In advanced systemic mastocytosis and mast cell sarcoma, symptoms may also arise from local infiltration and expansion of neoplastic mast cells in the digestive tract, liver, and spleen, leading to malabsorption, weight loss, hepatosplenomegaly, ascites, and even hypersplenism {1280,193}.

Macroscopic appearance

Not clinically relevant

Histopathology

In almost all cases of mastocytosis involving the digestive tract, the number of intramucosal mast cells is substantially increased {809,1828}. A tendency of the mast cells to group together is suspicious for, and formation of compact micronodular or band-like infiltrates is pathognomonic for, mastocytosis and never seen in mast cell hyperplasia. The diagnostic mast cell infiltrates may be small but should consist of at least 15 coherently clustering mast cells. Sometimes only very few small but diagnostic mast cell infiltrates are encountered within the villi, whereas most cases show predominant involvement of the basal portion of the mucosa. In advanced systemic mastocytosis, a more diffuse-compact involvement of the mucosa is seen, the microarchitecture of the glands is almost effaced, and a diagnosis of a neoplastic infiltrate is obvious. Sarcomatous destructive growth of highly atypical mast cells also involving the deeper layers of the digestive tract wall is only seen in the exceptionally rare mast cell sarcoma.

An increased number of eosinophils, which is a very common finding in mastocytosis, is also seen in the digestive tract. Rarely, eosinophilic mucositis may obscure the underlying mastocytosis, which can only be diagnosed after appropriate immunohistochemical staining. The association of microscopic colitis and chronic inflammatory bowel disease does occur, posing

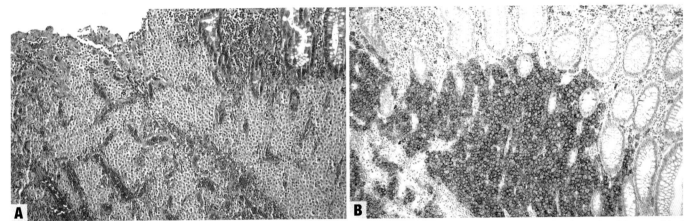

Fig. 11.54 Mast cell sarcoma involving the intestinal mucosa. **A** Sheets of medium-sized tumour cells with pale cytoplasm and almost complete destruction of the pre-existent glands/crypts dominate the picture in conventional H&E staining. There is ulceration overlying the neoplastic infiltrate. **B** Immunostaining with anti-CD117 (KIT) confirms the diagnosis of a localized mast cell sarcoma. Because the patient had a history of a systemic mastocytosis, the final diagnosis should read "secondary mast cell sarcoma infiltrating the large bowel".

considerable diagnostic problems for the histopathologist {282, 2676,3304}.

The main site of involvement of the liver is the portal triad. Mast cells may form subdiagnostic groups or even larger compact (diagnostic) infiltrates within the fibrotic portal triads. Because mast cells are normally virtually absent from the sinusoids, the presence of loosely scattered mast cells in liver sinusoids is also highly suspicious for systemic mastocytosis.

Immunohistochemically, mast cells show coexpression of tryptase and KIT (CD117) but also the typical aberrant expression of CD25 {1140}. However, in a considerable number of patients, mastocytosis lesions show an abnormal phenotype with weak expression of CD25 and almost-missing expression of tryptase. Therefore, screening for systemic mastocytosis involving the digestive tract mucosa should always be performed using anti-KIT antibodies. The aberrant immunophenotype of mast cells is also commonly found in other tissues/organs in patients with systemic mastocytosis.

Cytology
Not clinically relevant

Diagnostic molecular pathology
In most patients with systemic mastocytosis involving the digestive tract, neoplastic mast cells display the somatic activating *KIT* point mutation p.D816V. In advanced systemic mastocytosis, in particular systemic mastocytosis with associated haematological neoplasm, additional somatic mutations in other genes are detected in a considerable number of patients, and these are known to be associated with a poor prognosis.

Essential and desirable diagnostic criteria
Essential: mast cells occurring in clusters or bands; immunoreactivity for KIT (CD117), tryptase, and CD25.

Staging (TNM)
Not clinically relevant

Prognosis and prediction
Prognosis depends on the type of systemic mastocytosis and is accordingly very unfavourable in patients with advanced systemic mastocytosis, whereas those with indolent systemic mastocytosis usually have an almost normal life expectancy {1279}.

Langerhans cell histiocytosis

Chan JKC
Pileri SA

Definition

Langerhans cell histiocytosis (LCH) is a clonal proliferation of cells with morphological and immunophenotypic features of Langerhans cells.

ICD-O coding

9751/1 Langerhans cell histiocytosis NOS

ICD-11 coding

2B31.2 Langerhans cell histiocytosis

Related terminology

Acceptable: histiocytosis X; eosinophilic granuloma.
Not recommended: Langerhans cell granulomatosis.

Subtype(s)

Langerhans cell histiocytosis, disseminated (9751/3)

Localization

LCH can involve a single or multiple sites, most commonly bone and skin. Gastrointestinal and liver involvement is common in paediatric patients with multisystem LCH and uncommon in adults.

Clinical features

Children with multisystem LCH are usually aged < 2 years, and they present with failure to thrive, diarrhoea, vomiting, protein-losing enteropathy, and hepatomegaly. They have multiple ulcerative lesions throughout the intestines {845,1519,3060}. Adults with GI tract involvement are asymptomatic or present with constipation, anaemia, or dysphagia {3060}. They often have a solitary polypoid or ulcerative lesion in the large intestine or (less commonly) the stomach and oesophagus {3060,

285}. Liver involvement in adults usually occurs in the setting of multiorgan disease, and it manifests as hepatomegaly and abnormal liver biochemistry (in particular, evidence of cholestasis) {1519,3}.

Epidemiology

The annual incidence in children is 4.1–5.4 cases per million person-years, and the M:F ratio is 1.2:1 to 2.2:1 {2836,2361, 2350}. LCH has a wide age range at presentation, but is more common in children.

Etiology

Unknown

Pathogenesis

Unknown

Macroscopic appearance

Not clinically relevant

Histopathology

LCH is characterized by proliferation of oval cells with deeply grooved or contorted nuclei, thin nuclear membranes, fine chromatin, and generally inconspicuous nucleoli. Nuclei atypia is minimal. The cells have a moderate amount of lightly eosinophilic cytoplasm. There are variable numbers of admixed eosinophils and histiocytes. Immunophenotypically, LCH expresses S100, CD1a, and CD207 (langerin). In the GI tract, the LCH infiltrate is centred in the mucosa or submucosa {3060}. There are variable numbers of admixed eosinophils and lymphocytes. The mucosa may show ulceration. In the liver, parenchymal involvement takes the form of sinusoidal infiltrate, granulomatoid clusters, and confluent tumour masses {1519}. The portal tracts,

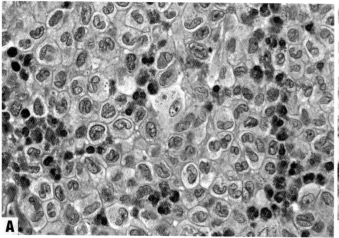
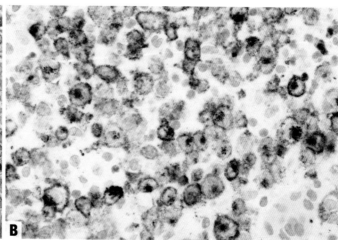

Fig. 11.55 Langerhans cell histiocytosis. **A** The Langerhans cells show grooved nuclei and thin nuclear membranes. There are admixed eosinophils. **B** Positive staining for CD207 (langerin) (immunoperoxidase).

including the bile ducts, are infiltrated by Langerhans cells, evolving to a pattern of sclerosing cholangitis with periductal fibrosis, ductopenia, and periportal ductular reaction. Langerhans cells may be sparse or absent in the late lesions.

Cytology
Not clinically relevant

Diagnostic molecular pathology
Almost all cases exhibit gain-of-function mutations in genes encoding proteins of the MAPK signalling pathway, most commonly *BRAF* p.V600E mutations (~50% of cases) and *MAP2K1* mutations {858,218}.

Essential and desirable diagnostic criteria
Essential: dense aggregates of uniform-appearing Langerhans cells with grooved nuclei and fine chromatin; immunoreactivity for S100, CD1a, and CD207.
Desirable: many admixed eosinophils.

Staging (TNM)
Not clinically relevant

Prognosis and prediction
Children with liver or GI tract involvement as part of multisystem LCH have a high mortality rate. Adults with localized gastrointestinal disease have an excellent prognosis, whereas those with liver involvement may die from complications of sclerosing cholangitis. Tumours with *BRAF* p.V600 mutations are treatable using BRAF inhibitors {777,176,1171}, and trial results are encouraging for this approach.

Follicular dendritic cell sarcoma

Chan JKC
Pileri SA

Definition

Follicular dendritic cell (FDC) sarcoma is a malignant neoplasm composed of spindled to ovoid cells showing morphological and immunophenotypic features of FDCs.

ICD-O coding

9758/3 Follicular dendritic cell sarcoma

ICD-11 coding

2B31.5 Follicular dendritic cell sarcoma

Related terminology

Acceptable: follicular dendritic cell tumour.

Subtype(s)

None

Localization

FDC sarcoma can occur in nodal or extranodal sites. In a literature review of 343 reported cases of FDC sarcoma, the liver was involved in 45 cases (with EBV-positive inflammatory FDC sarcoma probably accounting for a high proportion), the GI tract in 18 cases, and the pancreas in 5 cases {2876}.

Clinical features

Patients usually present with a mass lesion in the involved organ. Rare patients have paraneoplastic pemphigus.

Epidemiology

FDC sarcoma is rare. The patients are usually adults, and there is no sex predilection.

Etiology

Unknown

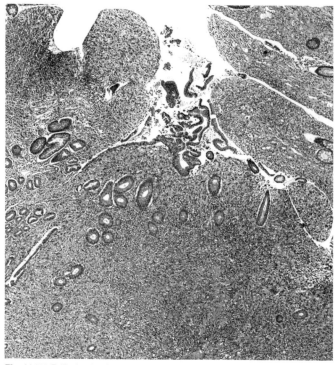

Fig. 11.57 Follicular dendritic cell sarcoma of the small intestine. A spindle cell tumour shows involvement of the mucosa and wall of the small intestine.

Pathogenesis

A proportion of cases have been reported to show IG gene rearrangement, a finding that requires further studies in light of the postulated mesenchymal derivation of normal FDCs {584}. EBV is negative, in contrast to the consistent EBV positivity in EBV-positive inflammatory FDC sarcoma.

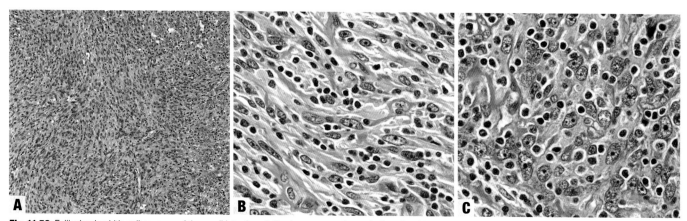

Fig. 11.56 Follicular dendritic cell sarcoma of the small intestine. **A** The tumour comprises spindly cells with a storiform growth pattern. There is a sprinkling of small lymphocytes. **B** The spindly tumour cells have indistinct cell borders, vesicular nuclei, and distinct nucleoli. There are intermingled small lymphocytes. **C** The tumour cells are ovoid, but cell borders are indistinct. The nuclei show distinct nucleoli and irregular clustering.

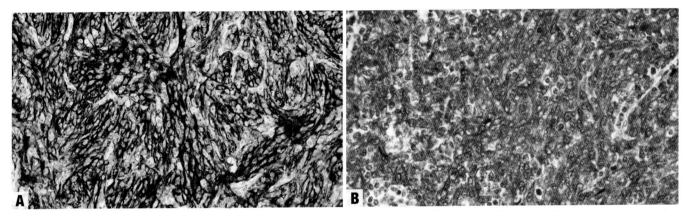

Fig. 11.58 Follicular dendritic cell sarcoma. **A** Positive immunostaining for CD21 (Immunoperoxidase). **B** Positive staining for PDL1 (immunoalkaline phosphatase).

Macroscopic appearance

FDC sarcomas are soft, bulky tumour masses.

Histopathology

The tumour comprises spindly to ovoid cells forming fascicles, storiform arrays, whorls, diffuse sheets, and vague nodules. The tumour cells show indistinct cell borders and a moderate amount of eosinophilic cytoplasm. The oval or elongated nuclei often show delicate nuclear membranes, vesicular chromatin, and distinct nucleoli, with variable degrees of pleomorphism. Binucleated and multinucleated forms are common. The tumour is typically lightly infiltrated by small lymphocytes, which can be aggregated around the blood vessels. FDC sarcoma shows immunoreactivity for one or more FDC markers, such as CD21, CD23, CD35, CXCL13, FDC-secreted protein, and serglycin {2584,1948}. PDL1 is often positive {1764}. Variable staining for EMA, S100, and CD68 can be present, whereas cytokeratin, CD1a, langerin, lysozyme, and myeloperoxidase are negative.

Cytology

Not clinically relevant

Diagnostic molecular pathology

Not clinically relevant

Essential and desirable diagnostic criteria

Essential: spindly to oval cell neoplasm with storiform, fascicular, or whorled growth pattern; neoplastic cells show indistinct cell borders, vesicular nuclei, and distinct nucleoli; sprinkling of small lymphocytes; positive immunostaining for one or more FDC markers.

Staging (TNM)

Not clinically relevant

Prognosis and prediction

FDC sarcoma is a low-grade to intermediate-grade malignancy. A pooled analysis of the literature shows local recurrence and distant metastasis rates of 28% and 27%, respectively {2876}. Large tumour size (≥ 6 cm), coagulative necrosis, high mitotic count, and substantial cytological atypia are associated with a worse prognosis {2876,545}.

Histiocytic sarcoma

Chan JKC
Pileri SA

Definition

Histiocytic sarcoma is a malignant proliferation of cells showing morphological and immunophenotypic features of tissue histiocytes.

ICD-O coding

9755/3 Histiocytic sarcoma

ICD-11 coding

2B31.1 Histiocytic sarcoma

Related terminology

None

Subtype(s)

None

Localization

Histiocytic sarcoma can occur in extranodal or nodal sites, and the GI tract is a common extranodal site of involvement {2584, 1277}. Occurrence in the liver, pancreas, gallbladder, or bile ducts is extremely rare.

Clinical features

The most common presentation is intestinal obstruction. Other patients present with abdominal pain or rectal bleeding.

Epidemiology

Histiocytic sarcoma is rare. It usually occurs in adults, without sex predilection.

Etiology

Unknown

Pathogenesis

A subset of cases show clonal IG gene rearrangement {584}, particularly when associated with low-grade B-cell lymphoma. This is postulated to represent a transdifferentiation process {430,913}.

Macroscopic appearance

Histiocytic sarcomas are usually solitary masses.

Histopathology

The tumour shows a diffuse proliferation of round to oval large cells with abundant cytoplasm. The nuclei are oval, grooved, or irregularly folded, often with vesicular chromatin and distinct nucleoli. They can exhibit variable degrees of pleomorphism. The cytoplasm is eosinophilic, often with some fine vacuoles. Haemophagocytosis is occasionally observed. The tumour cells can sometimes be spindly. Variable numbers of reactive cells may be admixed. The tumour shows expression of one or more histiocytic markers, including CD163, CD68, and lysozyme, whereas Langerhans cell (CD1a, CD207), follicular dendritic cell (CD21, CD35), and myeloid cell (myeloperoxidase, CD13) markers are negative. There can be heterogeneous expression of S100.

Cytology

Not clinically relevant

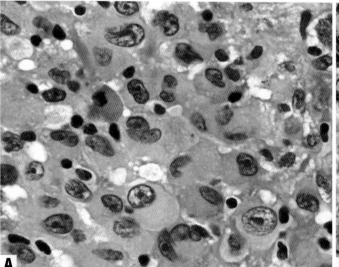 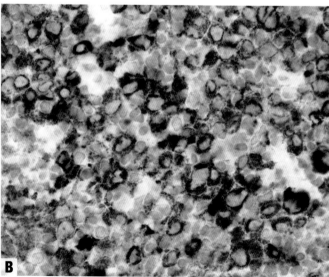

Fig. 11.59 Histiocytic sarcoma of the stomach. **A** The neoplastic cells are large and have abundant eosinophilic cytoplasm that occasionally contains small vacuoles. The nuclei are round, reniform, or grooved. **B** Positive staining for CD163 (immunoperoxidase).

Diagnostic molecular pathology

Not clinically relevant

Essential and desirable diagnostic criteria

Essential: tumour composed of non-cohesive large cells with abundant eosinophilic cytoplasm; neoplastic cells have reniform, grooved, or irregularly folded nuclei and distinct nucleoli; positive immunostaining for one or more histiocytic markers.

Staging (TNM)

Not clinically relevant

Prognosis and prediction

Histiocytic sarcoma is generally an aggressive neoplasm with poor response to therapy. Patients with localized disease and small primary tumours have a more favourable outcome {2584, 1277}.

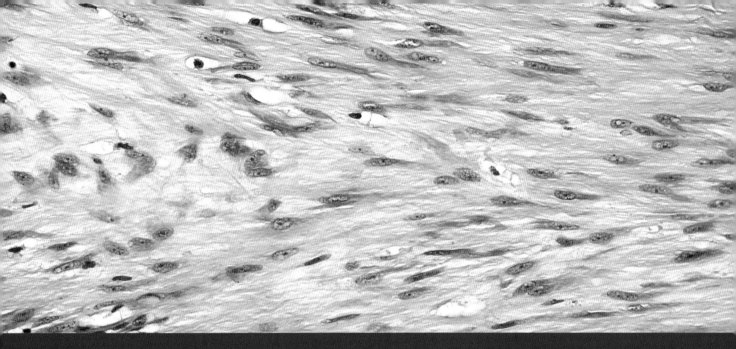

12

Mesenchymal tumours of the digestive system

Edited by: Fukayama M, Goldblum JR, Miettinen M, Lazar AJ

Gastrointestinal stromal tumour
Adipose tissue and (myo)fibroblastic tumours
   Inflammatory myofibroblastic tumour
   Desmoid fibromatosis
   Solitary fibrous tumour
   Lipoma
   Inflammatory fibroid polyp
   Plexiform fibromyxoma
Smooth muscle and skeletal muscle tumours
   Leiomyoma
   Leiomyosarcoma
   Rhabdomyosarcoma
Vascular and perivascular tumours
   Haemangioma
   Epithelioid haemangioendothelioma
   Kaposi sarcoma
   Angiosarcoma

Glomus tumour
Lymphangioma and lymphangiomatosis
Neural tumours
   Schwannoma
   Granular cell tumour
   Perineurioma
   Ganglioneuroma and ganglioneuromatosis
Tumours of uncertain differentiation
   PEComa, including angiomyolipoma
   Mesenchymal hamartoma of the liver
   Calcifying nested stromal-epithelial tumour of the
      liver
   Synovial sarcoma
   Gastrointestinal clear cell sarcoma / malignant
      gastrointestinal neuroectodermal tumour
   Embryonal sarcoma of the liver

WHO classification of mesenchymal tumours of the digestive system

Gastrointestinal stromal tumour
8936/3   Gastrointestinal stromal tumour
       Succinate dehydrogenase–deficient gastrointestinal stromal tumour

Adipose tissue and (myo)fibroblastic tumours
8825/1   Inflammatory myofibroblastic tumour
       Epithelioid inflammatory myofibroblastic sarcoma
8821/1   Desmoid-type fibromatosis
8822/1   Abdominal fibromatosis
8815/1   Solitary fibrous tumour NOS
8815/3   Solitary fibrous tumour, malignant
       Lipomatous solitary fibrous tumour
9160/0   Giant cell angiofibroma
8850/0   Lipoma NOS
8861/0   Angiolipoma NOS
8811/0   Plexiform fibromyxoma

Smooth muscle and skeletal muscle tumours
8890/0   Leiomyoma NOS
       Seedling leiomyomas
8890/1   Leiomyomatosis NOS
8890/3   Leiomyosarcoma NOS
8910/3   Embryonal rhabdomyosarcoma NOS
8912/3   Rhabdomyosarcoma, spindle cell / sclerosing type
8920/3   Alveolar rhabdomyosarcoma

Vascular and perivascular tumours
9120/0   Haemangioma NOS
       Dieulafoy lesion
       Gastric antral vascular ectasia (GAVE)
       Angiodysplasia
       Anastomosing haemangioma
       Infantile haemangioma
       Diffuse hepatic haemangiomatosis
       Hepatic small vessel neoplasm
9133/3   Epithelioid haemangioendothelioma NOS
9140/3   Kaposi sarcoma
9120/3   Angiosarcoma
       Epithelioid angiosarcoma
8711/0   Glomus tumour NOS
8711/1   Glomangiomatosis
8711/1   Glomus tumour of uncertain malignant potential
8711/3   Glomus tumour, malignant
9170/0   Lymphangioma NOS

Neural tumours
9560/0   Schwannoma NOS
       Microcystic/reticular schwannoma
       Mucosal Schwann cell hamartoma
9580/0   Granular cell tumour NOS
9580/3   Granular cell tumour, malignant
9571/0   Perineurioma NOS
9490/0   Ganglioneuroma
9491/0   Ganglioneuromatosis

Tumours of uncertain differentiation
8714/0   PEComa, benign
       Sclerosing PEComa
8860/0   Angiomyolipoma
       Inflammatory subtype of angiomyolipoma
8714/3   PEComa, malignant
8975/1   Calcifying nested stromal-epithelial tumour
9040/3   Synovial sarcoma NOS
9041/3   Synovial sarcoma, monophasic fibrous
9043/3   Synovial sarcoma, biphasic
9044/3   Clear cell sarcoma NOS
8991/3   Embryonal sarcoma

These morphology codes are from the International Classification of Diseases for Oncology, third edition, second revision (ICD-O-3.2) {1378A}. Behaviour is coded /0 for benign tumours; /1 for unspecified, borderline, or uncertain behaviour; /2 for carcinoma in situ and grade III intraepithelial neoplasia; /3 for malignant tumours, primary site; and /6 for malignant tumours, metastatic site. Behaviour code /6 is not generally used by cancer registries.

This classification is modified from the previous WHO classification, taking into account changes in our understanding of these lesions.

TNM staging of gastrointestinal stromal tumours

Gastrointestinal Stromal Tumour (GIST)

Rules for Classification

The classification applies only to gastrointestinal stromal tumours. There should be histological confirmation of the disease.

The following are the procedures for assessing the T, N, and M categories.

T categories	Physical examination, imaging, endoscopy, and/or surgical exploration
N categories	Physical examination, imaging, and/or surgical exploration
M categories	Physical examination, imaging, and/or surgical exploration

Anatomical Sites and Subsites

- Oesophagus (C15)
- Stomach (C16)
- Small intestine (C17)
  1. Duodenum (C17.0)
  2. Jejunum (C17.1)
  3. Ileum (C17.2)
- Colon (C18)
- Rectosigmoid junction (C19)
- Rectum (C20)
- Omentum (C48.1)
- Mesentery (C48.1)

Regional Lymph Nodes

The regional lymph nodes are those appropriate to the site of the primary tumour; see gastrointestinal sites for details.

TNM Clinical Classification

T – Primary Tumour

TX	Primary tumour cannot be assessed
T0	No evidence for primary tumour
T1	Tumour 2 cm or less
T2	Tumour more than 2 cm but not more than 5 cm
T3	Tumour more than 5 cm but not more than 10 cm
T4	Tumour more than 10 cm in greatest dimension

N – Regional Lymph Nodes

NX	Regional lymph nodes cannot be assessed*
N0	No regional lymph node metastasis
N1	Regional lymph node metastasis

Note
* NX: Regional lymph node involvement is rare for GISTs, so that cases in which the nodal status is not assessed clinically or pathologically could be considered N0 instead of NX or pNX.

M – Distant Metastasis

M0	No distant metastasis
M1	Distant metastasis

pTNM Pathological Classification

The pT and pN categories correspond to the T and N categories.

pM – Distant Metastasis*

pM1   Distant metastasis microscopically confirmed

Note
* pM0 and pMX are not valid categories

G Histopathological Grading

Grading for GIST is dependent on mitotic rate.*

Low mitotic rate:	5 or fewer per 50 hpf
High mitotic rate:	over 5 per 50 hpf

Note
* The mitotic rate of GIST is best expressed as the number of mitoses per 50 high power fields (hpf) using the 40× objective (total area 5 mm^2 in 50 fields).

Stage

Staging criteria for gastric tumours can be applied in primary, solitary omental GISTs. Staging criteria for intestinal tumours can be applied to GISTs in less common sites such as oesophagus, colon, rectum, and mesentery.

Gastric GIST

				Mitotic rate
Stage IA	T1,T2	N0	M0	Low
Stage IB	T3	N0	M0	Low
Stage II	T1,T2	N0	M0	High
	T4	N0	M0	Low
Stage IIIA	T3	N0	M0	High
Stage IIIB	T4	N0	M0	High
Stage IV	Any T	N1	M0	Any rate
	Any T	Any N	M1	Any rate

Small Intestinal GIST

				Mitotic rate
Stage I	T1,T2	N0	M0	Low
Stage II	T3	N0	M0	Low
Stage IIIA	T1	N0	M0	High
	T4	N0	M0	Low
Stage IIIB	T2,T3,T4	N0	M0	High
Stage IV	Any T	N1	M0	Any rate
	Any T	Any N	M1	Any rate

Note: The mitotic rates (counts) listed under the "G Histopathological Grading" heading above are based on a field area of 0.1 mm^2 as used in the original paper; modern microscopes are likely to have a field area of 0.2 mm^2, but measurement of field area is advisable, because instruments vary.

The information presented here has been excerpted from the 2017 *TNM classification of malignant tumours*, eighth edition (408,3385A). © 2017 UICC.
A help desk for specific questions about the TNM classification is available at https://www.uicc.org/tnm-help-desk.

Mesenchymal tumours of the digestive system: Introduction

Lazar AJ
Hornick JL

Although this chapter on mesenchymal tumours is restricted to the entities most relevant to the digestive system, a more general introduction to soft tissue pathology is presented here. Indeed, although characteristic patterns exist, virtually any soft tissue tumour can arise at any site on at least rare occasion. For example, there are descriptions of Ewing sarcoma arising in the liver and low-grade fibromyxoid sarcoma in the small intestine, but such involvement is not characteristic {2479,1802}.

Incidence

The incidence of soft tissue sarcoma is fairly consistent at 30–50 cases per million person-years {1016,1126,2074,920}. Benign soft tissue neoplasms as a group show an incidence of at least 100-fold higher. Individual benign mesenchymal entities range from frequent (e.g. lipoma) to rare (e.g. spindle cell haemangioma) {2257}. Sarcomas are a relatively rare subset of gastrointestinal tumours, far outnumbered by carcinomas and benign mesenchymal gastrointestinal neoplasms {808}. Gastrointestinal stromal tumour (GIST) is the most common sarcoma of the GI tract {2145,1907}, with an incidence of approximately 10 cases per million person-years {523, 3470}. Other primary gastrointestinal sarcomas are exceptionally rare. Subcentimetre, clinically occult GISTs are among the most common human neoplasms, identified in as many as 35% of gastrectomy specimens; most never progress to malignancy {1546}. Therefore, at both ends of its risk spectrum, GIST probably represents the most common sarcoma, as well as the most common effectively benign mesenchymal neoplasm of the GI tract. Other common benign mesenchymal tumours of the GI tract are lipomas, leiomyomas, vascular lesions, and nerve sheath tumours. Haemangiomas are by far the most common mesenchymal tumours of the liver; primary hepatic sarcomas are rare. The full breadth of deep soft tissue tumours is covered in the 2013 *WHO classification of tumours of soft tissue and bone* volume of the fourth edition of this series, which is due to be updated in 2019 {949}. More sarcomas (both numerically greater in aggregate and more sarcoma types) are seen in adults than in children, but sarcomas constitute only 1% of malignancies in adults {3033}. They arise mainly in the extremities (in particular the thighs), trunk, head and neck, and retroperitoneum. GISTs most often arise in the stomach (60%) followed by the small bowel (30%) {2145}. Sarcomas account for about 10–15% of paediatric malignancies, but their overall incidence rate in children is much lower than in adults, and fewer specific entities are encountered in childhood {1137,3568}.

Etiology and pathogenesis

Most soft tissue neoplasms arise spontaneously, with an unknown cause, but a clear etiology can be discerned for some cases. Viruses associated with soft tissue tumours include EBV (associated with some smooth muscle tumours

Box 12.01 The biological potential of mesenchymal tumours of the digestive system, based on the 2013 *WHO classification of tumours of soft tissue and bone*, which is due to be updated in 2019 {949}

Benign
- Ganglioneuroma/ganglioneuromatosis
- Glomus tumour (all forms)[a]
- Granular cell tumour
- Haemangioma
- Inflammatory fibroid polyp
- Leiomyoma
- Lipoma
- Lymphangioma/lymphangiomatosis
- Mesenchymal hamartoma of the liver
- PEComa[a]
- Perineurioma
- Plexiform fibromyxoma
- Schwannoma

Intermediate (locally aggressive)
- Desmoid fibromatosis

Intermediate (rarely metastasizing; < 2%)
- Inflammatory myofibroblastic tumour
- Kaposi sarcoma
- Solitary fibrous tumour

Malignant
- Angiosarcoma
- Embryonal sarcoma of the liver
- Gastrointestinal clear cell sarcoma
- Gastrointestinal stromal tumour[b]
- Leiomyosarcoma
- Rhabdomyosarcoma (all forms)
- Synovial sarcoma

[a]PEComa and glomus tumour have both benign (most common) and malignant (rare) forms. [b]Based on validated risk stratification, behaviour in gastrointestinal stromal tumour ranges from essentially benign to uncertain malignant potential to malignant (see *Gastrointestinal stromal tumour*, p. 439).

in immunosuppressed patients) {769} and HHV8 (associated with Kaposi sarcoma) {539}. Angiosarcoma can complicate longstanding lymphoedema, in particular after radical mastectomy (as seen in Stewart–Treves syndrome). Sarcomas can also arise in fields of prior therapeutic irradiation {2519}. Associations with chemical exposure, immunosuppression/transplantation, and chronic tissue irritation have been described in a subset of sarcoma cases {1765}. Soft tissue tumours (both benign and malignant) are also associated with several inherited syndromes, including Maffucci syndrome (associated with chondroid and vascular tumours), tuberous sclerosis (associated with angiomyolipomas of kidney and liver), and Cowden syndrome (associated with lipomas and haemangiomas). These syndromes are discussed in more detail in the *WHO classification of tumours of soft tissue and bone* volume {949}. Desmoid fibromatosis can be seen in the setting of familial adenomatous polyposis with germline *APC* mutations {737,1434}. GISTs are usually sporadic, although germline *KIT* or *PDGFRA* mutations (familial GIST), *NF1* mutations (neurofibromatosis type 1), and succinate dehydrogenase mutations (including Carney–Stratakis syndrome) account for a small subset of tumours {3194, 442,2706}. The cell of origin of most sarcomas is unknown, and precursor or in situ lesions are not recognized. The exception is GIST, where somatic alterations in *KIT* and *PDGFRA*, believed to arise in precursors to the interstitial cells of Cajal, are identified in the vast majority of GISTs, small precursor lesions can be seen, and hypertrophy of the interstitial cells of Cajal is noted in families with inherited predisposition to GIST {2881}. Somatic genetic factors such as recurrent chromosomal translocations drive the pathogenesis of some sarcomas, but how and in what cell these somatic genetic factors arise remains unknown.

Clinical features

Benign and malignant soft tissue and neural tumours typically present as painless masses, and their growth rates vary. GISTs and other gastrointestinal mesenchymal neoplasms may be detected incidentally or may present with abdominal pain, gastrointestinal bleeding, anaemia, or an abdominal mass. The vast majority of benign soft tissue tumours are < 5 cm {808}. Malignant tumours can grow to be much larger. Involvement of digestive system organs can be secondary, such as a retroperitoneal sarcoma extending to involve the pancreas.

Because of their rarity, gastrointestinal tumours favoured to be mesenchymal should be referred to a specialist multidisciplinary centre before biopsy or surgery for optimal management {712}.

Histopathology

Malignant soft tissue neoplasms generally exhibit nuclear pleomorphism, mitotic activity, and necrosis to varying degrees. Some benign tumours can also show one or more of these features; for example, nuclear atypia can be seen in schwannoma with ancient change. For GIST, mitotic activity is the main histological feature of malignancy. In contrast to many other malignant mesenchymal neoplasms, even aggressive GISTs generally show uniform nuclear morphology. Immunohistochemistry is often needed to confirm the tumour cell lineage and diagnosis.

Genetics

Benign soft tissue tumours feature simple genetic properties with diploid karyotypes perhaps adorned by a single characteristic chromosomal rearrangement. In malignancy, two genetic classes exist: simple-karyotype sarcomas associated with a recurrent mutation or translocation (e.g. synovial sarcoma) and complex-karyotype sarcomas with numerous chromosomal aberrations but generally lacking recurrent mutations (e.g. leiomyosarcoma) other than *TP53* {368}.

As an intermediate tumour that locally recurs but does not metastasize, desmoid fibromatosis is generally associated with a single somatic mutation in *CTNNB1* and much less commonly *APC* {3068,1534}. GIST shows a characteristic molecular progression usually initiated with activating mutations in *KIT* or *PDGFRA* followed by stepwise chromosomal deletions probably harbouring various tumour suppressors {2881}.

Diagnostic procedures

Investigation includes clinical assessment of the size and depth of the tumour, the use of endoscopy and imaging modalities (CT and MRI), and biopsy. Imaging can be used to assess the extent of a primary tumour, to determine its relationship to normal structures, and to identify metastases. Small lesions of ≤ 1–1.5 cm in diameter can be completely excised on endoscopy. Larger lesions (and all deeper-seated tumours) necessitate diagnostic sampling. Core needle biopsy (often image-guided and preferably using a larger-bore needle) can provide diagnostic information on malignancy, subtype, and grade, with high sensitivity and specificity {1223,3372}. Open biopsy and cytology are less commonly used but can be important modalities; endoscopic biopsy is often used for gastrointestinal mesenchymal tumours.

Tumour behaviour

The *WHO classification of tumours of soft tissue and bone* {949} recognizes four tumour behaviour categories: benign, intermediate (locally aggressive), intermediate (rarely metastasizing), and malignant (see Box 12.01). Benign tumours are usually cured by local excision and rarely recur locally (and any recurrences are non-destructive). Intermediate tumours can be either locally aggressive (e.g. desmoid fibromatosis, which locally infiltrates surrounding tissues) or rarely metastasizing (tumours with a very low [< 2%] but definite risk of metastasis; e.g. plexiform fibrohistiocytic tumour). Malignant tumours such as leiomyosarcoma infiltrate and recur locally and commonly metastasize (i.e. in > 20% of cases). GISTs range from clinically insignificant, small benign lesions to aggressive sarcomas.

Grading

Grading is an attempt to predict clinical behaviour on the basis of histological variables, but it can only be performed using material from primary untreated neoplasms. It is not applicable to all sarcomas; for example, angiosarcomas, clear cell sarcomas, and epithelioid sarcomas are always considered to be high-grade. The most widely used system for grading soft tissue sarcomas is the three-tiered system developed by the French Fédération Nationale des Centres de Lutte Contre le Cancer (FNCLCC) {650,2339}. It uses a combination of tumour differentiation, mitotic count, and necrosis to categorize tumours as being of low, intermediate, or high grade. However, this system is not applicable to GISTs. More broadly applicable molecular approaches are currently in development {607,1863}.

Staging

The American Joint Committee on Cancer (AJCC) and the Union for International Cancer Control (UICC) TNM staging systems are widely used {127,408}. Sarcoma staging incorporates histological grading and site of involvement along with histological type, tumour size, extent of lymph node involvement, and presence or absence of distant metastasis. Alternative staging and risk assessment approaches incorporating non-anatomical variables such as age and sex are also under consideration {402,2659}.

Prognosis and predictive factors

Complete excision is the most important factor in preventing local recurrence {3343,3729}. Factors generally associated with a greater risk of metastasis are larger tumour size and higher grade. In some instances, histological subtype alone is predictive, but one of the principal factors in assessing prognosis and determining management is histological grade. Site is also important, because low-grade sarcomas in sites where complete surgical excision is difficult (e.g. the retroperitoneum or head and neck) generally have a worse outcome than do similarly staged tumours in the extremities {1100}. A risk assessment system incorporating anatomical site, mitotic count, and tumour size is applied to GISTs in order to predict malignant behaviour and to select patients for adjuvant targeted therapy {287}.

Gastrointestinal stromal tumour

Dei Tos AP
Hornick JL
Miettinen M

Definition

Gastrointestinal stromal tumour (GIST) is a mesenchymal neoplasm with variable behaviour, characterized by differentiation towards the interstitial cells of Cajal.

ICD-O coding

8936/3 Gastrointestinal stromal tumour

ICD-11 coding

2B5B & XH9HQ1 Gastrointestinal stromal tumour, primary site & Gastrointestinal stromal sarcoma

Related terminology

Not recommended: leiomyoblastoma; gastrointestinal autonomic nerve sheath tumour (GANT); gastrointestinal pacemaker cell tumour (GIPACT).

Subtype(s)

Succinate dehydrogenase–deficient gastrointestinal stromal tumour

Localization

GIST can occur anywhere in the GI tract; however, approximately 54% of all GISTs arise in the stomach, 30% in the small bowel (including the duodenum), 5% in the colon and rectum, and about 1% in the oesophagus {2762}. Rarely, GISTs arise in the appendix. About 10% of cases are primarily disseminated, and the site of origin cannot be established with certainty. Extragastrointestinal GISTs occur predominantly in the mesentery, omentum, and retroperitoneum; most probably represent a metastasis from an unrecognized primary or a detached mass from the GI tract.

Clinical features

The most common presentations include vague abdominal symptoms, as well as symptoms related to mucosal ulceration, acute and chronic bleeding, an abdominal mass, and tumour perforation. Smaller GISTs are detected incidentally during endoscopy, surgery, or CT. Advanced GISTs spread into the peritoneal cavity and retroperitoneal space and often metastasize to the liver. Bone, skin, and soft tissue metastases are infrequently observed, whereas lung metastases are exceedingly rare. Systemic spread can occur years after detection of the primary tumour. Gastric GISTs exhibit a higher local recurrence rate than do small bowel GISTs, but the latter have a higher rate of abdominal dissemination and metastasis.

Epidemiology

Population-based studies in Scandinavia indicate an incidence of 1.1–1.5 cases per 100 000 person-years {2364}. However, incidental subcentimetre GISTs (called microGISTs) seem to be remarkably common. A frequency of 10% was reported in a study of oesophagogastric junction carcinoma resection specimens {11}, and even higher frequencies in autopsy and entirely embedded gastrectomy series (22.5% and 35%, respectively) {48,1546}. Approximately 25% of gastric GISTs (excluding microGISTs) are clinically malignant. SEER Program data (interpolated from data on leiomyosarcomas) indicate that GISTs account for 2.2% of all malignant gastric tumours {3299}.

Sporadic GISTs can occur at any age, with a peak incidence in the sixth decade of life (median age: 60–65 years) and a slight male predominance {2154}. A small fraction of GISTs affect

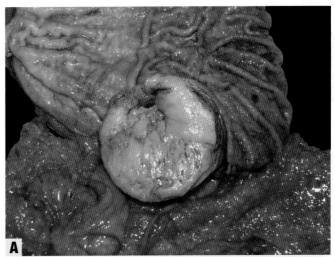

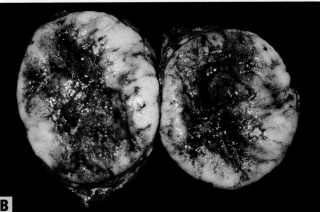

Fig. 12.01 Gastrointestinal stromal tumour (GIST). **A** Gross image of localized gastric GIST. Ulceration of the gastric mucosa is present. **B** Gross image of metastatic GIST to the liver. The cut surface features areas of haemorrhage and necrosis.

children and adolescents; such tumours are usually succinate dehydrogenase (SDH)-deficient (and *KIT/PDGFRA*-wildtype). SDH-deficient GISTs arise in the stomach, are more common in females, and affect younger patients {2144,1422}.

Etiology

Most GISTs are sporadic; 5–10% occur in association with a variety of syndromes. Most syndromic GISTs are SDH-deficient, including those associated with the non-hereditary Carney triad (GIST, pulmonary chondroma, paraganglioma) {509} and the autosomal dominant Carney–Stratakis syndrome (GIST and paraganglioma in the context of SDH germline mutations) {2538,3145}.

Rarely, GISTs are associated with neurofibromatosis type 1 (NF1); such cases are often multifocal, and most are located in the small bowel {2140,1015}. The extremely rare familial GISTs are caused by germline mutations of *KIT* or (far more rarely) *PDGFRA* {284,1881,2040}. Patients with these tumours tend to develop multiple GISTs, throughout the GI tract, that can behave aggressively.

Pathogenesis

Most GISTs harbour gain-of-function mutations of the *KIT* or *PDGFRA* oncogene and progress by the stepwise inactivation of tumour suppressor genes. See *Diagnostic molecular pathology*, below, for full details, which are of clinical significance.

Macroscopic appearance

Localized GIST presents as a well-circumscribed mass of highly variable size (ranging from incidental, submillimetre lesions to > 20 cm). In larger lesions, the cut surface may show foci of haemorrhage, cystic change, and/or necrosis. Gastric GISTs often feature an intraluminal component and may produce umbilicated mucosal ulcers. In the small bowel, GISTs more frequently present as external masses. Some GISTs feature a narrow pedicle linked to the serosal surface, the interruption of which may contribute to the generation of extragastrointestinal GISTs {2154,2148,2139}.

Advanced disease most often presents as a main lesion associated with multiple smaller nodules that may extend from the diaphragm to the pelvis. Invasion of surrounding organs such as the spleen and pancreas can be observed in aggressive tumours. SDH-deficient GISTs are often associated with a distinctive multinodular pattern of growth.

Histopathology

Microscopically, GISTs exhibit a broad morphological spectrum. Anatomical location (gastric vs small bowel) seems to influence the histological appearance. Most gastric GISTs are spindle cell tumours, with epithelioid morphology seen in approximately 20–25% of cases. Some cases feature a combination of spindle cell and epithelioid histology. Nuclear pleomorphism is uncommon. Distinctive histological patterns among spindle cell GISTs exist. One example is the sclerosing type, seen especially in small tumours that often contain calcifications. The palisaded-vacuolated subtype is one of the most common, whereas some examples show a diffuse hypercellular pattern. Very rarely, sarcomatoid features with substantial nuclear atypia and high mitotic activity can be observed. Epithelioid GISTs may show sclerosing, discohesive, hypercellular (sometimes with a pseudopapillary pattern), or sarcomatous morphology with substantial atypia and mitotic activity. Myxoid stroma is rarely observed {2154}.

Small intestinal and colonic GISTs are usually spindle cell tumours with diffuse sheets or vague storiform arrangements of tumour cells. Tumours with low biological potential often contain extracellular collagen globules (skeinoid fibres). Intestinal GISTs may feature anuclear areas (somewhat mimicking Verocay bodies or neuropil) composed of cell processes. Nuclear palisading, perivascular hyalinization, and regressive vascular

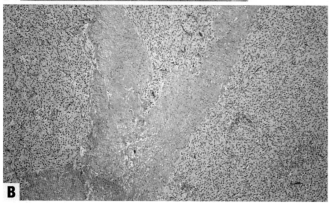

Fig. 12.02 Succinate dehydrogenase–deficient gastrointestinal stromal tumour. **A** The tumour shows a multinodular growth pattern through the wall of the stomach. **B** Muscularis propria separates tumour nodules.

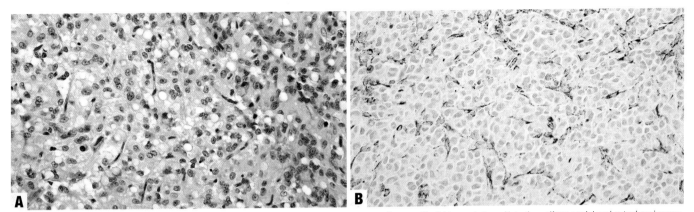

Fig. 12.03 Succinate dehydrogenase–deficient gastrointestinal stromal tumour. **A** The tumour shows epithelioid morphology. Note the uniform nuclei and cytoplasmic vacuoles. **B** The tumour cells show loss of staining for SDHB. Endothelial cells serve as an internal positive control.

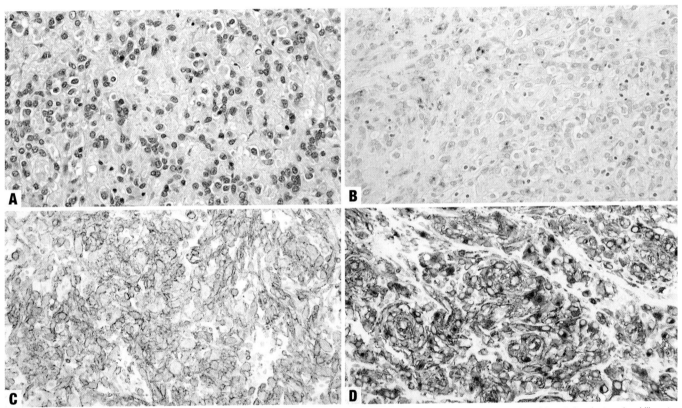

Fig. 12.04 Gastrointestinal stromal tumour (GIST), epithelioid type. **A** This tumour harbours a *PDGFRA* mutation. Note the round nuclei and abundant eosinophilic cytoplasm. **B** *PDGFRA*-mutant GISTs often show limited expression of KIT by immunohistochemistry (or are entirely KIT-negative). **C** Immunohistochemistry for DOG1 (ANO1) is helpful to confirm the diagnosis of *PDGFRA*-mutant GISTs. **D** *PDGFRA*-mutant GISTs typically show strong and diffuse expression of PDGFRA.

changes (e.g. dilated and thrombosed vessels, haemosiderin deposition, and fibrosis) similar to those in schwannomas can be seen. Rectal GISTs most often feature spindle cell morphology {1058,394,2142,2154,2148}.

SDH-deficient GISTs characteristically show epithelioid morphology and are typically multinodular with plexiform mural involvement. Unlike in conventional GISTs, lymphovascular invasion and lymph node metastases are common {2158,808A}.

Extremely rarely, morphological progression to high-grade (KIT-negative) sarcomatous morphology can be observed either de novo or after therapy with imatinib (dedifferentiated GIST). Dedifferentiation can also be associated with heterologous

epithelial, myogenic, or angiosarcomatous differentiation {1906, 164}.

Immunophenotypically, most GISTs show strong and diffuse expression of KIT (CD117), which appears as cytoplasmic, membrane-associated, or sometimes perinuclear dot-like staining. However, a small minority (< 5%), especially GISTs with *PDGFRA* mutations, may lack KIT expression or show very limited staining {2109}. The chloride-channel protein ANO1/DOG1 is an equally sensitive and specific marker and may rescue diagnostically as many as 50% of KIT-negative GISTs {3553, 877,2156,2391}. KIT and DOG1 are also expressed in the interstitial cells of Cajal, whose precursors are believed to be the

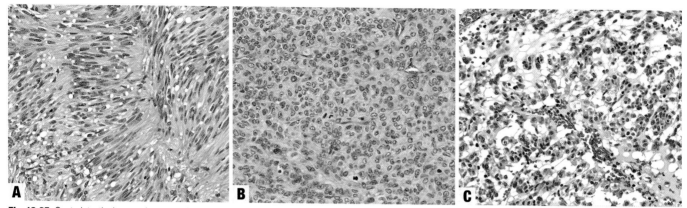

Fig. 12.05 Gastrointestinal stromal tumour (GIST). **A** GISTs are often composed of cytologically bland spindle cells that may feature distinctive paranuclear vacuolization. **B** Rarely, GIST may feature a high-grade morphology that is associated with high mitotic count. **C** The presence of myxoid change of the stroma is seen in this example of epithelioid GIST.

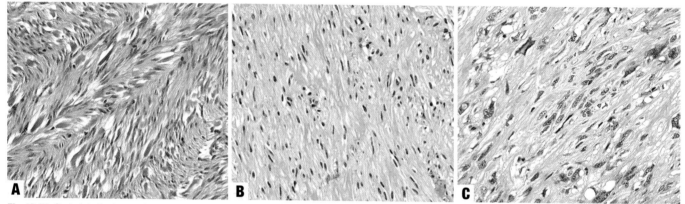

Fig. 12.06 Gastrointestinal stromal tumour (GIST). **A** Small bowel GISTs most often feature a spindle cell morphology that may be associated with the presence of skeinoid fibres. **B** GISTs sometimes appear microscopically hypocellular with neoplastic cells embedded in abundant fibrous stroma. **C** The presence of nuclear pleomorphism represents a rare morphological feature of GIST.

histogenetic origin of GISTs. Most spindle cell GISTs (especially gastric tumours) are positive for CD34, whereas epithelioid examples are less consistently positive. Some GISTs express h-caldesmon; a minority express SMA; and rare examples show positivity for desmin, keratins (CK18), or S100 {2148}. SDH-deficient GISTs exhibit loss of SDHB protein expression irrespective of which SDH gene is mutated {1041,2158,997}. SDHA loss is specific for *SDHA*-mutant tumours {3501}. Loss of expression of neurofibromin (NF1; using an antibody specific to the C-terminus) may help in identifying NF1-associated GISTs {2760}.

Cytology
Not clinically relevant

Diagnostic molecular pathology
About 85% of GISTs harbour gain-of-function mutations of the *KIT* or *PDGFRA* oncogene located on chromosome 4 (4q12), encoding for type III receptor tyrosine kinases {1242,1610, 1208,1469}. With exceedingly rare exceptions, they are mutually exclusive and result in the constitutive activation of either KIT or PDGFRA. Normally, KIT and PDGFRA are activated by the binding of their respective ligands (i.e. stem cell factor and PDGFA). Downstream oncogenic signalling involves the RAS/MAPK and PI3K/AKT/mTOR pathways {672,1468,2881}.

About 75% of GISTs harbour activating mutations of *KIT*, most often in exon 11 (66% overall) or exon 9 (6%); mutations in exons 13 and 17 are rare (~1% each) {1242,2774,859,1469}. *KIT* exon 11 mutations include deletions (45%), substitution mutations (30%), and insertion/deletion (indel) mutations (15%) including duplications. Nearly all *KIT* exon 9 mutations are duplications (p.A502_Y503); 80% of GISTs with such mutations arise in the small intestine. *KIT* exon 13 and 17 mutations are most often p.K642E and p.N822K, respectively {1612,1791}.

About 10% of GISTs harbour *PDGFRA* activating mutations (most often in the stomach), usually in exon 18 (8% overall); mutations in exons 12 and 14 are rare {1208,673}. The most common *PDGFRA* mutations are p.D842V (55%) and p.V561D (10%). Patients with *PDGFRA*-mutant tumours have a lower risk of metastasis than patients with *KIT*-mutant tumours {1469}. Given the differences in prognosis, nearly 85% of advanced GISTs harbour *KIT* mutations and only 2% harbour *PDGFRA* mutations {859}.

Many GISTs that are wildtype for *KIT* and *PDGFRA* harbour alterations in SDH subunit genes (5–10% overall) {1422,356}; 60% harbour inactivating mutations (nearly always germline); and 40% harbour *SDHC* promoter methylation (epimutation) {2158,1573}, leading to SDH dysfunction (SDH-deficient GIST). Patients with SDH-deficient GISTs are younger than those with tyrosine kinase receptor gene–mutant tumours; nearly all paediatric GISTs are SDH-deficient {356}. Tumours from patients with Carney triad usually show *SDHC* epimutation {1573}. *SDHA* is the most commonly mutated subunit gene (~35% of SDH-deficient GISTs) {3501}, followed by *SDHB*, *SDHC*, and *SDHD*. Rare GISTs are associated with mutations of *NF1* (which are usually germline alterations in patients with NF1 or rarely somatic mutations), *BRAF*, or *KRAS* {2173,290,1015}. Like *KIT* and *PDGFRA* mutations, these alterations also result in RAS/RAF/MEK pathway activation.

Most GISTs (with the exception of SDH-deficient tumours) progress through a stepwise acquisition of chromosomal alterations, each of which probably inactivates tumour suppressor genes: loss of 14q (as many as 70%), followed by loss of 22q (~50%), 1p (~50%), and 15q (~40%) {2881}. *MAX* is the 14q GIST tumour suppressor gene, inactivated early (in microscopic and low-risk tumours) {2882}. Inactivating mutations in *CDKN2A*, *TP53*, and *RB1* are found in GISTs of higher-risk categories {2901}. *DMD* inactivation is a late even in GIST progression, identified in nearly all metastatic GISTs {3522}. Very rare GISTs harbour *NTRK3* or *FGFR1* gene fusions {401,2990}.

Essential and desirable diagnostic criteria
Essential: an intramural, submucosal, or subserosal mass; spindle cell, epithelioid, or mixed morphology; KIT and/or DOG1 immunopositivity; SDHB loss in SDH-deficient GISTs.
Desirable: KIT or *PDGFRA* gene mutations in approximately 85% of tumours.

Staging (TNM)
Risk stratification is preferred to anatomical staging.

Prognosis and prediction
The best-documented prognostic parameters for GIST are mitotic activity, tumour size, and anatomical site (see Table 12.01). Mitotic counting is for an area of 5 mm², which in most modern microscopes corresponds to 20–25 fields with the 40× objective and standard eyepiece diameter {2146}. This prognostic assessment applies best to *KIT/PDGFRA*-mutant GISTs. In general, intestinal GISTs and SDH-deficient GISTs are more unpredictable {3755,2070}. Tumours with low mitotic counts can metastasize, whereas tumours with higher mitotic counts may remain indolent for extended periods. Many patients with SDH-deficient GISTs with liver metastases can survive for years or decades without specific treatment, in contrast to patients with *KIT/PDGFRA*-mutant GISTs, which are rapidly progressive when metastatic. Tumour rupture is an additional adverse factor in GIST {1256}. The grading principles for soft tissue sarcomas do not apply to GIST. In order to refine risk assessment for consideration of adjuvant therapy, it has been suggested to include size and mitotic counts as continuous variables to be incorporated along with anatomical site into prognostic tools such as nomograms {2762} or prognostic contour maps {1470}.

Mutation status also represents a prognostic as well as predictive factor {1792}. In general, *KIT*-mutant tumours tend to behave more aggressively than *PDGFRA*-mutant or triple-negative (*KIT*,

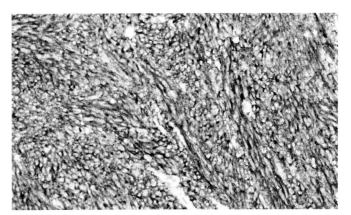

Fig. 12.07 Gastrointestinal stromal tumour. KIT (CD117)-positive gastrointestinal stromal tumour. Cytoplasmic immunopositivity is associated with perinuclear dot-like accentuation.

Table 12.01 Relationship of mitotic count and tumour size to prognosis of gastrointestinal stromal tumour (GIST), based on United States Armed Forces Institute of Pathology (AFIP) data from large long-term follow-up studies

Category	Mitotic count (mitoses/5 mm²)	Tumour size (cm)	% of progressive disease[a]	
			Stomach	Small bowel[b]
1	≤ 5	≤ 2	0	0
2		> 2 to ≤ 5	1.9	4.3
3a		> 5 to ≤ 10	3.6	24
3b		> 10	12	52
4	> 5	≤ 2	0	50
5		> 2 to ≤ 5	16	73
6a		> 5 to ≤ 10	55	85
6b		> 10	86	90

[a]Defined as metastasis or death due to disease. [b]Prognostic assessment of GISTs of all non-gastric sites can follow the criteria for small bowel GISTs.
Data are based on reference {2146}.

PDGFRA, *BRAF* wildtype) tumours. The best outcome seems to be associated with *PDGFRA* exon 12, *BRAF*, and *KIT* exon 11 mutations. The worst outcome seems to be associated with *KIT* exon 9 and 11 and *PDGFRA* exon 18 (non-D842V) mutated GISTs {2761}.

Mutation status also predicts response to imatinib, with *KIT* exon 11–mutant tumours exhibiting the highest rate of response and *PDGFRA* exon 18 (D842V) mutants showing primary resistance {1471}. Molecular status also influences imatinib dose selection, with *KIT* exon 9 mutants benefiting from a higher dosage (800 mg instead of 400 mg) {742}. Secondary mutations are associated with acquired resistance to imatinib. Secondary *KIT* gene mutations are most often found in the ATP-binding pocket of the kinase domain (exons 13 and 14) or in the kinase activation loop (exons 17 and 18) {162,1076}. Both *KIT/PDGFRA/BRAF*/SDH-wildtype and NF1-associated GISTs are also characterized by a lack of sensitivity to imatinib {520}.

Inflammatory myofibroblastic tumour

Fritchie KJ
Hornick JL
Rossi S

Definition

Inflammatory myofibroblastic tumour is a distinctive fibroblastic/myofibroblastic neoplasm of intermediate biological potential with a prominent inflammatory infiltrate, chiefly lymphocytes and plasma cells.

ICD-O coding

8825/1 Inflammatory myofibroblastic tumour

ICD-11 coding

2F70 & XH66Z0 Neoplasms of uncertain behaviour of oral cavity or digestive organs & Myofibroblastic tumour NOS

Related terminology

Not recommended: inflammatory pseudotumour; inflammatory fibrosarcoma; plasma cell granuloma.

Subtype(s)

Epithelioid inflammatory myofibroblastic sarcoma (8825/3)

Localization

The small intestine and colon are the most commonly involved gastrointestinal sites, followed by the stomach. The oesophagus, pancreas (direct extension from retroperitoneum), appendix, and liver are rare sites. The submucosa, muscularis propria, or mesentery may be involved {2019}. Epithelioid inflammatory myofibroblastic sarcoma has a marked predilection for the mesentery of the small intestine and omentum {2055}.

Clinical features

Patients may present with abdominal pain, bowel obstruction, or fever {2019,2113}. Leukocytosis, anaemia, elevated erythrocyte sedimentation rate, and hypergammaglobulinaemia are found in about half of affected patients {648,2019}.

Epidemiology

Children and young adults are most often affected, although the age range is broad {648,2019}. Epithelioid inflammatory myofibroblastic sarcoma shows a marked male predominance, but non-epithelioid–type tumours show no sex predilection {2055}.

Etiology

Unknown

Pathogenesis

About two thirds of inflammatory myofibroblastic tumours harbour tyrosine kinase receptor gene rearrangements, most often involving the *ALK* locus at 2p23, with diverse fusion partners {2054}. Epithelioid inflammatory myofibroblastic sarcoma usually has *RANBP2-ALK* fusion, or more rarely *RRBP1-ALK* fusion {2055,1825}. Approximately 5% of inflammatory myofibroblastic tumours harbour *ROS1* gene fusions; other rare gene fusions involve *NTRK3*, *PDGFRB*, and *RET* {1951,165,3650,80}.

Macroscopic appearance

Most tumours are 3–12 cm in size, with firm white or yellow cut surfaces.

Histopathology

Histological examination reveals loose fascicles of uniform, plump spindle cells with vesicular chromatin, small nucleoli, and pale cytoplasm {648}. The stroma may be myxoid or collagenous, typically containing an inflammatory infiltrate dominated by lymphocytes and plasma cells, with fewer eosinophils and neutrophils. Some tumours exhibit a compact, fascicular architecture with minimal stroma. A subset of tumour cells may resemble ganglion cells. Mitotic activity is low and necrosis is usually absent, but both may occasionally be present. Epithelioid inflammatory myofibroblastic sarcoma is composed of

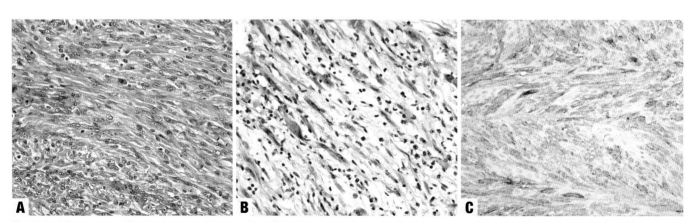

Fig. 12.08 Inflammatory myofibroblastic tumour of the stomach. **A** This cellular, fascicular tumour is composed of plump spindle cells with vesicular chromatin and eosinophilic cytoplasm. Note the occasional plasma cells and lymphocytes. **B** Some examples contain myxoid stroma. The tumour cells contain prominent nucleoli and amphophilic cytoplasm and are admixed with frequent lymphocytes. **C** Immunohistochemistry is positive for ALK in as many as 60% of cases, usually with a diffuse, cytoplasmic staining pattern.

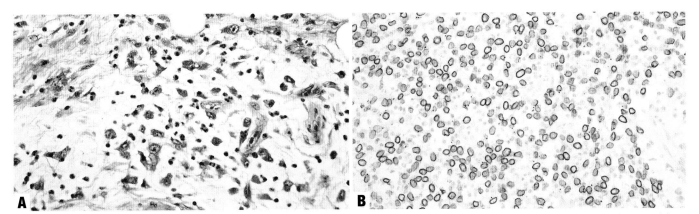

Fig. 12.09 Epithelioid inflammatory myofibroblastic sarcoma. **A** This tumour arose in the mesentery of the small intestine. The tumour is composed of loosely arranged, large polygonal cells with prominent nucleoli and amphophilic cytoplasm, embedded in abundant myxoid stroma with prominent neutrophils. **B** Most examples show a distinctive nuclear membrane pattern of ALK expression by immunohistochemistry, correlating with a *RANBP2-ALK* gene fusion.

epithelioid or round cells with large nucleoli and amphophilic or eosinophilic cytoplasm, embedded in an abundant myxoid stroma with prominent neutrophils {2055}.

Inflammatory myofibroblastic tumours are positive for SMA in nearly all cases, and in more than half of cases, also for desmin. Keratin expression is observed in 20–30% of cases. KIT, DOG1 (ANO1), CD34, S100, SOX10, and EMA are negative. Nearly 60% of inflammatory myofibroblastic tumours express ALK (usually with a diffuse cytoplasmic pattern) {664} and approximately 5% of cases express ROS1, correlating with underlying *ALK* and *ROS1* gene fusions, respectively {1278,165}. Epithelioid inflammatory myofibroblastic sarcomas show distinctive nuclear membrane or perinuclear ALK staining patterns {2055}.

Cytology
Not clinically relevant

Diagnostic molecular pathology
Positive immunohistochemistry for ALK, or more rarely ROS1, is sufficient for diagnosis, and demonstration of a fusion gene is not usually required.

Essential and desirable diagnostic criteria
Essential: loose fascicles of plump spindle cells without substantial pleomorphism (except epithelioid type); an inflammatory infiltrate of lymphocytes and plasma cells; SMA, often with ALK or (rarely) ROS1 expression.

Staging (TNM)
Not clinically relevant

Prognosis and prediction
Most conventional gastrointestinal inflammatory myofibroblastic tumours have a low rate of local recurrence {2019}. Distant metastases are rare (< 5%); histological features do not reliably predict clinical behaviour {647}. ALK-negative tumours may have a higher risk of metastases {647}. Epithelioid inflammatory myofibroblastic sarcoma is an aggressive subtype that recurs rapidly, with disseminated intra-abdominal disease, variable liver metastases, and a high mortality rate {2055}.

Desmoid fibromatosis

Fritchie KJ
Hornick JL
Rossi S

Definition

Desmoid fibromatosis is a locally aggressive, non-metastasizing myofibroblastic neoplasm with an infiltrative growth pattern.

ICD-O coding

8821/1 Desmoid-type fibromatosis
8822/1 Abdominal fibromatosis

ICD-11 coding

2F7C & XH13Z3 Neoplasms of uncertain behaviour of connective or other soft tissue & Desmoid-type fibromatosis (aggressive fibromatosis)
2F7C & XH6116 Neoplasms of uncertain behaviour of connective or other soft tissue & Abdominal (mesenteric) fibromatosis

Related terminology

Acceptable: desmoid tumour; aggressive fibromatosis.

Subtype(s)

None

Localization

Intra-abdominal desmoid fibromatosis arises most commonly in the mesentery of the small bowel, followed by the mesentery of the ileocolic region and the mesocolon. Less frequently involved sites include the pelvis, omentum, and retroperitoneum {444}.

Clinical features

Most patients present with an asymptomatic abdominal mass, whereas a minority report abdominal pain. Gastrointestinal bleeding and acute abdomen may rarely occur after intestinal perforation {1535}.

Epidemiology

The sexes are equally affected by intra-abdominal fibromatosis {1293}. The age range is broad, with a peak in the third decade

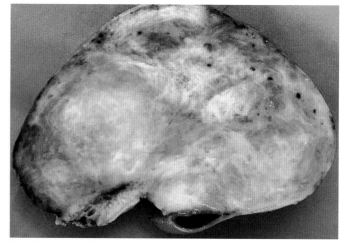

Fig. 12.11 Desmoid fibromatosis of the mesentery of the small bowel. Grossly, the tumour appears well circumscribed and features a whorled cut surface.

of life. Most cases are sporadic, but 10–15% are associated with germline mutations in the *APC* gene (i.e. familial adenomatous polyposis); such tumours tend to present at a younger age {1868,654}.

Etiology

There are multiple causes. There is a considerably increased prevalence of desmoid fibromatosis in patients with familial adenomatous polyposis (also known as Gardner syndrome). Physical factors are also relevant, because surgery increases the risk of tumour development {1077}.

Pathogenesis

The WNT/β-catenin signalling pathway is dysregulated in virtually all tumours {687,2564}. Somatic activating mutations in the *CTNNB1* gene and germline inactivating mutations in the *APC* gene are mutually exclusive and are likely to be the initiating

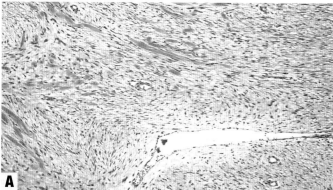
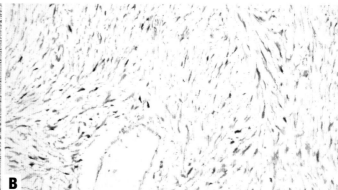

Fig. 12.10 Desmoid fibromatosis. **A** The tumour consists of long fascicles of uniform spindle cells with keloidal fibres and delicate blood vessels. **B** Most of the neoplastic nuclei express β-catenin.

events in the vast majority of sporadic and familial tumours, respectively. Rare sporadic tumours, wildtype for *CTNNB1*, carry somatic inactivation of *APC*. There is evidence that these mutations interfere with β-catenin proteasomal degradation, resulting in accumulation of β-catenin in the cytoplasm and in its subsequent translocation to the nucleus with consequent constitutive activation of the WNT pathway {2397}. In rare tumours with both *CTNNB1* and *APC* wildtype, the WNT pathway is impaired by other mechanisms {687}.

Macroscopic appearance
Intra-abdominal desmoid fibromatosis tends to present as a large mass, often as large as 10 cm in diameter, with a whorled cut surface.

Histopathology
Microscopically, the tumour consists of long sweeping fascicles of slender spindle or stellate cells harbouring tapering or ovoid nuclei and inconspicuous or small nucleoli. Nuclear hyperchromasia and cytological atypia are absent. Hypocellular areas with a myxoid background reminiscent of nodular fasciitis, abundant keloidal fibres, or zones of hyalinization may be seen. The vasculature is variably prominent, composed of delicate, sometimes dilated vessels, with perivascular oedema and microhaemorrhages. Although the gross appearance is circumscribed, extensive soft tissue infiltration is present microscopically {444}. Desmoid fibromatosis is usually positive for SMA and occasionally desmin. Nuclear expression of β-catenin is observed in at least 80% of tumours {323,502}.

Cytology
Not clinically relevant

Diagnostic molecular pathology
In 85–95% of sporadic cases, *CTNNB1* activating mutations are identified in exon 3, encoding the N-terminus of β-catenin (codons 32–45), with the most common mutations being c.121A>G (p.T41A), c.134C>T (p.S45F), and c.133T>C (p.S45P) {687,2564}. In desmoid-related familial adenomatous polyposis, *APC* germline mutations are often located beyond codon 1444 {2564}. The absence of *CTNNB1* mutations in an apparently sporadic tumour should raise concern for unrecognized familial forms of desmoid fibromatosis and should prompt colonoscopy and other clinical investigations {2564,1534}. Most cases have a balanced genomic profile, but a minority (~25%) show recurrent copy-number changes (loss of 6q, loss of 5q, gain of 20q, and gain of 8); the role of these changes is unclear {2829}.

Essential and desirable diagnostic criteria
Essential: long sweeping fascicles of myofibroblasts without substantial cytological atypia; infiltrative margins.
Desirable: nuclear β-catenin expression.

Staging (TNM)
Not clinically relevant

Prognosis and prediction
Desmoid fibromatosis is characterized by unpredictable behaviour, with phases of stabilization and rapid growth {1077}. Spontaneous regression, most often observed in abdominal

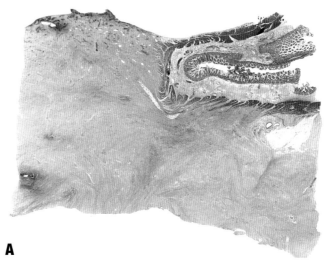

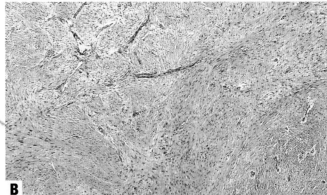

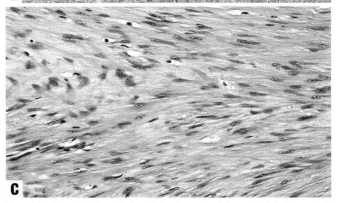

Fig. 12.12 Desmoid fibromatosis with involvement of the small intestine. **A** Full-thickness involvement. **B** Medium power shows irregular fascicles of hypocellular fibrous tissue with small vessels. **C** The cells are spindle-shaped with minimal nuclear irregularity.

wall lesions, is rarely seen at intra-abdominal sites. Recurrence occurs in 20–30% of patients {687,1534}, and it is associated with young age and larger tumour size {687,2829}. Intra-abdominal tumours are at lower risk for local recurrence than tumours in the extremities but at higher risk than abdominal wall lesions {687}. Incomplete resection does not correlate consistently with recurrence {687}. Recurrence-free survival appears to be worse with tumours harbouring *CTNNB1* p.S45F mutations {1810, 1534}. Very rare tumour-related deaths have been reported for patients with grossly incompletely resected intra-abdominal tumours, especially if syndromic {687,2564}.

Solitary fibrous tumour

Fritchie KJ
Hornick JL
Rossi S

Definition

Solitary fibrous tumour (SFT) is a fibroblastic tumour characterized by a prominent, thin-walled, dilated (staghorn) vasculature and *NAB2-STAT6* gene rearrangement.

ICD-O coding

8815/1 Solitary fibrous tumour NOS
8815/3 Solitary fibrous tumour, malignant

ICD-11 coding

2F7C & XH7E62 Neoplasms of uncertain behaviour of connective or other soft tissue & Solitary fibrous tumour NOS
2B5Y & XH1HP3 Other specified malignant mesenchymal neoplasms & Solitary fibrous tumour, malignant

Related terminology

Not recommended: haemangiopericytoma.

Subtype(s)

Lipomatous solitary fibrous tumour; giant cell angiofibroma (9160/0)

Localization

SFTs may arise at any anatomical location, including the oesophagus, gallbladder, liver and pancreas, and small bowel mesentery, as well as the serosal surfaces of the stomach and colon {2021,1812,2211,1978,1844,398,3753}. The lipomatous subtype has a predilection for abdominopelvic and retroperitoneal locations {2355,1824,951}.

Clinical features

SFTs usually present in adulthood as slow-growing masses. Tumours impinging on abdominal organs may cause symptoms, although most are painless. Rarely, hypoglycaemia develops secondary to tumour production of insulin-like growth factors, and serum IGF2 levels return to normal after resection {981, 2073,299}.

Epidemiology

SFTs are primarily seen in adults aged 20–70 years and are rare in children and adolescents. Generally, the sex incidence is equal, although the lipomatous form is slightly more common in males.

Etiology

Unknown

Pathogenesis

SFTs are characterized by *NAB2-STAT6* gene fusions resulting from an inversion at the 12q13 locus {2737,2193,615}. In the chimeric protein, the repressor domain of NAB2 is replaced with an activation domain from STAT6, creating a potent transcriptional activator of EGR1 and constitutive activation of EGR-mediated transcription.

Macroscopic appearance

The tumours are well circumscribed and unencapsulated, ranging up to 25 cm and appearing exophytic when arising from the serosal surfaces.

Histopathology

SFTs are usually composed of bland ovoid to spindled cells with pale eosinophilic cytoplasm organized in short poorly defined or haphazard fascicles around a prominent vascular network of thin-walled, dilated, and branching staghorn blood vessels. The degree of cellularity is variable, even within the same tumour,

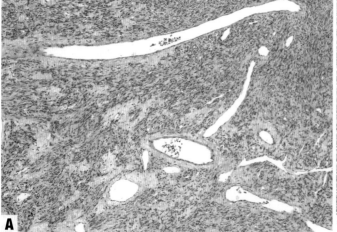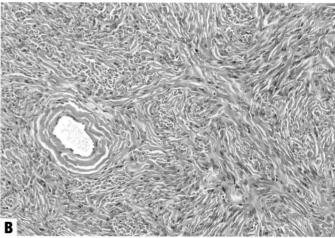

Fig. 12.13 Solitary fibrous tumour. **A** Solitary fibrous tumours harbour a prominent network of branching blood vessels with perivascular hyalinization. **B** Tumours are composed of uniform ovoid to spindled cells with variable stromal hyalinization.

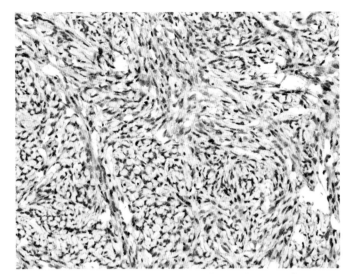
Fig. 12.14 Solitary fibrous tumour. STAT6 shows diffuse nuclear expression.

ranging from singly arranged or linear clusters of cells to densely cellular. Stromal and perivascular hyalinization is common and may be striking. Tumours may show myxoid change, cystic degeneration, or haemorrhage. A subset of SFTs harbour a component of mature adipose tissue (lipomatous SFT) and may mimic well-differentiated or dedifferentiated liposarcoma {2355,1824,951}. Giant cell–rich cases (giant cell angiofibroma) contain multinucleated stromal giant cells creating pseudovascular spaces {745}.

The vast majority of SFTs are positive for CD34 (90–95%) and STAT6 (98%; nuclear) {2918}. STAT6 is considered a highly sensitive and specific marker for this entity {810}. SFTs may be variably positive for EMA and SMA, and they rarely show focal staining for keratins and/or desmin {1156,2356,242}.

Cytology
Not clinically relevant

Diagnostic molecular pathology
Not clinically relevant

Essential and desirable diagnostic criteria
Essential: uniform ovoid to spindled cells arranged in short or haphazard fascicles; variable stromal hyalinization; prominent branching, staghorn vasculature.
Desirable: nuclear STAT6 expression.

Staging (TNM)
Not clinically relevant

Prognosis and prediction
Prognostication of SFT is notoriously difficult. The majority of tumours behave in a benign fashion, but approximately 10% act aggressively, resulting in local recurrence and distant metastasis. Features associated with higher risk of aggressive behaviour include older patient age, larger tumour size, high cellularity, cytological atypia, > 4 mitoses/2 mm^2, haemorrhage, necrosis, and frank sarcomatous transformation {1057,3402,754}.

Lipoma

Fritchie KJ
Hornick JL
Rossi S

Definition

Lipoma is a benign tumour composed of mature adipocytes, and may include other mesenchymal elements in subtypes.

ICD-O coding

8850/0 Lipoma NOS
8861/0 Angiolipoma NOS

ICD-11 coding

2E80.02 & XH1PL8 Deep internal or visceral lipoma & Lipoma NOS
2E80.02 & XH3C77 Deep internal or visceral lipoma & Angiolipoma

Related terminology

None

Subtype(s)

None

Localization

Lipomas may occur anywhere in the digestive system. The large intestine is the most commonly affected site, with most lipomas arising in the caecum and the ascending colon {2308, 693}. Less often, lipomas can be seen in the small intestine, most commonly in the ileum, followed by the stomach and the oesophagus {734,493,3206}. Lipomas typically arise in the submucosa; < 10% involve the subserosa. Intramucosal lipomas are rare, but they can rarely represent sentinel lesions for Cowden syndrome (*PTEN* hamartoma tumour syndrome) {2962,2961,464}.

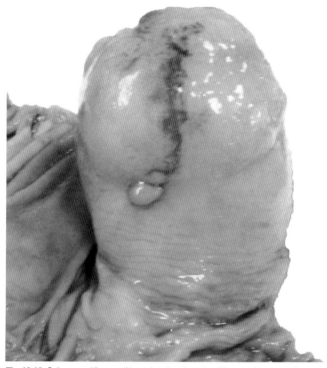

Fig. 12.16 Submucosal lipoma of the colon. A pedunculated lipoma of the ascending colon.

Clinical features

Gastrointestinal lipomas are usually asymptomatic and often incidental findings during endoscopy, surgery, or autopsy. A variety of symptoms may occur when these tumours reach a large size, usually > 2 cm for the small intestine and > 4 cm

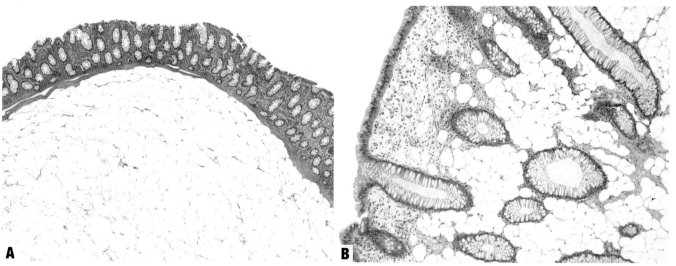

Fig. 12.15 Lipoma of the colon. **A** This submucosal lipoma shows adipocytes located below the muscularis mucosa. **B** Adipocytes are located in the lamina propria and surround the crypts in an intramucosal lipoma.

for the stomach and colon {2308,693,493}. The symptoms vary from mild abdominal pain and changes in bowel habits to life-threatening complications, because gastrointestinal lipomas may cause intestinal obstruction due to colocolonic intussusception, bleeding, and perforation {2308,693,493}.

Epidemiology
The prevalence of lipomas in the large bowel is estimated at 0.2–4.4% of patients undergoing endoscopy {693}. Peak incidence is within the sixth decade of life, with a possible female predilection {2308}.

Etiology
Unknown

Pathogenesis
As many as 75% of lipomas harbour simple chromosomal aberrations. Abnormalities of 12q13-q14 are most common, usually with rearrangements of the *HMGA2* gene, encoding a member of the high-mobility group of proteins {2904}.

Macroscopic appearance
Gastrointestinal lipomas vary considerably in size, from sub-centimetre lesions to tumours measuring > 10 cm. They may present as sessile or pedunculated masses.

Histopathology
Microscopically, lipomas consist of mature adipocytes of uniform size without substantial cytological atypia or atypical hyperchromatic stromal cells. Ulceration of the overlying mucosa may be observed, especially in large lesions. In intramucosal lipomas, the adipocytes are seen in the basal portion of the lamina propria, often surrounding the crypts. Intramucosal lipomas must be distinguished from pseudolipomatosis, which is caused by the infiltration of gas into the mucosa during endoscopy. Rarely, subtypes described in soft tissues (e.g. angiolipoma) can occur in digestive system sites. Angiolipomas show prominent capillary vessels with scattered fibrin microthrombi.

Cytology
Not clinically relevant

Diagnostic molecular pathology
Not clinically relevant

Essential and desirable diagnostic criteria
Essential: mature uniform adipocytes without cytological atypia.

Staging (TNM)
Not clinically relevant

Prognosis and prediction
Gastrointestinal lipomas are benign. Resection, either endoscopic or surgical, is reserved for symptomatic/complicated cases {2308,693}.

Inflammatory fibroid polyp

Fritchie KJ
Hornick JL
Rossi S

Definition
Inflammatory fibroid polyp is a benign, often polypoid, hypocellular fibroblastic neoplasm with a predilection for the stomach and ileum, containing a prominent inflammatory infiltrate, especially eosinophils.

ICD-O coding
None

ICD-11 coding
DA98.2 Inflammatory fibroid polyp of small intestine
DB35.4 Inflammatory fibroid polyp of large intestine
XA6452 Small intestine
XA9780 Duodenum
XA8UM1 Jejunum
XA0QT6 Ileum

Related terminology
None

Subtype(s)
None

Localization
The stomach (especially the antrum) is the most commonly affected site, followed by the ileum, although inflammatory fibroid polyps may arise throughout the GI tract {1476,1669}. Tumours are usually centred in the submucosa but can be restricted to the mucosa.

Clinical features
Small tumours in the upper GI tract can be discovered incidentally at endoscopy. Larger tumours may present with abdominal pain, bleeding, or obstruction; intussusception is a common presentation for small intestine tumours. Tumours may be sessile or polypoid in appearance.

Epidemiology
Inflammatory fibroid polyps are rare. There is a slight female predominance and a peak incidence in middle-aged adults {719}.

Etiology
Most tumours are sporadic, but rare cases are familial {158}, associated with germline *PDGFRA* mutations {2705}. Mutation carriers often develop multiple tumours, including gastrointestinal stromal tumours.

Pathogenesis
PDGFRA activating mutations are identified in many cases, most often in small intestine tumours {2883,1793,719}; exon 18 mutations, usually c.2525A>T (p.D842V), predominate in

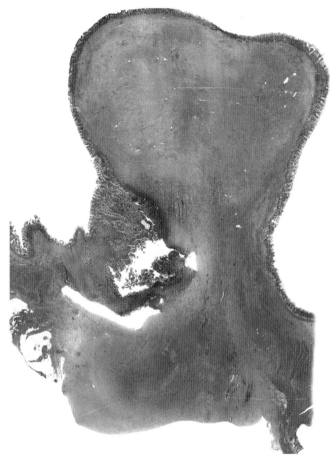

Fig. 12.17 Inflammatory fibroid polyp of the small intestine. As is characteristic of small/large bowel inflammatory fibroid polyp, this example shows transmural involvement.

gastric tumours, whereas exon 12 mutations are nearly always identified in small intestine tumours {1342}. Germline *PDGFRA* mutations have been found in the rare familial cases {2705}.

Macroscopic appearance
Inflammatory fibroid polyps range widely in size; gastric tumours are usually < 3 cm, whereas ileal tumours are often larger. The cut surface is white and often fleshy.

Histopathology
Histological features include a poorly marginated, hypocellular lesion containing a haphazard arrangement of short spindled and stellate cells with fine chromatin, small or indistinct nucleoli, and scant eosinophilic cytoplasm. The stroma is often oedematous and sometimes myxoid or collagenous, with a prominent mixed inflammatory infiltrate, often rich in eosinophils and lymphocytes. Small and intermediate-sized, rounded blood vessels, some with concentric (onion-skin) fibrosis, are a typical finding.

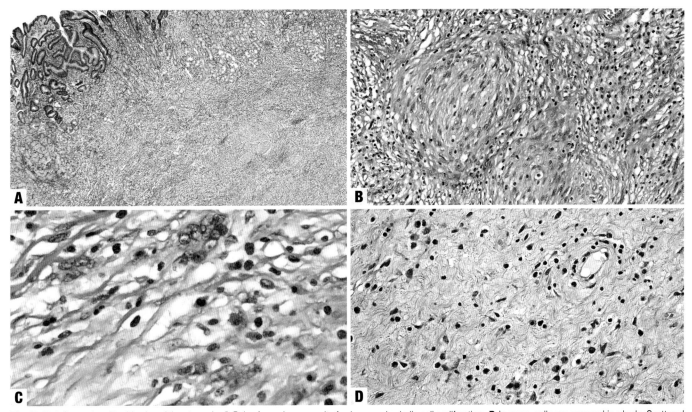

Fig. 12.18 Inflammatory fibroid polyp of the stomach. **A** Polyp formed as a result of submucosal spindle cell proliferation. **B** In areas, cells are arranged in whorls. Scattered multinucleated giant cells are characteristic. **C** Eosinophils are present in the background. **D** A less cellular example with fine, fibrillary collagenous stroma and prominent eosinophils.

By immunohistochemistry, CD34 and PDGFRA are positive in most cases {1182,1793}. More-limited SMA expression is observed in a small subset of tumours. KIT, DOG1 (ANO1), desmin, S100, SOX10, and keratins are negative.

Cytology
Not clinically relevant

Diagnostic molecular pathology
Not clinically relevant

Essential and desirable diagnostic criteria
Essential: a hypocellular appearance, with short spindled to stellate cells in an oedematous or myxoid stroma; an inflammatory infiltrate of eosinophils and lymphocytes.
Desirable: Expression of CD34.

Staging (TNM)
Not clinically relevant

Prognosis and prediction
Inflammatory fibroid polyps are benign.

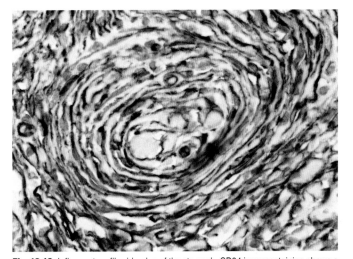

Fig. 12.19 Inflammatory fibroid polyp of the stomach. CD34 immunostaining shows a whorled pattern of positive staining.

Plexiform fibromyxoma

Fritchie KJ
Hornick JL
Rossi S

Definition

Plexiform fibromyxoma is a benign mesenchymal neoplasm that arises in the antrum and pyloric region.

ICD-O coding

8811/0 Plexiform fibromyxoma

ICD-11 coding

2E92.1 Benign neoplasm of stomach

Related terminology

Acceptable: plexiform angiomyxoid myofibroblastic tumour of the stomach.

Subtype(s)

None

Localization

Plexiform fibromyxoma is primarily gastric, but the duodenum can be involved.

Clinical features

Presenting symptoms include gastrointestinal bleeding, ulcer, weight loss, and pyloric obstruction.

Epidemiology

Males and females are affected equally, and tumours have been reported over a wide patient age distribution, including in childhood.

Etiology

Unknown

Pathogenesis

Recurrent *MALAT1-GLI1* fusions and *GLI1* polysomy have been identified in a subset of tumours that show GLI1 overexpression {3106}.

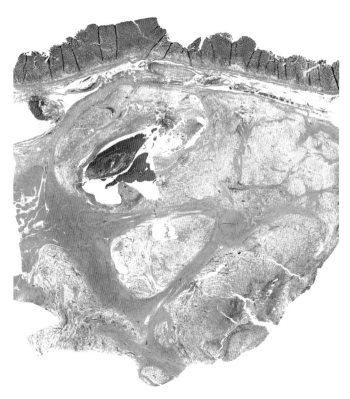

Fig. 12.20 Plexiform fibromyxoma. Low-power examination shows a plexiform arrangement of intramural myxoid nodules.

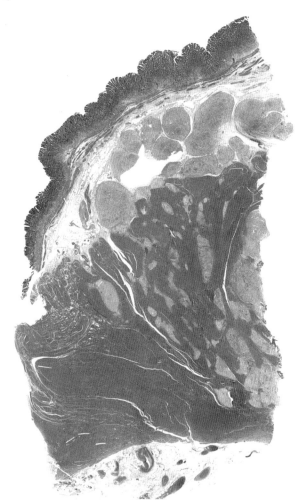

Fig. 12.21 Plexiform fibromyxoma. A nice scanning magnification to show the plexiform pattern.

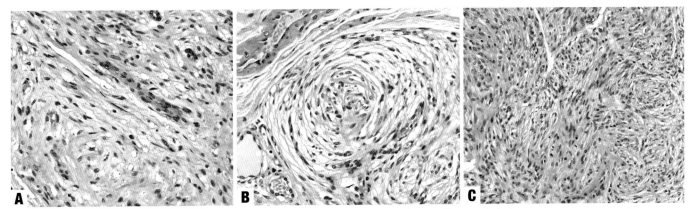

Fig. 12.22 Plexiform fibromyxoma. **A,B,C** High-power shows the spectrum of morphology: hypovascular, more fibrous, and whorls.

Macroscopic appearance
The tumours form gelatinous or haemorrhagic multinodular masses of 3–15 cm (median: 5.5 cm), sometimes protruding from the serosa {3211,2149} but centred in the muscularis propria. Extension into the mucosa with associated ulceration is noted in a subset of cases.

Histopathology
The nodules are composed of bland spindle cells, probably myofibroblasts, set in a myxoid, fibromyxoid, or collagenous matrix with a prominent arborizing thin-walled capillary network. Increased cellularity may be seen in tumours in the duodenal bulb or with extramural extension. Tumour nodules may extend into veins, which is of no clinical significance {2149}. Substantial cytological atypia is absent, and the mitotic count is low (median: 1 mitosis/10 mm^2) {2149}. The spindle cells are positive for SMA and occasionally for desmin, whereas ALK, CD34, keratins, KIT, and DOG1 are negative {2149,3211}.

Cytology
Not clinically relevant

Diagnostic molecular pathology
Not clinically relevant

Essential and desirable diagnostic criteria
Essential: multinodular and plexiform low-power architecture; uniform spindle cells in a myxoid, fibromyxoid, or collagenous stroma; delicate arborizing vasculature.

Staging (TNM)
Not clinically relevant

Prognosis and prediction
Plexiform fibromyxomas are benign, with no reports of recurrence or metastasis {3210,3211,2149}.

Leiomyoma

Dry SM
Kumarasinghe MP

Definition

Leiomyoma is a benign mesenchymal neoplasm showing smooth muscle differentiation.

ICD-O coding

8890/0 Leiomyoma NOS

ICD-11 coding

2E86.1 Leiomyoma of other or unspecified sites
XA0828 Oesophagus
XA9607 Gastrointestinal tract

Related terminology

None

Subtype(s)

Leiomyomatosis NOS (8890/1); seedling leiomyomas

Localization

Clinically relevant leiomyomas predominantly occur in the oesophagus, colon, and rectum and are rare in the stomach and small intestine. Typically, leiomyomas are intramural in the upper GI tract, whereas they occur in the muscularis mucosae in the colon and rectum. Leiomyoma is the most common benign intramural mesenchymal tumour of the oesophagus and tends to arise in the oesophagogastric junction and the mid-oesophagus. Smaller (< 7 mm) incidentally recognized leiomyomas have been reported in oesophagogastric resections (seedling leiomyomas) {3225}. Oesophageal leiomyomatosis is regarded as a hamartomatous disorder in children, but case reports of adult cases have been published in the literature {149,2660}.

Clinical features

Large tumours of the oesophagus may be symptomatic. However, most leiomyomas are discovered incidentally at endoscopy or surgery, often as a polyp.

Epidemiology

The prevalence is unknown. The incidence of leiomyoma varies according to site. Approximately 10% of all leiomyomas of the GI tract occur in the oesophagus {2143,2255,11}. However, even in the oesophagus, leiomyomas are relatively rare, with autopsy data showing an incidence of 0.006–8% {1833}.

Etiology

Some cases of leiomyomatosis may be familial, associated with Alport syndrome and deletions of the *COL4A5* and *COL4A6* genes {149}.

Pathogenesis

Unknown

Macroscopic appearance

Grossly, intramural leiomyomas are firm white tumours with a whorled appearance on cut surface.

Histopathology

Microscopically, the tumours are composed of bundles of well-differentiated spindled smooth muscle cells with blunt-ended nuclei. There is no clear demarcation or well-formed capsule. Mitotic activity is generally not detected. There may be focal nuclear atypia. By immunohistochemistry, lesional cells are typically positive for desmin, SMA, caldesmon, and calponin. A distinctive type of leiomyoma that occurs in the colon originates in the muscularis mucosae.

Leiomyoma must be differentiated from other spindle cell lesions of the GI tract. Throughout the GI tract, the main differential diagnosis is with gastrointestinal stromal tumour, which may show similar bland spindle cells. However, immunohistochemical stains diagnostic of gastrointestinal stromal tumour, such as KIT (CD117), DOG1, and CD34, are consistently negative in leiomyomas. Schwannomas are spindle cell tumours that show strong, diffuse positivity for S100 and are negative for desmin. Inflammatory fibroid polyps usually arise in the submucosa of the stomach and small bowel, and they show ovoid, spindled, or epithelioid cells with scant cytoplasm set in a myxoid to oedematous stroma with a marked inflammatory infiltrate consisting predominantly of eosinophils, as well as lymphocytes and histiocytes. These also are positive for CD34, and a minority of cases are positive for SMA, but they are negative for desmin, KIT (CD117), DOG1, and S100.

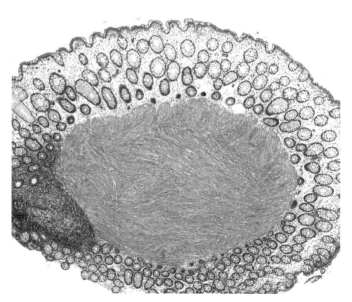

Fig. 12.23 Colonic mucosa-based leiomyoma.

Cytology

Large mass-forming leiomyomas of the GI tract may be sampled by EUS-guided FNA. Fragments of spindle cells with bland cytology are noted in adequate samples. Confirmatory immunohistochemical stains can be performed on cell block material {3132}.

Diagnostic molecular pathology

Not clinically relevant

Essential and desirable diagnostic criteria

Essential: fascicles of spindle cells with eosinophilic cytoplasm; lack of conspicuous mitotic activity and necrosis; expression of SMA and desmin; lack of KIT (CD117), DOG1, and CD34.

Staging (TNM)

Not clinically relevant

Prognosis and prediction

Leiomyomas are benign tumours, with virtually no risk of progression to leiomyosarcoma in the GI tract.

Leiomyosarcoma

Dry SM
Kumarasinghe MP

Definition
Leiomyosarcoma is a malignant neoplasm showing smooth muscle differentiation.

ICD-O coding
8890/3 Leiomyosarcoma NOS

ICD-11 coding
2B58.2 Leiomyosarcoma of stomach
2B58.Y Leiomyosarcoma "other specified primary site" (includes remainder of GI tract)
XA6452 Small intestine
XA1B13 Large intestine
XH7ED4 Leiomyosarcoma

Related terminology
None

Subtype(s)
None

Localization
The GI tract leiomyosarcomas reported since 2000 most commonly occurred in the small intestine (40%) and colorectum (40%) and more rarely in the stomach (10%) and oesophagus (10%) {3648,1232}.

Clinical features
Dysphagia, gastro-oesophageal reflux, gastrointestinal bleeding, abdominal pain, intestinal obstruction, weight loss, and anaemia have all been reported.

Epidemiology
Before the recognition of gastrointestinal stromal tumours (GISTs), leiomyosarcomas were commonly reported in the GI tract. They are now considered very rare, with only 76 cases reported since 2000 (before 2000, many GISTs were misclassified as leiomyosarcoma). Small intestine and colorectal cases are equally common in males and females, whereas oesophageal and gastric cases are more common in males, with an M:F ratio of 2.5:1. The median patient age at presentation is about 60 years, except for gastric tumours, which arise in younger patients (median age: 37 years) {1232}. The anorectum is the only site in the tubular gut where leiomyosarcoma is more common than GIST.

Etiology
Unknown

Pathogenesis
Unknown

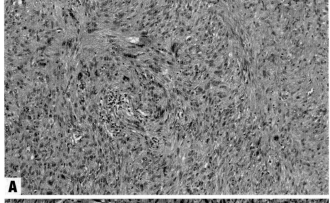
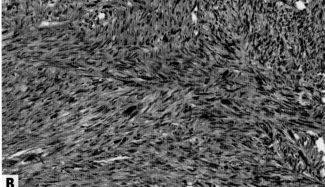
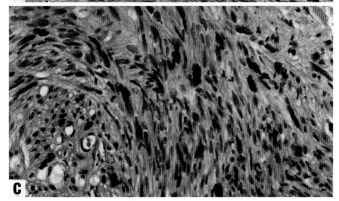

Fig. 12.24 Leiomyosarcoma. **A** Leiomyosarcomas show spindled cells with abundant eosinophilic cytoplasm in long intersecting fascicles. **B** Variable degrees of nuclear pleomorphism are seen. **C** Tumour cells show blunt-ended, so-called cigar-shaped nuclei and nuclear pleomorphism. Mitoses are present.

Macroscopic appearance
Leiomyosarcomas may present as polypoid or lobulated intraluminal tumours or as ulcerating, sessile, solid, or cystic masses {1232,2155,2142,2152}.

Histopathology

Leiomyosarcomas consist of long intersecting fascicles of spindle cells with ample eosinophilic cytoplasm and nuclei with blunt ends (cigar-shaped nuclei). Moderate nuclear pleomorphism with hyperchromatic enlarged nuclei is common, although nuclear pleomorphism can range from mild to marked. Mitoses are numerous in GI tract leiomyosarcomas, although rare tumours with low mitotic counts have been reported {1232, 2155}. Necrosis may be present. Leiomyosarcomas are positive for SMA, most are desmin-positive, and rare cases show staining for keratins and CD34 {2151,2142}. Other muscle markers (MSA, calponin, and caldesmon) are also typically positive {3648}. The main differential diagnosis is with GISTs, most of which show shorter and more haphazardly located fascicles of cells, more nuclear uniformity, and far fewer mitoses. GISTs are immunohistochemically positive for KIT (CD117) and DOG1, which are negative in leiomyosarcoma. EBV-associated smooth muscle tumours can show a range of histological appearances, from lesions mimicking leiomyomas to tumours composed entirely of small round to ovoid blue cells. These are positive for SMA, with variable desmin positivity. All show diffuse, strong staining for EBV-encoded small RNA (EBER), which is not seen in leiomyosarcoma. These should be considered in immunosuppressed patients and patients with multiple synchronous or metachronous tumours {769}. Schwannoma may also enter the differential diagnosis. In the GI tract, schwannomas tend to be cellular, with peripheral lymphoplasmacytic aggregates, and by immunohistochemistry they are strongly, diffusely positive for S100 and negative for SMA and desmin.

Cytology

Not clinically relevant

Diagnostic molecular pathology

Unlike GISTs, leiomyosarcomas do not carry KIT or PDGFRA mutations, but they often have aberrations in TP53 and RB1.

Essential and desirable diagnostic criteria

Essential: cellular tumours with long intersecting fascicles of spindle cells; pleomorphic, enlarged nuclei; increased mitoses, sometimes with tumour necrosis.

Staging (TNM)

Leiomyosarcoma should be staged using the sarcoma staging information from the eighth edition (2017) of the Union for International Cancer Control (UICC) TNM classification {408}

Prognosis and prediction

Leiomyosarcomas are aggressive neoplasms, with a 40–80% local recurrence rate and a 55–70% metastasis rate. The rate of death from disease is 25–50%, depending on the site. Tumour size > 5 cm appears to correlate with prognosis. Interestingly, mitotic counts and nuclear atypia do not correlate with prognosis, and leiomyosarcomas with low mitotic counts have recurred locally in the abdomen {3648,2155,1232}. Studies have proposed different classes of leiomyosarcomas (based on gene expression), which were associated with different outcomes; however, these are not currently used for clinical prognostication {1117,1406}.

Rhabdomyosarcoma

Dry SM
Kumarasinghe MP

Definition

Rhabdomyosarcoma is a malignant neoplasm composed of primitive muscle precursor–derived cells characterized by variable levels of skeletal muscle differentiation.

ICD-O coding

8900/3 Rhabdomyosarcoma NOS
8910/3 Embryonal rhabdomyosarcoma NOS
8912/3 Rhabdomyosarcoma, spindle cell / sclerosing type
8920/3 Alveolar rhabdomyosarcoma

ICD-11 coding

2B55.Y Rhabdomyosarcoma, other specified primary site
XH0GA1 Rhabdomyosarcoma NOS
XH83G1 Embryonal rhabdomyosarcoma NOS
XH7099 Alveolar rhabdomyosarcoma
XH7NM2 Spindle cell rhabdomyosarcoma

Related terminology

Embryonal rhabdomyosarcoma (ERMS)
Acceptable: myosarcoma; malignant rhabdomyoma; rhabdopoietic sarcoma; rhabdosarcoma; embryonal sarcoma; botryoid rhabdomyosarcoma; sarcoma botryoides.

Alveolar rhabdomyosarcoma (ARMS)
Acceptable: monomorphous round cell rhabdomyosarcoma.

Spindle cell / sclerosing rhabdomyosarcoma (SCSRMS)
Acceptable: spindle cell rhabdomyosarcoma; sclerosing rhabdomyosarcoma.
Note: Spindle cell / sclerosing rhabdomyosarcoma was included in the embryonal sarcoma category by WHO until 2013.

Subtype(s)

None

Localization

ERMS most commonly arises in the head and neck and the genitourinary system. The botryoid subtype affects epithelial-lined viscera, such as the biliary tract, bladder, pharynx, auditory canal, and conjunctiva. The soft tissues of the trunk and extremities are uncommonly involved, whereas this is the most common sites of involvement for ARMS. Other sites of involvement for ARMS include the perineal, paraspinal, and paranasal sinuses {3141,2518}.

SCSRMS sites of involvement vary by age at presentation. In infants, the paratesticular region is most often involved, whereas the head and neck is the most common location in older children and adults {3141,2476,609,1867}. SCSRMS may uncommonly involve bone, whereas bone involvement is extremely rare for ERMS and ARMS. Pleomorphic rhabdomyosarcoma usually affects the soft tissues of the extremities of older adults.

Clinical features

Clinical features of GI tract involvement include jaundice for ERMS affecting the biliary tree and constipation/obstruction for ARMS of the perineal area. Rhabdomyosarcomas arising at other sites typically present as a painless mass, which may or may not be rapidly growing and may or may not cause additional symptoms, depending on adjacent structures.

Epidemiology

Although rhabdomyosarcomas are exceedingly rare in the digestive tract, peribiliary ERMS is most frequent. All other types are exceptional.

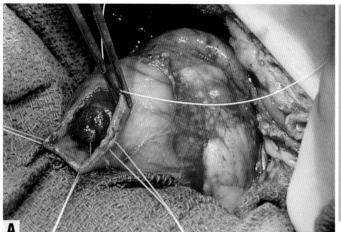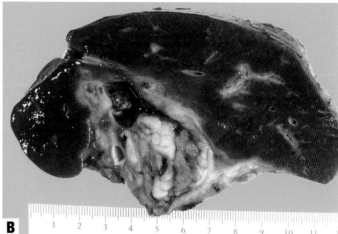

Fig. 12.25 Botryoid rhabdomyosarcoma. **A** Gross intraoperative photograph of a botryoid rhabdomyosarcoma involving the biliary tree. **B** Involving the biliary tree, with a fleshy cut surface.

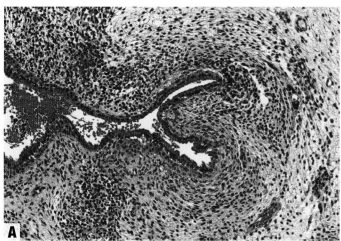
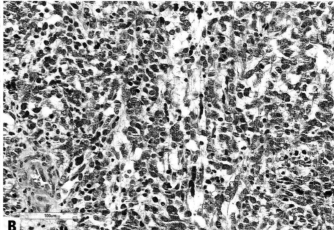

Fig. 12.26 Embryonal rhabdomyosarcoma. **A** Showing a condensation of tumour cells under the epithelial surface (cambium layer) and cells in a myxoid matrix. **B** Showing a combination of round cells, spindled cells, and pleomorphic cells. The spindled strap cells in the centre show cross-striations.

Etiology
Unknown

Pathogenesis
See *Diagnostic molecular pathology*, below.

Macroscopic appearance
Grossly, the botryoid subtype of ERMS shows polypoid nodules directly underlying the epithelial surface in hollow viscera, including the biliary tree. Other types of ERMS, ARMS, and pleomorphic rhabdomyosarcoma have a fleshy cut appearance, whereas SCSRMS has a whitish-grey and whorled cut surface.

Histopathology
The various types of rhabdomyosarcoma have different histological features, as described below.

ERMS shows features of embryonic skeletal muscle cells, with spindled or small round cells with scant eosinophilic cytoplasm in a myxoid stroma. Scattered pleomorphic cells may be seen, and some cases show cells with cytoplasmic cross-striations. Many cases show increased perivascular cellularity, and the botryoid subtype shows a condensation of neoplastic cells just under the epithelium (called a cambium layer).

ARMS is composed of round cells attached to fibrous septa with varying degrees of cystic change. The solid subtype presents as solid nests of tumour cells and is easily misdiagnosed. Some cases of ARMS show prominent wreath-like giant cells.

SCSRMS shows a range of histological features. The spindled subtype is composed of distinctly elongated, uniform, short spindled cells, often in long intersecting fascicles, forming fascicular, herringbone, or whorled patterns. The sclerosing subtype shows round, ovoid, or short spindled cells within an extensively hyalinized/collagenized or pseudochondroid stroma, with pseudoalveolar, pseudovascular, nested, or cord-like patterns present. Neither subtype tends to show strap cells, wreath-like giant cells, or marked nuclear atypia. Definite rhabdomyoblastic differentiation is usually limited to some paratesticular tumours.

Pleomorphic rhabdomyosarcoma is a high-grade sarcoma with pleomorphic polygonal, spindled, and round cells without any definite embryonal or alveolar components.

All rhabdomyosarcomas show relatively strong desmin positivity, although this can be patchy. Myogenin (nuclear) is typically diffusely positive in ARMS, but it is scattered in ERMS and SCSRMS. MYOD1 (nuclear) is diffusely positive. In SCSRMS, MYOD1 staining does not appear to correlate with *MYOD1* mutation status. Keratins, EMA, SMA, and CD34 may be positive in some cases {2518,2476,3141}.

Cytology
Not clinically relevant

Diagnostic molecular pathology
SCSRMS was previously considered a good-prognosis subtype, but recent work links its prognosis to the presence (poor prognosis, similar to that of ARMS) or absence of *MYOD1* mutations, which are associated with (but not unique to) sclerosing morphology {2476}. Tumours with *NCOA2* and *VGLL2* fusions, which usually arise congenitally or in infants, have a particularly favourable prognosis. Overall, the prognosis is better in the paediatric population, probably related to mutation status. ARMS typically shows *PAX3-FOXO1* or *PAX7-FOXO1* fusions {2518}. ERMS does not have a characteristic molecular aberration.

Essential and desirable diagnostic criteria
Essential: the features are dependent on type, but all cases show histological or immunohistochemical evidence of skeletal muscle differentiation.

Staging (TNM)
The Intergroup Rhabdomyosarcoma Study Group (IRSG) staging system {2652A} is commonly used.

Prognosis and prediction
Prognosis and prediction vary by subtype and stage. The 5-year overall survival rate is about 80% in ERMS and 65% in ARMS {2132}. As previously mentioned, the prognosis of SCSRMS depends on *MYOD1* (poor prognosis) or *NCOA2/VGLL2* {2476}.

Haemangioma

Thway K
Doyle LA

Definition
Haemangioma is a benign vascular tumour.

ICD-O coding
9120/0 Haemangioma NOS

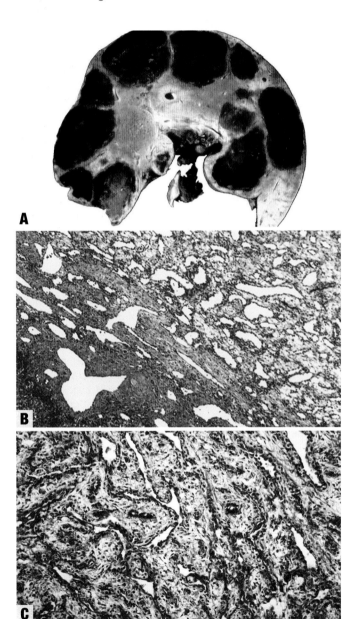

Fig. 12.27 Infantile haemangioma (infantile haemangioendothelioma). **A** Multiple brown cavitary lesions. **B** The tumour is well circumscribed but not encapsulated, and it consists of small vessels. **C** Vessels are lined by a single layer of plump endothelial cells surrounded by a scant fibrous stroma; note the scattered bile ducts (Masson's trichrome staining).

ICD-11 coding
2E81.0Y Other specified neoplastic haemangioma
XH5AW4 Haemangioma NOS

Related terminology
Acceptable: angioma; capillary haemangioma; cavernous haemangioma; venous malformation; arteriovenous malformation; venous or vascular ectasia; haemangiolymphangioma; infantile haemangioma; infantile haemangioendothelioma; juvenile capillary haemangioma; hepatic small vessel neoplasm.

Subtype(s)
Dieulafoy lesion; gastric antral vascular ectasia (GAVE); angiodysplasia; anastomosing haemangioma; infantile haemangioma; diffuse hepatic haemangiomatosis; hepatic small vessel neoplasm

Localization
GI tract haemangiomas and vascular malformations (VMs) can occur singly or multiply anywhere from the oesophagus to the colon {3707}. The small intestine is the most common site, with haemangiomas and VMs accounting for 10% of tumours arising in this location {3446}. Tumours of the colorectum are rarer, with 50% located in the rectum. Gastric lesions tend to be VMs more frequently than true haemangiomas {669,1158}.

Clinical features
Most patients with GI tract haemangiomas present with occult or acute gastrointestinal bleeding {1872}, followed by abdominal pain, bowel obstruction, perforation, or intussusception. Small polypoid lesions may be detected incidentally during screening endoscopy. Grossly, GI tract haemangiomas are either polypoid and intraluminal or poorly defined diffusely infiltrating submucosal lesions. They are purplish-red to blue, and soft and compressible unless containing a thrombus or phleboliths {1872, 3090}.

Malformations can manifest as ulcerating lesions with haemorrhage and thrombosis, and they can invade surrounding structures, particularly in the rectosigmoid region {3707}. Diagnosis is usually made endoscopically and/or by angiography or other imaging modalities. Biopsy is performed in some cases {1158}. Multiple lesions may arise in specific settings (e.g. Maffucci syndrome, Klippel–Trénaunay syndrome, congenital blue rubber bleb naevus syndrome, and hereditary haemorrhagic telangiectasia), and they may be associated with similar lesions in other organs, such as the skin and liver.

The presentation of hepatic infantile haemangioma is typically with abdominal distension (or more rarely with spontaneous or traumatic rupture with pain) and anaemia due to haemoperitoneum {2704}. Approximately 25% of patients have associated congestive heart failure, and about 10% have haemangiomas of the skin or other sites {2940}. Other associations are coagulopathy and hepatomegaly. Lesions may be solitary or multiple, with solitary tumours more common (ratio: 3:2).

Cavernous haemangiomas of the liver are usually asymptomatic and found incidentally on imaging, but they are often symptomatic when > 4 cm in size, precipitating pain or mass effect. These are often solitary, or less frequently multiple, lesions. They may enlarge or rupture in pregnancy, and they can also enlarge or recur in patients who are on estrogen therapy. However, rupture is very rare, as are other severe complications such as thrombosis and Kasabach–Merritt syndrome with consumptive coagulopathy. These lesions vary markedly in size, from millimetres to very large (giant) tumours measuring 15–31 cm {3480}, but they are usually < 5 cm.

Epidemiology

The age range for GI tract haemangiomas is from congenital to the eighth decade of life and beyond. Sex distribution varies from equal to an overall male preponderance for haemangiomas; gastrointestinal VMs appear more frequent in women {3623,1158}.

Hepatic infantile haemangiomas most frequently occur in infancy or early childhood, and they are the most common mesenchymal hepatic tumours in infants and children (accounting for ~20% of liver tumours from birth to the age of 21 years), but they are rare in adults. Most cases present by the age of 2 years {2940}, and there is a female predominance (M:F ratio: 0.5:1).

Cavernous haemangiomas of the liver are the most common benign hepatic tumours {332}, with a prevalence in the general population as high as 20% in autopsy studies {1527}. They can occur at all ages but arise most commonly in women in the third to fifth decades of life.

Etiology

Most lesions in the GI tract previously described as cavernous or venous haemangiomas are now considered to be venous malformations, as defined by the International Society for the Study of Vascular Anomalies classification {3535}.

Associations of GI tract VMs with autoimmune connective tissue or vascular disorders are described {817,2130}.

Hepatic infantile haemangiomas are rarely associated with congenital disorders such as hemihypertrophy {3599}.

Endogenous and exogenous estrogen exposure is a potential pathophysiological mechanism for the development and progression of hepatic cavernous haemangiomas {1048}.

Pathogenesis

See *Diagnostic molecular pathology*, below.

Macroscopic appearance

Haemangiomas have different macroscopic appearances depending on anatomical location and type. They may be present as polypoid or intraluminal lesions, or as poorly defined, infiltrative lesions in the GI tract wall, sometimes seen to invade surrounding structures. They are usually purplish-red and can have a spongy consistency, or they may be firmer when containing thrombi or phleboliths.

Histopathology

The multitude of names for gastrointestinal haemangiomas reflects the morphological heterogeneity of overlapping entities {1158}. Haemangiomas comprise proliferations of lymphatics, capillaries, or veins (with any predominating) within the mucosa or submucosa. There are often dilated vessels that can form irregular cavities, sometimes with thrombosis. Reactive congestion of normal mucosal capillaries away from the lesion is typical {1158}.

Capillary haemangiomas are proliferations of small, thin-walled vessels. Cavernous haemangiomas are relatively circumscribed proliferations of large, often dilated, thin-walled vessels or blood-filled sinuses lined by a single layer of endothelium. They can infiltrate large segments of the intestine and mesentery. Focal calcification, thrombi, stromal oedema, and hyalinization can be present {1872}.

Anastomosing haemangioma is a rare benign vascular neoplasm that is most frequently described in the genitourinary tract but can more rarely occur in the GI tract and liver. It is composed of anastomosing small capillary-like vessels with mild endothelial atypia and occasional endothelial cell hobnailing. Vascular thrombi are relatively frequent, and there can rarely be hyaline globules or extramedullary haematopoiesis. The anastomosing growth pattern can resemble angiosarcoma, but the lesions are typically relatively circumscribed and lack severe atypia or diffuse infiltration {1920}.

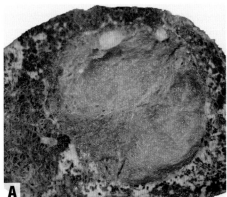 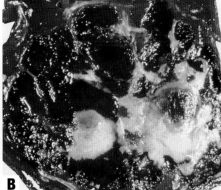 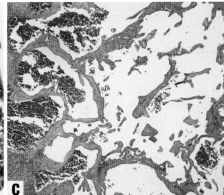

Fig. 12.28 Cavernous haemangioma. **A** Diffuse haemangiomatosis showing numerous dark blood-filled vessels extending beyond the central spongy mass and involving the whole liver lobe. **B** Multilocular blood-filled structures with pale solid areas. **C** Note the large thin-walled vascular spaces.

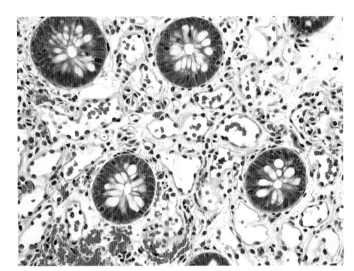

Fig. 12.29 Haemangioma of the colon involving lamina propria and composed of small thin-walled capillary-like vessels lined by bland endothelial cells.

VMs, which may be localized or diffuse (haemangiomatosis) are defined by submucosal or transmural clusters of irregular, distorted vessels with variable wall thickness, some indeterminate (vein vs artery), with or without feeder or shunt vessels. The predominant vessel type (artery, vein, mixed, or capillary) is variable. An identifiable feeder vessel may be present in the submucosa, muscularis propria, or subserosa. Intralesional haemorrhage, thrombosis, and fibrosis are common, and there can be aneurysm-like cavities or vessel abnormalities (e.g. shunt vessels), wall tufts (excrescences), and arterialized veins {1158}. Mucosal ulceration can be present. Dieulafoy lesion is a type of gastrointestinal VM. Gastric antral vascular ectasia (GAVE), also known as watermelon stomach, is another presentation at this site. The term "angiodysplasia" includes clinically/endoscopically defined entities that are histologically considered to be VMs.

GI tract haemangiomas show heterogeneous expression of the endothelial markers CD31 and ERG in the lining endothelium, and podoplanin can be variably expressed.

Hepatic infantile haemangioma (formerly often designated infantile haemangioendothelioma) is a benign vascular tumour with features similar to those of infantile haemangioma (juvenile capillary haemangioma) of the skin and/or superficial soft tissues in children. Hepatic infantile haemangiomas comprise well-defined proliferations of numerous small, capillary-like vascular channels that are particularly prominent at the periphery. The channels are lined by plump endothelial cells, which are usually present as single layers. The vessels are surrounded by small amounts of compact or loose fibrous stroma. More centrally, particularly in larger lesions, are frequent larger cavernous vessels lined by flattened endothelium with fibrosis of the surrounding stroma, corresponding to tumour regression. Characteristic findings include entrapment of hepatocytes and small bile ducts peripherally, as well as areas of extramedullary haematopoiesis. The lining endothelial cells express CD31, CD34, and factor VIII–related antigen. GLUT1 is typically diffusely and strongly positive and helps to exclude non-neoplastic vessels (including those of hepatic VMs), as well as most other benign vascular neoplasms that do not express this marker {2183, 3432}.

Cavernous haemangiomas of the liver typically comprise proliferations of blood-filled vascular channels of varying sizes, lined by single layers of flattened endothelial cells and separated by fibrous septa of varying thickness. The surrounding fibrous stroma may contain small, arborizing vessels. Although they are macroscopically well defined, there is frequently an irregular interface with the liver parenchyma and dilated, blood-filled haemangioma-like vessels present 0.1–2 cm beyond the confines of the main lesion {1578}. The vessel walls are predominantly composed of collagen, with some elastic fibres and smooth muscle. Associated organizing thrombi and infarction, with variable fibrosis and calcification, may be seen. The lining endothelium is underlined by collagen IV, and the lesions are negative for ER and PR {1578}.

In sclerosed hepatic haemangiomas, there is occlusion of most to all lesional vessels, with surrounding fibrosis, increased elastic fibres, and calcifications, and the vessels may only be discernible with elastic stains. Capillary haemangiomas of the liver are only rarely documented in adults. Diffuse hepatic haemangiomatosis is extremely rare, with extensive replacement of liver parenchyma by diffuse and multiple haemangiomas, and some cases involving multiple organs. Large vascular channels are not restricted to the areas of cavernous haemangioma, and they can be found in otherwise normal-looking liver parenchyma {1850}. Diffuse or multiple lesions must be distinguished from peliosis hepatis and haemorrhagic telangiectasia.

Hepatic small vessel neoplasm is a rare, apparently benign or low-grade entity described in adults. These neoplasms are relatively small (average: 2.1 cm), poorly defined, and infiltrative proliferations of small, thin-walled vessels lined by flattened to plump, ovoid hobnail endothelial cells, with luminal erythrocytes and occasional extramedullary haematopoiesis. These vessels can infiltrate around portal tracts and between hepatic plates. Papillary growth or multilayering, cellular atypia, mitotic activity, and necrosis are absent {1043}, as are features of cavernous haemangioma. The adjacent hepatic parenchyma may show some hepatocyte plate expansion, sometimes with areas of focal nodular hyperplasia–like changes.

The lining endothelium uniformly expresses CD31, CD34, and FLI1. The Ki-67 proliferation index appears to be the most helpful tool in discriminating these lesions from angiosarcoma, because lesions with 10% nuclear labelling have all been angiosarcomas (mean Ki-67 proliferation index for hepatic small vessel neoplasm and hepatic angiosarcoma: 3.7% and 42.8%, respectively). No cases of recurrence or metastasis have yet been reported, although close clinical follow-up is indicated because of the currently uncertain outcome {1043}.

Cytology
Not clinically relevant

Diagnostic molecular pathology
Most haemangiomas and VMs show no specific genetic abnormalities. Patients with syndromic associations may show corresponding germline mutations (e.g. *IDH1* mutations in Maffucci syndrome). *GNAQ* mutations occur in almost 70% of anastomosing haemangiomas {275}.

Essential and desirable diagnostic criteria

Essential: morphology is dependent on the characteristic type of haemangioma, with different types and calibres of lesional vessels, but the vessels are essentially well formed, without cellular atypia.

Desirable: immunohistochemical evidence of endothelial differentiation.

Staging (TNM)

Not clinically relevant

Prognosis and prediction

For localized GI tract haemangiomas and VMs, the treatment is surgical excision. Endoscopic treatment with banding and sclerotherapy can be successful when resection is not feasible {3707,3090}.

The typical course of infantile haemangioma is of postnatal proliferation followed by maturation and childhood involution, but these lesions can be life-threatening when associated with congestive heart failure and/or consumptive coagulopathy {1385,1729}. The overall survival rate is approximately 70%, with deaths tending to occur during the initial presenting episode. Adverse risk factors include associated congestive heart failure, jaundice, multiple lesional nodules, and the absence of cavernous differentiation {2940}. Steroid treatment has been commonly used, but 25% of patients are resistant {1729}. Propranolol, a non-selective β-blocker, has been shown to be a well-tolerated and effective treatment for infantile haemangiomas (although generally non-efficacious for other forms of vascular haemangiomas or malformations). Patients who do not respond to drugs may be treated with resection or transarterial embolization, with liver transplantation as a last resort {631}.

Cavernous haemangiomas have not been demonstrated to undergo malignant transformation, and surgical excision is necessary only for large, symptomatic tumours.

Epithelioid haemangioendothelioma

Hornick JL

Definition
Epithelioid haemangioendothelioma is a malignant endothelial neoplasm composed of epithelioid cells in a myxohyaline or fibrous stroma, most commonly with a *WWTR1-CAMTA1* or *YAP1-TFE3* fusion.

ICD-O coding
9133/3 Epithelioid haemangioendothelioma NOS

ICD-11 coding
2B5Y Other specified malignant mesenchymal neoplasms & XH9GF8 Epithelioid haemangioendothelioma

Related terminology
None

Subtype(s)
None

Localization
Epithelioid haemangioendothelioma may arise in the liver, lungs, bone, or soft tissue. Hepatic epithelioid haemangioendothelioma often presents with multifocal disease {1390,2016}. Some patients present with both liver and lung or spleen involvement.

Clinical features
Epithelioid haemangioendothelioma of the liver is often discovered incidentally {2016}. Other patients present with abdominal pain, weight loss, or ascites. Rarely the presentation may include haemoperitoneum, may be mistaken for Budd–Chiari syndrome, or may cause non-cirrhotic portal hypertension {3201}. Multifocal involvement of the liver is identified in > 75% of patients, often involving the right and left lobes {1390,2016, 2111}. Radiological findings are variable; in about 30% of cases, the nodules show a targetoid appearance on MRI, with peripheral high signal intensity on T1-weighted images and low signal intensity on T2-weighted images, referred to as the bright-dark ring sign {2111,847}.

Epidemiology
Epithelioid haemangioendothelioma is rare. There is a slight female predominance and a peak incidence in middle-aged adults, with a wide age range; children are rarely affected {2016}.

Etiology
Epithelioid haemangioendothelioma is sporadic.

Pathogenesis
See *Diagnostic molecular pathology*, below.

Macroscopic appearance
Hepatic epithelioid haemangioendothelioma ranges in size from small (subcentimetre) nodules to large coalescing masses > 10 cm. The cut surface is typically white and firm. Histological features include a variably nodular or infiltrative growth pattern with prominent myxohyaline or fibrous stroma.

Histopathology
The tumours are composed of epithelioid, stellate, and spindle cells with fine chromatin, small nucleoli, and eosinophilic cytoplasm, including occasional intracytoplasmic vacuoles, arranged in cords or as single cells. Invasion of sinusoids and portal and hepatic veins is a frequent feature, sometimes associated with necrosis. The fibrous stroma with lacunae is characteristic and may be useful to suggest epithelioid haemangioendothelioma (but is also seen in cholangiocarcinoma). Occasional tumours show nuclear atypia and variability, including pleomorphic and multinucleated cells. The mitotic count is highly variable; many tumours contain rare mitotic figures.

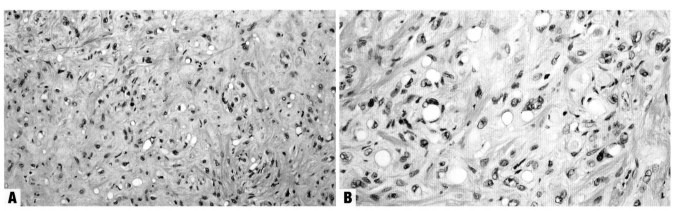

Fig. 12.30 Epithelioid haemangioendothelioma of the liver. **A** Composed of cords of epithelioid cells embedded within a hyaline stroma. **B** Some cases show nuclear atypia and contain occasional multinucleated cells. Note the myxohyaline stroma and prominent cytoplasmic vacuoles.

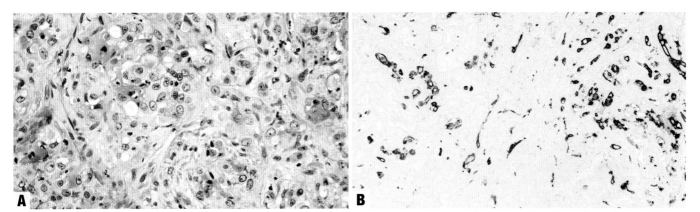

Fig. 12.31 Epithelioid haemangioendothelioma. **A** A cellular epithelioid haemangioendothelioma with less stroma. Such tumours may be mistaken for carcinomas. **B** Tumour cells often contain large vacuoles representing intracytoplasmic lumina, highlighted by CD34 immunostaining.

By immunohistochemistry, epithelioid haemangioendothelioma is positive for endothelial markers, including CD31, CD34, podoplanin (D2-40), and ERG {2157}. Immunoreactivity for keratins (CK8 and CK18) is observed in a subset of cells in many cases {2141}, potentially leading to confusion with carcinomas. CAMTA1 is positive in 85–90% of cases {3002,806}, correlating with underlying gene rearrangement.

Cytology
Not clinically relevant

Diagnostic molecular pathology
WWTR1-CAMTA1 gene fusion, resulting from a t(1;3)(p36;q25) translocation, is a characteristic feature of epithelioid haemangioendothelioma, found in as many as 90% of cases {2119,874,3249,2545}. Multifocal hepatic disease is monoclonal {873}. Rare hepatic tumours harbour a *YAP1-TFE3* fusion {163,1724}. Whether such tumours constitute a subtype of epithelioid haemangioendothelioma or a distinct tumour type is uncertain.

Essential and desirable diagnostic criteria
Essential: cords of epithelioid and spindle cells with cytoplasmic vacuolization set within a myxohyaline or fibrous stroma; expression of CD31, CD34, and/or ERG.
Desirable: *WWTR1-CAMTA1* gene fusion with CAMTA1 expression, or more rarely *YAP1-TFE3* gene fusion with TFE3 expression.

Staging (TNM)
This neoplasm is not formally staged according to the TNM soft tissue tumours classification system.

Prognosis and prediction
Epithelioid haemangioendothelioma of the liver pursues a variable clinical course; some patients have progressive disease, whereas others have indolent, stable disease {295}. The distant metastatic rate is 20–30% {1390,2016}. Histological features do not reliably predict outcome. Epithelioid haemangioendothelioma has a much better prognosis than angiosarcoma of the liver, although a substantial proportion of patients die of disease {2016,2111}.

Kaposi sarcoma

Thway K
Doyle LA

Definition
Kaposi sarcoma (KS) is an HHV8-associated vascular neoplasm characterized by disorganized endothelial cell growth, resulting in the formation of erythrocyte-containing clefts, organized neovascularization, and an associated inflammatory infiltrate.

ICD-O coding
9140/3 Kaposi sarcoma

ICD-11 coding
2B57.2 Kaposi sarcoma of gastrointestinal sites
XH36A5 Kaposi sarcoma

Related terminology
Acceptable: angiosarcoma multiplex; granuloma multiplex haemorrhagicum.

Subtype(s)
None

Localization
KS may occur in any site within the GI tract.

Clinical features
KS involves the mucosa of the upper and lower GI tract, usually at multiple sites. The upper tract is most commonly involved, particularly the stomach and duodenum {2270}. Disease can be clinically silent or symptomatic, with symptoms depending on site and extent but usually comprising occult or acute gastrointestinal bleeding, dysphagia, or epigastric pain {2514,1820, 2270}. Hepatic KS is usually clinically silent, but the lesions typically manifest as reddish-brown foci in portal and periportal areas.

Epidemiology
Gastrointestinal involvement occurs in two settings. Iatrogenic KS occurring after solid organ transplantation or immunosuppressive therapy for the treatment of other diseases shows visceral involvement in half of all cases {160,1820}. AIDS-associated KS {160}, which shows a predilection for men who have sex with men, typically presents as cutaneous lesions, but with disease progression the GI tract is the most common extracutaneous site {1389,1820,3128}; gastrointestinal involvement occurs in as many as 50% of patients with untreated AIDS. Disseminated hepatic KS is mostly associated with AIDS. Most patients with KS of the liver are asymptomatic and do not manifest evidence of hepatic injury, and KS is usually an incidental finding at autopsy, found in approximately 15% of patients with AIDS. Effective HIV therapy correlates with a decline in KS incidence {790}.

Etiology
HHV8 (also called KS-associated herpesvirus), a DNA virus underlying KS {561,2206}, encodes a latency-associated nuclear antigen (LANA), which is the product of the viral gene *ORF73*. HHV8 sequencing shows linkage of HHV8 genetic variants with specific populations {3330}. HHV8 is mainly sexually transmitted. HHV8 DNA is detected in all forms of KS (> 95% of AIDS-related and non–AIDS-related KS) {378,1879,160}. Antibodies against HHV8 nuclear antigens appear before clinical KS {1007}. Not all HHV8 infections lead to pathological manifestations, and most primary infections are asymptomatic {790}.

Pathogenesis
There is serological correlation between HHV8 infection and KS, although not all seropositive individuals have the disease. HHV8 infection is required but not sufficient for disease induction, which requires genetic, immunological, and environmental

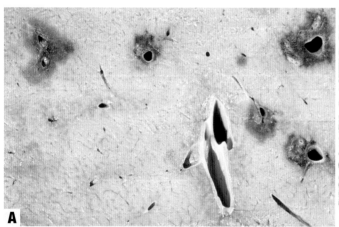
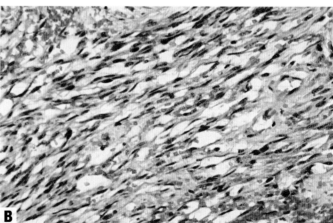

Fig. 12.32 Kaposi sarcoma. **A** Multiple dark-brown lesions are centred in large portal areas. **B** Spindle cells and slit-like vascular spaces.

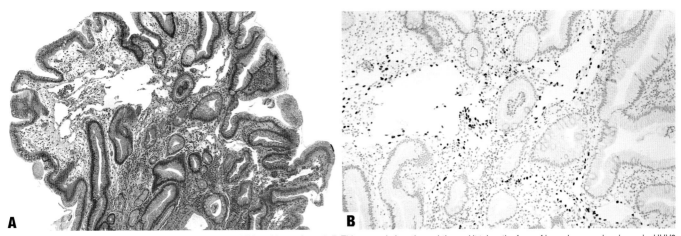

Fig. 12.33 Gastric lymphangioma-like Kaposi sarcoma in an HIV-positive patient. **A,B** This example is rather subtle, and it takes the form of irregular vascular channels. HHV8 is positive.

factors {864,2843}. KS is often linked with HIV infection and can develop at any disease stage, but is more frequent in advanced immune suppression {1871,303,1820}.

Macroscopic appearance

Gastrointestinal KS manifests as reddish-blue or brown flat macules, luminal polypoid nodules, or ulcerating and haemorrhagic lesions involving the mucosa, or rarely as a transmural mass.

Histopathology

Gastrointestinal KS is typically mucosally based, comprising infiltrative proliferations of small irregular vascular channels and fascicles of non-pleomorphic spindled endothelial cells within the lamina propria, sometimes with mucosal ulceration. Like in cutaneous lesions, intracellular or extracellular hyaline globules are characteristic. Similarly, lymphoplasmacytic infiltrates, erythrocyte extravasation, and haemosiderin deposition are seen {2516}. Rare subtypes are lymphangioma-like, intravascular {1965}, and anaplastic KS (which is aggressive) {3724}. Within the liver, KS typically involves the portal and periportal areas. It is present as poorly vasoformative streams of relatively uniform, mildly atypical spindle cells, often with cytoplasmic eosinophilic hyaline globules, with associated haemorrhage and haemosiderin deposition.

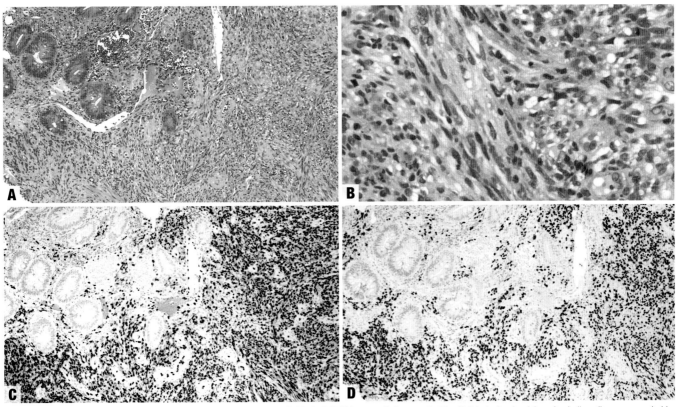

Fig. 12.34 Rectal involvement by Kaposi sarcoma in an HIV-positive individual. **A,B** This example is more florid, with interlacing fascicles of spindly cells, accompanied by extravasation of red cells and haemorrhage. **C,D** ERG and HHV8 are positive.

Mesenchymal tumours of the digestive system   469

Endothelial and spindle cells express CD31, CD34, ERG, and podoplanin. Nuclear HHV8 is immunohistochemically detectable in almost all lesions. KS shows diffuse nuclear expression of latency-associated nuclear antigen 1 (LANA-1), unlike spindle cell mimics, which are negative. In early KS, VEGFR3 is more extensively expressed than LANA-1 {2548,826}.

Cytology

Not clinically relevant

Diagnostic molecular pathology

PCR and in situ hybridization show HHV8 in the flat endothelial cells lining vascular spaces and in spindle cells {377}. Most advanced lesions are oligoclonal, with variably sized viral episomes, suggesting that KS represents reactive/non-neoplastic proliferations rather than neoplasms with metastases {827}.

Essential and desirable diagnostic criteria

Essential: clinical history of severe or HIV-associated immunosuppression; characteristic histological appearance of infiltrating small irregular vascular channels and fascicles of non-pleomorphic spindled endothelial cells.

Desirable: immunohistochemical evidence of endothelial differentiation; HHV8 expression.

Staging (TNM)

This neoplasm is not formally staged according to the TNM soft tissue tumours classification system.

Prognosis and prediction

Enteric KS has low morbidity. About 80% of lesions are clinically silent, and lesions sometimes regress spontaneously. Gastrointestinal involvement does not substantially influence survival {2566,2514}, for which the degree of immunosuppression at diagnosis is the most important determinant {2514}. Withdrawal of immunosuppression can sometimes cause disease resolution. Although most patients with hepatic KS are asymptomatic, the rare patients with clinically significant disease may undergo rapid progression to liver and multiorgan failure, which is often fatal {3424}. Combined highly active antiretroviral therapy (HAART) and systemic chemotherapy improves morbidity and mortality {2063}.

Angiosarcoma

Thway K
Doyle LA
Fukayama M
Hornick JL

Definition

Angiosarcoma is a malignant neoplasm showing endothelial differentiation and a variable degree of vessel formation.

ICD-O coding

9120/3 Angiosarcoma

ICD-11 coding

2B56.3 Angiosarcoma of liver
2B56.Y Angiosarcoma, other specified primary site
XH6264 Haemangiosarcoma

Related terminology

Acceptable: haemangiosarcoma; malignant angioendothelioma; malignant haemangioendothelioma; lymphangiosarcoma.

Subtype(s)

Epithelioid angiosarcoma

Localization

Primary angiosarcomas can (rarely) arise at any site within the GI tract, including the mesentery. Angiosarcoma can also be metastatic (e.g. from skin and subcutaneous sites from the head and neck of elderly patients, and from occult retroperitoneal, soft tissue, or visceral sites), and it may be multifocal {111}.

Clinical features

The presenting symptoms of gastrointestinal or hepatic angiosarcomas are nonspecific and may include abdominal pain, mass, or ascites {2939}. Acute abdomen can occur in hepatic angiosarcomas due to rupture, and in gastrointestinal tumours due to bleeding, bowel obstruction or perforation, intra-abdominal haemorrhage, and intussusception. Metastases can be multifocal (diffuse angiosarcomatosis) within the bowel wall. Hepatic angiosarcomas may rarely cause fulminant hepatic failure. On sectioning, angiosarcomas have a variable appearance, ranging from firm greyish-white tissue to markedly haemorrhagic tissue with cystic spaces.

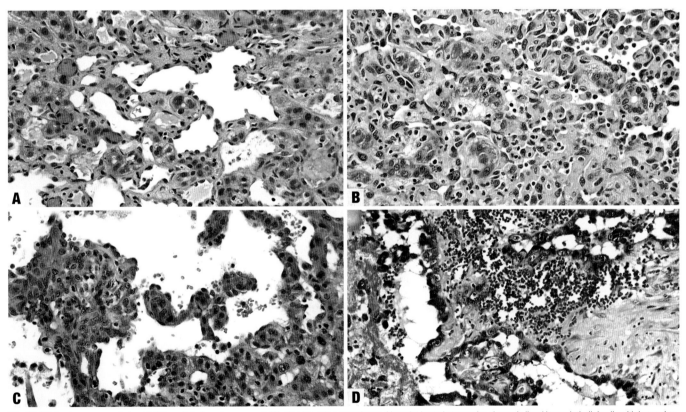

Fig. 12.35 Angiosarcoma. **A** A well-differentiated angiosarcoma infiltrating hepatic parenchyma. Note the irregular vascular channels lined by endothelial cells with hyperchromatic nuclei showing a hobnail appearance. **B** A poorly differentiated angiosarcoma showing marked nuclear atypia. The tumour infiltrates hepatic parenchyma and forms micropapillary structures. **C** The tumour cells surround hepatic cords and form solid sheets of spindle cells. **D** Small intestinal angiosarcoma contains irregularly shaped vascular lumina lined by highly atypical endothelial cells with mitotic activity.

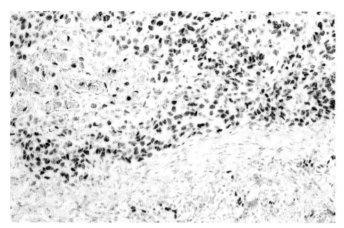

Fig. 12.36 Angiosarcoma. Nuclear expression of ERG helps confirm endothelial differentiation.

Epidemiology

Angiosarcoma has a peak incidence in the seventh decade of life, but it can rarely affect children {770,2939}. There is a male predominance. In the liver, angiosarcoma is the most common primary malignant mesenchymal neoplasm in adults and accounts for 2% of all primary hepatic malignancies {571}.

Etiology

Primary angiosarcomas of the GI tract arise de novo or in the field of prior therapeutic abdominopelvic irradiation, typically after several (usually > 10) years. Patients with hepatic angiosarcomas may have had exposure to carcinogens such as vinyl chloride monomer, arsenic, and anabolic–androgenic steroids. Historically, iatrogenic thorium oxide (Thorotrast) was an etiological factor, but this is now rare.

Pathogenesis

Most angiosarcomas harbour complex karyotypes, without recurrent chromosomal changes {1107,3461}, but unlike other sarcomas with complex genomics, angiosarcomas show low levels of alterations in *TP53* and PIK3CA/AKT/mTOR pathways, and *TP53* mutation and *PTEN* deletions are rare {1405,161}. Genes related to angiogenesis and endothelial cell receptors (including *TIE1*, *TEK*, *KDR*, and *FLT1*) are usually upregulated compared with other sarcomas {166,1404}. About 40% of cases harbour recurrent somatic mutations involving angiogenic signalling pathways (e.g. *KDR*, *PTPRB*, and *PLCG1* mutations), with rare mutations in RAS genes, *PIK3CA*, *TP53*, *FLT4*, and *TIE1* {166,1405,286}. Hepatic angiosarcomas have been found to be frequently ATRX-deficient, with an associated alternative lengthening of telomeres phenotype {1898}. Vinyl chloride–associated hepatic angiosarcomas are thought to harbour increased frequencies of *TP53* mutations compared with sporadic hepatic cases, with a *TP53* mutation spectrum distinct from those not associated with this agent {3093}.

Macroscopic appearance

Angiosarcomas are haemorrhagic, often ulcerating, diffuse or multinodular masses. In the GI tract they can extend transmurally, including into the mesentery. Within the liver, angiosarcomas are typically poorly defined neoplasms involving much of the organ, and many have splenic involvement.

Histopathology

Most soft tissue angiosarcomas are high-grade neoplasms with nuclear atypia, prominent mitotic activity, and coagulative necrosis, but there is a broad morphological spectrum ranging from well-formed, anastomosing vessels to solid sheets of high-grade epithelioid or spindled cells without clear vasoformation, often with multiple patterns in the same tumour. Vascular channels are often poorly formed, with a complex dissecting pattern into fibrous tissue, or compressed, with predominantly solid morphology and only subtle cleft-like spaces suggesting vascular differentiation. The endothelial cells lining the vascular structures are spindled or epithelioid and may form buds, hobnails, or papillary-like projections. Within hepatic parenchyma, tumour cells often line pre-existing vascular channels and hepatic sinusoids. Thorotrast-associated tumours often contain portal fibrosis, with Thorotrast granules present in these foci. Primary hepatic angiosarcomas should be distinguished from angiosarcomas metastatic to the liver (and also from rare primary splenic angiosarcomas with hepatic metastases).

Epithelioid morphology is common in GI tract angiosarcomas {111}. Epithelioid angiosarcomas show solid architecture and large atypical epithelioid or polygonal cells with ovoid vesicular nuclei, prominent large central nucleoli, and abundant cytoplasm, resembling carcinoma, melanoma, or lymphoma; vasoformative areas may be absent or subtle. Less frequently, angiosarcomas appear to be of low grade with well-formed vascular channels lined by minimally atypical spindled cells.

Angiosarcomas typically show membranous CD31 and nuclear ERG positivity, with variable expression of CD34 (~50%), factor VIII–related antigen {2147,2157,950}, FLI1 {950}, and the lymphatic endothelial marker podoplanin. Keratin and EMA expression may be seen, particularly in epithelioid subtypes, and may lead to an erroneous diagnosis of carcinoma {74,948}. Distinction from haemangioendothelioma is important. Immunohistochemistry should be interpreted in the context of a panel, because there can be aberrant expression of other markers, including KIT, CD30, synaptophysin, and chromogranin {3281}.

Cytology

Not clinically relevant

Diagnostic molecular pathology

Diagnostic molecular pathology is not required unless an inherited tumour syndrome is suspected (see *Pathogenesis*, above).

Essential and desirable diagnostic criteria

Essential: malignant endothelial histology; nuclear pleomorphism; vascular immunohistochemistry.

Staging (TNM)

Staging of angiosarcoma is not recommended, because its typically aggressive natural history is not consistent with soft tissue staging systems.

Prognosis and prediction

Most angiosarcomas of the GI tract or liver are highly aggressive, and survival time > 1 year is rare {3719,2939}. Poor prognostic factors include older age, large tumour size, and high Ki-67 proliferation index {2114,909}.

Glomus tumour

Thway K
Doyle LA
Fukayama M

Definition

Glomus tumour is a neoplasm composed of cells that resemble the perivascular modified smooth muscle cells of the normal glomus body.

ICD-O coding

8711/0 Glomus tumour NOS
8711/1 Glomangiomatosis
8711/1 Glomus tumour of uncertain malignant potential
8711/3 Glomus tumour, malignant

ICD-11 coding

2E92 & XH47J2 Benign neoplasm of digestive organs & Glomus tumour NOS
2F70 & XH7CP7 Neoplasms of uncertain behaviour of oral cavity or digestive organs & Glomangiomatosis
Malignant neoplasms of digestive organs
2C12.0 & XH21E6 Malignant neoplasm of liver & Glomus tumour, malignant

Related terminology

Glomus tumour
Acceptable: glomangioma; glomangiomyoma.

Malignant glomus tumour
Acceptable: glomangiosarcoma.

Subtype(s)

None

Localization

Although they occur far more commonly in superficial soft tissues, glomus tumours can rarely arise in viscera, including within the GI tract and the liver. Within the GI tract, they virtually always arise within the stomach (particularly the antrum) and rarely within the oesophagus or intestines {2150}.

Clinical features

The presentation of gastrointestinal glomus tumour is with symptoms of upper gastrointestinal bleeding (haematemesis or melaena) or epigastric pain, and less commonly, because of their antral-predominant location, symptoms of gastric outlet obstruction. Small tumours may be detected incidentally. Most tumours are solitary, but as many as 10% of patients have multiple lesions. Hepatic glomus tumours tend to be much larger than cutaneous lesions, possibly because they are less easily detectable in non-cutaneous sites {1571,1241}. They can present with epigastric fullness or pain, or as a mass lesion. Familial cases are rare.

Epidemiology

These can occur at any age, but glomus tumours within the GI tract have a strong female predominance, with a median patient age of 55 years (range: 19–90 years) {2150}. Hepatic glomus tumours tend to arise in patients in their fourth to seventh decades of life.

Etiology

Multiple familial glomus tumours occur due to inactivating mutations in the glomulin gene (*GLMN*), which is inherited in an autosomal dominant pattern. Most sporadic cases are associated with NOTCH family gene rearrangements.

Pathogenesis

NOTCH family and *BRAF* mutations are implicated: see *Diagnostic molecular pathology*, below.

Macroscopic appearance

Grossly, the tumours are well-circumscribed, often multinodular, 2–3 cm intramural masses. There may be extension into the mucosa or serosa. Cystic change and calcifications may be present.

Histopathology

Morphologically and immunohistochemically, GI tract glomus tumours are similar to those of peripheral soft tissue sites. They are composed of uniform, small rounded cells with central dark round nuclei and moderate amounts of eosinophilic to clear cytoplasm. Individual cells are surrounded by sharply defined basal lamina. The stroma may be focally myxoid or hyalinized. Cells rarely show epithelioid or oncocytic features {2621,3069}. Cases with epithelioid morphology have large polygonal to

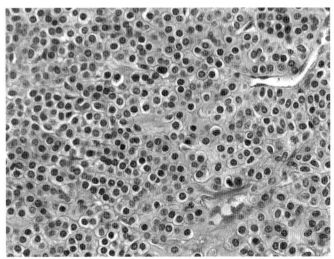

Fig. 12.37 Glomus tumour. The tumour cells are monotonous and round, with prominent cell borders and small central round nuclei.

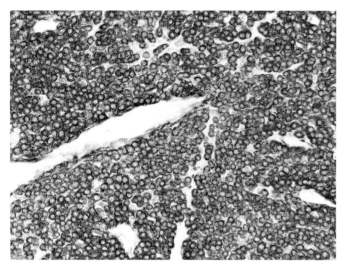

Fig. 12.38 Glomus tumour. Diffuse expression of SMA, with accentuation of cell borders, is characteristic.

spindle cells with abundant eosinophilic cytoplasm and large, irregular nuclei with atypia (in keeping with senescent/ancient change), but small areas of conventional glomus tumour can be present peripherally {2621}.

Gastric glomus tumours can show plexiform growth within the muscularis propria. Focal nuclear atypia and vascular invasion are relatively common, and vascular involvement is not prognostically adverse. Primary hepatic glomus tumours should be distinguished from tumours metastasizing from other sites. Most hepatic glomus tumours have shown typical features.

The criteria for malignancy in the GI tract are undefined, due to insufficient data, but the peripheral soft tissue criteria for malignancy are deep location and size > 2 cm, or atypical mitotic figures, or moderate to high nuclear grade and ≥ 5 mitoses/10 mm² {952}.

There is diffuse, strong expression of SMA in virtually all cases, and caldesmon in > 60%. Most cases express collagen IV and display net-like pericellular laminin {2150}. There can be focal synaptophysin expression, a potential diagnostic pitfall in the differential diagnosis with neuroendocrine tumours (NETs), particularly in small biopsy or cytological preparations {2150}. Cytoplasmic SIRT1 expression is also described {778}. Chromogranin, CD56, desmin, S100, keratin, CD34, KIT (CD117), and DOG1 are negative.

Cytology
Not clinically relevant

Diagnostic molecular pathology
About half of benign and malignant glomus tumours from a variety of sites harbour recurrent NOTCH family gene rearrangements, often with fusion of *NOTCH2* to *MIR143* {2229}.

BRAF p.V600E mutations have been detected in 6% of glomus tumours, all either malignant or of uncertain malignant potential. BRAF is a potential therapeutic target in patients with progressive disease {1523}.

Essential and desirable diagnostic criteria
Essential: round glomoid cells; sometimes plexiform growth in the GI tract.
Desirable: strong SMA expression.

Staging (TNM)
Not clinically relevant, unless the tumour is malignant.

Prognosis and prediction
Most glomus tumours are benign, and complete resection by wedge or segmental resection or partial gastrectomy is curative. Malignant behaviour is based on two reported cases of gastric glomus tumours that metastasized to the liver and resulted in patient death. Both were > 5 cm, and one showed mild atypia, spindle cell foci, and vascular invasion but had very low mitotic activity {2150,952}.

Lymphangioma and lymphangiomatosis

Thway K
Doyle LA

Definition
Lymphangioma is a benign tumour consisting of single-layer endothelial-lined lymphatic spaces containing chylous or serous material. Lymphangiomatosis is multicentric or extensively infiltrating lymphangioma.

ICD-O coding
9170/0 Lymphangioma NOS

ICD-11 coding
LA90.12 & XH9MR8 Lymphatic malformations of certain specified sites & Lymphangioma
2E81.10 Disseminated lymphangiomatosis

Related terminology
Acceptable: intra-abdominal cystic lymphangioma; haemangiolymphangioma.

Subtype(s)
None

Localization
Lymphangiomas can arise at all sites in the GI tract, but they are most common in the small intestine, followed by the large intestine and oesophagus. In the peritoneal cavity, most occur within the mesentery and retroperitoneum {3387,2222}. Diffuse lymphangiomatosis can involve either a single organ or multiple organs (e.g. the liver, spleen, lungs, and bones). Hepatic lymphangiomas are rare, with most reported cases arising as a component of diffuse lymphangiomatosis.

Clinical features
Patients can present with anaemia from bleeding, intussusception, or acute abdomen. Oesophageal lesions vary from small mucosal nodules to pedunculated polyps or large mass lesions that extend into surrounding structures. They usually involve the middle to lower third, although the upper oesophagus can be involved in some cystic lymphangiomas arising in infants.

Epidemiology
GI tract lymphangiomas are rare, accounting for < 1% of all lymphangiomas. Lymphangiomas primarily occur in children and young adults, although there is a wide age range, including older adults (particularly for mesenteric lesions) {3223,2713, 2222}; there is an overall slight male predominance.

Etiology
Unknown

Pathogenesis
Many of these lesions are present congenitally or appear in early childhood. Putative mechanisms for the development of

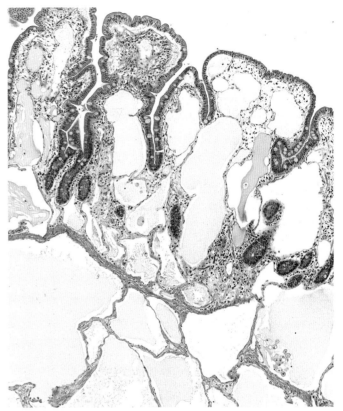

Fig. 12.39 Lymphangioma of the small intestine involving mucosa and submucosa. The lymphatic channels are dilated and lined by inconspicuous endothelium, and they contain lymphatic fluid and occasional lipid-laden macrophages.

lymphangiomas include abnormal budding of the lymphatic system from the cardinal vein and failure of the lymphatic system to separate from or connect with the venous system during embryonic development {3559A}. In the acquired setting, lymphatic obstructions, trauma, infections, and chronic inflammation have also been suggested {3559A}, with development potentiated by various lymphangiogenic cytokines or growth factors.

Macroscopic appearance
Lymphangiomas of the GI tract occur in two main forms: (1) small (< 2 cm) polypoid white or yellow mucosal lesions that are usually incidentally detected and (2) larger masses (as large as 20 cm) that may be transmural or that may arise in mesenteric fat. Cavernous lymphangiomas are polypoid and multinodular, with a soft, spongy consistency. Thick, gelatinous, or milky fluid may be expressed from the cystic spaces {1276}.

Histopathology
GI tract lesions show expansion of the mucosa, submucosa, or muscularis propria by dilated cystic spaces lined by a single simple layer of lymphatic endothelial cells, which are usually

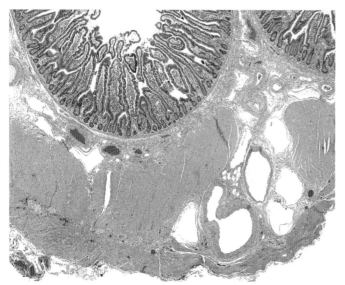

Fig. 12.40 Lymphangioma of the small intestine predominantly involving muscularis propria. Scattered thick-walled vessels with a smooth muscle wall, some with medial sclerosis, are also present.

attenuated without cytological atypia. Some dilated spaces are partially invested by a layer of smooth muscle and/or underlying fibromuscular lymphatic vessel walls. The lymphatic spaces contain clear fluid or prominent foamy histiocytes. Deeper lesions may be associated with overlying mucosal clusters of dilated small lymphatics {1276,1158}. There are often scattered lymphoid aggregates, granulation tissue, or (more rarely) foci of xanthogranulomatous inflammation, particularly in lesions occurring in the mesentery or retroperitoneum, where florid cellular reactive myofibroblastic proliferations can obscure the underlying lymphatic abnormality. Although lymphangioma is the predominant morphology, there can be associated complex

vascular malformations {1276}, aneurysm-like cavities, and vessel abnormalities such as shunt vessels and wall excrescences {1158}. Hepatic lesions are often multiloculated, and they show cystic dilatation of lymphatic vessels within hepatic parenchyma.

Haemangiolymphangiomas are composed of proliferations or networks of vascular spaces or vessels (lymphatics, capillaries, veins or venules, or arteries or arterioles), lined by bland endothelium with intervening connective tissue stroma {1158}. The endothelial cells are typically positive for CD31 and D2-40 and show variable CD34 expression. SMA is positive in smooth muscle cells surrounding the cysts. The lesions are negative for keratin. The smooth muscle component, where present, lacks melanocytic antigens, facilitating distinction from lymphangioleiomyomatosis (PEComa) {1276}.

Cytology
Not clinically relevant

Diagnostic molecular pathology
Not clinically relevant

Essential and desirable diagnostic criteria
Essential: tumour composed of thin-walled vascular spaces; immunohistochemistry for CD31 and D2-40, with variable CD34 expression.

Staging (TNM)
Not clinically relevant

Prognosis and prediction
These are benign tumours that typically do not recur {3223}, although diffuse lymphangiomatosis with visceral involvement can be fatal.

Schwannoma

Antonescu CR
Hornick JL

Definition
Schwannoma is a benign neoplasm of nerve sheath cells showing Schwannian differentiation.

ICD-O coding
9560/0 Schwannoma NOS

ICD-11 coding
2E92 & XH98Z3 Benign neoplasm of digestive organs & Schwannoma (neurilemmoma)

Related terminology
Not recommended: neurilemmoma; neurinoma.

Subtype(s)
Microcystic/reticular schwannoma; mucosal Schwann cell hamartoma

Localization
Gastrointestinal schwannomas form solid intramural masses centred in the submucosa. Schwannomas are far more prevalent in the stomach than in any other gastrointestinal location, with only rare occurrences in the lower oesophagus, colon, and rectum {2153}.

Clinical features
The tumours are homogeneously attenuating, well-defined mural masses on CT, typically lacking intratumoural haemorrhage, necrosis, and degeneration, features that may help distinguish these tumours from gastrointestinal stromal tumours {1873}. Depending on the tumour size, patients can be asymptomatic (with the lesions being discovered incidentally during endoscopic or other imaging work-up) or can present with gastrointestinal bleeding or mass-like symptoms (with sizable tumours).

Epidemiology
Schwannomas are rare gastrointestinal mesenchymal tumours; the incidence of gastrointestinal stromal tumour is 50 times that of gastrointestinal schwannoma. The tumours occur in older adults, with a marked female predominance.

Etiology
Gastrointestinal schwannomas may be associated with neurofibromatosis in some cases.

Pathogenesis
A substantial percentage of conventional schwannomas, whether sporadic or associated with neurofibromatosis type 2, show loss of heterozygosity at *NF2* and/or *NF2*-inactivating mutations, resulting in loss of merlin (the *NF2* gene product) expression. However, one molecular study focusing on gastrointestinal schwannomas of various anatomical sites showed that most cases lacked *NF2* gene alterations, suggesting that they may represent a morphologically and genetically distinct group of peripheral nerve sheath tumours that are different from conventional schwannomas {1794}.

Macroscopic appearance
The tumours are typically located within the submucosa or muscularis propria, but they may extend into overlying mucosa to protrude into the gastric/colonic lumen or may bulge into the serosal surface. The average size is approximately 3 cm, with a range of 0.5–11 cm reported. On cut surface, the tumours are well circumscribed, may be vaguely lobulated, and have a yellow fleshy appearance. Cystic change is occasionally seen.

Histopathology
Gastrointestinal schwannomas are uncommon mesenchymal neoplasms that show features distinct from those of their soft tissue and CNS counterparts. The typical histological features include a well-circumscribed, unencapsulated mural nodule mostly confined to the muscularis propria. The tumours have a spindle cell phenotype, usually with microtrabecular architecture and focal nuclear atypia, as well as peritumoural lymphoid cuffs, often containing germinal centres.

One histological subtype of schwannoma described in the GI tract is the microcystic/reticular subtype. It occurs as a well-circumscribed, unencapsulated submucosal lesion arising along the GI tract, including in the stomach, small bowel, and colon {1905}. Mucosal Schwann cell hamartoma, although of uncertain histogenesis, can also be considered a related schwannoma

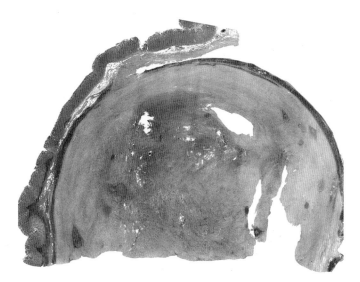

Fig. 12.41 Gastric schwannoma. This well-circumscribed tumour involves the muscularis propria and has a prominent peripheral lymphoid cuff.

Chapter 12

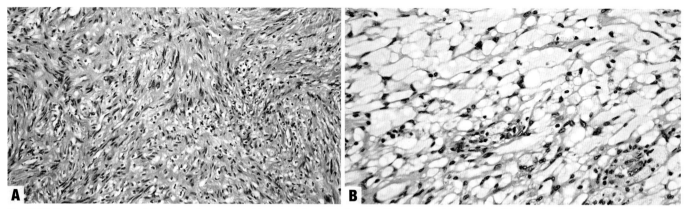

Fig. 12.42 Gastric schwannoma. **A** The tumour is composed of loose fascicles of spindle cells with tapering nuclei and eosinophilic cytoplasm. Note the stromal collagen and lymphocytes. **B** The microcystic/reticular subtype shows a net-like architecture with myxoid stroma.

subtype; it typically presents as neural colorectal polyps distinct from neurofibromas and mucosal neuromas {1038}.

Importantly, features commonly seen in soft tissue schwannomas, such as encapsulation, nuclear palisading, vascular hyalinization, and dilatation, are either absent or infrequent in the GI tract {2847,3488}. A low mitotic count is noted, and necrosis is typically absent. Gastrointestinal schwannomas are strongly and diffusely positive for S100 and in most cases GFAP and nestin {1289}. The tumours are rarely positive for CD34, and they are negative for HMB45, KIT, DOG1, SMA, desmin, and synaptophysin.

Cytology
Not clinically relevant

Diagnostic molecular pathology
Not clinically relevant

Essential and desirable diagnostic criteria
Essential: a well-circumscribed mass; areas of cellular and hypocellular spindle cells; strong S100 positivity.

Staging (TNM)
Not clinically relevant

Prognosis and prediction
Gastrointestinal schwannomas follow a benign clinical course, with no malignant subtypes recognized. Long-term follow-up shows no recurrences or metastases.

Granular cell tumour

Antonescu CR
Hornick JL

Definition
Granular cell tumour is a benign neoplasm showing neuroectodermal differentiation and composed of epithelioid cells of Schwannian derivation with distinctive lysosome-rich granular cytoplasm.

ICD-O coding
9580/0 Granular cell tumour NOS
9580/3 Granular cell tumour, malignant

ICD-11 coding
2E8Y & XH09A9 Benign neoplasm of mesothelial tissue, other specified organs & Granular cell tumour NOS
XH90D3 Granular cell tumour, malignant

Related terminology
Not recommended: granular cell schwannoma; granular cell nerve sheath tumour; granular cell myoblastoma; Abrikossoff tumour.

Subtype(s)
None

Localization
About 5–10% of granular cell tumours arise in the GI tract. Within the GI tract, the most common site is the oesophagus, followed by the large bowel and perianal region {131,2515,3059, 1060}. Within the oesophagus, about 60% of cases are located in the lower part, with the remainder evenly divided between the upper and middle portions. Examples in the large bowel arise throughout its length, most often in the right colon {3059}. Rare examples can also involve the stomach, small bowel, gallbladder, and bile ducts.

Clinical features
Most gastrointestinal granular cell tumours are relatively small and are discovered incidentally during endoscopy for other reasons. Most cases are solitary and involve the lamina propria or submucosa, but multifocal examples also occur.

Epidemiology
Granular cell tumours usually occur in adults in the fourth to sixth decades of life, but they can be encountered at any age. There is a predilection for females and for African-Americans.

Etiology
Multiple granular cell tumours have been reported in association with various syndromes, such as neurofibromatosis type 1, Noonan syndrome, and LEOPARD syndrome (multiple lentigines, electrocardiographic conduction abnormalities, ocular hypertelorism, pulmonic stenosis, abnormal genitalia, retardation of growth, and sensorineural deafness), mostly characterized by aberrant signalling within the RAS/MAPK pathways through inactivating mutations {2908}. However, most reported syndromic cases do not affect the GI tract.

Pathogenesis
Recent genomic studies have shown mutually exclusive, clonal, inactivating somatic mutations in the endosomal pH regulators *ATP6AP1* and *ATP6AP2* in 72% of granular cell tumours {2513A}. Inactivating mutations in these two genes are probably oncogenic drivers of granular cell tumours and underpin the genesis of the intracytoplasmic granules that characterize them, providing a genetic link between endosomal pH regulation and tumorigenesis.

Macroscopic appearance
The tumours typically appear as small yellowish nodules with an intact overlying mucosa. Tumour size ranges from 0.1 to 3.0 cm.

Histopathology
Gastrointestinal granular cell tumours are either poorly marginated or circumscribed, arranged in sheets, nests, lobules, or ribbons within a variably dense fibrous stroma. The overlying squamous epithelium in oesophageal tumours typically shows acanthosis, and sometimes pseudoepitheliomatous hyperplasia. The tumour cells are monotonous, plump, and polyhedral to somewhat elongated, with distinct cell borders. The cells show abundant eosinophilic cytoplasm that is granular in appearance. The nuclei are typically eccentrically located, small and regular, and somewhat hyperchromatic, with generally inconspicuous nucleoli. Occasional tumours, most commonly in the colon, feature degenerative nuclear changes. Multinucleation, nuclear pleomorphism, prominent nucleoli, and mitotic figures

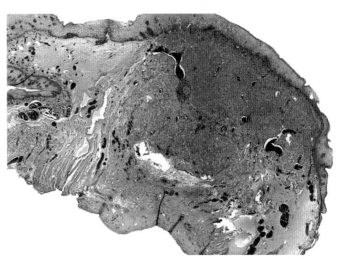

Fig. 12.43 Granular cell tumour. This oesophageal tumour involves the lamina propria and extends into the muscularis mucosae.

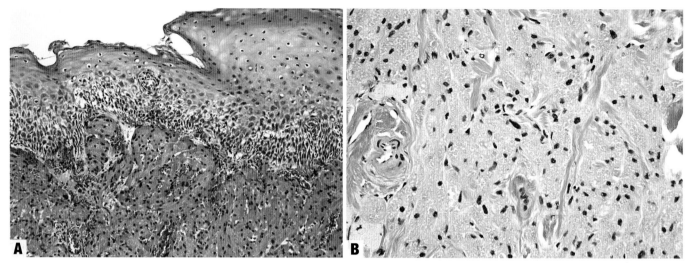

Fig. 12.44 Granular cell tumour. **A** The squamous epithelium overlying the tumour shows basal cell hyperplasia. **B** The tumour is composed of polygonal cells with hyperchromatic nuclei and abundant granular eosinophilic cytoplasm. Note the occasional cells with degenerative nuclear atypia.

are uncommon features. Malignant granular cell tumours are rare, and their features vary from overtly sarcomatous to morphologically bland. However, most malignant examples show vesicular nuclei with prominent nucleoli, increased mitotic activity (> 2 mitoses/2 mm²), and geographical necrosis.

Immunohistochemically, regardless of the degree of malignancy, the tumours are positive for S100, nestin, calretinin, and in a subset of cases CD57 {2515}. Because of their abundant lysosomal cytoplasmic content, the tumours are also positive for CD68.

Cytology
Not clinically relevant

Diagnostic molecular pathology
Not clinically relevant

Essential and desirable diagnostic criteria
Essential: plump cells with copious, distinctly granular cytoplasm; overlying squamous hyperplasia; strong S100 positivity.

Staging (TNM)
Not clinically relevant

Prognosis and prediction
The vast majority of gastrointestinal granular cell tumours are benign and do not recur, even after incomplete excision. Exceptionally rare oesophageal malignant granular cell tumours pursue a locally aggressive course and metastasize.

Perineurioma

Antonescu CR
Hornick JL

Definition
Perineurioma is a benign unencapsulated peripheral nerve sheath tumour composed entirely of cells with perineurial differentiation.

ICD-O coding
9571/0 Perineurioma NOS

ICD-11 coding
2F38 & XH0XF7 Benign neoplasm of other or unspecified sites & Perineurioma NOS

Related terminology
Acceptable: benign fibroblastic polyp.

Subtype(s)
None

Localization
Most gastrointestinal perineuriomas occur in the large bowel, with only rare occurrences in the small bowel or stomach.

Clinical features
Most intestinal perineuriomas are asymptomatic and discovered incidentally during colorectal cancer screening. The rectosigmoid colon is the most common site. Occasionally, the tumours can present with recurrent gastrointestinal bleeding (gastric location).

Epidemiology
Gastrointestinal perineuriomas occur in middle-aged adults, with a female predominance.

Etiology
Unknown

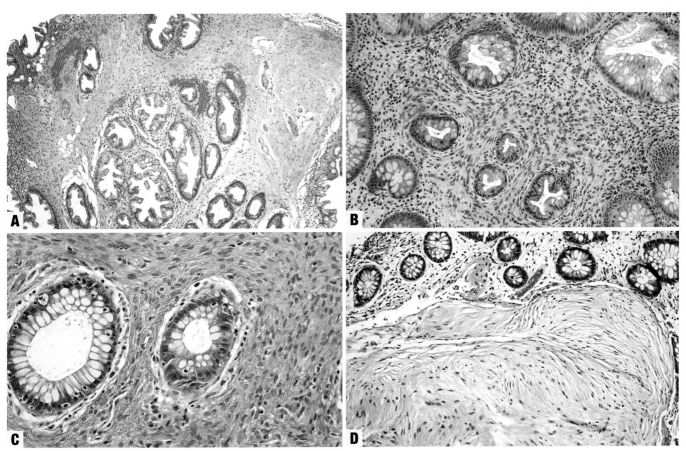

Fig. 12.45 Perineurioma. **A** Mucosal lesions involve the lamina propria and are often associated with serrated epithelial polyps. **B** The spindle cells whorl around crypts. Note the adjacent dilated crypts with serrated architecture. **C** The lesional cells contain slender nuclei and indistinct cytoplasm and are dispersed within a fine collagenous stroma. **D** This colonic tumour is composed of elongated spindle cells with slender nuclei arranged in a whorled growth pattern. Mural perineuriomas of the GI tract are identical to soft tissue perineuriomas.

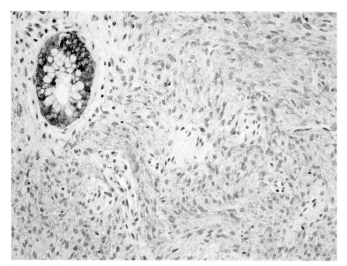

Fig. 12.46 Mucosal perineurioma. Immunohistochemistry for EMA is positive. Note the delicate pattern of staining.

Pathogenesis

Similar to schwannomas, most perineuriomas harbour chromosome 22 deletions or monosomies, probably targeting the *NF2* tumour suppressor gene. The molecular pathogenetic basis for colorectal mucosal perineuriomas is unknown, although associated serrated polyps harbour typical *BRAF* p.V600E mutations {47,2489}.

Macroscopic appearance

Most gastrointestinal perineuriomas present as small (0.2–0.6 cm) colonic polyps. Less commonly, they can present as non-polypoid lesions within the submucosa.

Histopathology

Intramucosal polypoid perineuriomas expand the lamina propria and uniformly entrap crypts. Colorectal mucosal perineuriomas are often associated with serrated epithelial polyps, including both hyperplastic polyps and sessile serrated lesions {1275,2489,1099}. Submucosal perineuriomas appear circumscribed but can focally infiltrate into the muscularis propria and subserosa {1099}. Similar to perineurioma of soft tissues, the gastrointestinal tumours are composed of uniform spindle cells with ovoid to elongated and tapering nuclei, as well as bipolar cytoplasmic processes. The cells are generally arranged in a diffuse solid growth, often showing a distinctive whorled architecture around crypts. Mitoses are rare or absent, and no necrosis is noted. The cells are positive for EMA (highlighting delicate cell processes), claudin-1, and/or GLUT1 {1275}. A subset of cases also express CD34. Gastrointestinal perineuriomas are negative for S100, GFAP, KIT, SMA, and keratins.

Cytology

Not clinically relevant

Diagnostic molecular pathology

Not clinically relevant

Essential and desirable diagnostic criteria

Essential: uniform spindle cells; S100-negative; EMA-positive.

Staging (TNM)

Not clinically relevant

Prognosis and prediction

Gastrointestinal perineuriomas are benign.

Ganglioneuroma and ganglioneuromatosis

Antonescu CR
Hornick JL

Definition

Ganglioneuroma is a benign neoplasm composed of mature ganglion cells, satellite cells, and numerous nerves (unmyelinated axons associated with Schwann cells). When ganglioneuroma is multiple and/or syndrome-associated, the term "ganglioneuromatosis" is used.

ICD-O coding

9490/0 Ganglioneuroma
9491/0 Ganglioneuromatosis

ICD-11 coding

2F38 & XH03L9 Benign neoplasm of other or unspecified sites & Ganglioneuroma
XH6LR5 Ganglioneuromatosis

Related terminology

None

Subtype(s)

None

Localization

Most cases of polypoid ganglioneuroma and ganglioneuromatosis occur within the large intestine (including the rectum), and occasionally cases arise within the appendix.

Clinical features

Most gastrointestinal lesions occur in the colon, with a predilection for the left side and the rectum, with few seen in the appendix. Ganglioneuromas typically present as small mucosal polyps, of < 1–2 cm, being detected incidentally during endoscopy work-up. The clinical presentation of ganglioneuromatosis is quite variable, including acute intestinal obstruction and intestinal motility disorders, or ganglioneuromatosis may be found incidentally during investigations for other pathology. Intestinal ganglioneuromas can be broadly divided into three groups: solitary ganglioneuroma, ganglioneuromatous polyposis, and diffuse ganglioneuromatosis. Most cases are sporadic and indolent; however, multiple lesions or lesions showing diffuse mural involvement have a strong association with multiple endocrine neoplasia (MEN) type 2B or (less commonly) neurofibromatosis type 1 {3308}.

Epidemiology

Patients have a wide age range and there is no sex predilection.

Etiology

Intestinal ganglioneuromatosis has a well-established association with MEN2B, and it is less commonly related to neurofibromatosis type 1. Ganglioneuromatosis polyposis is often associated with Cowden syndrome (*PTEN* hamartoma tumour

syndrome) {2331}. MEN2A and MEN2B are associated with germline mutations in the *RET* proto-oncogene {371}. MEN2A, familial medullary thyroid carcinoma, and MEN2B are collectively associated with a 70–100% risk of medullary thyroid carcinoma. Individuals with MEN2B often have distinct physical features including mucosal neuromas of the lips and tongue, ganglioneuromatosis of the GI tract, distinctive facies with enlarged lips, and a Marfanoid body habitus {508}. Approximately 40% of affected individuals have diffuse ganglioneuromatosis of the GI tract. Associated symptoms include abdominal distension, megacolon, constipation, and diarrhoea. Most patients with MEN2B report gastrointestinal symptoms starting in infancy or early childhood. Clinical recognition and accurate diagnosis of individuals who are at risk of harbouring a germline *RET* mutation are critical for the prevention and management of potentially life-threatening neoplasms.

Pathogenesis

See *Cowden syndrome* (p. 547).

Macroscopic appearance

Ganglioneuromas typically present as small mucosal polyps of < 1–2 cm.

Histopathology

The solitary lesions are typically polypoid, showing ganglion cells, spindled Schwann cells, and eosinophils within the lamina propria. Cystic glands can be present, reminiscent of juvenile polyps in some cases. In contrast, diffuse ganglioneuromatosis is characterized by an exuberant, poorly demarcated, nodular, or diffuse proliferation of nerve fibres, ganglion cells, and supporting cells of the enteric nervous system. Their growth

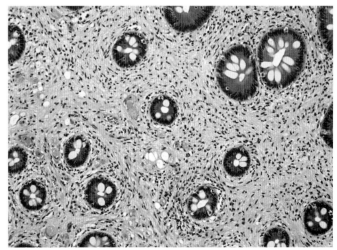

Fig. 12.47 Polypoid ganglioneuroma. The colonic crypts are surrounded by spindled Schwann cells and scattered ganglion cells.

Chapter 12

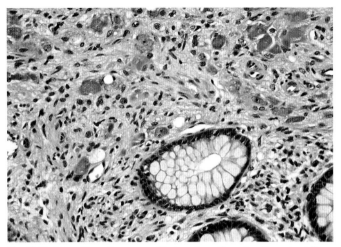

Fig. 12.48 Polypoid ganglioneuroma. Clusters of ganglion cells with amphophilic cytoplasm dispersed among Schwann cells.

pattern varies, from fusiform, hyperplastic expansions of the myenteric plexus to confluent transmural ganglioneuromatous proliferations that distort the myenteric plexus and infiltrate the adjacent bowel wall. Immunohistochemical markers of neural differentiation (neurofilament, neuron-specific enolase, synaptophysin, and PHOX2B) can be used to highlight the ganglion cells {2383}. S100 diffusely stains the Schwannian component and delineates the ganglion cells, which are S100-negative.

Cytology
Not clinically relevant

Diagnostic molecular pathology
Diagnostic molecular pathology is not clinically relevant, unless an inherited tumour syndrome is suspected.

Essential and desirable diagnostic criteria
Essential: a mixture of Schwannian and ganglion cells; Schwann cells S100-positive; ganglion cells S100-negative.

Staging (TNM)
Not clinically relevant

Prognosis and prediction
Both solitary and multifocal forms follow a benign course. Malignant transformation has not been documented in ganglioneuromatosis.

PEComa, including angiomyolipoma

Hornick JL
Miettinen M
Sciot R
Tsui WM

Definition

PEComa is a mesenchymal neoplasm composed of distinctive, predominantly epithelioid cells showing variable expression of smooth muscle and melanocytic markers. Angiomyolipoma is a PEComa subtype that also contains adipocytes and thick-walled, tortuous blood vessels.

ICD-O coding

8714/0 PEComa, benign
8714/3 PEComa, malignant
8860/0 Angiomyolipoma

ICD-11 coding

2E92 & XH4CC6 Benign neoplasm of digestive organs & Perivascular epithelioid tumour, benign
2B90 Malignant neoplasms of colon
2C12.0 Malignant neoplasm of liver
2B80 Malignant neoplasms of small intestine
2C10 Malignant neoplasm of pancreas
XH9WD1 Perivascular epithelioid tumour, malignant
XH4VB4 Angiomyolipoma

Related terminology

PEComa
Acceptable: monotypic epithelioid angiomyolipoma.

Subtype(s)

Sclerosing PEComa; inflammatory subtype of angiomyolipoma

Localization

PEComas of the digestive tract most commonly arise in the colon, liver, small intestine, and pancreas; origin in the stomach and other gastrointestinal sites is particularly rare {807,588, 1937}. PEComas may also involve the mesenteries and peritoneum (in the peritoneum most often as metastases).

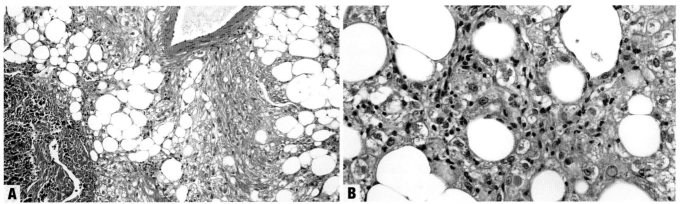

Fig. 12.49 Angiomyolipoma. **A** Hepatic angiomyolipoma showing characteristic components: adipocytes, thick-walled blood vessels, and epithelioid cells. **B** The epithelioid tumour cells contain abundant granular eosinophilic to clear cytoplasm. Note the admixed adipocytes.

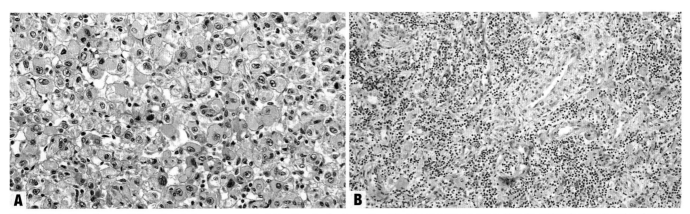

Fig. 12.50 Angiomyolipoma. **A** Some hepatic tumours are epithelioid, with cells showing eosinophilic (or oncocytic) cytoplasm. Note the mild nuclear atypia and nuclear pseudoinclusions. **B** Occasional hepatic angiomyolipomas contain a prominent inflammatory infiltrate of lymphocytes and plasma cells, which may obscure the neoplastic component. Note the epithelioid cells within the wall of a blood vessel.

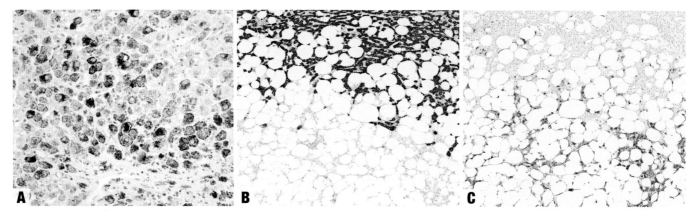

Fig. 12.51 Angiomyolipoma. **A** HMB45 is the best confirmatory diagnostic marker. **B** Angiomyolipoma dominated by adipocytes. This tumour might be mistaken for lipoma. However, the tumour margin shows invasion of hepatocellular plates (Hep Par-1 immunostaining). **C** Occasional HMB45-positive epithelioid cells are present, confirming the diagnosis of angiomyolipoma. Note that the invaded hepatocellular plates are HMB45-negative.

Angiomyolipoma is nearly exclusive to the kidney, liver, and pancreas. Some patients present with both hepatic and renal angiomyolipomas, most with tuberous sclerosis {3360}.

Clinical features

In the intestines and stomach, PEComas form a mural mass that may contain or entirely consist of a polypoid mucosal component. Tumours can become symptomatic, with abdominal pain or bleeding. In the mesenteries and liver, PEComas can form pedunculated nodular masses. Malignant PEComas of the GI tract often metastasize to the liver, peritoneum, lymph nodes, and lungs {807}.

Hepatic angiomyolipoma is usually discovered incidentally {3673}. Some patients present with vague abdominal symptoms or right upper quadrant pain. Most lesions are solitary; multifocal disease may be associated with tuberous sclerosis. Rarely, patients present with hepatic rupture and haemoperitoneum {785}.

On CT, hepatic angiomyolipomas are hypodense, with peripheral enhancement in the arterial phase; on MRI, the tumours are typically hypointense on T1-weighted images and hyperintense on T2-weighted images {1889}.

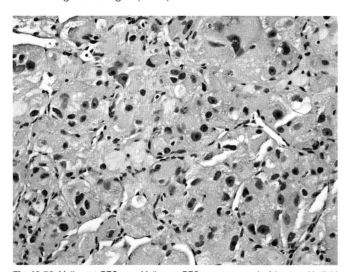

Fig. 12.52 Malignant PEComa. Malignant PEComa composed of large epithelioid cells with marked nuclear atypia, macronucleoli, and a trabecular architecture.

Epidemiology

Gastrointestinal and hepatic PEComas and angiomyolipomas are rare. PEComas in the GI tract affect children and adults over a wide age range, with a mean age of 35–40 years and a female predominance (M:F ratio: 1:1.5) {807,588}. Hepatic angiomyolipoma shows a marked female predominance and a peak incidence in middle-aged adults {1071,3360,3673}.

Etiology

Most hepatic angiomyolipomas are sporadic; 5–10% of patients have tuberous sclerosis {3360,341}. Other gastrointestinal PEComas are rarely associated with tuberous sclerosis {807}.

Pathogenesis

Unknown

Macroscopic appearance

Most gastrointestinal PEComas are circumscribed, unencapsulated masses that can extend into the adjacent mesenteric tissue. Tumour size ranges from < 1 cm to > 20 cm, with a median size of 6 cm {807}. The cut surface varies from pale tan to greyish-brown.

Hepatic angiomyolipomas also show a large range in size, from small lesions to large masses occupying much of the liver {1071,3360}. The cut surface is yellow or tan and often fleshy, with variable necrosis and haemorrhage.

Histopathology

The architecture of PEComas is often nested, alveolar, or trabecular, with a delicate capillary vascular network, although it can also be sheet-like. Most cases are dominated by epithelioid cells, with a spindle cell component seen in a minority of cases, rarely as a dominant feature. The cytoplasm ranges from granular eosinophilic to clear. Occasional pleomorphic cells are a common finding. Mitotic activity is usually low (< 1 mitosis/ mm²). In the sclerosing subtype, tumour cells are arranged in cords within a dense collagenous stroma.

Most hepatic angiomyolipomas contain an admixture of adipocytes, epithelioid cells, and thick-walled blood vessels; the relative proportions of these components vary considerably, although epithelioid cells are often a dominant component. The epithelioid cells are often intimately associated with the blood vessel walls. Some tumours contain a spindle cell component. The cytological features of the epithelioid and spindle cells are similar to those in other PEComas. Some tumours are dominated by adipocytes with a minor component of epithelioid cells; others contain a limited adipocytic component. Extramedullary haematopoiesis is frequently observed. The inflammatory subtype may be obscured by prominent chronic inflammatory cells {2991}. Necrosis and foci of haemorrhage are commonly found in large tumours. The mitotic count is usually low.

By immunohistochemistry, PEComas (including angiomyolipomas) are positive for both smooth muscle markers (desmin and/or SMA, each 60–75%) and melanocytic markers (HMB45, melan-A, PNL2, MITF, tyrosinase), with variable extent of staining {953,807,2384,3360,2017}. Epithelioid cells show more-extensive expression of melanocytic markers than the spindle cell component. Occasional KIT positivity should not lead to confusion with gastrointestinal stromal tumour {807,2018}. TFE3 positivity may be encountered {807}, especially in *TFE3*-rearranged subtypes {182}. These tumours are typically negative for keratins, S100, and SOX10.

Apparent lipomas in the liver should be stained with HMB45, because these lesions are often in fact angiomyolipomas. Positive staining for glutamine synthetase (GS) or negative staining for liver fatty-acid binding protein should not be mistaken for evidence of hepatic adenoma {3664}; Hep Par-1 (CPS1) and arginase-1 (ARG1) are negative.

Cytology
Not clinically relevant

Diagnostic molecular pathology
Specific molecular genetic information on GI tract PEComas is limited. PEComas (including hepatic angiomyolipomas) are known to harbour *TSC2* mutations (biallelic inactivation), resulting in activation of the mTOR signalling pathway; *TSC1* is rarely mutated {49,2494,1320,3664}. A minority of PEComas contain *TFE3* gene rearrangements {182,49}.

Essential and desirable diagnostic criteria
Essential: epithelioid and/or spindle cells with granular eosinophilic to clear cytoplasm; nested, trabecular, or sheet-like architecture; variable coexpression of melanocytic and smooth muscle markers; angiomyolipoma: variable admixture of adipocytes, thick-walled blood vessels, and epithelioid cells.

Staging (TNM)
Not clinically relevant

Prognosis and prediction
For GI tract PEComas, marked nuclear atypia, diffuse pleomorphism, and mitotic activity (> 1 mitosis/mm^2) are the strongest risk factors for metastatic behaviour {807}, but quantification of risk remains problematic due to the rarity of this entity.

Nearly all hepatic angiomyolipomas are benign {1071,3360, 3673}. Rare primary malignant hepatic PEComas have been reported, some with adipocytic and vascular components {2347, 757}. Histological atypia is not a reliable criterion for malignancy in hepatic angiomyolipomas {3664}; some borderline cases should be classified as angiomyolipoma of uncertain malignant potential, pending follow-up.

Mesenchymal hamartoma of the liver

Tsui WM
Miettinen M

Definition

Mesenchymal hamartoma (MH) of the liver is a benign liver tumour characterized by a commonly multicystic loose connective tissue mass accompanied by a ductal component with ductal plate malformation.

ICD-O coding

None

ICD-11 coding

2E92.7 Benign neoplasm of liver or intrahepatic bile ducts

Related terminology

None

Subtype(s)

None

Localization

Liver only: MHs occur in the right liver lobe in 75% of cases, the left lobe in 22%, and both lobes in 3%.

Clinical features

Clinically, MH typically presents with abdominal distension and an upper abdominal mass, although some cases are found incidentally. Pain is rarely a dominant feature, and only few patients show anorexia, vomiting, or failure to thrive {752}. Abdominal distension may rapidly progress and cause respiratory distress {3121}. Large MHs in neonates and infants may compromise blood circulation and evolve into life-threatening lesions. MH may be associated with mesenchymal stem villous hyperplasia of the placenta {515}. A subset of MHs are detectable prenatally (fetal MH), usually in the last trimester of pregnancy. Liver function is usually normal, but serum levels of AFP may be slightly elevated {359}; in exceptional cases, MH is associated with high levels of serum AFP {1113}.

Epidemiology

MH is the third most common hepatic tumour in childhood (after hepatoblastoma and infantile haemangioma). It accounts for 12% of all liver tumours during the first 2 years of life and 8% from birth to the age of 21 years. About 85% of affected children present before the age of 3 years, and < 5% of MHs are

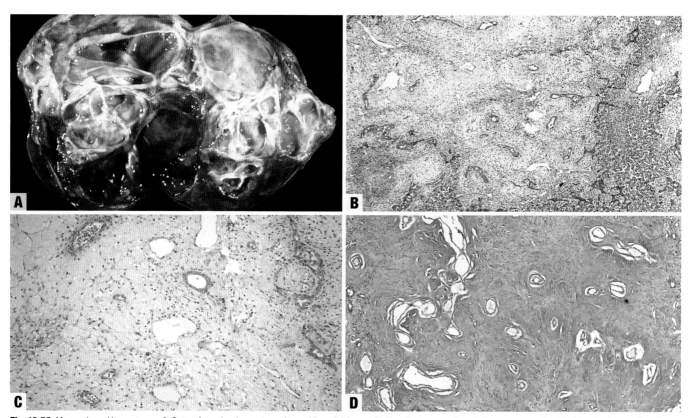

Fig. 12.53 Mesenchymal hamartoma. **A** Cut surface showing cysts and tan-white solid tissue. **B** Abundant mesenchymal stroma surrounding bile ducts in abnormal configuration and interposed islands of hepatocytes. **C** Myxoid stroma with spindle fibroblasts, vessels, and fluid-filled spaces; bile ducts displaying ductal plate malformation. **D** Collagenized stroma arranged concentrically around the ducts.

diagnosed after the age of 5 years {752}. About 15% of cases have been observed in the neonatal period {2243}. This lesion is slightly more common in boys than in girls. In contrast, the rare MHs occurring in adults are more frequent in women than in men {3701}.

Etiology
MH is primarily mesenchymal in origin, believed to arise from a developmental abnormality in the formation of ductal plates during late embryogenesis and related to disordered mesenchymal–epithelial transformation.

Pathogenesis
Based on cytogenetic and DNA analysis findings, there is some evidence that a neoplastic process may be involved {3227}. This is also supported by the observation of evolution of undifferentiated embryonal sarcoma from MH {1803}.

Recurrent genetic alterations found in MH include either chromosomal rearrangements involving chromosome 19q13.4 (in sporadic cases) {2972} or androgenetic/biparental mosaicism (in cases associated with placental mesenchymal dysplasia) {2675}. The breakpoint 19q13.4 is in the vicinity of the chromosome 19q microRNA cluster (C19MC), which is activated in both scenarios {1521}. Karyotype analyses of undifferentiated embryonal sarcoma also reveal chromosomal rearrangements involving 19q13.4, similar to those in MH {2646}.

Macroscopic appearance
Most MHs present as expanding, well-delimited masses without a capsule. Multiple cystic spaces lacking a communication with bile ducts are noted on cut surfaces in 85% of cases. Very young patients show fewer cysts and a more solid phenotype, suggesting that cysts develop in parallel with progressive tumour growth. In one series, 41% of tumours were solid and 59% cystic {557}. The cysts, ranging in size from a few millimetres to 15 cm, contain yellow fluid or gelatinous material.

Histopathology
Microscopically, the lesion is composed of loose connective tissue and epithelial bile ducts in varying proportions arranged in lobulated islands. The mesenchyme is typically loose, myxoid, and rich in glycosaminoglycans, and it contains spindle fibroblasts, dilated vessels, and fluid-filled spaces. It may be collagenous and arranged concentrically around the ducts. The biliary structures may be tortuous and occasionally dilated, and they are often arranged in a ductal plate malformation pattern. Islets of hepatocytes without an acinar architecture may be present. Non–epithelial-lined cysts develop within the mesenchyme due to accumulation of fluid. Foci of extramedullary haematopoiesis are observed in > 85% of cases.

Cytology
Not clinically relevant

Diagnostic molecular pathology
Not clinically relevant

Essential and desirable diagnostic criteria
None

Staging (TNM)
Not clinically relevant

Prognosis and prediction
As a rule, MH has a benign course in the absence of complications, with a good prognosis if the mass is resected {3695}. Exceptions are patients with severe cardiopulmonary complications and the rare instances of evolution into undifferentiated embryonal sarcoma {2649,1530}.

Calcifying nested stromal-epithelial tumour of the liver

Hornick JL

Definition

Calcifying nested stromal-epithelial tumour (CNSET) of the liver is a rare, low-grade hepatic neoplasm of uncertain lineage characterized by a distinctive nested architecture surrounded by a cellular myofibroblastic stroma and psammomatous calcifications.

ICD-O coding

8975/1 Calcifying nested stromal-epithelial tumour

ICD-11 coding

XH8X78 Calcifying nested epithelial stromal tumour

Related terminology

Acceptable: nested stromal-epithelial tumour; ossifying stromal-epithelial tumour; desmoplastic nested spindle cell tumour; ossifying malignant mixed epithelial and stromal tumour.

Subtype(s)

None

Localization

CNSET usually arises in the right hepatic lobe {1206,1234,2014}.

Clinical features

CNSET is often discovered incidentally, sometimes with a history of a calcified hepatic nodule. Occasional patients present with abdominal pain, a palpable mass, or nausea. Several reported patients have presented with Cushing syndrome {1206,2014}.

Epidemiology

CNSET is rare, with < 40 reported cases. There is a female predominance and a predilection for children, adolescents, and young adults {1206,1234,2014}.

Etiology

Most CNSETs are sporadic. Several cases have been associated with Beckwith–Wiedemann syndrome {2033,1567}.

Pathogenesis

CTNNB1 gene deletions have been identified in several cases {203}.

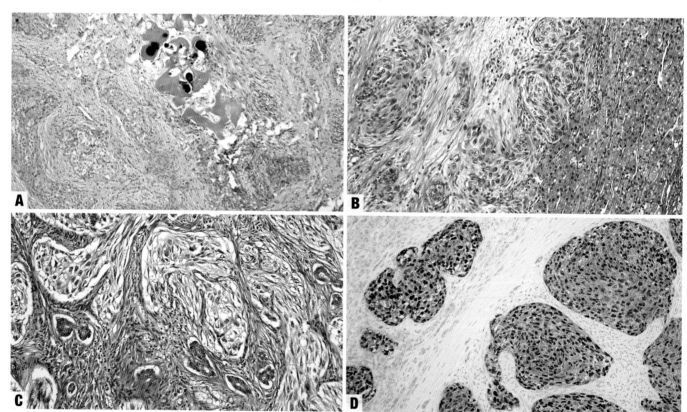

Fig. 12.54 Calcifying nested stromal-epithelial tumour. **A** This example shows psammomatous calcifications. Note the nested architecture and cellular stroma. **B** This tumour type shows a sharp interface with the adjacent liver parenchyma. **C** The tumour is composed of nests of epithelioid and spindle cells surrounded by a cellular stroma containing a bile ductular proliferation. **D** Immunohistochemistry for β-catenin shows aberrant nuclear and cytoplasmic staining.

Macroscopic appearance

CNSET is well circumscribed but unencapsulated, with a multi-nodular, sharp interface with adjacent liver. Tumours range from 2.8 to 30 cm; most are > 10 cm. The cut surface is yellow or white, homogeneous, and granular {2014}.

Histopathology

The tumours are composed of ovoid to irregular nests of variably spindled to epithelioid cells, cuffed by a cellular stroma. A focally trabecular architecture is sometimes observed. Occasional nests contain central necrosis. The tumour cells are bland and uniform, with vesicular chromatin, indistinct nucleoli, and eosinophilic cytoplasm with low mitotic activity. The nests often harbour psammomatous calcifications, and sometimes ossification. The stroma may contain a bile ductular proliferation.

By immunohistochemistry, the tumour cells are positive for broad-spectrum keratins and WT1 (usually nuclear but sometimes cytoplasmic or perinuclear dot-like), with aberrant nuclear and cytoplasmic β-catenin staining {1206,1234,2014,203}. Expression of CD56, EMA, PR, neuron-specific enolase, and KIT (CD117) is variable. Desmin, chromogranin, synaptophysin, Hep Par-1 (CPS1), and polyclonal CEA are negative. The spindle cells in the stroma are positive for SMA.

Cytology

Not clinically relevant

Diagnostic molecular pathology

Not clinically relevant

Essential and desirable diagnostic criteria

Essential: nested architecture surrounded by cellular myofibroblastic stroma; bland and uniform epithelioid and spindle cells; expression of keratins, WT1, and nuclear β-catenin.

Staging (TNM)

Not clinically relevant

Prognosis and prediction

Many patients with CNSET are cured by surgical excision, whereas several reported patients have developed locally recurrent disease, necessitating liver transplantation {1206, 1234,2014,411}. One reported patient had lymph node metastasis {2116}. Distant metastases have not been reported.

Synovial sarcoma

Miettinen M
Sciot R
Tsui WM

Definition

Synovial sarcoma is a malignant neoplasm with a spindle cell (monophasic) or epithelioid to glandular and spindle cell (biphasic) appearance and *SS18-SSX1/2/4* gene rearrangement.

ICD-O coding

9040/3 Synovial sarcoma NOS

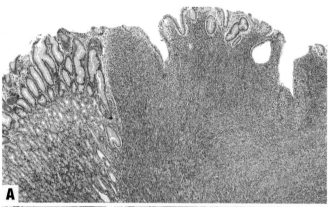
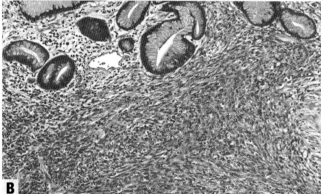
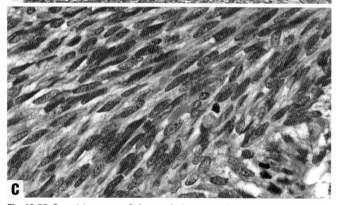

Fig. 12.55 Synovial sarcoma. **A** A case of primary synovial sarcoma of the stomach, with transmural involvement. **B** Higher power shows infiltration around gastric glands in this monophasic example. **C** A case of primary synovial sarcoma of the stomach, with transmural involvement.

ICD-11 coding

2B5A.Y & XH9B22 Synovial sarcoma, other specified primary site & Synovial sarcoma NOS

Related terminology

None

Subtype(s)

Synovial sarcoma, monophasic fibrous (9041/3); synovial sarcoma, biphasic (9043/3)

Localization

Primary synovial sarcoma is very rare in the GI tract and occurs primarily in the stomach, but a small number of cases have been reported in the oesophagus, small intestine, and colon.

Clinical features

In the GI tract, the reported occurrence is preferentially in middle-aged or older adults, with no sex predilection, although examples have been reported in children, especially in the oesophagus. Synovial sarcoma may occur as a polypoid or ulcerated mucosal lesion or a transmural mass lesion.

Epidemiology

None

Etiology

Unknown

Pathogenesis

Gene rearrangements are common and can be helpful for diagnosis (see *Diagnostic molecular pathology*, below).

Macroscopic appearance

The most common presentation in the oesophagus is a polypoid mucosal mass. In the stomach, cases with early diagnosis form a cup-like or plaque-like mucosal lesion or a subserosal mass of 1–2 cm. Mucosal tumours usually extend into the submucosa and often also involve the muscularis propria. More-advanced tumours form transmural masses of 5 cm to > 10 cm.

Histopathology

Most gastrointestinal synovial sarcomas are monophasic spindle cell tumours composed of relatively uniform spindle cells with almost no matrix or with a focal collagenous matrix. A minority of cases have a biphasic histology, with glandular elements and spindle cells, similar to the monophasic tumours. Mitotic counts vary, but most cases have a low-grade appearance with scarce mitoses. High-grade components with a round cell pattern and prominent mitotic activity may be present and portend a poorer prognosis. Immunohistochemically, the lesion shows patchy, focal positivity for keratin and EMA in the monophasic

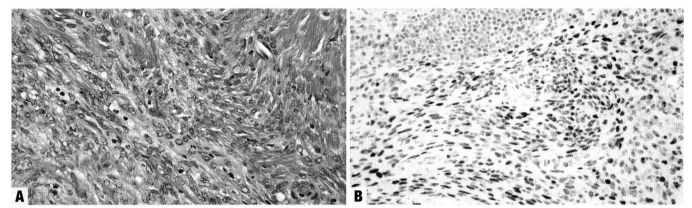

Fig. 12.56 Synovial sarcoma. **A** The tumours can be highly infiltrative. **B** Distinct nuclear expression of TLE1 in tumour cells is characteristic.

spindle cell tumours and strong positivity in the glandular elements. Positivity for calretinin, S100, DOG1, and rarely KIT (KIT usually being focal) can occur, and this raises the differential diagnostic consideration of gastrointestinal stromal tumour.

Cytology
Not clinically relevant

Diagnostic molecular pathology
Like other synovial sarcomas, those in the GI tract feature *SS18-SSX1* or *SS18-SSX2* gene fusions (rarely, *SS18-SSX4*).

Essential and desirable diagnostic criteria
Essential: spindle cells, sometimes with a biphasic epithelioid or glandular component; patchy expression of keratins and/or EMA in spindle cells; *SS18-SSX1/2/4* rearrangement.

Staging (TNM)
This neoplasm is not formally staged according to the TNM soft tissue tumours classification system.

Prognosis and prediction
The available follow-up data suggest that small mucosal synovial sarcomas with low-grade features have an excellent prognosis after complete excision, whereas smaller tumours with high-grade components and larger transmural tumours are associated with metastatic behaviour.

Chapter 12

Gastrointestinal clear cell sarcoma / malignant gastrointestinal neuroectodermal tumour

Miettinen M
Sciot R
Tsui WM

Definition

Gastrointestinal clear cell sarcoma (CCS) / malignant gastrointestinal neuroectodermal tumour (GNET) is a sarcoma involving the GI tract with neuroectodermal differentiation and gene fusion translocations involving *EWSR1*, usually *EWSR1-ATF1* or *EWSR1-CREB1*.

ICD-O coding

9044/3 Clear cell sarcoma NOS

ICD-11 coding

XH77N6 Clear cell sarcoma

Related terminology

None

Subtype(s)

None

Localization

The most common locations are the small intestine, stomach, and colon.

Clinical features

Gastrointestinal CCS-like tumour has a predilection for arising in young adults but can also occur in old age. It is an aggressive tumour that often metastasizes to regional lymph nodes and liver, and metastases are often detected at presentation.

Epidemiology

Tumours reported as GNET have a median patient age of 33 years (range: 10–81 years) and an even sex distribution, whereas tumours reported as GI tract CCS have a higher median age (57 years; range: 35–85 years) and 85% of the cases occur in males {1093}.

Etiology

Unknown

Pathogenesis

Most cases contain *EWSR1* gene aberrations, with *ATF1* or *CREB1* as the partner.

Macroscopic appearance

The tumours are 2–15 cm in size and variably form endophytic polypoid masses or mural lesions, often with ulceration resembling common carcinomas. The tumours are solid and often lobulated and tan-white on sectioning.

Histopathology

Most cases show round cell histology with uniform cells in vague nested or pseudopapillary patterns, but spindle cell

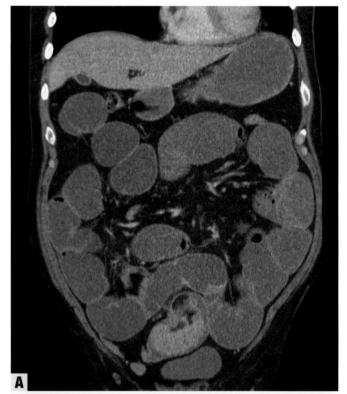

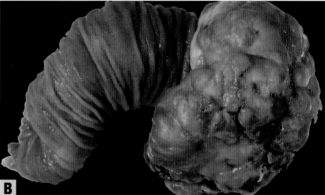

Fig. 12.57 Gastrointestinal clear cell sarcoma / malignant gastrointestinal neuroectodermal tumour. **A** CT image of clear cell sarcoma of the GI tract forming a mass within the wall of the ileum, with intussusception and small bowel obstruction. **B** This tumour involves the bowel.

histology is seen occasionally. The cells contain large round nuclei with vesicular chromatin and usually inconspicuous but occasionally prominent nucleoli. The cytoplasm is usually pale eosinophilic and shows clearing only in a minority of cases. Half of the cases contain osteoclastic giant cells. Mitotic activity is variable. Immunohistochemically, positivity for S100 and SOX10 is typical, whereas markers that are more melanocyte-specific

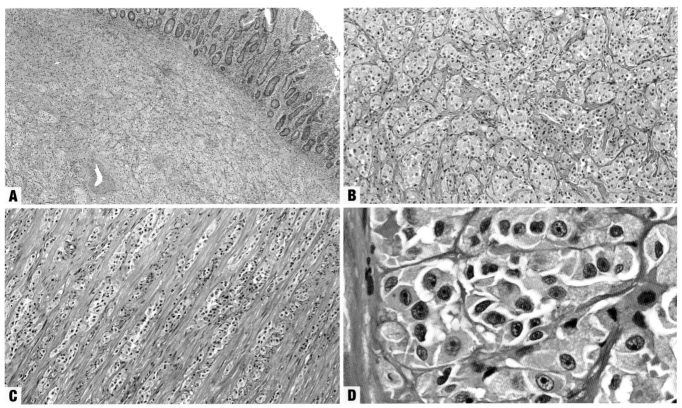

Fig. 12.58 Gastrointestinal clear cell sarcoma / malignant gastrointestinal neuroectodermal tumour. **A** This tumour arose in the small intestine. **B** A nested architecture is dominant here. **C** This area infiltrates smooth muscle of the bowel wall. **D** High power demonstrating nested architecture with epithelioid features.

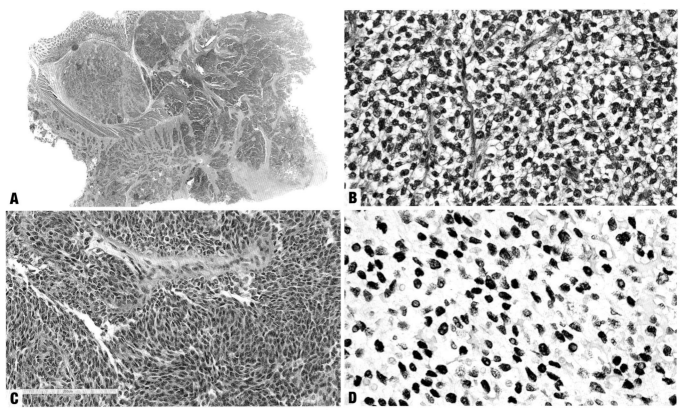

Fig. 12.59 Gastrointestinal clear cell sarcoma / malignant gastrointestinal neuroectodermal tumour. **A** Nodular and infiltrative patterns are present with extensive infiltration of the bowel wall. **B** Despite the name, distinct clear-cell change is relatively uncommon. **C** A more solid proliferation of spindle cells. **D** Immunoreactivity for both S100 and SOX10 (the latter depicted here) is characteristic, whereas more-specific melanocytic stains such as HMB45 or melan-A are very uncommon.

(HMB45, melan-A, and MITF) are negative. CD56 and synaptophysin positivity is a characteristic feature, and the neuroblastoma marker NB84 can also be expressed. Unlike gastrointestinal stromal tumour, these tumours are negative for KIT and DOG1. They are also negative for chromogranin, CD34, desmin, keratins, and SMA.

It is debated whether GI tract CCS and malignant GNET should be considered different tumours or the same tumour with different degrees of differentiation {1093}. Many authorities prefer the term "CCS" when there is expression of melan-A, HMB45, or MITF and the term "malignant GNET" when these markers are absent {1093,1378,118,3514}.

The primary differential diagnosis is with metastatic melanoma. The absence of a clinical history of melanoma is supportive, and the demonstration of *EWSR1* gene rearrangement is definitive. The distinction from other sarcomas harbouring *EWSR1* gene rearrangements is based on the combination of morphology and immunohistochemistry.

Cytology
Not clinically relevant

Diagnostic molecular pathology
Most cases contain *EWSR1* gene aberrations. Most have an *EWSR1-ATF1* fusion similar to that of peripheral CCS, and a minority of cases contain an *EWSR1-CREB1* fusion.

Essential and desirable diagnostic criteria
Essential: positivity for S100 and SOX10; *EWSR1* fusion gene.

Staging (TNM)
Not clinically relevant

Prognosis and prediction
Not clinically relevant

Embryonal sarcoma of the liver

Hornick JL
Miettinen M
Tsui WM

Definition
Embryonal sarcoma of the liver is a malignant hepatic neoplasm of children, composed of heterogeneous undifferentiated mesenchymal cells.

ICD-O coding
8991/3 Embryonal sarcoma

ICD-11 coding
XH42Q2 Embryonal sarcoma

Related terminology
Acceptable: undifferentiated embryonal sarcoma.
Not recommended: malignant mesenchymoma of the liver.

Subtype(s)
None

Localization
Embryonal sarcoma usually arises in the right hepatic lobe {1281,1401}.

Clinical features
Patients often present with abdominal distension, pain, fever, and weight loss; hepatic rupture with haemoperitoneum is uncommon {3142}. Leukocytosis and elevated serum alkaline phosphatase are common. Invasion of the inferior vena cava with extension to the right atrium may be observed {1762}.

Epidemiology
Embryonal sarcoma is rare, although it is the most common malignant hepatic mesenchymal neoplasm in the paediatric population. Children aged 5–15 years are typically affected, with no sex predilection {3142,2992}; presentation in adulthood is rare {1858}.

Etiology
Embryonal sarcoma is sporadic. Rarely, transformation from mesenchymal hamartoma has been reported {2978}.

Pathogenesis
Unknown

Macroscopic appearance
Embryonal sarcoma is well circumscribed but unencapsulated. Tumours are large (10–30 cm). The cut surface is heterogeneous, with alternating solid, fleshy, and mucoid areas and foci of cystic degeneration, necrosis, and haemorrhage {3142}.

Histopathology
The tumour is typically composed of variably spindled, stellate, and pleomorphic giant cells loosely arranged in a myxoid stroma; fibrotic areas with solid, fascicular, or storiform growth may be observed {3142,1762}. Cytoplasmic PAS-positive eosinophilic hyaline (lysosomal) globules in giant cells are a characteristic finding {3142}. Mitotic activity (including atypical mitoses) is easily detected. Peripheral entrapment of bile ducts is often seen, as is extramedullary haematopoiesis. Rare cases associated with mesenchymal hamartoma have been reported {1803,2405}.

Embryonal sarcoma shows no specific immunophenotype. Variable, often limited expression of keratins, desmin, and MSA may be seen {1762,2351,1570}; a subset of cases are positive

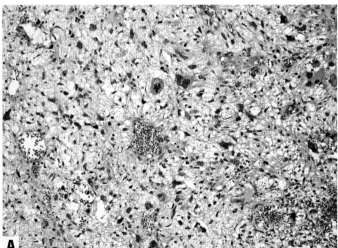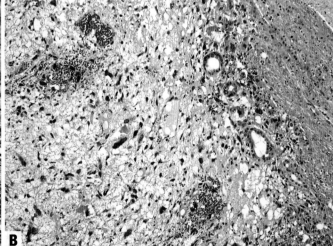

Fig. 12.60 Embryonal sarcoma of the liver. **A** The tumour is composed of variably spindled, stellate, and pleomorphic cells embedded in a myxoid strom. **B** Entrapment of bile ducts is often seen at the periphery of the tumour. Note the myxoid stroma.

Chapter 12

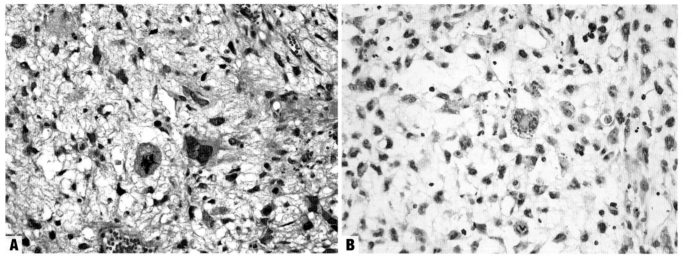

Fig. 12.61 Embryonal sarcoma of the liver. **A** There is a haphazard growth pattern. Note the multinucleated tumour giant cells and mitotic activity, including atypical mitotic figures. **B** Eosinophilic globules within the cytoplasm of tumour cells are a characteristic finding.

for glypican-3 (GPC3) {1874}. The tumour cells are negative for EMA, Hep Par-1 (CPS1), AFP, myogenin, and MYOD1 {2351}.

Cytology
Not clinically relevant

Diagnostic molecular pathology
Embryonal sarcoma typically shows a complex karyotype {3105}. The t(11;19)(q13;q13.4) characteristic of mesenchymal hamartoma has been detected in several cases {2646}.

Essential and desirable diagnostic criteria
Essential: spindled, stellate, and pleomorphic giant cells loosely arranged in a myxoid stroma.

Staging (TNM)
Not clinically relevant

Prognosis and prediction
Although embryonal sarcoma of the liver may pursue an aggressive clinical course, with metastases to the lung and peritoneum, patients with surgically resectable tumours often have a favourable outcome {1401,3267,2075}. Tumour size > 15 cm is an adverse prognostic indicator {2992}.

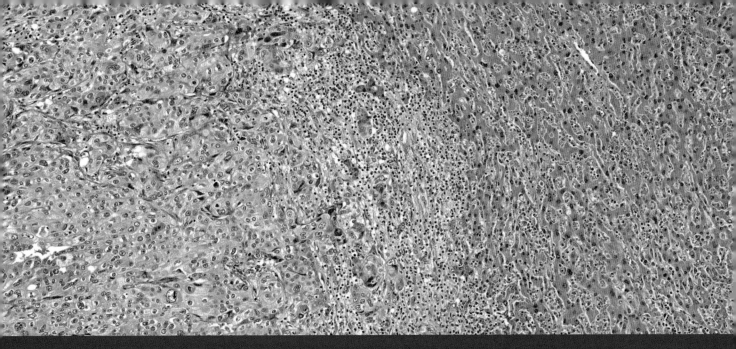

13

Other tumours of the digestive system

Edited by: Paradis V, Schirmacher P, Singh R

Mucosal melanoma
Germ cell tumours
Metastases

WHO classification of other tumours of the digestive system

8720/3	Melanoma NOS
8721/3	Nodular melanoma
8746/3	Mucosal lentiginous melanoma
9064/3	Germinoma
9070/3	Embryonal carcinoma NOS
9071/3	Yolk sac tumour NOS
9080/0	Teratoma, benign
9080/3	Teratoma, malignant, NOS
9084/0	Dermoid cyst NOS
9085/3	Mixed germ cell tumour
8140/6	Adenocarcinoma, metastatic, NOS
8010/6	Carcinoma, metastatic, NOS

These morphology codes are from the International Classification of Diseases for Oncology, third edition, second revision (ICD-O-3.2) {1378A}. Behaviour is coded /0 for benign tumours; /1 for unspecified, borderline, or uncertain behaviour; /2 for carcinoma in situ and grade III intraepithelial neoplasia; /3 for malignant tumours, primary site; and /6 for malignant tumours, metastatic site. Behaviour code /6 is not generally used by cancer registries.

This classification is modified from the previous WHO classification, taking into account changes in our understanding of these lesions.

Mucosal melanoma of the digestive system

Scolyer RA
Prieto VG

Definition
Mucosal melanoma of the digestive system is a malignant melanocytic neoplasm arising in the digestive tract, typically in the anorectal region.

ICD-O coding
8720/3 Melanoma NOS
8721/3 Nodular melanoma
8746/3 Mucosal lentiginous melanoma

ICD-11 coding
2C11.2 & XH4846 Other specified malignant neoplasms of other or ill-defined digestive organs & Malignant melanoma NOS
2C11.2 & XH5QP3 Other specified malignant neoplasms of other or ill-defined digestive organs & Mucosal lentiginous melanoma
2C11.2 & XH4QG5 Other specified malignant neoplasms of other or ill-defined digestive organs & Nodular melanoma

Related terminology
Acceptable: mucosal lentiginous melanoma; anal melanoma; anorectal melanoma.

Subtype(s)
None

Localization
In the digestive tract, these rare tumours typically arise in the anorectal region {338,552}. Less common locations include the oesophagus, stomach, intestine, and gallbladder {753,802}. Melanoma involving the small intestine or stomach most commonly represents metastasis rather than a primary tumour.

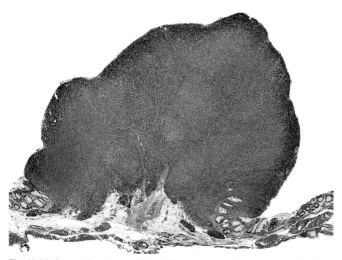

Fig. 13.01 Anorectal melanoma. Polypoid invasive anorectal melanoma arising in columnar rectal mucosa of a 59-year-old woman, with satellitosis in submucosa.

Clinical features
The clinical signs and symptoms depend on the anatomical location affected. Diagnosis is often delayed. Anorectal melanomas often present with rectal bleeding, a mass, pain, or a change in bowel habits, and they are often misdiagnosed as haemorrhoids because of their dark colour {1357,2023}. The median patient age at diagnosis is approximately 65 years – about a decade older than for cutaneous melanoma. There is no sex predilection.

Epidemiology
Primary melanoma involving the digestive tract accounts for < 1% of gastrointestinal malignancies and about 1% of anorectal malignancies overall. Mucosal melanomas account for approximately 1% of all melanomas in most European populations and for 25–50% of melanomas in dark-skinned populations {338}.

Etiology
The etiology of mucosal melanomas is unknown. Unlike cutaneous melanomas, they show no association with ultraviolet (UV) radiation exposure {1199}.

Pathogenesis
Unlike cutaneous melanomas, mucosal melanomas show a low mutation burden, with no UV signature. Instead, they are characterized by numerous chromosomal structural variants and abundant copy-number changes, including multiple high-level amplifications {1199,988}. The most common somatic mutations involve *KIT*, *SF3B1*, *ATRX*, *TP53*, *ARID2*, *SETD2*, and *BRAF*. Mutations in *BRAF* are found in about 10% of mucosal melanomas, which is much lower than the 35–40% rate seen in cutaneous melanomas {1211,1199,223,2692}.

Macroscopic appearance
Primary mucosal melanoma usually shows a lentiginous or nodular pattern {2550}. Anorectal melanomas usually present as large, expansive, nodular masses. Involvement of anal squamous epithelium or rectal mucosa is not always identifiable. An associated naevus is rarely seen.

Histopathology
The tumour is usually composed of sheets or expansive nodules of large pleomorphic epithelioid or (less commonly) malignant melanocytic spindle cells {2694A,2613}. Pigmentation is variable and may be absent. Necrosis is rare. The nuclei often have vesicular chromatin and prominent nucleoli. Occasionally, small or naevoid cells may predominate. Less frequently, a lentiginous growth of individual atypical melanocytes in the basal layer may occur, sometimes with nests or confluent growth. A subepithelial lymphocytic infiltrate is common.

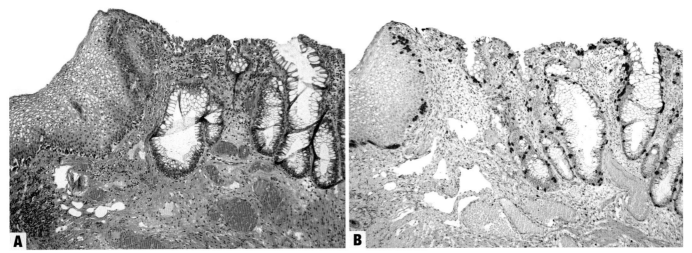

Fig. 13.02 Anorectal melanoma. **A** Anorectal melanoma in situ showing lentiginous growth involving the squamocolumnar junctional epithelium of a 73-year-old man. **B** SOX10 highlights the melanoma cells.

Cytology

FNA specimens are usually obtained from metastases. The typical cytological appearances include a dissociated population of large epithelioid (or sometimes spindle) cells {2250}. Isolated giant cells and intranuclear pseudoinclusions are often present. Cytoplasmic pigment is usually present in a minority of cells. Pigmented macrophages may be seen in the background.

Diagnostic molecular pathology

The characteristic mutations include several with clinical significance for treatment. Mucosal melanomas should be tested for *BRAF* and *KIT* mutations, in particular when systemic treatment with targeted therapy is being considered {1211,1199,223,2692}.

Essential and desirable diagnostic criteria

Essential: demonstrated malignancy and melanocytic differentiation; relation to the mucosa of the digestive tract; no evidence of previous or synchronous melanoma outside the digestive tract.

Staging (TNM)

There are no Union for International Cancer Control (UICC) staging criteria for gastrointestinal melanomas (including anorectal melanomas).

Prognosis and prediction

Unlike cutaneous melanoma, primary melanoma of the GI tract remains associated with relatively poor overall survival despite the use of multiple treatment modalities, including surgery, radiotherapy, and systemic therapies {700,1218,440,1357}. This is partly attributable to delayed detection. The reported 5-year survival rates for patients with anorectal melanoma are approximately 20% {167,1357}. Outcome after systemic immunotherapy for metastatic mucosal melanoma appears to be poorer than for cutaneous melanoma, but the data are limited {3025}.

Germer cell tumours of the digestive system

Quaglia A
Moch H
Oliva E

Definition
Germ cell tumours of the digestive system are tumours derived from extragonadal germ cells.

ICD-O coding
9064/3 Germinoma
9070/3 Embryonal carcinoma NOS
9071/3 Yolk sac tumour NOS
9080/0 Teratoma, benign
9080/3 Teratoma, malignant, NOS
9084/0 Dermoid cyst NOS
9085/3 Mixed germ cell tumour

ICD-11 coding
2C12.0Y & XH1E13 Other specified malignant neoplasm of liver & Germinoma, germ cell tumour, NOS
2C12.0Y & XH8MB9 Other specified malignant neoplasm of liver & Embryonal carcinoma NOS
2C12.0Y & XH09W7 Other specified malignant neoplasm of liver & Yolk sac tumour
2E92.7 & XH3GV5 Benign neoplasm of liver or intrahepatic bile ducts & Teratoma, benign
2C12.0Y & XH7YZ9 Other specified malignant neoplasm of liver & Teratoma, malignant, NOS
2E92.7 & XH9F67 Benign neoplasm of liver or intrahepatic bile ducts & Dermoid cyst NOS
2C12.0Y & XH2PS1 Other specified malignant neoplasm of liver & Mixed germ cell tumour

Related terminology
None

Subtype(s)
None

Localization
Extragonadal germ cell tumours arise mainly along the body midline, and very rarely in the liver {2104}. Most hepatic germ cell tumours form intrahepatic masses in the right, left, or both lobes. However, germ cell tumours at the porta hepatis {425} or around the common bile duct {2245,1603} have also been described. Extragonadal germ cell tumours originating at other sites in the digestive system are extremely rare.

Clinical features
As reported for extragonadal germ cell tumours at other sites, the presentation can vary depending on the patient's age – i.e. depending on whether the tumours have a congenital/neo-natal (birth to 6 months), childhood (prepubertal; 7 months to puberty), or adulthood (postpubertal) presentation {2104}. Like other primary liver tumours, intraparenchymal tumours may first present with weight loss, a palpable abdominal mass, upper quadrant pain, and general symptoms. Tumours at the porta hepatis or centred on the common bile duct can present with obstructive jaundice. High levels of serum AFP are character-istic of yolk sac tumours and mixed tumours containing a yolk sac component. Slight elevations of AFP levels can be related to embryonal carcinoma or teratoma. High levels of β-hCG may be seen in choriocarcinoma {2969}.

Epidemiology
Germ cell tumours of the digestive system are exceedingly rare. They can affect children and adults of any age, both males and females.

Etiology
There are no data to suggest a specific etiology, probably because of the rarity of these lesions.

Pathogenesis
The possible mechanisms underlying the development of extragonadal (including hepatic) germ cell tumours are arrest and survival of germ cell precursors at ectopic sites during embryological migration, as well as proliferation of pluripotent embryonic cells {2104}. The molecular data on hepatic germ cell tumours are limited to rare cases. In a hepatic malignant mixed germ cell tumour, chromosome 12p amplification and isochromosome 12p were demonstrated by FISH in immature teratoma and yolk sac components {3625}.

Macroscopic appearance
The macroscopic appearance is variable, but tumours may be solid or cystic with areas of haemorrhage.

Histopathology
In the GI tract, most germ cell tumours represent metastatic dis-ease from other sites {3537,1528,329}, sometimes from occult pri-maries (typically testicular). In rare cases in children and adults, primary germ cell tumours may arise within the liver; these are most commonly teratomas {3584,969,2366,2030,2642,3581} or (exceptionally) yolk sac tumours {1177,2321,2313,1112,1926, 3530,3595}. Malignant mixed germ cell tumours with various components, including yolk sac tumour, teratoma, embryonal carcinoma, and choriocarcinoma, have also been described {3625,3466,3288}. Hepatic germ cell tumours are histopatho-logically similar to those of primary gonadal origin {2184,1727}.

The immunohistochemical profile of germ cell tumours of the digestive system is similar to that of their gonadal counterparts. Yolk sac tumours stain for AFP, glypican-3 (GPC3), and SALL4. More-differentiated endodermal elements may express markers of their corresponding somatic tissues (e.g. CDX2 for intestinal elements, TTF1 for foregut epithelia, and Hep Par-1 for hepato-cytes). Dysgerminomas and seminomas express PLAP, KIT, podoplanin (as recognized by D2-40), OCT3/4, NANOG, and

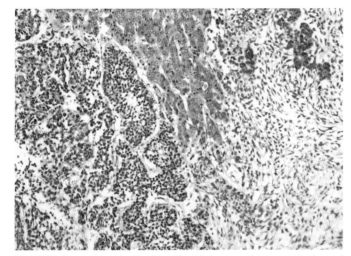

Fig. 13.03 Germ cell tumour of the liver. A liver hilum germ cell tumour centred around the common hepatic/bile duct in a 9-year-old girl. Serum AFP = 4000 µg/L. A mature hepatocellular component (centre) is admixed with an immature epithelial (left) and mesenchymal (right) component.

SALL4. Choriocarcinomas stain for broad-spectrum cytokeratins and hCG. Embryonal carcinomas express broad-spectrum cytokeratins, GPC3, SALL4, NANOG, OCT3/4, and (unlike other germ cell tumours) CD30.

The differential diagnosis depends on patient age at presentation and tumour location. The possibility of metastatic spread from an occult extrahepatic gonadal or extragonadal germ cell tumour should always be considered. The possibility of a carcinoma with secondary germ cell differentiation should also be considered, and sampling is important in such instances. Intraparenchymal lesions must be differentiated from other primary paediatric or adult liver tumours, in particular hepatocellular carcinoma and hepatoblastoma {2104,2419}. Nuclear β-catenin expression could be of help in distinguishing hepatocellular differentiation in a yolk sac tumour or teratoma from hepatoblastoma (which stains positively) {450}. Calcifying nested stromal-epithelial tumour can also be confused with intrahepatic teratoma, because of its biphasic appearance (see *Calcifying nested stromal-epithelial tumour of the liver*, p. 490) {2104}. GI tract carcinomas may show differentiation into yolk sac tumour or choriocarcinoma {1088,2618}.

Cytology
Not clinically relevant

Diagnostic molecular pathology
Not clinically relevant

Essential and desirable diagnostic criteria
Essential: no evidence of a previous or synchronous germ cell tumour outside the digestive system; the same diagnostic criteria as those for germ cell tumours of primary gonadal origin {2184,1727}.

Staging (TNM)
Because of the rarity of germ cell tumours of the digestive system, there are insufficient data in the literature to support a dedicated staging system.

Prognosis and prediction
Experience with these tumours is limited.

Digestive system metastases

Schirmacher P

Definition

Metastases are tumours arising at any site via the local or distant spread of carcinomas, neuroectodermal tumours (including melanoma), germ cell tumours, or sarcomas, discontinuous from the primary tumour.

"Carcinoma of unknown primary (CUP)" is a clinical and operational term that does not denote a distinct pathological entity; rather, it refers to a histologically proven malignant epithelial neoplasm for which the primary site cannot be convincingly determined despite exhaustive diagnostic efforts. CUP is a working diagnosis used in multidisciplinary settings; the term should be used restrictively, to avoid inadequate diagnostics and patient exclusion from treatment options.

ICD-O coding

8140/6 Adenocarcinoma, metastatic, NOS
8010/6 Carcinoma, metastatic, NOS

ICD-11 coding

2E2Z Malignant neoplasm metastasis, unspecified
2D8Y & XH8UE4 Malignant neoplasm metastasis in other specified digestive system organs & Adenocarcinoma, metastatic, NOS
Malignant neoplasm metastasis in digestive system
2D80.0 Malignant neoplasm metastasis in liver
2D80.1 Malignant neoplasm metastasis in bile duct
2D80.Y Other specified malignant neoplasm metastasis in liver or intrahepatic bile duct
2D80.Z Malignant neoplasm metastasis in liver or intrahepatic bile duct, unspecified
2D81 Malignant neoplasm metastasis in pancreas
2D82 Malignant neoplasm metastasis in extrahepatic bile ducts
2D83 Malignant neoplasm metastasis in ampulla of Vater
2D84 Malignant neoplasm metastasis in small intestine
2D85 Malignant neoplasm metastasis in large intestine
2D86 Malignant neoplasm metastasis in anus
2D8Y Malignant neoplasm metastasis in other specified digestive system organs
2D8Z Unspecified malignant neoplasm metastasis in digestive system

Related terminology

None

Subtype(s)

See the sections on the respective primary malignancies.

Localization

Metastatic tumours and CUP can involve any organ, but the liver is by far the most commonly involved organ site in the digestive tract {789}. In the liver and small intestine, metastatic tumours outnumber primary tumours; in other sites, metastases are far less common than primary tumours, and they typically occur late in disease as part of diffuse multiorgan involvement (see Table 13.01). Therefore, the frequency of metastatic involvement varies substantially between clinical and autopsy-related studies, with higher frequencies noted at autopsy {789,3533}. Metastatic disease in the GI tract can occur as a single tumour nodule, oligometastatic lesions (e.g. liver metastasis of colorectal cancer, renal cell carcinoma metastasis), or a multinodular or

Table 13.01 Characteristics of metastases in the digestive tract {789,3533}

Anatomical site	Relative frequency of metastasis (and autopsy frequency)	Most common primary sites	Typical appearance	References
Oesophagus	2.7% (6.1%)	Breast; lung; cutaneous melanoma	Submucosal nodule, can become ulcerated	{2182,2652, 3046}
Stomach	2.6% (1.7–5.4%)	Breast; lung; oesophagus; cutaneous melanoma	Submucosal nodule; linitis plastica appearance in lobular breast cancer	{473,2406}
Small intestine	~70%	Cutaneous melanoma; lung; breast; ovary; testis	Bowel wall thickening; submucosal nodule; ulcerated tumour	{1358}
Colorectum	5–10% (14%)	Stomach; breast; cervix; lung	Bowel wall thickening; submucosal nodule; ulcerated tumour	
Liver	70–97% (varies geographically and with primary liver cancer frequency)	Colorectum; breast; stomach; pancreas; melanoma	Multinodular; uninodular in colorectal and kidney cancers	
Biliary tract	Very low	Melanoma (accounting for 50%); stomach; breast	Mainly gallbladder, polypoid, and diffuse wall infiltration	
Pancreas	4% (15%)	Kidney; cutaneous melanoma; colorectum; breast; sarcomas	Circumscribed, haemorrhagic, or cystic masses	

diffuse multiorgan manifestation, depending on the tumour type and the organs involved {789}.

Haematolymphoid neoplasms may show diffuse organ involvement as part of primary systemic disease or discrete nodular involvement of organs, but the term "metastasis" is not used for these neoplasms.

Clinical features

Metastatic disease is the leading cause of tumour-related death. The clinical signs depend on the type and location of the tumorous manifestations. The most common symptoms include various degrees of abdominal pain and gastrointestinal bleeding, followed by weight loss, dysphagia, malabsorption, bowel obstruction, and bowel perforation, as well as haematemesis/haematochezia and resulting anaemia. Some metastatic malignancies are associated with defined paraneoplastic symptoms. Clinical and diagnostic consequences largely depend on the therapeutic options. A single metastasis or single-organ involvement, in particular of the liver, may be treated by resection or other locoregional therapies (e.g. endoradiotherapy for hepatic metastases of colorectal cancer). Otherwise, systemic therapies such as chemotherapy and immunotherapy, as well as molecularly targeted therapies, may be appropriate, depending on the tumour type. Specific molecular pathology diagnostics are often necessary {3131}.

Liver metastasis plays a specific role in gastrointestinal metastasis because of its anatomical, diagnostic, clinical, and therapeutic peculiarities. The liver is the most common and clinically relevant site of gastrointestinal metastasis. It is the primary site of haematogenous metastasis from all organs drained by the portal venous system (most prominently the colon). Cases of liver metastasis outnumber primary liver carcinomas by a factor of 2.5–40 {2309}, depending largely on the frequency of primary liver cancer in the population. They display the full spectrum of single-nodule, oligonodular, and diffuse metastasis. Intraorgan metastasis is a clinically relevant primary dissemination step for hepatocellular carcinoma (unlike for carcinomas of other organs). Depending on the extent of metastatic involvement and the type of underlying primary, liver metastasis may be treated locoregionally (i.e. by resection and endoradiotherapy; in particular for metastases of colorectal cancer) or systemically {3323}. Liver metastases are typically amenable to biopsy and further diagnostics for management purposes (including targeted therapies).

CUP accounts for 2–3% of all clinical cancer cases {3408,3026}. There is no sex predilection. History of smoking is a risk factor. CUP typically presents with a short history and progressed metastatic disease, which may show an atypical pattern of distribution. Neuroendocrine and squamous cell carcinomas are managed differently than most cases of adenocarcinoma and undifferentiated CUP, which are usually managed with platinum-based combination chemotherapy {945}.

Epidemiology

As diagnostic methods improve, most patients with CUP can eventually be successfully diagnosed, so incidence figures are unreliable. Metastases (of many tumour types) to the liver are common; the rest of the GI tract is less commonly affected, but the possibility of metastasis should always be considered.

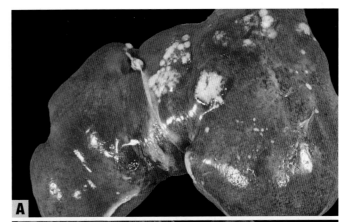
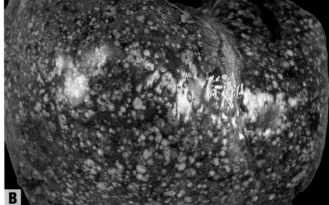
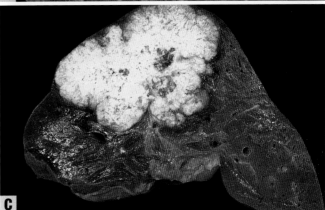

Fig. 13.04 Digestive system metastases. **A** Metastatic colon carcinoma showing umbilication and hyperaemic borders. **B** Metastatic small cell carcinoma of the lung forming innumerable small nodules. **C** Metastatic colon carcinoma; cut surface.

Etiology

See the sections on the respective primary tumours.

Pathogenesis

Depending on the type and localization of the primary tumour, metastatic spread to and within the GI tract follows the routes of lymphatics and venous blood flow or occurs along canalicular spaces (e.g. if the tumour infiltrates the peritoneal cavity). There are also entity-specific preferred metastatic conditions that cannot be readily explained by anatomical considerations. Lymphatic metastasis predominantly involves the locoregional lymph nodes (as reflected by the TNM classification), depending on the primary tumour localization. Skip metastases to

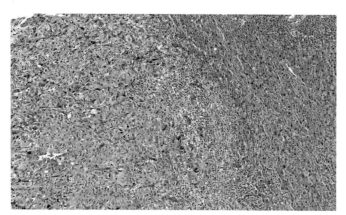

Fig. 13.05 Liver metastasis. Poorly differentiated salivary gland carcinoma metastatic to the liver.

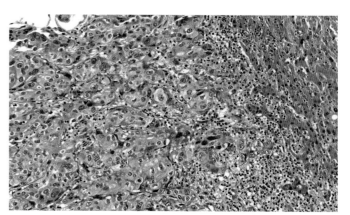

Fig. 13.06 Liver metastasis. Poorly differentiated salivary gland carcinoma metastatic to the liver.

distant lymph nodes in the absence of involvement of primary locoregional lymph node locations are rare. Lymphatic invasion, although not formally considered lymphatic metastasis, is a prerequisite and risk factor for lymph node metastasis. Lymphatic metastasis is usually not observed in sarcomas. Haematogenous metastasis commonly involves the venous system, following the flow of blood. Metastases from the gastrointestinal system preferentially occur in the liver because of drainage by the portal venous system. Several tumour entities are associated with unusual and more frequent than expected metastasis; for example, uveal melanomas frequently and preferentially spread to the liver, and cutaneous melanomas to the upper digestive tract.

Among the reasons for the clinical existence of CUP are the following: a small primary tumour may evade detection (e.g. neuroendocrine tumour [NET] or neuroendocrine carcinoma [NEC]) or may have regressed (e.g. testicular tumours), or a primary tumour may be equivalent to or indistinguishable among multiple intraorgan metastases. A primary tumour developing from ectopic tissue or monotypic differentiation of germ cell tumours may be mistakenly diagnosed as a metastasis. Diagnostic error, such as the mistyping of metastatic lesions or the failure to recognize the malignancy of a previously resected tumour, may rarely lead to a CUP diagnosis.

Macroscopic appearance

The size, number, location, and macroscopic appearance of metastatic lesions depend mainly on the type of tumour, the organ involved, the stage of disease, the type and extent of therapy administered, and the patient's condition (e.g. immune response).

Histopathology

Most metastatic lesions are histologically similar to the primary tumour, but loss and even changes of differentiation may occur in metastasis, especially under therapeutic pressure and hypoxic conditions. Metastases of tumours with mixed differentiation may show only part of the primary tumour's differentiation spectrum.

The vast majority (~80%) of CUPs are adenocarcinomas or undifferentiated carcinomas, about 2–4% are neuroendocrine neoplasms (NENs), and 5–8% are squamous cell carcinomas. Failure to identify the primary tumour on autopsy has been

reported in about 25% of CUP cases. Immunohistology and molecular diagnostics (including methylomic, transcriptomic, and proteomic analyses) can help narrow down or confirm a more specific diagnosis in some cases {2212,1746}. Molecular diagnostics may also help determine options for targeted and immuno-oncological treatments, depending on the available diagnostic technologies and drugs.

Cytology

Cytological evaluation follows the criteria for the respective primary tumours.

Diagnostic molecular pathology

Depending on the primary tumour type, metastatic disease in the GI tract may require molecular pathological analysis for various reasons. The typing of certain tumours, such as sarcomas and paediatric neoplasms, can critically depend on molecular analysis. If the link between a metastasis and one or more primary tumours is in question, molecular analysis may help to demonstrate a clonal relationship. Predictive molecular tumour analysis is a rapidly evolving field, with high relevance for metastatic lesions in the GI tract. The molecular markers to be analysed depend on the tumour type and the available therapeutic options. Entity-agnostic molecular testing (e.g. analysis of microsatellite instability, tumour mutation burden, and several translocations) is also evolving, in the context of various clinical trials and immuno-oncological therapies. Molecular pathological analysis can facilitate the detection of hereditary tumour syndromes, in particular in younger patients and in the setting of co-occurrence of different, especially uncommon tumour types.

Essential and desirable diagnostic criteria

In many cases, routine and special histological staining is sufficient for typing a metastasis or confirming its relation to a known primary tumour. Pertinent immunohistochemistry studies guided by morphology and clinical information (and in some cases molecular pathology) are helpful for determining or delineating the primary tumour entity of a given metastasis. Diagnostic necessity and procedures are related to the clinical options being considered by the multidisciplinary team. If a positive therapeutic consequence is potentially achievable, the available spectrum of diagnostic technologies (including routine and special staining, immunohistology, and molecular pathology) should be applied in an interdisciplinary setting. CUP with neuroendocrine or squamous differentiation has a better prognosis and is treated differently, so it is important to identify any such cases.

Staging (TNM)
The TNM staging of metastatic disease in the GI tract follows the criteria established for the respective tumour entities. There is no specific staging system for CUP.

Prognosis and prediction
Metastatic tumours usually indicate advanced tumour stage and therefore poor prognosis. Oligometastatic disease, resectability (e.g. of liver metastases of colorectal cancer), and the presence of specific molecular therapeutic target structures (depending on the tumour type) are positive prognostic and predictive factors. Microsatellite instability generally indicates better prognosis (even in metastatic disease) and favourable response to immuno-oncological treatment. The frequency of microsatellite instability in metastatic lesions varies widely among tumour entities, ranging from virtual absence (e.g. in hepatocellular carcinoma) to substantial proportions (e.g. in colorectal cancer).

Prognosis depends on the extent of metastatic involvement of the liver and other sites, the patient's general health condition, the treatment options available, and the response to therapy. A lower frequency of hepatic metastasis has been reported in the setting of cirrhosis, but it is unclear whether this is attributable to a higher frequency of primary liver tumours, increased mortality due to cirrhosis, surveillance bias, a protective effect of cirrhosis itself, or altered intrahepatic and portal venous blood flow {612}. Experimental evidence of metastasis promotion by steatohepatitis has been reported.

CUP has a poor prognosis, with reported median survival times of 6–9 months; mean survival times of 1–2 years, attributable to therapeutic progress, have been reported in selected cohorts. Prognostic factors include the Eastern Cooperative Oncology Group (ECOG) score, extent of organ involvement, amenability to locoregional treatment, and type of CUP. Neuroendocrine and squamous CUPs have a better prognosis than other types.

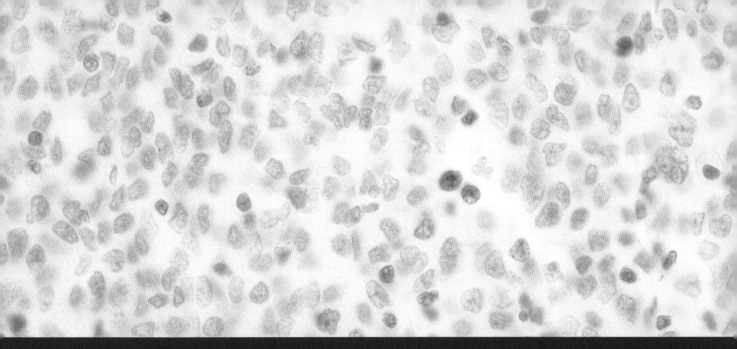

14

Genetic tumour syndromes of the digestive system

Edited by: Arends MJ, Carneiro F, Lax SF, Lazar AJ

Lynch syndrome
Familial adenomatous polyposis 1
GAPPS and other fundic gland polyposes
Other adenomatous polyposes
Serrated polyposis
Hereditary diffuse gastric cancer
Familial pancreatic cancer
Juvenile polyposis syndrome
Peutz–Jeghers syndrome
Cowden syndrome
Other genetic tumour syndromes

Genetic tumour syndromes of the digestive system: Introduction

Carneiro F
Arends MJ
Lax SF
Lazar AJ

Cancer is a disease of the genome, characterized by an accumulation of DNA perturbations selected for their malignant properties resulting in differential cellular survival, such as uncontrolled cell division, resistance to apoptosis, and the ability to migrate beyond the site of initiation and to survive and proliferate at metastatic sites. The study of familial cancer syndromes with simple Mendelian inheritance patterns has identified key genes that are critical not only because of the roles they play in genetic susceptibility to cancer, but also for the insight they provide into the molecular pathogenesis and classification of many sporadic cancers. Not all the syndromes described in this chapter are linked to cancer; some are associated with benign (and premalignant) proliferations whose study has contributed to our understanding of the function of their causative genes in important biological processes such as development and tissue homeostasis. Some of the syndromes covered in this chapter predominantly affect a single organ, such as the stomach (hereditary diffuse gastric cancer and gastric adenocarcinoma and proximal polyposis of the stomach [GAPPS]), the pancreas (familial pancreatic cancer), or the colorectum (familial adenomatous polyposis). Others involve several organs of the digestive system (Peutz–Jeghers syndrome and Lynch syndrome). Relevant data and new findings are presented throughout. The recognition of these syndromes and their features is critical for patient care.

Most syndromes are defined on the basis of a clinicopathological phenotype, but as more genes are identified and screening for them becomes increasingly routine in clinical practice, it is expected that conditions will increasingly be defined by their causative gene(s), rather than by simply lumping seemingly similar phenotypes together regardless of molecular derangements. Pathologists have a very important role in recognizing the syndromes addressed in this chapter. Clinicopathological classification remains crucial even in the current era (when broad genomic interrogation is often feasible), because there remain cases in which no germline mutations can be found, as the search for additional causative genes continues.

The section on Lynch syndrome (LS) includes a description of relevant new findings. There are now accurate data on LS-associated tumour types, and the risks thereof, stratified by gene, sex, age, and cancer status. The available resources include a comprehensive publicly accessible database of the pathogenic mutations in human mismatch repair genes that are causative of LS, curated by an internationally recognized expert group {1380}. Exploitation of the immune response in mismatch repair–deficient tumours has paved the way to more-effective immunotherapies based on PD1/PDL1 blockade. Lynch-like syndrome, i.e. the occurrence of colorectal cancers with loss of mismatch repair that is not due to LS, is now being investigated via the sequencing of such cancers. These investigations have demonstrated that the genes in which heritable mutations may predispose an individual to cancer are also prone to somatic mutation, in both LS and non-LS tumours.

Familial adenomatous polyposis 1 and GAPPS, because of their distinct phenotypic features (e.g. GAPPS predominantly affects the stomach), are described in their own separate sections, despite the fact that GAPPS is currently considered to be a subtype of familial adenomatous polyposis because of the shared genetic etiology of causative mutations localized in the promoter region of APC.

The section on other adenomatous polyposes describes several new conditions that are defined on the basis of their specific genetic aberrations.

The section on serrated polyposis presents new diagnostic criteria, updated from those included in the fourth edition. Only two clinical criteria are now included in the definition, corresponding to the two main phenotypes of serrated polyposis. The previous criterion of any number of serrated polyps occurring proximal to the sigmoid colon in an individual who has a first-degree relative with serrated polyposis has been discarded. Another change is the inclusion of the sigmoid colon in the criteria.

The section addressing hereditary diffuse gastric cancer includes an improved characterization of the syndrome's clinicopathological and genetic features. Recent findings have confirmed the existence of an indolent phenotype in asymptomatic carriers of CDH1 germline mutations, as well as an aggressive histological and immunohistochemical phenotype in aggressive, lethal cases.

The study of familial and hereditary pancreatic cancers demonstrates the importance of pathology in understanding genetics and vice versa, as well as the merits of including both descriptive names and gene names in syndrome designations when both types of information aid our understanding.

The three sections addressing hamartomatous polyps clearly demonstrate that colonic juvenile and Peutz–Jeghers polyps are quite distinctive, and that Cowden polyps are typically a mixture of various types of characteristic polyps; in contrast, gastric hamartomatous polyps are much less distinctive. In juvenile polyposis syndrome, SMAD4 immunohistochemistry can be used to guide additional testing and genetic counselling.

The final section of this chapter is dedicated to a group of miscellaneous syndromes involving the digestive system: Li–Fraumeni syndrome, hereditary haemorrhagic telangiectasia, syndromes associated with gastroenteropancreatic neuroendocrine tumours [NETs], and multilocus inherited neoplasia alleles syndrome – which is characterized by two or more inherited cancer predisposition alleles in the same individual and is increasingly recognized in the context of broad-panel germline testing for a variety of genes when a genetic syndrome is clinically suspected.

Table 14.01 lists each of the syndromes discussed in this chapter and summarizes key information about the disease/phenotype, pattern of inheritance, causative gene(s), and normal function of the encoded protein(s). Some of the syndromes included in the table are not discussed in detail in this chapter because of space limitations.

Table 14.01 The heritable syndromes currently understood to cause cancers in the digestive tract

Disease/phenotype	Syndrome MIM number	Inheritance	Locus	Gene(s)	Gene MIM number	Encoded protein(s)	Normal protein function
Lynch syndrome	609310	AD	3p22.2	MLH1	120436	MLH1	DNA mismatch repair
	120435	AD	2p21-p16.3	MSH2	609309	MSH2	
	614350	AD	2p16.3	MSH6	600678	MSH6	
	614337	AD	7p22.1	PMS2	600259	PMS2	
	613244	AD	2p21	EPCAM	185535	EpCAM	Calcium-independent cell–cell adhesion; mutation results in epigenetic silencing of MSH2
Muir–Torre syndrome	158320	AD	3p22.2	MLH1	120436	MLH1	DNA mismatch repair
			2p21-p16.3	MSH2	609309	MSH2	
			2p16.3	MSH6	600678	MSH6	
			7p22.1	PMS2	600259	PMS2	
	–	AR	1p34.1	MUTYH	604933	MUTYH	Repair of oxidative DNA damage
Constitutional mismatch repair deficiency syndrome	276300	AR	3p22.2	MLH1	120436	MLH1	DNA mismatch repair; this syndrome results from biallelic mismatch repair gene mutations
			2p21-p16.3	MSH2	609309	MSH2	
			2p16.3	MSH6	600678	MSH6	
			7p22.1	PMS2	600259	PMS2	
Familial adenomatous polyposis	175100	AD	5q22.2	APC	611731	APC	Negative regulation of β-catenin and WNT signalling
Gastric adenocarcinoma and proximal polyposis of the stomach (GAPPS)	175100	AD	5q22.2	APC	611731	APC	Negative regulation of β-catenin and WNT signalling (tumour suppressor)
Other adenomatous polyposes							
MUTYH-associated polyposis	608456	AR	1p34.1	MUTYH	604933	MUTYH	Repair of oxidative DNA damage
NTHL1-associated polyposis	616415	AR	16p13.3	NTHL1	602656	NTHL1	DNA repair
Polymerase proofreading–associated polyposis	615083	AD	12q24.33	POLE	174762	POLE	DNA repair and chromosomal DNA replication
Hereditary mixed polyposis syndrome	601228	AD	15q13.3	GREM1	603054	GREM1	BMP antagonism
AXIN2-associated polyposis (oligo-dontia-colorectal cancer syndrome)	608615	AD	17q24.1	AXIN2	604025	AXIN2	Negative regulation of β-catenin and WNT signalling
X-linked agammaglobulinaemia	300755	XLR	Xq22.1	BTK	300300	BTK	Development and maturation of B cells
Serrated polyposis	617108	AD	17q22	RNF43	612482	An E3 ubiquitin ligase	Negative regulation of WNT signalling
Familial diffuse gastric cancer with or without cleft lip and/or palate	137215	AD	16q22.1	CDH1	192090	E-cadherin	Calcium-dependent cell–cell adhesion
Familial pancreatic cancer							
Susceptibility to pancreatic cancer 4[a]	614320	Unknown	17q21.31	BRCA1	113705	BRCA1	DNA repair
Susceptibility to pancreatic cancer 2	613347	AD	13q13.1	BRCA2	600185	BRCA2	DNA repair
Pancreatic cancer	260350	AD, MF	17p13.1	TP53	191170	p53	Regulation of cell division and prevention of tumour formation
			19p13.3	STK11	602216	STK11	Suppression of cell division (tumour suppressor)

AD, autosomal dominant; AR, autosomal recessive; MF, multifactorial; XLR, X-linked recessive. [a]The degree of raised risk of pancreatic cancer with BRCA1 is uncertain.

(Continued on next page)

Table 14.01 The heritable syndromes currently understood to cause cancers in the digestive tract (continued)

Disease/phenotype	Syndrome MIM number	Inheritance	Locus	Gene(s)	Gene MIM number	Encoded protein(s)	Normal protein function
Juvenile polyposis syndrome							
Juvenile polyposis syndrome, infantile form	174900	AD	10q23.2	BMPR1A	601299	BMPR1A	Regulation of cell growth and division (proliferation)
Polyposis, juvenile intestinal	174900	AD	18q21.2	SMAD4	600993	SMAD4	A transcription factor and tumour suppressor
			10q23.2	RMPR1A	601299	BMPR1A	Regulation of cell growth and division (proliferation)
Juvenile polyposis / hereditary haemorrhagic telangiectasia syndrome	175050	AD	18q21.2	SMAD4	600993	SMAD4	A transcription factor and tumour suppressor
Chromosome 10q22.3-q23.2 deletion syndrome (including juvenile polyposis of infancy)	612242	AD	10q23.2	BMPR1A	601299	BMPR1A	Regulation of cell growth and division (proliferation)
Peutz–Jeghers syndrome	175200	AD	19p13.3	STK11	602216	STK11	Suppression of cell division (tumour suppressor)
Cowden syndrome							
Cowden syndrome 1	158350	AD	10q23.31	PTEN	601728	PTEN	A phosphatase; regulation of cell division (tumour suppressor)
Cowden syndrome 4	615107	AD	10q23.31	KLLN	612105	Killin	Triggers apoptosis
Cowden syndrome 5	615108	AD	3q26.32	PIK3CA	171834	PIK3CA (p110α)	A catalytic subunit of PI3K
Cowden syndrome 6	615109	AD	14q32.33	AKT1	164730	AKT1	Modulation of the AKT/mTOR signalling pathway
Cowden syndrome 7	616858	AD	20p11.23	SEC23B	610512	SEC23B	ER-associated protein secretion
Other genetic tumour syndromes							
Li–Fraumeni syndrome	151623	AD	17p13.1	TP53	191170	p53	Regulation of cell division (tumour suppressor)
Hereditary haemorrhagic telangiectasia	175050	AD	18q21.2	SMAD4	600993	SMAD4	A transcription factor and tumour suppressor
Multiple endocrine neoplasia type 1	131100	AD	11q13.1	MEN1	613733	Menin	DNA repair and regulation of apoptosis (tumour suppressor)
Multiple endocrine neoplasia type 2A	171400	AD	10q11.21	RET	164761	RET	Normal development of nerve cells
Multiple endocrine neoplasia type 2B	162300	AD	10q11.21	RET	164761	RET	Normal development of nerve cells
Multiple endocrine neoplasia type 4	610755	AD	12p13.1	CDKN1B	600778	p27	Prevention of aberrant cell division (tumour suppressor)
Neurofibromatosis type 1	162200	AD	17q11.2	NF1	613113	Neurofibromin (NF1)	Negative regulation of RAS
Tuberous sclerosis 1	191100	AD	9q34.13	TSC1	605284	Hamartin	Tumour suppression via interaction with and regulation of other proteins
Tuberous sclerosis 2	613254	AD	16p13.3	TSC2	191092	Tuberin	Tumour suppression via interaction with and regulation of other proteins
Von Hippel–Lindau syndrome	193300	AD	3p25.3	VHL	608537	VHL	Ubiquitination and degradation of HIF (tumour suppressor)
Multilocus inherited neoplasia alleles syndrome		MF					This syndrome results from the inheritance of mutated alleles associated with multiple syndromes (those listed above and others)

AD, autosomal dominant; AR, autosomal recessive; MF, multifactorial; XLR, X-linked recessive. [a]The degree of raised risk of pancreatic cancer with *BRCA1* is uncertain.

Lynch syndrome

Frankel WL
Arends MJ
Frayling IM
Nagtegaal ID

Definition
Lynch syndrome (LS) is an autosomal dominant disorder resulting from constitutional pathogenic mutations affecting the DNA mismatch repair genes *MLH1*, *MSH2*, *MSH6*, and *PMS2*.

MIM numbering
609310 Colorectal cancer, hereditary nonpolyposis, type 2
120435 Lynch syndrome I (colorectal cancer, hereditary non-polyposis, type 1)
614350 Colorectal cancer, hereditary nonpolyposis, type 5
614337 Colorectal cancer, hereditary nonpolyposis, type 4
613244 Colorectal cancer, hereditary nonpolyposis, type 8

ICD-11 coding
None

Related terminology
Not recommended: cancer family syndrome {1969}; hereditary non-polyposis colorectal cancer.

Subtype(s)
Muir–Torre syndrome (MIM number: 158320) {1970}; constitutional mismatch repair deficiency syndrome and Turcot syndrome (MIM number: 276300); allelic conditions due to biallelic mismatch repair gene mutations

Localization
Depending on which gene is involved, cancers occurring in LS can arise in the colon, rectum, endometrium, stomach, small bowel, gallbladder, hepatobiliary tract, pancreas, renal pelvis and/or ureter, bladder, kidney, ovary, brain, or prostate.

Clinical features
LS is characterized by predisposition to a wide variety of cancers. Tumours occurring in this setting can develop at any age, but often arise in young people. Some individuals with LS develop multiple tumours; others develop no tumours at all, so personal history is important. Family history alone has poor predictive value (both positive and negative). Cases of LS due to de novo germline mutations are well described.

The cancers that occur in LS include tumours of the colorectum, endometrium, stomach, small bowel, ovary, gallbladder, hepatobiliary tract, pancreas, urinary tract (renal pelvis, ureter, and bladder), kidney, brain, and prostate, as well as sebaceous skin tumours. Factors that affect the risk of an individual with LS include sex, age, the affected gene, and history of cancer (see Table 14.02, p. 515, and Table 14.03, p. 516) {2307,2261,2262,2263,2954}. The risk of cancer is highest with mutations of *MSH2* and *MLH1*, somewhat lower (and with later onset) when *MSH6* is affected, and lower still with *PMS2* mutations. Patients with LS can develop any cancer, which may or may not be due to their LS.

Table 14.02 Relative cumulative incidence of cancer by the age of 75 years in carriers of pathogenic mutations in mismatch repair genes, stratified by affected gene

Organ	ICD-9	Population incidence	Relative cumulative incidence, by affected gene (95% CI)			
			MLH1	MSH2	MSH6	PMS2
Any organ		24.4%	3.1 (2.8–3.4)	<u>3.3</u> (2.9–3.7)	2.5 (1.7–3.2)	2.1 (0.0–4.1)
By organ (in descending order of relative cumulative incidence)						
Duodenum	152	0.1%	**<u>64.7</u> (27.4–102.1)**	20.1 (0.6–39.6)	0	0
Colon	153	2.1%	**<u>22.3</u> (18.7–25.9)**	20.2 (15.6–24.7)	6.8 (1.5–12.1)	0
Bile duct and gallbladder	156	0.2%	**<u>18.7</u> (6.3–31.1)**	8.6 (0.0–25.4)	0	0
Sigmoid and rectum	154	1.4%	**8.4 (5.2–11.7)**	<u>13.0</u> (7.8–18.3)	3.3 (0.0–6.9)	0
Stomach	151	0.8%	**8.9 (4.4–13.4)**	<u>9.7</u> (2.3–17.0)	6.6 (0.0–16.4)	0
Pancreas	157	0.8%	**<u>7.8</u> (3.3–12.3)**	0.6 (0.0–1.9)	1.8 (0.0–5.2)	0
By anatomical region (in descending order of relative cumulative incidence)						
Gynaecological		2.6%	**19.1 (15.6–22.7)**	<u>25.3</u> (20.1–30.4)	20.8 (13.3–28.2)	10.1 (0.3–20.0)
Colorectal		3.8%	**<u>12.1</u> (10.0–14.2)**	11.3 (8.7–13.9)	3.9 (0.9–7.0)	0
Upper gastrointestinal		1.9%	**<u>11.2</u> (8.2–14.3)**	5.4 (2.1–8.6)	3.5 (0.0–7.8)	0
Urinary tract		2.3%	3.5 (1.9–5.1)	<u>10.8</u> (7.2–14.4)	4.8 (0.7–8.8)	0

Notes: **Bold** numbers indicate significantly increased (*P* < 0.05) relative cumulative incidence. <u>Underlining</u> indicates the maximum relative cumulative incidence by gene.

Table 14.03 Cumulative incidence of colon and rectosigmoid cancer stratified by age, pathogenically mutated mismatch repair gene, and sex (there was no observed colon or rectosigmoid cancer in carriers of a pathogenic *PMS2* mutation in any age group)

Organ (ICD-9 code)	Age (years)	Cumulative incidence (%) by age indicated, affected gene, and sex (95% CI)					
		MLH1		*MSH2*		*MSH6*	
		Females	Males	Females	Males	Females	Males
Colon (153)	40	10.4 (5.2–15.6)	15.4 (9.0–21.9)	10.1 (2.9–17.3)	7.4 (1.2–13.6)	0	0
	50	18.8 (12.6–25.0)	33.3 (25.5–41.1)	23.8 (14.8–32.8)	15.8 (7.2–24.3)	3.0 (0.0–8.7)[b]	0
	60	28.1 (20.9–35.2)	45.2 (36.6–53.8)[a]	31.4 (21.9–41.0)	21.5 (11.3–31.6)	5.7 (0.0–13.3)[b]	5.1 (0.0–15.0)[b]
	70	37.3 (28.5–46.1)	45.2 (36.6–53.8)	44.7 (33.7–55.7)	32.4 (17.7–47.2)	16.9 (0.8–33.0)[b]	11.0 (0.0–25.4)[b]
	75	42.1 (31.8–52.5)	50.8 (40.1–61.5)	44.7 (33.7–55.7)	42.6 (20.4–64.9)	16.9 (0.8–33.0)[b]	11.0 (0.0–25.4)[b]
Sigmoid and rectum (154)	40	1.4 (0.0–3.3)	1.9 (0.0–4.1)	0	1.3 (0.0–3.8)	0	0
	50	2.9 (0.3–5.4)	3.6 (0.8–6.4)	1.0 (0.0–3.0)	8.9 (3.0–14.7)	0	0
	60	6.1 (2.4–9.8)	6.5 (2.6–10.5)	4.0 (0.2–7.8)	17.9 (9.2–26.5)	4.6 (0.0–10.7)	0
	70	10.2 (4.9–15.6)	7.6 (3.2–12.1)	8.2 (2.2–14.3)	20.7 (10.7–30.7)	7.0 (0.0–14.6)	0
	75	11.7 (5.7–17.7)	11.7 (4.7–18.7)	12.9 (4.4–21.3)	26.0 (12.3–39.7)	7.0 (0.0–14.6)	0

[a]Significantly higher (*P* < 0.05) than among females of the same age. [b]Significantly lower (*P* < 0.05) than among carriers of a pathogenic *MLH1* or *MSH2* mutation of the same sex and age.

Note: Up-to-date estimates are available at http://www.lscarisk.org/.

Muir–Torre syndrome is the co-occurrence of a sebaceous skin tumour (i.e. sebaceous adenoma, sebaceoma, sebaceous carcinoma, or keratoacanthoma) with any internal cancer {2915}. Many patients with LS have such skin tumours {26} and therefore may be diagnosed with Muir–Torre syndrome, but not all patients with Muir–Torre syndrome have LS. Sebaceous skin tumours have been reported in some patients with *MUTYH*-associated adenomatous polyposis due to recessive *MUTYH* mutations.

Individuals with LS do not develop large numbers of colorectal adenomas, unless they have some other predisposing condition {3559}. However, individuals who inherit a mismatch repair mutation in the same gene from each parent, and therefore have constitutional mismatch repair deficiency syndrome (CMMRD) due to biallelic mismatch repair gene mutations, develop multiple adenomas at a very young age {194} (see also *Other adenomatous polyposes*, p. 529). CMMRD also predisposes individuals to colorectal cancer (CRC), brain tumours, leukaemia, lymphoma, neurofibromatosis type 1–like skin features, and a wide variety of other DNA repair deficiency–related abnormalities {3572}. Turcot described a syndrome of multiple colorectal adenomas and brain cancer {1152,3367}. Most cases are actually due to CMMRD; therefore, Turcot syndrome is an allelic variant of CMMRD. However, similar cases can be due to familial adenomatous polyposis (caused by inherited *APC* mutations).

Although Warthin was the first to describe what is now known as LS, Lynch redescribed it, calling it "the cancer family syndrome" {3531,1969}. Endeavours to study families with the syndrome in order to identify the responsible genes resulted in the Amsterdam criteria (AC), which were intended merely to identify families suitable for participation in research involving genetic linkage analysis (in ignorance of the spectrum and penetrance of the disease). The term "hereditary non-polyposis CRC" was then coined, as an umbrella term to help in the education of clinicians (still before the genes responsible for LS had been identified and the full clinical spectrum was apparent) {1967}. The subsequent Bethesda guidelines were developed in an attempt to help select tumours to test for possible LS, again in ignorance of

the syndrome's full clinical characteristics. Both the Amsterdam criteria and the Bethesda guidelines suffer from poor sensitivity. The Amsterdam criteria suffer from overly stringent specificity (excluding many individuals from testing), and the Bethesda guidelines suffer from nonspecificity at the cost of insensitivity. Later, the term "hereditary non-polyposis CRC" was no longer recommended (because it was inaccurate and confusing), and LS was defined as being caused by a constitutional pathogenic mismatch repair mutation {3448}.

Epidemiology

Systematic testing of CRC cases suggests that LS is a cause of CRC in approximately 1 in 30 cases. From the weighted mean extrapolated penetrance to age 85 years of LS as CRC (0.25) and the country-specific lifetime risks of CRC, the prevalence of LS in the general population can be estimated to be approximately 1 in 125 (1 in 100–180) {1445,3727,3078,2263}. Founder mutations causing LS have been found in many populations; for example, Finland has a higher prevalence of LS as a result of this effect {2398,1169,1095,3491,831}. In addition, certain mutations are relatively more common {760}.

Etiology

The primary cause of LS is a constitutional pathogenic mutation affecting a mismatch repair gene (*MLH1*, *MSH2*, *MSH6*, or *PMS2*). Some individuals with LS have mutations involving adjacent genes that affect or extend into a mismatch repair gene; for example a mutation in *EPCAM* (*TACSTD1*) affecting *MSH2* or in *LRRFIP2* affecting *MLH1* {3448,1910,1715,2209}. Some individuals may have epigenetic mechanisms (DNA methylation) affecting *MLH1* or *MSH2*, some of which may be caused by rearrangements involving adjacent genes {1246,1054,1910,1715,2209}.

The International Society for Gastrointestinal Hereditary Tumours (InSiGHT) curates a public database of mismatch repair genes {1380}, interprets genetic variants according to published criteria, and is recognized by ClinGen / the Global Alliance for

Genomics and Health as the sole definitive worldwide resource {3300,1381}.

A number of environmental and lifestyle factors have been identified as modifiers of LS. Cigarette smoking, increased body mass index, and alcohol consumption are associated with increased risk, whereas acetylsalicylic acid, ibuprofen, multivitamin and calcium supplements, hormone replacement therapy (but not oral contraceptive pill use), and increasing parity in women are associated with a reduction of cancer risk in LS {2499,3573,2235,67}.

Pathogenesis

Cells do not lose mismatch repair function unless both alleles of a given mismatch repair gene are inactivated. Therefore, it is not until a normal cell in a person with LS acquires a somatic hit in the corresponding normal mismatch repair allele that that cell becomes mismatch repair–deficient (dMMR). This deficiency has several important consequences. Firstly, dMMR cells escape from the normal control of apoptosis and gain a relative growth advantage, although this may be dependent on subsequent mutations in other genes {2610}. Secondly, mismatch repair deficiency leads to an increase in the point mutation rate, especially within repetitive stretches of DNA called microsatellites; this manifests as microsatellite instability (MSI). Thirdly, mismatch repair deficiency may also lead to abnormal mismatch repair protein expression, which is identifiable by immunohistochemistry.

In the normal colonic mucosa of people with LS, mismatch repair deficiency is present in approximately one crypt per 1 cm2 (i.e. in ~10 000 crypts per individual) {56}. These crypts can lead to immediately invasive lesions with mutations in *CTNNB1* (encoding β-catenin, which activates the WNT pathway) rather than *APC*, and with flat rather than polypoid morphology; such lesions are thought to account for the interval cancers that occur between seemingly normal colonoscopies. Patients with LS can undoubtedly develop CRC from adenomas, but some of the flat lesions can also acquire secondary *APC* mutations and become adenomatous and polypoid. Therefore, there are at least three pathways to CRC in LS: (1) dMMR crypts can give rise to flat lesions with mutations in *CTNNB1* rather than *APC*, which develop in flat cancers; (2) these flat lesions may then acquire secondary *APC* mutations and turn into adenomatous polypoid lesions; and (3) patients with LS can develop adenomas with primary *APC* mutations (as in the normal population), and these secondarily acquire mismatch repair deficiency during progression {55}. It is important to note that rectal cancers with MSI are usually due to LS, even though they do not harbour *CTNNB1* mutations, suggesting that pathway only occurs in the colon {2362,738,2363}.

A substantial proportion (~15%) of non-LS colon cancers have mismatch repair deficiency. Most are due to sporadic somatic biallelic hypermethylation of the *MLH1* gene promoter, as part of the right-sided sessile serrated lesion pathway. These tumours usually (in ~85% of cases) acquire specific *BRAF* oncogene mutations (*BRAF* p.V600E mutations), which can be used to distinguish them from CRCs that are not sporadic. The occasional CRC in patients with LS can arise along this other pathway; therefore, an age-dependent proportion of CRC shows sporadic mismatch repair deficiency (see Table 14.04) {3029,3425}. In some sporadic CRC cases, mismatch repair deficiency is due to two somatic mismatch repair gene mutations. In a proportion of these cases, this may be due to another predisposition to CRC from a hereditary condition affecting DNA repair, such as *MUTYH*-associated polyposis, or polymerase proofreading–associated polyposis (PPAP) {3443}. Because these tumours have the characteristics of LS and may occur in individuals with personal and family histories also consistent with LS, some authors use the term "Lynch-like syndrome" to describe such cases (see Table 14.05, p. 518) {782,498,2068}.

Constitutional hypermethylation of the *MLH1* promoter can also cause LS. This is usually sporadic and not heritable, but some cases have heritable chromosomal rearrangements that cause *MLH1* promoter methylation, by involving the *LRRFIP2* gene adjacent to *MLH1* on chromosome 3.

Recently, recessive inheritance of mutations in the mismatch repair gene *MSH3* has also been identified as a cause of adenomatous polyposis {24} (see also *Other adenomatous polyposes*, p. 529). With increasing gene panel sequence testing, individuals are also being found with mutations in more than one mismatch repair gene (called digenic LS) {2210,3559}, but it is unclear whether this is more severe than LS due to one mismatch repair mutation.

Macroscopic appearance

The gross appearance is related to the tumour type and is not distinctive.

Histopathology

The typical histological features in CRC with MSI include the presence of tumour-infiltrating lymphocytes, Crohn-like peritumoural lymphocytic reaction, poor differentiation, mucinous and signet-ring cell features, and a medullary growth pattern {102,1603A,3344,2994}. These features are identified in both sporadic cancers with MSI and those that occur in the setting of LS. Although these histological findings are commonly seen, they are not specific enough by themselves to distinguish microsatellite-stable from -unstable cases.

Limited data are available about non-colorectal LS-associated cancers. Most LS-associated gastric carcinomas are

Table 14.04 The proportions of colon cancers, by age, caused by microsatellite instability (MSI) overall, MSI due to Lynch syndrome (LS), and sporadic MSI, and the resulting probability that MSI in a colon cancer is due to LS

Age (years)	Proportion of colon cancers caused by MSI			Probability that MSI in a colon cancer is due to LS[a]
	Overall	Due to LS	Sporadic	
35	23%	22%	2%	92%
40	16%	14%	2%	90%
45	10%	9%	2%	87%
50	7%	6%	2%	79%
55	6%	4%	2%	60%
60	10%	3%	7%	28%
65	11%	3%	8%	32%
70	14%	3%	11%	23%

[a]Assuming that all LS tumours have MSI.
Derived from van Lier et al. {3425}.

Table 14.05 "Lynch-like syndrome (LLS)" is a term used to describe tumours with mismatch repair (MMR) deficiency (and therefore microsatellite instability and/or abnormal immunohistochemistry) due to somatic mutations in both alleles of the same MMR gene, occurring in the setting of other features suggestive of Lynch syndrome (LS), such as young age of onset, other LS-associated tumour types, and a related family history; patients with LLS may have heritable mutations in other (often DNA repair or maintenance) genes that have predisposed them to somatic MMR gene mutations; these are important to recognize and are listed below

Syndrome	Gene(s)	Mode of inheritance	Characteristic distinguishing clinical features
Polymerase proofreading–associated polyposis	*POLE* and *POLD1*	Autosomal dominant	Multiple colorectal adenomas; personal and/or family history of endometrial, brain, or other LS-associated tumours; hypermutant phenotype on DNA sequencing {1516}
MUTYH-associated polyposis	*MUTYH*	Autosomal recessive	Multiple colorectal adenomas; frequent G→T mutations on DNA sequencing {524}
NTHL1-associated polyposis	*NTHL1*	Autosomal recessive	{3549}
n/a	*FAN1*	Autosomal dominant	{2926,3443}
n/a	*BUB1* and *BUB3*	Autosomal dominant	{3443}
n/a	*SETD2*	Autosomal dominant	{3443}
None	None	None	Coincidental sporadic MMR mutations; no underlying cause

n/a, not applicable.

Notes: Synonyms for LLS include "LS mimic", "LS-like", and "mutation-negative LS". Patients with LLS may represent a heterogeneous group. LLS has a mean age of onset similar to that of LS. At least 50–60% of LLS-associated colorectal cancers exhibit biallelic somatic inactivation of the MMR genes within the tumour through somatic mutations (nonsense, missense, or frameshift mutations; splice-site deletions; gene deletions; or loss of heterozygosity). LS tumours may themselves have somatic mutations in the same genes in which heritable mutations cause the syndromes that in turn give rise to LLS. The overarching term "familial colorectal cancer X (FCC-X)" has been used for familial colorectal cancer in which the tumours are microsatellite-stable (i.e. do not have MMR deficiency). Mutations in LLS-associated genes can also be the cause of FCC-X. The potential value of multiple gene test panels and tumour DNA sequencing will be apparent.
Sources: {1516,524,3403,1160,499}

intestinal-type {1,1130,492}, < 13% are diffuse-type, and mucinous carcinomas are very rare. The presence of intraepithelial lymphocytes is not described. LS-associated small bowel carcinomas {3620} show frequently mucinous, signet-ring cell or medullary differentiation, often in combination with tumour-infiltrating lymphocytes and Crohn-like reaction, similar to ampullary carcinomas {3044}. Other types of LS-associated biliary carcinomas do not have any distinguishing features {3044}. Pancreatic cancers with a strong association with LS are acinar cell carcinomas {1931} and medullary carcinomas {3562}.

Although patients with these specific subtypes do present with an increased incidence of MSI and LS, the histological features of LS-associated cancers are not specific. Testing of (selections of) patients with CRC and/or other types of cancer is recommended by a large number of professional organizations, based on either the presence of MSI or the absence of mismatch repair proteins in the tumour. There is no consensus as to whether immunohistochemistry or molecular testing is the preferred first test, and they can be used in combination {2319,3078,3077,3029}. In cases with a low tumour cell percentage or intense inflammatory reaction, immunohistochemistry is the better option. Subsequent determination of hypermethylation and somatic mutations can be applied to estimate the risk of germline mutations in patients. *BRAF* mutation analysis is an alternative to *MLH1* hypermethylation testing. The use of larger targeted mutation panels that combine microsatellite testing and mutation analyses is under investigation.

Immunohistochemistry for the mismatch repair proteins (MLH1, PMS2, MSH2, and MSH6) is a common first step to screen CRCs for mismatch repair deficiency. The presence of all four proteins suggests microsatellite stability. Loss of nuclear staining for any of the proteins indicates MSI and suggests the most likely involved gene and the need for additional testing. Loss of MSH2 alone or loss of both MSH2 and MSH6 suggests a mutation in *MSH2*. Similarly, loss of MLH1 alone or loss of both MLH1 and PMS2 suggests an underlying mutation or methylation in *MLH1*. Concomitant loss of both MSH2 and MSH6 (or of both MLH1 and PMS2) reflects the heterodimeric binding of MSH2 with MSH6 (or of MLH1 with PMS2) in mismatch repair complexes, such that loss of the first partner leads to relative

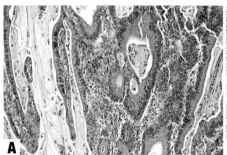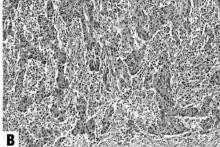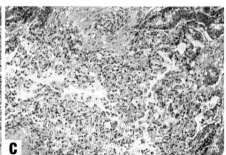

Fig. 14.01 Microsatellite-unstable colorectal adenocarcinoma. **A** Mucinous features with tumour-infiltrating lymphocytes. **B** Poorly differentiated tumour with tumour-infiltrating lymphocytes. **C** Signet-ring cells adjacent to well-differentiated tumour.

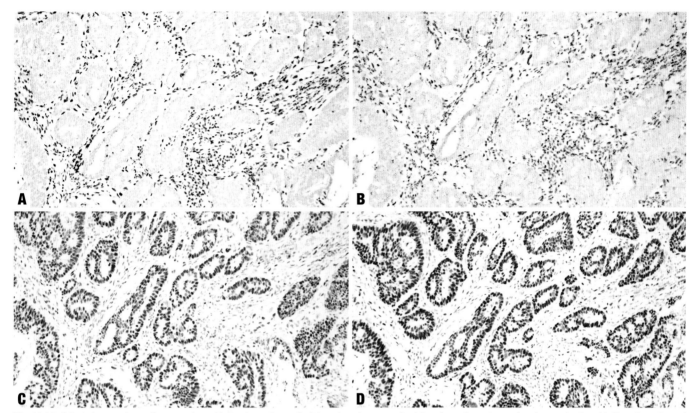

Fig. 14.02 Colon adenocarcinoma from a patient with Lynch syndrome. Serial sections immunostained for mismatch repair proteins; the neoplastic epithelium shows loss of expression of MLH1 (**A**) and PMS2 (**B**), whereas the stroma shows expression of both. The tumour expresses MSH2 (**C**) and MSH6 (**D**).

instability and loss of the second {1882}. The typical expression pattern includes diffuse staining in the tumour nuclei and many benign cells, including epithelial and stromal cells and lymphocytes. Fig. 14.02 shows a tumour with loss of nuclear expression of MLH1 and PMS2 and intact staining for MSH2 and MSH6. This pattern could be seen either in a sporadic tumour (most commonly due to methylation of the *MLH1* promoter) or in the setting of LS.

The interpretation of mismatch repair protein immunohistochemistry is typically straightforward, but it should always be performed with adequate internal control staining. Some pitfalls and unusual patterns of expression can occur, but awareness will prevent misinterpretation. Patchy intact staining can occur due to uneven antibody diffusion, variable fixation, or tissue hypoxia {553,2160}. Cytoplasmic staining may occur, but it is considered abnormal and therefore deficient, because there is no staining in the nuclei and cytoplasmic staining has been described with mutations {2934}. Weak, patchy, nucleolar, or even absent MSH6 expression has been reported in a substantial number of rectal tumours after neoadjuvant treatment without MSI or mutation confirmed by molecular testing {240,2638}. In occasional cases, heterogeneous staining or loss of MSH6 expression can be due to a secondary (non-germline) mutation in the *MSH6* coding mononucleotide tract {1082,2997}. Approximately 3–10% of LS tumours that have mismatch repair deficiency with MSI show no abnormality on immunohistochemistry (presumably because of mutations that disable protein function but leave the protein detectable by immunohistochemistry) {253}.

Diagnostic molecular pathology

LS results from autosomal dominant inheritance of a constitutional mutation affecting one of four DNA mismatch repair genes: *MSH2* (2p21), *MLH1* (3p22.2), *MSH6* (2p16.3, only 300 kb from *MSH2*), and *PMS2* (7p22.1) {1972}. InSiGHT curates a public database of mismatch repair genes {1380}, interprets genetic variants according to published criteria, and is recognized by ClinGen / the Global Alliance for Genomics and Health as the sole definitive worldwide resource {3300,1381}.

Patients with deletions of the 3′ (terminal) end of *EPCAM* that do not extend into *MSH2* are at risk of gastrointestinal cancers but seemingly not of the non-gastrointestinal cancers characteristic of LS {1553,1971,1910}. In contrast, patients with *EPCAM* deletions that extend into *MSH2* have a phenotype indistinguishable from that of patients with mutations in *MSH2*.

Defective mismatch repair in a tumour prevents recognition and repair of insertions or deletions that naturally occur during DNA replication within repetitive DNA sequences. This can be detected as MSI, which is defined as the presence of extra alleles at a microsatellite compared with normal DNA (from normal tissue or blood) from the same individual {967}. Microsatellites vary in their propensity to show instability, and therefore the frequency with which the same microsatellite is affected in different tumour types varies. Instability is best observed at mononucleotide repeats (e.g. AAAAAAAAA…), with this being more substantial than at dinucleotide repeats (e.g. CACACACA…). Like any laboratory test, MSI tests balance sensitivity against specificity. Current markers used in colon cancer MSI diagnosis are known to have reduced sensitivity at detecting MSI in non-colonic tumours, such as endometrial, small bowel, or gastric

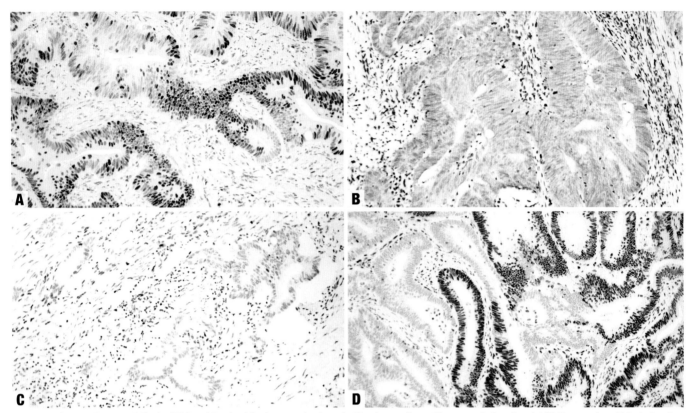

Fig. 14.03 Colorectal cancer. **A** Patchy MLH1 staining should be interpreted as intact in this microsatellite-stable cancer. **B** Cytoplasmic MSH2 expression with lack of nuclear staining should be interpreted as loss of expression. **C** Weak and patchy MSH6 immunoexpression in rectal cancer after neoadjuvant therapy should be interpreted as intact; no germline *MSH6* mutation identified. **D** A heterogeneous pattern of staining for MSH6 (present in one area and lost in another, with excellent internal control in both) should be interpreted as intact; no germline *MSH6* mutation in either area.

cancers, and in tumours from patients with *MSH6* mutations. Therefore, a small number of LS-associated tumours may not appear to have MSI using this test (although they might be recognized by abnormal mismatch repair immunohistochemistry).

It is important to note that dMMR tumours do not always have abnormal immunohistochemistry or test positive for MSI. Immunohistochemistry and MSI testing of carcinomas at sites other than the colon, or due to constitutional mutations in *MSH6* or *PMS2*, or adenomas, has reduced sensitivity. Immunohistochemistry and MSI tests must be interpreted bearing in mind the tumour type, the patient's personal and family history, and other test results (e.g. *BRAF* status); a multidisciplinary approach is recommended.

The value of mismatch repair immunohistochemistry and MSI is considerably enhanced by testing more than one tumour from the same family and/or individual, especially if the tumours are rare (e.g. rectal cancers, colorectal adenomas, small bowel cancers, and sebaceous skin tumours). Consistent immunohistochemical abnormality of one mismatch repair protein is excellent evidence for the pathogenicity of a mutation in that gene, which is important given the number of missense and other difficult-to-interpret mutations that occur in LS. MSI in rectal cancers is rare and strongly associated with LS; this can be exploited clinically because the finding therefore has an excellent positive predictive value for LS, and negative predictive value when not present. Similarly, MSI is rare in adenomas outside of LS, providing good positive and negative predictive values {1949}. Some CRCs due to *MUTYH*-associated polyposis or PPAP may exhibit both MSI and abnormal immunohistochemistry due to somatic mismatch repair gene mutations; they therefore appear to be due to LS, but are Lynch-like syndrome cases (see Table 14.05, p. 518).

About 15% of sporadic colon cancers have MSI, usually due to epigenetic silencing of *MLH1* by promoter hypermethylation at both alleles. Therefore, unselected colon cancers with MSI have a poor positive predictive value for LS, although lack of MSI has a good negative predictive value for LS. Further tests (*BRAF* mutation and *MLH1* methylation tests) are required for microsatellite-unstable cancers with loss of MLH1 on immunohistochemistry, to distinguish between LS and sporadic origin. Because sporadic *MLH1* promoter hypermethylation in colon cancers is strongly age-dependent, age is a useful discriminator in its interpretation.

Somatic mutations in CRCs in the proto-oncogene *BRAF*, usually resulting in activating missense p.V600E mutations or similar mutations at this codon, occur in at least 85% of sporadic colon cancers with MSI, but not in those due to LS; therefore, such mutations are highly predictive of the tumour being of sporadic origin and not due to LS. However, sporadic tumours harbouring *BRAF* mutations can occasionally occur in patients with LS, so the absence of *BRAF* p.V600E mutations does not definitively diagnose LS, although it does indicate that LS is more likely. Alternatively, detection of *MLH1* gene promoter hypermethylation in a tumour provides good, although not unequivocal, evidence that the tumour is sporadic in origin, for two reasons: (1) very occasional sporadic tumours do occur in LS and (2) constitutional *MLH1* promoter methylation can be found in a few patients with LS (in some cases, this constitutional *MLH1* methylation is due to a rearrangement and is therefore transmissible) {1246}. A good practice for testing of *MLH1* promoter methylation in tumours is to include testing of the patient's normal DNA (e.g. from normal tissue surrounding a cancer or from blood), then *MLH1* promoter methylation will be readily apparent when it occurs.

LS can be definitively diagnosed after tumour testing by constitutional mismatch repair gene sequencing to identify the pathogenic constitutional mutation. It is often useful to have samples from more than one individual in the family, because case segregation studies may be required in order to determine pathogenicity or whether an individual is a phenocopy. If the family is likely to have a mutation but no point mutation is found, then large-scale mutations, such as deletion of a whole exon (or more), should be considered. In cases with very young onset (e.g. < 35 years), LS is likely even in the absence of a family history, although mutations in genes (e.g. *BUB1* and *BUB3*) encoding mitotic spindle checkpoint proteins should be considered, especially in teenaged patients. Tumours from such individuals do not exhibit MSI, nor do those (usually) from families with specific *POLD1* and *POLE* proofreading mutations (in PPAP), although the family histories may be Lynch-like. In such cases, some tumours may acquire two mismatch repair gene mutations due to a non-LS underlying syndrome (including PPAP due to mutations in *POLD1* and/or *POLE*), and therefore appear to be due to LS on tumour testing. Rare, characteristic tumours, such as small bowel cancer, ureteric transitional cell carcinoma, or skin sebaceous adenoma/carcinoma, have a high positive predictive value for LS and are therefore clinically significant. Synchronous or metachronous bowel cancers are also clinically significant, as is the development of any two LS-related tumours (e.g. CRC and endometrial cancer).

Mismatch repair deficiency causes frequent insertion and deletion mutations. When these occur in the protein-coding regions of genes, they result in frameshifts, which in turn result in the expression of novel, antigenic frameshift peptides that stimulate the immune system {2698}. Local immune suppression in such tumours enables their survival; therefore, immune checkpoint inhibitors such as PD1/PDL1 blockade, which inhibit such suppression, are effective in dMMR tumours {1816}.

As tumour sequencing becomes more widespread, data on specific mutations in cancer-associated genes, as well as mutation spectra, are becoming available in individual cases. This will both guide treatment and diagnose more causes of hereditary

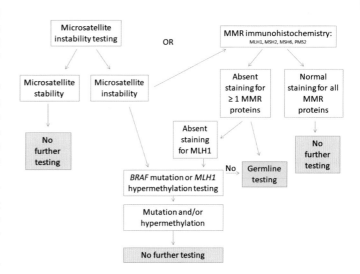

Fig. 14.04 A suggested algorithm for colorectal cancer tumour testing for Lynch syndrome. MMR, mismatch repair.

predisposition, including Lynch-like syndrome and multilocus inherited neoplasia alleles syndrome (multiple constitutional mutations in the same patient). It is also likely that mutation spectra (or signatures), being more sensitive and specific, will replace MSI testing. Although gene panel testing may remove the need for mismatch repair immunohistochemistry as a way of selecting which genes to test, mismatch repair immunohistochemistry will remain critically important in providing phenotypic data to enable the interpretation of genetic variants {3559,105}.

Essential and desirable diagnostic criteria
A suggested algorithm for CRC tumour testing for LS is shown in Fig. 14.04.

Staging (TNM)
Not clinically relevant

Prognosis and prediction
Not clinically relevant

Familial adenomatous polyposis 1

Arends MJ
Brosens LAA
Frayling IM
Tomlinson I

Definition

Classic familial adenomatous polyposis (FAP) 1 is an autosomal dominant syndrome caused by pathogenic *APC* mutations. It is typically characterized by > 100 adenomatous polyps in the colorectum, extracolonic manifestations (including polyps) elsewhere in the GI tract, and desmoid tumours.

MIM numbering

175100 Familial adenomatous polyposis

ICD-11 coding

2B90.Y Other specific malignant neoplasms of colon

Related terminology

Acceptable: adenomatous polyposis coli.

Not recommended: Gardner syndrome (obsolete term; almost all patients with FAP have such features); Turcot syndrome (in some cases, but most cases of Turcot syndrome are due to constitutional mismatch repair deficiency syndrome; see *Lynch syndrome*, p. 515).

Subtype(s)

Attenuated familial adenomatous polyposis

Localization

Classic FAP1 is characterized by the development during adolescence of hundreds of colorectal adenomas, a small proportion of which progress to colorectal adenocarcinoma. Most patients also develop gastric and duodenal polyps, leading to an increased risk of duodenal adenocarcinoma. Desmoid tumours occur in about 10% of patients with FAP, mostly in the small bowel mesentery, abdominal wall, or extremities. Less frequent extraintestinal malignancies are hepatoblastoma and cancers of the thyroid, biliary tree, pancreas, and CNS. Frequent benign extraintestinal features are osteomas, dental abnormalities (supernumerary teeth and odontomas), and congenital hypertrophy of the retinal pigment epithelium {417}.

Clinical features

In the GI tract, classic FAP is characterized by numerous (usually > 100 and as many as several thousand) adenomatous polyps of the large bowel. The onset of colorectal adenomatous polyps usually occurs in the second decade of life. If colectomy is not performed, patients have a near 100% risk of colorectal adenocarcinoma by the age of 45 years {3451}.

Attenuated FAP is distinguished from classic FAP by fewer (20–100) colorectal adenomas and a slightly reduced risk (of 80%) and later onset (at a mean age of 56 years) of colorectal cancer {3031,1658}.

Almost all patients with FAP develop duodenal adenomas, mostly in the periampullary region and distal duodenum. Small bowel polyps and cancer typically present a decade later than colon polyps and cancer. About 4–10% of patients develop duodenal adenocarcinoma {415}. More than 60% of patients with FAP develop gastric polyps, which are mainly benign fundic gland polyps (FGPs), but also adenomas {421}. Severe and predominant fundic gland polyposis without duodenal and colorectal polyposis is defined as gastric adenocarcinoma and proximal polyposis of the stomach (GAPPS), a syndrome currently considered a rare subtype of FAP (see *GAPPS and other fundic gland polyposes*, p. 526) {1883}. The severity of gastrointestinal features is variable {686}.

Desmoid tumours occur in about 10% of patients with FAP, mostly in the small intestinal mesentery, abdominal wall, or extremities. The risk of desmoid fibromatosis in FAP is increased by clinical features such as prior surgery and certain types of *APC* mutations {2821}. Although desmoid tumours have no metastatic potential, they cause severe morbidity and mortality in a substantial proportion of patients with FAP {2137,642}.

The presence of benign extragastrointestinal features is variable, but almost all patients with FAP have some on close inspection {3451}. Some benign extraintestinal manifestations can be used as a clinical marker for asymptomatic carriers in families with FAP. In addition, FAP has been associated with a slightly increased risk of papillary carcinoma of the thyroid gland, hepatobiliary tree tumours, childhood hepatoblastoma,

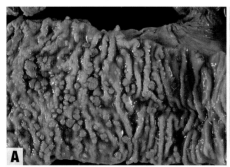
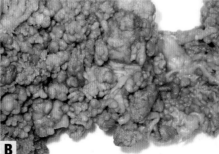
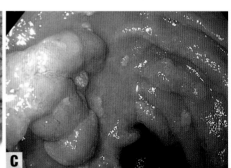

Fig. 14.05 Familial adenomatous polyposis. **A** The colon contains hundreds of polyps, which are histologically adenomas. **B** Adenocarcinoma of the colon arising in a 24-year-old female *APC* mutation carrier with multiple colonic adenomas. **C** Endoscopic picture showing duodenal adenomatosis.

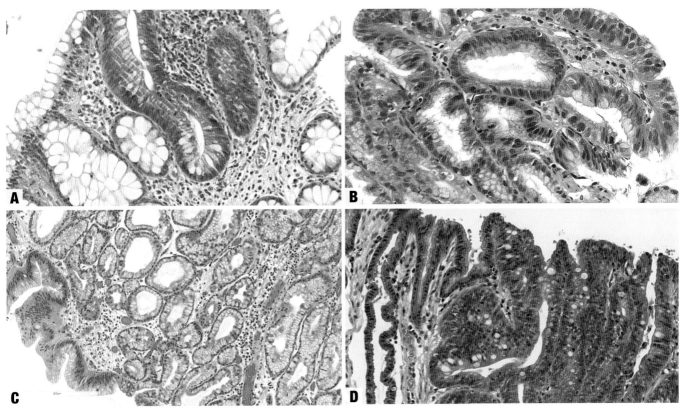

Fig. 14.06 Familial adenomatous polyposis (FAP) 1. **A** Oligocryptal adenoma. Microadenoma in otherwise normal-looking colorectal mucosa that is characteristic of FAP. **B** Gastric foveolar-type adenoma. The vast majority of gastric adenomas in FAP are foveolar-type adenomas with low-grade dysplasia, mainly located in the gastric body; distinction between a fundic gland polyp with low-grade dysplasia and a gastric foveolar-type adenoma can be difficult, but this is of little importance because the risk of neoplastic progression is very low for both lesions. **C** Gastric pyloric gland adenoma. Characteristic densely packed cuboidal to low columnar epithelium with pale or eosinophilic (ground-glass) cytoplasm. **D** Gastric intestinal-type adenomas. These polyps are rare and seem to be related to *Helicobacter pylori* infection and chronic atrophic gastritis; detection of *H. pylori* infection, gastric atrophy, and intestinal-type adenomas in patients with FAP seems to be important to identify patients at increased risk of gastric cancer.

adrenocortical adenomas and carcinomas, and brain tumours – i.e. medulloblastoma (Turcot syndrome) {2450,966,965}.

Epidemiology

The prevalence is 1 in 8000–10 000. It affects males and females equally and accounts for < 1% of all colorectal cancers {3451}.

Etiology

FAP is a Mendelian autosomal dominant syndrome caused by germline (constitutional) mutations in the *APC* gene (chromosome 5q22.2) that result in a truncated or absent APC protein. The severity of disease varies with the position of the mutation in the *APC* gene. Inherited *APC* mutations located in or around the mutation cluster region (around codon / amino acid 1309) are associated with the highest number of adenomas (thousands – severe polyposis) and the greatest risk of cancer at a younger age, whereas mutations outside this region are mostly associated with many hundreds of adenomas and a slightly lower cancer risk {1781,1101}. Attenuated FAP-associated inherited mutations (associated with < 100 adenomas) are located nearer to the N-terminus or within the alternatively spliced section of exon 9 (9a), and these patients develop fewer polyps at a later age {1658}. Desmoid tumours are associated with germline

mutations in *APC* involving codons 1310–2011 in the mid- to C-terminal portion of the encoded protein {3070}.

APC acts as a classic tumour suppressor gene, and a tumour phenotype arises when the non-mutant allele is spontaneously lost or mutated by a somatic event (second hit). When the inherited mutation is in the mutation cluster region, the second somatic mutation may be either a point mutation or a complete deletion or loss of heterozygosity of the second allele. However, loss of heterozygosity is never observed with inherited mutations outside the mutation cluster region, and in attenuated FAP second hits are only observed in the mutation cluster region. Therefore, for a colorectal adenoma/cancer to develop, at least one mutation must be within the mutation cluster region. Interestingly, patients with constitutional deletions of the entire *APC* gene do not always exhibit a low number of (i.e. < 100) colorectal adenomas.

In about 20–30% of FAP cases, there is no known family history of the condition, and most of these cases probably represent either de novo mutations or cases of the recessive syndrome *MUTYH*-associated polyposis (see *Other adenomatous polyposes*, p. 529). Despite the variations in phenotype, it is very rare for any carrier of a pathogenic *APC* mutation not to develop multiple bowel polyps and cancer if preventive measures are not taken. Mosaic de novo *APC* mutation carriers also exist, and they typically have milder and/or localized polyposis {1222}.

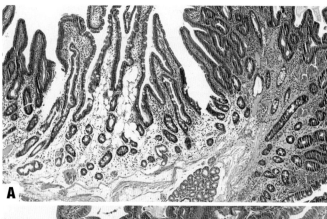

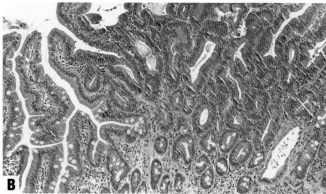

Fig. 14.07 Duodenal adenoma in familial adenomatous polyposis. **A** Low-power microphotograph showing low-grade dysplasia; because of the villous nature of the normal mucosa, there is often ambivalence as to whether to call an adenoma tubular or villous. **B** High-power view of the adenoma.

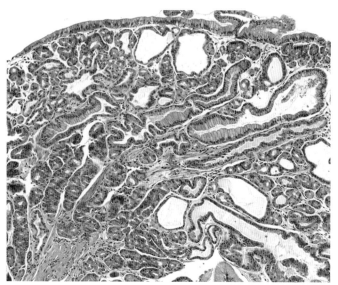

Fig. 14.08 Fundic gland polyp in familial adenomatous polyposis. Characteristic dilated oxyntic glands without dysplasia are observed; although low-grade dysplasia is frequently seen, malignant transformation is exceedingly rare.

Pathogenesis

The classic APC protein isoform is 2843 amino acids long (several isoforms exist as a result of alternative splicing), and it is centrally involved in regulating WNT signalling. Normal APC restrains colorectal epithelial cell proliferation through its role as a scaffold protein that binds critical components that tag (by phosphorylation and ubiquitination) the WNT effector protein β-catenin for proteasomal destruction. With APC protein truncation (or absence), the loss of critical APC functions (especially its binding of the AXIN and β-catenin proteins) results in greatly impaired degradation of β-catenin with upregulation of WNT signalling, effectively rendering the WNT pathway constitutively switched on {2559,2333}. Adenomas arise owing to somatically acquired second hits to the non-mutant *APC* gene. The adenomas subsequently progress in a very similar way to sporadic adenomas of the large bowel, through mutations in genes such as *KRAS*, *SMAD4*, and *TP53* (see *Colorectal adenocarcinoma*, p. 177) {1614}.

Macroscopic appearance

The classic appearance of the resected colon is illustrated in Fig. 14.05. There are large numbers of polypoid or villous adenomas. Most patients with FAP also develop duodenal adenomas.

Histopathology

The large bowel polyps are almost always classic adenomas of varying type (tubular, tubulovillous, or villous), grade (low or high), and size; they are similar to sporadic adenomas in appearance. The same features are observed in duodenal adenomas. However, characteristic of FAP is the frequent presence of monocryptal adenomas and oligocryptal adenomas (microadenomas) in otherwise normal-looking colorectal mucosa, including in the stalk mucosa of resected larger adenomatous polyps.

Most gastric polyps (80%) are FGPs. FGPs in FAP are often multiple and may cause fundic gland polyposis. Low-grade dysplasia has been described in nearly 40% of FAP-associated FGPs, but high-grade dysplasia and malignant transformation are rare {421}. About 20% of gastric polyps are adenomas, mostly foveolar-type adenomas (17%), some pyloric gland adenomas (3%), and rarely intestinal-type adenomas {421}.

Desmoid tumours appear as bland, indolent, invasive fibroblastic tumours of connective tissue that expand relentlessly and are difficult to excise completely (sometimes called aggressive fibromatosis). Immunohistochemistry reveals nuclear expression of β-catenin.

Diagnostic molecular pathology

About 80–90% of sporadic colorectal cancers carry acquired mutations in the *APC* gene, and this is considered to be the tumour-initiating event in most cases {1614}. Although APC has other functions (including regulation of cell polarity, cell–cell adhesion, cytoskeletal organization, and spindle formation), its WNT pathway function of controlling intracellular levels of β-catenin is key to its effects on adenomagenesis {1687}.

Essential and desirable diagnostic criteria

The presence of > 100 colorectal adenomas is indicative of a probable diagnosis of classic FAP. However, given the phenotypic variability of FAP, several other polyposis conditions can have near-identical features. These other conditions include *MUTYH*-associated polyposis, polymerase proofreading-associated polyposis, *NTHL1*-associated polyposis, hereditary mixed polyposis syndrome, constitutional mismatch repair deficiency syndrome, and multiple polyps associated with mutations in other genes (e.g. *MSH3*, *BUB1*, *AXIN2*, and *FAN1*) {24}, although the number of colorectal polyps is usually lower in these other syndromes and there may be a different pattern of inheritance and other extracolonic features to provide diagnostic clues (see *Other adenomatous polyposes*, p. 529). Another group of patients with a phenotype mimicking FAP have multiple colonic adenomas, usually without extracolonic features or a strong family history; these individuals may have a polygenic form of polyposis. The essential molecular criterion is the presence of a pathogenic germline (constitutional) *APC* mutation – and this is the gold standard for FAP diagnosis, although a small number of cases have undetectable *APC* mutations and may be regarded as presumed FAP if typical clinical features are present and molecular evidence of the other conditions is absent.

Staging (TNM)

FAP tumours are staged in the same way as equivalent sporadic tumours at each site.

Prognosis and prediction

Approaches to the management of FAP cases are guided by their clinical presentation and severity. Colorectal screening by endoscopy and chemoprevention are in use {21,1575,417}. Colectomy is often required to prevent the development of colorectal adenocarcinoma. Upper gastrointestinal endoscopy is indicated for FAP patients aged 25–30 years and is guided by the Spigelman stage of duodenal polyposis {3114,415}. Duodenal polyposis is treated endoscopically for as long as possible, but surgery is often required. In addition, screening for extraintestinal manifestations is recommended by some {21,3193}.

People with FAP have a 3.35-fold elevated risk of dying compared with the general population {2394}. The main causes of

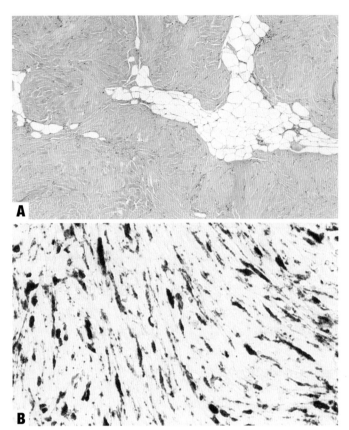

Fig. 14.09 Desmoid tumour. **A** The lesion is characterized by bland, indolent, invasive fibroblastic proliferation. **B** Immunohistochemical expression of β-catenin is observed in the nuclei of the fibroblasts.

death are upper gastrointestinal malignancy, perioperative complications, desmoid tumours, and suicide {2394,1003}.

GAPPS and other fundic gland polyposes

Carneiro F
Chenevix-Trench G
de Boer WB
Kumarasinghe MP
Wen X
Worthley DL

Definition
Gastric adenocarcinoma and proximal polyposis of the stomach (GAPPS) is an autosomal dominant cancer predisposition syndrome associated with an increased risk of gastric (but not colorectal) adenocarcinoma, together with proximal polyposis of the stomach. Because it involves *APC*, GAPPS is considered to be part of familial adenomatous polyposis (FAP), but it has a unique phenotype.

MIM numbering
175100 Gastric adenocarcinoma and proximal polyposis of the stomach

ICD-11 coding
None

Related terminology
None

Subtype(s)
None

Localization
The body and fundus of the stomach is involved by a carpeting of polyposis, with sparing of the antrum and relative sparing of the lesser curve. There is no involvement of the duodenum or large bowel.

Clinical features
Patients can present with nonspecific gastrointestinal symptoms such as abdominal pain, dyspepsia, and melaena. Polyposis may be asymptomatic, and asymptomatic patients present for screening endoscopy because they belong to a known GAPPS family. Patients with gastric adenocarcinoma may present with symptoms and signs of gastric malignancy. Endoscopy reveals a characteristic carpeting polyposis, with the polyps generally < 10 mm in diameter {3607}.

Epidemiology
This is an autosomal dominant syndrome with incomplete penetrance. Families have been identified in Australia, North America, Europe, and Japan {3607,3666,2697,283,730,1883}.

Etiology
GAPPS is caused by germline point mutations in the YY1 binding site of the *APC* promoter 1B. Such mutations also occur very rarely in families with FAP {1883}.

Pathogenesis
The point mutations that segregate with GAPPS (c.-191T>C, c.-192A>G and c.-195A>C) are all positioned within the YY1 binding motif of the *APC* gene, reducing the transcriptional level of APC.

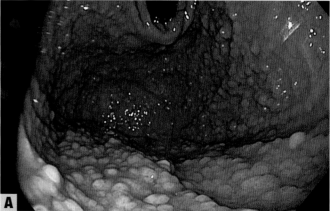
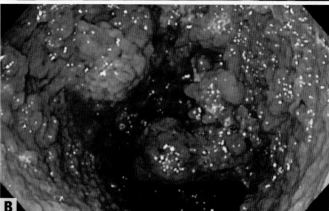

Fig. 14.10 Gastric adenocarcinoma and proximal polyposis of the stomach (GAPPS). **A** The characteristic carpeting polyposis is observed on endoscopy. **B** A dominant polyp in the setting of carpeting polyposis, corresponding to a typical gastric-type adenoma.

Macroscopic appearance
There are typically numerous polyps carpeting the gastric fundus and body. An arbitrary number of > 100 has been proposed as a diagnostic criterion, although some family members may have fewer polyps {3607,3666}. Polyps are predominantly < 10 mm in size {730,3607} and are sessile with a smooth surface. In some cases, larger, dominant polyps as large as 40 mm may be present {730,2697}, or there may be a malignant tumour.

Histopathology
A range of microscopic features have been described in the literature, including fundic gland polyps (FGPs), fundic gland–like polyps, hyperproliferative aberrant pits, hyperplastic polyps, gastric-type adenomas, and adenocarcinomas (tubular/intestinal and mixed with a poorly cohesive component). Some lesions show a mixture of the above features. The larger,

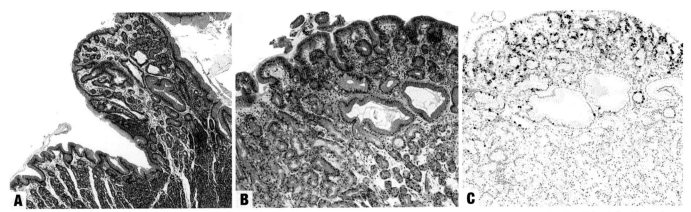

Fig. 14.11 Gastric adenocarcinoma and proximal polyposis of the stomach (GAPPS). **A** Fundic gland–type polyp; absence of typical cystically dilated glands lined by a mixture of mucinous and oxyntic cells and an expanded or inverted foveolar compartment. **B** Hyperproliferative aberrant pits. Disorganized proliferation of oxyntic glands in the superficial part of the mucosa, around the gastric pits. **C** Proliferative activity highlighted by Ki-67 immunostaining.

dominant polyps tend to show foci of dysplasia {2697} or may be adenomatous {730}.

FGPs: These polyps were described in all published reports, encompassing typical FGPs as well as fundic gland–like polyps {730,3607,3666}, which have atypical features such as the absence of typical cystically dilated glands lined by a mixture of mucinous and oxyntic cells and an expanded or inverted foveolar compartment {730}.

Hyperproliferative aberrant pits: These polypoid lesions typically show disorganized proliferation of specialized/oxyntic glands high up in the mucosa, involving the attenuated foveolar region around the gastric pits, with proliferative activity highlighted by Ki-67 immunoreactivity. Hyperproliferative aberrant pits appear to be the most frequent early pathological findings {730}, and there is a morphological continuum of these lesions progressing to dysplasia and adenomas {730}.

Hyperplastic polyps: Occasional hyperplastic polyps have been described {3607}. There may also be elongation, irregularity, dilatation, and branching of the foveolar compartment imparting an appearance of inverted foveolar hyperplasia {730}.

Preinvasive neoplastic lesions: Some of the FGPs are inherently neoplastic, showing focal dysplasia. There may also be discrete adenomas, which are often multifocal {730,3607,2697,283}. The dysplastic epithelium shows eosinophilic cytoplasm with mostly basally located, enlarged oval to round nuclei; conspicuous to prominent nucleoli; and an apical mucin cap. These are similar to the changes described in gastric foveolar dysplasia/adenomas. Both low-grade and high-grade dysplastic changes are reported. High-grade dysplasia is characterized by advanced architectural complexity and crowding coupled with high-grade nuclear features comprising loss of polarity, round to oval vesicular nuclei, and prominent nucleoli as focal change in a background of low-grade dysplasia.

Adenocarcinomas: All adenocarcinomas described to date have been of tubular (per the WHO classification) / intestinal (per the Laurén classification) or mixed type.

Immunohistochemistry: Dysplastic lesions in the GAPPS setting are of gastric foveolar phenotype (with immunoreactivity for MUC5AC) {730,14,188,3604}. The immunophenotype of adenocarcinoma is described in two reports. One describes

expression of MUC5AC, CK7, CDX2 (very focal, strong), and CD10 (moderate) in the absence of CK20, MUC2, and MUC6 {730}. The other report (of the analysis of different markers) describes increased expression of nuclear β-catenin, Ki-67, and p53 {2101}.

Differential diagnosis: The main differential diagnosis is fundic gland polyposis in the setting of FAP (classic and attenuated forms). The unique sparing of the antrum in patients with GAPPS, and the absence of a colonic polyposis phenotype, is an important clinical feature that distinguishes GAPPS from (attenuated) FAP. Prolonged use of proton-pump inhibitors may be the cause of FGPs/polyposis without dysplasia and should be considered in the differential diagnosis {2061}.

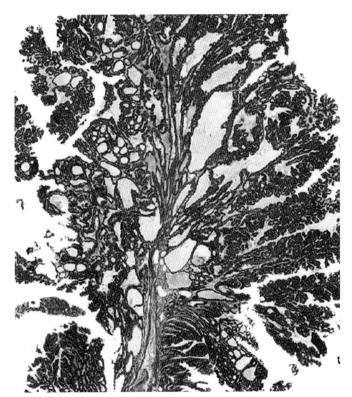

Fig. 14.12 Gastric adenocarcinoma and proximal polyposis of the stomach (GAPPS). Discrete foveolar-type adenoma.

Box 14.01 Gastric adenocarcinoma and proximal polyposis of the stomach (GAPPS) clinical criteria

Essential criteria
1. Phenotypic features:
   • Proximal (body and fundus) gastric polyposis with antral sparing; no evidence of colorectal or duodenal polyposis[a]
   • > 100 polyps carpeting the proximal stomach in the index patient or > 30 polyps in a first-degree relative of another patient
   • Predominantly fundic gland polyps and/or fundic gland–like polyps
2. Proband or family member with either dysplastic fundic gland polyps or gastric adenocarcinoma
3. Mutation in the chr5:112043220_112043224 region of promoter 1B of *APC*[b,c]

Supportive criteria (families in whom genetic testing could be considered)
1. Family history (autosomal dominant pattern of inheritance)
2. Spectrum of other histological lesions: hyperproliferative aberrant pits hyperplastic polyps, gastric-type adenomas

[a]Exclusions include other heritable gastric polyposis syndromes and use of proton-pump inhibitors; in patients on proton-pump inhibitors, it is recommended to repeat the endoscopy off therapy. [b]The point mutations that segregate with GAPPS (c.-191T>C, c.-192A>G, and c.-195A>C) are all positioned within the YY1 binding motif of the *APC* gene. [c]Familial adenomatous polyposis has also been caused by these mutations; although criteria for GAPPS mean there is no colorectal polyposis, testing for promoter 1B variants should still be considered for patients with familial adenomatous polyposis that are *APC* mutation–negative, especially if they also have fundic gland polyps.

Diagnostic molecular pathology

A second *APC* hit occurs in most FGPs in GAPPS by loss of wildtype allele or truncating mutations in the *APC* gene, but this appears to be a late event, occurring in only a subset of the polyp's epithelial cells.

Essential and desirable diagnostic criteria

The clinical criteria for genetic testing are presented in Box 14.01.

Staging (TNM)

Adenocarcinomas developed in the setting of GAPPS should be staged using the eighth editions (2017) of the Union for International Cancer Control (UICC) TNM classification {408} and the American Joint Committee on Cancer (AJCC) cancer staging manual {127}.

Prognosis and prediction

Prognosis is often poor in patients with gastric adenocarcinoma.

Other adenomatous polyposes

Arends MJ
Frayling IM
Morreau H
Tomlinson I

Definition
Other adenomatous polyposes are a heterogeneous group of generally, but not exclusively, inherited (genetic) conditions characterized by multiple colorectal adenomatous polyps.
The diagnostic algorithm for patients with adenomatous polyposis in whom FAP and Lynch syndrome have been excluded is shown in Fig. 14.13 (p. 530).

MIM numbering
608456 MUTYH-associated polyposis
616415 NTHL1-associated polyposis
615083 Polymerase proofreading–associated polyposis
601228 Hereditary mixed polyposis syndrome
608615 AXIN2-associated polyposis (oligodontia-colorectal cancer syndrome)
300755 X-linked agammaglobulinaemia

Subtype(s)
MUTYH-associated polyposis; NTHL1-associated polyposis; polymerase proofreading–associated polyposis; MSH3-associated polyposis; constitutional mismatch repair deficiency syndrome; AXIN2-associated polyposis

Localization
The adenomatous polyposes discussed in this section primarily affect the colorectum. Depending on the condition, the stomach, duodenum, and/or small bowel may also be involved.

Etiology
A database of mutations in MSH2, MLH1, MSH6, PMS2, MUTYH, POLD1, POLE, and MSH3, called the International Society for Gastrointestinal Hereditary Tumours (InSiGHT) Database, is available online {1380}.

MUTYH-associated polyposis
MUTYH-associated polyposis (MAP) {572} is a constitutional DNA repair disorder of base excision repair, caused by recessively inherited mutations in MUTYH. MUTYH is a DNA glycosylase enzyme that excises adenines misincorporated opposite 8-oxo-7,8-dihydro-2′-deoxyguanosine (8-oxoguanine), which is a stable product of oxidative DNA damage; 8-oxoguanine mispairs with adenine instead of cytosine, predisposing to G→T transversions. Several population-specific founder mutations have been identified: p.Y179C and p.G396D in northern Europeans, p.E480del in southern Europeans, p.Y104* in Pakistanis, and p.E480* in Indians. The prevalence is approximately 1 in 2000 {3574}. Patients with MAP develop multiple adenomatous polyps of the large bowel in adulthood; the number of adenomas is typically 10–100 but can be anywhere from zero to several hundred {181}. MAP accounts for 15–40% of cases in which a patient has 10–99 adenomas, and for about 15% of cases in which > 100 adenomas are present. About two thirds of patients with MAP develop colorectal cancer, and MAP accounts for 0.3–0.8% of all colorectal cancer cases {903,2358}. The number of adenomas does not correlate with the presence of carcinoma, which may indicate that pathways other than conventional adenoma–carcinoma progression are at play (as is the case in Lynch syndrome); this may also suggest that adenomas do not necessarily grow or progress more rapidly to cancer in the setting of MAP {2358}. Duodenal polyposis is observed in about 20% of cases, with a concomitant increased risk of duodenal adenocarcinoma {181}. Sebaceous skin tumours have also been described, indicating that MAP is a cause of Muir–Torre syndrome (see Lynch syndrome, p. 515). The colorectal adenomas and adenocarcinomas in MAP are similar to sporadic tumours macroscopically and microscopically, but they have a characteristic G→T somatic mutation spectrum and may be more likely to have some otherwise uncommon somatic KRAS mutations (e.g. c.34G>T p.G12C) {3030}; these rare KRAS mutations should therefore arouse suspicion of MAP. Adenomas arise as a result of the acquisition of somatic APC and mitochondrial gene mutations {3030,3456}. MAP may also be a cause of Lynch-like syndrome; the association with a family history, the relatively young onset of colorectal cancers (which may have acquired somatic mutations in mismatch repair genes causing microsatellite instability [MSI] and immunohistochemical abnormalities), and the similarity of the tumours' histopathological features to those of Lynch syndrome–associated cancers suggest that there may be molecular and pathological phenotypic overlap between MAP and Lynch syndrome {498}.

NTHL1-associated polyposis
NTHL1-associated polyposis (NAP) {3549} is a constitutional DNA repair disorder of base excision repair, caused by recessively inherited mutations in NTHL1. NTHL1 repairs a variety of DNA lesions, including 5-hydroxycytosine and 5-hydroxyuracil, two products of cytosine oxidation that are mutagenic because they mispair with adenine, resulting in C→T transitions {3548}. NTHL1 p.Q90* appears to be the most common mutation in northern Europe. NAP is thought to be rarer than MAP, although the exact prevalence is unknown. NAP is associated with adenomatous polyps of the large bowel arising in adulthood, generally by the age of 50 years {3549}. Tumours at other sites (e.g. endometrial cancer) are also seen, indicating that NAP is a cause of Lynch-like syndrome, given the clinical overlap and the occurrence of acquired somatic mismatch repair gene mutations resulting in MSI and immunohistochemical abnormalities {2722,289}. Like in MAP, sebaceous skin tumours have also been reported. The colorectal adenomas and adenocarcinomas in NAP are similar to sporadic tumours macroscopically and microscopically, but they have a characteristic C→T somatic mutation spectrum.

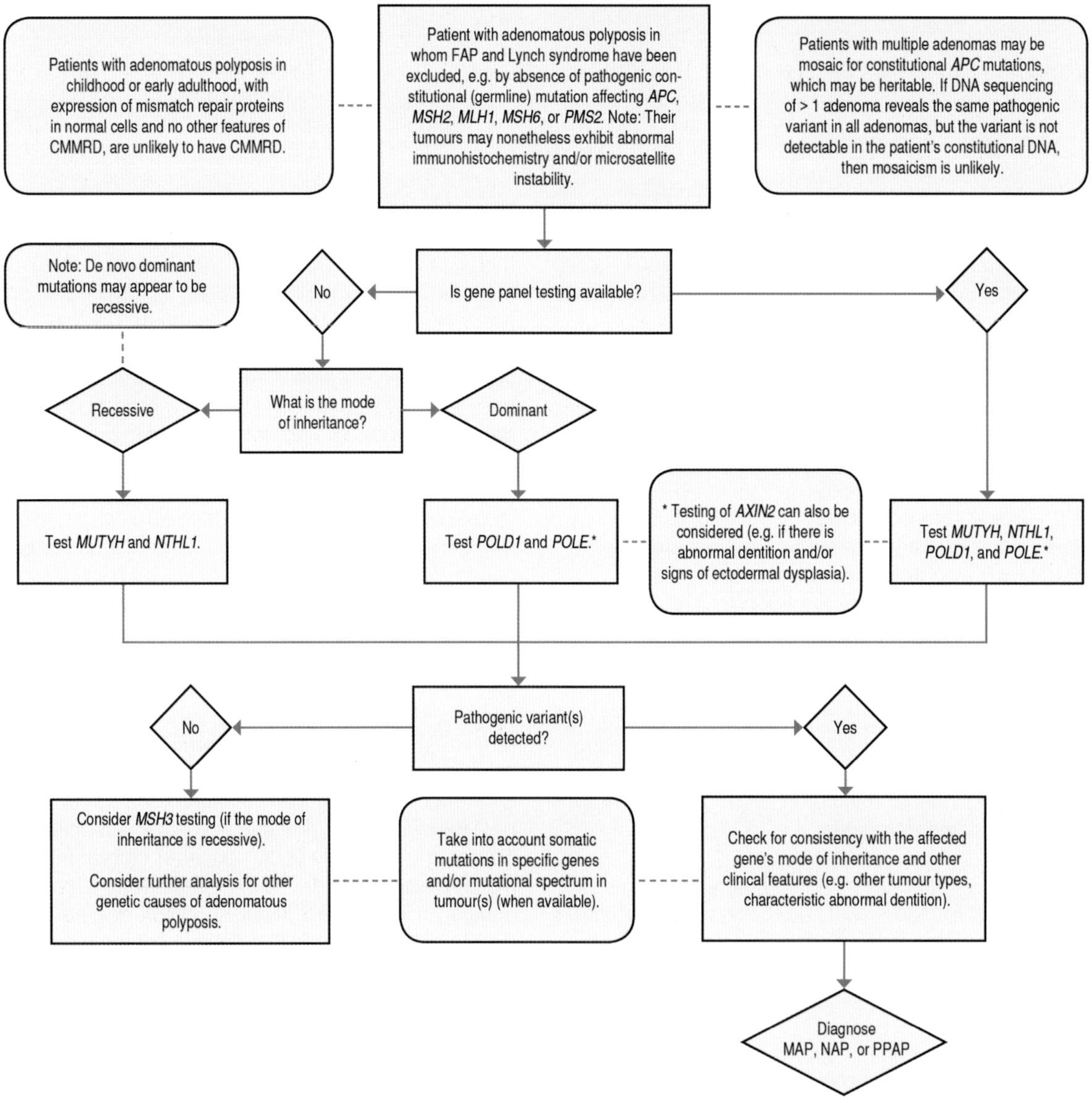
Patients with adenomatous polyposis in childhood or early adulthood, with expression of mismatch repair proteins in normal cells and no other features of CMMRD, are unlikely to have CMMRD.
Patient with adenomatous polyposis in whom FAP and Lynch syndrome have been excluded, e.g. by absence of pathogenic constitutional (germline) mutation affecting APC, MSH2, MLH1, MSH6, or PMS2. Note: Their tumours may nonetheless exhibit abnormal immunohistochemistry and/or microsatellite instability.
Patients with multiple adenomas may be mosaic for constitutional APC mutations, which may be heritable. If DNA sequencing of > 1 adenoma reveals the same pathogenic variant in all adenomas, but the variant is not detectable in the patient's constitutional DNA, then mosaicism is unlikely.
Note: De novo dominant mutations may appear to be recessive.
No
Is gene panel testing available?
Yes
Recessive
What is the mode of inheritance?
Dominant
Test MUTYH and NTHL1.
Test POLD1 and POLE.*
* Testing of AXIN2 can also be considered (e.g. if there is abnormal dentition and/or signs of ectodermal dysplasia).
Test MUTYH, NTHL1, POLD1, and POLE.*
No
Pathogenic variant(s) detected?
Yes
Consider MSH3 testing (if the mode of inheritance is recessive).
Consider further analysis for other genetic causes of adenomatous polyposis.
Take into account somatic mutations in specific genes and/or mutational spectrum in tumour(s) (when available).
Check for consistency with the affected gene's mode of inheritance and other clinical features (e.g. other tumour types, characteristic abnormal dentition).
Diagnose MAP, NAP, or PPAP

Fig. 14.13 Diagnostic algorithm for patients with adenomatous polyposis in whom familial adenomatous polyposis (FAP) and Lynch syndrome have been excluded. CMMRD, constitutional mismatch repair deficiency; MAP, *MUTYH*-associated polyposis; NAP, *NTHL1*-associated polyposis; PPAP, polymerase proofreading–associated polyposis.

Polymerase proofreading–associated polyposis

Polymerase proofreading–associated polyposis (PPAP) {2493} is caused by dominantly inherited mutations in the proofreading (exonuclease) domains of *POLD1* and *POLE* {2493,2661,409}. These proofreading mutations cause a defect in the correction of mispaired bases inserted during DNA replication, leading to a hypermutant phenotype with exceedingly numerous point mutations, without the normal polymerase allele itself needing to undergo somatic mutation {409}. PPAP is therefore an exception to the Knudson multiple-hit hypothesis; it is unique among the constitutional DNA repair disorders in that it is not recessively inherited. PPAP accounts for approximately 10% of all cases of FAP {436}. Adenomatous polyps of the large bowel occur in adulthood, generally by the age of 50 years. The risk of developing colorectal cancer by the age of 70 years is between 1 in 3 and 2 in 3 {436}. Duodenal adenomatous polyposis and adenocarcinoma also occur {3113}. The colorectal adenomas and adenocarcinomas in PPAP are similar to sporadic tumours macroscopically and microscopically, but they have a characteristic hypermutant somatic mutation spectrum. This form of polyposis is thought to be rarer than MAP, although the exact prevalence is unknown. Extraintestinal tumours (e.g. endometrial adenocarcinoma) can occur, and some may acquire somatic mismatch repair gene mutations resulting in MSI and immunohistochemical abnormalities suggestive of Lynch syndrome, indicating that PPAP is another cause of Lynch-like syndrome {1425,856}. Hypermutant cancers associated with PPAP, being rich in neoantigens such as those with MSI, appear to be good targets for PD1/PDL1 immune checkpoint inhibitor immunotherapy {798,2808}.

Constitutional mismatch repair deficiency syndrome

Constitutional mismatch repair deficiency syndrome (CMMRD) {194} is caused by recessive (biallelic) inheritance of mutations in one of the four DNA mismatch repair genes (*MSH2, MLH1, MSH6,* and *PMS2*), in contrast to the dominantly inherited (monoallelic) mutations that give rise to Lynch syndrome. CMMRD is therefore a classic recessive constitutional DNA repair disorder, with a complex and often severe phenotype {228,713}. The prevalence is uncertain, but may be as high as 1 in 40 000 {3450}. The tumour phenotype varies (with some patients succumbing to multiple malignancies), and it differs from that seen in Lynch syndrome; about half of all patients with CMMRD develop brain tumours (usually glioblastomas); half develop digestive tract cancers; and one third develop haematological malignancies. The brain tumours and haematological malignancies typically arise in the first and second decades of life; the colorectal and small intestinal cancers arise in the second, third, and fourth decades, with some adenomas {3450,1870,2695}. Some cases may include immunological abnormalities, as well as cutaneous features suggestive of neurofibromatosis (i.e. neurofibromas and café-au-lait patches), which can cause diagnostic confusion {3389}. Patients are prone to developing multiple adenomatous polyps and adenocarcinoma of the large bowel from early childhood to adulthood {1870}. On immunohistochemical analysis, all the cells of individuals with CMMRD show loss of a specific DNA mismatch repair protein (i.e. the protein encoded by whichever mismatch repair gene harbours the inherited mutations). Therefore, it is important to test for all four of the mismatch repair markers and to examine both normal and neoplastic tissue in order to diagnose this condition {228}. Some tumours, such as those in the brain, may not have MSI, but may have a hypermutant phenotype due to the acquisition of somatic POLD1 and/or POLE mutations.

Hereditary mixed polyposis syndrome

Hereditary mixed polyposis syndrome is caused by a 40 kb upstream duplication that leads to increased and ectopic expression of the BMP antagonist GREM1. Patients develop a variety of colorectal polyps, including adenomas, hyperplastic polyps, inflammatory polyps, prolapse-type polyps, and lymphoid aggregates, with a high risk of colorectal cancer. Therefore, it is unlikely that a case of pure adenomatous or serrated polyposis has hereditary mixed polyposis syndrome as its cause {1416,643}.

MSH3-associated polyposis

Biallelic inheritance of mutations in the DNA mismatch repair gene MSH3 causes recessive adenomatous polyposis {24}. Tumours arising in this setting do not have classic MSI at mononucleotide repeats, but rather at di-, tri-, tetra-, and pentanucleotide repeats – a phenomenon called elevated microsatellite alterations at selected tetranucleotides (EMAST) {500}. The phenotypes of the few cases reported to date include colorectal and duodenal adenomas, colorectal cancer, gastric cancer, and early-onset astrocytoma {24}.

AXIN2-associated polyposis

AXIN2 is a regulator of β-catenin degradation in the WNT signalling pathway, so it is functionally related to APC {2094}. Inherited AXIN2 mutations have been described in families with adenomatous polyposis and ectodermal dysplasia (including oligodontia), but they have also been described in individuals with adenomatous polyposis and no ectodermal dysplasia {1782,2067,2723}.

Immune deficiency–associated polyposis

An increased risk of colorectal adenomatous polyposis and cancer is associated with a variety of inherited immune deficiencies, including X-linked agammaglobulinaemia (caused by BTK mutations) and common variable immunodeficiency {3412,1989,418,22}. Gastric adenocarcinoma and paediatric colonic neuroendocrine carcinoma [NEC] can also occur {214,2859}.

Other conditions associated with multiple colorectal adenomas

Acromegalic patients are prone to having small numbers of colorectal adenomas and also colorectal cancers (but this is not a classic polyposis) {595}. Polyposis with no detectable cause, despite comprehensive gene panel testing, is a common finding, and there are other, as yet undiscovered, causes of adenomatous polyposis.

Serrated polyposis

Rosty C
Brosens LAA
Dekker E
Nagtegaal ID

Definition
Serrated polyposis is a condition of largely unknown etiology, characterized by multiple serrated polyps in the large intestine and associated with an increased risk of colorectal carcinoma.

MIM numbering
617108 Serrated polyposis

ICD-11 coding
2E92.40 Polyposis syndrome

Related terminology
Not recommended: hyperplastic polyposis (a historical term used before the recognition of different histological subtypes of serrated polyps).

Subtype(s)
None

Localization
Serrated polyposis affects the large intestine but not the upper GI tract or the small intestine {839}. Extracolonic manifestations have not been reported.

Clinical features
The clinical criteria for the diagnosis of serrated polyposis are presented in Box 14.02.

Males and females are almost equally affected. Most patients are diagnosed at 50–60 years of age, but the age range at diagnosis is wide, with some patients diagnosed in early adulthood

Box 14.02 Clinical criteria for the diagnosis of serrated polyposis

Criterion 1:	≥ 5 serrated lesions/polyps proximal to the rectum, all being ≥ 5 mm in size, with ≥ 2 being ≥ 10 mm in size
Criterion 2:	> 20 serrated lesions/polyps of any size distributed throughout the large bowel, with ≥ 5 being proximal to the rectum

Any histological subtype of serrated lesion/polyp (hyperplastic polyp, sessile serrated lesion without or with dysplasia, traditional serrated adenoma, and unclassified serrated adenoma) is included in the final polyp count. The polyp count is cumulative over multiple colonoscopies.

{839,494,1361,3575}. The first clinical presentation can be at the time of colorectal carcinoma diagnosis, during screening colonoscopy in symptomatic patients or for family history of colorectal cancer, or by population screening in asymptomatic patients. Faecal blood tests do not perform well in detecting serrated polyps, because serrated polyps are less likely to bleed than conventional adenomas. The phenotype of serrated polyposis is heterogeneous, representing a continuum between patients who barely meet the clinical definition and patients with high polyp burden and multiple large polyps fulfilling both criteria {1361,846}. About 25% of patients present with a type 1 phenotype (i.e. fulfilling only clinical criterion 1), 45% present with a type 2 phenotype (fulfilling only clinical criterion 2), and 30% have both phenotypes {494,1361}. The clinical phenotype in a given patient may evolve over time, depending on the findings from surveillance colonoscopies.

The median cumulative polyp number is most commonly 30–40, with a range as wide as 6–240 polyps and frequent pancolonic distribution {839,494,1361,2764}.

Epidemiology
The highest reported prevalence in primary screening colonoscopies is 0.1% {1363}. In faecal occult blood test–based screening cohorts, the rate of serrated polyposis ranged from 0.34% to 0.66% in initial colonoscopies; in the primary colonoscopy cohorts, the rate ranged from 0% to 0.09% {2724,3423}. The rate of serrated polyposis after follow-up colonoscopy was reported as 0.4–0.8% {1363}.

Environmental factors associated with serrated polyposis include cigarette smoking and high body mass index. Paradoxically, patients with a history of smoking have a lower risk of colorectal carcinoma {1361,437}. About one third of patients with serrated polyposis have at least one first-degree relative with colorectal carcinoma; 5% have a first-degree relative with serrated polyposis {494,1361}. The first-degree relatives of patients with serrated polyposis have 5 times the incidence of colorectal carcinoma as is seen in the general population {3575,366}.

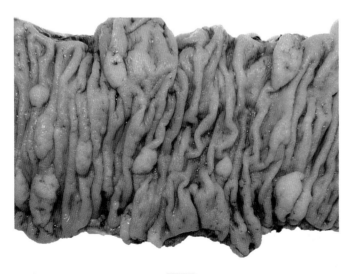

1 cm

Fig. 14.14 Serrated polyposis. Multiple colonic sessile polyps in the setting of serrated polyposis from a colectomy specimen.

Etiology

Genetic studies are currently underway to identify a genetic cause for at least a subset of serrated polyposis, but no high-penetrance candidate genes have yet been identified. Pathogenic germline variants in *RNF43* have been reported in 2% of patients with serrated polyposis {435,2630,3663}. In one study, no germline mutations in any of the well-known polyposis genes were found in 65 patients with serrated polyposis {643}.

Serrated polyposis can also be a component of well-defined genetic syndromes: *MUTYH*-associated polyposis {365} and hereditary mixed polyposis syndrome caused by a duplication upstream of *GREM1* {1416}. Although patients with *PTEN* hamartoma tumour syndrome / Cowden syndrome and juvenile polyposis may in rare cases strictly fulfil the criteria of serrated polyposis, they almost always have other polyp types or extraintestinal features, and expert pathology review is extremely important in the diagnostic work-up of these rare patients with polyposis for a correct clinicopathological classification.

Referral to clinical genetic services is recommended in order to test all possible underlying genetic defects in patients with unexplained polyposis.

Pathogenesis

The pathogenesis is largely unknown. A small subset of patients show autosomal dominant inheritance with germline inactivating mutations in *RNF43* (17q23.2), a gene involved in the WNT signalling pathway {1000,1700}.

Macroscopic appearance

The macroscopic appearances mimic those of the sporadic lesions associated with the syndrome.

Histopathology

Any patient fulfilling at least one of the clinical criteria (see Box 14.02) is diagnosed with serrated polyposis. Any subtype of serrated lesions/polyps (hyperplastic polyps, sessile serrated lesions with or without dysplasia, traditional serrated adenomas, and unclassified serrated adenomas; see *Colorectal serrated lesions and polyps*, p. 163) is included in the final count. The diagnosis may require more than one colonoscopy, and the polyp count is cumulative across multiple procedures.

In a series of 100 patients with polyp histology review, 45% of all lesions were hyperplastic polyps, 34% sessile serrated

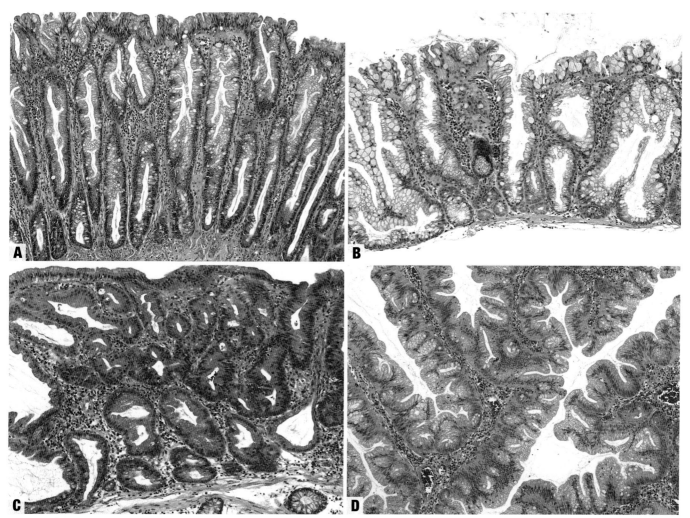

Fig. 14.15 Serrated polyposis. All subtypes of serrated polyp can occur in serrated polyposis. **A** Hyperplastic polyp with preserved crypt architecture and serration in upper part of the crypts. **B** Sessile serrated polyp showing distorted crypts with dilatation of the base. **C** Sessile serrated polyp with dysplasia showing crowding of crypts lined by dysplastic cells. **D** Exophytic traditional serrated adenoma with ectopic crypt formations, slit-like serration, and tall columnar eosinophilic cells.

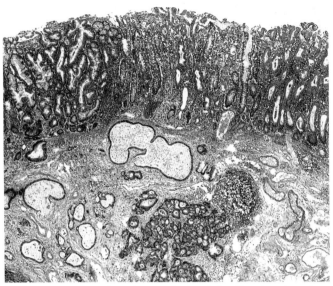

Fig. 14.16 Colorectal carcinoma in serrated polyposis. Small invasive colorectal carcinoma arising from a sessile serrated lesion in the setting of serrated polyposis.

lesions (including 7% with dysplasia), 17% conventional adenomas, and 4% traditional serrated adenomas {2764}. In two large retrospective studies without central histology review, 25–30% of patients presented with at least one serrated polyp with dysplasia, 76% with at least one serrated polyp ≥ 10 mm, 75–80% with at least one conventional adenoma, and 35–45% with at least one advanced conventional adenoma {494,1361}.

Diagnostic molecular pathology
Serrated polyps in the setting of serrated polyposis have molecular characteristics similar to those of sporadic polyps. In a systematic review and meta-analysis, *BRAF* mutation was found in 73% of serrated polyps and 0% of conventional adenomas. *KRAS* mutation was found in 8% of serrated polyps and 3% of conventional adenomas {1202}.

Approximately 50% of colorectal carcinomas in patients with serrated polyposis have a *BRAF* mutation, < 5% have a *KRAS* mutation, and 40% are *MLH1*-deficient {364,2766}. This molecular phenotype suggests that only half of all serrated polyposis–associated colorectal carcinomas develop from serrated polyps via the serrated neoplasia pathway. The other half presumably follow the conventional adenoma–carcinoma pathway.

Essential and desirable diagnostic criteria
The clinical criteria for the diagnosis of serrated polyposis are presented in Box 14.02 (p. 532).

Staging (TNM)
Not clinically relevant

Prognosis and prediction
Once dysplastic, the sessile serrated lesions may develop relatively rapidly into cancer {316}. The cancer risk differs depending on the phenotype, first clinical presentation, and polyp histology. In two large retrospective multicentre cohort studies, colorectal carcinoma was diagnosed in 16% and 29% of patients, most of them before or at the time of serrated polyposis diagnosis {494,1361}. As many as 50% of colorectal carcinomas were in the rectosigmoid. Synchronous or metachronous colorectal carcinomas occurred in 4% of patients. Reported risk factors for colorectal carcinoma included the fulfilment of both clinical criteria for serrated polyposis, more than two sessile serrated lesions proximal to splenic flexure, at least one serrated polyp with dysplasia, and at least one advanced conventional adenoma. Cases can be successfully managed by serial colonoscopies in tertiary centres with low rate of surgical referral {2536,837}. In a prospective study of 41 patients under annual surveillance after clearing colonoscopy, polyps were detected in 80% of patients at each surveillance colonoscopy, but none developed colorectal carcinoma during 5 years of follow-up {1201}. In a large retrospective Spanish study, the cumulative incidence of colorectal carcinoma detected during surveillance was 3.1% and 6.4% at 3 years and 5 years, respectively {2742}.

Hereditary diffuse gastric cancer

Carneiro F
Guilford P
Oliveira C
van der Post RS

Definition

Hereditary diffuse gastric cancer (HDGC) is an autosomal dominant cancer susceptibility syndrome characterized by diffuse-type gastric cancer (DGC) and invasive lobular breast cancer (LBC), principally caused by inactivating germline mutations in *CDH1* (encoding E-cadherin).

MIM numbering

137215 Familial diffuse gastric cancer with or without cleft lip and/or palate

ICD-11 coding

None

Related terminology

None

Subtype(s)

None

Localization

HDGC can affect all topographical regions of the gastric mucosa {1340,568,506,2498,1635}.

Clinical features

The age of clinical presentation of gastric cancer (GC) in index cases is extremely variable (14–85 years), even within families. The overall risk before the age of 20 years is low {1161}. Female *CDH1* mutation carriers have a 40% lifetime risk of developing LBC {1161}. However, DGC is the main cause of mortality in both sexes.

Epidemiology

It is estimated that about 10% of all GC cases (~100 000/year) present familial aggregation {2439}. Increased GC risk in families may be associated with shared genetic susceptibility, lifestyle, and environmental factors {2439}. The prevalence of HDGC is estimated to be < 1% of all GC cases (~10 000/year). Pathogenic germline *CDH1* mutations have been identified in families with HDGC from most countries and many ethnicities, although the incidence of HDGC is highly variable in different populations {1142,1592,3167}. In HDGC families clinically defined using either the 2010 {942} or 2015 {3415} criteria, *CDH1* mutations have been detected in 14–20% and 19% of cases, respectively {3416,1161,300}.

Etiology

CDH1 is located on the long arm of chromosome 16 (16q22.1), comprises 16 exons, and encodes E-cadherin, which is a transmembrane protein predominantly expressed at the basolateral membrane of epithelial cells and involved in homophilic cell–cell adhesion and transduction of mechanical force {407,1819}.

Its cytoplasmic domain interacts with numerous structural and regulatory proteins, including the catenin family {3730}. These interactions influence cell survival signalling, the microtubule network, and the organization of the cortical actin cytoskeleton

Box 14.03 Definitions of *CDH1*-related gastric cancer and precursor lesions

> **SRCC in situ (pTis):** Presence of signet-ring cells within the basal membrane, replacing normal epithelial cells
>
> **Pagetoid spread of signet-ring cells (pTis):** Pagetoid spread pattern is reflected by a second row of signet-ring cells beneath the normal epithelial cells in a gastric gland within the basal membrane
>
> **Intramucosal (pT1a) SRCC:** Invasive carcinoma showing signet-ring cells restricted to the mucosa
>
> **Advanced hereditary diffuse gastric cancer:** Poorly cohesive cancer with a minor SRCC component and sometimes precursor lesions or pT1a SRCC in surrounding gastric tissue

SRCC, signet-ring cell carcinoma.

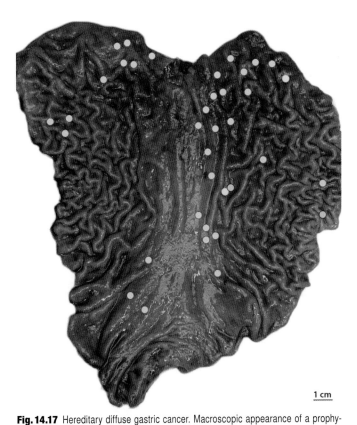

Fig. 14.17 Hereditary diffuse gastric cancer. Macroscopic appearance of a prophylactic gastrectomy specimen from a *CDH1* mutation carrier; the stomach appears normal to the naked eye; on histology, many microscopic lesions were observed, encompassing foci of intramucosal carcinoma (green dots), as well as carcinomas in situ (blue dots) and pagetoid spread lesions (yellow dots).

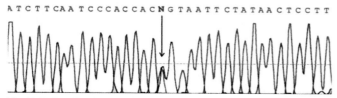

Fig. 14.18 Germline alterations described in hereditary diffuse gastric cancer. Example of a deleterious splice-site mutation.

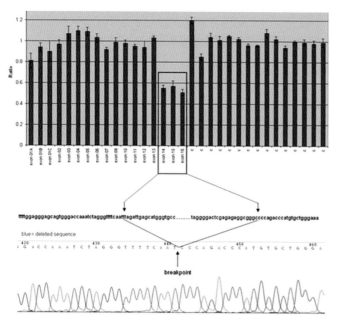

Fig. 14.19 Germline alterations described in hereditary diffuse gastric cancer. Example of a large deletion affecting the last 3 exons of the *CDH1* gene.

{407}, with a profound effect on cell shape, polarity, and motility {1819}.

More than 155 different *CDH1* germline mutations have been reported in HDGC families {1161}. Of these, approximately 80% are truncating and predicted to be pathogenic. These include large deletions and nonsense, splice-site, and frameshift mutations {1161,3168,3637,2440}. The remaining 20% are missense changes, some of which disrupt E-cadherin function, whereas others remain variants of unknown significance {2117}. HDGC mutations span the whole length of *CDH1*, and no major hotspots have been identified.

Germline mutations in *CTNNA1* (which encodes α-catenin) have been identified in at least five families with HDGC {1161,2012,3550}. Given the well-established interaction between E-cadherin and α-catenin in the adherens junction {3730}, it is likely that *CTNNA1* constitutes a genuine minor HDGC gene. No evidence for any other common HDGC genes has been found by exome sequencing {3482,936}, although multiple families meeting the HDGC clinical criteria carry pathogenic germline mutations in other cancer susceptibility genes, such as *PALB2*, *MSH2*, *RECQL5*, *ATM*, and *BRCA2* {1332,2441,678}.

Pathogenesis

Initiation of DGC and LBC in HDGC families requires inactivation of the second *CDH1* allele. *CDH1* promoter methylation is the most prevalent mechanism of second allele inactivation in primary tumours, and loss of heterozygosity is the most frequent mechanism in lymph node metastases {1332,2441,678}. Loss of E-cadherin in model systems results in misalignment of the mitotic spindle {1814,755,1334} and occasional displacement of cells out of the epithelial plane. In HDGC, displacement of proliferating E-cadherin–null cells into the lamina propria may be the initiating event for signet-ring cell carcinoma (SRCC) / DGC. The presence of hundreds of pT1a foci in some *CDH1* mutation carriers suggests that mutations in other genes are not required for the establishment of these early foci {568}. The lack of correlation between age and the number of SRCC foci detected in the total gastrectomy specimens in *CDH1* mutation carriers suggests that a proportion of the indolent foci may be transient.

Macroscopic appearance

Macroscopic features differ in the stomachs of asymptomatic *CDH1* mutation carriers submitted to prophylactic/risk-reducing gastrectomy and index patients with HDGC. In the former, the stomach nearly always appears normal to the naked eye and on palpation, and slicing shows normal mucosal thickness. Most index patients present with cancers that are indistinguishable from sporadic DGC, often with linitis plastica, which can involve all topographical regions within the stomach.

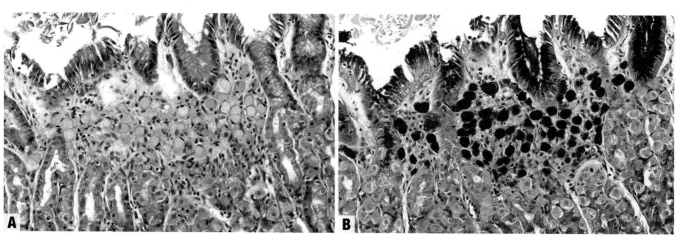

Fig. 14.20 Hereditary diffuse gastric cancer. **A** Intramucosal signet-ring cell carcinoma (pT1a). A small focus of loose signet-ring cells restricted to the mucosa. **B** The signet-ring cells are highlighted by PAS staining.

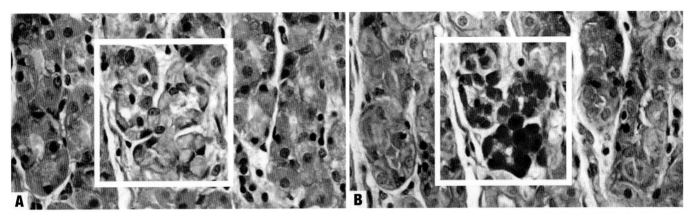

Fig. 14.21 Signet-ring cell carcinoma in situ (pTis). **A** Signet-ring cells are present within the basal membrane, replacing normal gastric epithelial cells. **B** The signet-ring cells are highlighted by PAS staining.

Histopathology

Early-stage HDGC in *CDH1* mutation carriers is character-ized by multiple foci of invasive (pT1a) SRCC (< 0.1–10 mm) in the superficial gastric mucosa, without nodal metastases {568,506,2743}. At the neck-zone level, neoplastic cells are small, and they usually enlarge towards the surface of the gastric mucosa. Less commonly, larger foci of intramucosal carcinoma can involve superficial and deep mucosa. In prophylactic gas-trectomy, histological examination of the entire gastric mucosa is recommended (one section per block) before the absence of neoplasia can be claimed. Because all topographical regions of the gastric mucosa can be affected, the surgical specimens should include a complete cuff of squamous oesophageal mucosa and distal duodenal mucosa. In most patients, there is no intestinal metaplasia or *Helicobacter pylori* infection. The International Gastric Cancer Linkage Consortium (IGCLC) has prepared a checklist for reporting the pathology of gastrectomy specimens from patients with HDGC {3415}.

Two precursors of pT1a SRCC are recognized: SRCC in situ (Tis) and pagetoid spread (not necessarily associated with an invasive carcinoma) of signet-ring cells (see Box 14.03, p. 535). Strictly following criteria for the identification of these precursors will diminish the risk of overdiagnosing nonspecific changes and distinguish precursors from mimics of SRCC in situ. On the basis

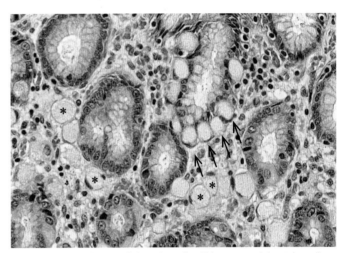

Fig. 14.23 Pagetoid spread of signet-ring cells with intramucosal signet-ring cell car-cinoma. Signet-ring cells grow as a second row beneath the normal epithelial cells in a gastric gland within the basal membrane (arrows); in this example, there are also a few intramucosal invasive tumour cells in the stroma between normal glands (asterisks).

of these precursors, a model for the development of DGC in carriers of deleterious germline *CDH1* mutations has been pro-posed (see Fig. 14.22) {506}.

Advanced HDGC shows the characteristic picture of diffuse-type, poorly cohesive GC. In most cases, there is at least a small component of typical signet-ring cells. However, most tumours are heterogeneous, displaying atypical cells with diffuse growth and also cords, (micro)glands, and small mucin lakes. Precursor lesions are an important clue for *CDH1*-related HDGC and may be found in surrounding non-neoplastic mucosa, distant from the tumour bulk.

Most pT1a SRCCs show absent or reduced staining for E-cad-herin {506,1333,243,2441,3414}, in keeping with a clonal origin of the cancer foci, indicating that the second *CDH1* allele has been downregulated or lost. E-cadherin immunohistochemistry is not recommended as a pre-screening test in HDGC, because E-cadherin immunoreactivity is often present to some level and is also often diminished in sporadic DGC.

Confirmation of carcinoma in situ and pagetoid spread of sig-net-ring cells by an independent pathologist with experience in the field is strongly recommended and will help distinguish pre-cursor lesions and tiny foci of early intramucosal carcinoma from

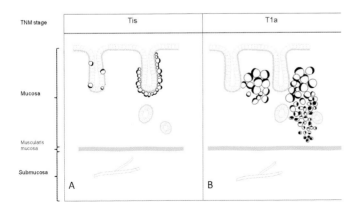

Fig. 14.22 Model of development of hereditary diffuse gastric cancer. Comparison of signet-ring cell carcinoma (SRCC) in situ, non-invasive SRCC, and early invasive SRCC. **A** Single signet-ring cells on left, pagetoid spread on right. **B** Early invasive SRCC, invasion into lamina propria.

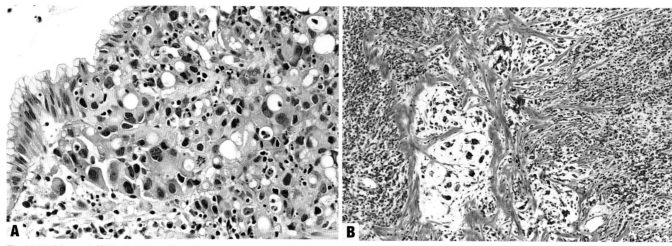

Fig. 14.24 Advanced *CDH1*-related hereditary diffuse gastric cancer. **A** Poorly cohesive gastric carcinoma. Biopsy from an 18-year-old patient who presented with advanced gastric cancer (proband); most cells are atypical and pleomorphic; very rare signet-ring cells are identified. **B** Poorly cohesive carcinoma with diffuse growth of polymorphic small tumour cells, presence of extracellular mucin with microglandular formation.

Box 14.04 Diagnostic criteria for *CDH1* testing and actionable causative genes in hereditary diffuse gastric cancer (HDGC)

Full clinical criteria {3415}

2 documented cases of gastric cancer at any age in first- or second-degree relatives, with ≥ 1 confirmed diffuse-type gastric cancer (DGC)
  or
Personal history of DGC < 40 years old
  or
Personal or family (first- or second-degree relatives) history of DGC and lobular breast cancer, one diagnosed < 50 years old

Supporting clinical criteria {3415}

Families with bilateral or multiple cases of lobular breast cancer < 50 years
  or
Families with clustering of DGC and cleft lip/palate
  or
Any patient that is diagnosed with signet-ring cell carcinoma in situ and/or pagetoid spread of signet-ring cells

Established genetic causes with clinical utility {2439}

Loss-of-function *CDH1* mutations (classified as pathogenic or likely pathogenic)

CDH1 deletions affecting the coding sequence and/or regulatory regions leading to loss of function

Novel candidate gene with likely clinical utility {2012,1161,3550}
Loss-of-function *CTNNA1* mutations

---

mimics of signet-ring cells (telescoped normal glands, globoid cells in hyperplastic lesions, clear/glassy-cell change of mucous glands, and xanthomatous cells) {3415}.

Diagnostic molecular pathology

The genetic/molecular landscape that follows somatic inactivation of the second *CDH1* allele in HDGC is poorly understood. Intramucosal carcinomas (pT1a) frequently show an indolent phenotype, characterized by signet-ring cells without immunoreactivity for Ki-67 or p53, whereas advanced carcinomas (pT > 1) usually have a more aggressive appearance, with pleomorphic cells immunoreactive for both proteins {3414,1333}. Aberrant expression of p16 has been associated with this aggressive phenotype {1822}, and progression of the intramucosal SRCCs is associated with the expression of SRC, fibronectin, PTK2, and STAT3, as well as with epithelial–mesenchymal transition {1333}.

Essential and desirable diagnostic criteria

Diagnostic criteria for *CDH1* testing and actionable causative genes are presented in Box 14.04.

Staging (TNM)

In most gastrectomy specimens from asymptomatic *CDH1* mutation carriers, only intramucosal cancers are diagnosed and staged as pT1apN0. Most index cases are diagnosed at an advanced stage.

Prognosis and prediction

The intramucosal SRCC/DGC may remain indolent for a long time and carry a very low risk for dissemination. Advanced HDGC has a poor prognosis.

The diagnosis of *CDH1*-related HDGC offers the opportunity for presymptomatic genetic screening of at-risk family members and lifesaving cancer risk-reduction gastrectomy for carriers. Enhanced screening to detect early LBC should be considered {3415}.

The clinical picture of *CTNNA1* mutation–positive HDGC families seems to be similar to that of *CDH1*-related HDGC, except that typical precursor lesions of SRCC/DGC and LBC have not been reported {3550,1161,2012}.

Familial pancreatic cancer

Hruban RH
Brosens LAA

Definition

Familial pancreatic cancer is a syndrome defined by pancreatic cancer in ≥ 2 first-degree relatives; this term is usually applied in the absence of a recognized germline mutation. Hereditary pancreatic cancer is a syndrome defined by pancreatic cancer due to an identified causative underlying germline mutation.

MIM numbering

614320 Susceptibility to pancreatic cancer 4
613347 Susceptibility to pancreatic cancer 2
260350 Pancreatic cancer

ICD-11 coding

None

Related terminology

None

Subtype(s)

None

Localization

The localization of familial and hereditary pancreatic cancers is the same as that of sporadic pancreatic cancers {3054}.

Clinical features

Having one, two, or three first-degree relatives with pancreatic cancer multiplies the risk of developing pancreatic cancer by 4.6, 6, and 32 times, respectively {1625,130}. In addition, having a family member with young-onset pancreatic cancer increases the risk of pancreatic cancer in kindreds with multiple family members with pancreatic cancer {429}. Anticipation, a trend towards younger age of onset and worse prognosis, has been suggested in some kindreds {2103}.

Familial pancreatic cancer shows a trend towards a slightly younger age of onset (58–68 years) than sporadic pancreatic cancer (61–74 years), and it is more common in certain groups, such as individuals of Ashkenazi Jewish ancestry {429,1968}. Otherwise, there are no differences in the clinical features of sporadic versus familial pancreatic cancers. In fact, 4–20% of pancreatic cancer patients without a family history of cancer have a deleterious germline mutation in a familial pancreatic cancer gene when sequenced {477,1954,224,3019}.

Several genetic syndromes confer an increased risk of pancreatic cancer with varying clinical features and associated extrapancreatic malignancies (see Table 14.06). For example, the risk of pancreatic cancer is substantially increased in individuals with Peutz–Jeghers syndrome, who typically have melanocytic macules on their lips and buccal mucosa, as well as hamartomatous polyps of the GI tract.

Epidemiology

Approximately 10–12% of patients with pancreatic cancer have a family history of the disease {543,2574,3019,2080,258,1212}. Some pancreatic cancers arise in patients with recognized genetic syndromes, but in most instances the genetic basis for

Table 14.06 Well-established hereditary pancreatic cancer genes and genetic syndromes

Affected gene(s)	Inherited syndrome	Prevalence in familial PDAC	Estimated lifetime risk of PDAC	Relative risk	Main extrapancreatic malignancies
BRCA2	Hereditary breast and ovarian cancer syndrome	6–12%	3–10%	3.5–10	Breast, ovarian, prostate
BRCA1[a]	Hereditary breast and ovarian cancer syndrome	0.7–1.2%	~2–5%	Uncertain	Breast, ovarian
PALB2	Hereditary breast and ovarian cancer syndrome	2–3%	7.5%	15	Breast, ovarian
ATM	None	2.6–3.2%	4%	9	None
Mismatch repair genes	Lynch syndrome	0.7%	6% (MSH2)	5–9	Colorectal, endometrial, etc.[b]
CDKN2A	Familial atypical multiple mole melanoma	0.7–2.5%	15–25%	13–22	Melanoma
STK11	Peutz–Jeghers syndrome	< 1%	30–60%	132	Many[c]
PRSS1	Hereditary pancreatitis	< 1%	≥ 30–40%	53–87	None
SPINK1, CPA1, or CPB1	Hereditary pancreatitis	Lower than for PRSS1	Lower than for PRSS1	Lower than for PRSS1	None

PDAC, pancreatic ductal adenocarcinoma.
[a]The degree of raised risk of pancreatic cancer with BRCA1 is uncertain. [b]See Lynch syndrome (p. 515). [c]See Peutz–Jeghers syndrome (p. 545).
Note: Up-to-date estimates are available at http://www.lscarisk.org/.

the familial aggregation of pancreatic carcinomas has not yet been identified. An autosomal dominant mode of inheritance has been suggested in familial pancreatic cancer {1624}.

Etiology
Germline mutations in a number of different genes predispose individuals to pancreatic cancer. A deleterious germline mutation can be identified in 4–19% of patients with apparently sporadic pancreatic cancers and 10–20% of patients with familial pancreatic cancer (see Table 14.06, p. 539) {3019,477,3500,1954}.

Well-established pancreatic cancer susceptibility genes include *BRCA2*, *ATM*, *BRCA1*, *PALB2*, *CDKN2A*, *STK11*, *PRSS1*, *SPINK1*, and the mismatch repair genes. Less common germline mutations in cancer susceptibility genes such as *TP53*, *BARD1*, *CHEK2*, *BUB1B*, *CPA1*, *CPB1*, and *BUB3* have also been reported {2736,3019,1187}.

The penetrance of these germline mutations is incomplete. For example, many patients with pancreatic ductal carcinoma who carry a germline *BRCA2* mutation do not have a strong family history of breast or pancreatic carcinoma {1056}. A number of patients with *BRCA2* mutations and pancreatic cancer are of Ashkenazi Jewish ancestry; a founder *BRCA2* mutation, c.6174delT, is present in about 1% of the Ashkenazi Jewish population {1056,2481}.

Together, the above genetic syndromes account for only a minority of familial pancreatic cancers. For most cases of familial aggregation of pancreatic cancer, the underlying genetic abnormality is currently unknown. With the advent of rapid and inexpensive whole-exome next-generation sequencing technologies, additional low-prevalence mutations responsible for familial aggregation of this disease are likely to be identified {2736,3229}.

In addition to rare but high-penetrance germline mutations, there are certain common polymorphisms that have been associated with either increased risk of or protection from pancreatic cancer in the general population. For example, genome-wide association studies have shown an association between risk for pancreatic cancer and ABO blood group: people with type O blood have a lower risk than people with type A or B {129}. A polymorphism on chromosome 5 that results in variable expression of the enzyme TERT is associated with increased risk for pancreatic cancer in the general population {898}.

Hereditary cancer syndromes related to increased risk of pancreatic cancer concern mainly pancreatic ductal adenocarcinoma, discussed above. There are also hereditary cancer syndromes related to increased risk of pancreatic acinar cell carcinoma (see *Pancreatic acinar cell carcinoma*, p. 333) and pancreatic neuroendocrine tumours (PanNETs; see *Pancreatic neuroendocrine neoplasms*, p. 343).

Pathogenesis
See *Pancreatic ductal adenocarcinoma* (p. 322).

Macroscopic appearance
See *Pancreatic ductal adenocarcinoma* (p. 322).

Histopathology
In general, there are no differences between invasive familial and invasive sporadic pancreatic cancers with regard to histological subtypes, mean tumour size, perineural invasion, angiolymphatic invasion, lymph node metastasis, and pathological stage {3054}. Microsatellite-unstable tumours in patients with Lynch syndrome can show a medullary phenotype {1055}, which is characterized by poor differentiation, a syncytial growth pattern, and pushing borders {1055}.

Compared with pancreatic resections from patients with sporadic pancreatic cancer, resections from patients with a strong family history of pancreatic cancer have a higher prevalence of non-invasive pancreatic cancer precursor lesions, including pancreatic intraepithelial neoplasia (2.75 times more) and intraductal papillary mucinous neoplasm, and these lesions are of higher grade than in patients with sporadic pancreatic cancer {428,2987,1336}.

Familial pancreatitis (primarily caused by germline mutations in *PRSS1* or *SPINK1*) is a risk factor for pancreatic cancer; affected pancreata are characterized by loss of the acinar parenchyma, fibrosis, and fatty replacement (lipomatous atrophy) {3062}.

Diagnostic molecular pathology
The germline alterations driving known causes of hereditary pancreatic cancer are summarized in Table 14.06 (p. 539). With the exception of cancers with mismatch repair defects, the somatic mutations in driver genes in familial pancreatic cancer are similar to those in sporadic pancreatic cancer {2388}.

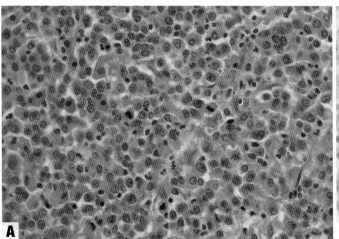 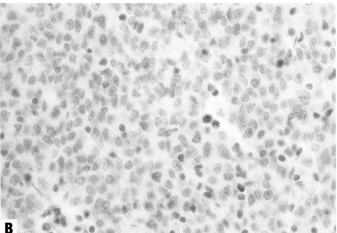

Fig. 14.25 Medullary carcinoma of the pancreas. **A** H&E staining. **B** There is loss of MSH2.

Essential and desirable diagnostic criteria

Essential: pancreatic cancer diagnosed in ≥ 2 first-degree relatives.

Staging (TNM)

TNM staging for sporadic and familial or hereditary pancreatic cancer is the same.

Prognosis and prediction

Screening of high-risk individuals (i.e. > 5% lifetime risk, or a 5-fold increased relative risk) for early disease has been reported, but screening has not been shown to save lives {481,1854}. With adjustment for stage, there are no clear differences in the prognosis of patients with familial or hereditary pancreatic cancer versus those with sporadic pancreatic cancer {1336}.

Patients with specific genetic defects may benefit from specific therapies, such as poly (ADP-ribose) polymerase (PARP) inhibitors or platinum-containing agents for BRCA-mutated tumours, immunotherapy for microsatellite-unstable tumours, and radiotherapy for *ATM*-mutated tumours {2581,1815}.

Juvenile polyposis syndrome

Brosens LAA
Jansen M

Definition
Juvenile polyposis syndrome (JPS) is an autosomal dominant cancer syndrome characterized by multiple juvenile polyps of the GI tract, predominantly of the colorectum, but also of the stomach and small intestine.

MIM numbering
174900 Juvenile polyposis syndrome, infantile form
174900 Polyposis, juvenile intestinal
175050 Juvenile polyposis / hereditary haemorrhagic telangiectasia syndrome
612242 Chromosome 10q22.3-q23.2 deletion syndrome (including juvenile polyposis of infancy)

ICD-11 coding
2B90.Y Other specified malignant neoplasms of colon
Juvenile polyposis of infancy
Juvenile gastrointestinal polyposis

Related terminology
Acceptable: generalized juvenile polyposis; juvenile polyposis coli; juvenile polyposis of infancy; chromosome 10q22.3-q23.2 deletion syndrome; juvenile polyposis of the stomach; familial juvenile polyposis; hamartomatous gastrointestinal polyposis; combined juvenile polyposis / hereditary haemorrhagic telangiectasia (Osler–Weber–Rendu) syndrome.

Subtype(s)
Colorectal or generalized juvenile polyposis; juvenile polyposis of infancy

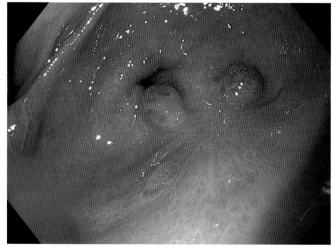

Fig. 14.26 Gastric juvenile polyps.

Localization
The polyps in JPS predominantly arise throughout the colon, ranging in number from 1 to > 100. Gastric and small intestinal polyps, respectively, are found in as many as 85% and 14–33% of patients {1491,1984,3605,421}.

Clinical features
The diagnostic criteria for JPS are summarized in Box 14.05. Patients usually present with gastrointestinal bleeding, manifesting as haematochezia. Melaena, prolapsed rectal polyp, passage of tissue through the anus, intussusception, abdominal pain, and anaemia are also common. Juvenile polyposis can present as either colorectal or generalized juvenile polyposis, or as juvenile polyposis of infancy, a subtype with severe symptoms (see Table 14.07) {751,2121,2807}.

JPS is associated with a 34-fold increased relative risk of colorectal cancer and a cumulative risk of colorectal cancer of 39–68% by the age of 60 years {419,3193}. The mean age at colon cancer diagnosis is 44 years (range: 15–68 years). Gastric duodenal and pancreatic cancers are also reported in JPS, but no formal risk analysis for these malignancies has been reported {1298}. Gastric cancer lifetime risk ranges from 10% to 30% {3193}. The median patient age of upper gastrointestinal carcinoma is 58 years (range: 21–73 years) {3193}. Gastric and small bowel carcinomas together are estimated to occur at about one fifth the frequency of colorectal cancer in patients with JPS {419}.

SMAD4 mutation carriers often have more severe gastric polyposis, a higher risk of gastric cancer {1806,2875,970,1157,180}, and hereditary haemorrhagic telangiectasia {1005}, whereas carriers of *BMPR1A* mutations are more likely to have cardiac defects.

Epidemiology
The incidence has been estimated to be 1 case per 100 000–160 000 person-years European populations. As many as half of all new cases arise in patients with no related family history {420,3193}.

Etiology
A germline mutation in *SMAD4* or *BMPR1A* is identified in 50–60% of JPS patients with colorectal or generalized juvenile polyposis {3421,180,1295,1299}. Most mutations are point mutations or small base-pair deletions, 5–15% of mutations are larger

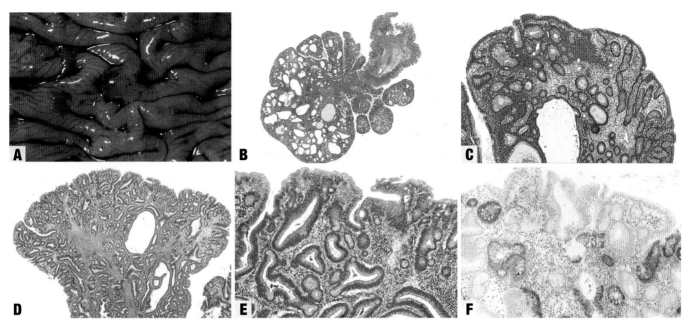

Fig. 14.27 Colonic juvenile polyp. **A** Juvenile polyps are typically spherical with a smooth surface due to erosion. **B** An example from a patient with juvenile polyposis syndrome, characterized by an increase of the stroma and cystically dilated crypts. **C** High-power magnification shows the increased stroma containing inflammatory cells and distorted and dilated crypts lined by non-dysplastic epithelium with reactive changes. **D** Juvenile polyp from a patient with a germline *SMAD4* mutation, with low-grade dysplasia. **E** At higher magnification. **F** SMAD4 loss in an example from a patient with a germline *SMAD4* mutation; note the abrupt and seemingly random loss of SMAD4 in the epithelium; although this polyp harbours low-grade dysplasia, SMAD4 loss is not necessarily associated with neoplastic progression – it can also be seen in non-dysplastic juvenile polyps.

deletions of one or more exons or the entire *SMAD4* or *BMPR1A* gene, and about 10% of mutations involve the gene promoter {3421,180,467}. Juvenile polyposis of infancy is associated with contiguous deletion of *BMPR1A* and *PTEN* genes at chromosome 10q23 {751,2121,2807,709}. Mutations in *ENG* have been found in patients fulfilling the diagnostic criteria for JPS, but the role of *ENG* remains unclear {1442,1296}. Either a family history of polyps, cancer, and extraintestinal findings, or a minimum of 3–5 juvenile polyps is important to ascertain before embarking on genetic testing {1442}.

Pathogenesis
Gastrointestinal cancer in JPS arises from adenomatous epithelium within the juvenile polyp. Neoplasia may develop through a landscaper mechanism, in which it is postulated that neoplastic transformation of the epithelium is the result of an abnormal stromal environment {1613,1170}. In contrast, homozygous *SMAD4* deletion was shown to be limited to the epithelium of juvenile polyps from patients with germline *SMAD4* mutations, suggesting that SMAD4 acts as a gatekeeper in JPS pathogenesis {3606,1788}, although these hypotheses are not mutually exclusive.

Macroscopic appearance
Juvenile polyps are typically spherical with a smooth surface due to erosion.

Histopathology
Smaller juvenile polyps are indistinguishable from sporadic juvenile polyps. They have an eroded surface, abundant oedematous stroma with inflammatory cells, and cystically dilated glands with reactive epithelium. In the multilobulated or atypical variety, the lobules may be either rounded or finger-like. There is a relative increase in the amount of epithelium over stroma. Glands show more budding and branching but less cystic change than in the classic solitary polyp {1436}. Foci of dysplasia are regularly seen, particularly in atypical or multilobulated juvenile polyps {1436,3422}.

Gastric juvenile polyps show irregular hyperplastic glands mostly lined by foveolar epithelium and abundant oedematous stroma. Dysplasia is seen in about 15% of these polyps, which

Table 14.07 Phenotypic subtypes of juvenile polyposis syndrome

Subtype	Clinical features	Associated genetic defects
Juvenile polyposis coli or generalized juvenile polyposis[a]	Polyps restricted to the colorectum Polyps in the stomach, small intestine, and colon	Germline mutation in *SMAD4* (in ~30% of patients) or *BMPR1A* (in ~20% of patients)
Juvenile polyposis of infancy or chromosome 10q22.3-q23.2 deletion syndrome	Generalized polyposis Often severe symptoms (diarrhoea, haemorrhage, malnutrition, intussusceptions) Often death at a young age Often congenital abnormalities	Contiguous *BMPR1A* and/or *PTEN* deletion

[a]Variable expressions of the same disease.

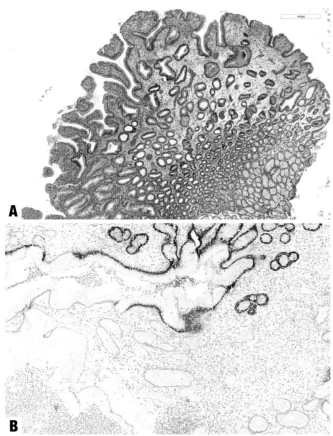

Fig. 14.28 Gastric juvenile polyp. **A** A small polyp from a patient with a germline *SMAD4* mutation, characterized by hyperplastic non-dysplastic foveolar epithelium and oedematous stroma. **B** SMAD4 loss in a polyp from a patient with a germline *SMAD4* mutation.

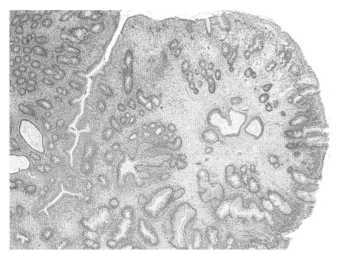

Fig. 14.29 Colonic juvenile polyp. An example from a *BMPR1A* mutation carrier.

can show intestinal or pyloric gland differentiation {1984}. It is difficult to reliably differentiate between gastric hyperplasic, juvenile, and Peutz–Jeghers polyps on the basis of histological features alone. It is therefore advisable to use more-inclusive terminology, such as "hamartomatous polyp NOS", and to recommend additional endoscopic examination with sampling of intestinal polyps and genetic testing in equivocal cases {1780,421}. Loss of SMAD4 immunostaining can be found in about half of all colonic and gastric juvenile polyps from patients with a germline *SMAD4* mutation, and it is indicative of somatic inactivation of the *SMAD4* wildtype allele. In contrast, loss of SMAD4 expression is never seen in sporadic juvenile polyps or juvenile polyps from *BMPR1A* mutation carriers. Loss of epithelial SMAD4 expression in the polyps of individuals with JPS is therefore specific for an underlying *SMAD4* germline mutation and can serve as a first screening for an underlying genetic defect. Loss of SMAD4 is not required for polyp formation or obligatory for neoplastic progression of a juvenile polyp {1788,1806}.

Diagnostic molecular pathology

Not clinically relevant

Essential and desirable diagnostic criteria

The diagnostic criteria for JPS are summarized in Box 14.05 (p. 542). Phenotypic subtypes of JPS and associated genetic defects are presented in Table 14.07 (p. 543).

Staging (TNM)

Not clinically relevant

Prognosis and prediction

Patients with juvenile polyposis of infancy rarely survive past 2 years of age, because of severe diarrhoea, anaemia, and hypoalbuminaemia. Patients with colorectal or generalized juvenile polyposis are mainly at risk of colorectal and upper gastrointestinal cancer. Treatment should focus on preventing malignancy by close surveillance. Prophylactic colorectal and/or gastric surgery should be considered for patients who have a polyp burden that cannot be managed endoscopically, polyps with high-grade dysplasia, or a strong family history of gastrointestinal cancer {416,3193}.

Peutz–Jeghers syndrome

Brosens LAA
Jansen M

Definition
Peutz–Jeghers syndrome (PJS) is an autosomal dominant polyp and cancer predisposition syndrome characterized by mucocutaneous melanin pigmentation and gastrointestinal polyposis.

MIM numbering
175200 Peutz–Jeghers syndrome

ICD-11 coding
LD2D.0 Peutz–Jeghers syndrome

Related terminology
None

Subtype(s)
None

Localization
About 95% of patients with PJS have polyps in the small intestine. A reported 25% of patients have polyps in the colon and stomach {421}, but this may be an underestimate, because

Box 14.06 Diagnostic criteria for Peutz–Jeghers syndrome (PJS)

1. ≥ 3 histologically confirmed Peutz–Jeghers polyps
2. Any number of Peutz–Jeghers polyps with a family history of PJS
3. Characteristic, prominent[a] mucocutaneous pigmentation with a family history of PJS
4. Any number of Peutz–Jeghers polyps and characteristic, prominent mucocutaneous pigmentation

[a]Some melanin pigmentation is also regularly seen in unaffected individuals, hence the emphasis on the prominence of the pigmentation; moreover, the pigmentation in patients with PJS may disappear with time and can in rare cases be absent altogether.

polyps in these sites are not as likely as small bowel polyps to be clinically prominent.

Clinical features
The diagnostic criteria are summarized in Box 14.06. Presenting symptoms include abdominal pain, intestinal bleeding, anaemia, and intussusception, which typically manifest in the first two decades of life {420}. If present, the characteristic mucocutaneous pigmentation facilitates diagnosis of asymptomatic patients in familial cases, but the characteristic Peutz–Jeghers polyps

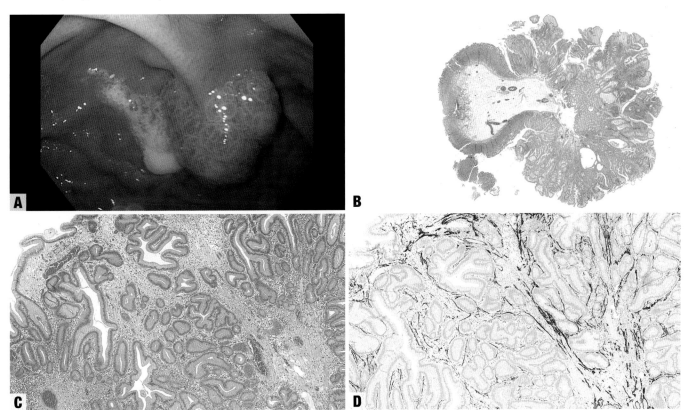

Fig. 14.30 Gastric Peutz–Jeghers polyp. **A** Endoscopic appearance. **B** Polyp with hyperplastic foveolar epithelium and inflammatory stroma with some cords of smooth muscle. **C** Polyp with inflammatory stroma, smooth muscle fibres, and non-dysplastic hyperplastic foveolar epithelium. **D** Caldesmon immunohistochemistry highlighting the smooth muscle fibres in the stroma.

Table 14.08 Peutz–Jeghers syndrome cancer risks for specific anatomical localizations at 65–70 years of age

Site	Cancer risk
Colorectum	39%
Small intestine	13%
Stomach	29%
Pancreas	11–36%
Breast	32–54%
Uterus	9%
Ovary	21%
Cervix	10%
Testis	9%
Lung	7–17%

are the main clinical hallmark. PJS is associated with a moderate or high risk of a range of malignancies, with an overall risk of any cancer by the age of 70 years of 81% (see Table 14.08) {1205,1034,1036}. Well-documented extraintestinal tumours include carcinomas of the breast and pancreas, as well as otherwise rare gonadal lesions, including sex cord tumour with annular tubules of the ovary and Sertoli cell tumour of the testis.

Epidemiology
The incidence of PJS is roughly one tenth that of FAP, with an estimated incidence of 1 case per 50 000–200 000 births.

Etiology
A germline mutation in the tumour suppressor gene *STK11* (formerly called *LKB1*), which encodes a serine/threonine kinase, can be found in > 90% of patients with PJS. Most germline defects are point mutations and small intragenic deletions, but some larger deletions of one or more exons have also been described {735}.

Pathogenesis
The direct precursor to gastrointestinal cancer in patients with PJS remains unknown {1426}. Peutz–Jeghers polyps are likely

an epiphenomenon to the cancer-prone condition and not obligate malignant precursors. Indeed, dysplasia in a Peutz–Jeghers polyp is exceedingly rare. In normal colonic crypts from patients with PJS, a protracted clonal evolution has been shown, allowing accumulation of mutations over time, which potentially explains the increased risk of colorectal cancer {1426,1787}.

Macroscopic appearance
The macroscopic appearance is not distinctive.

Histopathology
Colorectal Peutz–Jeghers polyps have a distinctive histology, with villous architecture and arborizing smooth muscle cores. Epithelial misplacement due to prolapse and peristaltic kneading is relatively common in Peutz–Jeghers polyps and may extend into the serosa, mimicking a well-differentiated invasive lesion {1426}. Gastric Peutz–Jeghers polyps often lack specific histology and are often not readily distinguishable from gastric juvenile polyps or sporadic hyperplastic polyps. Without knowledge of the clinical context, one should therefore be cautious about establishing a new diagnosis of PJS on the basis of gastric polyps alone {1780,421}.

Diagnostic molecular pathology
Not clinically relevant

Essential and desirable diagnostic criteria
The diagnostic criteria for PJS are presented in Box 14.06 (p. 545).

Staging (TNM)
Not clinically relevant

Prognosis and prediction
Small bowel intussusception can be a major source of mortality in PJS, but this can be prevented with push enteroscopy with clean-sweep polypectomy and treated by surgery {3554}. The prognosis for patients with PJS is now mainly determined by the risk of malignancy, and an increased cancer mortality has been shown in PJS {3426}. Patients with PJS should be surveilled to prevent gastrointestinal complications and cancer {3193}.

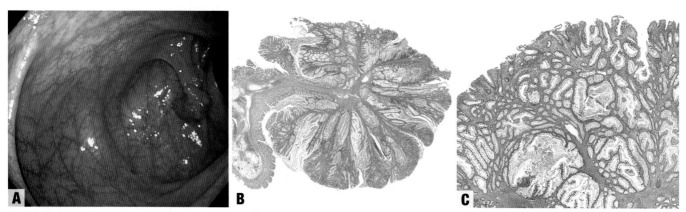

Fig. 14.31 Colonic Peutz–Jeghers polyp. **A** Endoscopic appearance. **B** Characterized by arborizing strands of smooth muscle and overlying non-neoplastic epithelium. **C** Detail of a polyp characterized by smooth muscle cores and non-neoplastic epithelium.

Cowden syndrome

Brosens LAA
Jansen M

Definition
Cowden syndrome (CS) is an autosomal dominant disorder characterized by multiple hamartomas involving organs derived from any of the three germ layers, with cancer predisposition.

MIM numbering
158350 Cowden syndrome 1
615107 Cowden syndrome 4
615108 Cowden syndrome 5
615109 Cowden syndrome 6
616858 Cowden syndrome 7

ICD-11 coding
LD2D.Y Cowden syndrome

Related terminology
Acceptable: Cowden disease; multiple hamartoma syndrome; *PTEN* hamartoma tumour syndrome.

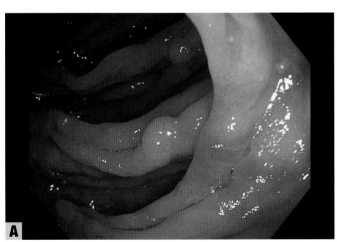

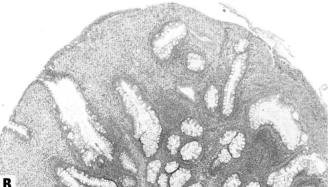

Fig. 14.32 Cowden syndrome. **A** Endoscopic appearance of small colonic Cowden polyps. **B** A juvenile polyp at medium power.

Box 14.07 The International Cowden Consortium (ICC) operational diagnostic criteria {3232}

Pathognomonic criteria
- Adult Lhermitte–Duclos disease (cerebellar tumours)
- Mucocutaneous lesions
    - Facial trichilemmomas, any number[a] (≥ 2 biopsy-proven trichilemmomas[b])
    - Acral keratoses
    - Papillomatous papules
- Mucosal lesions
- Autism spectrum disorder

Major criteria
- Breast cancer
- Non-medullary thyroid cancer
- Megalocephaly
- Endometrial carcinoma
- Mucocutaneous lesions[b]
    - 1 biopsy-proven trichilemmoma
    - Multiple palmoplantar keratoses
    - Multifocal cutaneous facial papules
    - Macular pigmentation of the glans penis
- Multiple gastrointestinal hamartomas or ganglioneuromas[b]

Minor criteria
- Other thyroid lesions (follicular adenomas, multinodular goitre)
- Mental retardation (i.e. IQ of ≤ 75)
- Gastrointestinal hamartomas[a] (single gastrointestinal hamartoma or ganglioneuroma[b])
- Fibrocystic breast disease
- Lipomas
- Fibromas
- Genitourinary tumours (especially renal cell carcinoma)
- Genitourinary malformations[a]
- Uterine fibroids
- Autism spectrum disorder[b]

Relaxed ICC operational diagnostic criteria for Cowden syndrome
≥ 1 pathognomonic criterion
   or
≥ 2 major or minor criteria

[a]Present in this section as defined by ICC criteria only. [b]Present in this section as defined by National Comprehensive Cancer Network (NCCN) 2010 criteria only.

Subtype(s)
PTEN hamartoma tumour syndrome (PHTS) is a heterogeneous group of disorders with autosomal dominant inheritance, caused by germline mutation of the *PTEN* gene. PHTS also includes Bannayan–Riley–Ruvalcaba syndrome and Proteus syndrome. However, most cases of PHTS correspond to CS, and the terms "PHTS" and "CS" are often used interchangeably {1253}.

Localization
Gastrointestinal polyps are present in virtually all patients with CS, occurring throughout the GI tract. Diffuse oesophageal glycogenic acanthosis is present in > 80% of CS cases.

Table 14.09 Lifetime cancer risks and general screening recommendations in *PTEN* hamartoma tumour syndrome {3233,2126,2582}

Cancer	Lifetime risk	Patient age at cancer diagnosis	Predominant histology	Recommended screening
Breast (female)	25–85%	38–50 years	Ductal adenocarcinoma	Starting at age 30 years: annual mammogram; consider MRI for patients with dense breasts
Thyroid	35%	Unknown	Follicular carcinoma	Annual ultrasound
Endometrial	19–28%	< 50 years	Endometrioid adenocarcinoma	Starting at age 30 years: annual endometrial biopsy or transvaginal ultrasound
Renal cell	34%	Unknown	Unknown	Starting at age 40 years: renal imaging every 2 years
Colon	9%	< 50 years	n/a	Starting at age 40 years: colonoscopy every 2 years
Melanoma	6%	Unknown	n/a	Annual dermatological examination

n/a, not applicable.

CS is associated with an increased risk of colorectal cancer {501,671,1869}.

Clinical features

CS is characterized by mucocutaneous lesions (multiple facial trichilemmomas, acral keratoses, papillomatous papules, and mucosal lesions are considered pathognomonic), an increased cancer risk, benign hamartomatous overgrowth of tissues (including gastrointestinal polyposis), and macrocephaly (see Box 14.07, p. 547, and Table 14.09) {2582}. Cancer risk is relatively broad, with risk of breast, thyroid, endometrial, renal cell, and colon cancers; melanoma; and other cancers {862}.

Epidemiology

The prevalence is estimated at about 1 in 200 000–250 000 in European populations, but this may be an underestimate, given the difficulty in diagnosing this syndrome {2329}.

Etiology

CS is an autosomal dominant disorder with age-related penetrance and variable expression. Germline mutation in *PTEN* (10q23.3) is found in about 85% of CS cases, as well as in subsets of other PHTS disorders (in 65% of Bannayan–Riley–Ruvalcaba syndrome cases, 20% of Proteus syndrome cases, and 50% of Proteus-like syndrome cases) {1253,2459,1900,2330}. Individualized risk calculation may aid assessment of a patient's risk of carrying a germline *PTEN* mutation based on clinical features {3232}.

Germline succinate dehydrogenase mutations have been found in about 5% of *PTEN* mutation–negative CS / CS-like individuals and are associated with increased frequencies of breast, thyroid, and renal cancers beyond those conferred by germline *PTEN* mutation {2349}.

Pathogenesis

PTEN is a virtually ubiquitously expressed tumour suppressor and a dual-specificity lipid and protein phosphatase that regulates cell proliferation, cell migration, and apoptosis through inhibition of AKT via the PI3K/AKT pathway {2126}. Inactivation of the second copy of the gene allows deregulation of the AKT pathway.

Macroscopic appearance

See the descriptions of the polyps within the relevant sections.

Histopathology

Gastrointestinal polyps in CS represent a mixture of histology {1204}. Hyperplastic polyps, hamartomatous/juvenile polyps, adenomas, and ganglioneuromas are the most frequent types of polyps in the colon {421}. Polyps typically measure between 3–10 mm, but they can be larger. Hyperplastic polyps are not part of the diagnostic criteria for PHTS. Colonic intramucosal lipomas have also been associated with CS {464}.

Polyps in the duodenum are mainly hamartomas and some ganglioneuromas and adenomas {421}. Most patients with CS

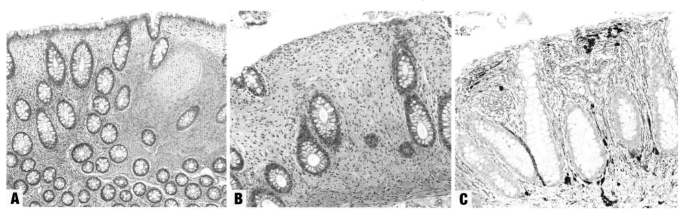

Fig. 14.33 Colonic ganglioneuroma in Cowden syndrome. **A,B** High-power views. **C** Neuron-specific enolase immunohistochemistry highlights ganglion cells in the lamina propria.

have gastric polyps {671,1869}, which are usually numerous, measure 1–20 mm, and are mostly diagnosed as hyperplastic or hamartomatous polyps. Dysplasia has not been reported in gastric CS polyps. Although incidental CS patients with gastric cancer have been reported, an increased gastric cancer risk has not been verified {1204,3233,421}. Diffuse oesophageal glycogenic acanthosis in combination with colonic polyposis may be diagnostic of CS {671,1869}.

Diagnostic molecular pathology
Not clinically relevant

Essential and desirable diagnostic criteria
The International Cowden Consortium (ICC) operational diagnostic criteria are listed in Box 14.07 (p. 547).

Staging (TNM)
Not clinically relevant

Prognosis and prediction
Patients with PHTS are at increased risk of several types of cancer, and interval screening is recommended (see Table 14.09) {3233,2126,434}.

Other genetic tumour syndromes

Frayling IM
Arends MJ
Tomlinson I

A number of genetic tumour predisposition syndromes confer a raised risk of various gastrointestinal tumours, including Li–Fraumeni syndrome (LFS), hereditary haemorrhagic telangiectasia (HHT), syndromes associated with gastroenteropancreatic neuroendocrine tumours (NETs), and multilocus inherited neoplasia alleles syndrome (MINAS).

MIM numbering

151623 Li–Fraumeni syndrome
175050 Hereditary haemorrhagic telangiectasia
131100 Multiple endocrine neoplasia type 1
171400 Multiple endocrine neoplasia type 2A
162300 Multiple endocrine neoplasia type 2B
610755 Multiple endocrine neoplasia type 4
162200 Neurofibromatosis type 1
191100 Tuberous sclerosis 1
613254 Tuberous sclerosis 2
193300 Von Hippel–Lindau syndrome

Li–Fraumeni syndrome

LFS is caused by dominantly inherited mutations in the tumour suppressor gene TP53 {2069}. Tumours characteristic of LFS include bone and soft tissue sarcomas; adrenocortical, brain, and breast cancers; and acute leukaemia. Recent analyses have shown that about one fifth of all families with LFS have young-onset gastric cancers and about one tenth have both gastric and colorectal cancers, but there was no association with the TP53 mutation location within the gene {2439,2069,183,679,3445}. There is only one published report of colorectal adenomatous polyposis and young-onset cancer in LFS, so that appears to have been an exceptional case {3711}; the increased risk of colorectal cancer in LFS appears to be low. In one large study (of 397 patients in 64 families), only 11 patients from 10 families developed colorectal cancer, albeit at a relatively young mean age (33 years), with 4 of the patients aged < 21 years {3598}. More recently, an increased risk of colon, gastric, and pancreatic cancer has been reported in LFS {2800,381,119}. The occurrence of both gastric and colorectal cancers at such young ages (at least in some cases) is good evidence of predisposition, but these studies were performed before the advent of cancer gene panel testing, so it is unknown whether the patients harboured mutations in other tumour-predisposing genes and therefore in fact had MINAS, in which patients have inherited mutations in more than one predisposing gene {3559}. Therefore, patients with LFS who develop GI tract tumours should be offered comprehensive cancer gene panel testing or exome/genome sequencing.

Hereditary haemorrhagic telangiectasia

HHT is a syndrome clinically distinct from juvenile polyposis syndrome (JPS). HHT is caused by mutations in ENG (encoding endoglin) and ACVRL1 (ALK1), with a few other genes also affected in some cases, whereas JPS is caused by mutations in SMAD4 and BMPR1A. HHT, which is also known as Osler–Weber–Rendu syndrome, has autosomal dominant inheritance and is characterized by recurrent epistaxis, mucocutaneous telangiectasia, and visceral arteriovenous malformations, including involvement of the GI tract. However, hamartomatous polyps (of JPS type) can also occur in HHT, and this may represent an allelic subtype of JPS (see Juvenile polyposis syndrome, p. 542). However, combined juvenile polyposis / HHT syndrome due to mutations in SMAD4 has also been described, with the mutations mostly clustering in the C-terminal MH2 domain of the SMAD4 protein. Therefore, SMAD4 mutations may increase the risk of gastrointestinal juvenile polyps, HHT-type visceral telangiectasia and arteriovenous malformations, early-onset gastrointestinal cancer, and juvenile idiopathic arthritis {1004,337}.

Syndromes associated with gastroenteropancreatic NETs

Approximately 5–10% of gastroenteropancreatic NETs may occur as part of a known predisposition syndrome, typically multiple endocrine neoplasia type 1, neurofibromatosis type 1, Cowden syndrome, tuberous sclerosis, or von Hippel–Lindau syndrome {3366,551,3127,1630,1993,152,70,1761}.

Multilocus inherited neoplasia alleles syndrome

MINAS is defined by the presence of two or more inherited cancer predisposition mutant alleles in the same individual. In the past, this syndrome has been underascertained, because standard clinical practice was to sequentially test for candidate inherited cancer genes until a pathogenic mutation was detected. Recently, the increased use of next-generation sequencing technologies for cancer gene panel testing and exome/genome sequencing has made it possible to test for many inherited cancer predisposition genes in parallel, facilitating the identification of patients with pathogenic mutations in more than one inherited cancer gene allele (i.e. with MINAS). Reported cases include the co-occurrence of a mutation in the mismatch repair gene MLH1 (causing Lynch syndrome) and a homozygous mutation in the nucleotide excision repair gene XPA (causing xeroderma pigmentosum) in an individual with two colon adenocarcinomas as well as skin lesions typical of xeroderma pigmentosum {3559}. For patients who show features of more than one condition, sequential genetic testing should not be stopped once a first pathogenic mutation has been identified.

Contributors

ADSAY, N. Volkan
Istanbul
TURKEY

AGAIMY, Abbas
Erlangen University Hospital
Krankenhausstraße 8-10
91054 Erlangen
GERMANY

AISHIMA, Shinichi
Saga University
5-1-1 Nabeshima
Saga 849-8501
JAPAN

ANTONESCU, Cristina R.
Memorial Sloan Kettering Cancer Center
1275 York Avenue
New York NY 10065
USA

ARENDS, Mark J.
Cancer Research UK Edinburgh Centre
MRC Institute of Genetics & Molecular Medicine
University of Edinburgh
Crewe Road South
Edinburgh EH4 2XR
UNITED KINGDOM

AROLA, Johanna
HUSLAB, University of Helsinki and
Helsinki University Hospital
Haartmaninkatu 3
00014 Helsinki
FINLAND

BASTURK, Olca
Memorial Sloan Kettering Cancer Center
1275 York Avenue
New York NY 10065
USA

BELLIZZI, Andrew M.
University of Iowa Hospitals and Clinics
200 Hawkins Drive
Iowa City IA 52242
USA

BHAGAT, Govind
Columbia University Medical Center
VC14-228, 630W 168th Street
New York NY 10032
USA

BIOULAC-SAGE, Paulette
Inserm, Université de Bordeaux
146 Rue Léo Saignat
33076 Bordeaux
FRANCE

BROSENS, Lodewijk A.A.
University Medical Center Utrecht
Heidelberglaan 100
3584 CX Utrecht
NETHERLANDS

BROWN, Ian S.
Envoi Pathology
5/38 Bishop Street
Kelvin Grove QLD 4059
AUSTRALIA

CAMPO, Elias*
Hospital Clinic of Barcelona
IDIBAPS
University of Barcelona
Carrer de Villarroel 170
08036 Barcelona
SPAIN

CARNEIRO, Fátima
Ipatimup/i3S
Rua Júlio Amaral de Carvalho 45
4200-135 Porto
PORTUGAL

CARR, Norman J.
Basingstoke and North Hampshire Hospital
Aldermaston Road
Basingstoke RG24 9NA
UNITED KINGDOM

CHADBURN, Amy
Weill Cornell Medicine
525 East 68th Street, ST-709
New York NY 10021
USA

CHAN, John K.C.
Queen Elizabeth Hospital
30 Gascoigne Road
Kowloon, Hong Kong SAR
CHINA

CHAN, Wing Chung*
City of Hope
1500 East Duarte Road
Duarte CA 91010
USA

CHENEVIX-TRENCH, Georgia
QIMR Berghofer
300 Herston Road
Brisbane QLD 4006
AUSTRALIA

CHEUK, Wah
Queen Elizabeth Hospital
30 Gascoigne Road
Kowloon, Hong Kong SAR
CHINA

CHEUNG, Nga-Yin Annie
University of Hong Kong
Queen Mary Hospital
Pok Fu Lam Road
Hong Kong SAR
CHINA

CHOTT, Andreas
Wilhelminenspital
Montleartstraße 37
1160 Vienna
AUSTRIA

COUVELARD, Anne*
Bichat Hospital AP-HP
46 Rue Henri Huchard
75018 PARIS
FRANCE

CREE, Ian A.
International Agency for Research on Cancer
150 Cours Albert Thomas
69372 Lyon
FRANCE

DE BOER, Willem Bastiaan
PathWest Laboratory Medicine WA
Fiona Stanley Hospital
Robin Warren Drive, Murdoch
Perth WA 6150
AUSTRALIA

DE LEVAL, Laurence
Institute of Pathology
Lausanne University Hospital
University of Lausanne
25 Rue du Bugnon
1011 Lausanne
SWITZERLAND

DEI TOS, Angelo Paolo*
University of Padua School of Medicine
Piazza Ospedale 1
31100 Treviso TV
ITALY

---

* Indicates disclosure of interests (see p. 557).

DEKKER, Evelien
Amsterdam UMC
Meibergdreef 9
1105 AZ Amsterdam
NETHERLANDS

DELABIE, Jan
University Health Network and
University of Toronto
200 Elizabeth Street
Toronto ON M5G 2C4
CANADA

DOYLE, Leona A.
Brigham and Women's Hospital
Harvard Medical School
75 Francis Street
Boston MA 02115
USA

DRY, Sarah M.
University of California, Los Angeles (UCLA)
13-222 CHS, 10833 Le Conte Avenue
Los Angeles CA 90095
USA

ESPOSITO, Irene
Institute of Pathology
Heinrich-Heine University and
University Hospital of Düsseldorf
Moorenstraße 5
40225 Düsseldorf
GERMANY

FERRY, Judith A.
Massachusetts General Hospital
55 Fruit Street
Boston MA 02114
USA

FITZGIBBONS, Patrick L.
St. Jude Medical Center
101 East Valencia Mesa Drive
Fullerton CA 92835
USA

FRANKEL, Wendy L.*
Ohio State University
Wexner Medical Center
1645 Neil Avenue, 129 Hamilton Hall
Columbus OH 43210
USA

FRAYLING, Ian M.
Institute of Medical Genetics
University Hospital of Wales
Cardiff CF14 4XW
UNITED KINGDOM

FRITCHIE, Karen J.
Mayo Clinic
200 First Street South-West
Rochester MN 55905
USA

FUJII, Satoshi
Exploratory Oncology Research &
Clinical Trial Center, National Cancer Center
6-5-1 Kashiwanoha
Kashiwa 277-8577
JAPAN

FUKAYAMA, Masashi
Graduate School of Medicine
University of Tokyo
7-3-1 Hongo, Bunkyo-ku
Tokyo 113-0033
JAPAN

FUKUSHIMA, Noriyoshi
Jichi Medical University
3311-1 Yakushiji, Shimotsuke
Tochigi 329-0498
JAPAN

FURUKAWA, Toru
Tohoku University Graduate School of Medicine
2-1 Seiryomachi, Aoba-ku
Sendai 980-8575
JAPAN

GASSON, Sophie
Independent Cancer Patients' Voice (ICPV)
17 Woodbridge Street
London EC1R 0LL
UNITED KINGDOM

GAULARD, Philippe
Hôpital Henri-Mondor
51 Avenue du Maréchal de Lattre de Tassigny
94010 Créteil
FRANCE

GENTA, Robert M.G.
Baylor College of Medicine
1 Baylor Plaza
Houston TX 77030
USA

GILL, Anthony J.
Royal North Shore Hospital
Pacific Highway
St Leonards NSW 2065
AUSTRALIA

GOLDBLUM, John R.
Cleveland Clinic
9500 Euclid Avenue L25
Cleveland OH 44195
USA

GRABSCH, Heike I.*
Department of Pathology
GROW School for Oncology and
Developmental Biology
Maastricht University Medical Center+
P. Debyelaan 25
6229 HX Maastricht
NETHERLANDS

GRAHAM, Rondell P.
Mayo Clinic
200 First Street South-West
Rochester MN 55905
USA

GUILFORD, Parry
University of Otago
PO Box 56
Dunedin 9016
NEW ZEALAND

HAMILTON, Stanley R.*
University of Texas
MD Anderson Cancer Center
1515 Holcombe Boulevard
Unit 85, Room G1.3540
Houston TX 77030
USA

HARPAZ, Noam
Icahn School of Medicine at Mount Sinai
1468 Madison Avenue
New York NY 10029
USA

HIRAOKA, Nobuyoshi*
National Cancer Center Hospital
5-1-1 Tsukiji, Chuo-ku
Tokyo 104-0045
JAPAN

HONG, Seung-Mo
Asan Medical Center
University of Ulsan College of Medicine
88 Olympic-ro 43 gil, Songpa-gu
Seoul 05505
REPUBLIC OF KOREA

HORNICK, Jason L.*
Brigham and Women's Hospital
Harvard Medical School
75 Francis Street
Boston MA 02115
USA

HORNY, Hans-Peter*
Institute of Pathology
Thalkirchnerstraße 36
72074 Munich
GERMANY

* Indicates disclosure of interests (see p. 557).

HRUBAN, Ralph H.*
Johns Hopkins University School of Medicine
Carnegie Room 415, 600 North Wolfe Street
Baltimore MD 21287-6417
USA

JAFFE, Elaine S.
National Cancer Institute
10 Center Drive, Room 3S 235
Bethesda MD 20892-1500
USA

JANSEN, Marnix*
University College London
21 University Street, Rockefeller Building
Room 410, Histopathology Department
London WC1E 6DE
UNITED KINGDOM

KAKAR, Sanjay
University of California San Francisco
505 Parnassus Avenue
San Francisco CA 94143
USA

KASAJIMA, Atsuko
Technical University of Munich
Ismaningerstraße 22
81675 Munich
GERMANY

KAWACHI, Hiroshi
Cancer Institute Hospital of
Japanese Foundation for Cancer Research
3-8-31 Ariake, Koto-ku
Tokyo 135-8550
JAPAN

KLIMSTRA, David S.
Memorial Sloan Kettering Cancer Center
1275 York Avenue
New York NY 10065
USA

KLÖPPEL, Günter
Technical University of Munich
Ismaningerstraße 22
81675 Munich
GERMANY

KO, Young Hyeh
Samsung Medical Center
Sungkyunkwan University School of Medicine
81 Irwon-ro, Gangnam-gu
Seoul 06351
REPUBLIC OF KOREA

KOMMINOTH, Paul
University of Zurich
Institute of Pathology
City Hospital Triemli
Birmensdorferstrasse 497
8063 Zurich
SWITZERLAND

KOMUTA, Mina
Cliniques Universitaires Saint-Luc
Avenue Hippocrate 10
1200 Brussels
BELGIUM

KONDO, Fukuo
Teikyo University Hospital
2-11-1, Kaga, Itabashi-ku
Tokyo 173-8606
JAPAN

KUMARASINGHE, M. Priyanthi
PathWest and University of Western Australia
J Block, QEII Medical Centre
Nedlands WA 6009
AUSTRALIA

KUSHIMA, Ryoji
Shiga University of Medical Science
Seta-Tsukinowa
Otsu 520-2192
JAPAN

LA ROSA, Stefano
Institute of Pathology
Lausanne University Hospital
University of Lausanne
25 Rue du Bugnon
1011 Lausanne
SWITZERLAND

LAI, Jinping
Kaiser Permanente, Permanente Medicine
Permanente Medical Group
KP Sacramento Medical Center
2025 Morse Avenue
Sacramento CA 95825
USA

LAKHANI, Sunil R.*
University of Queensland and
Pathology Queensland
Royal Brisbane and Women's Hospital Campus
Royal Brisbane and Women's Hospital
Herston QLD 4029
AUSTRALIA

LAM, Alfred King Yin
Griffith University School of Medicine
Gold Coast Campus
Gold Coast QLD 4222
AUSTRALIA

LAUWERS, Gregory Y.
H. Lee Moffitt Cancer Center and Research
Institute and University of South Florida,
Morsani College of Medicine
12902 USF Magnolia Drive
Tampa FL 33612-9416
USA

LAX, Sigurd F.
General Hospital Graz West
Göstinger Straße 22
8020 Graz
AUSTRIA

LAZAR, Alexander J.
University of Texas
MD Anderson Cancer Center
1515 Holcombe Boulevard, Unit 85
Houston TX 77030
USA

LEONCINI, Lorenzo
University of Siena
Department of Medical Biotechnology
Pathological Anatomy Division
Via dele Scotte
53100 Siena SI
ITALY

LI, Gan Di
West China Hospital, Sichuan University
37 Guoxuexiang
Chengdu 610041
CHINA

LI, Xiao-Qiu
Fudan University Shanghai Cancer Center
270 Dong-an Road
Shanghai 200032
CHINA

MAITRA, Anirban
MD Anderson Cancer Center
1515 Holcombe Boulevard
Houston TX 77030
USA

MÄKINEN, Markus J.*
University of Oulu
Aapistie 5
90220 Oulu
FINLAND

MIETTINEN, Markku
National Cancer Institute
National Institutes of Health
9000 Rockville Pike
Building 10, Room 2S235C
Bethesda MD 20892-0001
USA

* Indicates disclosure of interests (see p. 557).

MISDRAJI, Joseph
Massachusetts General Hospital
55 Fruit Street
Boston MA 02114
USA

MOCH, Holger
University of Zurich and
University Hospital Zurich
12 Schmelzbergstrasse
8091 Zurich
SWITZERLAND

MONTES-MORENO, Santiago
Hospital Universitario Marqués de
Valdecilla / IDIVAL
Avenida de Valdecilla 25
39008 Santander
SPAIN

MONTGOMERY, Elizabeth A.
Johns Hopkins Medical Institutions
Weinberg 2242, 401 North Broadway
Baltimore MD 21231
USA

MORREAU, Hans
Leiden University Medical Center
Albinusdreef 2
3000 DR Leiden
NETHERLANDS

NAGTEGAAL, Iris D.*
Radboud University Medical Center
PO Box 9101
6500 HB Nijmegen (812)
NETHERLANDS

NAKAMURA, Shigeo
Nagoya University Hospital
65 Tsurumai-cho, Showa-ku
Nagoya 466-8550
JAPAN

NAKANUMA, Yasuni
Kanazawa University Graduate School
of Medicine
13-1 Takaramachi
Kanazawa 820-8640
JAPAN

NAULT, Jean Charles
AP-HP
Avenue du 14 Juillet
93140 Bondy
FRANCE

NG, Irene O.L.
University of Hong Kong
Queen Mary Hospital
Hong Kong SAR
CHINA

NOTOHARA, Kenji
Kurashiki Central Hospital
1-1-1 Miwa
Kurashiki 710-8602
JAPAN

OCHIAI, Atsushi
National Cancer Center
6-5-1 Kashiwanoha
Kashiwa 277-8577
JAPAN

ODZE, Robert D.
Boston MA
USA

OFFERHAUS, G. Johan A.
University Medical Center Utrecht
PO Box 85500
3508 GA Utrecht
NETHERLANDS

OHASHI, Kenichi
Yokohama City University School of Medicine
3-9 Fukuura, Kanazawa-ku
Yokohama 236-0004
JAPAN

OHIKE, Nobuyuki
Showa University Fujigaoka Hospital
1-30 Fujigaoka, Aoba-ku
Yokohama 227-8501
JAPAN

OLIVA, Esther
Massachusetts General Hospital
55 Fruit Street
Boston MA 02114
USA

OLIVEIRA, Carla
i3S - Instituto de Investigação e Inovação em
Saúde & IPATIMUP - Institute of Molecular
Pathology and Immunology of the
University of Porto
Rua Alfredo Allen 208
4200-135 Porto
PORTUGAL

OTT, German
Department of Clinical Pathology
Robert-Bosch-Krankenhaus
Auerbachstraße 110
70376 Stuttgart
GERMANY

PAI, Reetesh K.
University of Pittsburgh Medical Center
200 Lothrop Street, Room A610, UPMC
Presbyterian Hospital, Department of Pathology
Pittsburgh PA 15213
USA

PAI, Rish K.
Mayo Clinic Arizona
13400 East Shea Boulevard
Scottsdale AZ 85259
USA

PARADIS, Valérie
Hôpital Beaujon
100 Boulevard du Général Leclerc
92118 Clichy
FRANCE

PARK, Young Nyun
Yonsei University College of Medicine
PO Box 8044
Seoul 03722
REPUBLIC OF KOREA

PERREN, Aurel*
University of Bern
31 Murtenstrasse
3008 Bern
SWITZERLAND

PILERI, Stefano A.
European Institute of Oncology
Via Giuseppe Ripamonti 435
20141 Milan MI
ITALY

PITMAN, Martha Bishop*
Harvard Medical School
Massachusetts General Hospital
55 Fruit Street
Boston MA 02114
USA

PRIETO, Victor G.*
University of Texas
MD Anderson Cancer Center
1515 Holcombe Boulevard
Houston TX 77030
USA

QUAGLIA, Alberto
Cellular Pathology
Royal Free London NHS Foundation Trust
University College London
Pond Street
London NW3 2QG
UNITED KINGDOM

REID, Michelle D.
Emory University Hospital
1364 Clifton Road North-East, Room G179B
Atlanta GA 30322
USA

---

* Indicates disclosure of interests (see p. 557).

RINDI, Guido*
Anatomic Pathology
Fondazione Policlinico Universitario
A. Gemelli IRCCS
Università Cattolica del Sacro Cuore
Largo Agostino Gemelli 8
00168 Rome RM
ITALY

ROA, Juan Carlos
Pontificia Universidad Católica de Chile
Marcoleta 377, 7th Floor
Santiago 8330024
CHILE

RONCALLI, Massimo
Humanitas University (Hunimed)
Via Rita Levi Montalcini 4
20090 Pieve Emanuele MI
ITALY

ROSENWALD, Andreas
Institute of Pathology
Josef-Schneider-Straße 2
97080 Würzburg
GERMANY

ROSSI, Sabrina
Bambino Gesù Children's Hospital
Piazza Sant'Onofrio 4
00165 Rome RM
ITALY

ROSTY, Christophe
Envoi Pathology
5/38 Bishop Street
Brisbane QLD 4059
AUSTRALIA

ROUS, Brian
Public Health England
Victoria House, Capital Park
Fulbourn, Cambridge CB21 XB
UNITED KINGDOM

RUGGE, Massimo
University of Padova
Via Aristide Gabelli 61
35100 Padua PD
ITALY

SAITO, Tsuyoshi
Juntendo University
3-1-1 Hongo, Bunkyo-ku
Tokyo 113-8421
JAPAN

SAKAMATO, Michiie
Keio University School of Medicine
35 Shinanomachi, Shinjuku-ku
Tokyo 160-8582
JAPAN

SALTO-TELLEZ, Manuel
Queen's University Belfast
97 Lisburn Road
Belfast BT9 7AE
UNITED KINGDOM

SASANO, Hironobu*
Tohoku University School of Medicine
2-1 Seiryou-machi, Aoba-ku
Sendai 980-8575
JAPAN

SAXENA, Romil
Indiana University
350 West 11th Street, Room 4014
Indianapolis IN 46202
USA

SCARPA, Aldo
ARC-Net Research Centre
University of Verona
Policlinico G.B. Rossi, Piazzale L.A. Scuro 10
37134 Verona VR
ITALY

SCHIRMACHER, Peter
Heidelberg University
Im Neuenheimer Feld 224
69120 Heidelberg
GERMANY

SCIOT, Raf
University Hospital Gasthuisberg, KULeuven
Herestraat 49
3000 Leuven
BELGIUM

SCOAZEC, Jean-Yves
Gustave Roussy Cancer Campus
114 Rue Edouard Vaillant
94805 Villejuif
FRANCE

SCOLYER, Richard A.
Royal Prince Alfred Hospital
Melanoma Institute Australia and
University of Sydney
Missenden Road Camperdown
Sydney NSW 2050
AUSTRALIA

SEKINE, Shigeki
National Cancer Center Hospital
5-1-1 Tsukiji, Chuo-ku
Tokyo 104-0045
JAPAN

SEMPOUX, Christine
Institute of Pathology
Lausanne University Hospital
University of Lausanne
25 Rue du Bugnon
1011 Lausanne
SWITZERLAND

SETO, Masao
Kurume University School of Medicine
67 Asahimachi
Kurume 830-0011
JAPAN

SHI, Chanjuan
Vanderbilt University Medical Center
1161 21st Avenue South, C-3321 MCN
Nashville TN 37232
USA

SHIA, Jinru
Memorial Sloan Kettering Cancer Center
1275 York Avenue
New York NY 10065
USA

SIEBERT, Reiner
Ulm University & Ulm University Medical Center
Albert-Einstein-Allee 11
89081 Ulm
GERMANY

SINGH, Rajendra
Icahn School of Medicine at Mount Sinai
1 Gustave L. Levy Place
New York NY 10029
USA

SINGHI, Aatur D.
University of Pittsburgh Medical Center
200 Lothrop Street, Room A616.2
Pittsburgh PA 15213
USA

SIPOS, Bence*
University Hospital Tübingen
Liebermeisterstraße 8
72076 Tübingen
GERMANY

SOARES, Fernando Augusto
Rede D'Or Hospitals
Rua das Perobas 266
São Paulo SP 04321-120
BRAZIL

SOLCIA, Enrico
Anatomic Pathology
University of Pavia
Via Forlanini 16
27100 Pavia PV
ITALY

SRIGLEY, John R.
Trillium Health Partners
Credit Valley Hospital Site
2200 Eglinton Avenue West
Mississauga ON L5M 2N1
CANADA

* Indicates disclosure of interests (see p. 557).

TAKEUCHI, Kengo
Japanese Foundation for Cancer Research
3-8-31 Ariake, Koto
Tokyo 135-8550
JAPAN

TAKUBO, Kaiyo
Tokyo Metropolitan Institute of Gerontology
35-2 Sakaecho, Itabashi-ku
Tokyo 173-0015
JAPAN

TAN, Puay Hoon*
Singapore General Hospital
20 College Road
Academia, Level 7, Diagnostics Tower
Singapore 169856
SINGAPORE

TAN, Soo Yong
National University of Singapore
NUH Main Building, Level 3
5 Lower Kent Ridge Road
Singapore 119074
SINGAPORE

TANG, Laura H.
Memorial Sloan Kettering Cancer Center
1275 York Avenue
New York NY 10065
USA

TERRIS, Benoit
Cochin Hospital, AP-HP
University Paris Descartes
Rue du Faubourg Saint-Jacques
75014 Paris
FRANCE

THOMPSON, Lester D.R.
Woodland Hills Medical Center
5601 De Soto Avenue
Woodland Hills CA 91365
USA

THWAY, Khin
Royal Marsden Hospital /
Institute of Cancer Research
203 Fulham Road
London SW3 6JJ
UNITED KINGDOM

TOMLINSON, Ian
Institute Of Cancer and
Genomic Science (ICGS)
Vincent Drive
Birmingham B15 2TT
UNITED KINGDOM

TORBENSON, Mickael S.
Mayo Clinic
100 First Street
Rochester MN 55905
USA

TSAO, Ming S.*
University Health Network
200 Elizabeth Street, 11th Floor
Toronto ON M5G 2C4
CANADA

TSUI, Wilson M.
Caritas Medical Centre
Wing Hong Street, Sham Shui Po
Kowloon, Hong Kong SAR
CHINA

TSUZUKI, Toyonori
Aichi Medical University Hospital
1-1 Yazakokarimata
Nagakute 480-1195
JAPAN

VALENT, Peter*
Medical University of Vienna
Währinger Gürtel 18–20
1090 Vienna
AUSTRIA

VAN DER POST, Rachel S.
Radboud University Medical Center
Geert Grooteplein Zuid 30, PO Box 824
6525 GA Nijmegen
NETHERLANDS

VIETH, Michael
Institute of Pathology
Preuschwitzer Straße 101
95445 Bayreuth
GERMANY

WASHINGTON, Mary K.
Vanderbilt University Medical Center
C-3321 MCN
Nashville TN 37232
USA

WATANABE, Reiko
National Cancer Center Hospital East
6-5-1 Kashiwanoha, Kashiwa-shi
Chiba 277-8577
JAPAN

WEN, Xiaogang
Centro Hospitalar de Vila Nova
de Gaia / Espinho
Rua Conceição Fernandes 1282
4434-502 Vila Nova de Gaia
PORTUGAL

WITTEKIND, Christian
University Hospital Leipzig
Liebigstraße 26
04103 Leipzig
GERMANY

WOOD, Laura D.*
Johns Hopkins University School of Medicine
CRB2 Room 345, 1550 Orleans Street
Baltimore MD 21231
USA

WORTHLEY, Daniel L.
South Australian Health and
Medical Research Institute
North Terrace
Adelaide SA 5000
AUSTRALIA

YAO, Takashi
Juntendo University Graduate School
of Medicine
2-1-1 Hongo, Bunkyo-ku
Tokyo 113-8421
JAPAN

YASUI, Wataru
Hiroshima University
1-2-3 Kasumi, Minami-ku
Hiroshima 734-8551
JAPAN

YOSHINO, Tadashi
Okayama University
2-5-1 Shikata-cho, Kita-ku
Okayama 700-8558
JAPAN

ZAMBONI, Giuseppe
University of Verona
IRCCS Sacro Cuore Don Calabria Hospital
Via Don Sempreboni 5
37024 Negrar VR
ITALY

ZEN, Yoh
Institute of Liver Studies
King's College Hospital
King's College London
London SE5 9RS
UNITED KINGDOM

* Indicates disclosure of interests (see p. 557).

Declaration of interests

Dr Campo reports receiving personal consultancy fees from Takeda and having benefited from research funding from Gilead Sciences and from personal consultancy fees from Celgene. He also reports holding patents on "methods for selecting and treating lymphoma types" and "evaluation of mantle cell lymphoma and methods related thereof".

Dr W.C. Chan reports having received support from Celgene.

Dr Couvelard reports benefiting from research funding from Ipsen, having received support for travel and accommodation from Novartis and Ipsen, and having received personal consultancy fees from Novartis.

Dr Dei Tos reports that his institute received non-monetary support from PharmaMar. He also reports having received honoraria from Lilly and Pfizer.

Dr Frankel reports that her unit at Ohio State University benefits from research funding from Myriad Genetics. She also reports having received honoraria from Cleveland Clinic and Memorial Sloan Kettering Cancer Center.

Dr Grabsch reports having received personal consultancy fees from Chugai.

Dr Hamilton reports receiving personal consultancy fees from Merck, Loxo Oncology, and HalioDx.

Dr Hiraoka reports having benefited from research funding from Ajinomoto.

Dr Hornick reports receiving personal consultancy fees from Epizyme and Eli Lilly.

Dr Horny reports having received personal consultancy fees from Novartis.

Dr Hruban reports having received personal consultancy fees in his capacity as a former member of the board of miDiagnostics.

Dr Jansen reports benefiting from research funding from Rosetrees Trust and the Engineering and Physical Sciences Research Council (EPSRC).

Dr Lakhani reports receiving personal consultancy fees from Sullivan Nicolaides Pathology and educational funding from Roche and Ventana Medical Systems.

Dr Mäkinen reports benefiting from support for travel from Roche Finland, Amgen, and Merck.

Dr Nagtegaal reports that her institute benefits from research funding from the Dutch Cancer Society (KWF) and the Dutch Digestive Foundation (MLDS).

Dr Perren reports having received honoraria from Novartis and Ipsen.

Dr Pitman reports receiving personal consultancy fees from Medtronic.

Dr Prieto reports having received honoraria from Myriad Genetics.

Dr Rindi reports receiving speaker honoraria from Novartis and Ipsen.

Dr Sasano reports receiving honoraria from Pfizer Oncology, Novartis Oncology, and Teijin Medical.

Dr Sipos reports having received personal consultancy fees and research funding from Novartis, and having received honoraria from Novartis, Roche, and Ipsen.

Dr P.H. Tan reports holding patents on "breast fibroadenoma susceptibility mutations and use thereof".

Dr Tsao reports that his institute receives research funding from Pfizer, Merck, and AstraZeneca. He also reports receiving personal consultancy fees from Merck, AstraZeneca, Bristol-Myers Squibb, Pfizer, Takeda, Bayer, and Hoffmann-La Roche.

Dr Valent reports having received personal consultancy fees and research funding from Novartis and Deciphera.

Dr Wood reports receiving personal consultancy fees from Personal Genome Diagnostics.

IARC/WHO Committee for the International Classification of Diseases for Oncology (ICD-O)

CREE, Ian A.
International Agency for Research on Cancer
150 Cours Albert Thomas
69372 Lyon
FRANCE

FERLAY, Jacques
International Agency for Research on Cancer
150 Cours Albert Thomas
69372 Lyon
FRANCE

JAKOB, Robert
Data Standards and Informatics
World Health Organization (WHO)
20 Avenue Appia
1211 Geneva
SWITZERLAND

ROUS, Brian
Public Health England
Victoria House, Capital Park
Fulbourn, Cambridge CB21 XB
UNITED KINGDOM

WATANABE, Reiko
National Cancer Center Hospital East
6-5-1 Kashiwanoha, Kashiwa-shi
Chiba 277-8577
JAPAN

WHITE, Valerie A.
International Agency for Research on Cancer
150 Cours Albert Thomas
69372 Lyon
FRANCE

ZNAOR, Ariana
International Agency for Research on Cancer
150 Cours Albert Thomas
69372 Lyon
FRANCE

Sources

Note: For all figures, tables, and boxes not listed below, the original source is this volume; the suggested source citation is

WHO Classification of Tumours Editorial Board. Digestive system tumours. Lyon (France): International Agency for Research on Cancer; 2019. (WHO classification of tumours series, 5th ed.; vol. 1). http://publications.iarc.fr/579.

TNM staging tables

Brierly JD, Gospodarowicz MK, Wittekind C, editors. TNM classification of malignant tumours. 8th ed. Oxford (UK): Wiley Blackwell; 2017.

This edition first published 2017 © 2017 UICC
Published 2017 by John Wiley & Sons, Ltd.

Figures

2.01	Lam AK
2.02A,B	Odze RD
2.03A–D	Odze RD
2.04	Kumarasinghe MP
2.05A–D	Fujii S
2.06	Fujii S
2.07	Fujii S
2.08A,B	Kumarasinghe MP
2.09	Kumarasinghe MP
2.10	Adapted, with permission from BMJ Publishing Group Limited, from: Arnold M, Soerjomataram I, Ferlay J, et al. Global incidence of oesophageal cancer by histological subtype in 2012. Gut. 2015 Mar;64(3):381–7. PMID:25320104.
2.11A	Lam AK
2.11B–D	Kumarasinghe MP
2.12	Kumarasinghe MP
2.13A,B	Kumarasinghe MP
2.14A	Gill AJ
2.14B	Lam AK
2.15	Tin-yan Elaine Cheung, Department of Pathology, Queen Elizabeth Hospital, Kowloon, Hong Kong SAR, China
2.16A,B	Tin-yan Elaine Cheung, Department of Pathology, Queen Elizabeth Hospital, Kowloon, Hong Kong SAR, China
2.17	Brown IS
2.18A–C	Brown IS
2.19	Adapted, with permission from BMJ Publishing Group Limited, from: Arnold M, Soerjomataram I, Ferlay J, et al. Global incidence of oesophageal cancer by histological subtype in 2012. Gut. 2015 Mar;64(3):381–7. PMID:25320104.
2.20A	Reprinted, with permission from Springer Nature, from: Japan Esophageal Society. Japanese classification of esophageal cancer, tenth edition: part I. Esophagus. 2009;6:1–25. doi:10.1007/s10388-009-0169-0. Copyright 2009.
2.20B	© Shimoda T Bosman FT, Carneiro F, Hruban RH, et al., editors. WHO classification of tumours of the digestive system. Lyon (France): International Agency for Research on Cancer; 2010. (WHO classification of tumours series, 4th ed.; vol. 3). http://publications.iarc.fr/13.
2.21A,B	Brown IS
2.22A,B	Brown IS
2.23A–C	Brown IS
2.24	Brown IS
2.25A,B	Fujii S
2.26A,B	Kawachi H
2.27A,B	Scoazec JY
2.28	Scoazec JY
2.29	Klöppel G
3.01A,B	Kushima R
3.02	Genta RMG
3.03	Genta RMG
3.04A,B	Kushima R
3.05A,B	Kushima R
3.06A–D	Kushima R
3.07A,B	Kushima R
3.08A,B	Lauwers GY
3.09	Kushima R
3.10A,B	Kushima R
3.11	Singhi AD
3.12A,B	Singhi AD
3.13	Montgomery EA
3.14	Montgomery EA
3.15	Montgomery EA
3.16	Montgomery EA
3.17A,B	Kushima R
3.18	Montgomery EA
3.19A–C	Sekine S
3.20A,B	Sekine S
3.21A–C	Montgomery EA
3.22	Montgomery EA
3.23A,B	Reprinted, with permission from Igaku-Shoin, from: Yao T et al. I to Cho, Stomach and Intestine. 2010;45(7):1192–202. Japanese.
3.23C,D	Carneiro F
3.23E,F	Tetsuo Ushiku, Department of Pathology, University of Tokyo, Tokyo, Japan
3.24A,B	Vieth M
3.25	Ferlay J, Ervik M, Lam F, et al. Global Cancer Observatory: Cancer Today [Internet]. Lyon (France): International Agency for Research on Cancer; 2018. Available from: https://gco.iarc.fr/today.
3.26	Reprinted, with permission from Springer Nature, from: Japanese Gastric Cancer Association. Japanese classification of gastric carcinoma: 3rd English edition. Gastric Cancer. 2011 Jun;14(2):101–12. PMID:21573743.

3.27A–C,E   Copyright 2011.
Mitsuhiro Fujishiro, Department of Gastroenterology & Hepatology, Nagoya University Graduate School of Medicine, Nagoya, Japan

3.27D,F–I   Fukayama M

3.28   Reprinted, with permission from Springer Nature, from: Japanese Gastric Cancer Association. Japanese classification of gastric carcinoma: 3rd English edition. Gastric Cancer. 2011 Jun;14(2):101–12. PMID:21573743. Copyright 2011.

3.29A–C   Fukayama M

3.30A,B   Fukayama M

3.31   Fukayama M

3.32   Fukayama M

3.33A,B   Fukayama M

3.34A,B   Fukayama M

3.35A–D   Carneiro F

3.36   Tetsuo Ushiku, Department of Pathology, University of Tokyo, Tokyo, Japan

3.37A–C   Hiroyuki Abe, Department of Pathology, Graduate School of Medicine, University of Tokyo, Tokyo, Japan

3.38   Tetsuo Ushiku, Department of Pathology, University of Tokyo, Tokyo, Japan

3.39   Tetsuo Ushiku, Department of Pathology, University of Tokyo, Tokyo, Japan

3.40A,B   Yao T

3.41   Reprinted, with permission from Taniguchi H, from: Taniguchi H. Squamous cell carcinoma and adenosquamous carcinoma. In: Fukayama M, Ohkura Y, editors. Tumor Pathology Atlas, Gastric Cancer. 2nd ed. Tokyo (Japan): Bunko-do Co.; 2015. Japanese. p. 124–8.

3.42A–C   Hirokazu Taniguchi, Department of Pathology and Clinical Laboratories, National Cancer Center Hospital, Tokyo, Japan

3.43A–C   Agaimy A

3.44A,C,D   Agaimy A

3.44B   Modified, with permission, from: Agaimy A, Rau TT, Hartmann A, et al. SMARCB1 (INI1)-negative rhabdoid carcinomas of the gastrointestinal tract: clinicopathologic and molecular study of a highly aggressive variant with literature review. Am J Surg Pathol. 2014 Jul;38(7):910–20. PMID:24503755.

3.45A–D   Montgomery EA

3.46A,B   Montgomery EA

3.47   Montgomery EA

3.48A,C–F   La Rosa S

3.48B   Rindi G

3.49A–H   La Rosa S

3.50A–D   La Rosa S

3.51A–C   Chan JKC

4.01   Rugge M

4.02   Sekine S

4.03A,B   Sekine S

4.04A,B   Adsay NV, Reid M

4.05A–D   Shia J

4.06A–C   Ohike N, Kim GE, Tajiri T, et al. Intra-ampullary papillary-tubular neoplasm (IAPN): characterization of tumoral intraepithelial neoplasia occurring within the ampulla: a clinicopathologic analysis of 82 cases. Am J Surg Pathol. 2010 Dec;34(12):1731–48. PMID:21084962. Available from: https://journals.lww.com/ajsp/Abstract/2010/12000/Intra_ampullary_Papillary_Tubular_Neoplasm__IAPN__.1.aspx

4.07   Ohike N, Kim GE, Tajiri T, et al. Intra-ampullary papillary-tubular neoplasm (IAPN): characterization of tumoral intraepithelial neoplasia occurring within the ampulla: a clinicopathologic analysis of 82 cases. Am J Surg Pathol. 2010 Dec;34(12):1731–48. PMID:21084962. Available from: https://journals.lww.com/ajsp/Abstract/2010/12000/Intra_ampullary_Papillary_Tubular_Neoplasm__IAPN__.1.aspx

4.08A   Paul Kelly, Histopathology Laboratory, Institute of Pathology, Royal Victoria Hospital, Belfast Health and Social Care Trust, Belfast, United Kingdom

4.08B   Adsay NV, Reid M

4.09A–C   Salto-Tellez M

4.10A,B   Adsay NV, Reid M

4.11   Adsay NV, Reid M

4.12   Adsay NV, Reid M

4.13   Sipos B

4.14   Reprinted, with permission, from: Rindi G, Klimstra DS, Abedi-Ardekani B, et al. A common classification framework for neuroendocrine neoplasms: an International Agency for Research on Cancer (IARC) and World Health Organization (WHO) expert consensus proposal. Mod Pathol. 2018 Dec;31(12):1770–86. PMID:30140036. doi:10.1038/s41379-018-0110-y. http://creativecommons.org/licenses/by/4.0/.

4.15   Perren A

4.16A–D   Chan JKC

4.17   Chan JKC

5.01A,B   Misdraji J

5.02   Pai RK (Reetesh)

5.03   Pai RK (Reetesh)

5.04A,C   Misdraji J

5.04B   Pai RK (Reetesh)

5.05A,B   Misdraji J

5.06   Misdraji J

5.07A,B   Misdraji J

5.08A,B   Misdraji J

5.09A   © Fenger C
Bosman FT, Carneiro F, Hruban RH, et al., editors. WHO classification of tumours of the digestive system. Lyon (France): International Agency for Research on Cancer; 2010. (WHO classification of tumours series, 4th ed.; vol. 3). http://publications.iarc.fr/13.

5.09B   Komminoth P

5.10   Couvelard A

5.11A,B   Tang LH, Klimstra DS

5.12   Rindi G

6.01   Rosty C

6.02A–C   Mäkinen MJ

6.03A–C   Mäkinen MJ

6.04A,B   Pai RK (Rish)

6.04C   Rosty C

6.05A–D   Rosty C

6.05E   Pai RK (Rish)

6.06A   Pai RK (Rish)

6.06B   Rosty C

6.07A,B   Rosty C

6.07C   Odze RD

6.08A–C   Rosty C

6.09A–C   Rosty C

6.10A,B   Rosty C

6.11   Odze RD

6.12   Jayan Mannath, University Hospitals Coventry & Warwickshire NHS Trust, Coventry, United Kingdom

6.13   Hamilton SR

6.14A   Hamilton SR

6.14B,C   Lax SF

6.15   Hamilton SR

6.16A,B   Lax SF

6.17A–C   Nagtegaal ID

6.18   Lax SF

6.19   Nagtegaal ID

6.20A,B   Odze RD

6.21   Odze RD

6.22A,B   Odze RD

6.23   Ferlay J, Ervik M, Lam F, et al. Global Cancer Observatory: Cancer Today [Internet]. Lyon (France): International Agency for Research on Cancer; 2018. Available from: https://gco.iarc.fr/today.

6.24A   © Kudo S
Bosman FT, Carneiro F, Hruban RH, et al., editors. WHO classification of tumours of the digestive system. Lyon (France): International Agency for Research on Cancer; 2010. (WHO classification of tumours series, 4th ed.; vol. 3). http://publications.iarc.fr/13.

6.24B	Shia J, Klimstra DS
6.24C	© Gabbert HE
	Bosman FT, Carneiro F, Hruban RH, et al., editors. WHO classification of tumours of the digestive system. Lyon (France): International Agency for Research on Cancer; 2010. (WHO classification of tumours series, 4th ed.; vol. 3). http://publications.iarc.fr/13.
6.25	Nagtegaal ID
6.26A	© Fogt F
	Bosman FT, Carneiro F, Hruban RH, et al., editors. WHO classification of tumours of the digestive system. Lyon (France): International Agency for Research on Cancer; 2010. (WHO classification of tumours series, 4th ed.; vol. 3). http://publications.iarc.fr/13.
6.26B	Nagtegaal ID
6.27A,B	Nagtegaal ID
6.28	Nagtegaal ID
6.29	Nagtegaal ID
6.30	Nagtegaal ID
6.31	Nagtegaal ID
6.32	Nagtegaal ID
6.33	Nagtegaal ID
6.34A–F	Nagtegaal ID
6.35	Reprinted from: Müller MF, Ibrahim AE, Arends MJ. Molecular pathological classification of colorectal cancer. Virchows Arch. 2016 Aug;469(2):125–34. PMID:27325016. http://creativecommons.org/licenses/by/4.0/
6.36A–C	Rindi G
6.37A–D	Rindi G
6.38A–C	Rindi G
6.39A–D	Rindi G
7.01	Lam AK
7.02	Lam AK
7.03	Lam AK
7.04A,B	Lam AK
7.05	Lam AK
7.06	Lam AK
7.07	Graham RP
7.08	Graham RP
7.09	Graham RP
7.10	Graham RP
7.11	Graham RP
7.12	© Fenger C
	Bosman FT, Carneiro F, Hruban RH, et al., editors. WHO classification of tumours of the digestive system. Lyon (France): International Agency for Research on Cancer; 2010. (WHO classification of tumours series, 4th ed.; vol. 3). http://publications.iarc.fr/13.
7.13A–C	Graham RP
7.14	© Fenger C
	Bosman FT, Carneiro F, Hruban RH, et al., editors. WHO classification of tumours of the digestive system. Lyon (France): International Agency for Research on Cancer; 2010. (WHO classification of tumours series, 4th ed.; vol. 3). http://publications.iarc.fr/13.
7.15A–C	Graham RP
7.16	Reprinted from: Lisovsky M, Patel K, Cymes K, et al. Immunophenotypic characterization of anal gland carcinoma: loss of p63 and cytokeratin 5/6. Arch Pathol Lab Med. 2007 Aug;131(8):1304–11. PMID:17683193
7.17	Shia J
7.18A,B	Shia J
7.19A–D	Shia J
7.20	Shia J
7.21	Adapted, with permission from Wolters Kluwer Health, Inc., from: Perez DR, Trakarnsanga A, Shia J, et al. Management and outcome of perianal Paget's disease: a 6-decade institutional experience. Dis Colon Rectum. 2014 Jun;57(6):747–51. PMID:24807600
7.22A,B	Klimstra DS
8.01A–C	Bioulac-Sage P
8.02A–C	Bioulac-Sage P
8.03A–C	Bioulac-Sage P
8.04A–F	Bioulac-Sage P
8.05A–F	Bioulac-Sage P
8.06A–E	Bioulac-Sage P
8.07A–C	Bioulac-Sage P
8.08	Ferlay J, Ervik M, Lam F, et al. Global Cancer Observatory: Cancer Today [Internet]. Lyon (France): International Agency for Research on Cancer; 2018. Available from: https://gco.iarc.fr/today.
8.09A,B	Park YN
8.10A–C	Torbenson MS
8.11A,B	Torbenson MS
8.12A–D	Torbenson MS
8.13A–C	Torbenson MS
8.14A,B	Torbenson MS
8.15A	Torbenson MS
8.15B–D	Park YN
8.16A–D	Park YN
8.17A,B	Sakamato M
8.18A–D	© Wee A
	Bosman FT, Carneiro F, Hruban RH, et al., editors. WHO classification of tumours of the digestive system. Lyon (France): International Agency for Research on Cancer; 2010. (WHO classification of tumours series, 4th ed.; vol. 3). http://publications.iarc.fr/13.
8.19	Saxena R
8.20A–C	Saxena R
8.21A,B	© Zimmerman A
	Bosman FT, Carneiro F, Hruban RH, et al., editors. WHO classification of tumours of the digestive system. Lyon (France): International Agency for Research on Cancer; 2010. (WHO classification of tumours series, 4th ed.; vol. 3). http://publications.iarc.fr/13.
8.22	Saxena R
8.23A,B	Tsui WM
8.24	Tsui WM
8.25A–D	Tsui WM
8.26A,B	Tsui WM
8.27	Tsui WM
8.28A	Klöppel G
8.28B	Nakanuma Y
8.29A–F	Nakanuma Y
8.30A,B	Tsui WM
8.30C,D	Nakanuma Y
8.31A,B	Nakanuma Y
8.32A–C	Tsui WM
8.33A,B	Tsui WM
8.34A–D	Nakanuma Y
8.35A–C	Nakanuma Y
8.36A–C	Nakanuma Y
8.37A–C	Nakanuma Y
8.38A,B	Nakanuma Y
8.39A–D	Nakanuma Y
8.40A–C	Nakanuma Y
8.41A–C	Park YN
8.42	Park YN
8.43	Park YN
8.44A–D	Park YN
8.45	Klimstra DS
8.46A,B	Klimstra DS
9.01	Basturk O
9.02	Basturk O
9.03A,B	Basturk O
9.03C	Aishima S
9.04A–F	Nakanuma Y
9.05A	Adsay V, Jang KT, Roa JC, et al. Intracholecystic papillary-tubular neoplasms (ICPN) of the gallbladder (neoplastic polyps, adenomas, and papillary neoplasms that are ≥1.0 cm): clinicopathologic and immunohistochemical analysis of 123 cases. Am J Surg Pathol. 2012 Sep;36(9):1279–301. PMID:22895264. Available from: https://journals.lww.com/ajsp/Abstract/2012/09000/Intracholecystic_Papillary_Tubular_Neoplasms.2.aspx
9.05B,C	Basturk O
9.06A–F	Basturk O
9.07A–C	Nakanuma Y
9.08	Adapted, with permission, from: Aishima S, Oda Y. Pathogenesis and classification of intrahepatic cholangiocarcinoma: different characters of perihilar large duct type versus peripheral small duct type. J Hepatobiliary Pancreat Sci. 2015 Feb;22(2):94–100. PMID:25181580
9.09A–E	Nakanuma Y
9.10A,B	Nakanuma Y

9.11	Nakanuma Y
9.12A,B	Nakanuma Y
9.13	Tsui WM
9.14	Nakanuma Y
9.15	Ferlay J, Ervik M, Lam F, et al. Global Cancer Observatory: Cancer Today [Internet]. Lyon (France): International Agency for Research on Cancer. Available from: https://gco.iarc.fr/today.
9.16	Modified, with permission, from: Shibata T, Arai Y, Totoki Y. Molecular genomic landscapes of hepatobiliary cancer. Cancer Sci. 2018 May;109(5):1282–91. PMID:29573058. Copyright Wiley Company.
9.17A–C	Roa JC
9.18A–C	Roa JC
9.19A–C	Roa JC
9.20A,B	Adsay NV
9.21A,B,D,E	Adsay NV
9.21C	Roa JC
9.22	Roa JC
9.23A,B	Roa JC
9.24A,B	Zen Y
9.25A–F	Zen Y
9.26A–B	Arola J
9.27A–E	Chan JKC
10.01	Anil Dasyam, Division of Abdominal Imaging, University of Pittsburgh, Pittsburgh PA, USA
10.02	Singhi AD
10.03A–C	Singhi AD
10.04A–D	Singhi AD
10.05A,B	Singhi AD
10.06A–D	Singhi AD
10.07	Singhi AD
10.08A,B	Basturk O
10.09	Basturk O
10.10A,B	Basturk O
10.11A,B	Basturk O
10.12A,B	Basturk O
10.13A,B	Basturk O
10.14A,B	Basturk O
10.15A,B	Basturk O
10.16	Reprinted, with permission, from: Basturk O, Adsay V, Askan G, et al. Intraductal tubulopapillary neoplasm of the pancreas: a clinicopathologic and immunohistochemical analysis of 33 cases. Am J Surg Pathol. 2017 Mar;41(3):313–25. PMID:27984235
10.17A,B	Basturk O
10.18	Basturk O
10.19A,B	Basturk O
10.20A,B	Esposito I
10.21	Ferlay J, Ervik M, Lam F, et al. Global Cancer Observatory: Cancer Today [Internet]. Lyon (France): International Agency for Research on Cancer; 2018. Available from: https://gco.iarc.fr/today.
10.22	Pitman MB
10.23A–D	Hruban RH
10.24A–D	Hruban RH
10.25A–D	Klöppel G
10.26A,B	Pitman MB
10.27A	Wood LD
10.27B	La Rosa S
10.28A–D	La Rosa S
10.29A–D	La Rosa S
10.30A,B	Klimstra DS
10.30C	La Rosa S
10.31A–C	Chan JKC
10.32A	Klimstra DS
10.32B	Zamboni G
10.33A	Reprinted, with permission from Elsevier, from: Ohike N, Morohoshi T. Exocrine pancreatic neoplasms of nonductal origin: acinar cell carcinoma, pancreatoblastoma, and solid-pseudopapillary neoplasm. Surg Pathol Clin. 2011 Jun;4(2):579–88. PMID:26837489. Copyright 2011.
10.33B	Ohike N
10.34A,B	Ohike N
10.35A–C	Ohike N
10.36A	Satomi Kawamoto, Russell H. Morgan Department of Radiology and Radiological Science, Johns Hopkins Medicine, Baltimore MD, USA
10.36B	Gill AJ
10.37	Klöppel G
10.38A–D	Klöppel G
10.39	Klöppel G
10.40A–D	Klöppel G
10.41A–D	Klöppel G
10.42A,B	Klöppel G
10.43A,B	Klöppel G
10.44A–D	Klöppel G
10.45A–C	Klöppel G
10.46A,B	Klöppel G
10.47A–C	Klöppel G
10.48A,B	Klöppel G
10.49A,B	Klöppel G
10.50	Damian Wild, Center of Neuroendocrine and Endocrine Tumors, Radiology & Nuclear Medicine, University Hospital Basel, Basel, Switzerland
10.51	Perren A
10.52	Singhi AD
10.53	Klöppel G
10.54A,B	Kasajima A
10.55A–D	La Rosa S
10.56	Couvelard A
10.57A–D	Couvelard A
10.58A,B	Singhi AD
10.59A–C	Singhi AD
10.60A–D	La Rosa S
10.61	Shi C
10.62A,B	Shi C
10.63A,C	Adsay NV
10.63B,D	Klöppel G
10.64	Adsay NV
10.65A	Klimstra DS
10.65B,C	Klöppel G
10.66A–C	Reprinted, with permission, from: Hruban RH, Pitman MB, Klimstra DS. Tumors of the pancreas. Washington, DC: American Registry of Pathology; 2007. (AFIP atlas of tumor pathology, series 4; fascicle 6).
10.67A–C	Ohike N
11.01A,B	Nakamura S
11.02A,B	Nakamura S
11.03A,B	Nakamura S
11.04A,B	Nakamura S
11.05A,B	Nakamura S
11.06A,B	Nakamura S
11.07A,B	Nakamura S
11.08A,B	Nakamura S
11.09A–D	Delabie J
11.10A–D	Adapted, with permission, from: Tari A, Kitadai Y, Mouri R, et al. Watch-and-wait policy versus rituximab-combined chemotherapy in Japanese patients with intestinal follicular lymphoma. J Gastroenterol Hepatol. 2018 Aug;33(8):1461–8. PMID:29377265
11.11A–D	Adapted, with permission, from: Tari A, Kitadai Y, Mouri R, et al. Watch-and-wait policy versus rituximab-combined chemotherapy in Japanese patients with intestinal follicular lymphoma. J Gastroenterol Hepatol. 2018 Aug;33(8):1461–8. PMID:29377265
11.12A	Chott A
11.12B	Bhagat G
11.13A–D	Chott A
11.14A–C	Bhagat G
11.15A	Chan JKC
11.15B	Tan SY
11.16A,B	Chan JKC
11.16C,D	de Leval L
11.17A–D	Tan SY
11.18	Tan SY
11.19A,B	Chan JKC
11.20A–F	Tan SY
11.21A	Reprinted, with permission from the American Society of Hematology, from: Perry AM, Warnke RA, Hu Q, et al. Indolent T-cell lymphoproliferative disease of the gastrointestinal tract. Blood. 2013 Nov 21; 122(22):3599–606. PMID:24009234. Permission conveyed through Copyright Clearance Center, Inc.; and Swerdlow SH, Campo E, Harris NL, et al., editors. WHO classification of tumours of haematopoietic and lymphoid tissues. Lyon (France): International Agency for Research on Cancer; 2017. (WHO classification of tumours series, 4th rev. ed.; vol. 2). http://publications.iarc.fr/556.
11.21B	Jaffe ES
11.22A–D	Jaffe ES

11.23A   Gaulard P
11.23B–D   Jaffe ES
11.24A,B   Chan JKC
11.25A–F   Chan JKC
11.26A,B   Chan JKC
11.27A–F   Nakamura S
11.28A   Lai J
11.28B   Chan WC
11.29A–E   Nakamura S
11.30A,B   Lai J
11.31A,B   Lai J
11.32   Nakamura S
11.33A   Ott G
11.33B   Chan JKC
11.34A   © Harris NL
Swerdlow SH, Campo E, Harris NL, et al., editors. WHO classification of tumours of haematopoietic and lymphoid tissues. Lyon (France): International Agency for Research on Cancer; 2017. (WHO classification of tumours series, 4th rev. ed.; vol. 2). http://publications.iarc.fr/556.
11.34B   © Sobin LH
Bosman FT, Carneiro F, Hruban RH, et al., editors. WHO classification of tumours of the digestive system. Lyon (France): International Agency for Research on Cancer; 2010. (WHO classification of tumours series, 4th ed.; vol. 3). http://publications.iarc.fr/13.
11.35A,B   © Sobin LH
Bosman FT, Carneiro F, Hruban RH, et al., editors. WHO classification of tumours of the digestive system. Lyon (France): International Agency for Research on Cancer; 2010. (WHO classification of tumours series, 4th ed.; vol. 3). http://publications.iarc.fr/13.
11.36A   © Jass JR (deceased)
Bosman FT, Carneiro F, Hruban RH, et al., editors. WHO classification of tumours of the digestive system. Lyon (France): International Agency for Research on Cancer; 2010. (WHO classification of tumours series, 4th ed.; vol. 3). http://publications.iarc.fr/13.
11.36B   Swerdlow SH
11.37   Nakamura S
11.38A,B   Leoncini L
11.39A,B   Leoncini L
11.40A,B   Kluin PM
11.41   Reproduced, with permission, from: Haralambieva E, Schuuring E, Rosati S, et al. Interphase fluorescence in situ hybridization for detection of 8q24/MYC breakpoints on routine histologic sections: validation in Burkitt lymphomas from three geographic regions. Genes Chromosomes Cancer. 2004 May;40(1):10–8. PMID:15034863; and Swerdlow SH, Campo E, Harris NL, et al., editors. WHO classification of tumours of haematopoietic and lymphoid tissues. Lyon (France): International Agency for Research on Cancer; 2017. (WHO classification of tumours series, 4th rev. ed.; vol. 2). http://publications.iarc.fr/556.
11.42   Jaffe ES
11.43A,B   Montes-Moreno S
11.44   Montes-Moreno S
11.45A–F   Montes-Moreno S
11.46A,B   Chadburn A
11.47A,B   Ferry JA
11.48A–C   Ko YH
11.49A,B   Ko YH
11.50A–D   Ko YH
11.51A   Reprinted, with permission from the American Society of Hematology, from: Takeuchi K, Yokoyama M, Ishizawa S, et al. Lymphomatoid gastropathy: a distinct clinicopathologic entity of self-limited pseudomalignant NK-cell proliferation. Blood. 2010 Dec 16;116(25):5631–7. PMID:20829373. Permission conveyed through Copyright Clearance Center, Inc.
11.51B   Chan JKC
11.52A,B   Horny H-P
11.53A–D   Horny H-P
11.54A,B   Horny H-P
11.55A,B   Chan JKC
11.56A–C   Chan JKC
11.57   Chan JKC
11.58A   Chan JKC
11.58B   Pileri SA
11.59A,B   Chan JKC

12.01A,B   A. Gronchi, Department of Surgery, Fondazione IRCCS Istituto Nazionale dei Tumori, Milan, Italy
12.02A,B   Hornick JL
12.03A,B   Hornick JL
12.04A–D   Hornick JL
12.05A–C   Dei Tos AP
12.06A–C   Dei Tos AP
12.07   Dei Tos AP
12.08A–C   Hornick JL
12.09A,B   Hornick JL
12.10A,B   Rossi S
12.11   Rossi S
12.12A–C   Chan JKC
12.13A,B   Fritchie KJ
12.14   Fritchie KJ
12.15A,B   Rossi S
12.16   Rossi S
12.17   Chan JKC
12.18A–C   Chan JKC
12.18D   Hornick JL
12.19   Chan JKC
12.20   Jorge Torres-Mora, Department of Laboratory Medicine and Pathology, Mayo Clinic College of Medicine, Rochester MN, USA
12.21   Chan JKC

12.22A–C   Chan JKC
12.23   Kumarasinghe MP
12.24A–C   Dry SM
12.25A,B   Dry SM
12.26A,B   Dry SM
12.27A–C   © Ishak K (deceased)
Bosman FT, Carneiro F, Hruban RH, et al., editors. WHO classification of tumours of the digestive system. Lyon (France): International Agency for Research on Cancer; 2010. (WHO classification of tumours series, 4th ed.; vol. 3). http://publications.iarc.fr/13.
12.28A   Tsui WM
12.28B,C   © Ishak K (deceased)
Bosman FT, Carneiro F, Hruban RH, et al., editors. WHO classification of tumours of the digestive system. Lyon (France): International Agency for Research on Cancer; 2010. (WHO classification of tumours series, 4th ed.; vol. 3). http://publications.iarc.fr/13.
12.29   Doyle LA
12.30A,B   Hornick JL
12.31A   Hornick JL
12.31B   Ian R. Wanless, Dalhousie University, Halifax NS, Canada
12.32A,B   © Ishak K (deceased)
Bosman FT, Carneiro F, Hruban RH, et al., editors. WHO classification of tumours of the digestive system. Lyon (France): International Agency for Research on Cancer; 2010. (WHO classification of tumours series, 4th ed.; vol. 3). http://publications.iarc.fr/13.
12.33A,B   Chan JKC
12.34A–D   Chan JKC
12.35A–C   Hornick JL
12.35D   Miettinen M
12.36   Doyle LA
12.37   Doyle LA
12.38   Doyle LA
12.39   Doyle LA
12.40   Doyle LA
12.41   Hornick JL
12.42A,B   Hornick JL
12.43   Hornick JL
12.44A,B   Hornick JL
12.45A–D   Hornick JL
12.46   Hornick JL
12.47   Hornick JL
12.48   Hornick JL
12.49A,B   Hornick JL
12.50A,B   Hornick JL
12.51A   Hornick JL
12.51B,C   Ian R. Wanless, Dalhousie University, Halifax NS, Canada
12.52   Hornick JL
12.53A   © Stocker JT
Bosman FT, Carneiro F, Hruban RH, et al., editors. WHO classification of tumours of the digestive system. Lyon (France): International Agency for Research on Cancer; 2010. (WHO classification of tumours series, 4th ed.; vol. 3).

http://publications.iarc.fr/13.
12.53B–D   Tsui WM
12.54A   Torbenson MS
12.54B–D   Hornick JL
12.55A,C   Chan JKC
12.55B   Wei-Lien Wang, Department of Pathology, MD Anderson Cancer Center, Houston TX, USA
12.56A,B   Hornick JL
12.57A,B   Daniel Wong, PathWest Laboratory Medicine, QEII Medical Centre, Nedlands WA, Australia
12.58A–D   Chan JKC
12.59A,C   Wei-Lien Wang, Department of Pathology, MD Anderson Cancer Center, Houston TX, USA
12.59B,D   Gill AJ
12.60A,B   Hornick JL
12.61A,B   Hornick JL

13.01   Priyadharsini Nagarajan, Department of Pathology, University of Texas MD Anderson Cancer Center, Houston TX, USA
13.02A,B   Priyadharsini Nagarajan, Department of Pathology, University of Texas MD Anderson Cancer Center, Houston TX, USA
13.03   Quaglia A
13.04A–C   © Anthony PP
Bosman FT, Carneiro F, Hruban RH, et al., editors. WHO classification of tumours of the digestive system. Lyon (France): International Agency for Research on Cancer; 2010. (WHO classification of tumours series, 4th ed.; vol. 3). http://publications.iarc.fr/13.
13.05   Singh R
13.06   Singh R

14.01A–C   Frankel WL
14.02A–D   Frankel WL
14.03A–D   Frankel WL
14.04   Nagtegaal ID
14.05A,B   Lax SF
14.05C   Brosens LAA
14.06A–D   Brosens LAA
14.07A,B   Brosens LAA
14.08   Brosens LAA
14.09A   Arends MJ
14.09B   Brosens LAA
14.10A   Kumarasinghe MP
14.10B   Adapted, with permission, from: de Boer WB, Ee H, Kumarasinghe MP. Neoplastic lesions of gastric adenocarcinoma and proximal polyposis syndrome (GAPPS) are gastric phenotype. Am J Surg Pathol. 2018 Jan;42(1):1–8. PMID:29112017
14.11A–C   Kumarasinghe MP
14.12   Kumarasinghe MP
14.13   Frayling IM
14.14   Rosty C
14.15A–D   Rosty C
14.16   Rosty C
14.17   Irene Gullo, Centro Hospitalar Universitário de São João; Institute of Molecular Pathology and Immunology of the University of Porto (Ipatimup), Instituto de Investigação e Inovação em Saúde (i3S), University of Porto, Porto, Portugal
14.18   Oliveira C
14.19   Oliveira C
14.20A,B   van der Post R
14.21A,B   Carneiro F
14.22   © Charlton A
Bosman FT, Carneiro F, Hruban RH, et al., editors. WHO classification of tumours of the digestive system. Lyon (France): International Agency for Research on Cancer; 2010. (WHO classification of tumours series, 4th ed.; vol. 3). http://publications.iarc.fr/13.
14.23   van der Post R
14.24A   Irene Gullo, Centro Hospitalar Universitário de São João; Institute of Molecular Pathology and Immunology of the University of Porto (Ipatimup), Instituto de Investigação e Inovação em Saúde (i3S), University of Porto, Porto, Portugal
14.24B   van der Post R
14.25A,B   Brosens LAA
14.26   Brosens LAA
14.27A–F   Brosens LAA
14.28A,B   Brosens LAA
14.29   Brosens LAA
14.30A–D   Brosens LAA
14.31A–C   Brosens LAA
14.32A,B   Brosens LAA
14.33A–C   Brosens LAA

Tables

3.04   Reprinted, with permission, from: Japanese Gastric Cancer Association. Japanese gastric cancer treatment guidelines. 5th ed. Tokyo (Japan): Kanehara Shuppan; 2018. Japanese.

4.01   Reproduced, with permission from Elsevier, from: Spigelman AD, Williams CB, Talbot IC, et al. Upper gastrointestinal cancer in patients with familial adenomatous polyposis. Lancet. 1989 Sep 30;2(8666):783–5. PMID:2571019. Copyright 1989.

8.13   Modified, with permission, from: Bosman FT, Carneiro F, Hruban RH, et al., editors. WHO classification of tumours of the digestive system. Lyon (France): International Agency for Research on Cancer; 2010. (WHO classification of tumours series, 4th ed.; vol. 3). http://publications.iarc.fr/13.

10.05   Modified from: Lloyd RV, Osamura RY, Klöppel G, et al., editors. WHO classification of tumours of endocrine organs. Lyon (France): International Agency for Research on Cancer; 2017. (WHO classification of tumours series, 4th ed.; vol. 10). http://publications.iarc.fr/554.

14.02   Reproduced, with permission from BMJ Publishing Group Ltd, from: Møller P, Seppälä TT, Bernstein I, et al. Cancer risk and survival in path_MMR carriers by gene and gender up to 75 years of age: a report from the Prospective Lynch Syndrome Database. Gut. 2018 Jul; 67(7):1306–16. PMID:28754778. Copyright 2018.

14.03   Reproduced, with permission from BMJ Publishing Group Ltd, from: Møller P, Seppälä TT, Bernstein I, et al. Cancer risk and survival in path_MMR carriers by gene and gender up to 75 years of age: a report from the Prospective Lynch Syndrome Database. Gut. 2018 Jul; 67(7):1306–16.
PMID:28754778. Copyright 2018.

14.04   Reprinted, with permission, from: Frayling I, Berry I, Wallace A, et al. (2016) ACGS best practice guidelines for genetic testing and diagnosis of Lynch syndrome. Association for Clinical Genetic Science. Available from: https://www.acgs.uk.com/quality/best-practice-guidelines/
Derived from: van Lier MG, Leenen CH, Wagner A, et al. Yield of routine molecular analyses in colorectal cancer patients ≤70 years to detect underlying Lynch syndrome. J Pathol. 2012 Apr;226(5):764–74. PMID:22081473

Boxes

3.02   IARC Monographs on the Evaluation of Carcinogenic Risks to Humans [Internet]. Lyon (France): International Agency for Research on Cancer; 2018. Agents classified by the IARC Monographs, Volumes 1–122; updated 2018 Jul 30. Available from: https://monographs.iarc.fr/agents-classified-by-the-iarc/.

3.03   Reprinted, with permission, from: The Paris endoscopic classification of superficial neoplastic lesions: esophagus, stomach, and colon: November 30 to December 1, 2002. Gastrointest Endosc. 2003 Dec;58(6 Suppl):S3–43. PMID:14652541; and Endoscopic Classification Review Group. Update on the Paris classification of superficial neoplastic lesions in the digestive tract. Endoscopy. 2005 Jun;37(6):570–8. PMID:15933932; and Japanese Gastric Cancer Association. Japanese classification of gastric carcinoma: 3rd English edition. Gastric Cancer. 2011 Jun;14(2):101–12. PMID:21573743

8.03   Adapted, with permission from Springer Nature, from: López-Terrada D, Alaggio R, de Dávila MT, et al. Towards an international pediatric liver tumor consensus classification: proceedings of the Los Angeles COG liver tumors symposium. Mod Pathol. 2014 Mar;27(3):472–91. PMID:24008558. Copyright 2014.

14.07   Adapted, with permission from Elsevier, from: Tan MH, Mester J, Peterson C, et al. A clinical scoring system for selection of patients for PTEN mutation testing is proposed on the basis of a prospective study of 3042 probands. Am J Hum Genet. 2011 Jan 7;88(1):42–56. PMID:21194675. Copyright 2011.

Images on the cover

Top left   Fig. 14.26: Brosens LAA
Top centre   Fig. 10.05B: Singhi AD
Top right   Fig. 14.17: Irene Gullo, Centro Hospitalar Universitário de São João; Institute of Molecular Pathology and Immunology of the University of Porto (Ipatimup), Instituto de Investigação e Inovação em Saúde (i3S), University of Porto, Porto, Portugal
Middle left   Fig. 14.27B: Brosens LAA
Middle centre   Fig. 11.43B: Montes-Moreno S
Middle right   Fig. 14.20B: van der Post R
Bottom left   Fig. 14.28B: Brosens LAA
Bottom centre   Fig. 10.55C: La Rosa S
Bottom right   Fig. 14.19: Oliveira C

Images on the chapter title pages

Chapter 1   Fig. 14.28B: Brosens LAA
Chapter 2   Fig. 2.26A: Kawachi H
Chapter 3   Fig. 3.13: Montgomery EA
Chapter 4   Fig. 4.05D: Shia J
Chapter 5   Fig. 5.01B: Misdraji J
Chapter 6   Fig. 6.10B: Rosty C
Chapter 7   Fig. 7.22B: Klimstra DS
Chapter 8   Fig. 8.20B: Saxena R
Chapter 9   Fig. 9.27C: Chan JKC
Chapter 10   Fig. 10.59A: Singhi AD
Chapter 11   Fig. 11.55A: Chan JKC
Chapter 12   Fig. 12.12C: Chan JKC
Chapter 13   Fig. 13.05: Singh R
Chapter 14   Fig. 14.25B: Brosens LAA

References

1. Aarnio M, Salovaara R, Aaltonen LA, et al. Features of gastric cancer in hereditary non-polyposis colorectal cancer syndrome. Int J Cancer. 1997 Oct 21;74(5):551–5. PMID:9355980

2. Abate F, Ambrosio MR, Mundo L, et al. Distinct viral and mutational spectrum of endemic Burkitt lymphoma. PLoS Pathog. 2015 Oct 15;11(10):e1005158. PMID:26468873

3. Abdallah M, Généreau T, Donadieu J, et al. Langerhans' cell histiocytosis of the liver in adults. Clin Res Hepatol Gastroenterol. 2011 Jun;35(6-7):475–81. PMID:21550330

4. Abe H, Hino R, Fukayama M. Platelet-derived growth factor-A and vascular endothelial growth factor-C contribute to the development of pulmonary tumor thrombotic microangiopathy in gastric cancer. Virchows Arch. 2013 May;462(5):523–31. PMID:23536282

5. Abe H, Saito R, Ichimura T, et al. CD47 expression in Epstein-Barr virus-associated gastric carcinoma: coexistence with tumor immunity lowering the ratio of CD8+/Foxp3+ T cells. Virchows Arch. 2018 Apr;472(4):643–51. PMID:29536167

6. Abe K, Suda K, Arakawa A, et al. Different patterns of p16INK4A and p53 protein expressions in intraductal papillary-mucinous neoplasms and pancreatic intraepithelial neoplasia. Pancreas. 2007 Jan;34(1):85–91. PMID:17198188

7. Abel ME, Chiu YS, Russell TR, et al. Adenocarcinoma of the anal glands. Results of a survey. Dis Colon Rectum. 1993 Apr;36(4):383–7. PMID:8458266

8. Abnet CC, Arnold M, Wei WQ. Epidemiology of esophageal squamous cell carcinoma. Gastroenterology. 2018 Jan;154(2):360–73. PMID:28823862

9. Abraham SC, Carney JA, Ooi A, et al. Achlorhydria, parietal cell hyperplasia, and multiple gastric carcinoids: a new disorder. Am J Surg Pathol. 2005 Jul;29(7):969–75. PMID:15958864

10. Abraham SC, Klimstra DS, Wilentz RE, et al. Solid-pseudopapillary tumors of the pancreas are genetically distinct from pancreatic ductal adenocarcinomas and almost always harbor beta-catenin mutations. Am J Pathol. 2002 Apr;160(4):1361–9. PMID:11943721

11. Abraham SC, Krasinskas AM, Hofstetter WL, et al. "Seedling" mesenchymal tumors (gastrointestinal stromal tumors and leiomyomas) are common incidental tumors of the esophagogastric junction. Am J Surg Pathol. 2007 Nov;31(11):1629–35. PMID:18059218

12. Abraham SC, Lee JH, Boitnott JK, et al. Microsatellite instability in intraductal papillary neoplasms of the biliary tract. Mod Pathol. 2002 Dec;15(12):1309–17. PMID:12481012

13. Abraham SC, Montgomery EA, Singh VK, et al. Gastric adenomas: intestinal-type and gastric-type adenomas differ in the risk of adenocarcinoma and presence of background mucosal pathology. Am J Surg Pathol. 2002 Oct;26(10):1276–85. PMID:12360042

14. Abraham SC, Nobukawa B, Giardiello FM, et al. Fundic gland polyps in familial adenomatous polyposis: neoplasms with frequent somatic adenomatous polyposis coli gene alterations. Am J Pathol. 2000 Sep;157(3):747–54. PMID:10980114

15. Abraham SC, Nobukawa B, Giardiello FM, et al. Sporadic fundic gland polyps: common gastric polyps arising through activating mutations in the beta-catenin gene. Am J Pathol. 2001 Mar;158(3):1005–10. PMID:11238048

16. Abraham SC, Park SJ, Cruz-Correa M, et al. Frequent CpG island methylation in sporadic and syndromic gastric fundic gland polyps. Am J Clin Pathol. 2004 Nov;122(5):740–6. PMID:15491970

17. Abraham SC, Park SJ, Lee JH, et al. Genetic alterations in gastric adenomas of intestinal and foveolar phenotypes. Mod Pathol. 2003 Aug;16(8):786–95. PMID:12920223

18. Abraham SC, Park SJ, Mugartegui L, et al. Sporadic fundic gland polyps with epithelial dysplasia: evidence for preferential targeting for mutations in the adenomatous polyposis coli gene. Am J Pathol. 2002 Nov;161(5):1735–42. PMID:12414520

19. Abraham SC, Wu TT, Klimstra DS, et al. Distinctive molecular genetic alterations in sporadic and familial adenomatous polyposis-associated pancreatoblastomas: frequent alterations in the APC/beta-catenin pathway and chromosome 11p. Am J Pathol. 2001 Nov;159(5):1619–27. PMID:11696422

20. Abrahams NA, Halverson A, Fazio VW, et al. Adenocarcinoma of the small bowel: a study of 37 cases with emphasis on histologic prognostic factors. Dis Colon Rectum. 2002 Nov;45(11):1496–502. PMID:12432298

21. Achatz MI, Porter CC, Brugières L, et al. Cancer screening recommendations and clinical management of inherited gastrointestinal cancer syndromes in childhood. Clin Cancer Res. 2017 Jul 1;23(13):e107–14. PMID:28674119

22. Adachi Y, Mori M, Kido A, et al. Multiple colorectal neoplasms in a young adult with hypogammaglobulinemia. Report of a case. Dis Colon Rectum. 1992 Feb;35(2):197–200. PMID:1735325

23. Adachi Y, Yasuda K, Inomata M, et al. Pathology and prognosis of gastric carcinoma: well versus poorly differentiated type. Cancer. 2000 Oct 1;89(7):1418–24. PMID:11013353

24. Adam R, Spier I, Zhao B, et al. Exome sequencing identifies biallelic MSH3 germline mutations as a recessive subtype of colorectal adenomatous polyposis. Am J Hum Genet. 2016 Aug 4;99(2):337–51. PMID:27476653

25. Adamson AR, Grahame-Smith DG, Bogomoletz V, et al. Malignant argentaffinoma with carcinoid syndrome and hypoglycaemia. Br Med J. 1971 Jul 10;3(5766):93–4. PMID:5314568

26. Adan F, Crijns MB, Zandstra WSE, et al. Cumulative risk of skin tumours in patients with Lynch syndrome. Br J Dermatol. 2018 Aug;179(2):522–3. PMID:29542113

27. Adesina AM, Lopez-Terrada D, Wong KK, et al. Gene expression profiling reveals signatures characterizing histologic subtypes of hepatoblastoma and global deregulation in cell growth and survival pathways. Hum Pathol. 2009 Jun;40(6):843–53. PMID:19200578

28. Adsay NV, Adair CF, Heffess CS, et al. Intraductal oncocytic papillary neoplasms of the pancreas. Am J Surg Pathol. 1996 Aug;20(8):980–94. PMID:8712298

29. Adsay NV, Andea A, Basturk O, et al. Secondary tumors of the pancreas: an analysis of a surgical and autopsy database and review of the literature. Virchows Arch. 2004 Jun;444(6):527–35. PMID:15057558

30. Adsay NV, Bagci P, Tajiri T, et al. Pathologic staging of pancreatic, ampullary, biliary, and gallbladder cancers: pitfalls and practical limitations of the current AJCC/UICC TNM staging system and opportunities for improvement. Semin Diagn Pathol. 2012 Aug;29(3):127–41. PMID:23062420

31. Adsay NV, Basturk O, Bonnett M, et al. A proposal for a new and more practical grading scheme for pancreatic ductal adenocarcinoma. Am J Surg Pathol. 2005 Jun;29(6):724–33. PMID:15897739

32. Adsay NV, Basturk O, Saka B, et al. Whipple made simple for surgical pathologists: orientation, dissection, and sampling of pancreaticoduodenectomy specimens for a more practical and accurate evaluation of pancreatic, distal common bile duct, and ampullary tumors. Am J Surg Pathol. 2014 Apr;38(4):480–93. PMID:24451278

33. Adsay NV, Conlon KC, Zee SY, et al. Intraductal papillary-mucinous neoplasms of the pancreas: an analysis of in situ and invasive carcinomas in 28 patients. Cancer. 2002 Jan 1;94(1):62–77. PMID:11815961

34. Adsay NV, Klimstra DS. Cystic forms of typically solid pancreatic tumors. Semin Diagn Pathol. 2000 Feb;17(1):81–8. PMID:10721809

35. Adsay NV, Longnecker DS, Klimstra DS. Pancreatic tumors with cystic dilatation of the ducts: intraductal papillary mucinous neoplasms and intraductal oncocytic papillary neoplasms. Semin Diagn Pathol. 2000 Feb;17(1):16–30. PMID:10721804

36. Adsay NV, Merati K, Andea A, et al. The dichotomy in the preinvasive neoplasia to invasive carcinoma sequence in the pancreas: differential expression of MUC1 and MUC2 supports the existence of two separate pathways of carcinogenesis. Mod Pathol. 2002 Oct;15(10):1087–95. PMID:12379756

37. Adsay NV, Merati K, Basturk O, et al. Pathologically and biologically distinct types of epithelium in intraductal papillary mucinous neoplasms: delineation of an "intestinal" pathway of carcinogenesis in the pancreas. Am J Surg Pathol. 2004 Jul;28(7):839–48. PMID:15223952

38. Adsay NV, Merati K, Nassar H, et al. Pathogenesis of colloid (pure mucinous) carcinoma of exocrine organs: coupling of gel-forming mucin (MUC2) production with altered cell polarity and abnormal cell-stroma interaction may be the key factor in the morphogenesis and indolent behavior of colloid carcinoma in the breast and pancreas. Am J Surg Pathol. 2003 May;27(5):571–8. PMID:12717243

39. Adsay NV, Pierson C, Sarkar F, et al. Colloid (mucinous noncystic) carcinoma of the pancreas. Am J Surg Pathol. 2001 Jan;25(1):26–42. PMID:11145249

40. Adsay V, Jang KT, Roa JC, et al. Intracholecystic papillary-tubular neoplasms (ICPN) of the gallbladder (neoplastic polyps, adenomas, and papillary neoplasms that are ≥1.0 cm): clinicopathologic and immunohistochemical analysis of 123 cases. Am J Surg Pathol. 2012 Sep;36(9):1279–301. PMID:22895264

41. Adsay V, Logani S, Sarkar F, et al. Foamy gland pattern of pancreatic ductal adenocarcinoma: a deceptively benign-appearing variant. Am J Surg Pathol. 2000 Apr;24(4):493–504. PMID:10757396

42. Adsay V, Mino-Kenudson M, Furukawa T, et al. Pathologic evaluation and reporting of intraductal papillary mucinous neoplasms of the pancreas and other tumoral intraepithelial neoplasms of pancreatobiliary tract: recommendations of Verona consensus meeting. Ann Surg. 2016 Jan;263(1):162–77. PMID:25775066

43. Adsay V, Ohike N, Tajiri T, et al. Ampullary region carcinomas: definition and site specific classification with delineation of four clinicopathologically and prognostically distinct subsets in an analysis of 249 cases. Am J Surg Pathol. 2012 Nov;36(11):1592–608. PMID:23026934

44. Agaimy A, Daum O, Märkl B, et al. SWI/SNF complex-deficient undifferentiated/rhabdoid carcinomas of the gastrointestinal tract: a series of 13 cases highlighting mutually exclusive loss of SMARCA4 and SMARCA2 and frequent co-inactivation of SMARCB1 and SMARCA2. Am J Surg Pathol. 2016 Apr;40(4):544–53. PMID:26551623

45. Agaimy A, Erlenbach-Wünsch K, Konukiewitz B, et al. ISL1 expression is not restricted to pancreatic well-differentiated neuroendocrine neoplasms, but is also commonly found in well and poorly differentiated neuroendocrine neoplasms of extrapancreatic origin. Mod Pathol. 2013 Jul;26(7):995–1003. PMID:23503646

46. Agaimy A, Rau TT, Hartmann A, et al. SMARCB1 (INI1)-negative rhabdoid carcinomas of the gastrointestinal tract: clinicopathologic and molecular study of a highly aggressive variant with literature review. Am J Surg Pathol. 2014 Jul;38(7):910–20. PMID:24503755

47. Agaimy A, Stoehr R, Vieth M, et al. Benign serrated colorectal fibroblastic polyps/intramucosal perineuriomas are true mixed epithelial-stromal polyps (hybrid hyperplastic polyp/mucosal perineurioma) with frequent BRAF mutations. Am J Surg Pathol. 2010 Nov;34(11):1663–71. PMID:20962618

48. Agaimy A, Wünsch PH, Hofstaedter F, et al. Minute gastric sclerosing stromal tumors (GIST tumorlets) are common in adults and frequently show c-KIT mutations. Am J Surg Pathol. 2007 Jan;31(1):113–20. PMID:17197927

49. Agaram NP, Sung YS, Zhang L, et al. Dichotomy of genetic abnormalities in PEComas with therapeutic implications. Am J Surg Pathol. 2015 Jun;39(6):813–25. PMID:25651471

50. Agarwal N, Kumar S, Dass J, et al. Diffuse pancreatic serous cystadenoma associated with neuroendocrine carcinoma: a case report and review of literature. JOP. 2009 Jan 8;10(1):55–8. PMID:19129617

51. Agnes A, Estrella JS, Badgwell B. The significance of a nineteenth century definition in the era of genomics: linitis plastica. World J Surg Oncol. 2017 Jul 5;15(1):123. PMID:28679451

52. Agoston AT, Odze RD. Evidence that gastric pit dysplasia-like atypia is a neoplastic precursor lesion. Hum Pathol. 2014 Mar;45(3):446–55. PMID:24529328

53. Agréus L, Kuipers EJ, Kupcinskas L, et al. Rationale in diagnosis and screening of

atrophic gastritis with stomach-specific plasma biomarkers. Scand J Gastroenterol. 2012 Feb;47(2):136–47. PMID:22242613
54. Aguilera N, Gru AA. Reexamining post-transplant lymphoproliferative disorders: newly recognized and enigmatic types. Semin Diagn Pathol. 2018 Jul;35(4):236–46. PMID:29615296
55. Ahadova A, Gallon R, Gebert J, et al. Three molecular pathways model colorectal carcinogenesis in Lynch syndrome. Int J Cancer. 2018 Jul 1;143(1):139–50. PMID:29424427
56. Ahadova A, von Knebel Doeberitz M, Bläker H, et al. CTNNB1-mutant colorectal carcinomas with immediate invasive growth: a model of interval cancers in Lynch syndrome. Fam Cancer. 2016 Oct;15(4):579–86. PMID:26960970
57. Ahls MG, Niedergethmann M, Dinter D, et al. Case report: intraductal tubulopapillary neoplasm of the pancreas with unique clear cell phenotype. Diagn Pathol. 2014 Jan 20;9:11. PMID:24443801
58. Ahn DW, Ryu JK, Kim J, et al. Endoscopic papillectomy for benign ampullary neoplasms: how can treatment outcome be predicted? Gut Liver. 2013 Mar;7(2):239–45. PMID:23560162
59. Ahn JS, Jeon JR, Yoo HS, et al. Hepatoid adenocarcinoma of the stomach: an unusual case of elevated alpha-fetoprotein with prior treatment for hepatocellular carcinoma. Clin Mol Hepatol. 2013 Jun;19(2):173–8. PMID:23837142
60. Ahn S, Bae GE, Kim KM. Exuberant squamous metaplasia of the gastric mucosa in a patient with gastric adenocarcinoma. Diagn Pathol. 2015 Apr 30;10:46. PMID:25925374
61. Ahn S, Lee SJ, Kim Y, et al. High-throughput protein and mRNA expression-based classification of gastric cancers can identify clinically distinct subtypes, concordant with recent molecular classifications. Am J Surg Pathol. 2017 Jan;41(1):106–15. PMID:27819872
63. Aishima S, Fujita N, Mano Y, et al. Different roles of S100P overexpression in intrahepatic cholangiocarcinoma: carcinogenesis of perihilar type and aggressive behavior of peripheral type. Am J Surg Pathol. 2011 Apr;35(4):590–8. PMID:21412073
64. Aishima S, Iguchi T, Fujita N, et al. Histological and immunohistological findings in biliary intraepithelial neoplasia arising from a background of chronic biliary disease compared with liver cirrhosis of non-biliary aetiology. Histopathology. 2011 Nov;59(5):867–75. PMID:22092398
65. Aishima S, Oda Y. Pathogenesis and classification of intrahepatic cholangiocarcinoma: different characters of perihilar large duct type versus peripheral small duct type. J Hepatobiliary Pancreat Sci. 2015 Feb;22(2):94–100. PMID:25181580
66. Aishima S, Tanaka Y, Kubo Y, et al. Bile duct adenoma and von Meyenburg complex-like duct arising in hepatitis and cirrhosis: pathogenesis and histological characteristics. Pathol Int. 2014 Nov;64(11):551–9. PMID:25329860
67. Ait Ouakrim D, Dashti SG, Chau R, et al. Aspirin, ibuprofen, and the risk of colorectal cancer in Lynch syndrome. J Natl Cancer Inst. 2015 Jun 24;107(9):djv170. PMID:26109217
68. Akagi T, Motegi M, Tamura A, et al. A novel gene, MALT1 at 18q21, is involved in t(11;18) (q21;q21) found in low-grade B-cell lymphoma of mucosa-associated lymphoid tissue. Oncogene. 1999 Oct 14;18(42):5785–94. PMID:10523859
69. Akazawa Y, Saito T, Hayashi T, et al. Next-generation sequencing analysis for gastric adenocarcinoma with enteroblastic differentiation: emphasis on the relationship with hepatoid adenocarcinoma. Hum Pathol. 2018 Aug;78:79–88. PMID:29751042
70. Akerström G, Hessman O, Hellman P, et al. Pancreatic tumours as part of the MEN-1 syndrome. Best Pract Res Clin Gastroenterol. 2005 Oct;19(5):819–30. PMID:16253903
71. Akita M, Fujikura K, Ajiki T, et al. Dichotomy in intrahepatic cholangiocarcinomas based on histologic similarities to hilar cholangiocarcinomas. Mod Pathol. 2017 Jul;30(7):986–97. PMID:28338651
72. Akiyama T, Shida T, Yoshitomi H, et al. Expression of sex determining region Y-box 2 and pancreatic and duodenal homeobox 1 in pancreatic neuroendocrine tumors. Pancreas. 2016 Apr;45(4):522–7. PMID:26491904
73. Al Efishat MA, Attiyeh MA, Eaton AA, et al. Multi-institutional validation study of pancreatic cyst fluid protein analysis for prediction of high-risk intraductal papillary mucinous neoplasms of the pancreas. Ann Surg. 2018 Aug;268(2):340–7. PMID:28700444
74. Al-Abbadi MA, Almasri NM, Al-Quran S, et al. Cytokeratin and epithelial membrane antigen expression in angiosarcomas: an immunohistochemical study of 33 cases. Arch Pathol Lab Med. 2007 Feb;131(2):288–92. PMID:17284115
75. Al-Saleem T, Al-Mondhiry H. Immunoproliferative small intestinal disease (IPSID): a model for mature B-cell neoplasms. Blood. 2005 Mar 15;105(6):2274–80. PMID:15542584
76. Al-Shoha M, Nadeem U, George N, et al. Verrucous carcinoma of the esophagus-remains a diagnostic enigma. Am J Gastroenterol. 2018 Jun;113(6):919–21. PMID:29748561
77. Al-Toma A, Goerres MS, Meijer JW, et al. Human leukocyte antigen-DQ2 homozygosity and the development of refractory celiac disease and enteropathy-associated T-cell lymphoma. Clin Gastroenterol Hepatol. 2006 Mar;4(3):315–9. PMID:16527694
78. Al-Toma A, Verbeek WH, Hadithi M, et al. Survival in refractory coeliac disease and enteropathy-associated T-cell lymphoma: retrospective evaluation of single-centre experience. Gut. 2007 Oct;56(10):1373–8. PMID:17470479
79. Alakus H, Babicky ML, Ghosh P, et al. Genome-wide mutational landscape of mucinous carcinomatosis peritonei of appendiceal origin. Genome Med. 2014 May 29;6(5):43. PMID:24944587
80. Alassiri AH, Ali RH, Shen Y, et al. ETV6-NTRK3 is expressed in a subset of ALK-negative inflammatory myofibroblastic tumors. Am J Surg Pathol. 2016 Aug;40(8):1051–61. PMID:27259007
81. Albores-Saavedra J, Batich K, Hossain S, et al. Carcinoid tumors and small-cell carcinomas of the gallbladder and extrahepatic bile ducts: a comparative study based on 221 cases from the Surveillance, Epidemiology, and End Results Program. Ann Diagn Pathol. 2009 Dec;13(6):378–83. PMID:19917473
82. Albores-Saavedra J, Chable-Montero F, Angeles-Albores D, et al. Early gallbladder carcinoma: a clinicopathologic study of 13 cases of intramucosal carcinoma. Am J Clin Pathol. 2011 Apr;135(4):637–42. PMID:21411787
83. Albores-Saavedra J, Chablé-Montero F, González-Romo MA, et al. Adenomas of the gallbladder. Morphologic features, expression of gastric and intestinal mucins, and incidence of high-grade dysplasia/carcinoma in situ and invasive carcinoma. Hum Pathol. 2012 Sep;43(9):1506–13. PMID:22386521
84. Albores-Saavedra J, Chablé-Montero F, Méndez-Sánchez N, et al. Adenocarcinoma with pyloric gland phenotype of the extrahepatic bile ducts: a previously unrecognized and distinctive morphologic variant of extrahepatic bile duct carcinoma. Hum Pathol. 2012 Dec;43(12):2292–8. PMID:22795356
85. Albores-Saavedra J, Córdova-Ramón JC, Chablé-Montero F, et al. Cystadenomas of the liver and extrahepatic bile ducts: morphologic and immunohistochemical characterization of the biliary and intestinal variants. Ann Diagn Pathol. 2015 Jun;19(3):124–9. PMID:25792461
86. Albores-Saavedra J, Hart A, Chablé-Montero F, et al. Carcinoids and high-grade neuroendocrine carcinomas of the ampulla of Vater: a comparative analysis of 139 cases from the Surveillance, Epidemiology, and End Results program-a population based study. Arch Pathol Lab Med. 2010 Nov;134(11):1692–6. PMID:21043824
87. Albores-Saavedra J, Henson DE, Klimstra DS. Tumors of the gallbladder, extrahepatic bile ducts and ampulla of Vater. Washington, DC: Armed Forces Institute of Pathology; 2000. (AFIP atlas of tumor pathology, series 3; fascicle 27).
88. Albores-Saavedra J, Henson DE, Klimstra DS. Tumors of the gallbladder, extrahepatic bile ducts, and Vaterian system. Washington, DC: American Registry of Pathology; 2015. (AFIP atlas of tumor pathology, series 4; fascicle 23).
89. Albores-Saavedra J, Hoang MP, Murakata LA, et al. Atypical bile duct adenoma, clear cell type: a previously undescribed tumor of the liver. Am J Surg Pathol. 2001 Jul;25(7):956–60. PMID:11420469
90. Albores-Saavedra J, Keenportz B, Bejarano PA, et al. Adenomyomatous hyperplasia of the gallbladder with perineural invasion: revisited. Am J Surg Pathol. 2007 Oct;31(10):1598–604. PMID:17895763
91. Albores-Saavedra J, Manivel C, Dorantes-Heredia R, et al. Nonmucinous cystadenomas of the pancreas with pancreatobiliary phenotype and ovarian-like stroma. Am J Clin Pathol. 2013 May;139(5):599–604. PMID:23596111
92. Albores-Saavedra J, Molberg K, Henson DE. Unusual malignant epithelial tumors of the gallbladder. Semin Diagn Pathol. 1996 Nov;13(4):326–38. PMID:8946610
93. Albores-Saavedra J, Schwartz AM, Batich K, et al. Cancers of the ampulla of Vater: demographics, morphology, and survival based on 5,625 cases from the SEER program. J Surg Oncol. 2009 Dec 1;100(7):598–605. PMID:19697352
94. Albores-Saavedra J, Shukla D, Carrick K, et al. In situ and invasive adenocarcinomas of the gallbladder extending into or arising from Rokitansky-Aschoff sinuses: a clinicopathologic study of 49 cases. Am J Surg Pathol. 2004 May;28(5):621–8. PMID:15105650
95. Albores-Saavedra J, Vardaman CJ, Vuitch F. Non-neoplastic polypoid lesions and adenomas of the gallbladder. Pathol Annu. 1993;28(Pt 1):145–77. PMID:8416136
96. Albores-Saavedra J, Wu J, Crook T, et al. Intestinal and oncocytic variants of pancreatic intraepithelial neoplasia. A morphological and immunohistochemical study. Ann Diagn Pathol. 2005 Apr;9(2):69–76. PMID:15806512
97. Albores-Saavedra J. Acinar cystadenoma of the pancreas: a previously undescribed tumor. Ann Diagn Pathol. 2002 Apr;6(2):113–5. PMID:12004359
98. Albuquerque A, Pessegueiro Miranda H, Lopes J, et al. Liver transplant recipients have a higher prevalence of anal squamous intraepithelial lesions. Br J Cancer. 2017 Dec 5;117(12):1761–7. PMID:29093575
99. Albuquerque A, Sheaff M, Stirrup O, et al. Performance of anal cytology compared with high-resolution anoscopy and histology in women with lower anogenital tract neoplasia. Clin Infect Dis. 2018 Sep 28;67(8):1262–8. PMID:29659752
100. Alcindor T, Tosikyan A, Vuong T, et al. Small-cell anal carcinoma and AIDS: case report and review of the literature. Int J Colorectal Dis. 2008 Jan;23(1):135–6. PMID:17279348
101. Aldaoud N, Joudeh A, Al-Momen S, et al. Anaplastic carcinoma arising in a mucinous cystic neoplasm masquerading as pancreatic pseudocyst. Diagn Cytopathol. 2016 Jun;44(6):538–42. PMID:27028547
102. Alexander J, Watanabe T, Wu TT, et al. Histopathological identification of colon cancer with microsatellite instability. Am J Pathol. 2001 Feb;158(2):527–35. PMID:11159189
103. Alexandraki KI, Grossman AB. The ectopic ACTH syndrome. Rev Endocr Metab Disord. 2010 Jun;11(2):117–26. PMID:20544290
104. Alexandraki KI, Kaltsas GA, Grozinsky-Glasberg S, et al. Appendiceal neuroendocrine neoplasms: diagnosis and management. Endocr Relat Cancer. 2016 Jan;23(1):R27–41. PMID:26483424
105. Alexandrov LB, Nik-Zainal S, Wedge DC, et al. Signatures of mutational processes in human cancer. Nature. 2013 Aug 22;500(7463):415–21. PMID:23945592
106. Allaire GS, Rabin L, Ishak KG, et al. Bile duct adenoma. A study of 152 cases. Am J Surg Pathol. 1988 Sep;12(9):708–15. PMID:3046396
107. Allan BJ, Parikh PP, Diaz S, et al. Predictors of survival and incidence of hepatoblastoma in the paediatric population. HPB (Oxford). 2013 Oct;15(10):741–6. PMID:23600968
108. Allanson BM, Bonavita J, Mirzai B, et al. Early Barrett esophagus-related neoplasia in segments 1 cm or longer is always associated with intestinal metaplasia. Mod Pathol. 2017 Aug;30(8):1170–6. PMID:28548120
109. Allemani C, Matsuda T, Di Carlo V, et al. Global surveillance of trends in cancer survival 2000-14 (CONCORD-3): analysis of individual records for 37 513 025 patients diagnosed with one of 18 cancers from 322 population-based registries in 71 countries. Lancet. 2018 Mar 17;391(10125):1023–75. PMID:29395269
110. Allen PJ, Kuk D, Castillo CF, et al. Multi-institutional validation study of the American Joint Commission on Cancer (8th edition) changes for T and N staging in patients with pancreatic adenocarcinoma. Ann Surg. 2017 Jan;265(1):185–91. PMID:27163957
111. Allison KH, Yoder BJ, Bronner MP, et al. Angiosarcoma involving the gastrointestinal tract: a series of primary and metastatic cases. Am J Surg Pathol. 2004 Mar;28(3):298–307. PMID:15104292
112. Allum W, Lordick F, Alsina M, et al. ECCO essential requirements for quality cancer care: oesophageal and gastric cancer. Crit Rev Oncol Hematol. 2018 Feb;122:179–93. PMID:29458786
113. Aloia TA, Járufe N, Javle M, et al. Gallbladder cancer: expert consensus statement. HPB (Oxford). 2015 Aug;17(8):681–90. PMID:26172135
114. Alpert LC, Truong LD, Bossart MI, et al. Microcystic adenoma (serous cystadenoma) of the pancreas. A study of 14 cases with immunohistochemical and electron-microscopic correlation. Am J Surg Pathol. 1988 Apr;12(4):251–63. PMID:3354751
115. Alvi MA, Loughrey MB, Dunne P, et al. Molecular profiling of signet ring cell colorectal cancer provides a strong rationale for genomic targeted and immune checkpoint inhibitor therapies. Br J Cancer. 2017 Jul 11;117(2):203–9. PMID:28595259
116. Alvi MA, McArt DG, Kelly P, et al. Comprehensive molecular pathology analysis of small bowel adenocarcinoma reveals novel targets with potential for clinical utility. Oncotarget. 2015 Aug 28;6(25):20863–74. PMID:26315110
117. Alvi MA, Wilson RH, Salto-Tellez M. Rare cancers: the greatest inequality in cancer

research and oncology treatment. Br J Cancer. 2017 Oct 24;117(9):1255–7. PMID:28934760

118. Alyousef MJ, Alratroot JA, ElSharkawy T, et al. Malignant gastrointestinal neuroectodermal tumor: a case report and review of the literature. Diagn Pathol. 2017 Mar 20;12(1):29. PMID:28320420

119. Amadou A, Waddington Achatz MI, Hainaut P. Revisiting tumor patterns and penetrance in germline TP53 mutation carriers: temporal phases of Li-Fraumeni syndrome. Curr Opin Oncol. 2018 Jan;30(1):23–9. PMID:29076966

120. Amato E, Molin MD, Mafficini A, et al. Targeted next-generation sequencing of cancer genes dissects the molecular profiles of intraductal papillary neoplasms of the pancreas. J Pathol. 2014 Jul;233(3):217–27. PMID:24604757

121. Amato T, Abate F, Piccaluga P, et al. Clonality analysis of immunoglobulin gene rearrangement by next-generation sequencing in endemic Burkitt lymphoma suggests antigen drive activation of BCR as opposed to sporadic Burkitt lymphoma. Am J Clin Pathol. 2016 Jan;145(1):116–27. PMID:26712879

122. Ambrosio MR, Lazzi S, Bello GL, et al. MYC protein expression scoring and its impact on the prognosis of aggressive B-cell lymphoma patients. Haematologica. 2019 Jan;104(1):e25–8. PMID:29954940

123. Ambrosio MR, Navari M, Di Lisio L, et al. The Epstein Barr-encoded BART-6-3p microRNA affects regulation of cell growth and immuno response in Burkitt lymphoma. Infect Agent Cancer. 2014 Apr 14;9:12. PMID:24731550

124. Ambrosio MR, Piccaluga PP, Ponzoni M, et al. The alteration of lipid metabolism in Burkitt lymphoma identifies a novel marker: adipophilin. PLoS One. 2012;7(8):e44315. PMID:22952953

125. Amieva MR, El-Omar EM. Host-bacterial interactions in Helicobacter pylori infection. Gastroenterology. 2008 Jan;134(1):306–23. PMID:18166359

126. Amin A, Epstein JI. Noninvasive micropapillary urothelial carcinoma: a clinicopathologic study of 18 cases. Hum Pathol. 2012 Dec;43(12):2124–8. PMID:22939957

127. Amin MB, Edge S, Greene F, et al., editors. AJCC cancer staging manual. 8th ed. New York (NY): Springer; 2017.

128. Ammann RW, Vetter D, Deyhle P, et al. Gastrointestinal involvement in systemic mastocytosis. Gut. 1976 Feb;17(2):107–12. PMID:1261881

129. Amundadottir L, Kraft P, Stolzenberg-Solomon RZ, et al. Genome-wide association study identifies variants in the ABO locus associated with susceptibility to pancreatic cancer. Nat Genet. 2009 Sep;41(9):986–90. PMID:19648918

130. Amundadottir LT. Pancreatic cancer genetics. Int J Biol Sci. 2016 Jan 28;12(3):314–25. PMID:26929738

131. An S, Jang J, Min K, et al. Granular cell tumor of the gastrointestinal tract: histologic and immunohistochemical analysis of 98 cases. Hum Pathol. 2015 Jun;46(6):813–9. PMID:25882927

132. Anagnostopoulos GK, Arvanitidis D, Sakorafas G, et al. Combined carcinoid-adenocarcinoma tumour of the anal canal. Scand J Gastroenterol. 2004 Feb;39(2):198–200. PMID:15000285

133. Andea A, Sarkar F, Adsay VN. Clinicopathological correlates of pancreatic intraepithelial neoplasia: a comparative analysis of 82 cases with and 152 cases without pancreatic ductal adenocarcinoma. Mod Pathol. 2003 Oct;16(10):996–1006. PMID:14559982

134. Anderson JC, Butterly LF, Robinson CM,

et al. Risk of metachronous high-risk adenomas and large serrated polyps in individuals with serrated polyps on index colonoscopy: data from the New Hampshire Colonoscopy Registry. Gastroenterology. 2018 Jan;154(1):117–27.e2. PMID:28927878

135. Anderson KE, Mack TM, Silverman DT. Cancer of the pancreas. In: Schottenfeld D, Fraumeni JF Jr, editors. Cancer epidemiology and prevention. 3rd ed. New York (NY): Oxford University Press; 2006. pp. 721–62.

136. Anderson MJ, Kwong CA, Atieh M, et al. Mixed acinar-neuroendocrine-ductal carcinoma of the pancreas: a tale of three lineages. BMJ Case Rep. 2016 Jun 2;2016. pii: bcr2015213661. PMID:27257019

137. Anderson WF, Rabkin CS, Turner N, et al. The changing face of noncardia gastric cancer incidence among US non-Hispanic whites. J Natl Cancer Inst. 2018 Jun 1;110(6):608–15. PMID:29361173

138. Andersson E, Arvidsson Y, Swärd C, et al. Expression profiling of small intestinal neuroendocrine tumors identifies subgroups with clinical relevance, prognostic markers and therapeutic targets. Mod Pathol. 2016 Jun;29(6):616–29. PMID:26965582

139. Andersson E, Swärd C, Stenman G, et al. High-resolution genomic profiling reveals gain of chromosome 14 as a predictor of poor outcome in ileal carcinoids. Endocr Relat Cancer. 2009 Sep;16(3):953–66. PMID:19458023

140. Ando N, Ozawa S, Kitagawa Y, et al. Improvement in the results of surgical treatment of advanced squamous esophageal carcinoma during 15 consecutive years. Ann Surg. 2000 Aug;232(2):225–32. PMID:10903602

141. Ando T, Hosokawa A, Yamawaki H, et al. Esophageal small-cell carcinoma with syndrome of inappropriate secretion of antidiuretic hormone. Intern Med. 2011;50(10):1099–103. PMID:21576835

142. Andrici J, Farzin M, Sioson L, et al. Mismatch repair deficiency as a prognostic factor in mucinous colorectal cancer. Mod Pathol. 2016 Mar;29(3):266–74. PMID:26769140

143. Andricovich J, Perkail S, Kai Y, et al. Loss of KDM6A activates super-enhancers to induce gender-specific squamous-like pancreatic cancer and confers sensitivity to BET inhibitors. Cancer Cell. 2018 Mar 12;33(3):512–26.e8. PMID:29533787

144. André TR, Brito M, Freire JG, et al. Rectal and anal canal neuroendocrine tumours. J Gastrointest Oncol. 2018 Apr;9(2):354–7. PMID:29755775

145. Anene C, Thompson JS, Saigh J, et al. Somatostatinoma: atypical presentation of a rare pancreatic tumor. Am J Gastroenterol. 1995 May;90(5):819–21. PMID:7733095

146. Ang DC, Shia J, Tang LH, et al. The utility of immunohistochemistry in subtyping adenocarcinoma of the ampulla of Vater. Am J Surg Pathol. 2014 Oct;38(10):1371–9. PMID:24832159

147. Angeles-Angeles A, Quintanilla-Martínez L, Larriva-Sahd J. Primary carcinoid of the common bile duct. Immunohistochemical characterization of a case and review of the literature. Am J Clin Pathol. 1991 Sep;96(3):341–4. PMID:1877530

148. Anjaneyulu V, Shankar-Swarnalatha G, Rao SC. Carcinoid tumor of the gall bladder. Ann Diagn Pathol. 2007 Apr;11(2):113–6. PMID:17349570

149. Anker MC, Arnemann J, Neumann K, et al. Alport syndrome with diffuse leiomyomatosis. Am J Med Genet A. 2003 Jun 15;119A(3):381–5. PMID:12784310

150. Anlauf M, Bauersfeld J, Raffel A, et al. Insulinomatosis: a multicentric insulinoma disease that frequently causes early

recurrent hyperinsulinemic hypoglycemia. Am J Surg Pathol. 2009 Mar;33(3):339–46. PMID:19011561

151. Anlauf M, Enosawa T, Henopp T, et al. Primary lymph node gastrinoma or occult duodenal microgastrinoma with lymph node metastases in a MEN1 patient: the need for a systematic search for the primary tumor. Am J Surg Pathol. 2008 Jul;32(7):1101–5. PMID:18520436

152. Anlauf M, Garbrecht N, Bauersfeld J, et al. Hereditary neuroendocrine tumors of the gastroenteropancreatic system. Virchows Arch. 2007 Aug;451 Suppl 1:S29–38. PMID:17684762

153. Anlauf M, Garbrecht N, Henopp T, et al. Sporadic versus hereditary gastrinomas of the duodenum and pancreas: distinct clinico-pathological and epidemiological features. World J Gastroenterol. 2006 Sep 14;12(34):5440–6. PMID:17006979

154. Anlauf M, Perren A, Henopp T, et al. Allelic deletion of the MEN1 gene in duodenal gastrin and somatostatin cell neoplasms and their precursor lesions. Gut. 2007 May;56(5):637–44. PMID:17135306

155. Anlauf M, Perren A, Meyer CL, et al. Precursor lesions in patients with multiple endocrine neoplasia type 1-associated duodenal gastrinomas. Gastroenterology. 2005 May;128(5):1187–98. PMID:15887103

156. Anlauf M, Schlenger R, Perren A, et al. Microadenomatosis of the endocrine pancreas in patients with and without the multiple endocrine neoplasia type 1 syndrome. Am J Surg Pathol. 2006 May;30(5):560–74. PMID:16699310

157. Anthony PP, James K. Pedunculated hepatocellular carcinoma. Is it an entity? Histopathology. 1987 Apr;11(4):403–14. PMID:3036680

158. Anthony PP, Morris DS, Vowles KD. Multiple and recurrent inflammatory fibroid polyps in three generations of a Devon family: a new syndrome. Gut. 1984 Aug;25(8):854–62. PMID:6745724

159. Anthony PP, Sarsfield P, Clarke T. Primary lymphoma of the liver: clinical and pathological features of 10 patients. J Clin Pathol. 1990 Dec;43(12):1007–13. PMID:2266172

160. Antman K, Chang Y. Kaposi's sarcoma. N Engl J Med. 2000 Apr 6;342(14):1027–38. PMID:10749966

161. Antonescu C. Malignant vascular tumors–an update. Mod Pathol. 2014 Jan;27 Suppl 1:S30–8. PMID:24384851

162. Antonescu CR, Besmer P, Guo T, et al. Acquired resistance to imatinib in gastrointestinal stromal tumor occurs through secondary gene mutation. Clin Cancer Res. 2005 Jun 1;11(11):4182–90. PMID:15930355

163. Antonescu CR, Le Loarer F, Mosquera JM, et al. Novel YAP1-TFE3 fusion defines a distinct subset of epithelioid hemangioendothelioma. Genes Chromosomes Cancer. 2013 Aug;52(8):775–84. PMID:23737213

164. Antonescu CR, Romeo S, Zhang L, et al. Dedifferentiation in gastrointestinal stromal tumor to an anaplastic KIT-negative phenotype: a diagnostic pitfall: morphologic and molecular characterization of 8 cases occurring either de novo or after imatinib therapy. Am J Surg Pathol. 2013 Mar;37(3):385–92. PMID:23348204

165. Antonescu CR, Suurmeijer AJ, Zhang L, et al. Molecular characterization of inflammatory myofibroblastic tumors with frequent ALK and ROS1 gene fusions and rare novel RET rearrangement. Am J Surg Pathol. 2015 Jul;39(7):957–67. PMID:25723109

166. Antonescu CR, Yoshida A, Guo T, et al. KDR activating mutations in human angiosarcomas are sensitive to specific kinase inhibitors.

Cancer Res. 2009 Sep 15;69(18):7175–9. PMID:19723655

167. Antoniuk PM, Tjandra JJ, Webb BW, et al. Anorectal malignant melanoma has a poor prognosis. Int J Colorectal Dis. 1993 Jul;8(2):81–6. PMID:8409692

168. Antwi SO, Mousa OY, Patel T. Racial, ethnic, and age disparities in incidence and survival of intrahepatic cholangiocarcinoma in the United States; 1995-2014. Ann Hepatol. 2018 Mar 1;17(2):274–85. PMID:29469047

169. Aoki Y, Tabuse K, Wada M, et al. Primary adenosquamous carcinoma of the stomach: experience of 11 cases and its clinical analysis. Gastroenterol Jpn. 1978;13(2):140–5. PMID:669198

170. Aparicio T, Zaanan A, Mary F, et al. Small bowel adenocarcinoma. Gastroenterol Clin North Am. 2016 Sep;45(3):447–57. PMID:27546842

171. Aparicio T, Zaanan A, Svrcek M, et al. Small bowel adenocarcinoma: epidemiology, risk factors, diagnosis and treatment. Dig Liver Dis. 2014 Feb;46(2):97–104. PMID:23796552

172. Appelman HD, Coopersmith N. Pleomorphic spindle-cell carcinoma of the gallbladder. Relation to sarcoma of the gallbladder. Cancer. 1970 Mar;25(3):535–41. PMID:5416826

173. Arai M, Shimizu S, Imai Y, et al. Mutations of the Ki-ras, p53 and APC genes in adenocarcinomas of the human small intestine. Int J Cancer. 1997 Feb 7;70(4):390–5. PMID:9033644

174. Arai T, Sakurai U, Sawabe M, et al. Frequent microsatellite instability in papillary and solid-type, poorly differentiated adenocarcinomas of the stomach. Gastric Cancer. 2013 Oct;16(4):505–12. PMID:23274922

175. Arcaini L, Zibellini S, Boveri E, et al. The BRAF V600E mutation in hairy cell leukemia and other mature B-cell neoplasms. Blood. 2012 Jan 5;119(1):188–91. PMID:22072557

176. Arceci RJ, Allen CE, Dunkel IJ, et al. A phase IIa study of afuresertib, an oral pan-AKT inhibitor, in patients with Langerhans cell histiocytosis. Pediatr Blood Cancer. 2017 May;64(5). PMID:27804235

177. Arena V, Arena E, Stigliano E, et al. Bile duct adenoma with oncocytic features. Histopathology. 2006 Sep;49(3):318–20. PMID:16918984

178. Arends MJ. Pathways of colorectal carcinogenesis. Appl Immunohistochem Mol Morphol. 2013 Mar;21(2):97–102. PMID:23417071

179. Arer IM, Yilmaz D, Ozek OC, et al. Unusual location of median raphe cyst presenting as perianal polyp: a case report. Dermatol Online J. 2016 Jun 15;22(6):13030/qt4f48g7jc. PMID:27617601

180. Aretz S, Stienen D, Uhlhaas S, et al. High proportion of large genomic deletions and a genotype phenotype update in 80 unrelated families with juvenile polyposis syndrome. J Med Genet. 2007 Nov;44(11):702–9. PMID:17873119

181. Aretz S, Uhlhaas S, Goergens H, et al. MUTYH-associated polyposis: 70 of 71 patients with biallelic mutations present with an attenuated or atypical phenotype. Int J Cancer. 2006 Aug 15;119(4):807–14. PMID:16557584

182. Argani P, Aulmann S, Illei PB, et al. A distinctive subset of PEComas harbors TFE3 gene fusions. Am J Surg Pathol. 2010 Oct;34(10):1395–406. PMID:20871214

183. Ariffin H, Chan AS, Oh L, et al. Frequent occurrence of gastric cancer in Asian kindreds with Li-Fraumeni syndrome. Clin Genet. 2015 Nov;88(5):450–5. PMID:25318593

184. Ariizumi S, Kotera Y, Katagiri S, et al. Combined hepatocellular-cholangiocarcinoma had poor outcomes after hepatectomy regardless of Allen and Lisa class or the predominance of intrahepatic cholangiocarcinoma

cells within the tumor. Ann Surg Oncol. 2012 May;19(5):1628–36. PMID:22113592
185. Arnaoutakis DJ, Kim Y, Pulitano C, et al. Management of biliary cystic tumors: a multi-institutional analysis of a rare liver tumor. Ann Surg. 2015 Feb;261(2):361–7. PMID:24509187
186. Arnason T, Borger DR, Corless C, et al. Biliary adenofibroma of liver: morphology, tumor genetics, and outcomes in 6 cases. Am J Surg Pathol. 2017 Apr;41(4):499–505. PMID:28266931
187. Arnason T, Fleming KE, Wanless IR. Peritumoral hyperplasia of the liver: a response to portal vein invasion by hypervascular neoplasms. Histopathology. 2013 Feb;62(3):458–64. PMID:23240735
188. Arnason T, Liang WY, Alfaro E, et al. Morphology and natural history of familial adenomatous polyposis-associated dysplastic fundic gland polyps. Histopathology. 2014 Sep;65(3):353–62. PMID:24548295
189. Arnold D, Lueza B, Douillard JY, et al. Prognostic and predictive value of primary tumour side in patients with RAS wild-type metastatic colorectal cancer treated with chemotherapy and EGFR directed antibodies in six randomized trials. Ann Oncol. 2017 Aug 1;28(8):1713–29. PMID:28407110
190. Arnold LD, Patel AV, Yan Y, et al. Are racial disparities in pancreatic cancer explained by smoking and overweight/obesity? Cancer Epidemiol Biomarkers Prev. 2009 Sep;18(9):2397–405. PMID:19723915
191. Arnold M, Sierra MS, Laversanne M, et al. Global patterns and trends in colorectal cancer incidence and mortality. Gut. 2017 Apr;66(4):683–91. PMID:26818619
192. Arnold M, Soerjomataram I, Ferlay J, et al. Global incidence of oesophageal cancer by histological subtype in 2012. Gut. 2015 Mar;64(3):381–7. PMID:25320104
193. Arock M, Valent P. Pathogenesis, classification and treatment of mastocytosis: state of the art in 2010 and future perspectives. Expert Rev Hematol. 2010 Aug;3(4):497–516. PMID:21083038
194. Aronson M, Gallinger S, Cohen Z, et al. Gastrointestinal findings in the largest series of patients with hereditary biallelic mismatch repair deficiency syndrome: report from the international consortium. Am J Gastroenterol. 2016 Feb;111(2):275–84. PMID:26729549
195. Arvey A, Ojesina AI, Pedamallu CS, et al. The tumor virus landscape of AIDS-related lymphomas. Blood. 2015 May 14;125(20):e14–22. PMID:25827832
196. Asare EA, Compton CC, Hanna NN, et al. The impact of stage, grade, and mucinous histology on the efficacy of systemic chemotherapy in adenocarcinomas of the appendix: analysis of the National Cancer Data Base. Cancer. 2016 Jan 15;122(2):213–21. PMID:26506400
197. Asayama M, Fuse N, Yoshino T, et al. Amrubicin for the treatment of neuroendocrine carcinoma of the gastrointestinal tract: a retrospective analysis of five cases. Cancer Chemother Pharmacol. 2011 Nov;68(5):1325–30. PMID:21461890
198. Ascolani M, Mescoli C, Palmieri G, et al. Colonic phenotype of the ileum in Crohn's disease: a prospective study before and after ileocolonic resection. Inflamm Bowel Dis. 2014 Sep;20(9):1555–61. PMID:25054336
199. Chathadi KV, Khashab MA, Acosta RD, et al. The role of endoscopy in ampullary and duodenal adenomas. Gastrointest Endosc. 2015 Nov;82(5):773–81. PMID:26260385
200. Askan G, Deshpande V, Klimstra DS, et al. Expression of markers of hepatocellular differentiation in pancreatic acinar cell neoplasms: a potential diagnostic pitfall. Am J Clin Pathol. 2016 Aug;146(2):163–9. PMID:27425386
201. Askling J, Dickman PW, Karlén P, et al. Family history as a risk factor for colorectal cancer in inflammatory bowel disease. Gastroenterology. 2001 May;120(6):1356–62. PMID:11313305
202. Aslan DL, Jessurun J, Gulbahce HE, et al. Endoscopic ultrasound-guided fine needle aspiration features of a pancreatic neoplasm with predominantly intraductal growth and prominent tubular cytomorphology: intraductal tubular carcinoma of the pancreas? Diagn Cytopathol. 2008 Nov;36(11):833–9. PMID:18831024
203. Assmann G, Kappler R, Zeindl-Eberhart E, et al. β-Catenin mutations in 2 nested stromal epithelial tumors of the liver–a neoplasia with defective mesenchymal-epithelial transition. Hum Pathol. 2012 Nov;43(11):1815–27. PMID:22749188
204. Atkin W, Brenner A, Martin J, et al. The clinical effectiveness of different surveillance strategies to prevent colorectal cancer in people with intermediate-grade colorectal adenomas: a retrospective cohort analysis, and psychological and economic evaluations. Health Technol Assess. 2017 Apr;21(25):1–536. PMID:28621643
205. Atkin WS, Edwards R, Kralj-Hans I, et al. Once-only flexible sigmoidoscopy screening in prevention of colorectal cancer: a multicentre randomised controlled trial. Lancet. 2010 May 8;375(9726):1624–33. PMID:20430429
206. Attygalle AD, Cabeçadas J, Gaulard P, et al. Peripheral T-cell and NK-cell lymphomas and their mimics; taking a step forward - report on the lymphoma workshop of the XVIth meeting of the European Association for Haematopathology and the Society for Hematopathology. Histopathology. 2014 Jan;64(2):171–99. PMID:24128129
207. Audard V, Cavard C, Richa H, et al. Impaired E-cadherin expression and glutamine synthetase overexpression in solid pseudopapillary neoplasm of the pancreas. Pancreas. 2008 Jan;36(1):80–3. PMID:18192886
208. Aung KL, Fischer SE, Denroche RE, et al. Genomics-driven precision medicine for advanced pancreatic cancer: early results from the COMPASS trial. Clin Cancer Res. 2018 Mar 15;24(6):1344–54. PMID:29288237
209. Avadhani V, Hacihasanoglu E, Memis B, et al. Cytologic predictors of malignancy in bile duct brushings: a multi-reviewer analysis of 60 cases. Mod Pathol. 2017 Sep;30(9):1273–86. PMID:28664934
210. Aydogdu I, Uzun E, Mirapoglu SL, et al. Buschke-Löwenstein tumor: three pediatric cases. Pediatr Int. 2016 Aug;58(8):769–72. PMID:27384409
211. Aytac E, Ozdemir Y, Ozuner G. Long term outcomes of neuroendocrine carcinomas (high-grade neuroendocrine tumors) of the colon, rectum, and anal canal. J Visc Surg. 2014 Feb;151(1):3–7. PMID:24412088
212. Azar C, Van de Stadt J, Rickaert F, et al. Intraductal papillary mucinous tumours of the pancreas. Clinical and therapeutic issues in 32 patients. Gut. 1996 Sep;39(3):457–64. PMID:8949654
213. Azimuddin K, Khubchandani IT, Stasik JJ, et al. Neoplasia after ureterosigmoidostomy. Dis Colon Rectum. 1999 Dec;42(12):1632–8. PMID:10613486
214. Bachmeyer C, Monge M, Cazier A, et al. Gastric adenocarcinoma in a patient with X-linked agammaglobulinaemia. Eur J Gastroenterol Hepatol. 2000 Sep;12(9):1033–5. PMID:11007143
215. Backes Y, Moons LM, Novelli MR, et al. Diagnosis of T1 colorectal cancer in pedunculated polyps in daily clinical practice: a multicenter study. Mod Pathol. 2017 Jan;30(1):104–12. PMID:27713422
216. Backes Y, Moss A, Reitsma JB, et al. Narrow band imaging, magnifying chromoendoscopy, and gross morphological features for the optical diagnosis of T1 colorectal cancer and deep submucosal invasion: a systematic review and meta-analysis. Am J Gastroenterol. 2017 Jan;112(1):54–64. PMID:27644737
217. Bacq Y, Jacquemin E, Balabaud C, et al. Familial liver adenomatosis associated with hepatocyte nuclear factor 1alpha inactivation. Gastroenterology. 2003 Nov;125(5):1470–5. PMID:14598263
218. Badalian-Very G, Vergilio JA, Degar BA, et al. Recurrent BRAF mutations in Langerhans cell histiocytosis. Blood. 2010 Sep 16;116(11):1919–23. PMID:20519626
219. Baek DH, Kim GH, Park DY, et al. Gastric epithelial dysplasia: characteristics and long-term follow-up results after endoscopic resection according to morphological categorization. BMC Gastroenterol. 2015 Feb 12;15:17. PMID:25886985
220. Baek SK, Han SW, Oh DY, et al. Clinicopathologic characteristics and treatment outcomes of hepatoid adenocarcinoma of the stomach, a rare but unique subtype of gastric cancer. BMC Gastroenterol. 2011 May 19;11:56. PMID:21592404
221. Baek SW, Kang HJ, Yoon JY, et al. Clinical study and review of articles (Korean) about retrorectal developmental cysts in adults. J Korean Soc Coloproctol. 2011 Dec;27(6):303–14. PMID:22259746
222. Bagg A, Dunphy CH. Immunosuppressive and immunomodulatory therapy-associated lymphoproliferative disorders. Semin Diagn Pathol. 2013 May;30(2):102–12. PMID:23541274
223. Bai X, Kong Y, Chi Z, et al. MAPK pathway and TERT promoter gene mutation pattern and its prognostic value in melanoma patients: a retrospective study of 2,793 cases. Clin Cancer Res. 2017 Oct 15;23(20):6120–7. PMID:28720667
224. Bailey P, Chang DK, Nones K, et al. Genomic analyses identify molecular subtypes of pancreatic cancer. Nature. 2016 Mar 3;531(7592):47–52. PMID:26909576
225. Baker HL, Caldwell DW. Lesions of the ampulla of Vater. Surgery. 1947 Apr;21(4):523–31. PMID:20290635
226. Baker KT, Salk JJ, Brentnall TA, et al. Precancer in ulcerative colitis: the role of the field effect and its clinical implications. Carcinogenesis. 2018 Jan 12;39(1):11–20. PMID:29087436
227. Baker ML, Seeley ES, Pai R, et al. Invasive mucinous cystic neoplasms of the pancreas. Exp Mol Pathol. 2012 Dec;93(3):345–9. PMID:22902940
228. Bakry D, Aronson M, Durno C, et al. Genetic and clinical determinants of constitutional mismatch repair deficiency syndrome: report from the constitutional mismatch repair deficiency consortium. Eur J Cancer. 2014 Mar;50(5):987–96. PMID:24440087
229. Balakrishnan M, George R, Sharma A, et al. Changing trends in stomach cancer throughout the world. Curr Gastroenterol Rep. 2017 Aug;19(8):36. PMID:28730504
230. Balci S, Basturk O, Saka B, et al. Substaging nodal status in ampullary carcinomas has significant prognostic value: proposed revised staging based on an analysis of 313 well-characterized cases. Ann Surg Oncol. 2015 Dec;22(13):4392–401. PMID:25783680
231. Balta Z, Sauerbruch T, Hirner A, et al. [Primary neuroendocrine carcinoma of the liver. From carcinoid tumor to small-cell hepatic carcinoma: case reports and review of the literature]. Pathologe. 2008 Feb;29(1):53–60. German. PMID:18210116
232. Ban S, Naitoh Y, Mino-Kenudson M, et al. Intraductal papillary mucinous neoplasm (IPMN) of the pancreas: its histopathologic difference between 2 major types. Am J Surg Pathol. 2006 Dec;30(12):1561–9. PMID:17122512
233. Banck MS, Kanwar R, Kulkarni AA, et al. The genomic landscape of small intestine neuroendocrine tumors. J Clin Invest. 2013 Jun;123(6):2502–8. PMID:23676460
234. Bandyopadhyay S, Basturk O, Coban I, et al. Isolated solitary ducts (naked ducts) in adipose tissue: a specific but underappreciated finding of pancreatic adenocarcinoma and one of the potential reasons of understaging and high recurrence rate. Am J Surg Pathol. 2009 Mar;33(3):425–9. PMID:19092633
235. Bang JY, Hebert-Magee S, Navaneethan U, et al. EUS-guided fine needle biopsy of pancreatic masses can yield true histology. Gut. 2018 Dec;67(12):2081–4. PMID:28988195
236. Bang UC, Benfield T, Hyldstrup L, et al. Mortality, cancer, and comorbidities associated with chronic pancreatitis: a Danish nationwide matched-cohort study. Gastroenterology. 2014 Apr;146(4):989–94. PMID:24389306
237. Bang YJ, Van Cutsem E, Feyereislova A, et al. Trastuzumab in combination with chemotherapy versus chemotherapy alone for treatment of HER2-positive advanced gastric or gastro-oesophageal junction cancer (ToGA): a phase 3, open-label, randomised controlled trial. Lancet. 2010 Aug 28;376(9742):687–97. PMID:20728210
238. Bano S, Upreti L, Puri SK, et al. Imaging of pancreatic serous cystadenocarcinoma. Jpn J Radiol. 2011 Dec;29(10):730–4. PMID:22009426
239. Banville N, Geraghty R, Fox E, et al. Medullary carcinoma of the pancreas in a man with hereditary nonpolyposis colorectal cancer due to a mutation of the MSH2 mismatch repair gene. Hum Pathol. 2006 Nov;37(11):1498–502. PMID:16996571
240. Bao F, Panarelli NC, Rennert H, et al. Neoadjuvant therapy induces loss of MSH6 expression in colorectal carcinoma. Am J Surg Pathol. 2010 Dec;34(12):1798–804. PMID:21107085
241. Bao Y, Giovannucci E, Fuchs CS, et al. Passive smoking and pancreatic cancer in women: a prospective cohort study. Cancer Epidemiol Biomarkers Prev. 2009 Aug;18(8):2292–6. PMID:19602702
242. Barak S, Wang Z, Miettinen M. Immunoreactivity for calretinin and keratins in desmoid fibromatosis and other myofibroblastic tumors: a diagnostic pitfall. Am J Surg Pathol. 2012 Sep;36(9):1404–9. PMID:22531174
243. Barber ME, Save V, Carneiro F, et al. Histopathological and molecular analysis of gastrectomy specimens from hereditary diffuse gastric cancer patients has implications for endoscopic surveillance of individuals at risk. J Pathol. 2008 Nov;216(3):286–94. PMID:18825658
244. Barbour AP, Jones M, Gonen M, et al. Refining esophageal cancer staging after neoadjuvant therapy: importance of treatment response. Ann Surg Oncol. 2008 Oct;15(10):2894–902. PMID:18663531
245. Bardales RH, Stelow EB, Mallery S, et al. Review of endoscopic ultrasound-guided fine-needle aspiration cytology. Diagn Cytopathol. 2006 Feb;34(2):140–75. PMID:16511852
246. Barghorn A, Komminoth P, Bachmann D, et al. Deletion at 3p25.3-p23 is frequently encountered in endocrine pancreatic tumours and is associated with metastatic progression. J Pathol. 2001 Aug;194(4):451–8. PMID:11523053
247. Barghorn A, Speel EJ, Farspour B, et al. Putative tumor suppressor loci at 6q22 and 6q23-q24 are involved in the malignant

progression of sporadic endocrine pancreatic tumors. Am J Pathol. 2001 Jun;158(6):1903–11. PMID:11395364
248. Barnes G Jr, Romero L, Hess KR, et al. Primary adenocarcinoma of the duodenum: management and survival in 67 patients. Ann Surg Oncol. 1994 Jan;1(1):73–8. PMID:7834432
249. Barr Fritcher EG, Voss JS, Brankley SM, et al. An optimized set of fluorescence in situ hybridization probes for detection of pancreatobiliary tract cancer in cytology brush samples. Gastroenterology. 2015 Dec;149(7):1813–24.e1. PMID:26327129
250. Barresi V, Reggiani Bonetti L, Ieni A, et al. Poorly differentiated clusters: clinical impact in colorectal cancer. Clin Colorectal Cancer. 2017 Mar;16(1):9–15. PMID:27444718
251. Barret M, Prat F. Diagnosis and treatment of superficial esophageal cancer. Ann Gastroenterol. 2018 May-Jun;31(3):256–65. PMID:29720850
252. Barth TF, Müller S, Pawlita M, et al. Homogeneous immunophenotype and paucity of secondary genomic aberrations are distinctive features of endemic but not of sporadic Burkitt's lymphoma and diffuse large B-cell lymphoma with MYC rearrangement. J Pathol. 2004 Aug;203(4):940–5. PMID:15258997
253. Bartley AN, Luthra R, Saraiya DS, et al. Identification of cancer patients with Lynch syndrome: clinically significant discordances and problems in tissue-based mismatch repair testing. Cancer Prev Res (Phila). 2012 Feb;5(2):320–7. PMID:22086678
254. Bartley AN, Washington MK, Colasacco C, et al. HER2 testing and clinical decision making in gastroesophageal adenocarcinoma: guideline from the College of American Pathologists, American Society for Clinical Pathology, and the American Society of Clinical Oncology. J Clin Oncol. 2017 Feb;35(4):446–64. PMID:28129524
255. Barton CM, Staddon SL, Hughes CM, et al. Abnormalities of the p53 tumour suppressor gene in human pancreatic cancer. Br J Cancer. 1991 Dec;64(6):1076–82. PMID:1764370
256. Barton JG, Barrett DA, Maricevich MA, et al. Intraductal papillary mucinous neoplasm of the biliary tract: a real disease? HPB (Oxford). 2009 Dec;11(8):684–91. PMID:20495637
257. Bartsch D, Hahn SA, Danichevski KD, et al. Mutations of the DPC4/Smad4 gene in neuroendocrine pancreatic tumors. Oncogene. 1999 Apr 8;18(14):2367–71. PMID:10327057
258. Bartsch DK, Kress R, Sina-Frey M, et al. Prevalence of familial pancreatic cancer in Germany. Int J Cancer. 2004 Jul 20;110(6):902–6. PMID:15170674
259. Bartsch DK, Slater EP, Albers M, et al. Higher risk of aggressive pancreatic neuroendocrine tumors in MEN1 patients with MEN1 mutations affecting the CHES1 interacting MENIN domain. J Clin Endocrinol Metab. 2014 Nov;99(11):E2387–91. PMID:25210877
260. Bartsch DK, Waldmann J, Fendrich V, et al. Impact of lymphadenectomy on survival after surgery for sporadic gastrinoma. Br J Surg. 2012 Sep;99(9):1234–40. PMID:22864882
261. Barugola G, Falconi M, Bettini R, et al. The determinant factors of recurrence following resection for ductal pancreatic cancer. JOP. 2007 Jan 9;8(1 Suppl):132–40. PMID:17228145
262. Bass J, Soucy P, Walton M, et al. Inflammatory cloacogenic polyps in children. J Pediatr Surg. 1995 Apr;30(4):585–8. PMID:7595840
263. Basturk O, Adsay V, Askan G, et al. Intraductal tubulopapillary neoplasm of the pancreas: a clinicopathologic and immunohistochemical analysis of 33 cases. Am J Surg Pathol. 2017 Mar;41(3):313–25. PMID:27984235
264. Basturk O, Berger MF, Yamaguchi H, et al. Pancreatic intraductal tubulopapillary neoplasm is genetically distinct from intraductal papillary mucinous neoplasm and ductal adenocarcinoma. Mod Pathol. 2017 Dec;30(12):1760–72. PMID:28776573
265. Basturk O, Chung SM, Hruban RH, et al. Distinct pathways of pathogenesis of intraductal oncocytic papillary neoplasms and intraductal papillary mucinous neoplasms of the pancreas. Virchows Arch. 2016 Nov;469(5):523–32. PMID:27591765
266. Basturk O, Coban I, Adsay NV. Pancreatic cysts: pathologic classification, differential diagnosis, and clinical implications. Arch Pathol Lab Med. 2009 Mar;133(3):423–38. PMID:19260748
267. Basturk O, Hong SM, Wood LD, et al. A revised classification system and recommendations from the Baltimore Consensus Meeting for Neoplastic Precursor Lesions in the Pancreas. Am J Surg Pathol. 2015 Dec;39(12):1730–41. PMID:26559377
268. Basturk O, Khayyata S, Klimstra DS, et al. Preferential expression of MUC6 in oncocytic and pancreatobiliary types of intraductal papillary neoplasms highlights a pyloropancreatic pathway, distinct from the intestinal pathway, in pancreatic carcinogenesis. Am J Surg Pathol. 2010 Mar;34(3):364–70. PMID:20139757
269. Basturk O, Saka B, Balci S, et al. Substaging of lymph node status in resected pancreatic ductal adenocarcinoma has strong prognostic correlations: proposal for a revised N classification for TNM staging. Ann Surg Oncol. 2015 Dec;22 Suppl 3:S1187–95. PMID:26362048
270. Basturk O, Tan M, Bhanot U, et al. The oncocytic subtype is genetically distinct from other pancreatic intraductal papillary mucinous neoplasm subtypes. Mod Pathol. 2016 Sep;29(9):1058–69. PMID:27282351
271. Basturk O, Tang L, Hruban RH, et al. Poorly differentiated neuroendocrine carcinomas of the pancreas: a clinicopathologic analysis of 44 cases. Am J Surg Pathol. 2014 Apr;38(4):437–47. PMID:24503751
272. Basturk O, Yang Z, Tang LH, et al. The high-grade (WHO G3) pancreatic neuroendocrine tumor category is morphologically and biologically heterogenous and includes both well differentiated and poorly differentiated neoplasms. Am J Surg Pathol. 2015 May;39(5):683–90. PMID:25723112
273. Basturk O, Zamboni G, Klimstra DS, et al. Intraductal and papillary variants of acinar cell carcinomas: a new addition to the challenging differential diagnosis of intraductal neoplasms. Am J Surg Pathol. 2007 Mar;31(3):363–70. PMID:17325477
274. Bauduer F, Marty F, Gemain MC, et al. Primary non-Hodgkin's lymphoma of the liver in a patient with hepatitis B, C, HIV infections. Am J Hematol. 1997 Mar;54(3):265. PMID:9067511
275. Bean GR, Joseph NM, Gill RM, et al. Recurrent GNAQ mutations in anastomosing hemangiomas. Mod Pathol. 2017 May;30(5):722–7. PMID:28084343
276. Bean SM, Chhieng DC. Anal-rectal cytology: a review. Diagn Cytopathol. 2010 Jul;38(7):538–46. PMID:19941374
277. Beasley MB, Lantuejoul S, Abbondanzo S, et al. The P16/cyclin D1/Rb pathway in neuroendocrine tumors of the lung. Hum Pathol. 2003 Feb;34(2):136–42. PMID:12612881
278. Beaugerie L, Carrat F, Nahon S, et al. High risk of anal and rectal cancer in patients with anal and/or perianal Crohn's disease. Clin Gastroenterol Hepatol. 2018 Jun;16(6):892–9.e2. PMID:29199142
279. Beaugerie L, Itzkowitz SH. Cancers complicating inflammatory bowel disease. N Engl J Med. 2015 Jul 9;373(2):195. PMID:26154801
280. Becker K, Mueller JD, Schulmacher C, et al. Histomorphology and grading of regression in gastric carcinoma treated with neoadjuvant chemotherapy. Cancer. 2003 Oct 1;98(7):1521–30. PMID:14508841
281. Becker WF. Pancreatoduodenectomy for carcinoma of the pancreas in an infant; report of a case. Ann Surg. 1957 Jun;145(6):864–70; discussion 870–2. PMID:13425296
282. Bedeir A, Jukic DM, Wang L, et al. Systemic mastocytosis mimicking inflammatory bowel disease: a case report and discussion of gastrointestinal pathology in systemic mastocytosis. Am J Surg Pathol. 2006 Nov;30(11):1478–82. PMID:17063092
283. Beer A, Streubel B, Asari R, et al. Gastric adenocarcinoma and proximal polyposis of the stomach (GAPPS) - a rare recently described gastric polyposis syndrome - report of a case. Z Gastroenterol. 2017 Nov;55(11):1131–4. PMID:29141268
284. Beghini A, Tibiletti MG, Roversi G, et al. Germline mutation in the juxtamembrane domain of the kit gene in a family with gastrointestinal stromal tumors and urticaria pigmentosa. Cancer. 2001 Aug 1;92(3):657–62. PMID:11505412
285. Behdad A, Owens SR. Langerhans cell histiocytosis involving the gastrointestinal tract. Arch Pathol Lab Med. 2014 Oct;138(10):1350–2. PMID:25268199
286. Behjati S, Tarpey PS, Sheldon H, et al. Recurrent PTPRB and PLCG1 mutations in angiosarcoma. Nat Genet. 2014 Apr;46(4):376–9. PMID:24633157
287. Belfiori G, Sartelli M, Cardinali L, et al. Risk stratification systems for surgically treated localized primary gastrointestinal stromal tumors (GIST). Review of literature and comparison of the three prognostic criteria: MSKCC Nomogramm, NIH-Fletcher and AFIP-Miettinen. Ann Ital Chir. 2015 May-Jun;86(3):219–27. PMID:26098671
288. Belhadj K, Reyes F, Farcet JP, et al. Hepatosplenic gammadelta T-cell lymphoma is a rare clinicopathologic entity with poor outcome: report on a series of 21 patients. Blood. 2003 Dec 15;102(13):4261–9. PMID:12907441
289. Belhadj S, Mur P, Navarro M, et al. Delineating the phenotypic spectrum of the NTHL1-associated polyposis. Clin Gastroenterol Hepatol. 2017 Mar;15(3):461–2. PMID:27720914
290. Belinsky MG, Rink L, Cai KQ, et al. Somatic loss of function mutations in neurofibromin 1 and MYC associated factor X genes identified by exome-wide sequencing in a wild-type GIST case. BMC Cancer. 2015 Nov 10;15:887. PMID:26555092
291. Bell D, Ranganathan S, Tao J, et al. Novel advances in understanding of molecular pathogenesis of hepatoblastoma: a Wnt/β-catenin perspective. Gene Expr. 2017 Feb 10;17(2):141–54. PMID:27938502
292. Bellizzi AM, Rock J, Marsh WL, et al. Serrated lesions of the appendix: a morphologic and immunohistochemical appraisal. Am J Clin Pathol. 2010 Apr;133(4):623–32. PMID:20231616
293. Bellizzi AM, Woodford RL, Moskaluk CA, et al. Basaloid squamous cell carcinoma of the esophagus: assessment for high-risk human papillomavirus and related molecular markers. Am J Surg Pathol. 2009 Nov;33(11):1608–14. PMID:19738459
294. Belsley NA, Pitman MB, Lauwers GY, et al. Serous cystadenoma of the pancreas: limitations and pitfalls of endoscopic ultrasound-guided fine-needle aspiration biopsy. Cancer. 2008 Apr 25;114(2):102–10. PMID:18260088
295. Ben-Haim M, Roayaie S, Ye MQ, et al. Hepatic epithelioid hemangioendothelioma: resection or transplantation, which and when? Liver Transpl Surg. 1999 Nov;5(6):526–31. PMID:10545542
296. Bende RJ, Smit LA, Bossenbroek JG, et al. Primary follicular lymphoma of the small intestine: alpha4beta7 expression and immunoglobulin configuration suggest an origin from local antigen-experienced B cells. Am J Pathol. 2003 Jan;162(1):105–13. PMID:12507894
297. Benedict MA, Lauwers GY, Jain D. Gastric adenocarcinoma of the fundic gland type: update and literature review. Am J Clin Pathol. 2018 Apr 25;149(6):461–73. PMID:29648578
298. Benhammane H, El M'rabet FZ, Idrissi Serhouchni K, et al. Small bowel adenocarcinoma complicating coeliac disease: a report of three cases and the literature review. Case Rep Oncol Med. 2012;2012:935183. PMID:23243535
299. Benn JJ, Firth RG, Sönksen PH. Metabolic effects of an insulin-like factor causing hypoglycaemia in a patient with a haemangiopericytoma. Clin Endocrinol (Oxf). 1990 Jun;32(6):769–80. PMID:2116946
300. Benusiglio PR, Colas C, Rouleau E, et al. Hereditary diffuse gastric cancer syndrome: improved performances of the 2015 testing criteria for the identification of probands with a CDH1 germline mutation. J Med Genet. 2015 Aug;52(8):563–5. PMID:26025002
301. Benya RV, Metz DC, Hijazi YJ, et al. Fine needle aspiration cytology of submucosal nodules in patients with Zollinger-Ellison syndrome. Am J Gastroenterol. 1993 Feb;88(2):258–65. PMID:8093826
302. Berardi RS. Carcinoid tumors of the colon (exclusive of the rectum): review of the literature. Dis Colon Rectum. 1972 Sep-Oct;15(5):383–91. PMID:4561188
303. Berberi A, Noujeim Z. Epidemiology and relationships between CD4+ counts and oral lesions among 50 patients infected with human immunodeficiency virus. J Int Oral Health. 2015 Jan;7(1):18–21. PMID:25709361
304. Berge T, Linell F. Carcinoid tumours. Frequency in a defined population during a 12-year period. Acta Pathol Microbiol Scand A. 1976 Jul;84(4):322–30. PMID:961424
305. Berger AC, Garcia M Jr, Hoffman JP, et al. Postresection CA 19-9 predicts overall survival in patients with pancreatic cancer treated with adjuvant chemoradiation: a prospective validation by RTOG 9704. J Clin Oncol. 2008 Dec 20;26(36):5918–22. PMID:19029412
306. Bergmann F, Aulmann S, Sipos B, et al. Acinar cell carcinomas of the pancreas: a molecular analysis in a series of 57 cases. Virchows Arch. 2014 Dec;465(6):661–72. PMID:25298229
307. Bergmann F, Aulmann S, Welsch T, et al. Molecular analysis of pancreatic acinar cell cystadenomas: evidence of a non-neoplastic nature. Oncol Lett. 2014 Aug;8(2):852–8. PMID:25009661
308. Bergmann F, Esposito I, Michalski CW, et al. Early undifferentiated pancreatic carcinoma with osteoclastlike giant cells: direct evidence for ductal evolution. Am J Surg Pathol. 2007 Dec;31(12):1919–25. PMID:18043049
309. Bergmann F, Singh S, Michel S, et al. Small bowel adenocarcinomas in celiac disease follow the CIM-MSI pathway. Oncol Rep. 2010 Dec;24(6):1535–9. PMID:21042749
309A. Bernick PE, Klimstra DS, Shia J, et al. Neuroendocrine carcinomas of the colon and rectum. Dis Colon Rectum. 2004 Feb;47(2):163–9. PMID:15043285
310. Bernstein CN, Blanchard JF, Kliewer E, et al. Cancer risk in patients with inflammatory bowel disease: a population-based study. Cancer. 2001 Feb 15;91(4):854–62. PMID:11241255

311. Bernstein CN, Shanahan F, Weinstein WM. Are we telling patients the truth about surveillance colonoscopy in ulcerative colitis? Lancet. 1994 Jan 8;343(8889):71–4. PMID:7903776

312. Bernstein H, Bernstein C, Payne CM, et al. Bile acids as carcinogens in human gastrointestinal cancers. Mutat Res. 2005 Jan;589(1):47–65. PMID:15652226

313. Bertani H, Mirante VG, Caruso A, et al. Successful treatment of diffuse esophageal papillomatosis with balloon-assisted radiofrequency ablation in a patient with Goltz syndrome. Endoscopy. 2014;46 Suppl 1 UCTN:E404–5. PMID:25314164

314. Bertoni F, Rossi D, Zucca E. Recent advances in understanding the biology of marginal zone lymphoma. F1000Res. 2018 Mar 28;7:406. PMID:29657712

315. Bertran E, Heise K, Andia ME, et al. Gallbladder cancer: incidence and survival in a high-risk area of Chile. Int J Cancer. 2010 Nov 15;127(10):2446–54. PMID:20473911

316. Bettington M, Walker N, Rosty C, et al. Clinicopathological and molecular features of sessile serrated adenomas with dysplasia or carcinoma. Gut. 2017 Jan;66(1):97–106. PMID:26475632

317. Bettington M, Walker N, Rosty C, et al. Critical appraisal of the diagnosis of the sessile serrated adenoma. Am J Surg Pathol. 2014 Feb;38(2):158–66. PMID:24418851

318. Bettington M, Walker NI, Rosty C, et al. Serrated tubulovillous adenoma of the large intestine. Histopathology. 2016 Mar;68(4):578–87. PMID:26212352

319. Bettington ML, Chetty R. Traditional serrated adenoma: an update. Hum Pathol. 2015 Jul;46(7):933–8. PMID:26001333

320. Bettington ML, Walker NI, Rosty C, et al. A clinicopathological and molecular analysis of 200 traditional serrated adenomas. Mod Pathol. 2015 Mar;28(3):414–27. PMID:25216220

321. Bhalla A, Mann SA, Chen S, et al. Histopathological evidence of neoplastic progression of von Meyenburg complex to intrahepatic cholangiocarcinoma. Hum Pathol. 2017 Sep;67:217–24. PMID:28823571

322. Bhathal PS, Hughes NR, Goodman ZD. The so-called bile duct adenoma is a peribiliary gland hamartoma. Am J Surg Pathol. 1996 Jul;20(7):858–64. PMID:8669534

323. Bhattacharya B, Dilworth HP, Iacobuzio-Donahue C, et al. Nuclear beta-catenin expression distinguishes deep fibromatosis from other benign and malignant fibroblastic and myofibroblastic lesions. Am J Surg Pathol. 2005 May;29(5):653–9. PMID:15832090

324. Bhattacharyya A, Chattopadhyay R, Mitra S, et al. Oxidative stress: an essential factor in the pathogenesis of gastrointestinal mucosal diseases. Physiol Rev. 2014 Apr;94(2):329–54. PMID:24692350

325. Bianchi G, Sohani AR. Heavy chain disease of the small bowel. Curr Gastroenterol Rep. 2018 Jan 25;20(1):3. PMID:29372346

326. Bianchi LK, Burke CA, Bennett AE, et al. Fundic gland polyp dysplasia is common in familial adenomatous polyposis. Clin Gastroenterol Hepatol. 2008 Feb;6(2):180–5. PMID:18237868

327. Biankin AV, Biankin SA, Kench JG, et al. Aberrant p16(INK4A) and DPC4/Smad4 expression in intraductal papillary mucinous tumours of the pancreas is associated with invasive ductal adenocarcinoma. Gut. 2002 Jun;50(6):861–8. PMID:12010891

328. Bilimoria KY, Bentrem DJ, Wayne JD, et al. Small bowel cancer in the United States: changes in epidemiology, treatment, and survival over the last 20 years. Ann Surg. 2009 Jan;249(1):63–71. PMID:19106677

329. Billmire D, Vinocur C, Rescorla F, et al. Malignant retroperitoneal and abdominal germ cell tumors: an intergroup study. J Pediatr Surg. 2003 Mar;38(3):315–8, discussion 315–8. PMID:12632341

330. Bioulac-Sage P, Cubel G, Taouji S, et al. Immunohistochemical markers on needle biopsies are helpful for the diagnosis of focal nodular hyperplasia and hepatocellular adenoma subtypes. Am J Surg Pathol. 2012 Nov;36(11):1691–9. PMID:23060349

331. Bioulac-Sage P, Laumonier H, Couchy G, et al. Hepatocellular adenoma management and phenotypic classification: the Bordeaux experience. Hepatology. 2009 Aug;50(2):481–9. PMID:19585623

332. Bioulac-Sage P, Laumonier H, Laurent C, et al. Benign and malignant vascular tumors of the liver in adults. Semin Liver Dis. 2008 Aug;28(3):302–14. PMID:18814083

333. Bioulac-Sage P, Rebouissou S, Sa Cunha A, et al. Over-expression of glutamine synthetase in focal nodular hyperplasia: a novel easy diagnostic tool in surgical pathology. Liver Int. 2009 Mar;29(3):459–65. PMID:18803590

334. Bioulac-Sage P, Rebouissou S, Sa Cunha A, et al. Clinical, morphologic, and molecular features defining so-called telangiectatic focal nodular hyperplasias of the liver. Gastroenterology. 2005 May;128(5):1211–8. PMID:15887105

335. Bioulac-Sage P, Rebouissou S, Thomas C, et al. Hepatocellular adenoma subtype classification using molecular markers and immunohistochemistry. Hepatology. 2007 Sep;46(3):740–8. PMID:17663417

336. Bioulac-Sage P, Taouji S, Possenti L, et al. Hepatocellular adenoma subtypes: the impact of overweight and obesity. Liver Int. 2012 Sep;32(8):1217–21. PMID:22429502

337. Bishop JC, Britton JF, Murphy AM, et al. Juvenile idiopathic arthritis associated with combined JP-HHT syndrome: a novel phenotype associated with a novel variant in SMAD4. J Pediatr Genet. 2018 Jun;7(2):78–82. PMID:29707409

338. Bishop KD, Olszewski AJ. Epidemiology and survival outcomes of ocular and mucosal melanomas: a population-based analysis. Int J Cancer. 2014 Jun 15;134(12):2961–71. PMID:24272143

339. Bismar TA, Basturk O, Gerald WL, et al. Desmoplastic small cell tumor in the pancreas. Am J Surg Pathol. 2004 Jun;28(6):808–12. PMID:15166674

340. Bizama C, García P, Espinoza JA, et al. Targeting specific molecular pathways holds promise for advanced gallbladder cancer therapy. Cancer Treat Rev. 2015 Mar;41(3):222–34. PMID:25639632

341. Black ME, Hedgire SS, Camposano S, et al. Hepatic manifestations of tuberous sclerosis complex: a genotypic and phenotypic analysis. Clin Genet. 2012 Dec;82(6):552–7. PMID:22251200

342. Blackford A, Parmigiani G, Kensler TW, et al. Genetic mutations associated with cigarette smoking in pancreatic cancer. Cancer Res. 2009 Apr 15;69(8):3681–8. PMID:19351817

343. Blackford A, Serrano OK, Wolfgang CL, et al. SMAD4 gene mutations are associated with poor prognosis in pancreatic cancer. Clin Cancer Res. 2009 Jul 15;15(14):4674–9. PMID:19584151

344. Blandamura S, Parenti A, Famengo B, et al. Three cases of pancreatic serous cystadenoma and endocrine tumour. J Clin Pathol. 2007 Mar;60(3):278–82. PMID:16644876

345. Blansfield JA, Choyke L, Morita SY, et al. Clinical, genetic and radiographic analysis of 108 patients with von Hippel-Lindau disease (VHL) manifested by pancreatic neuroendocrine neoplasms (PNETs). Surgery. 2007 Dec;142(6):814–8, discussion 818.e1–2. PMID:18063061

346. Blaydon DC, Etheridge SL, Risk JM, et al. RHBDF2 mutations are associated with tylosis, a familial esophageal cancer syndrome. Am J Hum Genet. 2012 Feb 10;90(2):340–6. PMID:22265016

347. Blinkenberg EO, Brendehaug A, Sandvik AK, et al. Angioma serpiginosum with oesophageal papillomatosis is an X-linked dominant condition that maps to Xp11.3-Xq12. Eur J Hum Genet. 2007 May;15(5):543–7. PMID:17342156

348. Blomberg M, Friis S, Munk C, et al. Genital warts and risk of cancer: a Danish study of nearly 50 000 patients with genital warts. J Infect Dis. 2012 May 15;205(10):1544–53. PMID:22427679

349. Bloomston M, Chanona-Vilchis J, Ellison EC, et al. Carcinosarcoma of the pancreas arising in a mucinous cystic neoplasm. Am Surg. 2006 Apr;72(4):351–5. PMID:16676863

350. Bluteau O, Jeannot E, Bioulac-Sage P, et al. Bi-allelic inactivation of TCF1 in hepatic adenomas. Nat Genet. 2002 Oct;32(2):312–5. PMID:12355088

351. Bläker H, Helmchen B, Bönisch A, et al. Mutational activation of the RAS-RAF-MAPK and the Wnt pathway in small intestinal adenocarcinomas. Scand J Gastroenterol. 2004 Aug;39(8):748–53. PMID:15513360

352. Boberg KM, Jebsen P, Clausen OP, et al. Diagnostic benefit of biliary brush cytology in cholangiocarcinoma in primary sclerosing cholangitis. J Hepatol. 2006 Oct;45(4):568–74. PMID:16879890

353. Boeckx N, Koukakis R, Op de Beeck K, et al. Primary tumor sidedness has an impact on prognosis and treatment outcome in metastatic colorectal cancer: results from two randomized first-line panitumumab studies. Ann Oncol. 2017 Aug 1;28(8):1862–8. PMID:28449055

354. Boffetta P, Hecht S, Gray N, et al. Smokeless tobacco and cancer. Lancet Oncol. 2008 Jul;9(7):667–75. PMID:18598931

355. Bogusz AM, Seegmiller AC, Garcia R, et al. Plasmablastic lymphomas with MYC/IgH rearrangement: report of three cases and review of the literature. Am J Clin Pathol. 2009 Oct;132(4):597–605. PMID:19762538

356. Boikos SA, Pappo AS, Killian JK, et al. Molecular subtypes of KIT/PDGFRA wild-type gastrointestinal stromal tumors: a report from the National Institutes of Health Gastrointestinal Stromal Tumor Clinic. JAMA Oncol. 2016 Jul 1;2(7):922–8. PMID:27011036

357. Boland PM, Ma WW. Immunotherapy for colorectal cancer. Cancers (Basel). 2017 May 11;9(5):E50. PMID:28492495

358. Bollard J, Couderc C, Blanc M, et al. Antitumor effect of everolimus in preclinical models of high-grade gastroenteropancreatic neuroendocrine carcinomas. Neuroendocrinology. 2013;97(4):331–40. PMID:23343749

359. Boman F, Bossard C, Fabre M, et al. Mesenchymal hamartomas of the liver may be associated with increased serum alpha foetoprotein concentrations and mimic hepatoblastomas. Eur J Pediatr Surg. 2004 Feb;14(1):63–6. PMID:15024683

361. Bonilla Guerrero R, Roberts LR. The role of hepatitis B virus integrations in the pathogenesis of human hepatocellular carcinoma. J Hepatol. 2005 May;42(5):760–77. PMID:15826727

362. Bonnavion R, Teinturier R, Gherardi S, et al. Foxa2, a novel protein partner of the tumour suppressor menin, is deregulated in mouse and human MEN1 glucagonomas. J Pathol. 2017 May;242(1):90–101. PMID:28188614

364. Boparai KS, Dekker E, Polak MM, et al. A serrated colorectal cancer pathway predominates over the classic WNT pathway in patients with hyperplastic polyposis syndrome. Am J Pathol. 2011 Jun;178(6):2700–7. PMID:21641392

365. Boparai KS, Dekker E, Van Eeden S, et al. Hyperplastic polyps and sessile serrated adenomas as a phenotypic expression of MYH-associated polyposis. Gastroenterology. 2008 Dec;135(6):2014–8. PMID:19013464

366. Boparai KS, Reitsma JB, Lemmens V, et al. Increased colorectal cancer risk in first-degree relatives of patients with hyperplastic polyposis syndrome. Gut. 2010 Sep;59(9):1222–5. PMID:20584785

367. Borazanci E, Millis SZ, Korn R, et al. Adenosquamous carcinoma of the pancreas: molecular characterization of 23 patients along with a literature review. World J Gastrointest Oncol. 2015 Sep 15;7(9):132–40. PMID:26380056

368. Borden EC, Baker LH, Bell RS, et al. Soft tissue sarcomas of adults: state of the translational science. Clin Cancer Res. 2003 Jun;9(6):1941–56. PMID:12796356

369. Bordi C. Neuroendocrine pathology of the stomach: the Parma contribution. Endocr Pathol. 2014 Jun;25(2):171–80. PMID:24782101

370. Borowsky J, Dumenil T, Bettington M, et al. The role of APC in WNT pathway activation in serrated neoplasia. Mod Pathol. 2018 Mar;31(3):495–504. PMID:29148535

371. Borrello MG, Smith DP, Pasini B, et al. RET activation by germline MEN2A and MEN2B mutations. Oncogene. 1995 Dec 7;11(11):2419–27. PMID:8570194

372. Borzio M, Fargion S, Borzio F, et al. Impact of large regenerative, low grade and high grade dysplastic nodules in hepatocellular carcinoma development. J Hepatol. 2003 Aug;39(2):208–14. PMID:12873817

373. Bosch SL, Teerenstra S, de Wilt JH, et al. Predicting lymph node metastasis in pT1 colorectal cancer: a systematic review of risk factors providing rationale for therapy decisions. Endoscopy. 2013 Oct;45(10):827–34. PMID:23884793

374. Bosetti C, Bertuccio P, Malvezzi M, et al. Cancer mortality in Europe, 2005-2009, and an overview of trends since 1980. Ann Oncol. 2013 Oct;24(10):2657–71. PMID:23921790

375. Bosetti C, Lucenteforte E, Bracci PM, et al. Ulcer, gastric surgery and pancreatic cancer risk: an analysis from the International Pancreatic Cancer Case-Control Consortium (PanC4). Ann Oncol. 2013 Nov;24(11):2903–10. PMID:23970016

376. Bosetti C, Rosato V, Li D, et al. Diabetes, antidiabetic medications, and pancreatic cancer risk: an analysis from the International Pancreatic Cancer Case-Control Consortium. Ann Oncol. 2014 Oct;25(10):2065–72. PMID:25057164

377. Boshoff C, Schulz TF, Kennedy MM, et al. Kaposi's sarcoma-associated herpesvirus infects endothelial and spindle cells. Nat Med. 1995 Dec;1(12):1274–8. PMID:7489408

378. Boshoff C, Whitby D, Hatziioannou T, et al. Kaposi's-sarcoma-associated herpesvirus in HIV-negative Kaposi's sarcoma. Lancet. 1995 Apr 22;345(8956):1043–4. PMID:7723505

379. Bosman FT, Carneiro F, Hruban RH, et al., editors. WHO classification of tumours of the digestive system. Lyon (France): International Agency for Research on Cancer; 2010. (WHO classification of tumours series, 4th ed.; vol. 3). http://publications.iarc.fr/13.

380. Boswell JT, Helwig EB. Squamous cell carcinoma and adenoacanthoma of the stomach. A clinicopathologic study. Cancer. 1965 Feb;18:181–92. PMID:14254074

381. Bougeard G, Renaux-Petel M, Flaman JM, et al. Revisiting Li-Fraumeni syndrome from

TP53 mutation carriers. J Clin Oncol. 2015 Jul 20;33(21):2345–52. PMID:26014290
382. Bourke MJ. Endoscopic resection in the duodenum: current limitations and future directions. Endoscopy. 2013;45(2):127–32. PMID:23364840
383. Bouvard V, Loomis D, Guyton KZ, et al. Carcinogenicity of consumption of red and processed meat. Lancet Oncol. 2015 Dec;16(16):1599–600. PMID:26514947
384. Bouvier AM, Belot A, Manfredi S, et al. Trends of incidence and survival in squamous-cell carcinoma of the anal canal in France: a population-based study. Eur J Cancer Prev. 2016 May;25(3):182–7. PMID:25973771
385. Bowman GA, Rosenthal D. Carcinoid tumors of the appendix. Am J Surg. 1983 Dec;146(6):700–3. PMID:6650751
386. Bowman SJ, Levison DA, Cotter FE, et al. Primary T cell lymphoma of the liver in a patient with Felty's syndrome. Br J Rheumatol. 1994 Feb;33(2):157–60. PMID:8162482
387. Boyar Cetinkaya R, Aagnes B, Thiis-Evensen E, et al. Trends in incidence of neuroendocrine neoplasms in Norway: a report of 16,075 cases from 1993 through 2010. Neuroendocrinology. 2017;104(1):1–10. PMID:26562558
388. Boyd CA, Benarroch-Gampel J, Sheffield KM, et al. 415 patients with adenosquamous carcinoma of the pancreas: a population-based analysis of prognosis and survival. J Surg Res. 2012 May 1;174(1):12–9. PMID:21816433
389. Boyd S, Mustonen H, Tenca A, et al. Surveillance of primary sclerosing cholangitis with ERC and brush cytology: risk factors for cholangiocarcinoma. Scand J Gastroenterol. 2017 Feb;52(2):242–9. PMID:27806633
390. Boyd S, Tenca A, Jokelainen K, et al. Screening primary sclerosing cholangitis and biliary dysplasia with endoscopic retrograde cholangiography and brush cytology: risk factors for biliary neoplasia. Endoscopy. 2016 May;48(5):432–9. PMID:26808393
391. Boyer SN, Wazer DE, Band V. E7 protein of human papilloma virus-16 induces degradation of retinoblastoma protein through the ubiquitin-proteasome pathway. Cancer Res. 1996 Oct 15;56(20):4620–4. PMID:8840974
392. Bradley CA, Salto-Tellez M, Laurent-Puig P, et al. Targeting c-MET in gastrointestinal tumours: rationale, opportunities and challenges. Nat Rev Clin Oncol. 2018 Jan 23;15(3):150. PMID:29358775
393. Bradley RF, Stewart JH 4th, Russell GB, et al. Pseudomyxoma peritonei of appendiceal origin: a clinicopathologic analysis of 101 patients uniformly treated at a single institution, with literature review. Am J Surg Pathol. 2006 May;30(5):551–9. PMID:16699309
394. Brainard JA, Goldblum JR. Stromal tumors of the jejunum and ileum: a clinicopathologic study of 39 cases. Am J Surg Pathol. 1997 Apr;21(4):407–16. PMID:9130987
395. Bramis K, Petrou A, Papalambros A, et al. Serous cystadenocarcinoma of the pancreas: report of a case and management reflections. World J Surg Oncol. 2012 Mar 8;10:51. PMID:22400805
396. Brancatelli G, Federle MP, Vullierme MP, et al. CT and MR imaging evaluation of hepatic adenoma. J Comput Assist Tomogr. 2006 Sep-Oct;30(5):745–50. PMID:16954922
397. Brat DJ, Lillemoe KD, Yeo CJ, et al. Progression of pancreatic intraductal neoplasias to infiltrating adenocarcinoma of the pancreas. Am J Surg Pathol. 1998 Feb;22(2):163–9. PMID:9500216
398. Bratton L, Salloum R, Cao W, et al. Solitary fibrous tumor of the sigmoid colon masquerading as an adnexal neoplasm. Case Rep Pathol. 2016;2016:4182026. PMID:27672467
399. Bray F, Ferlay J, Soerjomataram I, et al. Global cancer statistics 2018: GLOBOCAN estimates of incidence and mortality worldwide for 36 cancers in 185 countries. CA Cancer J Clin. 2018 Nov;68(6):394–424. PMID:30207593
400. Brcic I, Cathomas G, Vanoli A, et al. Medullary carcinoma of the small bowel. Histopathology. 2016 Jul;69(1):136–40. PMID:26599717
401. Brenca M, Rossi S, Polano M, et al. Transcriptome sequencing identifies ETV6-NTRK3 as a gene fusion involved in GIST. J Pathol. 2016 Mar;238(4):543–9. PMID:26606880
402. Brennan MF, Antonescu CR, Moraco N, et al. Lessons learned from the study of 10,000 patients with soft tissue sarcoma. Ann Surg. 2014 Sep;260(3):416–21, discussion 421–2. PMID:25115417
403. Bressac B, Kew M, Wands J, et al. Selective G to T mutations of p53 gene in hepatocellular carcinoma from southern Africa. Nature. 1991 Apr 4;350(6317):429–31. PMID:1672732
404. Bridge MF, Perzin KH. Primary adenocarcinoma of the jejunum and ileum. A clinicopathologic study. Cancer. 1975 Nov;36(5):1876–87. PMID:53095
405. Bridgewater J, Galle PR, Khan SA, et al. Guidelines for the diagnosis and management of intrahepatic cholangiocarcinoma. J Hepatol. 2014 Jun;60(6):1268–89. PMID:24681130
406. Bridgewater JA, Goodman KA, Kalyan A, et al. Biliary tract cancer: epidemiology, radiotherapy, and molecular profiling. Am Soc Clin Oncol Educ Book. 2016;35:e194–203. PMID:27249723
407. Brieher WM, Yap AS. Cadherin junctions and their cytoskeleton(s). Curr Opin Cell Biol. 2013 Feb;25(1):39–46. PMID:23127608
408. Brierly JD, Gospodarowicz MK, Wittekind C, editors. TNM classification of malignant tumours. 8th ed. Oxford (UK): Wiley Blackwell; 2017.
409. Briggs S, Tomlinson I. Germline and somatic polymerase ε and δ mutations define a new class of hypermutated colorectal and endometrial cancers. J Pathol. 2013 Jun;230(2):148–53. PMID:23447401
410. Brockmann D, Tries B, Esche H. Isolation and characterization of novel adenovirus type 12 E1A mRNAs by cDNA PCR technique. Virology. 1990 Dec;179(2):585–90. PMID:2146800
411. Brodsky SV, Sandoval C, Sharma N, et al. Recurrent nested stromal epithelial tumor of the liver with extrahepatic metastasis: case report and review of literature. Pediatr Dev Pathol. 2008 Nov-Dec;11(6):469–73. PMID:18338937
412. Brody JR, Costantino CL, Potoczek M, et al. Adenosquamous carcinoma of the pancreas harbors KRAS2, DPC4 and TP53 molecular alterations similar to pancreatic ductal adenocarcinoma. Mod Pathol. 2009 May;22(5):651–9. PMID:19270646
413. Bronowicki JP, Bineau C, Feugier P, et al. Primary lymphoma of the liver: clinical-pathological features and relationship with HCV infection in French patients. Hepatology. 2003 Apr;37(4):781–7. PMID:12668970
414. Brooks DD, Winawer SJ, Rex DK, et al. Colonoscopy surveillance after polypectomy and colorectal cancer resection. Am Fam Physician. 2008 Apr 1;77(7):995–1002. PMID:18441865
415. Brosens LA, Keller JJ, Offerhaus GJ, et al. Prevention and management of duodenal polyps in familial adenomatous polyposis. Gut. 2005 Jul;54(7):1034–43. PMID:15951555
416. Brosens LA, Langeveld D, van Hattem WA, et al. Juvenile polyposis syndrome. World J Gastroenterol. 2011 Nov 28;17(44):4839–44. PMID:22171123
417. Brosens LA, Offerhaus GJ, Giardiello FM. Hereditary colorectal cancer: genetics and screening. Surg Clin North Am. 2015 Oct;95(5):1067–80. PMID:26315524
418. Brosens LA, Tytgat KM, Morsink FH, et al. Multiple colorectal neoplasms in X-linked agammaglobulinemia. Clin Gastroenterol Hepatol. 2008 Jan;6(1):115–9. PMID:17967562
419. Brosens LA, van Hattem A, Hylind LM, et al. Risk of colorectal cancer in juvenile polyposis. Gut. 2007 Jul;56(7):965–7. PMID:17303595
420. Brosens LA, van Hattem WA, Jansen M, et al. Gastrointestinal polyposis syndromes. Curr Mol Med. 2007 Feb;7(1):29–46. PMID:17311531
421. Brosens LA, Wood LD, Offerhaus GJ, et al. Pathology and genetics of syndromic gastric polyps. Int J Surg Pathol. 2016 May;24(3):185–99. PMID:26721304
422. Brotto M, Finegold MJ. Distinct patterns of p27/KIP 1 gene expression in hepatoblastoma and prognostic implications with correlation before and after chemotherapy. Hum Pathol. 2002 Feb;33(2):198–205. PMID:11957145
423. Broughan TA, Leslie JD, Soto JM, et al. Pancreatic islet cell tumors. Surgery. 1986 Jun;99(6):671–8. PMID:2424108
424. Brousse N, Meijer JW. Malignant complications of coeliac disease. Best Pract Res Clin Gastroenterol. 2005 Jun;19(3):401–12. PMID:15925845
425. Brown B, Khalil B, Batra G, et al. Mature cystic teratoma arising at the porta hepatis: a diagnostic dilemma. J Pediatr Surg. 2008 Apr;43(4):e1–3. PMID:18405692
426. Brown IS, Whiteman DC, Lauwers GY. Foveolar type dysplasia in Barrett esophagus. Mod Pathol. 2010 Jun;23(6):834–43. PMID:20228780
427. Brown K, Kristopaitis T, Yong S, et al. Cystic glucagonoma: a rare variant of an uncommon neuroendocrine pancreas tumor. J Gastrointest Surg. 1998 Nov-Dec;2(6):533–6. PMID:10457311
428. Brune K, Abe T, Canto M, et al. Multifocal neoplastic precursor lesions associated with lobular atrophy of the pancreas in patients having a strong family history of pancreatic cancer. Am J Surg Pathol. 2006 Sep;30(9):1067–76. PMID:16931950
429. Brune KA, Lau B, Palmisano E, et al. Importance of age of onset in pancreatic cancer kindreds. J Natl Cancer Inst. 2010 Jan 20;102(2):119–26. PMID:20068195
430. Brunner P, Rufle A, Dirnhofer S, et al. Follicular lymphoma transformation into histiocytic sarcoma: indications for a common neoplastic progenitor. Leukemia. 2014 Sep;28(9):1937–40. PMID:24850291
431. Brunt E, Aishima S, Clavien PA, et al. cHCC-CCA: consensus terminology for primary liver carcinomas with both hepatocytic and cholangiocytic differentation. Hepatology. 2018 Jul;68(1):113–26. PMID:29360137
432. Brusselaers N, Engstrand L, Lagergren J. Maintenance proton pump inhibition therapy and risk of oesophageal cancer. Cancer Epidemiol. 2018 Apr;53:172–7. PMID:29477057
433. Bryant KL, Mancias JD, Kimmelman AC, et al. KRAS: feeding pancreatic cancer proliferation. Trends Biochem Sci. 2014 Feb;39(2):91–100. PMID:24388967
434. Bubien V, Bonnet F, Brouste V, et al. High cumulative risks of cancer in patients with PTEN hamartoma tumour syndrome. J Med Genet. 2013 Apr;50(4):255–63. PMID:23335809
435. Buchanan DD, Clendenning M, Zhuoer L, et al. Lack of evidence for germline RNF43 mutations in patients with serrated polyposis syndrome from a large multinational study. Gut. 2017 Jun;66(6):1170–2. PMID:27582512
436. Buchanan DD, Stewart JR, Clendenning M, et al. Risk of colorectal cancer for carriers of a germ-line mutation in POLE or POLD1. Genet Med. 2018 Aug;20(8):890–5. PMID:29120461
437. Buchanan DD, Sweet K, Drini M, et al. Risk factors for colorectal cancer in patients with multiple serrated polyps: a cross-sectional case series from genetics clinics. PLoS One. 2010 Jul 16;5(7):e11636. PMID:20661287
438. Buckle G, Maranda L, Skiles J, et al. Factors influencing survival among Kenyan children diagnosed with endemic Burkitt lymphoma between 2003 and 2011: a historical cohort study. Int J Cancer. 2016 Sep 15;139(6):1231–40. PMID:27136063
439. Buetow PC, Rao P, Thompson LD. From the Archives of the AFIP. Mucinous cystic neoplasms of the pancreas: radiologic-pathologic correlation. Radiographics. 1998 Mar-Apr;18(2):433–49. PMID:9536488
440. Bullard KM, Tuttle TM, Rothenberger DA, et al. Surgical therapy for anorectal melanoma. J Am Coll Surg. 2003 Feb;196(2):206–11. PMID:12595048
441. Burgos J, Curran A, Landolfi S, et al. Risk factors of high-grade anal intraepithelial neoplasia recurrence in HIV-infected MSM. AIDS. 2017 Jun 1;31(9):1245–52. PMID:28252530
442. Burgoyne AM, Somaiah N, Sicklick JK. Gastrointestinal stromal tumors in the setting of multiple tumor syndromes. Curr Opin Oncol. 2014 Jul;26(4):408–14. PMID:24840526
443. Burke AP, Sobin LH, Federspiel BH, et al. Goblet cell carcinoids and related tumors of the vermiform appendix. Am J Clin Pathol. 1990 Jul;94(1):27–35. PMID:2163192
444. Burke AP, Sobin LH, Shekitka KM, et al. Intra-abdominal fibromatosis. A pathologic analysis of 130 tumors with comparison of clinical subgroups. Am J Surg Pathol. 1990 Apr;14(4):335–41. PMID:2321698
445. Burke AP, Thomas RM, Elsayed AM, et al. Carcinoids of the jejunum and ileum: an immunohistochemical and clinicopathologic study of 167 cases. Cancer. 1997 Mar 15;79(6):1086–93. PMID:9070484
446. Burke M, Shepherd N, Mann CV. Carcinoid tumours of the rectum and anus. Br J Surg. 1987 May;74(5):358–61. PMID:3594122
447. Burkitt D. A sarcoma involving the jaws in African children. Br J Surg. 1958 Nov;46(197):218–23. PMID:13628987
448. Burns PN, Wilson SR. Focal liver masses: enhancement patterns on contrast-enhanced images–concordance of US scans with CT scans and MR images. Radiology. 2007 Jan;242(1):162–74. PMID:17090710
449. Burt AD, Alves V, Bedossa P, et al. Data set for the reporting of intrahepatic cholangiocarcinoma, perihilar cholangiocarcinoma and hepatocellular carcinoma: recommendations from the International Collaboration on Cancer Reporting (ICCR). Histopathology. 2018 Sep;73(3):369–85. PMID:29573451
450. Burt AD, Ferrell LD, Hübscher SG. MacSween's pathology of the liver. 7th ed. Philadelphia (PA): Elsevier; 2018.
451. Buttar NS, Wang KK, Sebo TJ, et al. Extent of high-grade dysplasia in Barrett's esophagus correlates with risk of adenocarcinoma. Gastroenterology. 2001 Jun;120(7):1630–9. PMID:11375945
452. Byun TJ, Han DS, Ahn SB, et al. Pseudoinvasion in an adenomatous polyp of the colon mimicking invasive colon cancer. Gut Liver. 2009 Jun;3(2):130–3. PMID:20431736
453. Büchler M, Malfertheiner P, Baczako K, et al. A metastatic endocrine-neurogenic tumor of the ampulla of Vater with multiple endocrine immunoreaction–malignant paraganglioma? Digestion. 1985;31(1):54–9. PMID:2858422
454. Bülow S, Björk J, Christensen IJ, et al. Duodenal adenomatosis in familial adenomatous polyposis. Gut. 2004 Mar;53(3):381–6. PMID:14960520
455. Cacheux W, Dangles-Marie V, Rouleau E, et al. Exome sequencing reveals

aberrant signalling pathways as hallmark of treatment-naive anal squamous cell carcinoma. Oncotarget. 2017 Dec 8;9(1):464–76. PMID:29416628

456. Cagir B, Nagy MW, Topham A, et al. Adenosquamous carcinoma of the colon, rectum, and anus: epidemiology, distribution, and survival characteristics. Dis Colon Rectum. 1999 Feb;42(2):258–63. PMID:10211505

458. Caillard S, Porcher R, Provot F, et al. Post-transplantation lymphoproliferative disorder after kidney transplantation: report of a nationwide French registry and the development of a new prognostic score. J Clin Oncol. 2013 Apr 1;31(10):1302–9. PMID:23423742

459. Cairo S, Armengol C, De Reyniès A, et al. Hepatic stem-like phenotype and interplay of Wnt/beta-catenin and Myc signaling in aggressive childhood liver cancer. Cancer Cell. 2008 Dec 9;14(6):471–84. PMID:19061838

460. Caldas C, Hahn SA, da Costa LT, et al. Frequent somatic mutations and homozygous deletions of the p16 (MTS1) gene in pancreatic adenocarcinoma. Nat Genet. 1994 Sep;8(1):27–32. PMID:7726912

461. Calderaro J, Couchy G, Imbeaud S, et al. Histological subtypes of hepatocellular carcinoma are related to gene mutations and molecular tumour classification. J Hepatol. 2017 Oct;67(4):727–38. PMID:28532995

462. Calderaro J, Nault JC, Balabaud C, et al. Inflammatory hepatocellular adenomas developed in the setting of chronic liver disease and cirrhosis. Mod Pathol. 2016 Jan;29(1):43–50. PMID:26516697

463. Calhoun ES, Jones JB, Ashfaq R, et al. BRAF and FBXW7 (CDC4, FBW7, AGO, SEL10) mutations in distinct subsets of pancreatic cancer: potential therapeutic targets. Am J Pathol. 2003 Oct;163(4):1255–60. PMID:14507635

464. Caliskan A, Kohlmann WK, Affolter KE, et al. Intramucosal lipomas of the colon implicate Cowden syndrome. Mod Pathol. 2018 Apr;31(4):643–51. PMID:29192650

465. Caliskan C, Makay O, Firat O, et al. McKittrick-Wheelock syndrome: is it really rare? Am J Emerg Med. 2010 Jan;28(1):105–6. PMID:20006212

466. Calle EE, Rodriguez C, Walker-Thurmond K, et al. Overweight, obesity, and mortality from cancer in a prospectively studied cohort of U.S. adults. N Engl J Med. 2003 Apr 24;348(17):1625–38. PMID:12711737

467. Calva-Cerqueira D, Chinnathambi S, Pechman B, et al. The rate of germline mutations and large deletions of SMAD4 and BMPR1A in juvenile polyposis. Clin Genet. 2009 Jan;75(1):79–85. PMID:18823382

468. Calvani J, Lopez P, Sarnacki S, et al. Solid pseudopapillary neoplasms of the pancreas do not express major pancreatic markers in pediatric patients. Hum Pathol. 2019 Jan;83:29–35. PMID:30130629

469. Camargo MC, Anderson WF, King JB, et al. Divergent trends for gastric cancer incidence by anatomical subsite in US adults. Gut. 2011 Dec;60(12):1644–9. PMID:21613644

470. Camargo MC, Murphy G, Koriyama C, et al. Determinants of Epstein-Barr virus-positive gastric cancer: an international pooled analysis. Br J Cancer. 2011 Jun 28;105(1):38–43. PMID:21654677

471. Campana JP, Pellegrini PA, Rossi GL, et al. Right versus left laparoscopic colectomy for colon cancer: does side make any difference? Int J Colorectal Dis. 2017 Jun;32(6):907–12. PMID:28204867

472. Campbell F, Verbeke CS. Pathology of the pancreas: a practical approach. London (UK): Springer-Verlag London; 2013.

473. Campoli PM, Ejima FH, Cardoso DM, et al.

Metastatic cancer to the stomach. Gastric Cancer. 2006;9(1):19–25. PMID:16557432

474. Cancer Genome Atlas Network. Comprehensive molecular characterization of human colon and rectal cancer. Nature. 2012 Jul 18;487(7407):330–7. PMID:22810696

475. Cancer Genome Atlas Research Network. Integrated genomic characterization of oesophageal carcinoma. Nature. 2017 Jan 12;541(7636):169–75. PMID:28052061

476. Cancer Genome Atlas Research Network. Comprehensive molecular characterization of gastric adenocarcinoma. Nature. 2014 Sep 11;513(7517):202–9. PMID:25079317

477. Cancer Genome Atlas Research Network. Integrated genomic characterization of pancreatic ductal adenocarcinoma. Cancer Cell. 2017 Aug 14;32(2):185–203.e13. PMID:28810144

478. Cancer Genome Atlas Research Network. Comprehensive and integrative genomic characterization of hepatocellular carcinoma. Cell. 2017 Jun 15;169(7):1327–41.e23. PMID:28622513

479. Candido JB, Morton JP, Bailey P, et al. CSF1R+ macrophages sustain pancreatic tumor growth through T cell suppression and maintenance of key gene programs that define the squamous subtype. Cell Rep. 2018 May 1;23(5):1448–60. PMID:29719257

480. Canto MI, Goggins M, Hruban RH, et al. Screening for early pancreatic neoplasia in high-risk individuals: a prospective controlled study. Clin Gastroenterol Hepatol. 2006 Jun;4(6):766–81, quiz 665. PMID:16682259

481. Canto MI, Harinck F, Hruban RH, et al. International Cancer of the Pancreas Screening (CAPS) Consortium summit on the management of patients with increased risk for familial pancreatic cancer. Gut. 2013 Mar;62(3):339–47. PMID:23135763

482. Canto MI, Hruban RH, Fishman EK, et al. Frequent detection of pancreatic lesions in asymptomatic high-risk individuals. Gastroenterology. 2012 Apr;142(4):796–804, quiz e14–5. PMID:22245846

483. Cao D, Antonescu C, Wong G, et al. Positive immunohistochemical staining of KIT in solid-pseudopapillary neoplasms of the pancreas is not associated with KIT/PDGFRA mutations. Mod Pathol. 2006 Sep;19(9):1157–63. PMID:16778826

484. Cao D, Maitra A, Saavedra JA, et al. Expression of novel markers of pancreatic ductal adenocarcinoma in pancreatic non-ductal neoplasms: additional evidence of different genetic pathways. Mod Pathol. 2005 Jun;18(6):752–61. PMID:15696124

485. Cao H, Wang B, Zhang Z, et al. Distribution trends of gastric polyps: an endoscopy database analysis of 24 121 northern Chinese patients. J Gastroenterol Hepatol. 2012 Jul;27(7):1175–80. PMID:22414211

486. Cao S, Cox K, Esquivel CO, et al. Post-transplant lymphoproliferative disorders and gastrointestinal manifestations of Epstein-Barr virus infection in children following liver transplantation. Transplantation. 1998 Oct 15;66(7):851–6. PMID:9798693

487. Cao XP, Liu YY, Xiao HP, et al. Pancreatic somatostatinoma characterized by extreme hypoglycemia. Chin Med J (Engl). 2009 Jul 20;122(14):1709–12. PMID:19719976

488. Cao Y, Gao Z, Li L, et al. Whole exome sequencing of insulinoma reveals recurrent T372R mutations in YY1. Nat Commun. 2013;4:2810. PMID:24326773

489. Capella C, Frigerio B, Cornaggia M, et al. Gastric parietal cell carcinoma–a newly recognized entity: light microscopic and ultrastructural features. Histopathology. 1984 Sep;8(5):813–24. PMID:6083970

490. Capella C, Marando A, Longhi E, et al.

Primary gastric Merkel cell carcinoma harboring DNA polyomavirus: first description of an unusual high-grade neuroendocrine carcinoma. Hum Pathol. 2014 Jun;45(6):1310–4. PMID:24709111

491. Capelle LG, de Vries AC, Haringsma J, et al. The staging of gastritis with the OLGA system by using intestinal metaplasia as an accurate alternative for atrophic gastritis. Gastrointest Endosc. 2010 Jun;71(7):1150–8. PMID:20381801

492. Capelle LG, Van Grieken NC, Lingsma HF, et al. Risk and epidemiological time trends of gastric cancer in Lynch syndrome carriers in the Netherlands. Gastroenterology. 2010 Feb;138(2):487–92. PMID:19900449

493. Cappell MS, Stevens CE, Amin M. Systematic review of giant gastric lipomas reported since 1980 and report of two new cases in a review of 117110 esophagogastroduodenoscopies. World J Gastroenterol. 2017 Aug 14;23(30):5619–33. PMID:28852321

494. Carballal S, Rodríguez-Alcalde D, Moreira L, et al. Colorectal cancer risk factors in patients with serrated polyposis syndrome: a large multicentre study. Gut. 2016 Nov;65(11):1829–37. PMID:26264224

495. Carbonnel F, d'Almagne H, Lavergne A, et al. The clinicopathological features of extensive small intestinal CD4 T cell infiltration. Gut. 1999 Nov;45(5):662–7. PMID:10517900

496. Cardinal LH, Carballo P, Lorenzo MC, et al. A six-year experience with anal cytology in women with HPV in the lower genital tract: utility, limitations, and clinical correlation. Diagn Cytopathol. 2014 May;42(5):396–400. PMID:24166879

497. Cardoso R, Coburn N, Seevaratnam R, et al. A systematic review and meta-analysis of the utility of EUS for preoperative staging for gastric cancer. Gastric Cancer. 2012 Sep;15 Suppl 1:S19–26. PMID:22237654

498. Carethers JM, Stoffel EM. Lynch syndrome and Lynch syndrome mimics: the growing complex landscape of hereditary colon cancer. World J Gastroenterol. 2015 Aug 21;21(31):9253–61. PMID:26309352

499. Carethers JM. Differentiating Lynch-like from Lynch syndrome. Gastroenterology. 2014 Mar;146(3):602–4. PMID:24468183

500. Carethers JM. Microsatellite instability pathway and EMAST in colorectal cancer. Curr Colorectal Cancer Rep. 2017 Feb;13(1):73–80. PMID:28367107

501. Carlson GJ, Nivatvongs S, Snover DC. Colorectal polyps in Cowden's disease (multiple hamartoma syndrome). Am J Surg Pathol. 1984 Oct;8(10):763–70. PMID:6496844

502. Carlson JW, Fletcher CD. Immunohistochemistry for beta-catenin in the differential diagnosis of spindle cell lesions: analysis of a series and review of the literature. Histopathology. 2007 Oct;51(4):509–14. PMID:17711447

503. Carmack SW, Genta RM, Graham DY, et al. Management of gastric polyps: a pathology-based guide for gastroenterologists. Nat Rev Gastroenterol Hepatol. 2009 Jun;6(6):331–41. PMID:19421245

504. Carmack SW, Genta RM, Schuler CM, et al. The current spectrum of gastric polyps: a 1-year national study of over 120,000 patients. Am J Gastroenterol. 2009 Jun;104(6):1524–32. PMID:19491866

505. Carmona-Bayonas A, Jiménez-Fonseca P, Echavarria I, et al. Surgery for metastases for esophageal-gastric cancer in the real world: data from the AGAMENON national registry. Eur J Surg Oncol. 2018 Aug;44(8):1191–8. PMID:29685755

506. Carneiro F, Huntsman DG, Smyrk TC, et al. Model of the early development of diffuse gastric cancer in E-cadherin mutation carriers and

its implications for patient screening. J Pathol. 2004 Jun;203(2):681–7. PMID:15141383

507. Carneiro F, Seixas M, Sobrinho-Simões M. New elements for an updated classification of the carcinomas of the stomach. Pathol Res Pract. 1995 Jul;191(6):571–84. PMID:7479380

508. Carney JA, Go VL, Sizemore GW, et al. Alimentary-tract ganglioneuromatosis. A major component of the syndrome of multiple endocrine neoplasia, type 2b. N Engl J Med. 1976 Dec 2;295(23):1287–91. PMID:980061

509. Carney JA. Gastric stromal sarcoma, pulmonary chondroma, and extra-adrenal paraganglioma (Carney triad): natural history, adrenocortical component, and possible familial occurrence. Mayo Clin Proc. 1999 Jun;74(6):543–52. PMID:10377927

510. Carpenter JB, Rennels MA. Immunophenotypic characteristics of anal gland carcinoma. Arch Pathol Lab Med. 2008 Oct;132(10):1547–8. PMID:18834205

511. Carr NJ, Cecil TD, Mohamed F, et al. A consensus for classification and pathologic reporting of pseudomyxoma peritonei and associated appendiceal neoplasia: the results of the Peritoneal Surface Oncology Group International (PSOGI) modified Delphi process. Am J Surg Pathol. 2016 Jan;40(1):14–26. PMID:26492181

512. Carr NJ, McCarthy WF, Sobin LH. Epithelial noncarcinoid tumors and tumor-like lesions of the appendix. A clinicopathologic study of 184 patients with a multivariate analysis of prognostic factors. Cancer. 1995 Feb 1;75(3):757–68. PMID:7828125

513. Carrera C, Kunk P, Rahma O. Small cell carcinoma of the gallbladder: case report and comprehensive analysis of published cases. J Oncol. 2015;2015:304909. PMID:26823665

514. Carstens PH, Cressman FK Jr. Malignant oncocytic carcinoid of the pancreas. Ultrastruct Pathol. 1989 Jan-Feb;13(1):69–75. PMID:2919439

515. Carta M, Maresi E, Giuffrè M, et al. Congenital hepatic mesenchymal hamartoma associated with mesenchymal stem villous hyperplasia of the placenta: case report. J Pediatr Surg. 2005 May;40(5):e37–9. PMID:15937805

516. Carvalho B, Buffart TE, Reis RM, et al. Mixed gastric carcinomas show similar chromosomal aberrations in both their diffuse and glandular components. Cell Oncol. 2006;28(5-6):283–94. PMID:17167181

517. Carvalho B, Sillars-Hardebol AH, Postma C, et al. Colorectal adenoma to carcinoma progression is accompanied by changes in gene expression associated with ageing, chromosomal instability, and fatty acid metabolism. Cell Oncol (Dordr). 2012 Feb;35(1):53–63. PMID:22278361

518. Cary NR, Barron DJ, McGoldrick JP, et al. Combined oesophageal adenocarcinoma and carcinoid in Barrett's oesophagitis: potential role of enterochromaffin-like cells in oesophageal malignancy. Thorax. 1993 Apr;48(4):404–5. PMID:8511743

519. Casadei R, D'Ambra M, Pezzilli R, et al. Solid serous microcystic tumor of the pancreas. JOP. 2008 Jul 10;9(4):538–40. PMID:18648150

520. Casali PG, Abecassis N, Bauer S, et al. Gastrointestinal stromal tumours: ESMO-EURACAN Clinical Practice Guidelines for diagnosis, treatment and follow-up. Ann Oncol. 2018 Oct;29(Supplement_4):iv68-iv78. PMID:29846513

521. Cassaro M, Rugge M, Gutierrez O, et al. Topographic patterns of intestinal metaplasia and gastric cancer. Am J Gastroenterol. 2000 Jun;95(6):1431–8. PMID:10894575

522. Cassaro M, Rugge M, Tieppo C, et al. Indefinite for non-invasive neoplasia lesions in gastric intestinal metaplasia: the

immunophenotype. J Clin Pathol. 2007 Jun;60(6):615–21. PMID:17557866
523. Cassier PA, Ducimetière F, Lurkin A, et al. A prospective epidemiological study of new incident GISTs during two consecutive years in Rhône Alpes region: incidence and molecular distribution of GIST in a European region. Br J Cancer. 2010 Jul 13;103(2):165–70. PMID:20588273
524. Castillejo A, Vargas G, Castillejo MI, et al. Prevalence of germline MUTYH mutations among Lynch-like syndrome patients. Eur J Cancer. 2014 Sep;50(13):2241–50. PMID:24953332
525. Castillo JJ, Bibas M, Miranda RN. The biology and treatment of plasmablastic lymphoma. Blood. 2015 Apr 9;125(15):2323–30. PMID:25636338
526. Castillo JJ, Furman M, Beltrán BE, et al. Human immunodeficiency virus-associated plasmablastic lymphoma: poor prognosis in the era of highly active antiretroviral therapy. Cancer. 2012 Nov 1;118(21):5270–7. PMID:22510767
527. Castillo JJ, Winer ES, Olszewski AJ. Population-based prognostic factors for survival in patients with Burkitt lymphoma: an analysis from the Surveillance, Epidemiology, and End Results database. Cancer. 2013 Oct 15;119(20):3672–9. PMID:23913575
528. Catena L, Bajetta E, Milione M, et al. Mammalian target of rapamycin expression in poorly differentiated endocrine carcinoma: clinical and therapeutic future challenges. Target Oncol. 2011 Jun;6(2):65–8. PMID:21468754
529. Caturelli E, Solmi L, Anti M, et al. Ultrasound guided fine needle biopsy of early hepatocellular carcinoma complicating liver cirrhosis: a multicentre study. Gut. 2004 Sep;53(9):1356–62. PMID:15306600
530. Cazals-Hatem D, Rebouissou S, Bioulac-Sage P, et al. Clinical and molecular analysis of combined hepatocellular-cholangiocarcinomas. J Hepatol. 2004 Aug;41(2):292–8. PMID:15288479
531. Celio MR, Pasi A, Bürgisser E, et al. 'Proopiocortin fragments' in normal human adult pituitary. Distribution and ultrastructural characterization of immunoreactive cells. Acta Endocrinol (Copenh). 1980 Sep;95(1):27–40. PMID:6257006
532. Cenaj O, Gibson J, Odze RD. Clinicopathologic and outcome study of sessile serrated adenomas/polyps with serrated versus intestinal dysplasia. Mod Pathol. 2018 Apr;31(4):633–42. PMID:29271414
533. Centeno BA, Stelow EB, Pitman MB. Pancreatic cytohistology: cytohistology of small tissue samples. Cambridge (UK): Cambridge University Press; 2015.
534. Ceppa EP, Burbridge RA, Rialon KL, et al. Endoscopic versus surgical ampullectomy: an algorithm to treat disease of the ampulla of Vater. Ann Surg. 2013 Feb;257(2):315–22. PMID:23059497
535. Cerar A, Jutersek A, Vidmar S. Adenoid cystic carcinoma of the esophagus. A clinicopathologic study of three cases. Cancer. 1991 Apr 15;67(8):2159–64. PMID:1706215
536. Cerri M, Capello D, Muti G, et al. Aberrant somatic hypermutation in post-transplant lymphoproliferative disorders. Br J Haematol. 2004 Nov;127(3):362–4. PMID:15491294
537. Cerwenka H, Bacher H, Mischinger HJ. Pyloric obstruction caused by prolapse of a hyperplastic gastric polyp. Hepatogastroenterology. 2002 Jul-Aug;49(46):958–60. PMID:12143253
538. Cesarman E, Chadburn A, Liu YF, et al. BCL-6 gene mutations in posttransplantation lymphoproliferative disorders predict response to therapy and clinical outcome. Blood. 1998 Oct 1;92(7):2294–302. PMID:9746767
539. Cesarman E, Knowles DM. Kaposi's sarcoma-associated herpesvirus: a lymphotropic human herpesvirus associated with Kaposi's sarcoma, primary effusion lymphoma, and multicentric Castleman's disease. Semin Diagn Pathol. 1997 Feb;14(1):54–66. PMID:9044510
540. Cha PC, Zembutsu H, Takahashi A, et al. A genome-wide association study identifies SNP in DCC is associated with gallbladder cancer in the Japanese population. J Hum Genet. 2012 Apr;57(4):235–7. PMID:22318345
541. Chadburn A, Cesarman E, Liu YF, et al. Molecular genetic analysis demonstrates that multiple posttransplantation lymphoproliferative disorders occurring in one anatomic site in a single patient represent distinct primary lymphoid neoplasms. Cancer. 1995 Jun 1;75(11):2747–56. PMID:7743481
542. Chadburn A, Chen JM, Hsu DT, et al. The morphologic and molecular genetic categories of posttransplantation lymphoproliferative disorders are clinically relevant. Cancer. 1998 May 15;82(10):1978–87. PMID:9587133
543. Chaffee KG, Oberg AL, McWilliams RR, et al. Prevalence of germ-line mutations in cancer genes among pancreatic cancer patients with a positive family history. Genet Med. 2018 Jan;20(1):119–27. PMID:28726808
544. Chan JK, Chan AC, Cheuk W, et al. Type II enteropathy-associated T-cell lymphoma: a distinct aggressive lymphoma with frequent γδ T-cell receptor expression. Am J Surg Pathol. 2011 Oct;35(10):1557–69. PMID:21921780
545. Chan JK, Fletcher CD, Nayler SJ, et al. Follicular dendritic cell sarcoma. Clinicopathologic analysis of 17 cases suggesting a malignant potential higher than currently recognized. Cancer. 1997 Jan 15;79(2):294–313. PMID:9010103
546. Chan K, Brown IS, Kyle T, et al. Chief cell-predominant gastric polyps: a series of 12 cases with literature review. Histopathology. 2016 May;68(6):825–33. PMID:26335020
547. Chan KW. Review of 253 cases of significant pathology in 7,910 cholecystectomies in Hong Kong. Pathology. 1988 Jan;20(1):20–3. PMID:3374970
548. Chan NG, Penswick JL, Labelle E, et al. Ectopic breast tissue presenting as an anal polyp. Can J Surg. 2007 Dec;50(6):E23–4. PMID:18067696
549. Chan-On W, Nairismägi ML, Ong CK, et al. Exome sequencing identifies distinct mutational patterns in liver fluke-related and non-infection-related bile duct cancers. Nat Genet. 2013 Dec;45(12):1474–8. PMID:24185513
550. Chand M, Siddiqui MR, Swift I, et al. Systematic review of prognostic importance of extramural venous invasion in rectal cancer. World J Gastroenterol. 2016 Jan 28;22(4):1721–6. PMID:26819536
551. Chandrasekharappa SC, Guru SC, Manickam P, et al. Positional cloning of the gene for multiple endocrine neoplasia-type 1. Science. 1997 Apr 18;276(5311):404–7. PMID:9103196
552. Chang AE, Karnell LH, Menck HR. The National Cancer Data Base report on cutaneous and noncutaneous melanoma: a summary of 84,836 cases from the past decade. Cancer. 1998 Oct 15;83(8):1664–78. PMID:9781962
553. Chang CL, Marra G, Chauhan DP, et al. Oxidative stress inactivates the human DNA mismatch repair system. Am J Physiol Cell Physiol. 2002 Jul;283(1):C148–54. PMID:12055083
554. Chang CY, Hernandez-Prera JC, Roayaie S, et al. Changing epidemiology of hepatocellular adenoma in the United States: review of the literature. Int J Hepatol. 2013;2013:604860. PMID:23509632
555. Chang DK, Jamieson NB, Johns AL, et al. Histomolecular phenotypes and outcome in adenocarcinoma of the ampulla of Vater. J Clin Oncol. 2013 Apr 1;31(10):1348–56. PMID:23439753
556. Chang HJ, Jee CD, Kim WH. Mutation and altered expression of beta-catenin during gallbladder carcinogenesis. Am J Surg Pathol. 2002 Jun;26(6):758–66. PMID:12023580
557. Chang HJ, Jin SY, Park C, et al. Mesenchymal hamartomas of the liver: comparison of clinicopathologic features between cystic and solid forms. J Korean Med Sci. 2006 Feb;21(1):63–8. PMID:16479067
558. Chang HK, Yu E, Kim J, et al. Adenocarcinoma of the small intestine: a multi-institutional study of 197 surgically resected cases. Hum Pathol. 2010 Aug;41(8):1087–96. PMID:20334897
559. Chang MS, Lee HS, Kim CW, et al. Clinicopathologic characteristics of Epstein-Barr virus-incorporated gastric cancers in Korea. Pathol Res Pract. 2001;197(6):395–400. PMID:11432666
560. Chang P, Attiyeh FF. Adenocarcinoma of the appendix. Dis Colon Rectum. 1981 Apr;24(3):176–80. PMID:6164526
561. Chang Y, Cesarman E, Pessin MS, et al. Identification of herpesvirus-like DNA sequences in AIDS-associated Kaposi's sarcoma. Science. 1994 Dec 16;266(5192):1865–9. PMID:7997879
562. Chang YC, Nagasue N, Abe S, et al. Comparison between the clinicopathologic features of AFP-positive and AFP-negative gastric cancers. Am J Gastroenterol. 1992 Mar;87(3):321–5. PMID:1371637
563. Chang YR, Park JK, Jang JY, et al. Incidental pancreatic cystic neoplasms in an asymptomatic healthy population of 21,745 individuals: large-scale, single-center cohort study. Medicine (Baltimore). 2016 Dec;95(51):e5535. PMID:28002329
563A. Chapman J, Gentles AJ, Sujoy V, et al. Gene expression analysis of plasmablastic lymphoma identifies downregulation of B-cell receptor signaling and additional unique transcriptional programs. Leukemia. 2015 Nov;29(11):2270–3. PMID:25921246
564. Chapuy B, Stewart C, Dunford AJ, et al. Molecular subtypes of diffuse large B cell lymphoma are associated with distinct pathogenic mechanisms and outcomes. Nat Med. 2018 May;24(5):679–90. PMID:29713087
565. Charalampakis N, Nogueras González GM, Elimova E, et al. The proportion of signet ring cell component in patients with localized gastric adenocarcinoma correlates with the degree of response to pre-operative chemoradiation. Oncology. 2016;90(5):239–47. PMID:27046280
566. Chari ST, Yadav D, Smyrk TC, et al. Study of recurrence after surgical resection of intraductal papillary mucinous neoplasm of the pancreas. Gastroenterology. 2002 Nov;123(5):1500–7. PMID:12404225
567. Charlesworth M, Verbeke CS, Falk GA, et al. Pancreatic lesions in von Hippel-Lindau disease? A systematic review and meta synthesis of the literature. J Gastrointest Surg. 2012 Jul;16(7):1422–8. PMID:22370733
568. Charlton A, Blair V, Shaw D, et al. Hereditary diffuse gastric cancer: predominance of multiple foci of signet ring cell carcinoma in distal stomach and transitional zone. Gut. 2004 Jun;53(6):814–20. PMID:15138207
569. Chatelain D, Paye F, Mourra N, et al. Unilocular acinar cell cystadenoma of the pancreas an unusual acinar cell tumor. Am J Clin Pathol. 2002 Aug;118(2):211–4. PMID:12162680
570. Chatterjee D, Katz MH, Rashid A, et al. Histologic grading of the extent of residual carcinoma following neoadjuvant chemoradiation in pancreatic ductal adenocarcinoma: a predictor for patient outcome. Cancer. 2012 Jun 15;118(12):3182–90. PMID:22028089
571. Chaudhary P, Bhadana U, Singh RA, et al. Primary hepatic angiosarcoma. Eur J Surg Oncol. 2015 Sep;41(9):1137–43. PMID:26008857
572. Cheadle JP, Sampson JR. MUTYH-associated polyposis–from defect in base excision repair to clinical genetic testing. DNA Repair (Amst). 2007 Mar 1;6(3):274–9. PMID:17161978
573. Chen AL, Misdraji J, Brugge WR, et al. Acinar cell cystadenoma: a challenging cytology diagnosis, facilitated by Moray® micro-forceps biopsy. Diagn Cytopathol. 2017 Jun;45(6):557–60. PMID:28236434
574. Chen C, Wang L, Liu X, et al. Gallbladder neuroendocrine carcinoma: report of 10 cases and comparision of clinicopathologic features with gallbladder adenocarcinoma. Int J Clin Exp Pathol. 2015 Jul 1;8(7):8218–26. PMID:26339390
575. Chen CN, Lin JJ, Chen JJ, et al. Gene expression profile predicts patient survival of gastric cancer after surgical resection. J Clin Oncol. 2005 Oct 10;23(29):7286–95. PMID:16145069
576. Chen H, Shen C, Yin R, et al. Clinicopathological characteristics, diagnosis, treatment, and outcomes of primary gastric adenosquamous carcinoma. World J Surg Oncol. 2015 Apr 2;13:136. PMID:25889482
577. Chen HW, Lu CH, Shun CT, et al. Gastric outlet obstruction due to giant hyperplastic gastric polyps. J Formos Med Assoc. 2005 Nov;104(11):852–5. PMID:16496067
578. Chen JN, He D, Tang F, et al. Epstein-Barr virus-associated gastric carcinoma: a newly defined entity. J Clin Gastroenterol. 2012 Apr;46(4):262–71. PMID:22392024
579. Chen RC, Wang J, Kuang XY, et al. Integrated analysis of microRNA and mRNA expression profiles in HBx-expressing hepatic cells. World J Gastroenterol. 2017 Mar 14;23(10):1787–95. PMID:28348484
580. Chen RW, Qiu MJ, Chen Y, et al. Analysis of the clinicopathological features and prognostic factors of primary hepatic neuroendocrine tumors. Oncol Lett. 2018 Jun;15(6):8604–10. PMID:30065788
581. Chen S, Chen Y, Yang J, et al. Primary mucoepidermoid carcinoma of the esophagus. J Thorac Oncol. 2011 Aug;6(8):1426–31. PMID:21587086
582. Chen SB, Weng HR, Wang G, et al. Primary adenosquamous carcinoma of the esophagus. World J Gastroenterol. 2013 Dec 7;19(45):8382–90. PMID:24363531
583. Chen TC, Kuo TT, Ng KF. Follicular dendritic cell tumor of the liver: a clinicopathologic and Epstein-Barr virus study of two cases. Mod Pathol. 2001 Apr;14(4):354–60. PMID:11301353
584. Chen W, Lau SK, Fong D, et al. High frequency of clonal immunoglobulin receptor gene rearrangements in sporadic histiocytic/dendritic cell sarcomas. Am J Surg Pathol. 2009 Jun;33(6):863–73. PMID:19145200
585. Chen Y, Shi H, Li H, et al. Clinicopathological features of inflammatory pseudotumour-like follicular dendritic cell tumour of the abdomen. Histopathology. 2016 May;68(6):858–65. PMID:26332157
586. Chen YW, Yen SH, Chen SY, et al. Anus-preservation treatment for anal cancer: retrospective analysis at a single institution. J Surg Oncol. 2007 Oct 1;96(5):374–80. PMID:17492635
587. Chen YY, Li AF, Huang KH, et al. Adenosquamous carcinoma of the stomach and review of the literature. Pathol Oncol Res. 2015

Jul;21(3):547–51. PMID:25567665
588. Chen Z, Han S, Wu J, et al. A systematic review: perivascular epithelioid cell tumor of gastrointestinal tract. Medicine (Baltimore). 2016 Jul;95(28):e3890. PMID:27428182
589. Chen Z, Xiao HE, Ramchandra P, et al. Imaging and pathological features of primary hepatic neuroendocrine carcinoma: an analysis of nine cases and review of the literature. Oncol Lett. 2014 Apr;7(4):956–62. PMID:24944650
590. Chen ZM, Scudiere JR, Abraham SC, et al. Pyloric gland adenoma: an entity distinct from gastric foveolar type adenoma. Am J Surg Pathol. 2009 Feb;33(2):186–93. PMID:18830123
591. Chen ZM, Wang HL. Alteration of cytokeratin 7 and cytokeratin 20 expression profile is uniquely associated with tumorigenesis of primary adenocarcinoma of the small intestine. Am J Surg Pathol. 2004 Oct;28(10):1352–9. PMID:15371952
592. Chene A, Donati D, Orem J, et al. Endemic Burkitt's lymphoma as a polymicrobial disease: new insights on the interaction between Plasmodium falciparum and Epstein-Barr virus. Semin Cancer Biol. 2009 Dec;19(6):411–20. PMID:19897039
593. Cheng DW, Sekhon HK, Toutounjian R, et al. Heterotopic gastric mucosa of the anus associated with anal ulcer. Tech Coloproctol. 2012 Apr;16(2):167–8. PMID:22124763
594. Cheng N, Hui DY, Liu Y, et al. Is gastric lymphoepithelioma-like carcinoma a special subtype of EBV-associated gastric carcinoma? New insight based on clinicopathological features and EBV genome polymorphisms. Gastric Cancer. 2015 Apr;18(2):246–55. PMID:24771002
595. Chesnokova V, Zonis S, Zhou C, et al. Growth hormone is permissive for neoplastic colon growth. Proc Natl Acad Sci U S A. 2016 Jun 7;113(23):E3250–9. PMID:27226307
596. Cheson BD, Fisher RI, Barrington SF, et al. Recommendations for initial evaluation, staging, and response assessment of Hodgkin and non-Hodgkin lymphoma: the Lugano classification. J Clin Oncol. 2014 Sep 20;32(27):3059–68. PMID:25113753
597. Chetty R, Bateman AC, Torlakovic E, et al. A pathologist's survey on the reporting of sessile serrated adenomas/polyps. J Clin Pathol. 2014 May;67(5):426–30. PMID:24399034
598. Chetty R, Clark SP, Pitson GA. Primary small cell carcinoma of the pancreas. Pathology. 1993 Jul;25(3):240–2. PMID:8265240
599. Chetty R, Hafezi-Bakhtiari S, Serra S, et al. Traditional serrated adenomas (TSAs) admixed with other serrated (so-called precursor) polyps and conventional adenomas: a frequent occurrence. J Clin Pathol. 2015 Apr;68(4):270–3. PMID:25589791
600. Chetty R, Serra S, Hsieh E. Basaloid squamous carcinoma of the anal canal with an adenoid cystic pattern: histologic and immunohistochemical reappraisal of an unusual variant. Am J Surg Pathol. 2005 Dec;29(12):1668–72. PMID:16327441
601. Chetty R, Serra S. Membrane loss and aberrant nuclear localization of E-cadherin are consistent features of solid pseudopapillary tumour of the pancreas. An immunohistochemical study using two antibodies recognizing different domains of the E-cadherin molecule. Histopathology. 2008 Feb;52(3):325–30. PMID:18269583
602. Cheuk W, Chan JK, Shek TW, et al. Inflammatory pseudotumor-like follicular dendritic cell tumor: a distinctive low-grade malignant intra-abdominal neoplasm with consistent Epstein-Barr virus association. Am J Surg Pathol. 2001 Jun;25(6):721–31. PMID:11395549
603. Cheuk W, Chan JK. Thyroid transcription factor-1 is of limited value in practical distinction between pulmonary and extrapulmonary small cell carcinomas. Am J Surg Pathol. 2001 Apr;25(4):545–6. PMID:11257635
604. Cheung R. Racial and social economic factors impact on the cause specific survival of pancreatic cancer: a SEER survey. Asian Pac J Cancer Prev. 2013;14(1):159–63. PMID:23534717
605. Chia NY, Tan P. Molecular classification of gastric cancer. Ann Oncol. 2016 May;27(5):763–9. PMID:26861606
606. Chiaravalli M, Reni M, O'Reilly EM. Pancreatic ductal adenocarcinoma: state-of-the-art 2017 and new therapeutic strategies. Cancer Treat Rev. 2017 Nov;60:32–43. PMID:28869888
607. Chibon F, Lagarde P, Salas S, et al. Validated prediction of clinical outcome in sarcomas and multiple types of cancer on the basis of a gene expression signature related to genome complexity. Nat Med. 2010 Jul;16(7):781–7. PMID:20581836
608. Chiche L, Dao T, Salamé E, et al. Liver adenomatosis: reappraisal, diagnosis, and surgical management: eight new cases and review of the literature. Ann Surg. 2000 Jan;231(1):74–81. PMID:10636105
609. Chiles MC, Parham DM, Qualman SJ, et al. Sclerosing rhabdomyosarcomas in children and adolescents: a clinicopathologic review of 13 cases from the Intergroup Rhabdomyosarcoma Study Group and Children's Oncology Group. Pediatr Dev Pathol. 2004 Nov-Dec;7(6):583–94. PMID:15630526
610. Chini P, Draganov PV. Diagnosis and management of ampullary adenoma: the expanding role of endoscopy. World J Gastrointest Endosc. 2011 Dec 16;3(12):241–7. PMID:22195233
611. Chino O, Kijima H, Shimada H, et al. Esophageal squamous cell carcinoma with lymphoid stroma: report of 3 cases with immunohistochemical analyses. Gastrointest Endosc. 2001 Oct;54(4):513–7. PMID:11577322
612. Chiou WY, Chang CM, Tseng KC, et al. Effect of liver cirrhosis on metastasis in colorectal cancer patients: a nationwide population-based cohort study. Jpn J Clin Oncol. 2015 Feb;45(2):160–8. PMID:25378650
613. Chirieac LR, Swisher SG, Correa AM, et al. Signet-ring cell or mucinous histology after preoperative chemoradiation and survival in patients with esophageal or esophagogastric junction adenocarcinoma. Clin Cancer Res. 2005 Mar 15;11(6):2229–36. PMID:15788671
614. Chlumská A, Waloschek T, Mukenšnabl P, et al. Pyloric gland adenoma: a histologic, immunohistochemical and molecular genetic study of 23 cases. Cesk Patol. 2015;51(3):137–43. PMID:26421956
615. Chmielecki J, Crago AM, Rosenberg M, et al. Whole-exome sequencing identifies a recurrent NAB2-STAT6 fusion in solitary fibrous tumors. Nat Genet. 2013 Feb;45(2):131–2. PMID:23313954
616. Chmielecki J, Hutchinson KE, Frampton GM, et al. Comprehensive genomic profiling of pancreatic acinar cell carcinomas identifies recurrent RAF fusions and frequent inactivation of DNA repair genes. Cancer Discov. 2014 Dec;4(12):1398–405. PMID:25266736
617. Cho C, Rullis I, Rogers LS. Bile duct adenomas as liver nodules. Arch Surg. 1978 Mar;113(3):272–4. PMID:205188
617A. Cho CJ, Kang HJ, Ryu YM, et al. Poor prognosis in Epstein-Barr virus-negative gastric cancer with lymphoid stroma is associated with immune phenotype. Gastric Cancer. 2018 Nov;21(6):925–35. PMID:29627937
618. Cho KJ, Jang JJ, Lee SS, et al. Basaloid squamous carcinoma of the oesophagus: a distinct neoplasm with multipotential differentiation. Histopathology. 2000 Apr;36(4):331–40. PMID:10759947
619. Choi AB, Maxwell JE, Keck KJ, et al. Is multifocality an indicator of aggressive behavior in small bowel neuroendocrine tumors? Pancreas. 2017 Oct;46(9):1115–20. PMID:28902780
620. Choi GH, Ann SY, Lee SI, et al. Collision tumor of hepatocellular carcinoma and neuroendocrine carcinoma involving the liver: case report and review of the literature. World J Gastroenterol. 2016 Nov 7;22(41):9229–34. PMID:27895410
621. Choi IJ, Kook MC, Kim YI, et al. Helicobacter pylori therapy for the prevention of metachronous gastric cancer. N Engl J Med. 2018 Mar 22;378(12):1085–95. PMID:29562147
622. Choi JI, Joo I, Lee JM. State-of-the-art preoperative staging of gastric cancer by MDCT and magnetic resonance imaging. World J Gastroenterol. 2014 Apr 28;20(16):4546–57. PMID:24782607
623. Choi JY, Kim MJ, Lee JY, et al. Typical and atypical manifestations of serous cystadenoma of the pancreas: imaging findings with pathologic correlation. AJR Am J Roentgenol. 2009 Jul;193(1):136–42. PMID:19542405
624. Choi PM. Predominance of rectosigmoid neoplasia in ulcerative colitis and its implication on cancer surveillance. Gastroenterology. 1993 Feb;104(2):666–7. PMID:8425717
625. Choi WT, Brown I, Ushiku T, et al. Gastric pyloric gland adenoma: a multicentre clinicopathological study of 67 cases. Histopathology. 2018 May;72(6):1007–14. PMID:29278427
626. Choi YY, Jeen YM, Kim YJ. Sarcomatoid carcinoma of colon: extremely poor prognosis. J Korean Surg Soc. 2011 Jun;80 Suppl 1:S26–30. PMID:22066078
627. Chopin-Laly X, Walter T, Hervieu V, et al. Neuroendocrine neoplasms of the jejunum: a heterogeneous group with distinctive proximal and distal subsets. Virchows Arch. 2013 May;462(5):489–99. PMID:23579432
628. Chott A, Haedicke W, Mosberger I, et al. Most CD56+ intestinal lymphomas are CD8+CD5-T-cell lymphomas of monomorphic small to medium size histology. Am J Pathol. 1998 Nov;153(5):1483–90. PMID:9811340
629. Chow JS, Chen CC, Ahsan H, et al. A population-based study of the incidence of malignant small bowel tumours: SEER, 1973-1990. Int J Epidemiol. 1996 Aug;25(4):722–8. PMID:8921448
630. Christ E, Wild D, Forrer F, et al. Glucagon-like peptide-1 receptor imaging for localization of insulinomas. J Clin Endocrinol Metab. 2009 Nov;94(11):4398–405. PMID:19820010
631. Christison-Lagay ER, Burrows PE, Alomari A, et al. Hepatic hemangiomas: subtype classification and development of a clinical practice algorithm and registry. J Pediatr Surg. 2007 Jan;42(1):62–7, discussion 67–8. PMID:17208542
632. Chu LC, Singhi AD, Haroun RR, et al. The many faces of pancreatic serous cystadenoma: radiologic and pathologic correlation. Diagn Interv Imaging. 2017 Mar;98(3):191–202. PMID:27614585
633. Chu YJ, Yang HI, Wu HC, et al. Aflatoxin B1 exposure increases the risk of hepatocellular carcinoma associated with hepatitis C virus infection or alcohol consumption. Eur J Cancer. 2018 May;94:37–46. PMID:29533866
634. Chuah SK, Hu TH, Kuo CM, et al. Upper gastrointestinal carcinoid tumors incidentally found by endoscopic examinations. World J Gastroenterol. 2005 Nov 28;11(44):7028–32. PMID:16437611
635. Chumbalkar V, Jennings TA, Ainechi S, et al. Extramammary Paget's disease of anal canal associated with rectal adenoma without invasive carcinoma. Gastroenterology Res. 2016 Dec;9(6):99–102. PMID:28058078
636. Chun YS, Pawlik TM, Vauthey JN. 8th Edition of the AJCC Cancer Staging Manual: pancreas and hepatobiliary cancers. Ann Surg Oncol. 2018 Apr;25(4):845–7. PMID:28752469
637. Chung JH, Sanford E, Johnson A, et al. Comprehensive genomic profiling of anal squamous cell carcinoma reveals distinct genomically defined classes. Ann Oncol. 2016 Jul;27(7):1336–41. PMID:27052656
638. Ciccocioppo R, Croci GA, Biagi F, et al. Intestinal T-cell lymphoma with enteropathy-associated T-cell lymphoma-like features arising in the setting of adult autoimmune enteropathy. Hematol Oncol. 2018 Apr;36(2):481–8. PMID:29446107
639. Cimino-Mathews A, Sharma R, Illei PB. Detection of human papillomavirus in small cell carcinomas of the anus and rectum. Am J Surg Pathol. 2012 Jul;36(7):1087–92. PMID:22531171
640. Cingolani N, Shaco-Levy R, Farruggio A, et al. Alpha-fetoprotein production by pancreatic tumors exhibiting acinar cell differentiation: study of five cases, one arising in a mediastinal teratoma. Hum Pathol. 2000 Aug;31(8):938–44. PMID:10987254
641. Cisco RM, Norton JA. Surgery for gastrinoma. Adv Surg. 2007;41:165–76. PMID:17972563
642. Clark SK, Phillips RK. Desmoids in familial adenomatous polyposis. Br J Surg. 1996 Nov;83(11):1494–504. PMID:9014661
643. Clendenning M, Young JP, Walsh MD, et al. Germline mutations in the polyposis-associated genes BMPR1A, SMAD4, PTEN, MUTYH and GREM1 are not common in individuals with serrated polyposis syndrome. PLoS One. 2013 Jun 21;8(6):e66705. PMID:23805267
644. Clot G, Jares P, Giné E, et al. A gene signature that distinguishes conventional and leukemic nonnodal mantle cell lymphoma helps predict outcome. Blood. 2018 Jul 26;132(4):413–22. PMID:29769262
645. Cloyd JM, Chun YS, Ikoma N, et al. Clinical and genetic implications of DNA mismatch repair deficiency in biliary tract cancers associated with Lynch syndrome. J Gastrointest Cancer. 2018 Mar;49(1):93–6. PMID:29238914
646. Coffey K, Beral V, Green J, et al. Lifestyle and reproductive risk factors associated with anal cancer in women aged over 50 years. Br J Cancer. 2015 Apr 28;112(9):1568–74. PMID:25867258
647. Coffin CM, Hornick JL, Fletcher CD. Inflammatory myofibroblastic tumor: comparison of clinicopathologic, histologic, and immunohistochemical features including ALK expression in atypical and aggressive cases. Am J Surg Pathol. 2007 Apr;31(4):509–20. PMID:17414097
648. Coffin CM, Watterson J, Priest JR, et al. Extrapulmonary inflammatory myofibroblastic tumor (inflammatory pseudotumor). A clinicopathologic and immunohistochemical study of 84 cases. Am J Surg Pathol. 1995 Aug;19(8):859–72. PMID:7611533
649. Cohen L, Taylor L. Beyond brochures: a systematic approach to prevention. Am J Public Health. 1991 Jul;81(7):929–30. PMID:2053677
650. Coindre JM. Grading of soft tissue sarcomas: review and update. Arch Pathol Lab Med. 2006 Oct;130(10):1448–53. PMID:17090186
651. Colecchia A, Scaioli E, Montrone L, et al. Pre-operative liver biopsy in cirrhotic patients with early hepatocellular carcinoma represents a safe and accurate diagnostic tool for tumour grading assessment. J Hepatol. 2011 Feb;54(2):300–5. PMID:21056498
652. Coleman HG, Xie SH, Lagergren J. The

epidemiology of esophageal adenocarcinoma. Gastroenterology. 2018 Jan;154(2):390–405. PMID:28780073
653. Collins MA, Bednar F, Zhang Y, et al. Oncogenic Kras is required for both the initiation and maintenance of pancreatic cancer in mice. J Clin Invest. 2012 Feb;122(2):639–53. PMID:22232209
654. Colombo C, Foo WC, Whiting D, et al. FAP-related desmoid tumors: a series of 44 patients evaluated in a cancer referral center. Histol Histopathol. 2012 May;27(5):641–9. PMID:22419028
655. Colombo P, Arizzi C, Roncalli M. Acinar cell cystadenocarcinoma of the pancreas: report of rare case and review of the literature. Hum Pathol. 2004 Dec;35(12):1568–71. PMID:15619219
656. Colonna J, Plaza JA, Frankel WL, et al. Serous cystadenoma of the pancreas: clinical and pathological features in 33 patients. Pancreatology. 2008;8(2):135–41. PMID:18382099
657. Compagno J, Oertel JE. Microcystic adenomas of the pancreas (glycogen-rich cystadenomas): a clinicopathologic study of 34 cases. Am J Clin Pathol. 1978 Mar;69(3):289–98. PMID:637043
658. Conlon KC, Klimstra DS, Brennan MF. Long-term survival after curative resection for pancreatic ductal adenocarcinoma. Clinicopathologic analysis of 5-year survivors. Ann Surg. 1996 Mar;223(3):273–9. PMID:8604907
659. Connell WR, Lennard-Jones JE, Williams CB, et al. Factors affecting the outcome of endoscopic surveillance for cancer in ulcerative colitis. Gastroenterology. 1994 Oct;107(4):934–44. PMID:7926483
660. Connolly MM, Dawson PJ, Michelassi F, et al. Survival in 1001 patients with carcinoma of the pancreas. Ann Surg. 1987 Sep;206(3):366–73. PMID:2820322
661. Connor AA, Denroche RE, Jang GH, et al. Association of distinct mutational signatures with correlates of increased immune activity in pancreatic ductal adenocarcinoma. JAMA Oncol. 2017 Jun 1;3(6):774–83. PMID:27768182
662. Conrad R, Cobb C, Raza A. Role of cytopathology in the diagnosis and management of gastrointestinal tract cancers. J Gastrointest Oncol. 2012 Sep;3(3):285–98. PMID:22943018
663. Conte B, George B, Overman M, et al. High-grade neuroendocrine colorectal carcinomas: a retrospective study of 100 patients. Clin Colorectal Cancer. 2016 Jun;15(2):e1–7. PMID:26810202
664. Cook JR, Dehner LP, Collins MH, et al. Anaplastic lymphoma kinase (ALK) expression in the inflammatory myofibroblastic tumor: a comparative immunohistochemical study. Am J Surg Pathol. 2001 Nov;25(11):1364–71. PMID:11684952
665. Cook JR, Harris NL, Isaacson PG, et al. Alpha heavy chain disease. In: Swerdlow SH, Campo E, Harris NL, et al., editors. WHO classification of tumours of haematopoietic and lymphoid tissues. Lyon (France): International Agency for Research on Cancer; 2017. p. 240. (WHO classification of tumours series, 4th rev. ed.; vol. 2). http://publications.iarc.fr/556.
666. Cook JR, Isaacson PG, Chott A, et al. Extranodal marginal zone lymphoma of mucosa-associated lymphoid tissue (MALT lymphoma). In: Swerdlow SH, Campo E, Harris NL, et al., editors. WHO classification of tumours of haematopoietic and lymphoid tissues. Lyon (France): International Agency for Research on Cancer; 2017. pp. 259–62. (WHO classification of tumours series, 4th rev. ed.; vol. 2). http://publications.iarc.fr/556.
667. Cooke CB, Krenacs L, Stetler-Stevenson M, et al. Hepatosplenic T-cell lymphoma: a distinct clinicopathologic entity of cytotoxic gamma delta T-cell origin. Blood. 1996 Dec 1;88(11):4265–74. PMID:8943863
668. Cooper WN, Luharia A, Evans GA, et al. Molecular subtypes and phenotypic expression of Beckwith-Wiedemann syndrome. Eur J Hum Genet. 2005 Sep;13(9):1025–32. PMID:15999116
669. Coppa GF, Eng K, Localio SA. Surgical management of diffuse cavernous hemangioma of the colon, rectum and anus. Surg Gynecol Obstet. 1984 Jul;159(1):17–22. PMID:6740459
670. Corcos O, Couvelard A, Giraud S, et al. Endocrine pancreatic tumors in von Hippel-Lindau disease: clinical, histological, and genetic features. Pancreas. 2008 Jul;37(1):85–93. PMID:18580449
671. Coriat R, Mozer M, Caux F, et al. Endoscopic findings in Cowden syndrome. Endoscopy. 2011 Aug;43(8):723–6. PMID:21437855
672. Corless CL, Barnett CM, Heinrich MC. Gastrointestinal stromal tumours: origin and molecular oncology. Nat Rev Cancer. 2011 Nov 17;11(12):865–78. PMID:22089421
673. Corless CL, Schroeder A, Griffith D, et al. PDGFRA mutations in gastrointestinal stromal tumors: frequency, spectrum and in vitro sensitivity to imatinib. J Clin Oncol. 2005 Aug 10;23(23):5357–64. PMID:15928335
674. Correa P, Piazuelo MB. The gastric precancerous cascade. J Dig Dis. 2012 Jan;13(1):2–9. PMID:22188910
675. Correa P. Gastric cancer: overview. Gastroenterol Clin North Am. 2013 Jun;42(2):211–7. PMID:23639637
676. Correa P. The biological model of gastric carcinogenesis. IARC Sci Publ. 2004;(157):301–10. PMID:15055303
677. Corrin B, Gilby ED, Jones NF, et al. Oat cell carcinoma of the pancreas with ectopic ACTH secretion. Cancer. 1973 Jun;31(6):1523–7. PMID:4350960
678. Corso G, Carvalho J, Marrelli D, et al. Somatic mutations and deletions of the E-cadherin gene predict poor survival of patients with gastric cancer. J Clin Oncol. 2013 Mar 1;31(7):868–75. PMID:23341533
679. Corso G, Pedrazzani C, Marrelli D, et al. Familial gastric cancer and Li-Fraumeni syndrome. Eur J Cancer Care (Engl). 2010 May;19(3):377–81. PMID:19674071
680. Cortina R, McCormick J, Kolm P, et al. Management and prognosis of adenocarcinoma of the appendix. Dis Colon Rectum. 1995 Aug;38(8):848–52. PMID:7634979
681. Corvalan A, Koriyama C, Akiba S, et al. Epstein-Barr virus in gastric carcinoma is associated with location in the cardia and with a diffuse histology: a study in one area of Chile. Int J Cancer. 2001 Nov;94(4):527–30. PMID:11745439
682. Costi R, Caruana P, Sarli L, et al. Ampullary adenocarcinoma in neurofibromatosis type 1. Case report and literature review. Mod Pathol. 2001 Nov;14(11):1169–74. PMID:11706080
683. Coulouarn C, Cavard C, Rubbia-Brandt L, et al. Combined hepatocellular-cholangiocarcinomas exhibit progenitor features and activation of Wnt and TGFβ signaling pathways. Carcinogenesis. 2012 Sep;33(9):1791–6. PMID:22696594
684. Courville EL, Yohe S, Chou D, et al. EBV-negative monomorphic B-cell post-transplant lymphoproliferative disorders are pathologically distinct from EBV-positive cases and frequently contain TP53 mutations. Mod Pathol. 2016 Oct;29(10):1200–11. PMID:27443517
685. Couvelard A, Terris B, Hammel P, et al. [Acinar cystic transformation of the pancreas (or acinar cell cystadenoma), a rare and recently described entity]. Ann Pathol. 2002 Oct;22(5):397–400. French. PMID:12483157
686. Crabtree MD, Tomlinson IP, Talbot IC, et al. Variability in the severity of colonic disease in familial adenomatous polyposis results from differences in tumour initiation rather than progression and depends relatively little on patient age. Gut. 2001 Oct;49(4):540–3. PMID:11559652
687. Crago AM, Chmielecki J, Rosenberg M, et al. Near universal detection of alterations in CTNNB1 and Wnt pathway regulators in desmoid-type fibromatosis by whole-exome sequencing and genomic analysis. Genes Chromosomes Cancer. 2015 Oct;54(10):606–15. PMID:26171757
688. Craig FE, Johnson LR, Harvey SA, et al. Gene expression profiling of Epstein-Barr virus-positive and -negative monomorphic B-cell posttransplant lymphoproliferative disorders. Diagn Mol Pathol. 2007 Sep;16(3):158–68. PMID:17721324
689. Creasy JM, Sadot E, Koerkamp BG, et al. The impact of primary tumor location on long-term survival in patients undergoing hepatic resection for metastatic colon cancer. Ann Surg Oncol. 2018 Feb;25(2):431–8. PMID:29181680
690. Crippa S, Fernández-Del Castillo C, Salvia R, et al. Mucin-producing neoplasms of the pancreas: an analysis of distinguishing clinical and epidemiologic characteristics. Clin Gastroenterol Hepatol. 2010 Feb;8(2):213–9. PMID:19835989
691. Crippa S, Salvia R, Warshaw AL, et al. Mucinous cystic neoplasm of the pancreas is not an aggressive entity: lessons from 163 resected patients. Ann Surg. 2008 Apr;247(4):571–9. PMID:18362619
692. Cristescu R, Lee J, Nebozhyn M, et al. Molecular analysis of gastric cancer identifies subtypes associated with distinct clinical outcomes. Nat Med. 2015 May;21(5):449–56. PMID:25894828
693. Crocetti D, Sapienza P, Sterpetti AV, et al. Surgery for symptomatic colon lipoma: a systematic review of the literature. Anticancer Res. 2014 Nov;34(11):6271–6. PMID:25368224
694. Cromwell I, Gaudet M, Peacock SJ, et al. Cost-effectiveness analysis of anal cancer screening in women with cervical neoplasia in British Columbia, Canada. BMC Health Serv Res. 2016 Jun 27;16:206. PMID:27349646
695. Crona J, Gustavsson T, Norlén O, et al. Somatic mutations and genetic heterogeneity at the CDKN1B locus in small intestinal neuroendocrine tumors. Ann Surg Oncol. 2015 Dec;22 Suppl 3:S1428–35. PMID:25586243
696. Crump M, Gospodarowicz M, Shepherd FA. Lymphoma of the gastrointestinal tract. Semin Oncol. 1999 Jun;26(3):324–37. PMID:10375089
697. Cruz-Correa M, Giardiello FM. Familial adenomatous polyposis. Gastrointest Endosc. 2003 Dec;58(6):885–94. PMID:14652558
698. Cubilla AL, Fitzgerald PJ. Morphological lesions associated with human primary invasive nonendocrine pancreas cancer. Cancer Res. 1976 Jul;36(7 PT 2):2690–8. PMID:1277176
699. Cubilla AL, Hajdu SI. Islet cell carcinoma of the pancreas. Arch Pathol. 1975 Apr;99(4):204–7. PMID:163633
700. Cui C, Lian B, Zhou L, et al. Multifactorial analysis of prognostic factors and survival rates among 706 mucosal melanoma patients. Ann Surg Oncol. 2018 Aug;25(8):2184–92. PMID:29748886
701. Cuilliere P, Lazure T, Bui M, et al. Solid adenoma with exclusive hepatocellular differentiation: a new variant among pancreatic benign neoplasms? Virchows Arch. 2002 Nov;441(5):519–22. PMID:12447684
702. Curia MC, Zuckermann M, De Lellis L, et al. Sporadic childhood hepatoblastomas show activation of beta-catenin, mismatch repair defects and p53 mutations. Mod Pathol. 2008 Jan;21(1):7–14. PMID:17962810
703. Czauderna P, Lopez-Terrada D, Hiyama E, et al. Hepatoblastoma state of the art: pathology, genetics, risk stratification, and chemotherapy. Curr Opin Pediatr. 2014 Feb;26(1):19–28. PMID:24322718
704. d'Amore F, Brincker H, Grønbaek K, et al. Non-Hodgkin's lymphoma of the gastrointestinal tract: a population-based analysis of incidence, geographic distribution, clinicopathologic presentation features, and prognosis. J Clin Oncol. 1994 Aug;12(8):1673–84. PMID:8040680
705. d'Huart MC, Chevaux JB, Bressenot AM, et al. Prevalence of esophageal squamous papilloma (ESP) and associated cancer in northeastern France. Endosc Int Open. 2015 Apr;3(2):E101–6. PMID:26135647
706. D'Onofrio M, De Robertis R, Tinazzi Martini P, et al. Oncocytic intraductal papillary mucinous neoplasms of the pancreas: imaging and histopathological findings. Pancreas. 2016 Oct;45(9):1233–42. PMID:27518461
707. Dabaja BS, Suki D, Pro B, et al. Adenocarcinoma of the small bowel: presentation, prognostic factors, and outcome of 217 patients. Cancer. 2004 Aug 1;101(3):518–26. PMID:15274064
708. Dabbs DJ. Diagnostic immunohistochemistry: theranostic and genomic applications. 5th ed. Philadelphia (PA): Elsevier; 2018.
709. Dahdaleh FS, Carr JC, Calva D, et al. Juvenile polyposis and other intestinal polyposis syndromes with microdeletions of chromosome 10q22-23. Clin Genet. 2012 Feb;81(2):110–6. PMID:21834858
710. Dal Molin M, Blackford AL, Siddiqui A, et al. Duodenal involvement is an independent prognostic factor for patients with surgically resected pancreatic ductal adenocarcinoma. Ann Surg Oncol. 2017 Aug;24(8):2379–86. PMID:28439733
711. Daling JR, Madeleine MM, Johnson LG, et al. Human papillomavirus, smoking, and sexual practices in the etiology of anal cancer. Cancer. 2004 Jul 15;101(2):270–80. PMID:15241823
712. Dangoor A, Seddon B, Gerrand C, et al. UK guidelines for the management of soft tissue sarcomas. Clin Sarcoma Res. 2016 Nov 15;6:20. PMID:27891213
713. Daou B, Zanello M, Varlet P, et al. An unusual case of constitutional mismatch repair deficiency syndrome with anaplastic ganglioglioma, colonic adenocarcinoma, osteosarcoma, acute myeloid leukemia, and signs of neurofibromatosis type 1: case report. Neurosurgery. 2015 Jul;77(1):E145–52, discussion E152. PMID:25850602
714. Darragh TM, Colgan TJ, Cox JT, et al. The lower anogenital squamous terminology standardization project for HPV-associated Lesions: background and consensus recommendations from the College of American Pathologists and the American Society for Colposcopy and Cervical Pathology. Arch Pathol Lab Med. 2012 Oct;136(10):1266–97. PMID:22742517
715. Das DK. Cytodiagnosis of hepatocellular carcinoma in fine-needle aspirates of the liver: its differentiation from reactive hepatocytes and metastatic adenocarcinoma. Diagn Cytopathol. 1999 Dec;21(6):370–7. PMID:10572267
716. Dasari A, Shen C, Halperin D, et al. Trends in the incidence, prevalence, and survival outcomes in patients with neuroendocrine tumors in the United States. JAMA Oncol. 2017 Oct 1;3(10):1335–42. PMID:28448665
717. Date K, Okabayashi T, Shima Y, et al. Clinicopathological features and surgical outcomes of intraductal tubulopapillary neoplasm of the pancreas: a systematic review. Langenbecks Arch Surg. 2016 Jun;401(4):439–47.

PMID:27001682

718. Daugule I, Sudraba A, Chiu HM, et al. Gastric plasma biomarkers and Operative Link for Gastritis Assessment gastritis stage. Eur J Gastroenterol Hepatol. 2011 Apr;23(4):302–7. PMID:21389862

719. Daum O, Hatlova J, Mandys V, et al. Comparison of morphological, immunohistochemical, and molecular genetic features of inflammatory fibroid polyps (Vanek's tumors). Virchows Arch. 2010 May;456(5):491–7. PMID:20393746

720. Daum S, Cellier C, Mulder CJ. Refractory coeliac disease. Best Pract Res Clin Gastroenterol. 2005 Jun;19(3):413–24. PMID:15925846

721. Daum S, Weiss D, Hummel M, et al. Frequency of clonal intraepithelial T lymphocyte proliferations in enteropathy-type intestinal T cell lymphoma, coeliac disease, and refractory sprue. Gut. 2001 Dec;49(6):804–12. PMID:11709515

722. Dave SS, Fu K, Wright GW, et al. Molecular diagnosis of Burkitt's lymphoma. N Engl J Med. 2006 Jun 8;354(23):2431–42. PMID:16760443

723. Davenport JR, Su T, Zhao Z, et al. Modifiable lifestyle factors associated with risk of sessile serrated polyps, conventional adenomas and hyperplastic polyps. Gut. 2018 Mar;67(3):456–65. PMID:27852795

724. Davison JM, Choudry HA, Pingpank JF, et al. Clinicopathologic and molecular analysis of disseminated appendiceal mucinous neoplasms: identification of factors predicting survival and proposed criteria for a three-tiered assessment of tumor grade. Mod Pathol. 2014 Nov;27(11):1521–39. PMID:24633196

725. Davison JM, Hartman DA, Singhi AD, et al. Loss of SMAD4 protein expression is associated with high tumor grade and poor prognosis in disseminated appendiceal mucinous neoplasms. Am J Surg Pathol. 2014 May;38(5):583–92. PMID:24618609

726. Dawsey SM, Lewin KJ, Wang GQ, et al. Squamous esophageal histology and subsequent risk of squamous cell carcinoma of the esophagus. A prospective follow-up study from Linxian, China. Cancer. 1994 Sep 15;74(6):1686–92. PMID:8082069

727. Dawson H, Novotny A, Becker K, et al. Macroscopy predicts tumor progression in gastric cancer: a retrospective patho-historical analysis based on Napoleon Bonaparte's autopsy report. Dig Liver Dis. 2016 Nov;48(11):1378–85. PMID:27522550

728. Dawson J, Bloom SR, Cockel R. A unique apudoma producing the glucagonoma and gastrinoma syndromes. Postgrad Med J. 1983 May;59(691):315–6. PMID:6878103

729. de Baaij LR, Berkhof J, van de Water JM, et al. A new and validated clinical prognostic model (epi) for enteropathy-associated t-cell lymphoma. Clin Cancer Res. 2015 Jul 1;21(13):3013–9. PMID:25779949

730. de Boer WB, Ee H, Kumarasinghe MP. Neoplastic lesions of gastric adenocarcinoma and proximal polyposis syndrome (GAPPS) are gastric phenotype. Am J Surg Pathol. 2018 Jan;42(1):1–8. PMID:29112017

731. De Herder WW, Lamberts SW. Octapeptide somatostatin-analogue therapy of Cushing's syndrome. Postgrad Med J. 1999 Feb;75(880):65–6. PMID:10448463

732. de Jonge PJ, van Blankenstein M, Looman CW, et al. Risk of malignant progression in patients with Barrett's oesophagus: a Dutch nationwide cohort study. Gut. 2010 Aug;59(8):1030–6. PMID:20639249

733. de Lambert G, Lardy H, Martelli H, et al. Surgical management of neuroendocrine tumors of the appendix in children and adolescents: a retrospective French multicenter study of 114 cases. Pediatr Blood Cancer. 2016

Apr;63(4):598–603. PMID:26663900

734. de Latour RA, Kilaru SM, Gross SA. Management of small bowel polyps: a literature review. Best Pract Res Clin Gastroenterol. 2017 Aug;31(4):401–8. PMID:28842049

735. de Leng WW, Jansen M, Carvalho R, et al. Genetic defects underlying Peutz-Jeghers syndrome (PJS) and exclusion of the polarity-associated MARK/Par1 gene family as potential PJS candidates. Clin Genet. 2007 Dec;72(6):568–73. PMID:17924967

736. de Leval L, Parrens M, Le Bras F, et al. Angioimmunoblastic T-cell lymphoma is the most common T-cell lymphoma in two distinct French information data sets. Haematologica. 2015 Sep;100(9):e361–4. PMID:26045291

737. DE Marchis ML, Tonelli F, Quaresmini D, et al. Desmoid tumors in familial adenomatous polyposis. Anticancer Res. 2017 Jul;37(7):3357–66. PMID:28668823

738. de Rosa N, Rodriguez-Bigas MA, Chang GJ, et al. DNA mismatch repair deficiency in rectal cancer: benchmarking its impact on prognosis, neoadjuvant response prediction, and clinical cancer genetics. J Clin Oncol. 2016 Sep 1;34(25):3039–46. PMID:27432916

739. de Sanjosé S, Brotons M, Pavón MA. The natural history of human papillomavirus infection. Best Pract Res Clin Obstet Gynaecol. 2018 Feb;47:2–13. PMID:28964706

740. De Vito C, Sarker D, Ross P, et al. Histological heterogeneity in primary and metastatic classic combined hepatocellular-cholangiocarcinoma: a case series. Virchows Arch. 2017 Nov;471(5):619–29. PMID:28707055

741. de-Thé G, Geser A, Day NE, et al. Epidemiological evidence for causal relationship between Epstein-Barr virus and Burkitt's lymphoma from Ugandan prospective study. Nature. 1978 Aug 24;274(5673):756–61. PMID:210392

742. Debiec-Rychter M, Sciot R, Le Cesne A, et al. KIT mutations and dose selection for imatinib in patients with advanced gastrointestinal stromal tumours. Eur J Cancer. 2006 May;42(8):1093–103. PMID:16624552

743. Deepak P, Sifuentes H, Sherid M, et al. T-cell non-Hodgkin's lymphomas reported to the FDA AERS with tumor necrosis factor-alpha (TNF-α) inhibitors: results of the REFURBISH study. Am J Gastroenterol. 2013 Jan;108(1):99–105. PMID:23032984

744. Degasperi E, Colombo M. Distinctive features of hepatocellular carcinoma in non-alcoholic fatty liver disease. Lancet Gastroenterol Hepatol. 2016 Oct;1(2):156–64. PMID:28404072

745. Dei Tos AP, Seregard S, Calonje E, et al. Giant cell angiofibroma. A distinctive orbital tumor in adults. Am J Surg Pathol. 1995 Nov;19(11):1286–93. PMID:7573691

746. Delabie J, Holte H, Vose JM, et al. Enteropathy-associated T-cell lymphoma: clinical and histological findings from the international peripheral T-cell lymphoma project. Blood. 2011 Jul 7;118(1):148–55. PMID:21566094

747. Delaunoit T, Neczyporenko F, Limburg PJ, et al. Pathogenesis and risk factors of small bowel adenocarcinoma: a colorectal cancer sibling? Am J Gastroenterol. 2005 Mar;100(3):703–10. PMID:15743371

748. Delcore R Jr, Cheung LY, Friesen SR. Outcome of lymph node involvement in patients with the Zollinger-Ellison syndrome. Ann Surg. 1988 Sep;208(3):291–8. PMID:3421754

749. Deleeuw RJ, Zettl A, Klinker E, et al. Whole-genome analysis and HLA genotyping of enteropathy-type T-cell lymphoma reveals 2 distinct lymphoma subtypes. Gastroenterology. 2007 May;132(5):1902–11. PMID:17484883

750. Delle Fave G, O'Toole D, Sundin A, et al. ENETS consensus guidelines update for

gastroduodenal neuroendocrine neoplasms. Neuroendocrinology. 2016;103(2):119–24. PMID:26784901

751. Delnatte C, Sanlaville D, Mougenot JF, et al. Contiguous gene deletion within chromosome arm 10q is associated with juvenile polyposis of infancy, reflecting cooperation between the BMPR1A and PTEN tumor-suppressor genes. Am J Hum Genet. 2006 Jun;78(6):1066–74. PMID:16685657

752. DeMaioribus CA, Lally KP, Sim K, et al. Mesenchymal hamartoma of the liver. A 35-year review. Arch Surg. 1990 May;125(5):598–600. PMID:2331217

753. DeMatos P, Wolfe WG, Shea CR, et al. Primary malignant melanoma of the esophagus. J Surg Oncol. 1997 Nov;66(3):201–6. PMID:9369967

754. Demicco EG, Wagner MJ, Maki RG, et al. Risk assessment in solitary fibrous tumors: validation and refinement of a risk stratification model. Mod Pathol. 2017 Oct;30(10):1433–42. PMID:28731041

755. den Elzen N, Buttery CV, Maddugoda MP, et al. Cadherin adhesion receptors orient the mitotic spindle during symmetric cell division in mammalian epithelia. Mol Biol Cell. 2009 Aug;20(16):3740–50. PMID:19553471

756. Deng N, Goh LK, Wang H, et al. A comprehensive survey of genomic alterations in gastric cancer reveals systematic patterns of molecular exclusivity and co-occurrence among distinct therapeutic targets. Gut. 2012 May;61(5):673–84. PMID:22315472

757. Deng YF, Lin Q, Zhang SH, et al. Malignant angiomyolipoma in the liver: a case report with pathological and molecular analysis. Pathol Res Pract. 2008;204(12):911–8. PMID:18723294

758. Deniz K, Moreira RK, Yeh MM, et al. Steatohepatitis-like changes in focal nodular hyperplasia, a finding to distinguish from steatohepatitic variant of hepatocellular carcinoma. Am J Surg Pathol. 2017 Feb;41(2):277–81. PMID:28079599

759. DeOliveira ML, Cunningham SC, Cameron JL, et al. Cholangiocarcinoma: thirty-one-year experience with 564 patients at a single institution. Ann Surg. 2007 May;245(5):755–62. PMID:17457168

759A. Derks S, Liao X, Chiaravalli AM, et al. Abundant PD-L1 expression in Epstein-Barr Virus-infected gastric cancers. Oncotarget. 2016 May 31;7(22):32925–32. PMID:27147580

760. Desai DC, Lockman JC, Chadwick RB, et al. Recurrent germline mutation in MSH2 arises frequently de novo. J Med Genet. 2000 Sep;37(9):646–52. PMID:10978353

761. Deshpande V, Fernandez-del Castillo C, Muzikansky A, et al. Cytokeratin 19 is a powerful predictor of survival in pancreatic endocrine tumors. Am J Surg Pathol. 2004 Sep;28(9):1145–53. PMID:15316313

762. Deshpande V, Mino-Kenudson M, Brugge WR, et al. Endoscopic ultrasound guided fine needle aspiration biopsy of autoimmune pancreatitis: diagnostic criteria and pitfalls. Am J Surg Pathol. 2005 Nov;29(11):1464–71. PMID:16224213

763. Detlefsen S, Fagerberg CR, Ousager LB, et al. Histiocytic disorders of the gastrointestinal tract. Hum Pathol. 2013 May;44(5):683–96. PMID:23063502

764. Detlefsen S, Sipos B, Feyerabend B, et al. Pancreatic fibrosis associated with age and ductal papillary hyperplasia. Virchows Arch. 2005 Nov;447(5):800–5. PMID:16021508

765. Deugnier YM, Charalambous P, Le Quilleuc D, et al. Preneoplastic significance of hepatic iron-free foci in genetic hemochromatosis: a study of 185 patients. Hepatology. 1993 Dec;18(6):1363–9. PMID:7902316

766. Devaney K, Goodman ZD, Ishak KG. Hepatobiliary cystadenoma and cystadenocarcinoma. A light microscopic and immunohistochemical study of 70 patients. Am J Surg Pathol. 1994 Nov;18(11):1078–91. PMID:7943529

767. Dewald GW, Smyrk TC, Thorland EC, et al. Fluorescence in situ hybridization to visualize genetic abnormalities in interphase cells of acinar cell carcinoma, ductal adenocarcinoma, and islet cell carcinoma of the pancreas. Mayo Clin Proc. 2009 Sep;84(9):801–10. PMID:19720778

769. Deyrup AT, Lee VK, Hill CE, et al. Epstein-Barr virus-associated smooth muscle tumors are distinctive mesenchymal tumors reflecting multiple infection events: a clinicopathologic and molecular analysis of 29 tumors from 19 patients. Am J Surg Pathol. 2006 Jan;30(1):75–82. PMID:16330945

770. Deyrup AT, Miettinen M, North PE, et al. Angiosarcomas arising in the viscera and soft tissue of children and young adults: a clinicopathologic study of 15 cases. Am J Surg Pathol. 2009 Feb;33(2):264–9. PMID:18987547

771. Dharnidharka VR, Lamb KE, Gregg JA, et al. Associations between EBV serostatus and organ transplant type in PTLD risk: an analysis of the SRTR National Registry Data in the United States. Am J Transplant. 2012 Apr;12(4):976–83. PMID:22226225

772. Dharnidharka VR, Webster AC, Martinez OM, et al. Post-transplant lymphoproliferative disorders. Nat Rev Dis Primers. 2016 Jan 28;2:15088. PMID:27189056

773. Dharnidharka VR. Comprehensive review of post-organ transplant hematologic cancers. Am J Transplant. 2018 Mar;18(3):537–49. PMID:29178667

774. Dhebri AR, Connor S, Campbell F, et al. Diagnosis, treatment and outcome of pancreatoblastoma. Pancreatology. 2004;4(5):441–51, discussion 452–3. PMID:15256806

775. di Pietro M, Canto MI, Fitzgerald RC. Endoscopic management of early adenocarcinoma and squamous cell carcinoma of the esophagus: screening, diagnosis, and therapy. Gastroenterology. 2018 Jan;154(2):421–36. PMID:28778650

776. Di Tommaso L, Destro A, Seok JY, et al. The application of markers (HSP70 GPC3 and GS) in liver biopsies is useful for detection of hepatocellular carcinoma. J Hepatol. 2009 Apr;50(4):746–54. PMID:19231003

777. Diamond EL, Subbiah V, Lockhart AC, et al. Vemurafenib for BRAF V600-mutant Erdheim-Chester disease and Langerhans cell histiocytosis: analysis of data from the histology-independent, phase 2, open-label VE-BASKET study. JAMA Oncol. 2018 Mar 1;4(3):384–8. PMID:29188284

778. Dickson BC, Riddle ND, Brooks JS, et al. Sirtuin 1 (SIRT1): a potential immunohistochemical marker and therapeutic target in soft tissue neoplasms with myoid differentiation. Hum Pathol. 2013 Jun;44(6):1125–30. PMID:23332867

779. Dieckhoff P, Runkel H, Daniel H, et al. Well-differentiated neuroendocrine neoplasia: relapse-free survival and predictors of recurrence after curative intended resections. Digestion. 2014;90(2):89–97. PMID:25196446

780. Diehm C, Abri O, Baitsch G, et al. [Iloprost, a stable prostacyclin derivative, in stage 4 arterial occlusive disease. A placebo-controlled multicenter study]. Dtsch Med Wochenschr. 1989 May 19;114(20):783–8. German. PMID:2470569

781. Dierickx D, Tousseyn T, Gheysens O. How I treat posttransplant lymphoproliferative disorders. Blood. 2015 Nov 12;126(20):2274–83. PMID:26384356

782. Dillon JL, Gonzalez JL, DeMars L, et al.

Universal screening for Lynch syndrome in endometrial cancers: frequency of germline mutations and identification of patients with Lynch-like syndrome. Hum Pathol. 2017 Dec;70:121–8. PMID:29107668
783. Din S, Wong K, Mueller MF, et al. Mutational analysis identifies therapeutic biomarkers in inflammatory bowel disease-associated colorectal cancers. Clin Cancer Res. 2018 Oct 15;24(20):5133–42. PMID:29950348
784. Dinesh U, Pervatikar SK, Rao R. FNAC diagnosis of pancreatic somatostatinoma. J Cytol. 2009 Oct;26(4):153–5. PMID:21938182
785. Ding GH, Liu Y, Wu MC, et al. Diagnosis and treatment of hepatic angiomyolipoma. J Surg Oncol. 2011 Jun;103(8):807–12. PMID:21283992
786. Ding W, Zhao S, Wang J, et al. Gastrointestinal lymphoma in southwest China: subtype distribution of 1,010 cases using the WHO (2008) classification in a single institution. Acta Haematol. 2016;135(1):21–8. PMID:26303279
787. Dinis-Ribeiro M, Areia M, de Vries AC, et al. Management of precancerous conditions and lesions in the stomach (MAPS): guideline from the European Society of Gastrointestinal Endoscopy (ESGE), European Helicobacter Study Group (EHSG), European Society of Pathology (ESP), and the Sociedade Portuguesa de Endoscopia Digestiva (SPED). Endoscopy. 2012 Jan;44(1):74–94. PMID:22198778
788. Disanto MG, Ambrosio MR, Rocca BJ, et al. Optimal minimal panels of immunohistochemistry for diagnosis of B-cell lymphoma for application in countries with limited resources and for triaging cases before referral to specialist centers. Am J Clin Pathol. 2016 May;145(5):687–95. PMID:27247372
789. Disibio G, French SW. Metastatic patterns of cancers: results from a large autopsy study. Arch Pathol Lab Med. 2008 Jun;132(6):931–9. PMID:18517275
790. Dittmer DP, Damania B. Kaposi sarcoma-associated herpesvirus: immunobiology, oncogenesis, and therapy. J Clin Invest. 2016 Sep 1;126(9):3165–75. PMID:27584730
791. Dixon MF, Genta RM, Yardley JH, et al. Classification and grading of gastritis. The updated Sydney System. International Workshop on the Histopathology of Gastritis, Houston 1994. Am J Surg Pathol. 1996 Oct;20(10):1161–81. PMID:8827022
792. Dixon MF, O'Connor HJ, Axon AT, et al. Reflux gastritis: distinct histopathological entity? J Clin Pathol. 1986 May;39(5):524–30. PMID:3722405
793. Dixon MF. Gastrointestinal epithelial neoplasia: Vienna revisited. Gut. 2002 Jul;51(1):130–1. PMID:12077106
794. Dobashi A, Tsuyama N, Asaka R, et al. Frequent BCOR aberrations in extranodal NK/T-cell lymphoma, nasal type. Genes Chromosomes Cancer. 2016 May;55(5):460–71. PMID:26773734
795. Doglioni C, Wotherspoon AC, Moschini A, et al. High incidence of primary gastric lymphoma in northeastern Italy. Lancet. 1992 Apr 4;339(8797):834–5. PMID:1347858
796. Doi M, Imai T, Shichiri M, et al. Octreotide-sensitive ectopic ACTH production by islet cell carcinoma with multiple liver metastases. Endocr J. 2003 Apr;50(2):135–43. PMID:12803233
797. Dokmak S, Paradis V, Vilgrain V, et al. A single-center surgical experience of 122 patients with single and multiple hepatocellular adenomas. Gastroenterology. 2009 Nov;137(5):1698–705. PMID:19664629
798. Domingo E, Freeman-Mills L, Rayner E, et al. Somatic POLE proofreading domain mutation, immune response, and prognosis in colorectal cancer: a retrospective, pooled biomarker study. Lancet Gastroenterol Hepatol. 2016 Nov;1(3):207–16. PMID:28404093
799. Domizio P, Owen RA, Shepherd NA, et al. Primary lymphoma of the small intestine. A clinicopathological study of 119 cases. Am J Surg Pathol. 1993 May;17(5):429–42. PMID:8470758
800. Domoto H, Terahata S, Senoh A, et al. Clear cell change in colorectal adenomas: its incidence and histological characteristics. Histopathology. 1999 Mar;34(3):250–6. PMID:10217566
801. Dong S, Chen L, Chen Y, et al. Primary hepatic extranodal marginal zone B-cell lymphoma of mucosa-associated lymphoid tissue type: a case report and literature review. Medicine (Baltimore). 2017 Mar;96(13):e6305. PMID:28353562
802. Dong XD, DeMatos P, Prieto VG, et al. Melanoma of the gallbladder: a review of cases seen at Duke University Medical Center. Cancer. 1999 Jan 1;85(1):32–9. PMID:9921971
802A. Donow C, Baisch H, Heitz PU, et al. Nuclear DNA content in 27 pancreatic endocrine tumours: correlation with malignancy, survival and expression of glycoprotein hormone alpha chain. Virchows Arch A Pathol Anat Histopathol. 1991;419(6):463–8. PMID:1750193
803. Donow C, Pipeleers-Marichal M, Schröder S, et al. Surgical pathology of gastrinoma. Site, size, multicentricity, association with multiple endocrine neoplasia type 1, and malignancy. Cancer. 1991 Sep 15;68(6):1329–34. PMID:1678681
804. Doubrovina E, Oflaz-Sozmen B, Prockop SE, et al. Adoptive immunotherapy with unselected or EBV-specific T cells for biopsy-proven EBV+ lymphomas after allogeneic hematopoietic cell transplantation. Blood. 2012 Mar 15;119(11):2644–56. PMID:22138512
805. Dowen SE, Crnogorac-Jurcevic T, Gangeswaran R, et al. Expression of S100P and its novel binding partner S100PBPR in early pancreatic cancer. Am J Pathol. 2005 Jan;166(1):81–92. PMID:15632002
806. Doyle LA, Fletcher CD, Hornick JL. Nuclear expression of CAMTA1 distinguishes epithelioid hemangioendothelioma from histologic mimics. Am J Surg Pathol. 2016 Jan;40(1):94–102. PMID:26414223
807. Doyle LA, Hornick JL, Fletcher CD. PEComa of the gastrointestinal tract: clinicopathologic study of 35 cases with evaluation of prognostic parameters. Am J Surg Pathol. 2013 Dec;37(12):1769–82. PMID:24061520
808. Doyle LA, Hornick JL. Mesenchymal tumors of the gastrointestinal tract other than GIST. Surg Pathol Clin. 2013 Sep;6(3):425–73. PMID:26839096
808A. Doyle LA, Nelson D, Heinrich MC, et al. Loss of succinate dehydrogenase subunit B (SDHB) expression is limited to a distinctive subset of gastric wild-type gastrointestinal stromal tumours: a comprehensive genotype-phenotype correlation study. Histopathology. 2012 Nov;61(5):801-9. PMID:22804613
809. Doyle LA, Sepehr GJ, Hamilton MJ, et al. A clinicopathologic study of 24 cases of systemic mastocytosis involving the gastrointestinal tract and assessment of mucosal mast cell density in irritable bowel syndrome and asymptomatic patients. Am J Surg Pathol. 2014 Jun;38(6):832–43. PMID:24618605
810. Doyle LA, Vivero M, Fletcher CD, et al. Nuclear expression of STAT6 distinguishes solitary fibrous tumor from histologic mimics. Mod Pathol. 2014 Mar;27(3):390–5. PMID:24030747
811. Dreijerink KM, Derks JL, Cataldo I, et al. Genetics and epigenetics of pancreatic neuroendocrine tumors and pulmonary carcinoids. Front Horm Res. 2015;44:115–38. PMID:26303708
812. Driessen A, Nafteux P, Lerut T, et al. Identical cytokeratin expression pattern CK7+/CK20- in esophageal and cardiac cancer: etiopathological and clinical implications. Mod Pathol. 2004 Jan;17(1):49–55. PMID:14631371
813. Drut R, Jones MC. Congenital pancreatoblastoma in Beckwith-Wiedemann syndrome: an emerging association. Pediatr Pathol. 1988;8(3):331–9. PMID:2845376
814. Du MQ. MALT lymphoma: recent advances in aetiology and molecular genetics. J Clin Exp Hematop. 2007 Nov;47(2):31–42. PMID:18040143
815. Dubourdeau M, Miyamura T, Matsuura Y, et al. Infection of HepG2 cells with recombinant adenovirus encoding the HCV core protein induces p21(WAF1) down-regulation – effect of transforming growth factor beta. J Hepatol. 2002 Oct;37(4):486–92. PMID:12217602
816. Dubé C, Yakubu M, McCurdy BR, et al. Risk of advanced adenoma, colorectal cancer, and colorectal cancer mortality in people with low-risk adenomas at baseline colonoscopy: a systematic review and meta-analysis. Am J Gastroenterol. 2017 Dec;112(12):1790–801. PMID:29087393
817. Duchini A, Sessoms SL. Gastrointestinal hemorrhage in patients with systemic sclerosis and CREST syndrome. Am J Gastroenterol. 1998 Sep;93(9):1453–6. PMID:9732924
818. Dudley JC, Lin MT, Le DT, et al. Microsatellite instability as a biomarker for PD-1 blockade. Clin Cancer Res. 2016 Feb 15;22(4):813–20. PMID:26880610
819. Dudley JC, Zheng Z, McDonald T, et al. Next-generation sequencing and fluorescence in situ hybridization have comparable performance characteristics in the analysis of pancreaticobiliary brushings for malignancy. J Mol Diagn. 2016 Jan;18(1):124–30. PMID:26596524
820. Dulai PS, Sandborn WJ, Gupta S. Colorectal cancer and dysplasia in inflammatory bowel disease: a review of disease epidemiology, pathophysiology, and management. Cancer Prev Res (Phila). 2016 Dec;9(12):887–94. PMID:27679553
821. Dulai PS, Singh S, Marquez E, et al. Chemoprevention of colorectal cancer in individuals with previous colorectal neoplasia: systematic review and network meta-analysis. BMJ. 2016 Dec 5;355:i6188. PMID:27919915
822. Dulak AM, Stojanov P, Peng S, et al. Exome and whole-genome sequencing of esophageal adenocarcinoma identifies recurrent driver events and mutational complexity. Nat Genet. 2013 May;45(5):478–86. PMID:23525077
823. Dumitrascu T, Dima S, Herlea V, et al. Neuroendocrine tumours of the ampulla of Vater: clinico-pathological features, surgical approach and assessment of prognosis. Langenbecks Arch Surg. 2012 Aug;397(6):933–43. PMID:22476195
824. Dunne PD, Alderdice M, O'Reilly PG, et al. Cancer-cell intrinsic gene expression signatures overcome intratumoural heterogeneity bias in colorectal cancer patient classification. Nat Commun. 2017 May 31;8:15657. PMID:28561046
825. Dunne PD, McArt DG, Bradley CA, et al. Challenging the cancer molecular stratification dogma: intratumoral heterogeneity undermines consensus molecular subtypes and potential diagnostic value in colorectal cancer. Clin Cancer Res. 2016 Aug 15;22(16):4095–104. PMID:27151745
826. Dupin N, Fisher C, Kellam P, et al. Distribution of human herpesvirus-8 latently infected cells in Kaposi's sarcoma, multicentric Castleman's disease, and primary effusion lymphoma. Proc Natl Acad Sci U S A. 1999 Apr 13;96(8):4546–51. PMID:10200299
827. Duprez R, Lacoste V, Brière J, et al. Evidence for a multiclonal origin of multicentric advanced lesions of Kaposi sarcoma. J Natl Cancer Inst. 2007 Jul 18;99(14):1086–94. PMID:17623796
828. Durot C, Dohan A, Boudiaf M, et al. Cancer of the anal canal: diagnosis, staging and follow-up with MRI. Korean J Radiol. 2017 Nov-Dec;18(6):946–56. PMID:29089827
829. Dursun N, Escalona OT, Roa JC, et al. Mucinous carcinomas of the gallbladder: clinicopathologic analysis of 15 cases identified in 606 carcinomas. Arch Pathol Lab Med. 2012 Nov;136(11):1347–58. PMID:23106580
830. Dursun N, Feng J, Basturk O, et al. Vacuolated cell pattern of pancreatobiliary adenocarcinoma: a clinicopathological analysis of 24 cases of a poorly recognized distinctive morphologic variant important in the differential diagnosis. Virchows Arch. 2010 Dec;457(6):643–9. PMID:20931225
831. Dymerska D, Gołębiewska K, Kuświk M, et al. New EPCAM founder deletion in Polish population. Clin Genet. 2017 Dec;92(6):649–53. PMID:28369810
832. Dziadzio M, Chee R, McNamara C, et al. EBV-driven diffuse large B-cell lymphoma confined to the liver in a patient with a history of idiopathic CD4 lymphocytopenia. BMJ Case Rep. 2013 Aug 21;2013. PMID:23966455
833. Därr R, Nambuba J, Del Rivero J, et al. Novel insights into the polycythemia-paraganglioma-somatostatinoma syndrome. Endocr Relat Cancer. 2016 Dec;23(12):899–908. PMID:27679736
834. Défachelles AS, Martin De Lassalle E, Boutard P, et al. Pancreatoblastoma in childhood: clinical course and therapeutic management of seven patients. Med Pediatr Oncol. 2001 Jul;37(1):47–52. PMID:11466723
835. D'Souza G, Wentz A, Wiley D, et al. Anal cancer screening in men who have sex with men in the multicenter AIDS cohort study. J Acquir Immune Defic Syndr. 2016 Apr 15;71(5):570–6. PMID:26656784
836. Eaden JA, Abrams KR, Mayberry JF. The risk of colorectal cancer in ulcerative colitis: a meta-analysis. Gut. 2001 Apr;48(4):526–35. PMID:11247898
837. East JE, Atkin WS, Bateman AC, et al. British Society of Gastroenterology position statement on serrated polyps in the colon and rectum. Gut. 2017 Jul;66(7):1181–96. PMID:28450390
838. Ebata T, Kosuge T, Hirano S, et al. Proposal to modify the International Union Against Cancer staging system for perihilar cholangiocarcinomas. Br J Surg. 2014 Jan;101(2):79–88. PMID:24375300
839. Edelstein DL, Axilbund JE, Hylind LM, et al. Serrated polyposis: rapid and relentless development of colorectal neoplasia. Gut. 2013 Mar;62(3):404–8. PMID:22490521
840. Edfeldt K, Ahmad T, Åkerström G, et al. TCEB3C a putative tumor suppressor gene of small intestinal neuroendocrine tumors. Endocr Relat Cancer. 2014 Feb 27;21(2):275–84. PMID:24351681
841. Egan L, D'Inca R, Jess T, et al. Non-colorectal intestinal tract carcinomas in inflammatory bowel disease: results of the 3rd ECCO Pathogenesis Scientific Workshop (II). J Crohns Colitis. 2014 Jan;8(1):19–30. PMID:23664498
842. Egan LJ, Walsh SV, Stevens FM, et al. Celiac-associated lymphoma. A single institution experience of 30 cases in the combination chemotherapy era. J Clin Gastroenterol. 1995 Sep;21(2):123–9. PMID:8583077
843. Egawa N, Egawa K, Griffin H, et al. Human

papillomaviruses; epithelial tropisms, and the development of neoplasia. Viruses. 2015 Jul 16;7(7):3863–90. PMID:26193301
844. Egawa N, Fukayama M, Kawaguchi K, et al. Relapsing oral and colonic ulcers with monoclonal T-cell infiltration. A low grade mucosal T-lymphoproliferative disease of the digestive tract. Cancer. 1995 Apr 1;75(7):1728–33. PMID:8826934
845. Egeler RM, Schipper ME, Heymans HS. Gastrointestinal involvement in Langerhans' cell histiocytosis (histiocytosis X): a clinical report of three cases. Eur J Pediatr. 1990 Feb;149(5):325–9. PMID:2178934
846. Egoavil C, Juárez M, Guarinos C, et al. Increased risk of colorectal cancer in patients with multiple serrated polyps and their first-degree relatives. Gastroenterology. 2017 Jul;153(1):106–12.e2. PMID:28400194
847. Ehman EC, Torbenson MS, Wells ML, et al. Hepatic tumors of vascular origin: imaging appearances. Abdom Radiol (NY). 2018 Aug;43(8):1978–90. PMID:29159525
849. Ekbom A, Helmick C, Zack M, et al. Ulcerative colitis and colorectal cancer. A population-based study. N Engl J Med. 1990 Nov 1;323(18):1228–33. PMID:2215606
850. El Rassi ZS, Mohsine RM, Berger F, et al. Endocrine tumors of the extrahepatic bile ducts. Pathological and clinical aspects, surgical management and outcome. Hepatogastroenterology. 2004 Sep-Oct;51(59):1295–300. PMID:15362737
851. El-Fattah MA. Non-Hodgkin lymphoma of the liver: a US population-based analysis. J Clin Transl Hepatol. 2017 Jun 28;5(2):83–91. PMID:28660145
852. El-Naggar AK, Chan JKC, Grandis JR, et al., editors. WHO classification of head and neck tumours. Lyon (France): International Agency for Research on Cancer; 2017. (WHO classification of tumours series, 4th ed.; vol. 9). http://publications.iarc.fr/548.
853. El-Serag HB, Rudolph KL. Hepatocellular carcinoma: epidemiology and molecular carcinogenesis. Gastroenterology. 2007 Jun;132(7):2557–76. PMID:17570226
854. El-Zimaity HM, Graham DY. Evaluation of gastric mucosal biopsy site and number for identification of Helicobacter pylori or intestinal metaplasia: role of the Sydney System. Hum Pathol. 1999 Jan;30(1):72–7. PMID:9923930
855. Eldor R, Glaser B, Fraenkel M, et al. Glucagonoma and the glucagonoma syndrome - cumulative experience with an elusive endocrine tumour. Clin Endocrinol (Oxf). 2011 May;74(5):593–8. PMID:21470282
856. Elsayed FA, Kets CM, Ruano D, et al. Germline variants in POLE are associated with early onset mismatch repair deficient colorectal cancer. Eur J Hum Genet. 2015 Aug;23(8):1080–4. PMID:25370038
857. Elstrom RL, Andreadis C, Aqui NA, et al. Treatment of PTLD with rituximab or chemotherapy. Am J Transplant. 2006 Mar;6(3):569–76. PMID:16468968
858. Emile JF, Abla O, Fraitag S, et al. Revised classification of histiocytoses and neoplasms of the macrophage-dendritic cell lineages. Blood. 2016 Jun 2;127(22):2672–81. PMID:26966089
859. Emile JF, Brahimi S, Coindre JM, et al. Frequencies of KIT and PDGFRA mutations in the MolecGIST prospective population-based study differ from those of advanced GISTs. Med Oncol. 2012 Sep;29(3):1765–72. PMID:21953054
860. Endo Y, Marusawa H, Kou T, et al. Activation-induced cytidine deaminase links between inflammation and the development of colitis-associated colorectal cancers. Gastroenterology. 2008 Sep;135(3):889–98, 898.e1–3. PMID:18691581
861. Endoscopic Classification Review Group. Update on the Paris classification of superficial neoplastic lesions in the digestive tract. Endoscopy. 2005 Jun;37(6):570–8. PMID:15933932
862. Eng C. PTEN hamartoma tumor syndrome. In: Adam MP, Ardinger HH, Pagon RA, et al., editors. GeneReviews. Seattle (WA): University of Washington, Seattle; 2001 Nov 29 [updated 2016 Jun 2]. PMID:20301661
863. Engelsgjerd M, Farraye FA, Odze RD. Polypectomy may be adequate treatment for adenoma-like dysplastic lesions in chronic ulcerative colitis. Gastroenterology. 1999 Dec;117(6):1288–94, discussion 1488–91. PMID:10579969
864. Ensoli B, Sgadari C, Barillari G, et al. Biology of Kaposi's sarcoma. Eur J Cancer. 2001 Jul;37(10):1251–69. PMID:11423257
865. Enzinger PC, Mayer RJ. Esophageal cancer. N Engl J Med. 2003 Dec 4;349(23):2241–52. PMID:14657432
866. Eom DW, Kang GH, Han SH, et al. Gastric micropapillary carcinoma: a distinct subtype with a significantly worse prognosis in TNM stages I and II. Am J Surg Pathol. 2011 Jan;35(1):84–91. PMID:21164291
867. Epstein JI, Sears DL, Tucker RS, et al. Carcinoma of the esophagus with adenoid cystic differentiation. Cancer. 1984 Mar 1;53(5):1131–6. PMID:6318960
868. Erichsen R, Baron JA, Hamilton-Dutoit SJ, et al. Increased risk of colorectal cancer development among patients with serrated polyps. Gastroenterology. 2016 Apr;150(4):895–902.e5. PMID:26677986
869. Erickson LA, Papouchado B, Dimashkieh H, et al. Cdx2 as a marker for neuroendocrine tumors of unknown primary sites. Endocr Pathol. 2004 Fall;15(3):247–52. PMID:15640551
870. Eriguchi N, Aoyagi S, Nakayama T, et al. Serous cystadenocarcinoma of the pancreas with liver metastases. J Hepatobiliary Pancreat Surg. 1998;5(4):467–70. PMID:9931400
871. Eriksson B, Orlefors H, Oberg K, et al. Developments in PET for the detection of endocrine tumours. Best Pract Res Clin Endocrinol Metab. 2005 Jun;19(2):311–24. PMID:15763703
872. Erlenbach-Wünsch K, Bihl M, Hartmann A, et al. Serrated epithelial colorectal polyps (hyperplastic polyps, sessile serrated adenomas) with perineurial stroma: Clinicopathological and molecular analysis of a new series. Ann Diagn Pathol. 2018 Aug;35:48–52. PMID:29747061
873. Errani C, Sung YS, Zhang L, et al. Monoclonality of multifocal epithelioid hemangioendothelioma of the liver by analysis of WWTR1-CAMTA1 breakpoints. Cancer Genet. 2012 Jan-Feb;205(1-2):12–7. PMID:22429593
874. Errani C, Zhang L, Sung YS, et al. A novel WWTR1-CAMTA1 gene fusion is a consistent abnormality in epithelioid hemangioendothelioma of different anatomic sites. Genes Chromosomes Cancer. 2011 Aug;50(8):644–53. PMID:21584898
875. Eskelund CW, Dahl C, Hansen JW, et al. TP53 mutations identify younger mantle cell lymphoma patients who do not benefit from intensive chemoimmunotherapy. Blood. 2017 Oct 26;130(17):1903–10. PMID:28819011
876. Espinet B, Ferrer A, Bellosillo B, et al. Distinction between asymptomatic monoclonal B-cell lymphocytosis with cyclin D1 overexpression and mantle cell lymphoma: from molecular profiling to flow cytometry. Clin Cancer Res. 2014 Feb 15;20(4):1007–19. PMID:24352646
877. Espinosa I, Lee CH, Kim MK, et al. A novel monoclonal antibody against DOG1 is a sensitive and specific marker for gastrointestinal stromal tumors. Am J Surg Pathol. 2008 Feb;32(2):210–8. PMID:18223323
878. Espinoza JA, Bizama C, García P, et al. The inflammatory inception of gallbladder cancer. Biochim Biophys Acta. 2016 Apr;1865(2):245–54. PMID:26980625
879. Esposito I, Bauer A, Hoheisel JD, et al. Microcystic tubulopapillary carcinoma of the pancreas: a new tumor entity? Virchows Arch. 2004 May;444(5):447–53. PMID:15014986
880. Esposito I, Kleeff J, Bergmann F, et al. Most pancreatic cancer resections are R1 resections. Ann Surg Oncol. 2008 Jun;15(6):1651–60. PMID:18351300
881. Esposito I, Segler A, Steiger K, et al. Pathology, genetics and precursors of human and experimental pancreatic neoplasms: an update. Pancreatology. 2015 Nov-Dec;15(6):598–610. PMID:26365060
881A. Estrella JS, Broaddus RR, Mathews A, et al. Progesterone receptor and PTEN expression predict survival in patients with low- and intermediate-grade pancreatic neuroendocrine tumors. Arch Pathol Lab Med. 2014 Aug;138(8):1027–36. PMID:25076292
882. Estrozi B, Bacchi CE. Neuroendocrine tumors involving the gastroenteropancreatic tract: a clinicopathological evaluation of 773 cases. Clinics (Sao Paulo). 2011;66(10):1671–5. PMID:22012036
883. Ettersperger J, Montcuquet N, Malamut G, et al. Interleukin-15-dependent T-cell-like innate intraepithelial lymphocytes develop in the intestine and transform into lymphomas in celiac disease. Immunity. 2016 Sep 20;45(3):610–25. PMID:27612641
884. European Association for the Study of the Liver (EASL). EASL Clinical Practice Guidelines on the management of benign liver tumours. J Hepatol. 2016 Aug;65(2):386–98. PMID:27085809
885. European Association for the Study of the Liver. EASL Clinical Practice Guidelines: Management of hepatocellular carcinoma. J Hepatol. 2018 Jul;69(1):182–236. PMID:29628281
886. European Study Group on Cystic Tumours of the Pancreas. European evidence-based guidelines on pancreatic cystic neoplasms. Gut. 2018 May;67(5):789–804. PMID:29574408
887. Evans M, Liu Y, Chen C, et al. Adenosquamous carcinoma of the esophagus: an NCDB-based investigation on comparative features and overall survival in a rare tumor. Oncology. 2017;93(5):336–42. PMID:28848104
888. Evason KJ, Grenert JP, Ferrell LD, et al. Atypical hepatocellular adenoma-like neoplasms with β-catenin activation show cytogenetic alterations similar to well-differentiated hepatocellular carcinomas. Hum Pathol. 2013 May;44(5):750–8. PMID:23084586
889. Fagih M, Serra S, Chetty R. Paucicellular infiltrating ductal carcinoma of pancreas: an unusual variant. Ann Diagn Pathol. 2007 Feb;11(1):46–8. PMID:17240307
890. Fahrenkrug J. Transmitter role of vasoactive intestinal peptide. Pharmacol Toxicol. 1993 Jun;72(6):354–63. PMID:8103215
891. Faivre J, Trama A, De Angelis R, et al. Incidence, prevalence and survival of patients with rare epithelial digestive cancers diagnosed in Europe in 1995-2002. Eur J Cancer. 2012 Jul;48(10):1417–24. PMID:22169462
892. Fakhruddin N, Bahmad HF, Aridi T, et al. Hepatoid adenocarcinoma of the stomach: a challenging diagnostic and therapeutic disease through a case report and review of the literature. Front Med (Lausanne). 2017 Sep 28;4:164. PMID:29034239
893. Falchook GS, Vega F, Dang NH, et al. Hepatosplenic gamma-delta T-cell lymphoma: clinicopathological features and treatment. Ann Oncol. 2009 Jun;20(6):1080–5. PMID:19237479
894. Falconi M, Bartsch DK, Eriksson B, et al. ENETS Consensus Guidelines for the management of patients with digestive neuroendocrine neoplasms of the digestive system: well-differentiated pancreatic non-functioning tumors. Neuroendocrinology. 2012;95(2):120–34. PMID:22261872
895. Falconi M, Eriksson B, Kaltsas G, et al. ENETS consensus guidelines update for the management of patients with functional pancreatic neuroendocrine tumors and non-functional pancreatic neuroendocrine tumors. Neuroendocrinology. 2016;103(2):153–71. PMID:26742109
896. Falini B, Agostinelli C, Bigerna B, et al. IRTA1 is selectively expressed in nodal and extranodal marginal zone lymphomas. Histopathology. 2012 Nov;61(5):930–41. PMID:22716304
897. Fan B, Malato Y, Calvisi DF, et al. Cholangiocarcinomas can originate from hepatocytes in mice. J Clin Invest. 2012 Aug;122(8):2911–5. PMID:22797301
898. Fang J, Jia J, Makowski M, et al. Functional characterization of a multi-cancer risk locus on chr5p15.33 reveals regulation of TERT by ZNF148. Nat Commun. 2017 May 2;8:15034. PMID:28447668
899. Fang Y, Su Z, Xie J, et al. Genomic signatures of pancreatic adenosquamous carcinoma (PASC). J Pathol. 2017 Oct;243(2):155–9. PMID:28722109
900. Farinha P, Gascoyne RD. Molecular pathogenesis of mucosa-associated lymphoid tissue lymphoma. J Clin Oncol. 2005 Sep 10;23(26):6370–8. PMID:16155022
901. Farraye FA, Odze RD, Eaden J, et al. AGA technical review on the diagnosis and management of colorectal neoplasia in inflammatory bowel disease. Gastroenterology. 2010 Feb;138(2):746–74, 774.e1–4, quiz e12–3. PMID:20141809
902. Farrell JM, Pang JC, Kim GE, et al. Pancreatic neuroendocrine tumors: accurate grading with Ki-67 index on fine-needle aspiration specimens using the WHO 2010/ENETS criteria. Cancer Cytopathol. 2014 Oct;122(10):770–8. PMID:25044931
903. Farrington SM, Tenesa A, Barnetson R, et al. Germline susceptibility to colorectal cancer due to base-excision repair gene defects. Am J Hum Genet. 2005 Jul;77(1):112–9. PMID:15931596
904. Farris AB, Misdraji J, Srivastava A, et al. Sessile serrated adenoma: challenging discrimination from other serrated colonic polyps. Am J Surg Pathol. 2008 Jan;32(1):30–5. PMID:18162767
905. Farris MS, Mosli MH, McFadden AA, et al. The association between leisure time physical activity and pancreatic cancer risk in adults: a systematic review and meta-analysis. Cancer Epidemiol Biomarkers Prev. 2015 Oct;24(10):1462–73. PMID:26174790
906. Fassan M, Pizzi M, Farinati F, et al. Lesions indefinite for intraepithelial neoplasia and OLGA staging for gastric atrophy. Am J Clin Pathol. 2012 May;137(5):727–32. PMID:22523210
907. Fassan M, Saraggi D, Balsamo L, et al. Early miR-223 upregulation in gastroesophageal carcinogenesis. Am J Clin Pathol. 2017 Mar 1;147(3):301–8. PMID:28395057
908. Fassan M, Simbolo M, Bria E, et al. High-throughput mutation profiling identifies novel molecular dysregulation in high-grade intraepithelial neoplasia and early gastric cancers. Gastric Cancer. 2014;17(3):442–9. PMID:24272205
909. Fayette J, Martin E, Piperno-Neumann S, et al. Angiosarcomas, a heterogeneous group of sarcomas with specific behavior depending on primary site: a retrospective study of 161

cases. Ann Oncol. 2007 Dec;18(12):2030–6. PMID:17974557
910. Feakins RM. Obesity and metabolic syndrome: pathological effects on the gastrointestinal tract. Histopathology. 2016 Apr;68(5):630–40. PMID:26599607
911. Fearon ER, Vogelstein B. A genetic model for colorectal tumorigenesis. Cell. 1990 Jun 1;61(5):759–67. PMID:2188735
912. Federspiel BH, Burke AP, Sobin LH, et al. Rectal and colonic carcinoids. A clinicopathologic study of 84 cases. Cancer. 1990 Jan 1;65(1):135–40. PMID:2293859
913. Feldman AL, Arber DA, Pittaluga S, et al. Clonally related follicular lymphomas and histiocytic/dendritic cell sarcomas: evidence for transdifferentiation of the follicular lymphoma clone. Blood. 2008 Jun 15;111(12):5433–9. PMID:18272816
914. Feldmann G, Beaty R, Hruban RH, et al. Molecular genetics of pancreatic intraepithelial neoplasia. J Hepatobiliary Pancreat Surg. 2007;14(3):224–32. PMID:17520196
915. Fels Elliott DR, Perner J, Li X, et al. Impact of mutations in Toll-like receptor pathway genes on esophageal carcinogenesis. PLoS Genet. 2017 May 22;13(5):e1006808. PMID:28531216
916. Feng F, Zheng G, Qi J, et al. Clinicopathological features and prognosis of gastric adenosquamous carcinoma. Sci Rep. 2017 Jul 4;7(1):4597. PMID:28676632
917. Fenger C, Filipe MI. Mucin histochemistry of the anal canal epithelium. Studies of normal anal mucosa and mucosa adjacent to carcinoma. Histochem J. 1981 Nov;13(6):921–30. PMID:7338481
918. Fenger C, Frisch M, Jass JJ, et al. Anal cancer subtype reproducibility study. Virchows Arch. 2000 Mar;436(3):229–33. PMID:10782881
919. Fenoglio LM, Severini S, Ferrigno D, et al. Primary hepatic carcinoid: a case report and literature review. World J Gastroenterol. 2009 May 21;15(19):2418–22. PMID:19452590
920. Ferlay J, Colombet M, Bray F. Cancer Incidence in Five Continents, CI5plus: IARC CancerBase No. 9 [Internet]. Lyon (France): International Agency for Research on Cancer; 2018. Available from: http://ci5.iarc.fr.
921. Ferlay J, Ervik M, Lam F, et al. Global Cancer Observatory: Cancer Today [Internet]. Lyon (France): International Agency for Research on Cancer; 2018. Available from: https://gco.iarc.fr/today.
922. Ferlay J, Partensky C, Bray F. More deaths from pancreatic cancer than breast cancer in the EU by 2017. Acta Oncol. 2016 Sep-Oct;55(9-10):1158–60. PMID:27551890
923. Ferlay J, Soerjomataram I, Dikshit R, et al. Cancer incidence and mortality worldwide: sources, methods and major patterns in GLOBOCAN 2012. Int J Cancer. 2015 Mar 1;136(5):E359–86. PMID:25220842
924. Fernandes T, Silva R, Devesa V, et al. AIRP best cases in radiologic-pathologic correlation: gastroblastoma: a rare biphasic gastric tumor. Radiographics. 2014 Nov-Dec;34(7):1929–33. PMID:25384293
925. Fernández-del Castillo C, Adsay NV. Intraductal papillary mucinous neoplasms of the pancreas. Gastroenterology. 2010 Sep;139(3):708–13, 713.e1–2. PMID:20650278
926. Fernández-Sordo JO, Konda VJ, Chennat J, et al. Is endoscopic ultrasound (EUS) necessary in the pre-therapeutic assessment of Barrett's esophagus with early neoplasia? J Gastrointest Oncol. 2012 Dec;3(4):314–21. PMID:23205307
927. Ferrari AP, Martins FP. Endoscopic surveillance of extensive esophageal papillomatosis not amenable to endoscopic therapy. Einstein (Sao Paulo). 2017 Jul-Sep;15(3):363–5. PMID:28746592
928. Ferreiro JF, Morscio J, Dierickx D, et al. EBV-positive and EBV-negative posttransplant diffuse large B cell lymphomas have distinct genomic and transcriptomic features. Am J Transplant. 2016 Feb;16(2):414–25. PMID:26780579
929. Ferreiro JF, Morscio J, Dierickx D, et al. Post-transplant molecularly defined Burkitt lymphomas are frequently MYC-negative and characterized by the 11q-gain/loss pattern. Haematologica. 2015 Jul;100(7):e275–9. PMID:25795716
930. Ferrell LD, Beckstead JH. Paneth-like cells in an adenoma and adenocarcinoma in the ampulla of Vater. Arch Pathol Lab Med. 1991 Sep;115(9):956–8. PMID:1929795
931. Ferreri AJ, Govi S, Ponzoni M. Marginal zone lymphomas and infectious agents. Semin Cancer Biol. 2013 Dec;23(6):431–40. PMID:24090976
932. Ferrone CR, Finkelstein DM, Thayer SP, et al. Perioperative CA19-9 levels can predict stage and survival in patients with resectable pancreatic adenocarcinoma. J Clin Oncol. 2006 Jun 20;24(18):2897–902. PMID:16782929
933. Ferrone CR, Tang LH, D'Angelica M, et al. Extrahepatic bile duct carcinoid tumors: malignant biliary obstruction with a good prognosis. J Am Coll Surg. 2007 Aug;205(2):357–61. PMID:17660084
934. Ferrone CR, Tang LH, Tomlinson J, et al. Determining prognosis in patients with pancreatic endocrine neoplasms: can the WHO classification system be simplified? J Clin Oncol. 2007 Dec 10;25(35):5609–15. PMID:18065733
935. Fertig RM, Alperstein A, Diaz C, et al. Metastatic neuroendocrine tumor of the esophagus with features of medullary thyroid carcinoma. Intractable Rare Dis Res. 2017 Aug;6(3):224–9. PMID:28944148
936. Fewings E, Larionov A, Redman J, et al. Germline pathogenic variants in PALB2 and other cancer-predisposing genes in families with hereditary diffuse gastric cancer without CDH1 mutation: a whole-exome sequencing study. Lancet Gastroenterol Hepatol. 2018 Jul;3(7):489–98. PMID:29706558
938. Filipe MI, Muñoz N, Matko I, et al. Intestinal metaplasia types and the risk of gastric cancer: a cohort study in Slovenia. Int J Cancer. 1994 May 1;57(3):324–9. PMID:8168991
939. Finalet Ferreiro J, Rouhigharabaei L, Urbankova H, et al. Integrative genomic and transcriptomic analysis identified candidate genes implicated in the pathogenesis of hepatosplenic T-cell lymphoma. PLoS One. 2014 Jul 24;9(7):e102977. PMID:25057852
940. Fiocca R, Rindi G, Capella C, et al. Glucagon, glicentin, proglucagon, PYY, PP and proPP-icosapeptide immunoreactivities of rectal carcinoid tumors and related non-tumor cells. Regul Pept. 1987 Jan;17(1):9–29. PMID:2882565
941. Fitzgerald RC, di Pietro M, Ragunath K, et al. British Society of Gastroenterology guidelines on the diagnosis and management of Barrett's oesophagus. Gut. 2014 Jan;63(1):7–42. PMID:24165758
942. Fitzgerald RC, Hardwick R, Huntsman D, et al. Hereditary diffuse gastric cancer: updated consensus guidelines for clinical management and directions for future research. J Med Genet. 2010 Jul;47(7):436–44. PMID:20591882
943. Fitzgerald TL, Hickner ZJ, Schmitz M, et al. Changing incidence of pancreatic neoplasms: a 16-year review of statewide tumor registry. Pancreas. 2008 Aug;37(2):134–8. PMID:18665072
944. Fitzmaurice GJ, Hurreiz H, McGalie CE, et al. Ectopic breast tissue at the anal verge–an unusual finding. Int J Colorectal Dis. 2010 Aug;25(8):1031–2. PMID:20198478
945. Fizazi K, Greco FA, Pavlidis N, et al. Cancers of unknown primary site: ESMO Clinical Practice Guidelines for diagnosis, treatment and follow-up. Ann Oncol. 2015 Sep;26 Suppl 5:v133–8. PMID:26314775
946. Flaherty KT, Puzanov I, Kim KB, et al. Inhibition of mutated, activated BRAF in metastatic melanoma. N Engl J Med. 2010 Aug 26;363(9):809–19. PMID:20818844
947. Fleming JB, Gonzalez RJ, Petzel MQ, et al. Influence of obesity on cancer-related outcomes after pancreatectomy to treat pancreatic adenocarcinoma. Arch Surg. 2009 Mar;144(3):216–21. PMID:19289659
948. Fletcher CD, Beham A, Bekir S, et al. Epithelioid angiosarcoma of deep soft tissue: a distinctive tumor readily mistaken for an epithelial neoplasm. Am J Surg Pathol. 1991 Oct;15(10):915–24. PMID:1718176
949. Fletcher CDM, Bridge JA, Hogendoorn PCW, et al., editors. WHO classification of tumours of soft tissue and bone. Lyon (France): International Agency for Research on Cancer; 2013. (WHO classification of tumours series, 4th ed.; vol. 5). http://publications.iarc.fr/15.
950. Folpe AL, Chand EM, Goldblum JR, et al. Expression of Fli-1, a nuclear transcription factor, distinguishes vascular neoplasms from potential mimics. Am J Surg Pathol. 2001 Aug;25(8):1061–6. PMID:11474291
951. Folpe AL, Devaney K, Weiss SW. Lipomatous hemangiopericytoma: a rare variant of hemangiopericytoma that may be confused with liposarcoma. Am J Surg Pathol. 1999 Oct;23(10):1201–7. PMID:10524520
952. Folpe AL, Fanburg-Smith JC, Miettinen M, et al. Atypical and malignant glomus tumors: analysis of 52 cases, with a proposal for the reclassification of glomus tumors. Am J Surg Pathol. 2001 Jan;25(1):1–12. PMID:11145243
953. Folpe AL, Mentzel T, Lehr HA, et al. Perivascular epithelioid cell neoplasms of soft tissue and gynecologic origin: a clinicopathologic study of 26 cases and review of the literature. Am J Surg Pathol. 2005 Dec;29(12):1558–75. PMID:16327428
954. Fong Y, Wagman L, Gonen M, et al. Evidence-based gallbladder cancer staging: changing cancer staging by analysis of data from the National Cancer Database. Ann Surg. 2006 Jun;243(6):767–71, discussion 771–4. PMID:16772780
955. Fossmark R, Calvete O, Mjønes P, et al. ECL-cell carcinoids and carcinoma in patients homozygous for an inactivating mutation in the gastric H(+) K(+) ATPase alpha subunit. APMIS. 2016 Jul;124(7):561–6. PMID:27150581
956. Foster DR, Foster DB. Gall-bladder polyps in Peutz-Jeghers syndrome. Postgrad Med J. 1980 May;56(655):373–6. PMID:7003570
957. Foukas PG, de Leval L. Recent advances in intestinal lymphomas. Histopathology. 2015 Jan;66(1):112–36. PMID:25639480
958. Fowler KJ, Sheybani A, Parker RA 3rd, et al. Combined hepatocellular and cholangiocarcinoma (biphenotypic) tumors: imaging features and diagnostic accuracy of contrast-enhanced CT and MRI. AJR Am J Roentgenol. 2013 Aug;201(2):332–9. PMID:23883213
959. Fraga M, Lloret E, Sanchez-Verde L, et al. Mucosal mantle cell (centrocytic) lymphomas. Histopathology. 1995 May;26(5):413–22. PMID:7657310
960. Francis A, Johnson DW, Teixeira-Pinto A, et al. Incidence and predictors of post-transplant lymphoproliferative disease after kidney transplantation during adulthood and childhood: a registry study. Nephrol Dial Transplant. 2018 May 1;33(5):881–9. PMID:29342279
961. Francis JM, Kiezun A, Ramos AH, et al. Somatic mutation of CDKN1B in small intestine neuroendocrine tumors. Nat Genet. 2013 Dec;45(12):1483–6. PMID:24185511
962. Franko J, Cole K, Pezzi CM, et al. Serous cystadenocarcinoma of the pancreas with metachronous hepatic metastasis. Am J Clin Oncol. 2008 Dec;31(6):624–5. PMID:19060596
963. Franko J, Feng W, Yip L, et al. Non-functional neuroendocrine carcinoma of the pancreas: incidence, tumor biology, and outcomes in 2,158 patients. J Gastrointest Surg. 2010 Mar;14(3):541–8. PMID:19997980
964. Frantz VK. Tumors of the pancreas. Washington, DC: Armed Forces Institute of Pathology; 1959. (AFIP atlas of tumor pathology, series 1, section 7; fascicles 27 and 28).
965. Frayling IM, Arends M. Adenomatous polyposis coli. In: Maloy S, Hughes K, editors. Brenner's encyclopedia of genetics. Volume 1. 2nd ed. San Diego (CA): Academic Press; 2013. pp. 27–9.
966. Frayling IM. Familial adenomatous polyposis (FAP) and adenomatous polyposis (due to MUTYH, NTHL1, POLE & POLD1). In: Firth HV, Hurst JA, editors. Oxford Desk Reference: Clinical genetics & genomics. 2nd ed. Oxford (UK): Oxford University Press; 2017.
967. Frayling IM. Microsatellite instability. Gut. 1999 Jul;45(1):1–4. PMID:10369691
968. Freeman C, Berg JW, Cutler SJ. Occurrence and prognosis of extranodal lymphomas. Cancer. 1972 Jan;29(1):252–60. PMID:5007387
969. Fried I, Rom-Gross E, Finegold M, et al. An infant with a diagnostically challenging hepatic teratoma, hypofibrinogenemia, and adrenal neuroblastoma: case report. Pediatr Dev Pathol. 2015 May-Jun;18(3):251–6. PMID:25756389
970. Friedl W, Uhlhaas S, Schulmann K, et al. Juvenile polyposis: massive gastric polyposis is more common in MADH4 mutation carriers than in BMPR1A mutation carriers. Hum Genet. 2002 Jul;111(1):108–11. PMID:12136244
971. Friedman HD. Nonmucinous, glycogen-poor cystadenocarcinoma of the pancreas. Arch Pathol Lab Med. 1990 Aug;114(8):888–91. PMID:2375664
972. Frilling A, Modlin IM, Kidd M, et al. Recommendations for management of patients with neuroendocrine liver metastases. Lancet Oncol. 2014 Jan;15(1):e8–21. PMID:24384494
973. Frisch M, Glimelius B, van den Brule AJ, et al. Sexually transmitted infection as a cause of anal cancer. N Engl J Med. 1997 Nov 6;337(19):1350–8. PMID:9358129
974. Fujii H, Aotake T, Horiuchi T, et al. Small cell carcinoma of the gallbladder: a case report and review of 53 cases in the literature. Hepatogastroenterology. 2001 Nov-Dec;48(42):1588–93. PMID:11813580
975. Fujikura K, Akita M, Abe-Suzuki S, et al. Mucinous cystic neoplasms of the liver and pancreas: relationship between KRAS driver mutations and disease progression. Histopathology. 2017 Oct;71(4):591–600. PMID:28570009
976. Fujikura K, Fukumoto T, Ajiki T, et al. Comparative clinicopathological study of biliary intraductal papillary neoplasms and papillary cholangiocarcinomas. Histopathology. 2016 Dec;69(6):950–61. PMID:27410028
977. Fujimoto A, Furuta M, Shiraishi Y, et al. Whole-genome mutational landscape of liver cancers displaying biliary phenotype reveals hepatitis impact and molecular diversity. Nat Commun. 2015 Jan 30;6:6120. PMID:25636086
978. Fujishiro M, Yoshida S, Matsuda R, et al. Updated evidence on endoscopic resection of early gastric cancer from Japan. Gastric Cancer. 2017 Mar;20 Suppl 1:39–44. PMID:27704225
979. Fujiya M, Tanaka K, Dokoshi T, et al. Efficacy and adverse events of EMR and endoscopic submucosal dissection for the treatment

of colon neoplasms: a meta-analysis of studies comparing EMR and endoscopic submucosal dissection. Gastrointest Endosc. 2015 Mar;81(3):583–95. PMID:25592748
980. Fukasawa M, Maguchi H, Takahashi K, et al. Clinical features and natural history of serous cystic neoplasm of the pancreas. Pancreatology. 2010;10(6):695–701. PMID:21242709
981. Fukasawa Y, Takada A, Tateno M, et al. Solitary fibrous tumor of the pleura causing recurrent hypoglycemia by secretion of insulin-like growth factor II. Pathol Int. 1998 Jan;48(1):47–52. PMID:9589464
982. Fukushima N, Fukayama M. Mucinous cystic neoplasms of the pancreas: pathology and molecular genetics. J Hepatobiliary Pancreat Surg. 2007;14(3):238–42. PMID:17520198
983. Fukushima N, Zamboni G. Mucinous cystic neoplasms of the pancreas: update on the surgical pathology and molecular genetics. Semin Diagn Pathol. 2014 Nov;31(6):467–74. PMID:25441310
984. Fung AD, Cohen C, Kavuri S, et al. Phosphohistone H3 and Ki-67 labeling indices in cytologic specimens from well-differentiated neuroendocrine tumors of the gastrointestinal tract and pancreas: a comparative analysis using automated image cytometry. Acta Cytol. 2013;57(5):501–8. PMID:24021213
985. Furlan D, Cerutti R, Genasetti A, et al. Microallelotyping defines the monoclonal or the polyclonal origin of mixed and collision endocrine-exocrine tumors of the gut. Lab Invest. 2003 Jul;83(7):963–71. PMID:12861036
986. Furlan D, Cerutti R, Uccella S, et al. Different molecular profiles characterize well-differentiated endocrine tumors and poorly differentiated endocrine carcinomas of the gastroenteropancreatic tract. Clin Cancer Res. 2004 Feb 1;10(3):947–57. PMID:14871972
987. Furlan D, Sahnane N, Bernasconi B, et al. APC alterations are frequently involved in the pathogenesis of acinar cell carcinoma of the pancreas, mainly through gene loss and promoter hypermethylation. Virchows Arch. 2014 May;464(5):553–64. PMID:24590585
988. Furney SJ, Turajlic S, Stamp G, et al. Genome sequencing of mucosal melanomas reveals that they are driven by distinct mechanisms from cutaneous melanoma. J Pathol. 2013 Jul;230(3):261–9. PMID:23620124
989. Furuhata A, Minamiguchi S, Mikami Y, et al. Intraductal tubulopapillary neoplasm with expansile invasive carcinoma of the pancreas diagnosed by endoscopic ultrasonography-guided fine needle aspiration: a case report. Diagn Cytopathol. 2014 Apr;42(4):314–20. PMID:24339429
990. Furukawa S, Uota S, Yamana T, et al. Distribution of human papillomavirus genotype in anal condyloma acuminatum among Japanese men: the higher prevalence of high risk human papillomavirus in men who have sex with men with HIV infection. AIDS Res Hum Retroviruses. 2018 Apr;34(4):375–81. PMID:29183133
991. Furukawa T, Fujisaki R, Yoshida Y, et al. Distinct progression pathways involving the dysfunction of DUSP6/MKP-3 in pancreatic intraepithelial neoplasia and intraductal papillary-mucinous neoplasms of the pancreas. Mod Pathol. 2005 Aug;18(8):1034–42. PMID:15832194
992. Furukawa T, Hatori T, Fujita I, et al. Prognostic relevance of morphological types of intraductal papillary mucinous neoplasms of the pancreas. Gut. 2011 Apr;60(4):509–16. PMID:21193453
993. Furukawa T, Klöppel G, Volkan Adsay N, et al. Classification of types of intraductal papillary-mucinous neoplasm of the pancreas: a consensus study. Virchows Arch. 2005 Nov;447(5):794–9. PMID:16088402
994. Furukawa T, Kuboki Y, Tanji E, et al. Whole-exome sequencing uncovers frequent GNAS mutations in intraductal papillary mucinous neoplasms of the pancreas. Sci Rep. 2011;1:161. PMID:22355676
995. Furukawa T, Oohashi K, Yamao K, et al. Intraductal ultrasonography of the pancreas: development and clinical potential. Endoscopy. 1997 Aug;29(6):561–9. PMID:9342572
996. Fuse N, Kuboki Y, Kuwata T, et al. Prognostic impact of HER2, EGFR, and c-MET status on overall survival of advanced gastric cancer patients. Gastric Cancer. 2016 Jan;19(1):183–91. PMID:25682441
997. Gaal J, Stratakis CA, Carney JA, et al. SDHB immunohistochemistry: a useful tool in the diagnosis of Carney-Stratakis and Carney triad gastrointestinal stromal tumors. Mod Pathol. 2011 Jan;24(1):147–51. PMID:20890271
998. Gaidano G, Cerri M, Capello D, et al. Molecular histogenesis of plasmablastic lymphoma of the oral cavity. Br J Haematol. 2002 Dec;119(3):622–8. PMID:12437635
999. Gaisa M, Sigel K, Hand J, et al. High rates of anal dysplasia in HIV-infected men who have sex with men, women, and heterosexual men. AIDS. 2014 Jan 14;28(2):215–22. PMID:24072194
1000. Gala MK, Mizukami Y, Le LP, et al. Germline mutations in oncogene-induced senescence pathways are associated with multiple sessile serrated adenomas. Gastroenterology. 2014 Feb;146(2):520–9. PMID:24512911
1001. Galandiuk S, Rodriguez-Justo M, Jeffery R, et al. Field cancerization in the intestinal epithelium of patients with Crohn's ileocolitis. Gastroenterology. 2012 Apr;142(4):855–64.e8. PMID:22178590
1002. Galanis C, Zamani A, Cameron JL, et al. Resected serous cystic neoplasms of the pancreas: a review of 158 patients with recommendations for treatment. J Gastrointest Surg. 2007 Jul;11(7):820–6. PMID:17440789
1003. Galle TS, Juel K, Bülow S. Causes of death in familial adenomatous polyposis. Scand J Gastroenterol. 1999 Aug;34(8):808–12. PMID:10499482
1004. Gallione C, Aylsworth AS, Beis J, et al. Overlapping spectra of SMAD4 mutations in juvenile polyposis (JP) and JP-HHT syndrome. Am J Med Genet A. 2010 Feb;152A(2):333–9. PMID:20101697
1005. Gallione CJ, Repetto GM, Legius E, et al. A combined syndrome of juvenile polyposis and hereditary haemorrhagic telangiectasia associated with mutations in MADH4 (SMAD4). Lancet. 2004 Mar 13;363(9412):852–9. PMID:15031030
1006. Gao S, Chen D, Huang L, et al. Primary squamous cell carcinoma of the stomach: a case report and literature review. Int J Clin Exp Pathol. 2015 Aug 1;8(8):9667–71. PMID:26464735
1007. Gao SJ, Kingsley L, Hoover DR, et al. Seroconversion to antibodies against Kaposi's sarcoma-associated herpesvirus-related latent nuclear antigens before the development of Kaposi's sarcoma. N Engl J Med. 1996 Jul 25;335(4):233–41. PMID:8657239
1008. Gao YB, Chen ZL, Li JG, et al. Genetic landscape of esophageal squamous cell carcinoma. Nat Genet. 2014 Oct;46(10):1097–102. PMID:25151357
1009. Garbrecht N, Anlauf M, Schmitt A, et al. Somatostatin-producing neuroendocrine tumors of the duodenum and pancreas: incidence, types, biological behavior, association with inherited syndromes, and functional activity. Endocr Relat Cancer. 2008 Mar;15(1):229–41. PMID:18310290
1010. Garby L, Caron P, Claustrat F, et al. Clinical characteristics and outcome of acromegaly induced by ectopic secretion of growth hormone-releasing hormone (GHRH): a French nationwide series of 21 cases. J Clin Endocrinol Metab. 2012 Jun;97(6):2093–104. PMID:22442262
1011. Garcia-Herrera A, Song JY, Chuang SS, et al. Nonhepatosplenic γδ T-cell lymphomas represent a spectrum of aggressive cytotoxic T-cell lymphomas with a mainly extranodal presentation. Am J Surg Pathol. 2011 Aug;35(8):1214–25. PMID:21753698
1012. García-Solano J, Pérez-Guillermo M, Conesa-Zamora P, et al. Clinicopathologic study of 85 colorectal serrated adenocarcinomas: further insights into the full recognition of a new subset of colorectal carcinoma. Hum Pathol. 2010 Oct;41(10):1359–68. PMID:20594582
1013. Garske U, Sandström M, Johansson S, et al. Lessons on tumour response: imaging during therapy with (177)Lu-DOTA-octreotate. A case report on a patient with a large volume of poorly differentiated neuroendocrine carcinoma. Theranostics. 2012;2(5):459–71. PMID:22768026
1014. Garud SS, Willingham FF. Molecular analysis of cyst fluid aspiration in the diagnosis and risk assessment of cystic lesions of the pancreas. Clin Transl Sci. 2012 Feb;5(1):102–7. PMID:22376266
1015. Gasparotto D, Rossi S, Polano M, et al. Quadruple-negative GIST is a sentinel for unrecognized neurofibromatosis type 1 syndrome. Clin Cancer Res. 2017 Jan 1;23(1):273–82. PMID:27390349
1016. Gatta G, van der Zwan JM, Casali PG, et al. Rare cancers are not so rare: the rare cancer burden in Europe. Eur J Cancer. 2011 Nov;47(17):2493–511. PMID:22033323
1017. Gaujoux S, Tissier F, Ragazzon B, et al. Pancreatic ductal and acinar cell neoplasms in Carney complex: a possible new association. J Clin Endocrinol Metab. 2011 Nov;96(11):E1888–95. PMID:21900385
1018. Gaulard P, Belhadj K, Reyes F. Gammadelta T-cell lymphomas. Semin Hematol. 2003 Jul;40(3):233–43. PMID:12876672
1019. Ge PS, Wani S, Watson RR, et al. Per-pass performance characteristics of endoscopic ultrasound-guided fine-needle aspiration of malignant solid pancreatic masses in a large multicenter cohort. Pancreas. 2018 Mar;47(3):296–301. PMID:29401169
1020. Ge R, Liu C, Yin X, et al. Clinicopathologic characteristics of inflammatory pseudotumor-like follicular dendritic cell sarcoma. Int J Clin Exp Pathol. 2014 Apr 15;7(5):2421–9. PMID:24966952
1021. Genkinger JM, Kitahara CM, Bernstein L, et al. Central adiposity, obesity during early adulthood, and pancreatic cancer mortality in a pooled analysis of cohort studies. Ann Oncol. 2015 Nov;26(11):2257–66. PMID:26347100
1022. Genkinger JM, Spiegelman D, Anderson KE, et al. Alcohol intake and pancreatic cancer risk: a pooled analysis of fourteen cohort studies. Cancer Epidemiol Biomarkers Prev. 2009 Mar;18(3):765–76. PMID:19258474
1023. Genta RM, Feagins LA. Advanced precancerous lesions in the small bowel mucosa. Best Pract Res Clin Gastroenterol. 2013 Apr;27(2):225–33. PMID:23809242
1024. Genta RM, Rugge M. Gastric precancerous lesions: heading for an international consensus. Gut. 1999 Jul;45 Suppl 1:I5–8. PMID:10457028
1025. Genta RM, Schuler CM, Robiou CI, et al. No association between gastric fundic gland polyps and gastrointestinal neoplasia in a study of over 100,000 patients. Clin Gastroenterol Hepatol. 2009 Aug;7(8):849–54. PMID:19465154
1026. Genç CG, Falconi M, Partelli S, et al. Recurrence of pancreatic neuroendocrine tumors and survival predicted by Ki67. Ann Surg Oncol. 2018 Aug;25(8):2467–74. PMID:29789972
1027. George DH, Murphy F, Michalski R, et al. Serous cystadenocarcinoma of the pancreas: a new entity? Am J Surg Pathol. 1989 Jan;13(1):61–6. PMID:2909198
1028. Gerada J, Savic A, Vassallo M. Squamous papilloma of the anal canal. Endoscopy. 2013;45 Suppl 2 UCTN:E42–3. PMID:23526509
1029. Gerson JN, Witteles RM, Chang DT, et al. Carcinoid syndrome complicating a pancreatic neuroendocrine tumor: a case report. Pancreas. 2017 Nov/Dec;46(10):1381–5. PMID:29040196
1030. Ghaferi AA, Chojnacki KA, Long WD, et al. Pancreatic VIPomas: subject review and one institutional experience. J Gastrointest Surg. 2008 Feb;12(2):382–93. PMID:17510774
1031. Ghosh Roy S, Robertson ES, Saha A. Epigenetic impact on EBV associated B-cell lymphomagenesis. Biomolecules. 2016 Nov 24;6(4):E46. PMID:27886133
1032. Ghotli ZA, Serra S, Chetty R. Clear cell (glycogen rich) gastric adenocarcinoma: a distinct tubulo-papillary variant with a predilection for the cardia/gastro-oesophageal region. Pathology. 2007 Oct;39(5):466–9. PMID:17886094
1033. Giannitrapani L, Soresi M, La Spada E, et al. Sex hormones and risk of liver tumor. Ann N Y Acad Sci. 2006 Nov;1089:228–36. PMID:17261770
1034. Giardiello FM, Brensinger JD, Tersmette AC, et al. Very high risk of cancer in familial Peutz-Jeghers syndrome. Gastroenterology. 2000 Dec;119(6):1447–53. PMID:11113065
1035. Giardiello FM, Hamilton SR, Kern SE, et al. Colorectal neoplasia in juvenile polyposis or juvenile polyps. Arch Dis Child. 1991 Aug;66(8):971–5. PMID:1656892
1036. Giardiello FM, Welsh SB, Hamilton SR, et al. Increased risk of cancer in the Peutz-Jeghers syndrome. N Engl J Med. 1987 Jun 11;316(24):1511–4. PMID:3587280
1037. Gibril F, Jensen RT. Zollinger-Ellison syndrome revisited: diagnosis, biologic markers, associated inherited disorders, and acid hypersecretion. Curr Gastroenterol Rep. 2004 Dec;6(6):454–63. PMID:15527675
1038. Gibson JA, Hornick JL. Mucosal Schwann cell "hamartoma": clinicopathologic study of 26 neural colorectal polyps distinct from neurofibromas and mucosal neuromas. Am J Surg Pathol. 2009 May;33(5):781–7. PMID:19065103
1039. Gibson SE, Swerdlow SH, Craig FE, et al. EBV-positive extranodal marginal zone lymphoma of mucosa-associated lymphoid tissue in the posttransplant setting: a distinct type of posttransplant lymphoproliferative disorder? Am J Surg Pathol. 2011 Jun;35(6):807–15. PMID:21552113
1040. Gigek CO, Calcagno DQ, Rasmussen LT, et al. Genetic variants in gastric cancer: risks and clinical implications. Exp Mol Pathol. 2017 Aug;103(1):101–11. PMID:28736214
1041. Gill AJ, Chou A, Vilain R, et al. Immunohistochemistry for SDHB divides gastrointestinal stromal tumors (GISTs) into 2 distinct types. Am J Surg Pathol. 2010 May;34(5):636–44. PMID:20305538
1042. Gill PS, Wong NACS. Primary perianal adenocarcinoma of intestinal type - a new proposed entity. Histopathology. 2018 Jul;73(1):157–61. PMID:29464744
1043. Gill RM, Buelow B, Mather C, et al. Hepatic small vessel neoplasm, a rare infiltrative vascular neoplasm of uncertain malignant

potential. Hum Pathol. 2016 Aug;54:143–51. PMID:27090685

1044. Giulino-Roth L, Wang K, MacDonald TY, et al. Targeted genomic sequencing of pediatric Burkitt lymphoma identifies recurrent alterations in antiapoptotic and chromatin-remodeling genes. Blood. 2012 Dec 20;120(26):5181–4. PMID:23091298

1045. Glazer ES, Tseng JF, Al-Refaie W, et al. Long-term survival after surgical management of neuroendocrine hepatic metastases. HPB (Oxford). 2010 Aug;12(6):427–33. PMID:20662794

1046. Gleeson EM, Feldman R, Mapow BL, et al. Appendix-derived pseudomyxoma peritonei (PMP): molecular profiling toward treatment of a rare malignancy. Am J Clin Oncol. 2018 Aug;41(8):777–83. PMID:28263231

1047. Glenn ST, Jones CA, Sexton S, et al. Conditional deletion of p53 and Rb in the renin-expressing compartment of the pancreas leads to a highly penetrant metastatic pancreatic neuroendocrine carcinoma. Oncogene. 2014 Dec 11;33(50):5706–15. PMID:24292676

1048. Glinkova V, Shevah O, Boaz M, et al. Hepatic haemangiomas: possible association with female sex hormones. Gut. 2004 Sep;53(9):1352–5. PMID:15306599

1049. Akinyemiju T, Abera S, Ahmed M, et al. The burden of primary liver cancer and underlying etiologies from 1990 to 2015 at the global, regional, and national level: results from the Global Burden of Disease Study 2015. JAMA Oncol. 2017 Dec 1;3(12):1683–91. PMID:28983565

1050. Glynne-Jones R, Nilsson PJ, Aschele C, et al. Anal cancer: ESMO-ESSO-ESTRO clinical practice guidelines for diagnosis, treatment and follow-up. Eur J Surg Oncol. 2014 Oct;40(10):1165–76. PMID:25239441

1051. Glynne-Jones R, Sebag-Montefiore D, Meadows HM, et al. Best time to assess complete clinical response after chemoradiotherapy in squamous cell carcinoma of the anus (ACT II): a post-hoc analysis of randomised controlled phase 3 trial. Lancet Oncol. 2017 Mar;18(3):347–56. PMID:28209296

1052. Godambe A, Brunt EM, Fulling KH, et al. Biliary adenofibroma with invasive carcinoma: case report and review of the literature. Case Rep Pathol. 2016;2016:8068513. PMID:26885426

1053. Goddard MJ, Lonsdale RN. The histogenesis of appendiceal carcinoid tumours. Histopathology. 1992 Apr;20(4):345–9. PMID:1577412

1054. Goel A, Nguyen TP, Leung HC, et al. De novo constitutional MLH1 epimutations confer early-onset colorectal cancer in two new sporadic Lynch syndrome cases, with derivation of the epimutation on the paternal allele in one. Int J Cancer. 2011 Feb 15;128(4):869–78. PMID:20473912

1055. Goggins M, Offerhaus GJ, Hilgers W, et al. Pancreatic adenocarcinomas with DNA replication errors (RER+) are associated with wild-type K-ras and characteristic histopathology. Poor differentiation, a syncytial growth pattern, and pushing borders suggest RER+. Am J Pathol. 1998 Jun;152(6):1501–7. PMID:9626054

1056. Goggins M, Schutte M, Lu J, et al. Germline BRCA2 gene mutations in patients with apparently sporadic pancreatic carcinomas. Cancer Res. 1996 Dec 1;56(23):5360–4. PMID:8968085

1057. Gold JS, Antonescu CR, Hajdu C, et al. Clinicopathologic correlates of solitary fibrous tumors. Cancer. 2002 Feb 15;94(4):1057–68. PMID:11920476

1058. Goldblum JR, Appelman HD. Stromal tumors of the duodenum. A histologic and immunohistochemical study of 20 cases. Am J Surg Pathol. 1995 Jan;19(1):71–80. PMID:7528472

1059. Goldblum JR, Hart WR. Perianal Paget's disease: a histologic and immunohistochemical study of 11 cases with and without associated rectal adenocarcinoma. Am J Surg Pathol. 1998 Feb;22(2):170–9. PMID:9500217

1060. Goldblum JR, Rice TW, Zuccaro G, et al. Granular cell tumors of the esophagus: a clinical and pathologic study of 13 cases. Ann Thorac Surg. 1996 Sep;62(3):860–5. PMID:8784020

1061. Goldenring JR, Nam KT, Wang TC, et al. Spasmolytic polypeptide-expressing metaplasia and intestinal metaplasia: time for reevaluation of metaplasias and the origins of gastric cancer. Gastroenterology. 2010 Jun;138(7):2207–10, 2210.e1. PMID:20450866

1062. Goldfarb WB, Bennett D, Monafo W. Carcinoma in heterotopic gastric pancreas. Ann Surg. 1963 Jul;158:56–8. PMID:14042636

1063. Goldstone R, Itzkowitz S, Harpaz N, et al. Dysplasia is more common in the distal than proximal colon in ulcerative colitis surveillance. Inflamm Bowel Dis. 2012 May;18(5):832–7. PMID:21739534

1064. Gomyo H, Kagami Y, Kato H, et al. Primary hepatic follicular lymphoma: a case report and discussion of chemotherapy and favorable outcomes. J Clin Exp Hematop. 2007 Nov;47(2):73–7. PMID:18040146

1065. Gonda TA, Glick MP, Sethi A, et al. Polysomy and p16 deletion by fluorescence in situ hybridization in the diagnosis of indeterminate biliary strictures. Gastrointest Endosc. 2012 Jan;75(1):74–9. PMID:22100297

1066. Gong S, Auer I, Duggal R, et al. Epstein-Barr virus-associated inflammatory pseudotumor presenting as a colonic mass. Hum Pathol. 2015 Dec;46(12):1956–61. PMID:26477709

1067. Gong Y, Zhou Q, Zhou Y, et al. Gastrectomy and risk of pancreatic cancer: systematic review and meta-analysis of observational studies. Cancer Causes Control. 2012 Aug;23(8):1279–88. PMID:22674223

1068. Gonzalez RS, Cates JM, Washington MK, et al. Adenoma-like adenocarcinoma: a subtype of colorectal carcinoma with good prognosis, deceptive appearance on biopsy and frequent KRAS mutation. Histopathology. 2016 Jan;68(2):183–90. PMID:25913616

1069. Gonzalez RS, Messing S, Tu X, et al. Immunohistochemistry as a surrogate for molecular subtyping of gastric adenocarcinoma. Hum Pathol. 2016 Oct;56:16–21. PMID:27342907

1070. Gonzalez-Obeso E, Fujita H, Deshpande V, et al. Gastric hyperplastic polyps: a heterogeneous clinicopathologic group including a distinct subset best categorized as mucosal prolapse polyp. Am J Surg Pathol. 2011 May;35(5):670–7. PMID:21451363

1071. Goodman ZD, Ishak KG. Angiomyolipomas of the liver. Am J Surg Pathol. 1984 Oct;8(10):745–50. PMID:6496843

1072. Goodsell DS. The molecular perspective: the ras oncogene. Oncologist. 1999;4(3):263–4. PMID:10394594

1073. Gopal DV, Lieberman DA, Magaret N, et al. Risk factors for dysplasia in patients with Barrett's esophagus (BE): results from a multicenter consortium. Dig Dis Sci. 2003 Aug;48(8):1537–41. PMID:12924649

1074. Gordjani N, Herdeg S, Ross UH, et al. Focal dermal hypoplasia (Goltz-Gorlin syndrome) associated with obstructive papillomatosis of the larynx and hypopharynx. Eur J Dermatol. 1999 Dec;9(8):618–20. PMID:10586128

1075. Gordon-Dseagu VL, Devesa SS, Goggins M, et al. Pancreatic cancer incidence trends: evidence from the Surveillance, Epidemiology, and End Results (SEER) population-based data. Int J Epidemiol. 2018 Apr 1;47(2):427–39. PMID:29149259

1076. Gounder MM, Maki RG. Molecular basis for primary and secondary tyrosine kinase inhibitor resistance in gastrointestinal stromal tumor. Cancer Chemother Pharmacol. 2011 Jan;67 Suppl 1:S25–43. PMID:21116624

1077. Gounder MM, Thomas DM, Tap WD. Locally aggressive connective tissue tumors. J Clin Oncol. 2018 Jan 10;36(2):202–9. PMID:29220303

1078. Grabowski P, Schönfelder J, Ahnert-Hilger G, et al. Expression of neuroendocrine markers: a signature of human undifferentiated carcinoma of the colon and rectum. Virchows Arch. 2002 Sep;441(3):256–63. PMID:12242522

1079. Grabsch H, Sivakumar S, Gray S, et al. HER2 expression in gastric cancer: rare, heterogeneous and of no prognostic value - conclusions from 924 cases of two independent series. Cell Oncol. 2010;32(1-2):57–65. PMID:20208134

1080. Graham RP, Arnold CA, Naini BV, et al. Basaloid squamous cell carcinoma of the anus revisited. Am J Surg Pathol. 2016 Mar;40(3):354–60. PMID:26866355

1081. Graham RP, Barr Fritcher EG, Pestova E, et al. Fibroblast growth factor receptor 2 translocations in intrahepatic cholangiocarcinoma. Hum Pathol. 2014 Aug;45(8):1630–8. PMID:24837095

1082. Graham RP, Kerr SE, Butz ML, et al. Heterogenous MSH6 loss is a result of microsatellite instability within MSH6 and occurs in sporadic and hereditary colorectal and endometrial carcinomas. Am J Surg Pathol. 2015 Oct;39(10):1370–6. PMID:26099011

1083. Graham RP, Nair AA, Davila JI, et al. Gastroblastoma harbors a recurrent somatic MALAT1-GLI1 fusion gene. Mod Pathol. 2017 Oct;30(10):1443–52. PMID:28731043

1084. Graham RP, Shrestha B, Caron BL, et al. Islet-1 is a sensitive but not entirely specific marker for pancreatic neuroendocrine neoplasms and their metastases. Am J Surg Pathol. 2013 Mar;37(3):399–405. PMID:23348208

1085. Graham RP, Torbenson MS. Fibrolamellar carcinoma: a histologically unique tumor with unique molecular findings. Semin Diagn Pathol. 2017 Mar;34(2):146–52. PMID:28110996

1086. Graham RP, Yeh MM, Lam-Himlin D, et al. Molecular testing for the clinical diagnosis of fibrolamellar carcinoma. Mod Pathol. 2018 Jan;31(1):141–9. PMID:28862261

1087. Granados R, Aramburu JA, Rodríguez JM, et al. Cytopathology of a primary follicular dendritic cell sarcoma of the liver of the inflammatory pseudotumor-like type. Diagn Cytopathol. 2008 Jan;36(1):42–6. PMID:18064686

1088. Granier G, Marty-Double C. [Gastrointestinal adenocarcinomas with a choriocarcinomatous component: 2 cases and a review of 120 cases in the literature]. Gastroenterol Clin Biol. 2007 Oct;31(10):854–7. French. PMID:18166865

1089. Grant CS. Insulinoma. Best Pract Res Clin Gastroenterol. 2005 Oct;19(5):783–98. PMID:16253900

1090. Gravante G, De Liguori Carino N, Overton J, et al. Primary carcinoids of the liver: a review of symptoms, diagnosis and treatments. Dig Surg. 2008;25(5):364–8. PMID:18984960

1091. Gray SG, Eriksson T, Ekström C, et al. Altered expression of members of the IGF-axis in hepatoblastomas. Br J Cancer. 2000 May;82(9):1561–7. PMID:10789725

1092. Grazioli L, Bondioni MP, Haradome H, et al. Hepatocellular adenoma and focal nodular hyperplasia: value of gadoxetic acid-enhanced MR imaging in differential diagnosis. Radiology. 2012 Feb;262(2):520–9. PMID:22282184

1093. Green C, Spagnolo DV, Robbins PD, et al. Clear cell sarcoma of the gastrointestinal tract and malignant gastrointestinal neuroectodermal tumour: distinct or related entities? A review. Pathology. 2018 Aug;50(5):490–8. PMID:29970252

1094. Green J, Czanner G, Reeves G, et al. Menopausal hormone therapy and risk of gastrointestinal cancer: nested case-control study within a prospective cohort, and meta-analysis. Int J Cancer. 2012 May 15;130(10):2387–96. PMID:21671473

1095. Green RC, Green JS, Buehler SK, et al. Very high incidence of familial colorectal cancer in Newfoundland: a comparison with Ontario and 13 other population-based studies. Fam Cancer. 2007;6(1):53–62. PMID:17039269

1096. Greene FL. Epithelial misplacement in adenomatous polyps of the colon and rectum. Cancer. 1974 Jan;33(1):206–17. PMID:4810096

1097. Griffin JF, Page AJ, Samaha GJ, et al. Patients with a resected pancreatic mucinous cystic neoplasm have a better prognosis than patients with an intraductal papillary mucinous neoplasm: a large single institution series. Pancreatology. 2017 May-Jun;17(3):490–6. PMID:28416122

1098. Grillo F, Fassan M, Sarocchi F, et al. HER2 heterogeneity in gastric/gastroesophageal cancers: from benchside to practice. World J Gastroenterol. 2016 Jul 14;22(26):5879–87. PMID:27468182

1099. Groisman GM, Hershkovitz D, Vieth M, et al. Colonic perineuriomas with and without crypt serration: a comparative study. Am J Surg Pathol. 2013 May;37(5):745–51. PMID:23588369

1100. Gronchi A, Miceli R, Shurell E, et al. Outcome prediction in primary resected retroperitoneal soft tissue sarcoma: histology-specific overall survival and disease-free survival nomograms built on major sarcoma center data sets. J Clin Oncol. 2013 May 1;31(13):1649–55. PMID:23530096

1101. Groves C, Lamlum H, Crabtree M, et al. Mutation cluster region, association between germline and somatic mutations and genotype-phenotype correlation in upper gastrointestinal familial adenomatous polyposis. Am J Pathol. 2002 Jun;160(6):2055–61. PMID:12057910

1102. Grozinsky-Glasberg S, Alexandraki KI, Barak D, et al. Current size criteria for the management of neuroendocrine tumors of the appendix: are they valid? Clinical experience and review of the literature. Neuroendocrinology. 2013;98(1):31–7. PMID:23051855

1103. Grulich AE, Poynten IM, Machalek DA, et al. The epidemiology of anal cancer. Sex Health. 2012 Dec;9(6):504–8. PMID:22958581

1104. Grützmann R, Lüttges J, Sipos B, et al. ADAM9 expression in pancreatic cancer is associated with tumour type and is a prognostic factor in ductal adenocarcinoma. Br J Cancer. 2004 Mar 8;90(5):1053–8. PMID:14997207

1105. Gschwantler M, Kriwanek S, Langner E, et al. High-grade dysplasia and invasive carcinoma in colorectal adenomas: a multivariate analysis of the impact of adenoma and patient characteristics. Eur J Gastroenterol Hepatol. 2002 Feb;14(2):183–8. PMID:11981343

1106. Guan H, Gurda G, Lennon AM, et al. Intraductal tubulopapillary neoplasm of the pancreas on fine needle aspiration: case report with differential diagnosis. Diagn Cytopathol. 2014 Feb;42(2):156–60. PMID:22807417

1107. Guillou L, Aurias A. Soft tissue sarcomas with complex genomic profiles. Virchows Arch. 2010 Feb;456(2):201–17. PMID:20217954

1108. Guinney J, Dienstmann R, Wang X, et al. The consensus molecular subtypes of colorectal

cancer. Nat Med. 2015 Nov;21(11):1350–6. PMID:26457759
1109. Gullo I, Carvalho J, Martins D, et al. The transcriptomic landscape of gastric cancer: insights into Epstein-Barr virus infected and microsatellite unstable tumors. Int J Mol Sci. 2018 Jul 17;19(7):E2079. PMID:30018250
1110. Gullo I, Oliveira P, Athelogou M, et al. New insights into the inflamed tumor immune microenvironment of gastric cancer with lymphoid stroma: from morphology and digital analysis to gene expression. Gastric Cancer. 2019 Jan;22(1):77–90. PMID:29779068
1111. Gumbs AA, Moore PS, Falconi M, et al. Review of the clinical, histological, and molecular aspects of pancreatic endocrine neoplasms. J Surg Oncol. 2002 Sep;81(1):45–53, discussion 54. PMID:12210027
1112. Gunawardena SA, Siriwardana HP, Wickramasinghe SY, et al. Primary endodermal sinus (yolk sac) tumour of the liver. Eur J Surg Oncol. 2002 Feb;28(1):90–1. PMID:11869022
1113. Gunes D, Uysal KM, Cecen E, et al. Stromal-predominant mesenchymal hamartoma of the liver with elevated serum alpha-fetoprotein level. Pediatr Hematol Oncol. 2008 Sep;25(7):685–92. PMID:18850482
1114. Guo KJ, Yamaguchi K, Enjoji M. Undifferentiated carcinoma of the gallbladder. A clinicopathologic, histochemical, and immunohistochemical study of 21 patients with a poor prognosis. Cancer. 1988 May 1;61(9):1872–9. PMID:2451557
1115. Guo L, Kuroda N, Miyazaki E, et al. Anal canal neuroendocrine carcinoma with Pagetoid extension. Pathol Int. 2004 Aug;54(8):630–5. PMID:15260855
1116. Guo M, Jia Y, Yu Z, et al. Epigenetic changes associated with neoplasms of the exocrine and endocrine pancreas. Discov Med. 2014 Feb;17(92):67–73. PMID:24534469
1117. Guo X, Jo VY, Mills AM, et al. Clinically relevant molecular subtypes in leiomyosarcoma. Clin Cancer Res. 2015 Aug 1;21(15):3501–11. PMID:25896974
1118. Guo XF, Mao T, Gu ZT, et al. Adenoid cystic carcinoma of the esophagus: report of two cases and review of the Chinese literature. Diagn Pathol. 2012 Dec 13;7:179. PMID:23236991
1119. Gupta A, Dixon E. Epidemiology and risk factors: intrahepatic cholangiocarcinoma. Hepatobiliary Surg Nutr. 2017 Apr;6(2):101–4. PMID:28503557
1120. Gupta NM, Goenka MK, Jindal A, et al. Primary lymphoma of the esophagus. J Clin Gastroenterol. 1996 Oct;23(3):203–6. PMID:8899502
1121. Gupta R, Dinda AK, Singh MK, et al. Macrocystic serous cystadenocarcinoma of the pancreas: the first report of a new pattern of pancreatic carcinoma. J Clin Pathol. 2008 Mar;61(3):396–8. PMID:18305183
1122. Gupta RB, Harpaz N, Itzkowitz S, et al. Histologic inflammation is a risk factor for progression to colorectal neoplasia in ulcerative colitis: a cohort study. Gastroenterology. 2007 Oct;133(4):1099–105, quiz 1340–1. PMID:17919486
1123. Gupta S, Wang F, Holly EA, et al. Risk of pancreatic cancer by alcohol dose, duration, and pattern of consumption, including binge drinking: a population-based study. Cancer Causes Control. 2010 Jul;21(7):1047–59. PMID:20349126
1124. Gurrera A, Alaggio R, Leone G, et al. Biliary adenofibroma of the liver: report of a case and review of the literature. Patholog Res Int. 2010 Oct 28;2010:504584. PMID:21151526
1125. Gusani NJ, Marsh JW, Nalesnik MA, et al. Carcinoid of the extra-hepatic bile duct: a case report with long-term follow-up and review of literature. Am Surg. 2008 Jan;74(1):87–90. PMID:18274439
1126. Gustafson P. Soft tissue sarcoma. Epidemiology and prognosis in 508 patients. Acta Orthop Scand Suppl. 1994 Jun;259:1–31. PMID:8042499
1127. Gustafsson BI, Siddique L, Chan A, et al. Uncommon cancers of the small intestine, appendix and colon: an analysis of SEER 1973-2004, and current diagnosis and therapy. Int J Oncol. 2008 Dec;33(6):1121–31. PMID:19020744
1128. Gut P, Waligórska-Stachura J, Czarnywojtek A, et al. Hindgut neuroendocrine neoplasms - characteristics and prognosis. Arch Med Sci. 2017 Oct;13(6):1427–32. PMID:29181074
1129. Guzińska-Ustymowicz K, Niewiarowska K, Pryczynicz A. Invasive micropapillary carcinoma: a distinct type of adenocarcinomas in the gastrointestinal tract. World J Gastroenterol. 2014 Apr 28;20(16):4597–606. PMID:24782612
1130. Gylling A, Abdel-Rahman WM, Juhola M, et al. Is gastric cancer part of the tumour spectrum of hereditary non-polyposis colorectal cancer? A molecular genetic study. Gut. 2007 Jul;56(7):926–33. PMID:17267619
1131. Ha C, Regan J, Cetindag IB, et al. Benign esophageal tumors. Surg Clin North Am. 2015 Jun;95(3):491–514. PMID:25965126
1132. Haas JE, Feusner JH, Finegold MJ. Small cell undifferentiated histology in hepatoblastoma may be unfavorable. Cancer. 2001 Dec 15;92(12):3130–4. PMID:11753992
1133. Hachiya H, Kita J, Shiraki T, et al. Intraductal papillary neoplasm of the bile duct developing in a patient with primary sclerosing cholangitis: a case report. World J Gastroenterol. 2014 Nov 14;20(42):15925–30. PMID:25400480
1134. Hacihasanoglu E, Memis B, Pehlivanoglu B, et al. Factors impacting the performance characteristics of bile duct brushings: a clinico-cytopathologic analysis of 253 patients. Arch Pathol Lab Med. 2018 Jul;142(7):863–70. PMID:29582676
1135. Hackeng WM, Montgomery EA, Giardiello FM, et al. Morphology and genetics of pyloric gland adenomas in familial adenomatous polyposis. Histopathology. 2017 Mar;70(4):549–57. PMID:27767239
1136. Hadjiliadis D, Khoruts A, Zauber AG, et al. Cystic fibrosis colorectal cancer screening consensus recommendations. Gastroenterology. 2018 Feb;154(3):736–45.e14. PMID:29289528
1137. HaDuong JH, Martin AA, Skapek SX, et al. Sarcomas. Pediatr Clin North Am. 2015 Feb;62(1):179–200. PMID:25435119
1138. Haggitt RC, Glotzbach RE, Soffer EE, et al. Prognostic factors in colorectal carcinomas arising in adenomas: implications for lesions removed by endoscopic polypectomy. Gastroenterology. 1985 Aug;89(2):328–36. PMID:4007423
1139. Hagiwara N, Tajiri T, Tajiri T, et al. Biological behavior of mucoepidermoid carcinoma of the esophagus. J Nippon Med Sch. 2003 Oct;70(5):401–7. PMID:14578940
1140. Hahn HP, Hornick JL. Immunoreactivity for CD25 in gastrointestinal mucosal mast cells is specific for systemic mastocytosis. Am J Surg Pathol. 2007 Nov;31(11):1669–76. PMID:18059223
1141. Hahn SA, Schutte M, Hoque AT, et al. DPC4, a candidate tumor suppressor gene at human chromosome 18q21.1. Science. 1996 Jan 19;271(5247):350–3. PMID:8553070
1142. Hakkaart C, Ellison-Loschmann L, Day R, et al. Germline CDH1 mutations are a significant contributor to the high frequency of early-onset diffuse gastric cancer cases in New Zealand Māori. Fam Cancer. 2019 Jan;18(1):83–90. PMID:29589180
1143. Hale G, Liu X, Hu J, et al. Correlation of exon 3 β-catenin mutations with glutamine synthetase staining patterns in hepatocellular adenoma and hepatocellular carcinoma. Mod Pathol. 2016 Nov;29(11):1370–80. PMID:27469330
1144. Halfdanarson TR, Bamlet WR, McWilliams RR, et al. Risk factors for pancreatic neuroendocrine tumors: a clinic-based case-control study. Pancreas. 2014 Nov;43(8):1219–22. PMID:25291526
1145. Halfdanarson TR, Rabe KG, Rubin J, et al. Pancreatic neuroendocrine tumors (PNETs): incidence, prognosis and recent trend toward improved survival. Ann Oncol. 2008 Oct;19(10):1727–33. PMID:18515795
1146. Halfdanarson TR, Rubin J, Farnell MB, et al. Pancreatic endocrine neoplasms: epidemiology and prognosis of pancreatic endocrine tumors. Endocr Relat Cancer. 2008 Jun;15(2):409–27. PMID:18508996
1148. Hamashige N, Doi Y, Yonezawa Y, et al. [Noninvasive detection and prognosis of coronary artery disease in elderly patients; usefulness of dipyridamole-loading myocardial scintigraphy]. Nihon Naika Gakkai Zasshi. 1987 Aug;76(8):1230–7. Japanese. PMID:3681095
1149. Hamashima C, Okamoto M, Shabana M, et al. Sensitivity of endoscopic screening for gastric cancer by the incidence method. Int J Cancer. 2013 Aug 1;133(3):653–9. PMID:23364866
1150. Hameed O, Xu H, Saddeghi S, et al. Hepatoid carcinoma of the pancreas: a case report and literature review of a heterogeneous group of tumors. Am J Surg Pathol. 2007 Jan;31(1):146–52. PMID:17197931
1151. Hamilton NA, Liu TC, Cavatiao A, et al. Ki-67 predicts disease recurrence and poor prognosis in pancreatic neuroendocrine neoplasms. Surgery. 2012 Jul;152(1):107–13. PMID:22503317
1152. Hamilton SR, Liu B, Parsons RE, et al. The molecular basis of Turcot's syndrome. N Engl J Med. 1995 Mar 30;332(13):839–47. PMID:7661930
1153. Hamilton-Dutoit SJ, Raphael M, Audouin J, et al. In situ demonstration of Epstein-Barr virus small RNAs (EBER 1) in acquired immunodeficiency syndrome-related lymphomas: correlation with tumor morphology and primary site. Blood. 1993 Jul 15;82(2):619–24. PMID:8392401
1154. Hammel PR, Vilgrain V, Terris B, et al. Pancreatic involvement in von Hippel-Lindau disease. The Groupe Francophone d'Etude de la Maladie de von Hippel-Lindau. Gastroenterology. 2000 Oct;119(4):1087–95. PMID:11040195
1155. Han DH, Choi GH, Kim KS, et al. Prognostic significance of the worst grade in hepatocellular carcinoma with heterogeneous histologic grades of differentiation. J Gastroenterol Hepatol. 2013 Aug;28(8):1384–90. PMID:23517197
1156. Hanau CA, Miettinen M. Solitary fibrous tumor: histological and immunohistochemical spectrum of benign and malignant variants presenting at different sites. Hum Pathol. 1995 Apr;26(4):440–9. PMID:7705824
1157. Handra-Luca A, Condroyer C, de Moncuit C, et al. Vessels' morphology in SMAD4 and BMPR1A-related juvenile polyposis. Am J Med Genet A. 2005 Oct 1;138A(2):113–7. PMID:16152648
1158. Handra-Luca A, Montgomery E. Vascular malformations and hemangiolymphangiomas of the gastrointestinal tract: morphological features and clinical impact. Int J Clin Exp Pathol. 2011 Jun 20;4(5):430–43. PMID:21738815
1159. Hang XF, Xin HG, Wang L, et al. Nonleukemic myeloid sarcoma of the liver: a case report and review of literature. Hepatol Int. 2011 Jun;5(2):747–50. PMID:21484146
1160. Hansen MF, Johansen J, Sylvander AE, et al. Use of multigene-panel identifies pathogenic variants in several CRC-predisposing genes in patients previously tested for Lynch syndrome. Clin Genet. 2017 Oct;92(4):405–14. PMID:28195393
1161. Hansford S, Kaurah P, Li-Chang H, et al. Hereditary diffuse gastric cancer syndrome: CDH1 mutations and beyond. JAMA Oncol. 2015 Apr;1(1):23–32. PMID:26182300
1162. Hanson IM, Armstrong GR. Anal intraepithelial neoplasia in an inflammatory cloacogenic polyp. J Clin Pathol. 1999 May;52(5):393–4. PMID:10560365
1164. Hao Y, Samuels Y, Li Q, et al. Oncogenic PIK3CA mutations reprogram glutamine metabolism in colorectal cancer. Nat Commun. 2016 Jun 20;7:11971. PMID:27321283
1165. Hara K, Saito T, Hayashi T, et al. A mutation spectrum that includes GNAS, KRAS and TP53 may be shared by mucinous neoplasms of the appendix. Pathol Res Pract. 2015 Sep;211(9):657–64. PMID:26160192
1166. Hara T, Ikebe D, Odaka A, et al. Preoperative histological subtype classification of intraductal papillary mucinous neoplasms (IPMN) by pancreatic juice cytology with MUC stain. Ann Surg. 2013 Jun;257(6):1103–11. PMID:23364699
1167. Harada K, Mizrak Kaya D, Lopez A, et al. Personalized therapy based on image for esophageal or gastroesophageal junction adenocarcinoma. Ann Transl Med. 2018 Feb;6(4):80. PMID:29666803
1168. Haralambieva E, Schuuring E, Rosati S, et al. Interphase fluorescence in situ hybridization for detection of 8q24/MYC breakpoints on routine histologic sections: validation in Burkitt lymphomas from three geographic regions. Genes Chromosomes Cancer. 2004 May;40(1):10–8. PMID:15034863
1169. Haraldsdottir S, Rafnar T, Frankel WL, et al. Comprehensive population-wide analysis of Lynch syndrome in Iceland reveals founder mutations in MSH6 and PMS2. Nat Commun. 2017 May 3;8:14755. PMID:28466842
1170. Haramis AP, Begthel H, van den Born M, et al. De novo crypt formation and juvenile polyposis on BMP inhibition in mouse intestine. Science. 2004 Mar 12;303(5664):1684–6. PMID:15017003
1171. Haroche J, Cohen-Aubart F, Emile JF, et al. Reproducible and sustained efficacy of targeted therapy with vemurafenib in patients with BRAF(V600E)-mutated Erdheim-Chester disease. J Clin Oncol. 2015 Feb 10;33(5):411–8. PMID:25422482
1172. Harpaz N, Ward SC, Mescoli C, et al. Precancerous lesions in inflammatory bowel disease. Best Pract Res Clin Gastroenterol. 2013 Apr;27(2):257–67. PMID:23809244
1173. Harsha HC, Kandasamy K, Ranganathan P, et al. A compendium of potential biomarkers of pancreatic cancer. PLoS Med. 2009 Apr 7;6(4):e1000046. PMID:19360088
1174. Hart M, Thakral B, Yohe S, et al. EBV-positive mucocutaneous ulcer in organ transplant recipients: a localized indolent posttransplant lymphoproliferative disorder. Am J Surg Pathol. 2014 Nov;38(11):1522–9. PMID:25007145
1175. Hart PA, Bellin MD, Andersen DK, et al. Type 3c (pancreatogenic) diabetes mellitus secondary to chronic pancreatitis and pancreatic cancer. Lancet Gastroenterol Hepatol. 2016 Nov;1(3):226–37. PMID:28404095
1176. Hart S, Horsman JM, Radstone CR, et al. Localised extranodal lymphoma of the head and neck: the Sheffield Lymphoma Group experience (1971-2000). Clin Oncol (R Coll Radiol). 2004 May;16(3):186–92. PMID:15191005

1177. Hart WR. Primary endodermal sinus (yolk sac) tumor of the liver. First reported case. Cancer. 1975 May;35(5):1453–8. PMID:47264
1178. Hartman DJ, Binion DG, Regueiro MD, et al. Distinct histopathologic and molecular alterations in inflammatory bowel disease-associated intestinal adenocarcinoma: c-MYC amplification is common and associated with mucinous/signet ring cell differentiation. Inflamm Bowel Dis. 2018 Jul 12;24(8):1780–90. PMID:29788391
1179. Hasebe T, Sakamoto M, Mukai K, et al. Cholangiocarcinoma arising in bile duct adenoma with focal area of bile duct hamartoma. Virchows Arch. 1995;426(2):209–13. PMID:7757293
1180. Hasegawa H, Ueda M, Furukawa K, et al. p53 gene mutations in early colorectal carcinoma. De novo vs. adenoma-carcinoma sequence. Int J Cancer. 1995 Feb 20;64(1):47–51. PMID:7665248
1181. Hasegawa S, Mitsuyama K, Kawano H, et al. Endoscopic discrimination of sessile serrated adenomas from other serrated lesions. Oncol Lett. 2011 Sep 1;2(5):785–9. PMID:22866127
1182. Hasegawa T, Yang P, Kagawa N, et al. CD34 expression by inflammatory fibroid polyps of the stomach. Mod Pathol. 1997 May;10(5):451–6. PMID:9160309
1183. Haselkorn T, Whittemore AS, Lilienfeld DE. Incidence of small bowel cancer in the United States and worldwide: geographic, temporal, and racial differences. Cancer Causes Control. 2005 Sep;16(7):781–7. PMID:16132788
1184. Hashimoto T, Ogawa R, Matsubara A, et al. Familial adenomatous polyposis-associated and sporadic pyloric gland adenomas of the upper gastrointestinal tract share common genetic features. Histopathology. 2015 Nov;67(5):689–98. PMID:25832318
1185. Hashimoto T, Yamashita S, Yoshida H, et al. WNT pathway gene mutations are associated with the presence of dysplasia in colorectal sessile serrated adenoma/polyps. Am J Surg Pathol. 2017 Sep;41(9):1188–97. PMID:28614199
1186. Hassan C, Gimeno-García A, Kalager M, et al. Systematic review with meta-analysis: the incidence of advanced neoplasia after polypectomy in patients with and without low-risk adenomas. Aliment Pharmacol Ther. 2014 May;39(9):905–12. PMID:24593121
1187. Hata T, Suenaga M, Marchionni L, et al. Genome-wide somatic copy number alterations and mutations in high-grade pancreatic intraepithelial neoplasia. Am J Pathol. 2018 Jul;188(7):1723–33. PMID:29684357
1188. Hatano B, Ohshima K, Tsuchiya T, et al. Clinicopathological features of gastric B-cell lymphoma: a series of 317 cases. Pathol Int. 2002 Nov;52(11):677–82. PMID:12685544
1189. Hatipoglu BA. Cushing's syndrome. J Surg Oncol. 2012 Oct 1;106(5):565–71. PMID:22740318
1190. Hattori N, Ushijima T. Epigenetic impact of infection on carcinogenesis: mechanisms and applications. Genome Med. 2016 Jan 28;8(1):10. PMID:26823082
1191. Hattori T, Sentani K, Hattori Y, et al. Pure invasive micropapillary carcinoma of the esophagogastric junction with lymph nodes and liver metastasis. Pathol Int. 2016 Oct;66(10):583–6. PMID:27553658
1192. Haug U, Knudsen AB, Brenner H, et al. Is fecal occult blood testing more sensitive for left- versus right-sided colorectal neoplasia? A systematic literature review. Expert Rev Mol Diagn. 2011 Jul;11(6):605–16. PMID:21745014
1193. Haupt B, Ro JY, Schwartz MR, et al. Colorectal adenocarcinoma with micropapillary pattern and its association with lymph node metastasis. Mod Pathol. 2007 Jul;20(7):729–33. PMID:17464318
1194. Hausmann S, Kong B, Michalski C, et al. The role of inflammation in pancreatic cancer. Adv Exp Med Biol. 2014;816:129–51. PMID:24818722
1195. Hauso O, Gustafsson BI, Kidd M, et al. Neuroendocrine tumor epidemiology: contrasting Norway and North America. Cancer. 2008 Nov 15;113(10):2655–64. PMID:18853416
1196. Haverkos BM, Coleman C, Gru AA, et al. Emerging insights on the pathogenesis and treatment of extranodal NK/T cell lymphomas (ENKTL). Discov Med. 2017 Mar;23(126):189–99. PMID:28472613
1197. Hayakawa M, Nishikura K, Ajioka Y, et al. Re-evaluation of phenotypic expression in differentiated-type early adenocarcinoma of the stomach. Pathol Int. 2017 Mar;67(3):131–40. PMID:28088838
1198. Hayashi I, Muto Y, Fujii Y, et al. Mucoepidermoid carcinoma of the stomach. J Surg Oncol. 1987 Feb;34(2):94–9. PMID:3807383
1199. Hayward NK, Wilmott JS, Waddell N, et al. Whole-genome landscapes of major melanoma subtypes. Nature. 2017 May 11;545(7653):175–80. PMID:28467829
1200. Hazewinkel Y, López-Cerón M, East JE, et al. Endoscopic features of sessile serrated adenomas: validation by international experts using high-resolution white-light endoscopy and narrow-band imaging. Gastrointest Endosc. 2013 Jun;77(6):916–24. PMID:23433877
1201. Hazewinkel Y, Tytgat KM, van Eeden S, et al. Incidence of colonic neoplasia in patients with serrated polyposis syndrome who undergo annual endoscopic surveillance. Gastroenterology. 2014 Jul;147(1):88–95. PMID:24657624
1202. He EY, Wyld L, Sloane MA, et al. The molecular characteristics of colonic neoplasms in serrated polyposis: a systematic review and meta-analysis. J Pathol Clin Res. 2016 Apr 22;2(3):127–37. PMID:27499922
1203. He J, Ahuja N, Makary MA, et al. 2564 resected periampullary adenocarcinomas at a single institution: trends over three decades. HPB (Oxford). 2014 Jan;16(1):83–90. PMID:23472829
1204. Heald B, Mester J, Rybicki L, et al. Frequent gastrointestinal polyps and colorectal adenocarcinomas in a prospective series of PTEN mutation carriers. Gastroenterology. 2010 Dec;139(6):1927–33. PMID:20600018
1205. Hearle N, Schumacher V, Menko FH, et al. Frequency and spectrum of cancers in the Peutz-Jeghers syndrome. Clin Cancer Res. 2006 May 15;12(10):3209–15. PMID:16707622
1206. Heerema-McKenney A, Leuschner I, Smith N, et al. Nested stromal epithelial tumor of the liver: six cases of a distinctive pediatric neoplasm with frequent calcifications and association with Cushing syndrome. Am J Surg Pathol. 2005 Jan;29(1):10–20. PMID:15613852
1207. Heetfeld M, Chougnet CN, Olsen IH, et al. Characteristics and treatment of patients with G3 gastroenteropancreatic neuroendocrine neoplasms. Endocr Relat Cancer. 2015 Aug;22(4):657–64. PMID:26113608
1208. Heinrich MC, Corless CL, Duensing A, et al. PDGFRA activating mutations in gastrointestinal stromal tumors. Science. 2003 Jan 31;299(5607):708–10. PMID:12522257
1209. Heitz PU, Kasper M, Polak JM, et al. Pancreatic endocrine tumors. Hum Pathol. 1982 Mar;13(3):263–71. PMID:7076209
1210. Hellan M, Sun CL, Artinyan A, et al. The impact of lymph node number on survival in patients with lymph node-negative pancreatic cancer. Pancreas. 2008 Jul;37(1):19–24. PMID:18580439
1211. Helmke BM, Mollenhauer J, Herold-Mende C, et al. BRAF mutations distinguish anorectal from cutaneous melanoma at the molecular level. Gastroenterology. 2004 Dec;127(6):1815–20. PMID:15578519
1212. Hemminki K, Li X. Familial and second primary pancreatic cancers: a nationwide epidemiologic study from Sweden. Int J Cancer. 2003 Feb 10;103(4):525–30. PMID:12478670
1213. Hempen PM, Zhang L, Bansal RK, et al. Evidence of selection for clones having genetic inactivation of the activin A type II receptor (ACVR2) gene in gastrointestinal cancers. Cancer Res. 2003 Mar 1;63(5):994–9. PMID:12615714
1214. Henderson L, Fehily C, Folaranmi S, et al. Management and outcome of neuroendocrine tumours of the appendix-a two centre UK experience. J Pediatr Surg. 2014 Oct;49(10):1513–7. PMID:25280658
1215. Hennedige TP, Neo WT, Venkatesh SK. Imaging of malignancies of the biliary tract- an update. Cancer Imaging. 2014 Apr 22;14:14. PMID:25608662
1216. Henriet E, Abou Hammoud A, Dupuy JW, et al. Argininosuccinate synthase 1 (ASS1): a marker of unclassified hepatocellular adenoma and high bleeding risk. Hepatology. 2017 Dec;66(6):2016–28. PMID:28646562
1217. Henson DE, Schwartz AM, Nsouli H, et al. Carcinomas of the pancreas, gallbladder, extrahepatic bile ducts, and ampulla of Vater share a field for carcinogenesis: a population-based study. Arch Pathol Lab Med. 2009 Jan;133(1):67–71. PMID:19123739
1218. Heppt MV, Roesch A, Weide B, et al. Prognostic factors and treatment outcomes in 444 patients with mucosal melanoma. Eur J Cancer. 2017 Aug;81:36–44. PMID:28600969
1219. Herfs M, Roncarati P, Koopmansch B, et al. A dualistic model of primary anal canal adenocarcinoma with distinct cellular origins, etiologies, inflammatory microenvironments and mutational signatures: implications for personalised medicine. Br J Cancer. 2018 May;118(10):1302–12. PMID:29700411
1220. Herman JM, Swartz MJ, Hsu CC, et al. Analysis of fluorouracil-based adjuvant chemotherapy and radiation after pancreaticoduodenectomy for ductal adenocarcinoma of the pancreas: results of a large, prospectively collected database at the Johns Hopkins Hospital. J Clin Oncol. 2008 Jul 20;26(21):3503–10. PMID:18640931
1221. Hermann G, Konukiewitz B, Schmitt A, et al. Hormonally defined pancreatic and duodenal neuroendocrine tumors differ in their transcription factor signatures: expression of ISL1, PDX1, NGN3, and CDX2. Virchows Arch. 2011 Aug;459(2):147–54. PMID:21739268
1222. Hes FJ, Nielsen M, Bik EC, et al. Somatic APC mosaicism: an underestimated cause of polyposis coli. Gut. 2008 Jan;57(1):71–6. PMID:17604324
1223. Heslin MJ, Lewis JJ, Woodruff JM, et al. Core needle biopsy for diagnosis of extremity soft tissue sarcoma. Ann Surg Oncol. 1997 Jul-Aug;4(5):425–31. PMID:9259971
1224. Hetzel JT, Huang CS, Coukos JA, et al. Variation in the detection of serrated polyps in an average risk colorectal cancer screening cohort. Am J Gastroenterol. 2010 Dec;105(12):2656–64. PMID:20717107
1225. Hibdon ES, Samuelson LC. Cellular plasticity in the stomach: insights into the cellular origin of gastric metaplasia. Gastroenterology. 2018 Mar;154(4):801–3. PMID:29425924
1226. Hibi Y, Fukushima N, Tsuchida A, et al. Pancreatic juice cytology and subclassification of intraductal papillary mucinous neoplasms of the pancreas. Pancreas. 2007 Mar;34(2):197–204. PMID:17312458
1227. Hidaka Y, Mitomi H, Saito T, et al. Alteration in the Wnt/β-catenin signaling pathway in gastric neoplasias of fundic gland (chief cell predominant) type. Hum Pathol. 2013 Nov;44(11):2438–48. PMID:24011952
1228. Higa E, Rosai J, Pizzimbono CA, et al. Mucosal hyperplasia, mucinous cystadenoma, and mucinous cystadenocarcinoma of the appendix. A re-evaluation of appendiceal "mucocele". Cancer. 1973 Dec;32(6):1525–41. PMID:4757938
1229. Higaki E, Yanagi S, Gotohda N, et al. Intraoperative peritoneal lavage cytology offers prognostic significance for gastric cancer patients with curative resection. Cancer Sci. 2017 May;108(5):978–86. PMID:28256061
1230. Higashi H, Tsutsumi R, Muto S, et al. SHP-2 tyrosine phosphatase as an intracellular target of Helicobacter pylori CagA protein. Science. 2002 Jan 25;295(5555):683–6. PMID:11743164
1231. Hijioka S, Hosoda W, Matsuo K, et al. Rb loss and KRAS mutation are predictors of the response to platinum-based chemotherapy in pancreatic neuroendocrine neoplasm with grade 3: a Japanese multicenter pancreatic NEN-G3 study. Clin Cancer Res. 2017 Aug 15;23(16):4625–32. PMID:28455360
1232. Hilal L, Barada K, Mukherji D, et al. Gastrointestinal (GI) leiomyosarcoma (LMS) case series and review on diagnosis, management, and prognosis. Med Oncol. 2016 Feb;33(2):20. PMID:26786155
1233. Hilgers W, Groot Koerkamp B, Geradts J, et al. Genomic FHIT analysis in RER+ and RER- adenocarcinomas of the pancreas. Genes Chromosomes Cancer. 2000 Mar;27(3):239–43. PMID:10679912
1234. Hill DA, Swanson PE, Anderson K, et al. Desmoplastic nested spindle cell tumor of liver: report of four cases of a proposed new entity. Am J Surg Pathol. 2005 Jan;29(1):1–9. PMID:15613851
1235. Hingorani SR, Petricoin EF, Maitra A, et al. Preinvasive and invasive ductal pancreatic cancer and its early detection in the mouse. Cancer Cell. 2003 Dec;4(6):437–50. PMID:14706336
1236. Hingorani SR, Wang L, Multani AS, et al. Trp53R172H and KrasG12D cooperate to promote chromosomal instability and widely metastatic pancreatic ductal adenocarcinoma in mice. Cancer Cell. 2005 May;7(5):469–83. PMID:15894267
1237. Hinoi T, Tani M, Lucas PC, et al. Loss of CDX2 expression and microsatellite instability are prominent features of large cell minimally differentiated carcinomas of the colon. Am J Pathol. 2001 Dec;159(6):2239–48. PMID:11733373
1238. Hirakawa K, Fuchigami T, Nakamura S, et al. Primary gastrointestinal T-cell lymphoma resembling multiple lymphomatous polyposis. Gastroenterology. 1996 Sep;111(3):778–82. PMID:8780585
1239. Hirji SA, Senturk JC, Hornick J, et al. A rare case of interdigitating dendritic cell sarcoma of the rectum: review of histopathology and management strategy. BMJ Case Rep. 2017 Aug 7;2017. PMID:28784918
1240. Hirono S, Tani M, Kawai M, et al. The carcinoembryonic antigen level in pancreatic juice and mural nodule size are predictors of malignancy for branch duct type intraductal papillary mucinous neoplasms of the pancreas. Ann Surg. 2012 Mar;255(3):517–22. PMID:22301608
1241. Hirose K, Matsui T, Nagano H, et al. Atypical glomus tumor arising in the liver: a case report. Diagn Pathol. 2015 Jul 19;10:112. PMID:26187280
1242. Hirota S, Isozaki K, Moriyama Y, et al. Gain-of-function mutations of c-kit in human

gastrointestinal stromal tumors. Science. 1998 Jan 23;279(5350):577–80. PMID:9438854
1243. Hirschman BA, Pollock BH, Tomlinson GE. The spectrum of APC mutations in children with hepatoblastoma from familial adenomatous polyposis kindreds. J Pediatr. 2005 Aug;147(2):263–6. PMID:16126064
1244. Hisa T, Nobukawa B, Suda K, et al. Intraductal carcinoma with complex fusion of tubular glands without macroscopic mucus in main pancreatic duct: dilemma in classification. Pathol Int. 2007 Nov;57(11):741–5. PMID:17922686
1245. Hissong E, Ramrattan G, Zhang P, et al. Gastric carcinomas with lymphoid stroma: an evaluation of the histopathologic and molecular features. Am J Surg Pathol. 2018 Apr;42(4):453–62. PMID:29438172
1246. Hitchins MP, Ward RL. Constitutional (germline) MLH1 epimutation as an aetiological mechanism for hereditary non-polyposis colorectal cancer. J Med Genet. 2009 Dec;46(12):793–802. PMID:19564652
1247. Hiyama T, Yoshihara M, Tanaka S, et al. Genetic polymorphisms and esophageal cancer risk. Int J Cancer. 2007 Oct 15;121(8):1643–58. PMID:17674367
1248. Hleyhel M, Belot A, Bouvier AM, et al. Trends in survival after cancer diagnosis among HIV-infected individuals between 1992 and 2009. Results from the FHDH-ANRS CO4 cohort. Int J Cancer. 2015 Nov 15;137(10):2443–53. PMID:25976897
1249. Hoang MP, Hobbs CM, Sobin LH, et al. Carcinoid tumor of the esophagus: a clinicopathologic study of four cases. Am J Surg Pathol. 2002 Apr;26(4):517–22. PMID:11914632
1250. Hoang MP, Hruban RH, Albores-Saavedra J. Clear cell endocrine pancreatic tumor mimicking renal cell carcinoma: a distinctive neoplasm of von Hippel-Lindau disease. Am J Surg Pathol. 2001 May;25(5):602–9. PMID:11342771
1251. Hoang MP, Murakata LA, Katabi N, et al. Invasive papillary carcinomas of the extrahepatic bile ducts: a clinicopathologic and immunohistochemical study of 13 cases. Mod Pathol. 2002 Dec;15(12):1251–8. PMID:12481004
1252. Hobbs CM, Lowry MA, Owen D, et al. Anal gland carcinoma. Cancer. 2001 Oct 15;92(8):2045–9. PMID:11596018
1253. Hobert JA, Eng C. PTEN hamartoma tumor syndrome: an overview. Genet Med. 2009 Oct;11(10):687–94. PMID:19668082
1254. Hochwald SN, Zee S, Conlon KC, et al. Prognostic factors in pancreatic endocrine neoplasms: an analysis of 136 cases with a proposal for low-grade and intermediate-grade groups. J Clin Oncol. 2002 Jun 1;20(11):2633–42. PMID:12039924
1255. Hoff PM, Coudry R, Moniz CM. Pathology of anal cancer. Surg Oncol Clin N Am. 2017 Jan;26(1):57–71. PMID:27889037
1256. Hohenberger P, Ronellenfitsch U, Oladeji O, et al. Pattern of recurrence in patients with ruptured primary gastrointestinal stromal tumour. Br J Surg. 2010 Dec;97(12):1854–9. PMID:20730857
1257. Holen KD, Klimstra DS, Hummer A, et al. Clinical characteristics and outcomes from an institutional series of acinar cell carcinoma of the pancreas and related tumors. J Clin Oncol. 2002 Dec 15;20(24):4673–8. PMID:12488412
1258. Hollowood K, Stamp G, Zouvani I, et al. Extranodal follicular dendritic cell sarcoma of the gastrointestinal tract. Morphologic, immunohistochemical and ultrastructural analysis of two cases. Am J Clin Pathol. 1995 Jan;103(1):90–7. PMID:7817952
1259. Holme Ø, Bretthauer M, Eide TJ, et al. Long-term risk of colorectal cancer in individuals with serrated polyps. Gut. 2015 Jun;64(6):929–36. PMID:25399542
1260. Holmes GK, Prior P, Lane MR, et al. Malignancy in coeliac disease–effect of a gluten free diet. Gut. 1989 Mar;30(3):333–8. PMID:2707633
1261. Holster IL, Aarts MJ, Tjwa ET, et al. Trend breaks in incidence of non-cardia gastric cancer in the Netherlands. Cancer Epidemiol. 2014 Feb;38(1):9–15. PMID:24309073
1262. Honda M, Furuta Y, Naoe H, et al. Primary mucosa-associated lymphoid tissue (MALT) lymphoma of the gallbladder and review of the literature. BMJ Case Rep. 2017 May 27;2017. PMID:28551602
1263. Honda M, Wong SL, Healy MA, et al. Long-term trends in primary sites of gastric adenocarcinoma in Japan and the United States. J Cancer. 2017 Jul 5;8(11):1935–42. PMID:28819392
1264. Honda S, Arai Y, Haruta M, et al. Loss of imprinting of IGF2 correlates with hypermethylation of the H19 differentially methylated region in hepatoblastoma. Br J Cancer. 2008 Dec 2;99(11):1891–9. PMID:19034281
1265. Honda S, Haruta M, Sugawara W, et al. The methylation status of RASSF1A promoter predicts responsiveness to chemotherapy and eventual cure in hepatoblastoma patients. Int J Cancer. 2008 Sep 1;123(5):1117–25. PMID:18537155
1266. Honda S, Miyagi H, Suzuki H, et al. RASSF1A methylation indicates a poor prognosis in hepatoblastoma patients. Pediatr Surg Int. 2013 Nov;29(11):1147–52. PMID:23989600
1267. Hong GS, Byun JH, Kim JH, et al. Thread sign in biliary intraductal papillary mucinous neoplasm: a novel specific finding for MRI. Eur Radiol. 2016 Sep;26(9):3112–20. PMID:26694060
1268. Hong SM, Goggins M, Wolfgang CL, et al. Vascular invasion in infiltrating ductal adenocarcinoma of the pancreas can mimic pancreatic intraepithelial neoplasia: a histopathologic study of 209 cases. Am J Surg Pathol. 2012 Feb;36(2):235–41. PMID:22082604
1269. Hong SM, Pawlik TM, Cho H, et al. Depth of tumor invasion better predicts prognosis than the current American Joint Committee on Cancer T classification for distal bile duct carcinoma. Surgery. 2009 Aug;146(2):250–7. PMID:19628081
1270. Hoorens A, Lemoine NR, McLellan E, et al. Pancreatic acinar cell carcinoma. An analysis of cell lineage markers, p53 expression, and Ki-ras mutation. Am J Pathol. 1993 Sep;143(3):685–98. PMID:8362971
1271. Hoorens A, Prenzel K, Lemoine NR, et al. Undifferentiated carcinoma of the pancreas: analysis of intermediate filament profile and Ki-ras mutations provides evidence of a ductal origin. J Pathol. 1998 May;185(1):53–60. PMID:9713360
1272. Hoots BE, Palefsky JM, Pimenta JM, et al. Human papillomavirus type distribution in anal cancer and anal intraepithelial lesions. Int J Cancer. 2009 May 15;124(10):2375–83. PMID:19189402
1273. Horie A, Yano Y, Kotoo Y, et al. Morphogenesis of pancreatoblastoma, infantile carcinoma of the pancreas: report of two cases. Cancer. 1977 Jan;39(1):247–54. PMID:188539
1274. Horiguchi H, Matsui-Horiguchi M, Sakata H, et al. Inflammatory pseudotumor-like follicular dendritic cell tumor of the spleen. Pathol Int. 2004 Feb;54(2):124–31. PMID:14720144
1275. Hornick JL, Fletcher CD. Intestinal perineuriomas: clinicopathologic definition of a new anatomic subset in a series of 10 cases. Am J Surg Pathol. 2005 Jul;29(7):859–65. PMID:15958849
1276. Hornick JL, Fletcher CD. Intraabdominal cystic lymphangiomas obscured by marked superimposed reactive changes: clinicopathological analysis of a series. Hum Pathol. 2005 Apr;36(4):426–32. PMID:15892005
1277. Hornick JL, Jaffe ES, Fletcher CD. Extranodal histiocytic sarcoma: clinicopathologic analysis of 14 cases of a rare epithelioid malignancy. Am J Surg Pathol. 2004 Sep;28(9):1133–44. PMID:15316312
1278. Hornick JL, Sholl LM, Dal Cin P, et al. Expression of ROS1 predicts ROS1 gene rearrangement in inflammatory myofibroblastic tumors. Mod Pathol. 2015 May;28(5):732–9. PMID:25612511
1279. Horny H-P, Akin C, Arber DA, et al. Mastocytosis. In: Swerdlow SH, Campo E, Harris NL, et al., editors. WHO classification of tumours of haematopoietic and lymphoid tissues. Lyon (France): International Agency for Research on Cancer; 2017. pp. 62–9. (WHO classification of tumours series, 4th rev. ed.; vol. 2). http://publications.iarc.fr/556.
1280. Horny HP, Sotlar K, Valent P. Evaluation of mast cell activation syndromes: impact of pathology and immunohistology. Int Arch Allergy Immunol. 2012;159(1):1–5. PMID:22555026
1281. Horowitz ME, Etcubanas E, Webber BL, et al. Hepatic undifferentiated (embryonal) sarcoma and rhabdomyosarcoma in children. Results of therapy. Cancer. 1987 Feb 1;59(3):396–402. PMID:3791152
1283. Hoshimoto S, Aiura K, Shito M, et al. Adenosquamous carcinoma of the ampulla of Vater: a case report and literature review. World J Surg Oncol. 2015 Sep 29;13:287. PMID:26420726
1284. Hosoda W, Chianchiano P, Griffin JF, et al. Genetic analyses of isolated high-grade pancreatic intraepithelial neoplasia (HG-PanIN) reveal paucity of alterations in TP53 and SMAD4. J Pathol. 2017 May;242(1):16–23. PMID:28188630
1285. Hosoda W, Wood LD. Molecular genetics of pancreatic neoplasms. Surg Pathol Clin. 2016 Dec;9(4):685–703. PMID:27926367
1286. Hosonuma K, Sato K, Honma M, et al. Small-cell carcinoma of the extrahepatic bile duct: a case report and review of the literature. Hepatol Int. 2008 Mar;2(1):129–32. PMID:19669289
1287. Hoster E, Dreyling M, Klapper W, et al. A new prognostic index (MIPI) for patients with advanced-stage mantle cell lymphoma. Blood. 2008 Jan 15;111(2):558–65. PMID:17962512
1288. Hoster E, Rosenwald A, Berger F, et al. Prognostic value of Ki-67 index, cytology, and growth pattern in mantle-cell lymphoma: results from randomized trials of the European Mantle Cell Lymphoma Network. J Clin Oncol. 2016 Apr 20;34(12):1386–94. PMID:26926679
1289. Hou YY, Tan YS, Xu JF, et al. Schwannoma of the gastrointestinal tract: a clinicopathological, immunohistochemical and ultrastructural study of 33 cases. Histopathology. 2006 Apr;48(5):536–45. PMID:16623779
1290. Houard C, Pinaquy JB, Mesguich C, et al. Role of 18F-FDG PET/CT in posttreatment evaluation of anal carcinoma. J Nucl Med. 2017 Sep;58(9):1414–20. PMID:28280225
1291. House MG, Gönen M, Jarnagin WR, et al. Prognostic significance of pathologic nodal status in patients with resected pancreatic cancer. J Gastrointest Surg. 2007 Nov;11(11):1549–55. PMID:17786531
1292. How-Kit A, Dejeux E, Dousset B, et al. DNA methylation profiles distinguish different subtypes of gastroenteropancreatic neuroendocrine tumors. Epigenomics. 2015;7(8):1245–58. PMID:26360914
1293. Howard JH, Pollock RE. Intra-abdominal and abdominal wall desmoid fibromatosis. Oncol Ther. 2016;4(1):57–72. PMID:28261640
1294. Howdle PD, Jalal PK, Holmes GK, et al. Primary small-bowel malignancy in the UK and its association with coeliac disease. QJM. 2003 May;96(5):345–53. PMID:12702783
1295. Howe JR, Bair JL, Sayed MG, et al. Germline mutations of the gene encoding bone morphogenetic protein receptor 1A in juvenile polyposis. Nat Genet. 2001 Jun;28(2):184–7. PMID:11381269
1296. Howe JR, Haidle JL, Lal G, et al. ENG mutations in MADH4/BMPR1A mutation negative patients with juvenile polyposis. Clin Genet. 2007 Jan;71(1):91–2. PMID:17204053
1297. Howe JR, Karnell LH, Menck HR, et al. The American College of Surgeons Commission on Cancer and the American Cancer Society. Adenocarcinoma of the small bowel: review of the National Cancer Data Base, 1985-1995. Cancer. 1999 Dec 15;86(12):2693–706. PMID:10594865
1298. Howe JR, Mitros FA, Summers RW. The risk of gastrointestinal carcinoma in familial juvenile polyposis. Ann Surg Oncol. 1998 Dec;5(8):751–6. PMID:9869523
1299. Howe JR, Roth S, Ringold JC, et al. Mutations in the SMAD4/DPC4 gene in juvenile polyposis. Science. 1998 May 15;280(5366):1086–8. PMID:9582123
1300. Howell WM, Leung ST, Jones DB, et al. HLA-DRB, -DQA, and -DQB polymorphism in celiac disease and enteropathy-associated T-cell lymphoma. Common features and additional risk factors for malignancy. Hum Immunol. 1995 May;43(1):29–37. PMID:7558926
1301. Hruban RH, Adsay NV, Albores-Saavedra J, et al. Pancreatic intraepithelial neoplasia: a new nomenclature and classification system for pancreatic duct lesions. Am J Surg Pathol. 2001 May;25(5):579–86. PMID:11342768
1302. Hruban RH, Klimstra DS. Adenocarcinoma of the pancreas. Semin Diagn Pathol. 2014 Nov;31(6):443–51. PMID:25441308
1303. Hruban RH, Maitra A, Kern SE, et al. Precursors to pancreatic cancer. Gastroenterol Clin North Am. 2007 Dec;36(4):831–49, vi. PMID:17996793
1304. Hruban RH, Pitman MB, Klimstra DS. Tumors of the pancreas. Washington, DC: American Registry of Pathology; 2007. (AFIP atlas of tumor pathology, series 4; fascicle 6).
1305. Hruban RH, Takaori K, Canto M, et al. Clinical importance of precursor lesions in the pancreas. J Hepatobiliary Pancreat Surg. 2007;14(3):255–63. PMID:17520200
1306. Hruban RH, Takaori K, Klimstra DS, et al. An illustrated consensus on the classification of pancreatic intraepithelial neoplasia and intraductal papillary mucinous neoplasms. Am J Surg Pathol. 2004 Aug;28(8):977–87. PMID:15252303
1307. Hruban RH, van Mansfeld AD, Offerhaus GJ, et al. K-ras oncogene activation in adenocarcinoma of the human pancreas. A study of 82 carcinomas using a combination of mutant-enriched polymerase chain reaction analysis and allele-specific oligonucleotide hybridization. Am J Pathol. 1993 Aug;143(2):545–54. PMID:8342602
1308. Hsing AW, Gao YT, Han TQ, et al. Gallstones and the risk of biliary tract cancer: a population-based study in China. Br J Cancer. 2007 Dec 3;97(11):1577–82. PMID:18000509
1309. Hsu C, Rashid A, Xing Y, et al. Varying malignant potential of appendiceal neuroendocrine tumors: importance of histologic subtype. J Surg Oncol. 2013 Feb;107(2):136–43. PMID:22767417
1310. Hsu HC, Thiam TK, Lu YJ, et al. Mutations of KRAS/NRAS/BRAF predict cetuximab resistance in metastatic colorectal cancer patients. Oncotarget. 2016 Apr 19;7(16):22257–70. PMID:26989027

1311. Hsu IC, Metcalf RA, Sun T, et al. Mutational hotspot in the p53 gene in human hepatocellular carcinomas. Nature. 1991 Apr 4;350(6317):427–8. PMID:1849234
1312. Hsu JT, Yeh CN, Chen YR, et al. Adenosquamous carcinoma of the pancreas. Digestion. 2005;72(2-3):104–8. PMID:16172546
1313. Hsu M, Sasaki M, Igarashi S, et al. KRAS and GNAS mutations and p53 overexpression in biliary intraepithelial neoplasia and intrahepatic cholangiocarcinomas. Cancer. 2013 May 1;119(9):1669–74. PMID:23335286
1314. Hsu M, Terris B, Wu TT, et al. Endometrial cysts within the liver: a rare entity and its differential diagnosis with mucinous cystic neoplasms of the liver. Hum Pathol. 2014 Apr;45(4):761–7. PMID:24491354
1315. Hsu M, Young RH, Misdraji J. Ruptured appendiceal diverticula mimicking low-grade appendiceal mucinous neoplasms. Am J Surg Pathol. 2009 Oct;33(10):1515–21. PMID:19623035
1316. Hu G, Qin L, Zhang X, et al. Epigenetic silencing of the MLH1 promoter in relation to the development of gastric cancer and its use as a biomarker for patients with microsatellite instability: a systematic analysis. Cell Physiol Biochem. 2018;45(1):148–62. PMID:29334683
1317. Hu S, Xu-Monette ZY, Balasubramanyam A, et al. CD30 expression defines a novel subgroup of diffuse large B-cell lymphoma with favorable prognosis and distinct gene expression signature: a report from the International DLBCL Rituximab-CHOP Consortium Program Study. Blood. 2013 Apr 4;121(14):2715–24. PMID:23343832
1318. Huang CC, Frankel WL, Doukides T, et al. Prolapse-related changes are a confounding factor in misdiagnosis of sessile serrated adenomas in the rectum. Hum Pathol. 2013 Apr;44(4):480–6. PMID:23069257
1319. Huang Q, Wu H, Nie L, et al. Primary high-grade neuroendocrine carcinoma of the esophagus: a clinicopathologic and immunohistochemical study of 42 resection cases. Am J Surg Pathol. 2013 Apr;37(4):467–83. PMID:23426118
1320. Huang SC, Chuang HC, Chen TD, et al. Alterations of the mTOR pathway in hepatic angiomyolipoma with emphasis on the epithelioid variant and loss of heterogeneity of TSC1/TSC2. Histopathology. 2015 Apr;66(5):695–705. PMID:25234729
1321. Hubert C, Sempoux C, Berquin A, et al. Bile duct carcinoid tumors: an uncommon disease but with a good prognosis? Hepatogastroenterology. 2005 Jul-Aug;52(64):1042–7. PMID:16001626
1322. Huebner M, Kendrick M, Reid-Lombardo KM, et al. Number of lymph nodes evaluated: prognostic value in pancreatic adenocarcinoma. J Gastrointest Surg. 2012 May;16(5):920–6. PMID:22421988
1323. Hugen N, Brown G, Glynne-Jones R, et al. Advances in the care of patients with mucinous colorectal cancer. Nat Rev Clin Oncol. 2016 Jun;13(6):361–9. PMID:26323388
1324. Hugen N, van Beek JJ, de Wilt JH, et al. Insight into mucinous colorectal carcinoma: clues from etiology. Ann Surg Oncol. 2014 Sep;21(9):2963–70. PMID:24728741
1325. Hugen N, van de Velde CJ, de Wilt JH, et al. Metastatic pattern in colorectal cancer is strongly influenced by histological subtype. Ann Oncol. 2014 Mar;25(3):651–7. PMID:24504447
1326. Hugen N, Verhoeven RH, Lemmens VE, et al. Colorectal signet-ring cell carcinoma: benefit from adjuvant chemotherapy but a poor prognostic factor. Int J Cancer. 2015 Jan 15;136(2):333–9. PMID:24841868
1327. Hughes K, Kelty S, Martin R. Hepatoid carcinoma of the pancreas. Am Surg. 2004 Nov;70(11):1030–3. PMID:15586521
1328. Hughes NR, Goodman ZD, Bhathal PS. An immunohistochemical profile of the so-called bile duct adenoma: clues to pathogenesis. Am J Surg Pathol. 2010 Sep;34(9):1312–8. PMID:20679879
1329. Huh CW, Jung DH, Kim H, et al. Clinicopathologic features of gastric carcinoma with lymphoid stroma in early gastric cancer. J Surg Oncol. 2016 Nov;114(6):769–72. PMID:27450278
1330. Huh J, Byun JH, Hong SM, et al. Malignant pancreatic serous cystic neoplasms: systematic review with a new case. BMC Gastroenterol. 2016 Aug 22;16(1):97. PMID:27549181
1331. Hui CK. Collision adenoma-carcinoid tumour of the colon complicated by carcinoid syndrome. Singapore Med J. 2012 Sep;53(9):e195–7. PMID:23023914
1332. Humar B, Blair V, Charlton A, et al. E-cadherin deficiency initiates gastric signet-ring cell carcinoma in mice and man. Cancer Res. 2009 Mar 1;69(5):2050–6. PMID:19223545
1333. Humar B, Fukuzawa R, Blair V, et al. Destabilized adhesion in the gastric proliferative zone and c-Src kinase activation mark the development of early diffuse gastric cancer. Cancer Res. 2007 Mar 15;67(6):2480–9. PMID:17363565
1334. Humar B, Guilford P. Hereditary diffuse gastric cancer: a manifestation of lost cell polarity. Cancer Sci. 2009 Jul;100(7):1151–7. PMID:19432899
1335. Hummel M, Bentink S, Berger H, et al. A biologic definition of Burkitt's lymphoma from transcriptional and genomic profiling. N Engl J Med. 2006 Jun 8;354(23):2419–30. PMID:16760442
1336. Humphris JL, Johns AL, Simpson SH, et al. Clinical and pathologic features of familial pancreatic cancer. Cancer. 2014 Dec 1;120(23):3669–75. PMID:25313458
1337. Hundal R, Shaffer EA. Gallbladder cancer: epidemiology and outcome. Clin Epidemiol. 2014 Mar 7;6:99–109. PMID:24634588
1338. Hunt RH, Camilleri M, Crowe SE, et al. The stomach in health and disease. Gut. 2015 Oct;64(10):1650–68. PMID:26342014
1339. Hunter J, Harmston C, Hughes P, et al. What is the nature of polyps detected by the NHS bowel cancer screening pilots? Colorectal Dis. 2011 May;13(5):538–41. PMID:20088957
1340. Huntsman DG, Carneiro F, Lewis FR, et al. Early gastric cancer in young, asymptomatic carriers of germ-line E-cadherin mutations. N Engl J Med. 2001 Jun 21;344(25):1904–9. PMID:11419427
1341. Hurley JJ, Thomas LE, Walton SJ, et al. The impact of chromoendoscopy for surveillance of the duodenum in patients with MUTYH-associated polyposis and familial adenomatous polyposis. Gastrointest Endosc. 2018 Oct;88(4):665–73. PMID:29702101
1342. Huss S, Wardelmann E, Goltz D, et al. Activating PDGFRA mutations in inflammatory fibroid polyps occur in exons 12, 14 and 18 and are associated with tumour localization. Histopathology. 2012 Jul;61(1):59–68. PMID:22394371
1343. Hussein S, Gindin T, Lagana SM, et al. Clonal T cell receptor gene rearrangements in coeliac disease: implications for diagnosing refractory coeliac disease. J Clin Pathol. 2018 Sep;71(9):825–31. PMID:29703761
1344. Hussell T, Isaacson PG, Crabtree JE, et al. The response of cells from low-grade B-cell gastric lymphomas of mucosa-associated lymphoid tissue to Helicobacter pylori. Lancet. 1993 Sep 4;342(8871):571–4. PMID:8102718
1344A. Hutchings D, Waters KM, Weiss MJ, et al. Cancerization of the pancreatic ducts: demonstration of a common and under-recognized process using immunolabeling of paired duct lesions and invasive pancreatic ductal adenocarcinoma for p53 and Smad4 expression. Am J Surg Pathol. 2018 Nov;42(11):1556–61. PMID:30212393
1345. Hwang S, Lee SG, Lee YJ, et al. Radical surgical resection for carcinoid tumors of the ampulla. J Gastrointest Surg. 2008 Apr;12(4):713–7. PMID:17992565
1346. Hyngstrom JR, Hu CY, Xing Y, et al. Clinicopathology and outcomes for mucinous and signet ring colorectal adenocarcinoma: analysis from the National Cancer Data Base. Ann Surg Oncol. 2012 Sep;19(9):2814–21. PMID:22476818
1347. Hyun JS, Kim GB, Choi BS, et al. Giant anal condyloma (giant condyloma acuminatum of anus) after allogeneic bone marrow transplantation associated with human papillomavirus: a case report. J Med Case Rep. 2015 Jan 19;9:9. PMID:25597932
1348. Iacobuzio-Donahue CA, Klimstra DS, Adsay NV, et al. Dpc-4 protein is expressed in virtually all human intraductal papillary mucinous neoplasms of the pancreas: comparison with conventional ductal adenocarcinomas. Am J Pathol. 2000 Sep;157(3):755–61. PMID:10980115
1349. Iacobuzio-Donahue CA, Wilentz RE, Argani P, et al. Dpc4 protein in mucinous cystic neoplasms of the pancreas: frequent loss of expression in invasive carcinomas suggests a role in genetic progression. Am J Surg Pathol. 2000 Nov;24(11):1544–8. PMID:11075857
1350. Iacovazzo D, Flanagan SE, Walker E, et al. MAFA missense mutation causes familial insulinomatosis and diabetes mellitus. Proc Natl Acad Sci U S A. 2018 Jan 30;115(5):1027–32. PMID:29339498
1351. IARC Monographs on the Evaluation of Carcinogenic Risks to Humans [Internet]. Lyon (France): International Agency for Research on Cancer; 2018. Agents classified by the IARC Monographs, Volumes 1–122; updated 2018 Jul 30. Available from: https://monographs.iarc.fr/agents-classified-by-the-iarc/.
1352. IARC Working Group on the Evaluation of Carcinogenic Risks to Humans. Tobacco smoke and involuntary smoking. IARC Monogr Eval Carcinog Risks Hum. 2004;83:1–1438. PMID:15285078
1353. Iavarone M, Manini MA, Sangiovanni A, et al. Contrast-enhanced computed tomography and ultrasound-guided liver biopsy to diagnose dysplastic liver nodules in cirrhosis. Dig Liver Dis. 2013 Jan;45(1):43–9. PMID:23022425
1354. Ibrahim AE, Arends MJ, Silva AL, et al. Sequential DNA methylation changes are associated with DNMT3B overexpression in colorectal neoplastic progression. Gut. 2011 Apr;60(4):499–508. PMID:21068132
1355. Ichihara S, Uedo N, Gotoda T. Considering the esophagogastric junction as a 'zone'. Dig Endosc. 2017 Apr;29 Suppl 2:3–10. PMID:28425656
1356. Ichimura T, Abe H, Morikawa T, et al. Low density of CD204-positive M2-type tumor-associated macrophages in Epstein-Barr virus-associated gastric cancer: a clinicopathologic study with digital image analysis. Hum Pathol. 2016 Oct;56:74–80. PMID:27342912
1357. Iddings DM, Fleisig AJ, Chen SL, et al. Practice patterns and outcomes for anorectal melanoma in the USA, reviewing three decades of treatment: is more extensive surgical resection beneficial in all patients? Ann Surg Oncol. 2010 Jan;17(1):40–4. PMID:19774417
1358. Idelevich E, Kashtan H, Mavor E, et al. Small bowel obstruction caused by secondary tumors. Surg Oncol. 2006 Jul;15(1):29–32. PMID:16905310
1359. Ideno N, Ohtsuka T, Kono H, et al. Intraductal papillary mucinous neoplasms of the pancreas with distinct pancreatic ductal adenocarcinomas are frequently of gastric subtype. Ann Surg. 2013 Jul;258(1):141–51. PMID:23532108
1360. Igarashi H, Ito T, Nishimori I, et al. Pancreatic involvement in Japanese patients with von Hippel-Lindau disease: results of a nationwide survey. J Gastroenterol. 2014 Mar;49(3):511–6. PMID:23543325
1361. IJspeert JE, Rana SA, Atkinson NS, et al. Clinical risk factors of colorectal cancer in patients with serrated polyposis syndrome: a multicentre cohort analysis. Gut. 2017 Feb;66(2):278–84. PMID:26603485
1362. IJspeert JE, Tutein Nolthenius CJ, Kuipers EJ, et al. CT-colonography vs. colonoscopy for detection of high-risk sessile serrated polyps. Am J Gastroenterol. 2016 Apr;111(4):516–22. PMID:27021193
1363. IJspeert JEG, Bevan R, Senore C, et al. Detection rate of serrated polyps and serrated polyposis syndrome in colorectal cancer screening cohorts: a European overview. Gut. 2017 Jul;66(7):1225–32. PMID:26911398
1364. Ikenberg H, Gissmann L, Gross G, et al. Human papillomavirus type-16-related DNA in genital Bowen's disease and in Bowenoid papulosis. Int J Cancer. 1983 Nov 15;32(5):563–5. PMID:6315601
1365. Ikoma N, Blum M, Chiang YJ, et al. Yield of staging laparoscopy and lavage cytology for radiologically occult peritoneal carcinomatosis of gastric cancer. Ann Surg Oncol. 2016 Dec;23(13):4332–7. PMID:27384751
1366. Ilardi G, Caroppo D, Varricchio S, et al. Anal melanoma with neuroendocrine differentiation: report of a case. Int J Surg Pathol. 2015 Jun;23(4):329–32. PMID:25722317
1367. Ilbawi AM, Simianu VV, Millie M, et al. Wide local excision of perianal mucinous adenocarcinoma. J Clin Oncol. 2015 Feb 1;33(4):e16–8. PMID:24590647
1368. Ilus T, Kaukinen K, Virta LJ, et al. Refractory coeliac disease in a country with a high prevalence of clinically-diagnosed coeliac disease. Aliment Pharmacol Ther. 2014 Feb;39(4):418–25. PMID:24387637
1369. Imaoka H, Shimizu Y, Mizuno N, et al. Clinical characteristics of adenosquamous carcinoma of the pancreas: a matched case-control study. Pancreas. 2014 Mar;43(2):287–90. PMID:24518509
1370. Imaoka H, Shimizu Y, Mizuno N, et al. Ring-enhancement pattern on contrast-enhanced CT predicts adenosquamous carcinoma of the pancreas: a matched case-control study. Pancreatology. 2014 May-Jun;14(3):221–6. PMID:24854619
1371. Inagawa S, Shimazaki J, Hori M, et al. Hepatoid adenocarcinoma of the stomach. Gastric Cancer. 2001;4(1):43–52. PMID:11706627
1372. Inai K, Kobuke T, Yonehara S, et al. Duodenal gangliocytic paraganglioma with lymph node metastasis in a 17-year-old boy. Cancer. 1989 Jun 15;63(12):2540–5. PMID:2655873
1373. Inayat F, Hassan GU, Tayyab GUN, et al. Post-transplantation lymphoproliferative disorder with gastrointestinal involvement. Ann Gastroenterol. 2018 Mar-Apr;31(2):248–51. PMID:29507477
1374. Ingkakul T, Warshaw AL, Fernández-Del Castillo C. Epidemiology of intraductal papillary mucinous neoplasms of the pancreas: sex differences between 3 geographic regions. Pancreas. 2011 Jul;40(5):779–80. PMID:21673537
1375. Inoue H, Furukawa T, Sunamura M, et al. Exclusion of SMAD4 mutation as an early genetic change in human pancreatic ductal tumorigenesis. Genes Chromosomes Cancer. 2001 Jul;31(3):295–9. PMID:11391801
1376. Inoue H, Kaga M, Ikeda H, et al.

Magnification endoscopy in esophageal squamous cell carcinoma: a review of the intrapapillary capillary loop classification. Ann Gastroenterol. 2015 Jan-Mar;28(1):41–8. PMID:25608626

1377. Inoue T, Nishi Y, Okumura F, et al. Solid pseudopapillary neoplasm of the pancreas associated with familial adenomatous polyposis. Intern Med. 2015;54(11):1349–55. PMID:26027985

1378. Insabato L, Guadagno E, Natella V, et al. An unusual association of malignant gastrointestinal neuroectodermal tumor (clear cell sarcoma-like) and Ewing sarcoma. Pathol Res Pract. 2015 Sep;211(9):688–92. PMID:26163185

1378A. International Association of Cancer Registries (IACR) [Internet]. Lyon (France): International Agency for Research on Cancer; 2019. ICD-O-3.2; updated 2019 Apr 23 [cited 2019 May 10]. Available from: http://www.iacr.com.fr/index.php?option=com_content&view=article&id=149:icd-o-3-2&catid=80&Itemid=545

1379. International Consensus Group for Hepatocellular Neoplasia. Pathologic diagnosis of early hepatocellular carcinoma: a report of the International Consensus Group for Hepatocellular Neoplasia. Hepatology. 2009 Feb;49(2):658–64. PMID:19177576

1380. International Society for Gastrointestinal Hereditary Tumours Database [Internet]. Leiden (Netherlands): Leiden University Medical Center; 2018. Available from: https://www.insight-database.org.

1381. International Society for Gastrointestinal Hereditary Tumours [Internet]. Middlesex (UK): International Society for Gastrointestinal Hereditary Tumours; 2018. MMR gene variant classification criteria. Available from: https://www.insight-group.org/criteria/.

1382. Iodice S, Gandini S, Maisonneuve P, et al. Tobacco and the risk of pancreatic cancer: a review and meta-analysis. Langenbecks Arch Surg. 2008 Jul;393(4):535–45. PMID:18193270

1383. Iqbal J, Greiner TC, Patel K, et al. Distinctive patterns of BCL6 molecular alterations and their functional consequences in different subgroups of diffuse large B-cell lymphoma. Leukemia. 2007 Nov;21(11):2332–43. PMID:17625604

1384. Iqbal J, Neppalli VT, Wright G, et al. BCL2 expression is a prognostic marker for the activated B-cell-like type of diffuse large B-cell lymphoma. J Clin Oncol. 2006 Feb 20;24(6):961–8. PMID:16418494

1385. Isaacs H Jr. Fetal and neonatal hepatic tumors. J Pediatr Surg. 2007 Nov;42(11):1797–803. PMID:18022426

1386. Isaacson PG, Dogan A, Price SK, et al. Immunoproliferative small-intestinal disease. An immunohistochemical study. Am J Surg Pathol. 1989 Dec;13(12):1023–33. PMID:2512818

1387. Isaacson PG, Du MQ. Gastrointestinal lymphoma: where morphology meets molecular biology. J Pathol. 2005 Jan;205(2):255–74. PMID:15643667

1388. Isaji S, Kawarada Y, Uemoto S. Classification of pancreatic cancer: comparison of Japanese and UICC classifications. Pancreas. 2004 Apr;28(3):231–4. PMID:15084962

1389. Iscovich J, Boffetta P, Franceschi S, et al. Classic Kaposi sarcoma: epidemiology and risk factors. Cancer. 2000 Feb 1;88(3):500–17. PMID:10649240

1390. Ishak KG, Sesterhenn IA, Goodman ZD, et al. Epithelioid hemangioendothelioma of the liver: a clinicopathologic and follow-up study of 32 cases. Hum Pathol. 1984 Sep;15(9):839–52. PMID:6088383

1391. Ishibashi H, Nimura S, Kayashima Y, et al. Multiple lesions of gastrointestinal tract invasion by monomorphic epitheliotropic intestinal T-cell lymphoma, accompanied by duodenal and intestinal enteropathy-like lesions and microscopic lymphocytic proctocolitis: a case series. Diagn Pathol. 2016 Jul 25;11(1):66. PMID:27457239

1392. Ishibashi Y, Matsuzono E, Yokoyama F, et al. A case of lymphomatoid gastropathy: a self-limited pseudomalignant natural killer (NK)-cell proliferative disease mimicking NK/T-cell lymphomas. Clin J Gastroenterol. 2013 Aug;6(4):287–90. PMID:26181731

1393. Ishida K, Sasano H, Moriya T, et al. Immunohistochemical analysis of steroidogenic enzymes in ovarian-type stroma of pancreatic mucinous cystic neoplasms: comparative study of subepithelial stromal cells in intraductal papillary mucinous neoplasms of the pancreas. Pathol Int. 2016 May;66(5):281–7. PMID:27060902

1394. Ishii M, Ota M, Saito S, et al. Lymphatic vessel invasion detected by monoclonal antibody D2-40 as a predictor of lymph node metastasis in T1 colorectal cancer. Int J Colorectal Dis. 2009 Sep;24(9):1069–74. PMID:19387662

1395. Ishii Y, Sasaki T, Serikawa M, et al. Elevated expression of cyclooxygenase-2 and microsomal prostaglandin E synthase-1 in primary sclerosing cholangitis: implications for cholangiocarcinogenesis. Int J Oncol. 2013 Oct;43(4):1073–9. PMID:23900502

1396. Ishikawa E, Tanaka T, Shimada K, et al. A prognostic model, including the EBV status of tumor cells, for primary gastric diffuse large B-cell lymphoma in the rituximab era. Cancer Med. 2018 Jun 1. PMID:29856127

1397. Ishikawa T, Nakao A, Nomoto S, et al. Immunohistochemical and molecular biological studies of serous cystadenoma of the pancreas. Pancreas. 1998 Jan;16(1):40–4. PMID:9436861

1398. Isikdogan A, Ayyildiz O, Buyukcelik A, et al. Non-Hodgkin's lymphoma in southeast Turkey: clinicopathologic features of 490 cases. Ann Hematol. 2004 May;83(5):265–9. PMID:15060744

1399. Islam F, Tang JC, Gopalan V, et al. Epigenetics: DNA methylation analysis in esophageal adenocarcinoma. Methods Mol Biol. 2018;1756:247–56. PMID:29600375

1400. Islami F, Ferlay J, Lortet-Tieulent J, et al. International trends in anal cancer incidence rates. Int J Epidemiol. 2017 Jun 1;46(3):924–38. PMID:27789668

1401. Ismail H, Dembowska-Bagińska B, Broniszczak D, et al. Treatment of undifferentiated embryonal sarcoma of the liver in children–single center experience. J Pediatr Surg. 2013 Nov;48(11):2202–6. PMID:24210186

1402. Isom JA, Arroyo MR, Reddy D, et al. NK cell enteropathy: a case report with 10 years of indolent clinical behaviour. Histopathology. 2018 Aug;73(2):345–50. PMID:29474745

1403. Isomoto H, Maeda T, Akashi T, et al. Multiple lymphomatous polyposis of the colon originating from T-cells: a case report. Dig Liver Dis. 2004 Mar;36(3):218–21. PMID:15046193

1404. Itakura E, Yamamoto H, Oda Y, et al. Detection and characterization of vascular endothelial growth factors and their receptors in a series of angiosarcomas. J Surg Oncol. 2008 Jan 1;97(1):74–81. PMID:18041747

1405. Italiano A, Chen CL, Thomas R, et al. Alterations of the p53 and PIK3CA/AKT/mTOR pathways in angiosarcomas: a pattern distinct from other sarcomas with complex genomics. Cancer. 2012 Dec 1;118(23):5878–87. PMID:22648906

1406. Italiano A, Lagarde P, Brulard C, et al. Genetic profiling identifies two classes of soft-tissue leiomyosarcomas with distinct clinical characteristics. Clin Cancer Res. 2013 Mar 1;19(5):1190–6. PMID:23329812

1407. Ito H, Hann LE, D'Angelica M, et al. Polypoid lesions of the gallbladder: diagnosis and followup. J Am Coll Surg. 2009 Apr;208(4):570–5. PMID:19476792

1408. Ito T, Igarashi H, Nakamura K, et al. Epidemiological trends of pancreatic and gastrointestinal neuroendocrine tumors in Japan: a nationwide survey analysis. J Gastroenterol. 2015 Jan;50(1):58–64. PMID:24499825

1409. Ito T, Sasano H, Tanaka M, et al. Epidemiological study of gastroenteropancreatic neuroendocrine tumors in Japan. J Gastroenterol. 2010 Feb;45(2):234–43. PMID:20058030

1410. Iwama T, Mishima Y, Utsunomiya J. The impact of familial adenomatous polyposis on the tumorigenesis and mortality at the several organs. Its rational treatment. Ann Surg. 1993 Feb;217(2):101–8. PMID:8382467

1411. Iwao M, Nakamuta M, Enjoji M, et al. Primary hepatic carcinoid tumor: case report and review of 53 cases. Med Sci Monit. 2001 Jul-Aug;7(4):746–50. PMID:11433205

1412. Iyomasa S, Kato H, Tachimori Y, et al. Carcinosarcoma of the esophagus: a twenty-case study. Jpn J Clin Oncol. 1990 Mar;20(1):99–106. PMID:2319703

1413. Iype S, Mirza TA, Propper DJ, et al. Neuroendocrine tumours of the gallbladder: three cases and a review of the literature. Postgrad Med J. 2009 Apr;85(1002):213–8. PMID:19417172

1414. Izadi M, Taheri S. Features, predictors and prognosis of lymphoproliferative disorders post-liver transplantation regarding disease presentation time: report from the PTLD.Int. survey. Ann Transplant. 2011 Jan-Mar;16(1):39–47. PMID:21436773

1415. Izumo A, Yamaguchi K, Eguchi T, et al. Mucinous cystic tumor of the pancreas: immunohistochemical assessment of "ovarian-type stroma". Oncol Rep. 2003 May-Jun;10(3):515–25. PMID:12684617

1416. Jaeger E, Leedham S, Lewis A, et al. Hereditary mixed polyposis syndrome is caused by a 40-kb upstream duplication that leads to increased and ectopic expression of the BMP antagonist GREM1. Nat Genet. 2012 May 6;44(6):699–703. PMID:22561515

1417. Jaffe ES, Harris NL, Swerdlow SH, et al. Follicular lymphoma. In: Swerdlow SH, Campo E, Harris NL, et al., editors. WHO classification of tumours of haematopoietic and lymphoid tissues. Lyon (France): International Agency for Research on Cancer; 2017. pp. 266–77. (WHO classification of tumours series, 4th rev. ed.; vol. 2). http://publications.iarc.fr/556.

1418. Jagelman DG, DeCosse JJ, Bussey HJ. Upper gastrointestinal cancer in familial adenomatous polyposis. Lancet. 1988 May 21;1(8595):1149–51. PMID:2896968

1419. Jais B, Rebours V, Malleo G, et al. Serous cystic neoplasm of the pancreas: a multinational study of 2622 patients under the auspices of the International Association of Pancreatology and European Pancreatic Club (European Study Group on Cystic Tumors of the Pancreas). Gut. 2016 Feb;65(2):305–12. PMID:26045140

1420. Jamel S, Markar SR, Malietzis G, et al. Prognostic significance of peritoneal lavage cytology in staging gastric cancer: systematic review and meta-analysis. Gastric Cancer. 2018 Jan;21(1):10–8. PMID:28779261

1421. James RD, Glynne-Jones R, Meadows HM, et al. Mitomycin or cisplatin chemoradiation with or without maintenance chemotherapy for treatment of squamous-cell carcinoma of the anus (ACT II): a randomised, phase 3, open-label, 2 × 2 factorial trial. Lancet Oncol. 2013 May;14(6):516–24. PMID:23578724

1422. Janeway KA, Kim SY, Lodish M, et al. Defects in succinate dehydrogenase in gastrointestinal stromal tumors lacking KIT and PDGFRA mutations. Proc Natl Acad Sci U S A. 2011 Jan 4;108(1):314–8. PMID:21173220

1423. Jang JY, Kim SW, Ahn YJ, et al. Multicenter analysis of clinicopathologic features of intraductal papillary mucinous tumor of the pancreas: is it possible to predict the malignancy before surgery? Ann Surg Oncol. 2005 Feb;12(2):124–32. PMID:15827792

1424. Jang KT, Park SM, Basturk O, et al. Clinicopathologic characteristics of 29 invasive carcinomas arising in 178 pancreatic mucinous cystic neoplasms with ovarian-type stroma: implications for management and prognosis. Am J Surg Pathol. 2015 Feb;39(2):179–87. PMID:25517958

1425. Jansen AM, van Wezel T, van den Akker BE, et al. Combined mismatch repair and POLE/POLD1 defects explain unresolved suspected Lynch syndrome cancers. Eur J Hum Genet. 2016 Jul;24(7):1089–92. PMID:26648449

1426. Jansen M, de Leng WW, Baas AF, et al. Mucosal prolapse in the pathogenesis of Peutz-Jeghers polyposis. Gut. 2006 Jan;55(1):1–5. PMID:16344569

1427. Japan Esophageal Society. Japanese Classification of Esophageal Cancer, 11th Edition: part I. Esophagus. 2017;14(1):1–36. PMID:28111535

1428. Japan Esophageal Society. Japanese Classification of Esophageal Cancer, 11th Edition: part II and III. Esophagus. 2017;14(1):37–65. PMID:28111536

1429. Japanese Gastric Cancer Association [Internet]. Kyoto (Japan): Japanese Gastric Cancer Association; 2018. [Japanese Gastric Cancer Association report of national registration analysis results: surgical cases in 2009]. Japanese. Available from: http://www.jgca.jp/entry/iganhtml/doc/2009_report.pdf.

1430. Japanese Gastric Cancer Association. Japanese classification of gastric carcinoma. 15th ed. Tokyo (Japan): Kanehara Shuppan; 2017. Japanese.

1431. Japanese Gastric Cancer Association. Japanese classification of gastric carcinoma: 3rd English edition. Gastric Cancer. 2011 Jun;14(2):101–12. PMID:21573743

1432. Japanese Gastric Cancer Association. Japanese gastric cancer treatment guidelines 2014 (ver. 4). Gastric Cancer. 2017 Jan;20(1):1–19. PMID:27342689

1433. Japanese Gastric Cancer Association. Japanese gastric cancer treatment guidelines. 5th ed. Tokyo (Japan): Kanehara Shuppan; 2018. Japanese.

1434. Jasperson KW, Patel SG, Ahnen DJ. APC-associated polyposis conditions. In: Adam MP, Ardinger HH, Pagon RA, et al., editors. GeneReviews. Seattle (WA): University of Washington, Seattle; 1998 Dec 18 [updated 2017 Feb 2]. PMID:20301519

1435. Jass JR, Atkin WS, Cuzick J, et al. The grading of rectal cancer: historical perspectives and a multivariate analysis of 447 cases. Histopathology. 1986 May;10(5):437–59. PMID:3721406

1436. Jass JR, Williams CB, Bussey HJ, et al. Juvenile polyposis–a precancerous condition. Histopathology. 1988 Dec;13(6):619–30. PMID:2853131

1437. Jass JR. Intestinal metaplasia and gastric cancer. Histopathology. 1987 Aug;11(8):881. PMID:3623443

1438. Javle M, Bekaii-Saab T, Jain A, et al. Biliary cancer: utility of next-generation sequencing for clinical management. Cancer. 2016 Dec 15;122(24):3838–47. PMID:27622582

1439. Jaworski RC, Biankin SA, Baird PJ.

Squamous cell carcinoma in situ arising in inflammatory cloacogenic polyps: report of two cases with PCR analysis for HPV DNA. Pathology. 2001 Aug;33(3):312–4. PMID:11523931

1440. Jeannot E, Poussin K, Chiche L, et al. Association of CYP1B1 germ line mutations with hepatocyte nuclear factor 1alpha-mutated hepatocellular adenoma. Cancer Res. 2007 Mar 15;67(6):2611–6. PMID:17363580

1441. Jederán É, Lővey J, Szentirmai Z, et al. The role of MRI in the assessment of the local status of anal carcinomas and in their management. Pathol Oncol Res. 2015 Jul;21(3):571–9. PMID:25354914

1442. Jelsig AM, Brusgaard K, Hansen TP, et al. Germline variants in hamartomatous polyposis syndrome-associated genes from patients with one or few hamartomatous polyps. Scand J Gastroenterol. 2016 Sep;51(9):1118–25. PMID:27146957

1443. Jemal A, Ward EM, Johnson CJ, et al. Annual report to the nation on the status of cancer, 1975-2014, featuring survival. J Natl Cancer Inst. 2017 Sep 1;109(9). PMID:28376154

1444. Jenkins MA, Hayashi S, O'Shea AM, et al. Pathology features in Bethesda guidelines predict colorectal cancer microsatellite instability: a population-based study. Gastroenterology. 2007 Jul;133(1):48–56. PMID:17631130

1445. Jensen LH, Bojesen A, Byriel L, et al. Implementing population-based screening for Lynch syndrome [abstract]. J Clin Oncol. 2013 May 20;31(15_suppl). Abstract no. 6600. doi:10.1200/jco.2013.31.15_suppl.6600.

1446. Jensen RT, Cadiot G, Brandi ML, et al. ENETS Consensus Guidelines for the management of patients with digestive neuroendocrine neoplasms: functional pancreatic endocrine tumor syndromes. Neuroendocrinology. 2012;95(2):98–119. PMID:22261919

1447. Jensen RT. Gastrointestinal abnormalities and involvement in systemic mastocytosis. Hematol Oncol Clin North Am. 2000 Jun;14(3):579–623. PMID:10909042

1448. Jeong D, Jiang K, Anaya DA. Mucinous cystic neoplasm of the liver masquerading as an echinococcal cyst: radiologic-pathologic differential of complex cystic liver lesions. J Clin Imaging Sci. 2016 Mar 30;6:12. PMID:27195178

1449. Jesinghaus M, Konukiewitz B, Foersch S, et al. Appendiceal goblet cell carcinoids and adenocarcinomas ex-goblet cell carcinoid are genetically distinct from primary colorectal-type adenocarcinoma of the appendix. Mod Pathol. 2018 May;31(5):829–39. PMID:29327707

1450. Jesinghaus M, Konukiewitz B, Keller G, et al. Colorectal mixed adenoneuroendocrine carcinomas and neuroendocrine carcinomas are genetically closely related to colorectal adenocarcinomas. Mod Pathol. 2017 Apr;30(4):610–9. PMID:28059096

1451. Jess T, Gamborg M, Matzen P, et al. Increased risk of intestinal cancer in Crohn's disease: a meta-analysis of population-based cohort studies. Am J Gastroenterol. 2005 Dec;100(12):2724–9. PMID:16393226

1452. Jess T, Loftus EV Jr, Velayos FS, et al. Risk factors for colorectal neoplasia in inflammatory bowel disease: a nested case-control study from Copenhagen County, Denmark and Olmsted County, Minnesota. Am J Gastroenterol. 2007 Apr;102(4):829–36. PMID:17222314

1453. Jess T, Rungoe C, Peyrin-Biroulet L. Risk of colorectal cancer in patients with ulcerative colitis: a meta-analysis of population-based cohort studies. Clin Gastroenterol Hepatol. 2012 Jun;10(6):639–45. PMID:22289873

1454. Jetmore AB, Ray JE, Gathright JB Jr, et al. Rectal carcinoids: the most frequent carcinoid tumor. Dis Colon Rectum. 1992 Aug;35(8):717–25. PMID:1643994

1455. Jha HC, Pei Y, Robertson ES. Epstein-Barr virus: diseases linked to infection and transformation. Front Microbiol. 2016 Oct 25;7:1602. PMID:27826287

1456. Jiang BG, Sun LL, Yu WL, et al. Retrospective analysis of histopathologic prognostic factors after hepatectomy for intrahepatic cholangiocarcinoma. Cancer J. 2009 May-Jun;15(3):257–61. PMID:19556914

1457. Jiang L, Gu ZH, Yan ZX, et al. Exome sequencing identifies somatic mutations of DDX3X in natural killer/T-cell lymphoma. Nat Genet. 2015 Sep;47(9):1061–6. PMID:26192917

1458. Jiang M, Chen X, Yi Z, et al. Prognostic characteristics of gastrointestinal tract NK/T-cell lymphoma: an analysis of 47 patients in China. J Clin Gastroenterol. 2013 Sep;47(8):e74–9. PMID:23948755

1459. Jiang W, Shadrach B, Carver P, et al. Histomorphologic and molecular features of pouch and peripouch adenocarcinoma: a comparison with ulcerative colitis-associated adenocarcinoma. Am J Surg Pathol. 2012 Sep;36(9):1385–94. PMID:22895272

1461. Jiao L, Chen L, White DL, et al. Low-fat dietary pattern and pancreatic cancer risk in the Women's Health Initiative Dietary Modification randomized controlled trial. J Natl Cancer Inst. 2018 Jan 1;110(1). PMID:28922784

1462. Jiao Y, Pawlik TM, Anders RA, et al. Exome sequencing identifies frequent inactivating mutations in BAP1, ARID1A and PBRM1 in intrahepatic cholangiocarcinomas. Nat Genet. 2013 Dec;45(12):1470–3. PMID:24185509

1463. Jiao Y, Shi C, Edil BH, et al. DAXX/ATRX, MEN1, and mTOR pathway genes are frequently altered in pancreatic neuroendocrine tumors. Science. 2011 Mar 4;331(6021):1199–203. PMID:21252315

1464. Jiao Y, Yonescu R, Offerhaus GJ, et al. Whole-exome sequencing of pancreatic neoplasms with acinar differentiation. J Pathol. 2014 Mar;232(4):428–35. PMID:24293293

1465. Jideh B, Weltman M, Wu Y, et al. Esophageal squamous papilloma lacks clear clinicopathological associations. World J Clin Cases. 2017 Apr 16;5(4):134–9. PMID:28470005

1466. Jing H, Geng M, Meng Q, et al. Sarcomatoid carcinoma of the stomach with osteoclast-like giant cells. Tumori. 2012 May-Jun;98(3):82e–5e. PMID:22825525

1467. Jo YS, Kim MS, Lee JH, et al. Frequent frameshift mutations in 2 mononucleotide repeats of RNF43 gene and its regional heterogeneity in gastric and colorectal cancers. Hum Pathol. 2015 Nov;46(11):1640–6. PMID:26297255

1468. Joensuu H, Hohenberger P, Corless CL. Gastrointestinal stromal tumour. Lancet. 2013 Sep 14;382(9896):973–83. PMID:23623056

1469. Joensuu H, Rutkowski P, Nishida T, et al. KIT and PDGFRA mutations and the risk of GI stromal tumor recurrence. J Clin Oncol. 2015 Feb 20;33(6):634–42. PMID:25605837

1470. Joensuu H, Vehtari A, Riihimäki J, et al. Risk of recurrence of gastrointestinal stromal tumour after surgery: an analysis of pooled population-based cohorts. Lancet Oncol. 2012 Mar;13(3):265–74. PMID:22153892

1471. Joensuu H, Wardelmann E, Sihto H, et al. Effect of KIT and PDGFRA mutations on survival in patients with gastrointestinal stromal tumors treated with adjuvant imatinib: an exploratory analysis of a randomized clinical trial. JAMA Oncol. 2017 May 1;3(5):602–9. PMID:28334365

1472. Johncilla M, Stachler M, Misdraji J, et al. Mutational landscape of goblet cell carcinoids and adenocarcinoma ex goblet cell carcinoids of the appendix is distinct from typical carcinoids and colorectal adenocarcinomas. Mod Pathol.

2018 Jun;31(6):989–96. PMID:29422640

1473. Johnson CM, Wei C, Ensor JE, et al. Meta-analyses of colorectal cancer risk factors. Cancer Causes Control. 2013 Jun;24(6):1207–22. PMID:23563998

1474. Johnson NA, Slack GW, Savage KJ, et al. Concurrent expression of MYC and BCL2 in diffuse large B-cell lymphoma treated with rituximab plus cyclophosphamide, doxorubicin, vincristine, and prednisone. J Clin Oncol. 2012 Oct 1;30(28):3452–9. PMID:22851565

1475. Johnston WT, Mutalima N, Sun D, et al. Relationship between Plasmodium falciparum malaria prevalence, genetic diversity and endemic Burkitt lymphoma in Malawi. Sci Rep. 2014 Jan 17;4:3741. PMID:24434689

1476. Johnstone JM, Morson BC. Inflammatory fibroid polyp of the gastrointestinal tract. Histopathology. 1978 Sep;2(5):349–61. PMID:721077

1477. Jonas S, Bechstein WO, Steinmüller T, et al. Vascular invasion and histopathologic grading determine outcome after liver transplantation for hepatocellular carcinoma in cirrhosis. Hepatology. 2001 May;33(5):1080–6. PMID:11343235

1478. Jones EA, Morson BC. Mucinous adenocarcinoma in anorectal fistulae. Histopathology. 1984 Mar;8(2):279–92. PMID:6327491

1479. Jones M, Zheng Z, Wang J, et al. Impact of next-generation sequencing on the clinical diagnosis of pancreatic cysts. Gastrointest Endosc. 2016 Jan;83(1):140–8. PMID:26253016

1480. Jones S, Hruban RH, Kamiyama M, et al. Exomic sequencing identifies PALB2 as a pancreatic cancer susceptibility gene. Science. 2009 Apr 10;324(5924):217. PMID:19264984

1481. Jones S, Zhang X, Parsons DW, et al. Core signaling pathways in human pancreatic cancers revealed by global genomic analyses. Science. 2008 Sep 26;321(5897):1801–6. PMID:18772397

1482. Joo M, Shahsafaei A, Odze RD. Paneth cell differentiation in colonic epithelial neoplasms: evidence for the role of the Apc/beta-catenin/Tcf pathway. Hum Pathol. 2009 Jun;40(6):872–80. PMID:19269007

1484. Joseph NM, Ferrell LD, Jain D, et al. Diagnostic utility and limitations of glutamine synthetase and serum amyloid-associated protein immunohistochemistry in the distinction of focal nodular hyperplasia and inflammatory hepatocellular adenoma. Mod Pathol. 2014 Jan;27(1):62–72. PMID:23807780

1485. Jukić Z, Limani R, Luci LG, et al. hGH and GHR expression in large cell neuroendocrine carcinoma of the colon and rectum. Anticancer Res. 2012 Aug;32(8):3377–81. PMID:22843918

1486. Jun JK, Choi KS, Lee HY, et al. Effectiveness of the Korean national cancer screening program in reducing gastric cancer mortality. Gastroenterology. 2017 May;152(6):1319–28. e7. PMID:28147224

1487. Jun SR, Lee JM, Han JK, et al. High-grade neuroendocrine carcinomas of the gallbladder and bile duct: report of four cases with pathological correlation. J Comput Assist Tomogr. 2006 Jul-Aug;30(4):604–9. PMID:16845291

1488. Jun SY, Son D, Kim MJ, et al. Heterotopic pancreas of the gastrointestinal tract and associated precursor and cancerous lesions: systematic pathologic studies of 165 cases. Am J Surg Pathol. 2017 Jun;41(6):833–48. PMID:28368927

1489. Jung G, Park KM, Lee SS, et al. Long-term clinical outcome of the surgically resected intraductal papillary neoplasm of the bile duct. J Hepatol. 2012 Oct;57(4):787–93. PMID:22634127

1490. Jäkel C, Bergmann F, Toth R, et al. Genome-wide genetic and epigenetic analyses of pancreatic acinar cell carcinomas reveal aberrations in genome stability. Nat Commun. 2017 Nov 6;8(1):1323. PMID:29109526

1491. Järvinen HJ, Sipponen P. Gastroduodenal polyps in familial adenomatous and juvenile polyposis. Endoscopy. 1986 Nov;18(6):230–4. PMID:3024956

1492. Kadota T, Fujii S, Oono Y, et al. Adenocarcinoma arising from heterotopic gastric mucosa in the cervical esophagus and upper thoracic esophagus: two case reports and literature review. Expert Rev Gastroenterol Hepatol. 2016;10(3):405–14. PMID:26610162

1493. Kaerlev L, Teglbjaerg PS, Sabroe S, et al. Occupation and small bowel adenocarcinoma: a European case-control study. Occup Environ Med. 2000 Nov;57(11):760–6. PMID:11024200

1494. Kaerlev L, Teglbjaerg PS, Sabroe S, et al. Occupational risk factors for small bowel carcinoid tumor: a European population-based case-control study. J Occup Environ Med. 2002 Jun;44(6):516–22. PMID:12085477

1495. Kahaleh M, Shami VM, Brock A, et al. Factors predictive of malignancy and endoscopic resectability in ampullary neoplasia. Am J Gastroenterol. 2004 Dec;99(12):2335–9. PMID:15571579

1496. Kai K, Yakabe T, Kohya N, et al. A case of unclassified multicystic biliary tumor with biliary adenofibroma features. Pathol Int. 2012 Jul;62(7):506–10. PMID:22726072

1497. Kaiho T, Tanaka T, Tsuchiya S, et al. A case of classical carcinoid tumor of the gallbladder: review of the Japanese published works. Hepatogastroenterology. 1999 Jul-Aug;46(28):2189–95. PMID:10521965

1498. Kakar S, Aksoy S, Burgart LJ, et al. Mucinous carcinoma of the colon: correlation of loss of mismatch repair enzymes with clinicopathologic features and survival. Mod Pathol. 2004 Jun;17(6):696–700. PMID:15017435

1499. Kakar S, Deng G, Smyrk TC, et al. Loss of heterozygosity, aberrant methylation, BRAF mutation and KRAS mutation in colorectal signet ring cell carcinoma. Mod Pathol. 2012 Jul;25(7):1040–7. PMID:22522845

1500. Kakar S, Muir T, Murphy LM, et al. Immunoreactivity of Hep Par 1 in hepatic and extrahepatic tumors and its correlation with albumin in situ hybridization in hepatocellular carcinoma. Am J Clin Pathol. 2003 Mar;119(3):361–6. PMID:12645337

1501. Kakiuchi M, Nishizawa T, Ueda H, et al. Recurrent gain-of-function mutations of RHOA in diffuse-type gastric carcinoma. Nat Genet. 2014 Jun;46(6):583–7. PMID:24816255

1502. Kalb B, Sarmiento JM, Kooby DA, et al. MR imaging of cystic lesions of the pancreas. Radiographics. 2009 Oct;29(6):1749–65. PMID:19959519

1503. Kamboj M, Gandhi JS, Gupta G, et al. Neuroendocrine carcinoma of gall bladder: a series of 19 cases with review of literature. J Gastrointest Cancer. 2015 Dec;46(4):356–64. PMID:26208508

1504. Kamdar KY, Rooney CM, Heslop HE. Posttransplant lymphoproliferative disease following liver transplantation. Curr Opin Organ Transplant. 2011 Jun;16(3):274–80. PMID:21467936

1505. Kaminsky P, Preiss J, Sasatomi E, et al. Biliary adenofibroma: a rare hepatic lesion with malignant features. Hepatology. 2017 Jan;65(1):380–3. PMID:27631648

1506. Kamisawa T, Tu Y, Egawa N, et al. Ductal and acinar differentiation in pancreatic endocrine tumors. Dig Dis Sci. 2002 Oct;47(10):2254–61. PMID:12395898

1507. Kamp K, Feelders RA, van Adrichem RC, et al. Parathyroid hormone-related peptide

(PTHrP) secretion by gastroenteropancreatic neuroendocrine tumors (GEP-NETs): clinical features, diagnosis, management, and follow-up. J Clin Endocrinol Metab. 2014 Sep;99(9):3060–9. PMID:24905065

1508. Kanai N, Nagaki S, Tanaka T. Clear cell carcinoma of the pancreas. Acta Pathol Jpn. 1987 Sep;37(9):1521–6. PMID:3687432

1509. Kanai T, Hirohashi S, Upton MP, et al. Pathology of small hepatocellular carcinoma. A proposal for a new gross classification. Cancer. 1987 Aug 15;60(4):810–9. PMID:2439190

1510. Kanda M, Matthaei H, Wu J, et al. Presence of somatic mutations in most early-stage pancreatic intraepithelial neoplasia. Gastroenterology. 2012 Apr;142(4):730–3.e9. PMID:22226782

1511. Kanda M, Sadakari Y, Borges M, et al. Mutant TP53 in duodenal samples of pancreatic juice from patients with pancreatic cancer or high-grade dysplasia. Clin Gastroenterol Hepatol. 2013 Jun;11(6):719–30.e5. PMID:23200980

1512. Kaneda A, Matsusaka K, Aburatani H, et al. Epstein-Barr virus infection as an epigenetic driver of tumorigenesis. Cancer Res. 2012 Jul 15;72(14):3445–50. PMID:22761333

1513. Kanellis G, Roncador G, Arribas A, et al. Identification of MNDA as a new marker for nodal marginal zone lymphoma. Leukemia. 2009 Oct;23(10):1847–57. PMID:19474799

1514. Kanetkar AV, Patkar S, Khobragade KH, et al. Neuroendocrine carcinoma of gallbladder: a step beyond palliative therapy, experience of 25 cases. J Gastrointest Cancer. 2018 Feb 13. PMID:29435905

1515. Kang JH, Lim YJ, Kang JH, et al. Prevalence of precancerous conditions and gastric cancer based upon the National Cancer Screening Program in Korea for 7 years, single center experience. Gastroenterol Res Pract. 2015;2015:571965. PMID:25642244

1516. Kang SY, Park CK, Chang DK, et al. Lynch-like syndrome: characterization and comparison with EPCAM deletion carriers. Int J Cancer. 2015 Apr 1;136(7):1568–78. PMID:25110875

1517. Kano Y, Kakinuma S, Goto F, et al. Primary hepatic neuroendocrine carcinoma with a cholangiocellular carcinoma component in one nodule. Clin J Gastroenterol. 2014 Oct;7(5):449–54. PMID:26184027

1518. Kanwal F, Kramer JR, Ilyas J, et al. HCV genotype 3 is associated with an increased risk of cirrhosis and hepatocellular cancer in a national sample of U.S. veterans with HCV. Hepatology. 2014 Jul;60(1):98–105. PMID:24615981

1519. Kaplan KJ, Goodman ZD, Ishak KG. Liver involvement in Langerhans' cell histiocytosis: a study of nine cases. Mod Pathol. 1999 Apr;12(4):370–8. PMID:10229501

1520. Kapran Y, Bauersfeld J, Anlauf M, et al. Multihormonality and entrapment of islets in pancreatic endocrine tumors. Virchows Arch. 2006 Apr;448(4):394–8. PMID:16418841

1521. Kapur RP, Berry JE, Tsuchiya KD, et al. Activation of the chromosome 19q microRNA cluster in sporadic and androgenetic-biparental mosaicism-associated hepatic mesenchymal hamartoma. Pediatr Dev Pathol. 2014 Mar-Apr;17(2):75–84. PMID:24555441

1522. Karamurzin Y, Zeng Z, Stadler ZK, et al. Unusual DNA mismatch repair-deficient tumors in Lynch syndrome: a report of new cases and review of the literature. Hum Pathol. 2012 Oct;43(10):1677–87. PMID:22516243

1523. Karamzadeh Dashti N, Bahrami A, Lee SJ, et al. BRAF V600E mutations occur in a subset of glomus tumors, and are associated with malignant histologic characteristics. Am J Surg Pathol. 2017 Nov;41(11):1532–41. PMID:28834810

1524. Karanjawala ZE, Illei PB, Ashfaq R, et al. New markers of pancreatic cancer identified through differential gene expression analyses: claudin 18 and annexin A8. Am J Surg Pathol. 2008 Feb;32(2):188–96. PMID:18223320

1525. Karaoglanoglu N, Eroglu A, Turkyilmaz A, et al. Oesophageal adenoid cystic carcinoma and its management options. Int J Clin Pract. 2005 Sep;59(9):1101–3. PMID:16115189

1526. Kardon DE, Thompson LD, Przygodzki RM, et al. Adenosquamous carcinoma of the pancreas: a clinicopathologic series of 25 cases. Mod Pathol. 2001 May;14(5):443–51. PMID:11353055

1527. Karhunen PJ. Benign hepatic tumours and tumour like conditions in men. J Clin Pathol. 1986 Feb;39(2):183–8. PMID:3950039

1528. Karlo C, Leschka S, Dettmer M, et al. Hepatic teratoma and peritoneal gliomatosis: a case report. Cases J. 2009 Dec 10;2:9302. PMID:20062626

1529. Karpathakis A, Dibra H, Pipinikas C, et al. Prognostic impact of novel molecular subtypes of small intestinal neuroendocrine tumor. Clin Cancer Res. 2016 Jan 1;22(1):250–8. PMID:26169971

1530. Karpelowsky JS, Pansini A, Lazarus C, et al. Difficulties in the management of mesenchymal hamartomas. Pediatr Surg Int. 2008 Oct;24(10):1171–5. PMID:18751987

1531. Karube K, Scarfò L, Campo E, et al. Monoclonal B cell lymphocytosis and "in situ" lymphoma. Semin Cancer Biol. 2014 Feb;24:3–14. PMID:23999128

1532. Kasenda B, Bass A, Koeberle D, et al. Survival in overweight patients with advanced pancreatic carcinoma: a multicentre cohort study. BMC Cancer. 2014 Sep 29;14:728. PMID:25266049

1533. Kashyap P, Sweetser S, Farrugia G. Esophageal papillomas and skin abnormalities. Focal dermal hypoplasia (Goltz syndrome) manifesting with esophageal papillomatosis. Gastroenterology. 2011 Mar;140(3):784, 1111. PMID:21272558

1534. Kasper B, Baumgarten C, Garcia J, et al. An update on the management of sporadic desmoid-type fibromatosis: a European Consensus Initiative between Sarcoma PAtients EuroNet (SPAEN) and European Organization for Research and Treatment of Cancer (EORTC)/ Soft Tissue and Bone Sarcoma Group (STBSG). Ann Oncol. 2017 Oct 1;28(10):2399–408. PMID:28961825

1535. Kasper B, Ströbel P, Hohenberger P. Desmoid tumors: clinical features and treatment options for advanced disease. Oncologist. 2011;16(5):682–93. PMID:21478276

1536. Katabi N, Albores-Saavedra J. The extrahepatic bile duct lesions in end-stage primary sclerosing cholangitis. Am J Surg Pathol. 2003 Mar;27(3):349–55. PMID:12604891

1537. Katabi N, Torres J, Klimstra DS. Intraductal tubular neoplasms of the bile ducts. Am J Surg Pathol. 2012 Nov;36(11):1647–55. PMID:23073323

1538. Katabi N. Neoplasia of gallbladder and biliary epithelium. Arch Pathol Lab Med. 2010 Nov;134(11):1621–7. PMID:21043815

1539. Katai H, Ishikawa T, Akazawa K, et al. Five-year survival analysis of surgically resected gastric cancer cases in Japan: a retrospective analysis of more than 100,000 patients from the nationwide registry of the Japanese Gastric Cancer Association (2001-2007). Gastric Cancer. 2018 Jan;21(1):144–54. PMID:28417260

1540. Katoh H, Ishikawa S. Genomic pathobiology of gastric carcinoma. Pathol Int. 2017 Feb;67(2):63–71. PMID:28004449

1541. Kawamoto K, Nakamura S, Iwashita A, et al. Clinicopathological characteristics of primary gastric T-cell lymphoma. Histopathology. 2009 Dec;55(6):641–53. PMID:20002766

1542. Kawamoto S, Hiraoka T, Kanemitsu K, et al. Alpha-fetoprotein-producing pancreatic cancer–a case report and review of 28 cases. Hepatogastroenterology. 1992 Jun;39(3):282–6. PMID:1380476

1543. Kawamoto S, Shi C, Hruban RH, et al. Small serotonin-producing neuroendocrine tumor of the pancreas associated with pancreatic duct obstruction. AJR Am J Roentgenol. 2011 Sep;197(3):W482-8. PMID:21862776

1544. Kawamoto Y, Ome Y, Terada K, et al. Undifferentiated carcinoma with osteoclast-like giant cells of the ampullary region: short term survival after pancreaticoduodenectomy. Int J Surg Case Rep. 2016;24:199–202. PMID:27281360

1545. Kawanaka Y, Kitajima K, Fukushima K, et al. Added value of pretreatment (18) F-FDG PET/CT for staging of advanced gastric cancer: comparison with contrast-enhanced MDCT. Eur J Radiol. 2016 May;85(5):989–95. PMID:27130061

1546. Kawanowa K, Sakuma Y, Sakurai S, et al. High incidence of microscopic gastrointestinal stromal tumors in the stomach. Hum Pathol. 2006 Dec;37(12):1527–35. PMID:16996566

1547. Kawazoe A, Kuwata T, Kuboki Y, et al. Clinicopathological features of programmed death ligand 1 expression with tumor-infiltrating lymphocyte, mismatch repair, and Epstein-Barr virus status in a large cohort of gastric cancer patients. Gastric Cancer. 2017 May;20(3):407–15. PMID:27629881

1548. Kayahara M, Nakagawara H, Kitagawa H, et al. The nature of neural invasion by pancreatic cancer. Pancreas. 2007 Oct;35(3):218–23. PMID:17895841

1549. Kaye PV, Haider SA, Ilyas M, et al. Barrett's dysplasia and the Vienna classification: reproducibility, prediction of progression and impact of consensus reporting and p53 immunohistochemistry. Histopathology. 2009 May;54(6):699–712. PMID:19438745

1550. Kedrin D, Gala MK. Genetics of the serrated pathway to colorectal cancer. Clin Transl Gastroenterol. 2015 Apr 9;6:e84. PMID:25856207

1551. Kelly GL, Stylianou J, Rasaiyaah J, et al. Different patterns of Epstein-Barr virus latency in endemic Burkitt lymphoma (BL) lead to distinct variants within the BL-associated gene expression signature. J Virol. 2013 Mar;87(5):2882–94. PMID:23269792

1552. Kelly PJ, Shinagare S, Sainani N, et al. Cystic papillary pattern in pancreatic ductal adenocarcinoma: a heretofore undescribed morphologic pattern that mimics intraductal papillary mucinous carcinoma. Am J Surg Pathol. 2012 May;36(5):696–701. PMID:22367300

1553. Kempers MJ, Kuiper RP, Ockeloen CW, et al. Risk of colorectal and endometrial cancers in EPCAM deletion-positive Lynch syndrome: a cohort study. Lancet Oncol. 2011 Jan;12(1):49–55. PMID:21145788

1554. Kennedy RD, Bylesjo M, Kerr P, et al. Development and independent validation of a prognostic assay for stage II colon cancer using formalin-fixed paraffin-embedded tissue. J Clin Oncol. 2011 Dec 10;29(35):4620–6. PMID:22067406

1555. Kenney B, Singh G, Salem RR, et al. Pseudointraductal papillary mucinous neoplasia caused by microscopic periductal endocrine tumors of the pancreas: a report of 3 cases. Hum Pathol. 2011 Jul;42(7):1034–41. PMID:21292301

1556. Kern MA, Breuhahn K, Schirmacher P. Molecular pathogenesis of human hepatocellular carcinoma. Adv Cancer Res. 2002;86:67–112. PMID:12374281

1557. Kerr NJ, Fukuzawa R, Reeve AE, et al. Beckwith-Wiedemann syndrome, pancreatoblastoma, and the wnt signaling pathway. Am J Pathol. 2002 Apr;160(4):1541–2, author reply 1542. PMID:11943738

1558. Keutgen XM, Nilubol N, Kebebew E. Malignant-functioning neuroendocrine tumors of the pancreas: a survival analysis. Surgery. 2016 May;159(5):1382–9. PMID:26704781

1559. Khalil MO, Morton LM, Devesa SS, et al. Incidence of marginal zone lymphoma in the United States, 2001-2009 with a focus on primary anatomic site. Br J Haematol. 2014 Apr;165(1):67–77. PMID:24417667

1560. Khan M, Dirweesh A, Alvarez C, et al. Anal neuroendocrine tumor masquerading as external hemorrhoids: a case report. Gastroenterology Res. 2017 Feb;10(1):56–8. PMID:28270879

1561. Khan MS, Luong TV, Watkins J, et al. A comparison of Ki-67 and mitotic count as prognostic markers for metastatic pancreatic and midgut neuroendocrine neoplasms. Br J Cancer. 2013 May 14;108(9):1838–45. PMID:23579216

1562. Khashab MA, Shin EJ, Amateau S, et al. Tumor size and location correlate with behavior of pancreatic serous cystic neoplasms. Am J Gastroenterol. 2011 Aug;106(8):1521–6. PMID:21468008

1563. Khawja SN, Mohammed S, Silberfein EJ, et al. Pancreatic cancer disparities in African Americans. Pancreas. 2015 May;44(4):522–7. PMID:25872128

1564. Khayyata S, Basturk O, Adsay NV. Invasive micropapillary carcinomas of the ampullo-pancreatobiliary region and their association with tumor-infiltrating neutrophils. Mod Pathol. 2005 Nov;18(11):1504–11. PMID:16007065

1565. Khor TS, Alfaro EE, Ooi EM, et al. Divergent expression of MUC5AC, MUC6, MUC2, CD10, and CDX-2 in dysplasia and intramucosal adenocarcinomas with intestinal and foveolar morphology: is this evidence of distinct gastric and intestinal pathways to carcinogenesis in Barrett esophagus? Am J Surg Pathol. 2012 Mar;36(3):331–42. PMID:22261707

1566. Khor TS, Badizadegan K, Ferrone C, et al. Acinar cystadenoma of the pancreas: a clinicopathologic study of 10 cases including multilocular lesions with mural nodules. Am J Surg Pathol. 2012 Nov;36(11):1579–91. PMID:23060352

1567. Khoshnam N, Robinson H, Clay MR, et al. Calcifying nested stromal-epithelial tumor (CNSET) of the liver in Beckwith-Wiedemann syndrome. Eur J Med Genet. 2017 Feb;60(2):136–9. PMID:27965001

1568. Khoury RE, Kabir C, Maker VK, et al. What is the incidence of malignancy in resected intraductal papillary mucinous neoplasms? An analysis of over 100 US institutions in a single year. Ann Surg Oncol. 2018 Jun;25(6):1746–51. PMID:29560572

1569. Khunamornpong S, Lerwill MF, Siriaunkgul S, et al. Carcinoma of extrahepatic bile ducts and gallbladder metastatic to the ovary: a report of 16 cases. Int J Gynecol Pathol. 2008 Jul;27(3):366–79. PMID:18580314

1570. Kiani B, Ferrell LD, Qualman S, et al. Immunohistochemical analysis of embryonal sarcoma of the liver. Appl Immunohistochem Mol Morphol. 2006 Jun;14(2):193–7. PMID:16785789

1571. Kihara A, Fukushima J, Horiuchi H. Glomus tumor of the liver presenting as a cystic lesion. Pathol Int. 2014 Jun;64(6):295–7. PMID:24965114

1572. Kikuma K, Watanabe J, Oshiro Y, et al. Etiological factors in primary hepatic B-cell lymphoma. Virchows Arch. 2012 Apr;460(4):379–87. PMID:22395482

1573. Killian JK, Miettinen M, Walker RL, et al. Recurrent epimutation of SDHC in gastrointestinal stromal tumors. Sci Transl Med. 2014 Dec 24;6(268):268ra177. PMID:25540324
1574. Kim A, Ahn SJ, Park DY, et al. Gastric crypt dysplasia: a distinct subtype of gastric dysplasia with characteristic endoscopic features and immunophenotypic and biological anomalies. Histopathology. 2016 May;68(6):843–9. PMID:26336971
1575. Kim B, Giardiello FM. Chemoprevention in familial adenomatous polyposis. Best Pract Res Clin Gastroenterol. 2011 Aug;25(4-5):607–22. PMID:22122775
1576. Kim DH, Shin N, Kim GH, et al. Mucin expression in gastric cancer: reappraisal of its clinicopathologic and prognostic significance. Arch Pathol Lab Med. 2013 Aug;137(8):1047–53. PMID:23899060
1577. Kim DH, Song MH, Kim DH. Malignant carcinoid tumor of the common bile duct: report of a case. Surg Today. 2006;36(5):485–9. PMID:16633759
1578. Kim GE, Thung SN, Tsui WM, et al. Hepatic cavernous hemangioma: underrecognized associated histologic features. Liver Int. 2006 Apr;26(3):334–8. PMID:16584396
1579. Kim H, Choi GH, Na DC, et al. Human hepatocellular carcinomas with "stemness"-related marker expression: keratin 19 expression and a poor prognosis. Hepatology. 2011 Nov;54(5):1707–17. PMID:22045674
1580. Kim H, Lim JH, Jang KT, et al. Morphology of intraductal papillary neoplasm of the bile ducts: radiologic-pathologic correlation. Abdom Imaging. 2011 Aug;36(4):438–46. PMID:20623279
1581. Kim H, Oh BK, Roncalli M, et al. Large liver cell change in hepatitis B virus-related liver cirrhosis. Hepatology. 2009 Sep;50(3):752–62. PMID:19585549
1582. Kim H, Park C, Han KH, et al. Primary liver carcinoma of intermediate (hepatocyte-cholangiocyte) phenotype. J Hepatol. 2004 Feb;40(2):298–304. PMID:14739102
1583. Kim HG, Kesey JE, Griswold JA. Giant anorectal condyloma acuminatum of Buschke-Löwenstein presents difficult management decisions. J Surg Case Rep. 2018 Apr 3;2018(4):rjy058. PMID:29644039
1584. Kim HN, Kim KM, Shin JU, et al. Prediction of carcinoma after resection in subjects with ampullary adenomas on endoscopic biopsy. J Clin Gastroenterol. 2013 Apr;47(4):346–51. PMID:23442830
1585. Kim JM, Cho MY, Sohn JH, et al. Diagnosis of gastric epithelial neoplasia: dilemma for Korean pathologists. World J Gastroenterol. 2011 Jun 7;17(21):2602–10. PMID:21677827
1586. Kim JY, Brosnan-Cashman JA, An S, et al. Alternative lengthening of telomeres in primary pancreatic neuroendocrine tumors is associated with aggressive clinical behavior and poor survival. Clin Cancer Res. 2017 Mar 15;23(6):1598–606. PMID:27663587
1587. Kim JY, Kim MS, Kim KS, et al. Clinicopathologic and prognostic significance of multiple hormone expression in pancreatic neuroendocrine tumors. Am J Surg Pathol. 2015 May;39(5):592–601. PMID:25602797
1588. Kim KM, Kim MJ, Cho BK, et al. Genetic evidence for the multi-step progression of mixed glandular-neuroendocrine gastric carcinomas. Virchows Arch. 2002 Jan;440(1):85–93. PMID:11942581
1589. Kim KM, Lee JK, Shin JU, et al. Clinicopathologic features of intraductal papillary neoplasm of the bile duct according to histologic subtype. Am J Gastroenterol. 2012 Jan;107(1):118–25. PMID:21946282
1590. Kim MJ, Lee EJ, Kim DS, et al. Composite intestinal adenoma-microcarcinoid in the colon and rectum: a case series and historical review. Diagn Pathol. 2017 Nov 7;12(1):78. PMID:29116005
1591. Kim MJ, Lee EJ, Suh JP, et al. Traditional serrated adenoma of the colorectum: clinicopathologic implications and endoscopic findings of the precursor lesions. Am J Clin Pathol. 2013 Dec;140(6):898–911. PMID:24225759
1592. Kim S, Chung JW, Jeong TD, et al. Searching for E-cadherin gene mutations in early onset diffuse gastric cancer and hereditary diffuse gastric cancer in Korean patients. Fam Cancer. 2013 Sep;12(3):503–7. PMID:23264079
1593. Kim SG, Wu TT, Lee JH, et al. Comparison of epigenetic and genetic alterations in mucinous cystic neoplasm and serous microcystic adenoma of pancreas. Mod Pathol. 2003 Nov;16(11):1086–94. PMID:14614047
1594. Kim SH, Park YN, Yoon DS, et al. Composite neuroendocrine and adenocarcinoma of the common bile duct associated with Clonorchis sinensis: a case report. Hepatogastroenterology. 2000 Jul-Aug;47(34):942–4. PMID:11020854
1595. Kim SJ, Akita M, Sung YN, et al. MDM2 amplification in intrahepatic cholangiocarcinomas: its relationship with large-duct type morphology and uncommon KRAS mutations. Am J Surg Pathol. 2018 Apr;42(4):512–21. PMID:29309301
1596. Kim SJ, Choi CW, Mun YC, et al. Multicenter retrospective analysis of 581 patients with primary intestinal non-hodgkin lymphoma from the Consortium for Improving Survival of Lymphoma (CISL). BMC Cancer. 2011 Jul 29;11:321. PMID:21798075
1597. Kim SJ, Jung HA, Chuang SS, et al. Extranodal natural killer/T-cell lymphoma involving the gastrointestinal tract: analysis of clinical features and outcomes from the Asia Lymphoma Study Group. J Hematol Oncol. 2013 Nov 16;6:86. PMID:24238138
1598. Kim SS, Kays DW, Larson SD, et al. Appendiceal carcinoids in children–management and outcomes. J Surg Res. 2014 Dec;192(2):250–3. PMID:25039014
1599. Kim ST, Ha SY, Lee J, et al. The clinicopathologic features and treatment of 607 hindgut neuroendocrine tumor (NET) patients at a single institution. Medicine (Baltimore). 2016 May;95(19):e3534. PMID:27175651
1600. Kim TH, Shivdasani RA. Stomach development, stem cells and disease. Development. 2016 Feb 15;143(4):554–65. PMID:26884394
1601. Kim TK, Jang HJ, Burns PN, et al. Focal nodular hyperplasia and hepatic adenoma: differentiation with low-mechanical-index contrast-enhanced sonography. AJR Am J Roentgenol. 2008 Jan;190(1):58–66. PMID:18094294
1602. Kim WJ, Hwang S, Lee YJ, et al. Clinicopathological features and long-term outcomes of intraductal papillary neoplasms of the intrahepatic bile duct. J Gastrointest Surg. 2016 Jul;20(7):1368–75. PMID:26873016
1603. Kim WS, Choi BI, Lee YS, et al. Endodermal sinus tumour associated with benign teratoma of the common bile duct. Pediatr Radiol. 1993;23(1):59–60. PMID:8469596
1603A. Kim Y, Wen X, Bae JM, et al. The distribution of intratumoral macrophages correlates with molecular phenotypes and impacts prognosis in colorectal carcinoma. Histopathology. 2018 Oct;73(4):663–71. PMID:29906313
1604. Kim YJ, Park JC, Kim JH, et al. Histologic diagnosis based on forceps biopsy is not adequate for determining endoscopic treatment of gastric adenomatous lesions. Endoscopy. 2010 Aug;42(8):620–6. PMID:20623445
1606. Kimura T, Yamamoto E, Yamano HO, et al. A novel pit pattern identifies the precursor of colorectal cancer derived from sessile serrated adenoma. Am J Gastroenterol. 2012 Mar;107(3):460–9. PMID:22233696
1607. Kimura W, Kuroda A, Morioka Y. Clinical pathology of endocrine tumors of the pancreas. Analysis of autopsy cases. Dig Dis Sci. 1991 Jul;36(7):933–42. PMID:2070707
1608. Kimura W, Moriya T, Hirai I, et al. Multicenter study of serous cystic neoplasm of the Japan Pancreas Society. Pancreas. 2012 Apr;41(3):380–7. PMID:22415666
1609. Kinch A, Cavelier L, Bengtsson M, et al. Donor or recipient origin of posttransplant lymphoproliferative disorders following solid organ transplantation. Am J Transplant. 2014 Dec;14(12):2838–45. PMID:25307322
1610. Kindblom LG, Remotti HE, Aldenborg F, et al. Gastrointestinal pacemaker cell tumor (GIPACT): gastrointestinal stromal tumors show phenotypic characteristics of the interstitial cells of Cajal. Am J Pathol. 1998 May;152(5):1259–69. PMID:9588894
1611. Kindmark H, Sundin A, Granberg D, et al. Endocrine pancreatic tumors with glucagon hypersecretion: a retrospective study of 23 cases during 20 years. Med Oncol. 2007;24(3):330–7. PMID:17873310
1612. Kinoshita K, Isozaki K, Hirota S, et al. c-kit gene mutation at exon 17 or 13 is very rare in sporadic gastrointestinal stromal tumors. J Gastroenterol Hepatol. 2003 Feb;18(2):147–51. PMID:12542597
1613. Kinzler KW, Vogelstein B. Landscaping the cancer terrain. Science. 1998 May 15;280(5366):1036–7. PMID:9616081
1614. Kinzler KW, Vogelstein B. Lessons from hereditary colorectal cancer. Cell. 1996 Oct 18;87(2):159–70. PMID:8861899
1615. Kipp BR, Fritcher EG, Clayton AC, et al. Comparison of KRAS mutation analysis and FISH for detecting pancreatobiliary tract cancer in cytology specimens collected during endoscopic retrograde cholangiopancreatography. J Mol Diagn. 2010 Nov;12(6):780–6. PMID:20864634
1616. Kirkwood KS, Debas HT. Neuroendocrine tumors: common presentations of uncommon diseases. Compr Ther. 1995 Dec;21(12):719–25. PMID:8789136
1617. Kirsch R, Messenger DE, Riddell RH, et al. Venous invasion in colorectal cancer: impact of an elastin stain on detection and interobserver agreement among gastrointestinal and nongastrointestinal pathologists. Am J Surg Pathol. 2013 Feb;37(2):200–10. PMID:23108018
1618. Kitagawa H, Nakamura M, Tani T, et al. A pure invasive micropapillary carcinoma of the pancreatic head: long disease-free survival after pancreatoduodenectomy and adjuvant chemotherapy with gemcitabine. Pancreas. 2007 Aug;35(2):190–2. PMID:17632330
1619. Kitagawa H, Ohta T, Makino I, et al. Carcinomas of the ventral and dorsal pancreas exhibit different patterns of lymphatic spread. Front Biosci. 2008 Jan 1;13:2728–35. PMID:17981748
1620. Kitai S, Kudo M, Minami Y, et al. Validation of a new prognostic staging system for hepatocellular carcinoma: a comparison of the biomarker-combined Japan Integrated Staging Score, the conventional Japan Integrated Staging Score and the BALAD Score. Oncology. 2008;75 Suppl 1:83–90. PMID:19092276
1622. Klas JV, Rothenberger DA, Wong WD, et al. Malignant tumors of the anal canal: the spectrum of disease, treatment, and outcomes. Cancer. 1999 Apr 15;85(8):1686–93. PMID:10223561
1623. Kleeff J, Korc M, Apte M, et al. Pancreatic cancer. Nat Rev Dis Primers. 2016 Apr 21;2:16022. PMID:27158978
1624. Klein AP, Beaty TH, Bailey-Wilson JE, et al. Evidence for a major gene influencing risk of pancreatic cancer. Genet Epidemiol. 2002 Aug;23(2):133–49. PMID:12214307
1625. Klein AP, Brune KA, Petersen GM, et al. Prospective risk of pancreatic cancer in familial pancreatic cancer kindreds. Cancer Res. 2004 Apr 1;64(7):2634–8. PMID:15059921
1626. Klein WM, Hruban RH, Klein-Szanto AJ, et al. Direct correlation between proliferative activity and dysplasia in pancreatic intraepithelial neoplasia (PanIN): additional evidence for a recently proposed model of progression. Mod Pathol. 2002 Apr;15(4):441–7. PMID:11950919
1627. Kletter GB, Sweetser DA, Wallace SF, et al. Adrenocorticotropin-secreting pancreatoblastoma. J Pediatr Endocrinol Metab. 2007 May;20(5):639–42. PMID:17642425
1628. Klimstra DS, Adsay V. Acinar neoplasms of the pancreas-a summary of 25 years of research. Semin Diagn Pathol. 2016 Sep;33(5):307–18. PMID:27320062
1629. Klimstra DS, Heffess CS, Oertel JE, et al. Acinar cell carcinoma of the pancreas. A clinicopathologic study of 28 cases. Am J Surg Pathol. 1992 Sep;16(9):815–37. PMID:1384374
1630. Klimstra DS, Modlin IR, Adsay NV, et al. Pathology reporting of neuroendocrine tumors: application of the Delphic consensus process to the development of a minimum pathology data set. Am J Surg Pathol. 2010 Mar;34(3):300–13. PMID:20118772
1631. Klimstra DS, Pitman MB, Hruban RH. An algorithmic approach to the diagnosis of pancreatic neoplasms. Arch Pathol Lab Med. 2009 Mar;133(3):454–64. PMID:19260750
1632. Klimstra DS, Rosai J, Heffess CS. Mixed acinar-endocrine carcinomas of the pancreas. Am J Surg Pathol. 1994 Aug;18(8):765–78. PMID:8037290
1633. Klimstra DS, Wenig BM, Heffess CS. Solid-pseudopapillary tumor of the pancreas: a typically cystic carcinoma of low malignant potential. Semin Diagn Pathol. 2000 Feb;17(1):66–80. PMID:10721808
1634. Klimstra DS. Nonductal neoplasms of the pancreas. Mod Pathol. 2007 Feb;20 Suppl 1:S94–112. PMID:17486055
1635. Kluijt I, Siemerink EJ, Ausems MG, et al. CDH1-related hereditary diffuse gastric cancer syndrome: clinical variations and implications for counseling. Int J Cancer. 2012 Jul 15;131(2):367–76. PMID:22020549
1636. Klöppel G, Adsay NV. Chronic pancreatitis and the differential diagnosis versus pancreatic cancer. Arch Pathol Lab Med. 2009 Mar;133(3):382–7. PMID:19260744
1637. Klöppel G, Adsay V, Konukiewitz B, et al. Precancerous lesions of the biliary tree. Best Pract Res Clin Gastroenterol. 2013 Apr;27(2):285–97. PMID:23809246
1638. Klöppel G, Anlauf M, Perren A, et al. Hyperplasia to neoplasia sequence of duodenal and pancreatic neuroendocrine diseases and pseudohyperplasia of the PP-cells in the pancreas. Endocr Pathol. 2014 Jun;25(2):181–5. PMID:24718881
1639. Klöppel G, Anlauf M. Gastrinoma–morphological aspects. Wien Klin Wochenschr. 2007;119(19-20):579–84. PMID:17985091
1640. Klöppel G, Basturk O, Schlitter AM, et al. Intraductal neoplasms of the pancreas. Semin Diagn Pathol. 2014 Nov;31(6):452–66. PMID:25282472
1641. Klöppel G, Couvelard A, Perren A, et al. ENETS Consensus Guidelines for the Standards of Care in Neuroendocrine Tumors: towards a standardized approach to the diagnosis of gastroenteropancreatic neuroendocrine tumors and their prognostic stratification. Neuroendocrinology. 2009;90(2):162–6. PMID:19060454

1642. Klöppel G, Heitz PU. Morphology and functional activity of gastroenteropancreatic neuroendocrine tumours. Recent Results Cancer Res. 1990;118:27–36. PMID:1978380
1643. Klöppel G, Heitz PU. Pancreatic endocrine tumors. Pathol Res Pract. 1988 Apr;183(2):155–68. PMID:2898775
1643A. Klöppel G, La Rosa S. Ki67 labeling index: assessment and prognostic role in gastroenteropancreatic neuroendocrine neoplasms. Virchows Arch. 2018 Mar;472(3):341–9. PMID:29134440
1644. Klöppel G, Lohse T, Bosslet K, et al. Ductal adenocarcinoma of the head of the pancreas: incidence of tumor involvement beyond the Whipple resection line. Histological and immunocytochemical analysis of 37 total pancreatectomy specimens. Pancreas. 1987;2(2):170–5. PMID:2819857
1645. Klöppel G, Maurer R, Hofmann E, et al. Solid-cystic (papillary-cystic) tumours within and outside the pancreas in men: report of two patients. Virchows Arch A Pathol Anat Histopathol. 1991;418(2):179–83. PMID:1705067
1646. Klöppel G, Morohoshi T, John HD, et al. Solid and cystic acinar cell tumour of the pancreas. A tumour in young women with favourable prognosis. Virchows Arch A Pathol Anat Histol. 1981;392(2):171–83. PMID:7281507
1647. Klöppel G, Rindi G, Anlauf M, et al. Site-specific biology and pathology of gastroenteropancreatic neuroendocrine tumors. Virchows Arch. 2007 Aug;451 Suppl 1:S9–27. PMID:17684761
1648. Klöppel G, Willemer S, Stamm B, et al. Pancreatic lesions and hormonal profile of pancreatic tumors in multiple endocrine neoplasia type I. An immunocytochemical study of nine patients. Cancer. 1986 May 1;57(9):1824–32. PMID:2420439
1649. Klöppel G. Clinicopathologic view of intraductal papillary-mucinous tumor of the pancreas. Hepatogastroenterology. 1998 Nov-Dec;45(24):1981–5. PMID:9951851
1650. Klöppel G. Mixed exocrine-endocrine tumors of the pancreas. Semin Diagn Pathol. 2000 May;17(2):104–8. PMID:10839610
1651. Klöppel G. Pseudocysts and other non-neoplastic cysts of the pancreas. Semin Diagn Pathol. 2000 Feb;17(1):7–15. PMID:10721803
1652. Knight JS, Tsodikov A, Cibrik DM, et al. Lymphoma after solid organ transplantation: risk, response to therapy, and survival at a transplantation center. J Clin Oncol. 2009 Jul 10;27(20):3354–62. PMID:19451438
1653. Knijn N, Mogk SC, Teerenstra S, et al. Perineural invasion is a strong prognostic factor in colorectal cancer: a systematic review. Am J Surg Pathol. 2016 Jan;40(1):103–12. PMID:26426380
1654. Knijn N, van Exsel UEM, de Noo ME, et al. The value of intramural vascular invasion in colorectal cancer - a systematic review and meta-analysis. Histopathology. 2018 Apr;72(5):721–8. PMID:28960400
1655. Knowles DM, Cesarman E, Chadburn A, et al. Correlative morphologic and molecular genetic analysis demonstrates three distinct categories of posttransplantation lymphoproliferative disorders. Blood. 1995 Jan 15;85(2):552–65. PMID:7812011
1656. Knox CD, Anderson CD, Lamps LW, et al. Long-term survival after resection for primary hepatic carcinoid tumor. Ann Surg Oncol. 2003 Dec;10(10):1171–5. PMID:14654473
1657. Knox RD, Luey N, Sioson L, et al. Medullary colorectal carcinoma revisited: a clinical and pathological study of 102 cases. Ann Surg Oncol. 2015 Sep;22(9):2988–96. PMID:25572685
1658. Knudsen AL, Bülow S, Tomlinson I, et al. Attenuated familial adenomatous polyposis: results from an international collaborative study. Colorectal Dis. 2010 Oct;12(10 Online):e243–9. PMID:20105204
1659. Ko HM, Harpaz N, McBride RB, et al. Serrated colorectal polyps in inflammatory bowel disease. Mod Pathol. 2015 Dec;28(12):1584–93. PMID:26403785
1660. Ko YH, Cho EY, Kim JE, et al. NK and NK-like T-cell lymphoma in extranasal sites: a comparative clinicopathological study according to site and EBV status. Histopathology. 2004 May;44(5):480–9. PMID:15139996
1661. Ko YH, Karnan S, Kim KM, et al. Enteropathy-associated T-cell lymphoma–a clinicopathologic and array comparative genomic hybridization study. Hum Pathol. 2010 Sep;41(9):1231–7. PMID:20399483
1662. Ko YH, Kim CW, Park CS, et al. REAL classification of malignant lymphomas in the Republic of Korea: incidence of recently recognized entities and changes in clinicopathologic features. Hematolymphoreticular Study Group of the Korean Society of Pathologists. Revised European-American lymphoma. Cancer. 1998 Aug 15;83(4):806–12. PMID:9708949
1663. Kobari M, Egawa S, Shibuya K, et al. Intraductal papillary mucinous tumors of the pancreas comprise 2 clinical subtypes: differences in clinical characteristics and surgical management. Arch Surg. 1999 Oct;134(10):1131–6. PMID:10522860
1664. Koch P, del Valle F, Berdel WE, et al. Primary gastrointestinal non-Hodgkin's lymphoma: I. Anatomic and histologic distribution, clinical features, and survival data of 371 patients registered in the German Multicenter Study GIT NHL 01/92. J Clin Oncol. 2001 Sep 15;19(18):3861–73. PMID:11559724
1665. Koffron A, Rao S, Ferrario M, et al. Intrahepatic biliary cystadenoma: role of cyst fluid analysis and surgical management in the laparoscopic era. Surgery. 2004 Oct;136(4):926–36. PMID:15467680
1666. Koga A, Tabata M, Kido H, et al. [Successful treatment of ectopic insulinoma. Report of a case (author's transl)]. Nihon Shokakibyo Gakkai Zasshi. 1979 Feb;76(2):279–84. Japanese. PMID:220443
1667. Koito K, Namieno T, Nagakawa T, et al. Pancreas: imaging diagnosis with color/power Doppler ultrasonography, endoscopic ultrasonography, and intraductal ultrasonography. Eur J Radiol. 2001 May;38(2):94–104. PMID:11335091
1668. Kojima M, Ikeda K, Saito N, et al. Neuroendocrine tumors of the large intestine: clinicopathological features and predictive factors of lymph node metastasis. Front Oncol. 2016 Jul 18;6:173. PMID:27486567
1669. Kolodziejczyk P, Yao T, Tsuneyoshi M. Inflammatory fibroid polyp of the stomach. A special reference to an immunohistochemical profile of 42 cases. Am J Surg Pathol. 1993 Nov;17(11):1159–68. PMID:8214261
1670. Komatsu H, Egawa S, Motoi F, et al. Clinicopathological features and surgical outcomes of adenosquamous carcinoma of the pancreas: a retrospective analysis of patients with resectable stage tumors. Surg Today. 2015 Mar;45(3):297–304. PMID:24973941
1671. Kominami A, Fujino M, Murakami H, et al. β-catenin mutation in ovarian solid pseudopapillary neoplasm. Pathol Int. 2014 Sep;64(9):460–4. PMID:25186079
1672. Komuta M, Spee B, Vander Borght S, et al. Clinicopathological study on cholangiolocellular carcinoma suggesting hepatic progenitor cell origin. Hepatology. 2008 May;47(5):1544–56. PMID:18393293
1673. Kondo E, Furukawa T, Yoshinaga K, et al. Not hMSH2 but hMLH1 is frequently silenced by hypermethylation in endometrial cancer but rarely silenced in pancreatic cancer with microsatellite instability. Int J Oncol. 2000 Sep;17(3):535–41. PMID:10938395
1674. Kondo F, Wada K, Nagato Y, et al. Biopsy diagnosis of well-differentiated hepatocellular carcinoma based on new morphologic criteria. Hepatology. 1989 May;9(5):751–5. PMID:2540084
1675. Kondo K. Duodenogastric reflux and gastric stump carcinoma. Gastric Cancer. 2002;5(1):16–22. PMID:12021855
1676. Konishi E, Nakashima Y, Smyrk TC, et al. Clear cell carcinoid tumor of the gallbladder. A case without von Hippel-Lindau disease. Arch Pathol Lab Med. 2003 Jun;127(6):745–7. PMID:12741904
1677. Konomi K, Chijiiwa K, Katsuta T, et al. Pancreatic somatostatinoma: a case report and review of the literature. J Surg Oncol. 1990 Apr;43(4):259–65. PMID:1969977
1678. Konstantinidis IT, Vinuela EF, Tang LH, et al. Incidentally discovered pancreatic intraepithelial neoplasia: what is its clinical significance? Ann Surg Oncol. 2013 Oct;20(11):3643–7. PMID:23748606
1679. Konstantinova AM, Michal M, Kacerovska D, et al. Hidradenoma papilliferum: a clinicopathologic study of 264 tumors from 261 patients, with emphasis on mammary-type alterations. Am J Dermatopathol. 2016 Aug;38(8):598–607. PMID:26863059
1680. Konukiewitz B, Enosawa T, Klöppel G. Glucagon expression in cystic pancreatic neuroendocrine neoplasms: an immunohistochemical analysis. Virchows Arch. 2011 Jan;458(1):47–53. PMID:20922407
1681. Konukiewitz B, Jesinghaus M, Steiger K, et al. Pancreatic neuroendocrine carcinomas reveal a closer relationship to ductal adenocarcinomas than to neuroendocrine tumors G3. Hum Pathol. 2018 Jul;77:70–9. PMID:29596894
1682. Konukiewitz B, Schlitter AM, Jesinghaus M, et al. Somatostatin receptor expression related to TP53 and RB1 alterations in pancreatic and extrapancreatic neuroendocrine neoplasms with a Ki67-index above 20. Mod Pathol. 2017 Apr;30(4):587–98. PMID:28059098
1683. Koo GC, Tan SY, Tang T, et al. Janus kinase 3-activating mutations identified in natural killer/T-cell lymphoma. Cancer Discov. 2012 Jul;2(7):591–7. PMID:22705984
1684. Koopman T, Louwen M, Hage M, et al. Pathologic diagnostics of HER2 positivity in gastroesophageal adenocarcinoma. Am J Clin Pathol. 2015 Feb;143(2):257–64. PMID:25596252
1685. Kooy-Winkelaar YM, Bouwer D, Janssen GM, et al. CD4 T-cell cytokines synergize to induce proliferation of malignant and nonmalignant innate intraepithelial lymphocytes. Proc Natl Acad Sci U S A. 2017 Feb 7;114(6):E980–9. PMID:28049849
1686. Koplin S, Agni R. Hepatic composite tumor in a patient with primary sclerosing cholangitis. Pathol Res Pract. 2009;205(5):361–4. PMID:19155146
1687. Korinek V, Barker N, Morin PJ, et al. Constitutive transcriptional activation by a beta-catenin-Tcf complex in APC-/- colon carcinoma. Science. 1997 Mar 21;275(5307):1784–7. PMID:9065401
1688. Kosmahl M, Pauser U, Anlauf M, et al. Pancreatic ductal adenocarcinomas with cystic features: neither rare nor uniform. Mod Pathol. 2005 Sep;18(9):1157–64. PMID:15920540
1689. Kosmahl M, Pauser U, Peters K, et al. Cystic neoplasms of the pancreas and tumor-like lesions with cystic features: a review of 418 cases and a classification proposal. Virchows Arch. 2004 Aug;445(2):168–78. PMID:15185076
1690. Kosmahl M, Seada LS, Jänig U, et al. Solid-pseudopapillary tumor of the pancreas: its origin revisited. Virchows Arch. 2000 May;436(5):473–80. PMID:10881741
1691. Kosmahl M, Wagner J, Peters K, et al. Serous cystic neoplasms of the pancreas: an immunohistochemical analysis revealing alpha-inhibin, neuron-specific enolase, and MUC6 as new markers. Am J Surg Pathol. 2004 Mar;28(3):339–46. PMID:15104296
1692. Koulos J, Symmans F, Chumas J, et al. Human papillomavirus detection in adenocarcinoma of the anus. Mod Pathol. 1991 Jan;4(1):58–61. PMID:1850518
1693. Koushik A, Spiegelman D, Albanes D, et al. Intake of fruits and vegetables and risk of pancreatic cancer in a pooled analysis of 14 cohort studies. Am J Epidemiol. 2012 Sep 1;176(5):373–86. PMID:22875754
1694. Kozaka K, Sasaki M, Fujii T, et al. A subgroup of intrahepatic cholangiocarcinoma with an infiltrating replacement growth pattern and a resemblance to reactive proliferating bile ductules: 'bile ductular carcinoma'. Histopathology. 2007 Sep;51(3):390–400. PMID:17553067
1695. Kozuka S, Sassa R, Taki T, et al. Relation of pancreatic duct hyperplasia to carcinoma. Cancer. 1979 Apr;43(4):1418–28. PMID:445339
1697. Kozuka S, Tsubone N, Yasui A, et al. Relation of adenoma to carcinoma in the gallbladder. Cancer. 1982 Nov 15;50(10):2226–34. PMID:7127263
1698. Krampitz GW, Norton JA. Current management of the Zollinger-Ellison syndrome. Adv Surg. 2013;47:59–79. PMID:24298844
1699. Krasinskas AM, Oakley GJ, Bagci P, et al. "Simple mucinous cyst" of the pancreas: a clinicopathologic analysis of 39 examples of a diagnostically challenging entity distinct from intraductal papillary mucinous neoplasms and mucinous cystic neoplasms. Am J Surg Pathol. 2017 Jan;41(1):121–7. PMID:27740966
1700. Krausova M, Korinek V. Wnt signaling in adult intestinal stem cells and cancer. Cell Signal. 2014 Mar;26(3):570–9. PMID:24308963
1701. Krausz Y, Freedman N, Rubinstein R, et al. 68Ga-DOTA-NOC PET/CT imaging of neuroendocrine tumors: comparison with ^{111}In-DTPA-octreotide (OctreoScan®). Mol Imaging Biol. 2011 Jun;13(3):583–93. PMID:20652423
1702. Krejs GJ. VIPoma syndrome. Am J Med. 1987 May 29;82 5B:37–48. PMID:3035922
1703. Kremer BE, Reshef R, Misleh JG, et al. Post-transplant lymphoproliferative disorder after lung transplantation: a review of 35 cases. J Heart Lung Transplant. 2012 Mar;31(3):296–304. PMID:22112992
1704. Krishna NB, Mehra M, Reddy AV, et al. EUS/EUS-FNA for suspected pancreatic cancer: influence of chronic pancreatitis and clinical presentation with or without obstructive jaundice on performance characteristics. Gastrointest Endosc. 2009 Jul;70(1):70–9. PMID:19249774
1705. Krishna SG, Brugge WR, Dewitt JM, et al. Needle-based confocal laser endomicroscopy for the diagnosis of pancreatic cystic lesions: an international external interobserver and intraobserver study (with videos). Gastrointest Endosc. 2017 Oct;86(4):644–54.e2. PMID:28286093
1706. Kruger S, Haas M, Burkl C, et al. Incidence, outcome and risk stratification tools for venous thromboembolism in advanced pancreatic cancer - a retrospective cohort study. Thromb Res. 2017 Sep;157:9–15. PMID:28675831
1707. Kubo T, Kiryu S, Akai H, et al. Hepatic involvement of histiocytic sarcoma: CT and MRI findings. Korean J Radiol. 2016

Sep-Oct;17(5):758–62. PMID:27587965
1708. Kubo Y, Aishima S, Tanaka Y, et al. Different expression of glucose transporters in the progression of intrahepatic cholangiocarcinoma. Hum Pathol. 2014 Aug;45(8):1610–7. PMID:24824030
1709. Kuboki Y, Shimizu K, Hatori T, et al. Molecular biomarkers for progression of intraductal papillary mucinous neoplasm of the pancreas. Pancreas. 2015 Mar;44(2):227–35. PMID:25423558
1710. Kuboki Y, Yamashita S, Niwa T, et al. Comprehensive analyses using next-generation sequencing and immunohistochemistry enable precise treatment in advanced gastric cancer. Ann Oncol. 2016 Jan;27(1):127–33. PMID:26489445
1711. Kubota K, Nakanuma Y, Kondo F, et al. Clinicopathological features and prognosis of mucin-producing bile duct tumor and mucinous cystic tumor of the liver: a multi-institutional study by the Japan Biliary Association. J Hepatobiliary Pancreat Sci. 2014 Mar;21(3):176–85. PMID:23908126
1712. Kudo S, Tamura S, Nakajima T, et al. Diagnosis of colorectal tumorous lesions by magnifying endoscopy. Gastrointest Endosc. 1996 Jul;44(1):8–14. PMID:8836710
1713. Kudo S. Endoscopic mucosal resection of flat and depressed types of early colorectal cancer. Endoscopy. 1993 Sep;25(7):455–61. PMID:8261988
1714. Kuhlmann KF, de Castro SM, Wesseling JG, et al. Surgical treatment of pancreatic adenocarcinoma; actual survival and prognostic factors in 343 patients. Eur J Cancer. 2004 Mar;40(4):549–58. PMID:14962722
1715. Kuiper RP, Vissers LE, Venkatachalam R, et al. Recurrence and variability of germline EPCAM deletions in Lynch syndrome. Hum Mutat. 2011 Apr;32(4):407–14. PMID:21309036
1716. Kulke MH, Anthony LB, Bushnell DL, et al. NANETS treatment guidelines: well-differentiated neuroendocrine tumors of the stomach and pancreas. Pancreas. 2010 Aug;39(6):735–52. PMID:20664472
1717. Kumagai S, Sobue T, Makiuchi T, et al. Relationship between cumulative exposure to 1,2-dichloropropane and incidence risk of cholangiocarcinoma among offset printing workers. Occup Environ Med. 2016 Aug;73(8):545–52. PMID:27371662
1718. Kumar S, Krenacs L, Otsuki T, et al. Bc1-1 rearrangement and cyclin D1 protein expression in multiple lymphomatous polyposis. Am J Clin Pathol. 1996 Jun;105(6):737–43. PMID:8659449
1719. Kumarasinghe G, Lavee O, Parker A, et al. Post-transplant lymphoproliferative disease in heart and lung transplantation: defining risk and prognostic factors. J Heart Lung Transplant. 2015 Nov;34(11):1406–14. PMID:26279197
1720. Kumarasinghe MP, Brown I, Raftopoulos S, et al. Standardised reporting protocol for endoscopic resection for Barrett oesophagus associated neoplasia: expert consensus recommendations. Pathology. 2014 Oct;46(6):473–80. PMID:25158823
1721. Kumaravel A, Lopez R, Brainard J, et al. Brush cytology vs. endoscopic biopsy for the surveillance of Barrett's esophagus. Endoscopy. 2010 Oct;42(10):800–5. PMID:20821361
1722. Kummar S, Ciesielski TE, Fogarasi MC. Management of small bowel adenocarcinoma. Oncology (Williston Park). 2002 Oct;16(10):1364–9, discussion 1370, 1372–3. PMID:12435206
1723. Kunisaki C, Makino H, Kimura J, et al. Impact of lymphovascular invasion in patients with stage I gastric cancer. Surgery. 2010 Feb;147(2):204–11. PMID:19878963
1724. Kuo FY, Huang HY, Chen CL, et al. TFE3-rearranged hepatic epithelioid hemangioendothelioma-a case report with immunohistochemical and molecular study. APMIS. 2017 Sep;125(9):849–53. PMID:28585251
1725. Kuo YH, Wang JH, Lu SN, et al. Natural course of hepatic focal nodular hyperplasia: a long-term follow-up study with sonography. J Clin Ultrasound. 2009 Mar-Apr;37(3):132–7. PMID:18855931
1726. Kuraoka K, Taniyama K, Fujitaka T, et al. Small cell carcinoma of the extrahepatic bile duct: case report and immunohistochemical analysis. Pathol Int. 2003 Dec;53(12):887–91. PMID:14629756
1727. Kurman RJ, Carcangiu ML, Herrington CS, et al., editors. WHO classification of tumours of female reproductive organs. Lyon (France): International Agency for Research on Cancer; 2014. (WHO classification of tumours series, 4th ed.; vol. 6). http://publications.iarc.fr/16.
1728. Kuroda N, Tanida N, Ohara M, et al. Anal canal adenocarcinoma with MUC5AC expression suggestive of anal gland origin. Med Mol Morphol. 2007 Mar;40(1):50–3. PMID:17384991
1729. Kuroda T, Hoshino K, Nosaka S, et al. Critical hepatic hemangioma in infants: recent nationwide survey in Japan. Pediatr Int. 2014 Jun;56(3):304–8. PMID:24689756
1730. Kurokawa Y, Matsuura N, Kimura Y, et al. Multicenter large-scale study of prognostic impact of HER2 expression in patients with resectable gastric cancer. Gastric Cancer. 2015 Oct;18(4):691–7. PMID:25224659
1731. Kushima R, Kim KM. Interobserver variation in the diagnosis of gastric epithelial dysplasia and carcinoma between two pathologists in Japan and Korea. J Gastric Cancer. 2011 Sep;11(3):141–5. PMID:22076218
1732. Kushima R, Müller W, Stolte M, et al. Differential p53 protein expression in stomach adenomas of gastric and intestinal phenotypes: possible sequences of p53 alteration in stomach carcinogenesis. Virchows Arch. 1996 Jul;428(4-5):223–7. PMID:8764930
1733. Kushima R, Remmele W, Stolte M, et al. Pyloric gland type adenoma of the gallbladder with squamoid spindle cell metaplasia. Pathol Res Pract. 1996 Sep;192(9):963–9, discussion 970–1. PMID:8950764
1734. Kushima R, Sekine S, Matsubara A, et al. Gastric adenocarcinoma of the fundic gland type shares common genetic and phenotypic features with pyloric gland adenoma. Pathol Int. 2013 Jun;63(6):318–25. PMID:23782334
1735. Kushima R, Vieth M, Borchard F, et al. Gastric-type well-differentiated adenocarcinoma and pyloric gland adenoma of the stomach. Gastric Cancer. 2006;9(3):177–84. PMID:16952035
1736. Kwak MS, Chung SJ, Yang JI, et al. Long-term outcome of small, incidentally detected rectal neuroendocrine tumors removed by simple excisional biopsy compared with the advanced endoscopic resection during screening colonoscopy. Dis Colon Rectum. 2018 Mar;61(3):338–46. PMID:29369898
1737. Kwon CH, Kim YK, Lee S, et al. Gastric poorly cohesive carcinoma: a correlative study of mutational signatures and prognostic significance based on histopathological subtypes. Histopathology. 2018 Mar;72(4):556–68. PMID:28873240
1738. Kwon HJ, Kim JW, Kim H, et al. Combined hepatocellular carcinoma and neuroendocrine carcinoma with ectopic secretion of parathyroid hormone: a case report and review of the literature. J Pathol Transl Med. 2018 Jul;52(4):232–7. PMID:29794961
1739. Kwon MJ, Kim JW, Jung JP, et al. Low incidence of KRAS, BRAF, and PIK3CA mutations in adenocarcinomas of the ampulla of Vater and their prognostic value. Hum Pathol. 2016 Apr;50:90–100. PMID:26997442
1740. Kwon MJ, Min BH, Lee SM, et al. Serrated adenoma of the stomach: a clinicopathologic, immunohistochemical, and molecular study of nine cases. Histol Histopathol. 2013 Apr;28(4):453–62. PMID:23404616
1741. Kytölä S, Höög A, Nord B, et al. Comparative genomic hybridization identifies loss of 18q22-qter as an early and specific event in tumorigenesis of midgut carcinoids. Am J Pathol. 2001 May;158(5):1803–8. PMID:11337378
1742. Kyu HH, Bachman VF, Alexander LT, et al. Physical activity and risk of breast cancer, colon cancer, diabetes, ischemic heart disease, and ischemic stroke events: systematic review and dose-response meta-analysis for the Global Burden of Disease Study 2013. BMJ. 2016 Aug 9;354:i3857. PMID:27510511
1743. Königsrainer I, Glatzle J, Klöppel G, et al. Intraductal and cystic tubulopapillary adenocarcinoma of the pancreas–a possible variant of intraductal tubular carcinoma. Pancreas. 2008 Jan;36(1):92–5. PMID:18192889
1744. Körner M, Waser B, Schonbrunn A, et al. Somatostatin receptor subtype 2A immunohistochemistry using a new monoclonal antibody selects tumors suitable for in vivo somatostatin receptor targeting. Am J Surg Pathol. 2012 Feb;36(2):242–52. PMID:22251942
1745. Küppers F, Jongen J, Bock JU, et al. Keratoacanthoma in the differential diagnosis of anal carcinoma: difficult diagnosis, easy therapy. Report of three cases. Dis Colon Rectum. 2000 Mar;43(3):427–9. PMID:10733129
1746. Küsters-Vandevelde HV, Kruse V, Van Maerken T, et al. Copy number variation analysis and methylome profiling of a GNAQ-mutant primary meningeal melanocytic tumor and its liver metastasis. Exp Mol Pathol. 2017 Feb;102(1):25–31. PMID:27974237
1747. Küçük C, Jiang B, Hu X, et al. Activating mutations of STAT5B and STAT3 in lymphomas derived from γδ-T or NK cells. Nat Commun. 2015 Jan 14;6:6025. PMID:25586472
1748. La Rosa S, Adsay V, Albarello L, et al. Clinicopathologic study of 62 acinar cell carcinomas of the pancreas: insights into the morphology and immunophenotype and search for prognostic markers. Am J Surg Pathol. 2012 Dec;36(12):1782–95. PMID:23026929
1749. La Rosa S, Bernasconi B, Frattini M, et al. TP53 alterations in pancreatic acinar cell carcinoma: new insights into the molecular pathology of this rare cancer. Virchows Arch. 2016 Mar;468(3):289–96. PMID:26586531
1750. La Rosa S, Bernasconi B, Vanoli A, et al. c-MYC amplification and c-myc protein expression in pancreatic acinar cell carcinomas. New insights into the molecular signature of these rare cancers. Virchows Arch. 2018 Oct;473(4):435–41. PMID:29721608
1751. La Rosa S, Franzi F, Albarello L, et al. Serotonin-producing enterochromaffin cell tumors of the pancreas: clinicopathologic study of 15 cases and comparison with intestinal enterochromaffin cell tumors. Pancreas. 2011 Aug;40(6):883–95. PMID:21705949
1752. La Rosa S, Franzi F, Marchet S, et al. The monoclonal anti-BCL10 antibody (clone 331.1) is a sensitive and specific marker of pancreatic acinar cell carcinoma and pancreatic metaplasia. Virchows Arch. 2009 Feb;454(2):133–42. PMID:19066953
1753. La Rosa S, Inzani F, Vanoli A, et al. Histologic characterization and improved prognostic evaluation of 209 gastric neuroendocrine neoplasms. Hum Pathol. 2011 Oct;42(10):1373–84. PMID:21531442
1754. La Rosa S, Marando A, Sessa F, et al. Mixed adenoneuroendocrine carcinomas (MANECs) of the gastrointestinal tract: an update. Cancers (Basel). 2012 Jan 16;4(1):11–30. PMID:24213223
1755. La Rosa S, Pariani D, Calandra C, et al. Ectopic duodenal insulinoma: a very rare and challenging tumor type. Description of a case and review of the literature. Endocr Pathol. 2013 Dec;24(4):213–9. PMID:24006218
1756. La Rosa S, Rigoli E, Uccella S, et al. CDX2 as a marker of intestinal EC-cells and related well-differentiated endocrine tumors. Virchows Arch. 2004 Sep;445(3):248–54. PMID:15517368
1757. La Rosa S, Sessa F, Capella C. Acinar cell carcinoma of the pancreas: overview of clinicopathologic features and insights into the molecular pathology. Front Med (Lausanne). 2015 Jun 15;2:41. PMID:26137463
1758. La Rosa S, Sessa F, Uccella S. Mixed neuroendocrine-nonneuroendocrine neoplasms (MiNENs): unifying the concept of a heterogeneous group of neoplasms. Endocr Pathol. 2016 Dec;27(4):284–311. PMID:27169712
1759. La Rosa S, Uccella S, Molinari F, et al. Mixed adenoma well-differentiated neuroendocrine tumor (MANET) of the digestive system: an indolent subtype of mixed neuroendocrine-nonneuroendocrine neoplasm (MiNEN). Am J Surg Pathol. 2018 Nov;42(11):1503–12. PMID:30001239
1760. La Rosa S, Vanoli A. Gastric neuroendocrine neoplasms and related precursor lesions. J Clin Pathol. 2014 Nov;67(11):938–48. PMID:25053544
1761. Lachlan KL, Lucassen AM, Bunyan D, et al. Cowden syndrome and Bannayan Riley Ruvalcaba syndrome represent one condition with variable expression and age-related penetrance: results of a clinical study of PTEN mutation carriers. J Med Genet. 2007 Sep;44(9):579–85. PMID:17526800
1762. Lack EE, Schloo BL, Azumi N, et al. Undifferentiated (embryonal) sarcoma of the liver. Clinical and pathologic study of 16 cases with emphasis on immunohistochemical features. Am J Surg Pathol. 1991 Jan;15(1):1–16. PMID:1702267
1763. Lage J, Uedo N, Dinis-Ribeiro M, et al. Surveillance of patients with gastric precancerous conditions. Best Pract Res Clin Gastroenterol. 2016 Dec;30(6):913–22. PMID:27938786
1764. Laginestra MA, Tripodo C, Agostinelli C, et al. Distinctive histogenesis and immunological microenvironment based on transcriptional profiles of follicular dendritic cell sarcomas. Mol Cancer Res. 2017 May;15(5):541–52. PMID:28130401
1765. Lahat G, Lazar A, Lev D. Sarcoma epidemiology and etiology: potential environmental and genetic factors. Surg Clin North Am. 2008 Jun;88(3):451–81, v. PMID:18514694
1766. Lahaye MJ, Engelen SM, Nelemans PJ, et al. Imaging for predicting the risk factors–the circumferential resection margin and nodal disease–of local recurrence in rectal cancer: a meta-analysis. Semin Ultrasound CT MR. 2005 Aug;26(4):259–68. PMID:16152740
1767. Lai JP, Mertens RB, Mirocha J, et al. Comparison of PAX6 and PAX8 as immunohistochemical markers for pancreatic neuroendocrine tumors. Endocr Pathol. 2015 Mar;26(1):54–62. PMID:25433656
1768. Lai R, Weiss LM, Chang KL, et al. Frequency of CD43 expression in non-Hodgkin lymphoma. A survey of 742 cases and further characterization of rare CD43+ follicular lymphomas. Am J Clin Pathol. 1999 Apr;111(4):488–94. PMID:10191768
1769. Laine L, Kaltenbach T, Barkun A, et al.

SCENIC international consensus statement on surveillance and management of dysplasia in inflammatory bowel disease. Gastrointest Endosc. 2015 Mar;81(3):489–501.e26. PMID:25708752
1770. Lam AK. Application of pathological staging in esophageal adenocarcinoma. Methods Mol Biol. 2018;1756:93–103. PMID:29600363
1771. Lam AK. Histopathological assessment for esophageal adenocarcinoma. Methods Mol Biol. 2018;1756:67–76. PMID:29600360
1772. Lam AK. Introduction: esophageal adenocarcinoma: updates of Current Status. Methods Mol Biol. 2018;1756:1–6. PMID:29600355
1773. Lam KY, Dickens P, Loke SL, et al. Squamous cell carcinoma of the oesophagus with mucin-secreting component (muco-epidermoid carcinoma and adenosquamous carcinoma): a clinicopathologic study and a review of literature. Eur J Surg Oncol. 1994 Feb;20(1):25–31. PMID:8131864
1774. Lam KY, Law S, Tin L, et al. The clinicopathological significance of p21 and p53 expression in esophageal squamous cell carcinoma: an analysis of 153 patients. Am J Gastroenterol. 1999 Aug;94(8):2060–8. PMID:10445528
1775. Lam KY, Law SY, Loke SL, et al. Double sarcomatoid carcinomas of the oesophagus. Pathol Res Pract. 1996 Jun;192(6):604–9. PMID:8857649
1776. Lam KY, Leung CY, Ho JW. Sarcomatoid carcinoma of the small intestine. Aust N Z J Surg. 1996 Sep;66(9):636–9. PMID:8859167
1777. Lam KY, Loke SL, Ma LT. Histochemistry of mucin secreting components in mucoepidermoid and adenosquamous carcinoma of the oesophagus. J Clin Pathol. 1993 Nov;46(11):1011–5. PMID:7504701
1778. Lam KY, Ma L. Pathology of esophageal cancers: local experience and current insights. Chin Med J (Engl). 1997 Jun;110(6):459–64. PMID:9594248
1779. Lam KY, Ma LT, Wong J. Measurement of extent of spread of oesophageal squamous carcinoma by serial sectioning. J Clin Pathol. 1996 Feb;49(2):124–9. PMID:8655677
1780. Lam-Himlin D, Park JY, Cornish TC, et al. Morphologic characterization of syndromic gastric polyps. Am J Surg Pathol. 2010 Nov;34(11):1656–62. PMID:20924281
1781. Lamlum H, Ilyas M, Rowan A, et al. The type of somatic mutation at APC in familial adenomatous polyposis is determined by the site of the germline mutation: a new facet to Knudson's 'two-hit' hypothesis. Nat Med. 1999 Sep;5(9):1071–5. PMID:10470088
1782. Lammi L, Arte S, Somer M, et al. Mutations in AXIN2 cause familial tooth agenesis and predispose to colorectal cancer. Am J Hum Genet. 2004 May;74(5):1043–50. PMID:15042511
1783. Lan KH, Sheu ML, Hwang SJ, et al. HCV NS5A interacts with p53 and inhibits p53-mediated apoptosis. Oncogene. 2002 Jul 18;21(31):4801–11. PMID:12101418
1784. Landen S, Elens M, Vrancken C, et al. Giant hepatic carcinoid: a rare tumor with a favorable prognosis. Case Rep Surg. 2014;2014:456509. PMID:24653852
1785. Lang H, Sotiropoulos GC, Brokalaki EI, et al. Survival and recurrence rates after resection for hepatocellular carcinoma in noncirrhotic livers. J Am Coll Surg. 2007 Jul;205(1):27–36. PMID:17617329
1786. Langer R, Becker K. Tumor regression grading of gastrointestinal cancers after neoadjuvant therapy. Virchows Arch. 2018 Feb;472(2):175–86. PMID:28918544
1787. Langeveld D, Jansen M, de Boer DV, et al. Aberrant intestinal stem cell lineage dynamics in Peutz-Jeghers syndrome and familial adenomatous polyposis consistent with protracted clonal evolution in the crypt. Gut. 2012 Jun;61(6):839–46. PMID:21940722
1788. Langeveld D, van Hattem WA, de Leng WW, et al. SMAD4 immunohistochemistry reflects genetic status in juvenile polyposis syndrome. Clin Cancer Res. 2010 Aug 15;16(16):4126–34. PMID:20682711
1789. Lanza G, Gafà R, Matteuzzi M, et al. Medullary-type poorly differentiated adenocarcinoma of the large bowel: a distinct clinicopathologic entity characterized by microsatellite instability and improved survival. J Clin Oncol. 1999 Aug;17(8):2429–38. PMID:10561306
1790. Larsson LI, Hirsch MA, Holst JJ, et al. Pancreatic somatostatinoma. Clinical features and physiological implications. Lancet. 1977 Mar 26;1(8013):666–8. PMID:66472
1791. Lasota J, Corless CL, Heinrich MC, et al. Clinicopathologic profile of gastrointestinal stromal tumors (GISTs) with primary KIT exon 13 or exon 17 mutations: a multicenter study on 54 cases. Mod Pathol. 2008 Apr;21(4):476–84. PMID:18246046
1792. Lasota J, Miettinen M. Clinical significance of oncogenic KIT and PDGFRA mutations in gastrointestinal stromal tumours. Histopathology. 2008 Sep;53(3):245–66. PMID:18312355
1793. Lasota J, Wang ZF, Sobin LH, et al. Gain-of-function PDGFRA mutations, earlier reported in gastrointestinal stromal tumors, are common in small intestinal inflammatory fibroid polyps. A study of 60 cases. Mod Pathol. 2009 Aug;22(8):1049–56. PMID:19448595
1794. Lasota J, Wasag B, Dansonka-Mieszkowska A, et al. Evaluation of NF2 and NF1 tumor suppressor genes in distinctive gastrointestinal nerve sheath tumors traditionally diagnosed as benign schwannomas: s study of 20 cases. Lab Invest. 2003 Sep;83(9):1361–71. PMID:13679444
1795. Lauby-Secretan B, Scoccianti C, Loomis D, et al. Body fatness and cancer–viewpoint of the IARC Working Group. N Engl J Med. 2016 Aug 25;375(8):794–8. PMID:27557308
1796. Lauby-Secretan B, Vilahur N, Bianchini F, et al. The IARC perspective on colorectal cancer screening. N Engl J Med. 2018 May 3;378(18):1734–40. PMID:29580179
1797. Laumonier H, Bioulac-Sage P, Laurent C, et al. Hepatocellular adenomas: magnetic resonance imaging features as a function of molecular pathological classification. Hepatology. 2008 Sep;48(3):808–18. PMID:18688875
1798. Lauren P. The two histological main types of gastric carcinoma: diffuse and so-called intestinal-type carcinoma. An attempt at a histo-clinical classification. Acta Pathol Microbiol Scand. 1965;64:31–49. PMID:14320675
1799. Laurent C, Fabiani B, Do C, et al. Immune-checkpoint expression in Epstein-Barr virus positive and negative plasmablastic lymphoma: a clinical and pathological study in 82 patients. Haematologica. 2016 Aug;101(8):976–84. PMID:27175027
1800. Laurent C, Trillaud H, Lepreux S, et al. Association of adenoma and focal nodular hyperplasia: experience of a single French academic center. Comp Hepatol. 2003 Apr 23;2(1):6. PMID:12812524
1801. Laurini JA, Perry AM, Boilesen E, et al. Classification of non-Hodgkin lymphoma in Central and South America: a review of 1028 cases. Blood. 2012 Dec 6;120(24):4795–801. PMID:23086753
1802. Laurini JA, Zhang L, Goldblum JR, et al. Low-grade fibromyxoid sarcoma of the small intestine: report of 4 cases with molecular cytogenetic confirmation. Am J Surg Pathol. 2011 Jul;35(7):1069–73. PMID:21677541
1803. Lauwers GY, Grant LD, Donnelly WH, et al. Hepatic undifferentiated (embryonal) sarcoma arising in a mesenchymal hamartoma. Am J Surg Pathol. 1997 Oct;21(10):1248–54. PMID:9331300
1804. Lauwers GY, Shimizu M, Correa P, et al. Evaluation of gastric biopsies for neoplasia: differences between Japanese and Western pathologists. Am J Surg Pathol. 1999 May;23(5):511–8. PMID:10328081
1805. Lauwers GY, Terris B, Balis UJ, et al. Prognostic histologic indicators of curatively resected hepatocellular carcinomas: a multi-institutional analysis of 425 patients with definition of a histologic prognostic index. Am J Surg Pathol. 2002 Jan;26(1):25–34. PMID:11756766
1806. Lawless ME, Toweill DL, Jewell KD, et al. Massive gastric juvenile polyposis: a clinicopathologic study using SMAD4 immunohistochemistry. Am J Clin Pathol. 2017 Apr 1;147(4):390. PMID:28340255
1807. Lawrence B, Gustafsson BI, Chan A, et al. The epidemiology of gastroenteropancreatic neuroendocrine tumors. Endocrinol Metab Clin North Am. 2011 Mar;40(1):1–18, vii. PMID:21349409
1808. Layfield LJ, Bentz J. Giant-cell containing neoplasms of the pancreas: an aspiration cytology study. Diagn Cytopathol. 2008 Apr;36(4):238–44. PMID:18335561
1809. Layfield LJ, Gopez EV. Percutaneous image-guided fine-needle aspiration of peritoneal lesions. Diagn Cytopathol. 2003 Jan;28(1):6–12. PMID:12508175
1810. Lazar AJ, Tuvin D, Hajibashi S, et al. Specific mutations in the beta-catenin gene (CTNNB1) correlate with local recurrence in sporadic desmoid tumors. Am J Pathol. 2008 Nov;173(5):1518–27. PMID:18832571
1811. Lazcano-Ponce EC, Miquel JF, Muñoz N, et al. Epidemiology and molecular pathology of gallbladder cancer. CA Cancer J Clin. 2001 Nov-Dec;51(6):349–64. PMID:11760569
1812. Lazure T, Dimet S, Ndiaye N, et al. Giant cell-rich solitary fibrous tumour of the gallbladder. First case report. Histopathology. 2007 May;50(6):805–7. PMID:17355274
1813. Le Bodic MF, Heymann MF, Lecomte M, et al. Immunohistochemical study of 100 pancreatic tumors in 28 patients with multiple endocrine neoplasia, type I. Am J Surg Pathol. 1996 Nov;20(11):1378–84. PMID:8898842
1814. Le Borgne R, Bellaïche Y, Schweisguth F. Drosophila E-cadherin regulates the orientation of asymmetric cell division in the sensory organ lineage. Curr Biol. 2002 Jan 22;12(2):95–104. PMID:11818059
1815. Le DT, Durham JN, Smith KN, et al. Mismatch repair deficiency predicts response of solid tumors to PD-1 blockade. Science. 2017 Jul 28;357(6349):409–13. PMID:28596308
1816. Le DT, Uram JN, Wang H, et al. PD-1 blockade in tumors with mismatch-repair deficiency. N Engl J Med. 2015 Jun 25;372(26):2509–20. PMID:26028255
1817. Le Roux C, Lombard-Bohas C, Delmas C, et al. Relapse factors for ileal neuroendocrine tumours after curative surgery: a retrospective French multicentre study. Dig Liver Dis. 2011 Oct;43(10):828–33. PMID:21641888
1818. Lechner MS, Laimins LA. Inhibition of p53 DNA binding by human papillomavirus E6 proteins. J Virol. 1994 Jul;68(7):4262–73. PMID:8207801
1819. Lecuit T, Yap AS. E-cadherin junctions as active mechanical integrators in tissue dynamics. Nat Cell Biol. 2015 May;17(5):533–9. PMID:25925582
1820. Lee AJ, Brenner L, Mourad B, et al. Gastrointestinal Kaposi's sarcoma: case report and review of the literature. World J Gastrointest Pharmacol Ther. 2015 Aug 6;6(3):89–95. PMID:26261737
1821. Lee CW, Tsai HI, Lin YS, et al. Intrahepatic biliary mucinous cystic neoplasms: clinicoradiological characteristics and surgical results. BMC Gastroenterol. 2015 Jun 10;15:67. PMID:26058559
1822. Lee HE, Smyrk TC, Zhang L. Histologic and immunohistochemical differences between hereditary and sporadic diffuse gastric carcinoma. Hum Pathol. 2018 Apr;74:64–72. PMID:29307626
1823. Lee HJ, Eom DW, Kang GH, et al. Colorectal micropapillary carcinomas are associated with poor prognosis and enriched in markers of stem cells. Mod Pathol. 2013 Aug;26(8):1123–31. PMID:23060121
1824. Lee JC, Fletcher CD. Malignant fat-forming solitary fibrous tumor (so-called "lipomatous hemangiopericytoma"): clinicopathologic analysis of 14 cases. Am J Surg Pathol. 2011 Aug;35(8):1177–85. PMID:21716088
1825. Lee JC, Li CF, Huang HY, et al. ALK oncoproteins in atypical inflammatory myofibroblastic tumours: novel RRBP1-ALK fusions in epithelioid inflammatory myofibroblastic sarcoma. J Pathol. 2017 Feb;241(3):316–23. PMID:27874193
1826. Lee JH, Abraham SC, Kim HS, et al. Inverse relationship between APC gene mutation in gastric adenomas and development of adenocarcinoma. Am J Pathol. 2002 Aug;161(2):611–8. PMID:12163385
1827. Lee JH, Kim MG, Jung MS, et al. Prognostic significance of lymphovascular invasion in node-negative gastric cancer. World J Surg. 2015 Mar;39(3):732–9. PMID:25376868
1828. Lee JK, Whittaker SJ, Enns RA, et al. Gastrointestinal manifestations of systemic mastocytosis. World J Gastroenterol. 2008 Dec 7;14(45):7005–8. PMID:19058339
1829. Lee JY, Chung H, Cho H, et al. Clinical characteristics and treatment outcomes of isolated myeloid sarcoma without bone marrow involvement: a single-institution experience. Blood Res. 2017 Sep;52(3):184–92. PMID:29043233
1830. Lee KB. Histopathology of a benign bile duct lesion in the liver: morphologic mimicker or precursor of intrahepatic cholangiocarcinoma. Clin Mol Hepatol. 2016 Sep;22(3):400–5. PMID:27729636
1831. Lee KTW, Gopalan V, Lam AK. Somatic DNA copy-number alterations detection for esophageal adenocarcinoma using digital polymerase chain reaction. Methods Mol Biol. 2018;1756:195–212. PMID:29600372
1832. Lee KTW, Smith RA, Gopalan V, et al. Targeted single gene mutation in esophageal adenocarcinoma. Methods Mol Biol. 2018;1756:213–29. PMID:29600373
1833. Lee LS, Singhal S, Brinster CJ, et al. Current management of esophageal leiomyoma. J Am Coll Surg. 2004 Jan;198(1):136–46. PMID:14698321
1834. Lee M, Pellegata NS. Multiple endocrine neoplasia syndromes associated with mutation of p27. J Endocrinol Invest. 2013 Oct;36(9):781–7. PMID:23800691
1836. Lee PN, Thornton AJ, Hamling JS. Epidemiological evidence on environmental tobacco smoke and cancers other than lung or breast. Regul Toxicol Pharmacol. 2016 Oct;80:134–63. PMID:27321059
1837. Lee RT, Ferreira J, Friedman K, et al. A rare cause of constipation: obstructing small cell neuroendocrine carcinoma of the anal canal. Int J Colorectal Dis. 2015 Sep;30(9):1291–2. PMID:26198995
1838. Lee S, Kim J, Soh JS, et al. Recurrence rate of lateral margin-positive cases after en bloc endoscopic submucosal dissection of colorectal neoplasia. Int J Colorectal Dis. 2018 Jun;33(6):735–43. PMID:29532207

1839. Lee S, Park HY, Kang SY, et al. Genetic alterations of JAK/STAT cascade and histone modification in extranodal NK/T-cell lymphoma nasal type. Oncotarget. 2015 Jul 10;6(19):17764–76. PMID:25980440
1840. Lee SE, Jang JY, Lee YJ, et al. Choledochal cyst and associated malignant tumors in adults: a multicenter survey in South Korea. Arch Surg. 2011 Oct;146(10):1178–84. PMID:22006877
1841. Lee SE, Kang SY, Cho J, et al. Pyloric gland adenoma in Lynch syndrome. Am J Surg Pathol. 2014 Jun;38(6):784–92. PMID:24518125
1842. Lee SY, Saito T, Mitomi H, et al. Mutation spectrum in the Wnt/β-catenin signaling pathway in gastric fundic gland-associated neoplasms/polyps. Virchows Arch. 2015 Jul;467(1):27–38. PMID:25820416
1843. Lee TY, Wu JC, Yu SH, et al. The occurrence of hepatocellular carcinoma in different risk stratifications of clinically noncirrhotic nonalcoholic fatty liver disease. Int J Cancer. 2017 Oct 1;141(7):1307–14. PMID:28509327
1844. Lee WA, Lee MK, Jeen YM, et al. Solitary fibrous tumor arising in gastric serosa. Pathol Int. 2004 Jun;54(6):436–9. PMID:15144403
1845. Lee WS, Koh YS, Kim JC, et al. Zollinger-Ellison syndrome associated with neurofibromatosis type 1: a case report. BMC Cancer. 2005 Jul 21;5:85. PMID:16042772
1846. Lee YC, Chiang TH, Chou CK, et al. Association between Helicobacter pylori eradication and gastric cancer incidence: a systematic review and meta-analysis. Gastroenterology. 2016 May;150(5):1113–24.e5. PMID:26836587
1847. Lee YC, Hsieh CC, Chuang JP. Prognostic significance of partial tumor regression after preoperative chemoradiotherapy for rectal cancer: a meta-analysis. Dis Colon Rectum. 2013 Sep;56(9):1093–101. PMID:23929020
1848. Lee YH, Oh BK, Yoo JE, et al. Chromosomal instability, telomere shortening, and inactivation of p21(WAF1/CIP1) in dysplastic nodules of hepatitis B virus-associated multistep hepatocarcinogenesis. Mod Pathol. 2009 Aug;22(8):1121–31. PMID:19465904
1849. Leggett B. FAP: another indication to treat H pylori. Gut. 2002 Oct;51(4):463–4. PMID:12235061
1850. Lehmann FS, Beglinger C, Schnabel K, et al. Progressive development of diffuse liver hemangiomatosis. J Hepatol. 1999 May;30(5):951–4. PMID:10365825
1851. Lei Z, Tan IB, Das K, et al. Identification of molecular subtypes of gastric cancer with different responses to PI3-kinase inhibitors and 5-fluorouracil. Gastroenterology. 2013 Sep;145(3):554–65. PMID:23684942
1852. Leng C, Li Y, Qin J, et al. Relationship between expression of PD-L1 and PD-L2 on esophageal squamous cell carcinoma and the antitumor effects of CD8+ T cells. Oncol Rep. 2016 Feb;35(2):699–708. PMID:26718132
1853. Lennon AM, Ahuja N, Wolfgang CL. AGA guidelines for the management of pancreatic cysts. Gastroenterology. 2015 Sep;149(3):825. PMID:26231607
1854. Lennon AM, Wolfgang CL, Canto MI, et al. The early detection of pancreatic cancer: what will it take to diagnose and treat curable pancreatic neoplasia? Cancer Res. 2014 Jul 1;74(13):3381–9. PMID:24924775
1855. Lenz G, Wright G, Dave SS, et al. Stromal gene signatures in large-B-cell lymphomas. N Engl J Med. 2008 Nov 27;359(22):2313–23. PMID:19038878
1856. Lenz G, Wright GW, Emre NC, et al. Molecular subtypes of diffuse large B-cell lymphoma arise by distinct genetic pathways. Proc Natl Acad Sci U S A. 2008 Sep 9;105(36):13520–5. PMID:18765795
1857. Lenze D, Leoncini L, Hummel M, et al. The different epidemiologic subtypes of Burkitt lymphoma share a homogenous micro RNA profile distinct from diffuse large B-cell lymphoma. Leukemia. 2011 Dec;25(12):1869–76. PMID:21701491
1858. Lenze F, Birkfellner T, Lenz P, et al. Undifferentiated embryonal sarcoma of the liver in adults. Cancer. 2008 May 15;112(10):2274–82. PMID:18361435
1859. Leonard D, Beddy D, Dozois EJ. Neoplasms of anal canal and perianal skin. Clin Colon Rectal Surg. 2011 Mar;24(1):54–63. PMID:22379406
1860. Leoncini E, Boffetta P, Shafir M, et al. Increased incidence trend of low-grade and high-grade neuroendocrine neoplasms. Endocrine. 2017 Nov;58(2):368–79. PMID:28303513
1861. Leoncini E, Carioli G, La Vecchia C, et al. Risk factors for neuroendocrine neoplasms: a systematic review and meta-analysis. Ann Oncol. 2016 Jan;27(1):68–81. PMID:26487581
1862. Lepage C, Rachet B, Coleman MP. Survival from malignant digestive endocrine tumors in England and Wales: a population-based study. Gastroenterology. 2007 Mar;132(3):899–904. PMID:17383419
1863. Lesluyes T, Pérot G, Largeau MR, et al. RNA sequencing validation of the Complexity INdex in SARComas prognostic signature. Eur J Cancer. 2016 Apr;57:104–11. PMID:26916546
1864. Leszczyszyn J, Łebski I, Łysenko L, et al. Anal warts (condylomata acuminata) - current issues and treatment modalities. Adv Clin Exp Med. 2014 Mar-Apr;23(2):307–11. PMID:24913124
1865. Leucci E, Cocco M, Onnis A, et al. MYC translocation-negative classical Burkitt lymphoma cases: an alternative pathogenetic mechanism involving miRNA deregulation. J Pathol. 2008 Dec;216(4):440–50. PMID:18802929
1866. Leung WK, Lin SR, Ching JY, et al. Factors predicting progression of gastric intestinal metaplasia: results of a randomised trial on Helicobacter pylori eradication. Gut. 2004 Sep;53(9):1244–9. PMID:15306578
1867. Leuschner I, Newton WA Jr, Schmidt D, et al. Spindle cell variants of embryonal rhabdomyosarcoma in the paratesticular region. A report of the Intergroup Rhabdomyosarcoma Study. Am J Surg Pathol. 1993 Mar;17(3):221–30. PMID:8434703
1868. Lev D, Kotilingam D, Wei C, et al. Optimizing treatment of desmoid tumors. J Clin Oncol. 2007 May 1;25(13):1785–91. PMID:17470870
1869. Levi Z, Baris HN, Kedar I, et al. Upper and lower gastrointestinal findings in PTEN mutation-positive Cowden syndrome patients participating in an active surveillance program. Clin Transl Gastroenterol. 2011 Nov 17;2:e5. PMID:23238744
1870. Levi Z, Kariv R, Barnes-Kedar I, et al. The gastrointestinal manifestation of constitutional mismatch repair deficiency syndrome: from a single adenoma to polyposis-like phenotype and early onset cancer. Clin Genet. 2015 Nov;88(5):474–8. PMID:25307252
1871. Levine AM, Tulpule A. Clinical aspects and management of AIDS-related Kaposi's sarcoma. Eur J Cancer. 2001 Jul;37(10):1288–95. PMID:11423260
1872. Levy AD, Abbott RM, Rohrmann CA Jr, et al. Gastrointestinal hemangiomas: imaging findings with pathologic correlation in pediatric and adult patients. AJR Am J Roentgenol. 2001 Nov;177(5):1073–81. PMID:11641173
1873. Levy AD, Quiles AM, Miettinen M, et al. Gastrointestinal schwannomas: CT features with clinicopathologic correlation. AJR Am J Roentgenol. 2005 Mar;184(3):797–802. PMID:15728600
1874. Levy M, Trivedi A, Zhang J, et al. Expression of glypican-3 in undifferentiated embryonal sarcoma and mesenchymal hamartoma of the liver. Hum Pathol. 2012 May;43(5):695–701. PMID:21937079
1875. Lewandrowski K, Warshaw A, Compton C. Macrocystic serous cystadenoma of the pancreas: a morphologic variant differing from microcystic adenoma. Hum Pathol. 1992 Aug;23(8):871–5. PMID:1644432
1875A. Lewin M, Handra-Luca A, Arrivé L, et al. Liver adenomatosis: classification of MR imaging features and comparison with pathologic findings. Radiology. 2006 Nov;241(2):433–40. PMID:16966481
1876. Lewis JT, Gaffney RL, Casey MB, et al. Inflammatory pseudotumor of the spleen associated with a clonal Epstein-Barr virus genome. Case report and review of the literature. Am J Clin Pathol. 2003 Jul;120(1):56–61. PMID:12866373
1877. Lewis JT, Talwalkar JA, Rosen CB, et al. Precancerous bile duct pathology in end-stage primary sclerosing cholangitis, with and without cholangiocarcinoma. Am J Surg Pathol. 2010 Jan;34(1):27–34. PMID:19898228
1878. Lewis JT, Talwalkar JA, Rosen CB, et al. Prevalence and risk factors for gallbladder neoplasia in patients with primary sclerosing cholangitis: evidence for a metaplasia-dysplasia-carcinoma sequence. Am J Surg Pathol. 2007 Jun;31(6):907–13. PMID:17527079
1879. Leão JC, Caterino-De-Araújo A, Porter SR, et al. Human herpesvirus 8 (HHV-8) and the etiopathogenesis of Kaposi's sarcoma. Rev Hosp Clin Fac Med Sao Paulo. 2002 Jul-Aug;57(4):175–86. PMID:12244338
1880. Li D, Bautista MC, Jiang SF, et al. Risks and predictors of gastric adenocarcinoma in patients with gastric intestinal metaplasia and dysplasia: a population-based study. Am J Gastroenterol. 2016 Aug;111(8):1104–13. PMID:27185078
1881. Li FP, Fletcher JA, Heinrich MC, et al. Familial gastrointestinal stromal tumor syndrome: phenotypic and molecular features in a kindred. J Clin Oncol. 2005 Apr 20;23(12):2735–43. PMID:15837988
1882. Li GM. Mechanisms and functions of DNA mismatch repair. Cell Res. 2008 Jan;18(1):85–98. PMID:18157157
1883. Li J, Woods SL, Healey S, et al. Point mutations in exon 1B of APC reveal gastric adenocarcinoma and proximal polyposis of the stomach as a familial adenomatous polyposis variant. Am J Hum Genet. 2016 May 5;98(5):830–42. PMID:27087319
1884. Li L, Qian M, Chen IH, et al. Acquisition of cholangiocarcinoma traits during advanced hepatocellular carcinoma development in mice. Am J Pathol. 2018 Mar;188(3):656–71. PMID:29248454
1885. Li M, Liu F, Zhang Y, et al. Whole-genome sequencing reveals the mutational landscape of metastatic small-cell gallbladder neuroendocrine carcinoma (GB-SCNEC). Cancer Lett. 2017 Apr 10;391:20–7. PMID:28040546
1886. Li M, Zhao H, Zhang X, et al. Inactivating mutations of the chromatin remodeling gene ARID2 in hepatocellular carcinoma. Nat Genet. 2011 Aug 7;43(9):828–9. PMID:21822264
1887. Li S, Tian B. Acute pancreatitis in patients with pancreatic cancer: timing of surgery and survival duration. Medicine (Baltimore). 2017 Jan;96(3):e5908. PMID:28099352
1888. Li T, Fan J, Qin LX, et al. Risk factors, prognosis, and management of early and late intrahepatic recurrence after resection of primary clear cell carcinoma of the liver. Ann Surg Oncol. 2011 Jul;18(7):1955–63. PMID:21240562
1889. Li T, Wang L, Yu HH, et al. Hepatic angiomyolipoma: a retrospective study of 25 cases. Surg Today. 2008;38(6):529–35. PMID:18516533
1890. Li TJ, Zhang YX, Wen J, et al. Basaloid squamous cell carcinoma of the esophagus with or without adenoid cystic features. Arch Pathol Lab Med. 2004 Oct;128(10):1124–30. PMID:15387711
1891. Li X, Shi Z, You R, et al. Inflammatory pseudotumor-like follicular dendritic cell sarcoma of the spleen: computed tomography imaging characteristics in 5 patients. J Comput Assist Tomogr. 2018 May/Jun;42(3):399–404. PMID:29287022
1892. Li X, Zhang Y, Zhang Y, et al. Survival prediction of gastric cancer by a seven-microRNA signature. Gut. 2010 May;59(5):579–85. PMID:19951901
1893. Li Y, Fu L, Li JB, et al. Increased expression of EIF5A2, via hypoxia or gene amplification, contributes to metastasis and angiogenesis of esophageal squamous cell carcinoma. Gastroenterology. 2014 Jun;146(7):1701–13.e9. PMID:24561231
1894. Li Z, Xia Y, Feng LN, et al. Genetic risk of extranodal natural killer T-cell lymphoma: a genome-wide association study. Lancet Oncol. 2016 Sep;17(9):1240–7. PMID:27470079
1895. Liang R, Todd D, Chan TK, et al. Prognostic factors for primary gastrointestinal lymphoma. Hematol Oncol. 1995 May-Jun;13(3):153–63. PMID:7622145
1896. Liang W, He W, Li Z. Extranodal follicular dendritic cell sarcoma originating in the pancreas: a case report. Medicine (Baltimore). 2016 Apr;95(15):e3377. PMID:27082603
1897. Liao X, Lochhead P, Nishihara R, et al. Aspirin use, tumor PIK3CA mutation, and colorectal-cancer survival. N Engl J Med. 2012 Oct 25;367(17):1596–606. PMID:23094721
1898. Liau JY, Tsai JH, Yang CY, et al. Alternative lengthening of telomeres phenotype in malignant vascular tumors is highly associated with loss of ATRX expression and is frequently observed in hepatic angiosarcomas. Hum Pathol. 2015 Sep;46(9):1360–6. PMID:26190196
1899. Liau JY, Tsai JH, Yuan RH, et al. Morphological subclassification of intrahepatic cholangiocarcinoma: etiological, clinicopathological, and molecular features. Mod Pathol. 2014 Aug;27(8):1163–73. PMID:24406866
1900. Liaw D, Marsh DJ, Li J, et al. Germline mutations of the PTEN gene in Cowden disease, an inherited breast and thyroid cancer syndrome. Nat Genet. 1997 May;16(1):64–7. PMID:9140396
1901. Libbrecht L, Cassiman D, Verslype C, et al. Clinicopathological features of focal nodular hyperplasia-like nodules in 130 cirrhotic explant livers. Am J Gastroenterol. 2006 Oct;101(10):2341–6. PMID:17032200
1902. Lichtenauer UD, Di Dalmazi G, Slater EP, et al. Frequency and clinical correlates of somatic Ying Yang 1 mutations in sporadic insulinomas. J Clin Endocrinol Metab. 2015 May;100(5):E776–82. PMID:25763608
1903. Lieberman DA, Rex DK, Winawer SJ, et al. Guidelines for colonoscopy surveillance after screening and polypectomy: a consensus update by the US Multi-Society Task Force on Colorectal Cancer. Gastroenterology. 2012 Sep;143(3):844–57. PMID:22763141
1904. Liebig C, Ayala G, Wilks JA, et al. Perineural invasion in cancer: a review of the literature. Cancer. 2009 Aug 1;115(15):3379–91. PMID:19484787
1905. Liegl B, Bennett MW, Fletcher CD. Microcystic/reticular schwannoma: a distinct

variant with predilection for visceral locations. Am J Surg Pathol. 2008 Jul;32(7):1080–7. PMID:18520439
1906. Liegl B, Hornick JL, Antonescu CR, et al. Rhabdomyosarcomatous differentiation in gastrointestinal stromal tumors after tyrosine kinase inhibitor therapy: a novel form of tumor progression. Am J Surg Pathol. 2009 Feb;33(2):218–26. PMID:18830121
1907. Liegl B, Hornick JL, Lazar AJ. Contemporary pathology of gastrointestinal stromal tumors. Hematol Oncol Clin North Am. 2009 Feb;23(1):49–68, vii–viii. PMID:19248970
1908. Ligato S, Furmaga W, Cartun RW, et al. Primary carcinoid tumor of the common hepatic duct: a rare case with immunohistochemical and molecular findings. Oncol Rep. 2005 Mar;13(3):543–6. PMID:15706430
1909. Ligneau B, Lombard-Bohas C, Partensky C, et al. Cystic endocrine tumors of the pancreas: clinical, radiologic, and histopathologic features in 13 cases. Am J Surg Pathol. 2001 Jun;25(6):752–60. PMID:11395552
1910. Ligtenberg MJ, Kuiper RP, Geurts van Kessel A, et al. EPCAM deletion carriers constitute a unique subgroup of Lynch syndrome patients. Fam Cancer. 2013 Jun;12(2):169–74. PMID:23264089
1911. Lilo MT, VandenBussche CJ, Allison DB, et al. Serous cystadenoma of the pancreas: potentials and pitfalls of a preoperative cytopathologic diagnosis. Acta Cytol. 2017;61(1):27–33. PMID:27889754
1912. Lim CH, Cho YK, Kim SW, et al. The chronological sequence of somatic mutations in early gastric carcinogenesis inferred from multiregion sequencing of gastric adenomas. Oncotarget. 2016 Jun 28;7(26):39758–67. PMID:27175599
1913. Lim H, Park YS, Lee JH, et al. Features of gastric carcinoma with lymphoid stroma associated with Epstein-Barr virus. Clin Gastroenterol Hepatol. 2015 Oct;13(10):1738–44.e2. PMID:25912839
1914. Lim JE, Chien MW, Earle CC. Prognostic factors following curative resection for pancreatic adenocarcinoma: a population-based, linked database analysis of 396 patients. Ann Surg. 2003 Jan;237(1):74–85. PMID:12496533
1915. Lin CC, Chiang JH, Li CI, et al. Independent and joint effect of type 2 diabetes and gastric and hepatobiliary diseases on risk of pancreatic cancer risk: 10-year follow-up of population-based cohort. Br J Cancer. 2014 Nov 25;111(11):2180–6. PMID:25275365
1916. Lin CW, Lai CH, Hsu CC, et al. Primary hepatic carcinoid tumor: a case report and review of the literature. Cases J. 2009 Jan 27;2(1):90. PMID:19173727
1917. Lin DC, Hao JJ, Nagata Y, et al. Genomic and molecular characterization of esophageal squamous cell carcinoma. Nat Genet. 2014 May;46(5):467–73. PMID:24686850
1918. Lin DC, Wang MR, Koeffler HP. Genomic and epigenomic aberrations in esophageal squamous cell carcinoma and implications for patients. Gastroenterology. 2018 Jan;154(2):374–89. PMID:28757263
1919. Lin H, van den Esschert J, Liu C, et al. Systematic review of hepatocellular adenoma in China and other regions. J Gastroenterol Hepatol. 2011 Jan;26(1):28–35. PMID:21175790
1920. Lin J, Bigge J, Ulbright TM, et al. Anastomosing hemangioma of the liver and gastrointestinal tract: an unusual variant histologically mimicking angiosarcoma. Am J Surg Pathol. 2013 Nov;37(11):1761–5. PMID:23887160
1921. Lin Y, Ueda J, Kikuchi S, et al. Comparative epidemiology of gastric cancer between Japan and China. World J Gastroenterol. 2011 Oct 21;17(39):4421–8. PMID:22110269
1923. Lindberg B, Arnelo U, Bergquist A, et al. Diagnosis of biliary strictures in conjunction with endoscopic retrograde cholangiopancreaticography, with special reference to patients with primary sclerosing cholangitis. Endoscopy. 2002 Nov;34(11):909–16. PMID:12430077
1924. Lisker-Melman M, Pittaluga S, Pluda JM, et al. Primary lymphoma of the liver in a patient with acquired immune deficiency syndrome and chronic hepatitis B. Am J Gastroenterol. 1989 Nov;84(11):1445–8. PMID:2683745
1925. Lisovsky M, Patel K, Cymes K, et al. Immunophenotypic characterization of anal gland carcinoma: loss of p63 and cytokeratin 5/6. Arch Pathol Lab Med. 2007 Aug;131(8):1304–11. PMID:17683193
1926. Littooij AS, McHugh K, McCarville MB, et al. Yolk sac tumour: a rare cause of raised serum alpha-foetoprotein in a young child with a large liver mass. Pediatr Radiol. 2014 Jan;44(1):18–22. PMID:23982265
1927. Liu C, Karam R, Zhou Y, et al. The UPF1 RNA surveillance gene is commonly mutated in pancreatic adenosquamous carcinoma. Nat Med. 2014 Jun;20(6):596–8. PMID:24859531
1928. Liu C, McKeone DM, Walker NI, et al. GNAS mutations are present in colorectal traditional serrated adenomas, serrated tubulovillous adenomas and serrated adenocarcinomas with adverse prognostic features. Histopathology. 2017 Jun;70(7):1079–88. PMID:28164369
1929. Liu C, Walker NI, Leggett BA, et al. Sessile serrated adenomas with dysplasia: morphological patterns and correlations with MLH1 immunohistochemistry. Mod Pathol. 2017 Dec;30(12):1728–38. PMID:28752838
1930. Liu H, Ye H, Ruskone-Fourmestraux A, et al. t(11;18) is a marker for all stage gastric MALT lymphomas that will not respond to H. pylori eradication. Gastroenterology. 2002 May;122(5):1286–94. PMID:11984515
1931. Liu W, Shia J, Gönen M, et al. DNA mismatch repair abnormalities in acinar cell carcinoma of the pancreas: frequency and clinical significance. Pancreas. 2014 Nov;43(8):1264–70. PMID:25058881
1932. Liu X, Mody K, de Abreu FB, et al. Molecular profiling of appendiceal epithelial tumors using massively parallel sequencing to identify somatic mutations. Clin Chem. 2014 Jul;60(7):1004–11. PMID:24821835
1933. Liu ZH, Lian BF, Dong QZ, et al. Whole-exome mutational and transcriptional landscapes of combined hepatocellular cholangiocarcinoma and intrahepatic cholangiocarcinoma reveal molecular diversity. Biochim Biophys Acta Mol Basis Dis. 2018 Jun;1864 6 Pt B:2360–8. PMID:29408647
1934. Lièvre A, Bachet JB, Le Corre D, et al. KRAS mutation status is predictive of response to cetuximab therapy in colorectal cancer. Cancer Res. 2006 Apr 15;66(8):3992–5. PMID:16618717
1935. Llovet JM, Brú C, Bruix J. Prognosis of hepatocellular carcinoma: the BCLC staging classification. Semin Liver Dis. 1999;19(3):329–38. PMID:10518312
1936. Lloyd RV, Osamura RY, Klöppel G, et al., editors. WHO classification of tumours of endocrine organs. Lyon (France): International Agency for Research on Cancer; 2017. (WHO classification of tumours series, 4th ed.; vol. 10). http://publications.iarc.fr/554.
1937. Lo RC. Epithelioid angiomyolipoma of the liver: a clinicopathologic study of 5 cases. Ann Diagn Pathol. 2013 Oct;17(5):412–5. PMID:23786777
1938. Loane J, Kealy WF, Mulcahy G. Perianal hidradenoma papilliferum occurring in a male: a case report. Ir J Med Sci. 1998 Jan-Mar;167(1):26–7. PMID:9540295
1939. Loftus EV Jr, Olivares-Pakzad BA, Batts KP, et al. Intraductal papillary-mucinous tumors of the pancreas: clinicopathologic features, outcome, and nomenclature. Members of the Pancreas Clinic, and Pancreatic Surgeons of Mayo Clinic. Gastroenterology. 1996 Jun;110(6):1909–18. PMID:8964418
1940. Loghavi S, Alayed K, Aladily TN, et al. Stage, age, and EBV status impact outcomes of plasmablastic lymphoma patients: a clinicopathologic analysis of 61 patients. J Hematol Oncol. 2015 Jun 10;8:65. PMID:26055271
1941. Logroño R, Rampy BA, Adegboyega PA. Fine needle aspiration cytology of hepatobiliary cystadenoma with mesenchymal stroma. Cancer. 2002 Feb 25;96(1):37–42. PMID:11836701
1942. Lohse I, Borgida A, Cao P, et al. BRCA1 and BRCA2 mutations sensitize to chemotherapy in patient-derived pancreatic cancer xenografts. Br J Cancer. 2015 Jul 28;113(3):425–32. PMID:26180923
1943. Lokko C, Turner J, Yoo W, et al. Anal squamous cell carcinoma in African Americans with and without HIV: a comparative study. J Cancer Epidemiol Treat. 2015;1(1):6–10. PMID:27774311
1944. Lomberk G, Blum Y, Nicolle R, et al. Distinct epigenetic landscapes underlie the pathobiology of pancreatic cancer subtypes. Nat Commun. 2018 May 17;9(1):1978. PMID:29773832
1945. Lomo LC, Blount PL, Sanchez CA, et al. Crypt dysplasia with surface maturation: a clinical, pathologic, and molecular study of a Barrett's esophagus cohort. Am J Surg Pathol. 2006 Apr;30(4):423–35. PMID:16625087
1946. Longacre TA, Kong CS, Welton ML. Diagnostic problems in anal pathology. Adv Anat Pathol. 2008 Sep;15(5):263–78. PMID:18724100
1947. Loos M, Bergmann F, Bauer A, et al. Solid type clear cell carcinoma of the pancreas: differential diagnosis of an unusual case and review of the literature. Virchows Arch. 2007 Jun;450(6):719–26. PMID:17453235
1948. Lorenzi L, Döring C, Rausch T, et al. Identification of novel follicular dendritic cell sarcoma markers, FDCSP and SRGN, by whole transcriptome sequencing. Oncotarget. 2017 Mar 7;8(10):16463–72. PMID:28145886
1949. Loukola A, Salovaara R, Kristo P, et al. Microsatellite instability in adenomas as a marker for hereditary nonpolyposis colorectal cancer. Am J Pathol. 1999 Dec;155(6):1849–53. PMID:10595914
1950. Love C, Sun Z, Jima D, et al. The genetic landscape of mutations in Burkitt lymphoma. Nat Genet. 2012 Dec;44(12):1321–5. PMID:23143597
1951. Lovly CM, Gupta A, Lipson D, et al. Inflammatory myofibroblastic tumors harbor multiple potentially actionable kinase fusions. Cancer Discov. 2014 Aug;4(8):889–95. PMID:24875859
1952. Lowenfels AB, Maisonneuve P, DiMagno EP, et al. Hereditary pancreatitis and the risk of pancreatic cancer. J Natl Cancer Inst. 1997 Mar 19;89(6):442–6. PMID:9091646
1953. Lowery MA, Klimstra DS, Shia J, et al. Acinar cell carcinoma of the pancreas: new genetic and treatment insights into a rare malignancy. Oncologist. 2011;16(12):1714–20. PMID:22042785
1954. Lowery MA, Wong W, Jordan EJ, et al. Prospective evaluation of germline alterations in patients with exocrine pancreatic neoplasms. J Natl Cancer Inst. 2018 Oct 1;110(10):1067–74. PMID:29506128
1955. Loy TS, Kaplan PA. Villous adenocarcinoma of the colon and rectum: a clinicopathologic study of 36 cases. Am J Surg Pathol. 2004 Nov;28(11):1460–5. PMID:15489649
1956. Lu DW, El-Mofty SK, Wang HL. Expression of p16, Rb, and p53 proteins in squamous cell carcinomas of the anorectal region harboring human papillomavirus DNA. Mod Pathol. 2003 Jul;16(7):692–9. PMID:12861066
1957. Ludvigsson JF, Bai JC, Biagi F, et al. Diagnosis and management of adult coeliac disease: guidelines from the British Society of Gastroenterology. Gut. 2014 Aug;63(8):1210–28. PMID:24917550
1958. Lugli A, Kirsch R, Ajioka Y, et al. Recommendations for reporting tumor budding in colorectal cancer based on the International Tumor Budding Consensus Conference (ITBCC) 2016. Mod Pathol. 2017 Sep;30(9):1299–311. PMID:28548122
1959. Lukás Z, Dvorák K, Kroupová I, et al. Immunohistochemical and genetic analysis of osteoclastic giant cell tumor of the pancreas. Pancreas. 2006 Apr;32(3):325–9. PMID:16628090
1960. Luminari S, Cesaretti M, Marcheselli L, et al. Decreasing incidence of gastric MALT lymphomas in the era of anti-Helicobacter pylori interventions: results from a population-based study on extranodal marginal zone lymphomas. Ann Oncol. 2010 Apr;21(4):855–9. PMID:19850642
1961. Lunniss PJ, Sheffield JP, Talbot IC, et al. Persistence of idiopathic anal fistula may be related to epithelialization. Br J Surg. 1995 Jan;82(1):32–3. PMID:7881949
1962. Luu C, Thapa R, Woo K, et al. Does histology really influence gastric cancer prognosis? J Gastrointest Oncol. 2017 Dec;8(6):1026–36. PMID:29299363
1963. Luvira V, Pugkhem A, Bhudhisawasdi V, et al. Long-term outcome of surgical resection for intraductal papillary neoplasm of the bile duct. J Gastroenterol Hepatol. 2017 Feb;32(2):527–33. PMID:27356284
1964. Luvira V, Somsap K, Pugkhem A, et al. Morphological classification of intraductal papillary neoplasm of the bile duct with survival correlation. Asian Pac J Cancer Prev. 2017 Jan 1;18(1):207–13. PMID:28240521
1965. Luzar B, Antony F, Ramdial PK, et al. Intravascular Kaposi's sarcoma - a hitherto unrecognized phenomenon. J Cutan Pathol. 2007 Nov;34(11):861–4. PMID:17944727
1966. Lymphoma Study Group of Japanese Pathologists. The World Health Organization classification of malignant lymphomas in Japan: incidence of recently recognized entities. Pathol Int. 2000 Sep;50(9):696–702. PMID:11012982
1967. Lynch HT, Cristofaro G, Rozen P, et al. History of the International Collaborative Group on Hereditary Non Polyposis Colorectal Cancer. Fam Cancer. 2003;2 Suppl 1:3–5. PMID:14574154
1968. Lynch HT, Deters CA, Lynch JF, et al. Familial pancreatic carcinoma in Jews. Fam Cancer. 2004;3(3-4):233–40. PMID:15516847
1969. Lynch HT, Krush AJ. Cancer family "G" revisited: 1895-1970. Cancer. 1971 Jun;27(6):1505–11. PMID:5088221
1970. Lynch HT, Lynch PM, Pester J, et al. The cancer family syndrome. Rare cutaneous phenotypic linkage of Torre's syndrome. Arch Intern Med. 1981 Apr;141(5):607–11. PMID:7224741
1971. Lynch HT, Riegert-Johnson DL, Snyder C, et al. Lynch syndrome-associated extracolonic tumors are rare in two extended families with the same EPCAM deletion. Am J Gastroenterol. 2011 Oct;106(10):1829–36. PMID:21769135
1972. Lynch HT, Smyrk T, Lynch JF. Molecular genetics and clinical-pathology features of hereditary nonpolyposis colorectal carcinoma (Lynch syndrome): historical journey from pedigree anecdote to molecular genetic confirmation. Oncology. 1998 Mar-Apr;55(2):103–8. PMID:9499183
1973. Lynch SM, Vrieling A, Lubin JH, et al.

Cigarette smoking and pancreatic cancer: a pooled analysis from the pancreatic cancer cohort consortium. Am J Epidemiol. 2009 Aug 15;170(4):403–13. PMID:19561064
1974. Lévy-Bohbot N, Merle C, Goudet P, et al. Prevalence, characteristics and prognosis of MEN 1-associated glucagonomas, VIPomas, and somatostatinomas: study from the GTE (Groupe des Tumeurs Endocrines) registry. Gastroenterol Clin Biol. 2004 Nov;28(11):1075–81. PMID:15657529
1975. López-Terrada D, Alaggio R, de Dávila MT, et al. Towards an international pediatric liver tumor consensus classification: proceedings of the Los Angeles COG liver tumors symposium. Mod Pathol. 2014 Mar;27(3):472–91. PMID:24008558
1976. López-Terrada D, Gunaratne PH, Adesina AM, et al. Histologic subtypes of hepatoblastoma are characterized by differential canonical Wnt and Notch pathway activation in DLK+ precursors. Hum Pathol. 2009 Jun;40(6):783–94. PMID:19200579
1977. Lüttges J, Feyerabend B, Buchelt T, et al. The mucin profile of noninvasive and invasive mucinous cystic neoplasms of the pancreas. Am J Surg Pathol. 2002 Apr;26(4):466–71. PMID:11914624
1978. Lüttges J, Mentzel T, Hübner G, et al. Solitary fibrous tumour of the pancreas: a new member of the small group of mesenchymal pancreatic tumours. Virchows Arch. 1999 Jul;435(1):37–42. PMID:10431844
1979. Lüttges J, Schemm S, Vogel I, et al. The grade of pancreatic ductal carcinoma is an independent prognostic factor and is superior to the immunohistochemical assessment of proliferation. J Pathol. 2000 Jun;191(2):154–61. PMID:10861575
1980. Lüttges J, Stigge C, Pacena M, et al. Rare ductal adenocarcinoma of the pancreas in patients younger than age 40 years. Cancer. 2004 Jan 1;100(1):173–82. PMID:14692038
1981. Lüttges J, Vogel I, Menke M, et al. Clear cell carcinoma of the pancreas: an adenocarcinoma with ductal phenotype. Histopathology. 1998 May;32(5):444–8. PMID:9639120
1983. Lüttges J, Zamboni G, Longnecker D, et al. The immunohistochemical mucin expression pattern distinguishes different types of intraductal papillary mucinous neoplasms of the pancreas and determines their relationship to mucinous noncystic carcinoma and ductal adenocarcinoma. Am J Surg Pathol. 2001 Jul;25(7):942–8. PMID:11420467
1984. Ma C, Giardiello FM, Montgomery EA. Upper tract juvenile polyps in juvenile polyposis patients: dysplasia and malignancy are associated with foveolar, intestinal, and pyloric differentiation. Am J Surg Pathol. 2014 Dec;38(12):1618–26. PMID:25390638
1985. Ma J, Siegel R, Jemal A. Pancreatic cancer death rates by race among US men and women, 1970-2009. J Natl Cancer Inst. 2013 Nov 20;105(22):1694–700. PMID:24203988
1986. Ma MX, Bourke MJ. Management of duodenal polyps. Best Pract Res Clin Gastroenterol. 2017 Aug;31(4):389–99. PMID:28842048
1987. Ma Q, Zhang C, Fang S, et al. Primary esophageal mucosa-associated lymphoid tissue lymphoma: a case report and review of literature. Medicine (Baltimore). 2017 Mar;96(13):e6478. PMID:28353588
1988. Ma Y, Zheng J, Zhu H, et al. Gastroblastoma in a 12-year-old Chinese boy. Int J Clin Exp Pathol. 2014 May 15;7(6):3380–4. PMID:25031764
1989. Maarschalk-Ellerbroek LJ, Oldenburg B, Mombers IM, et al. Outcome of screening endoscopy in common variable immunodeficiency disorder and X-linked agammaglobulinemia. Endoscopy. 2013;45(4):320–3. PMID:23325698
1990. Maas M, Nelemans PJ, Valentini V, et al. Long-term outcome in patients with a pathological complete response after chemoradiation for rectal cancer: a pooled analysis of individual patient data. Lancet Oncol. 2010 Sep;11(9):835–44. PMID:20692872
1991. Machado JC, Soares P, Carneiro F, et al. E-cadherin gene mutations provide a genetic basis for the phenotypic divergence of mixed gastric carcinomas. Lab Invest. 1999 Apr;79(4):459–65. PMID:10211998
1992. Machado MC, Machado MA. Solid serous adenoma of the pancreas: an uncommon but important entity. Eur J Surg Oncol. 2008 Jul;34(7):730–3. PMID:18440191
1993. Machens A, Schaaf L, Karges W, et al. Age-related penetrance of endocrine tumours in multiple endocrine neoplasia type 1 (MEN1): a multicentre study of 258 gene carriers. Clin Endocrinol (Oxf). 2007 Oct;67(4):613–22. PMID:17590169
1994. Mackey AC, Green L, Liang LC, et al. Hepatosplenic T cell lymphoma associated with infliximab use in young patients treated for inflammatory bowel disease. J Pediatr Gastroenterol Nutr. 2007 Feb;44(2):265–7. PMID:17255842
1995. Macon WR, Levy NB, Kurtin PJ, et al. Hepatosplenic alphabeta T-cell lymphomas: a report of 14 cases and comparison with hepatosplenic gammadelta T-cell lymphomas. Am J Surg Pathol. 2001 Mar;25(3):285–96. PMID:11224598
1996. Macon WR, Williams ME, Greer JP, et al. Paracortical nodular T-cell lymphoma. Identification of an unusual variant of peripheral T-cell lymphoma. Am J Surg Pathol. 1995 Mar;19(3):297–303. PMID:7872427
1997. Madura JA, Jarman BT, Doherty MG, et al. Adenosquamous carcinoma of the pancreas. Arch Surg. 1999 Jun;134(6):599–603. PMID:10367867
1998. Maejima T, Kono T, Orii F, et al. Anal canal adenocarcinoma in a patient with longstanding Crohn's disease arising from rectal mucosa that migrated from a previously treated rectovaginal fistula. Am J Case Rep. 2016 Jul 4;17:448–53. PMID:27373845
1999. Maffione AM, Marzola MC, Capirci C, et al. Value of (18)F-FDG PET for predicting response to neoadjuvant therapy in rectal cancer: systematic review and meta-analysis. AJR Am J Roentgenol. 2015 Jun;204(6):1261–8. PMID:26001237
2000. Magrath I. Epidemiology: clues to the pathogenesis of Burkitt lymphoma. Br J Haematol. 2012 Mar;156(6):744–56. PMID:22260300
2001. Maguilnik I, Neumann WL, Sonnenberg A, et al. Reactive gastropathy is associated with inflammatory conditions throughout the gastrointestinal tract. Aliment Pharmacol Ther. 2012 Oct;36(8):736–43. PMID:22928604
2002. Maguire A, Sheahan K. Primary small bowel adenomas and adenocarcinomas-recent advances. Virchows Arch. 2018 Sep;473(3):265–73. PMID:29998424
2003. Mahmud A, Poon R, Jonker D. PET imaging in anal canal cancer: a systematic review and meta-analysis. Br J Radiol. 2017 Dec;90(1080):20170370. PMID:28972796
2004. Mahon M, Xu J, Yi X, et al. Paneth cell in adenomas of the distal colorectum is inversely associated with synchronous advanced adenoma and carcinoma. Sci Rep. 2016 May 18;6:26129. PMID:27188450
2005. Mahurkar S, Reddy DN, Rao GV, et al. Genetic mechanisms underlying the pathogenesis of tropical calcific pancreatitis. World J Gastroenterol. 2009 Jan 21;15(3):264–9. PMID:19140225
2006. Maire F, Hammel P, Terris B, et al. Intraductal papillary and mucinous pancreatic tumour: a new extracolonic tumour in familial adenomatous polyposis. Gut. 2002 Sep;51(3):446–9. PMID:12171972
2007. Maire F, Hammel P, Terris B, et al. Prognosis of malignant intraductal papillary mucinous tumours of the pancreas after surgical resection. Comparison with pancreatic ductal adenocarcinoma. Gut. 2002 Nov;51(5):717–22. PMID:12377813
2008. Maitra A, Adsay NV, Argani P, et al. Multicomponent analysis of the pancreatic adenocarcinoma progression model using a pancreatic intraepithelial neoplasia tissue microarray. Mod Pathol. 2003 Sep;16(9):902–12. PMID:13679454
2009. Maitra A, Hruban RH. Pancreatic cancer. Annu Rev Pathol. 2008;3:157–88. PMID:18039136
2010. Maitra A, Krueger JE, Tascilar M, et al. Carcinoid tumors of the extrahepatic bile ducts: a study of seven cases. Am J Surg Pathol. 2000 Nov;24(11):1501–10. PMID:11075851
2011. Maitra A, Tascilar M, Hruban RH, et al. Small cell carcinoma of the gallbladder: a clinicopathologic, immunohistochemical, and molecular pathology study of 12 cases. Am J Surg Pathol. 2001 May;25(5):595–601. PMID:11342770
2012. Majewski IJ, Kluijt I, Cats A, et al. An α-E-catenin (CTNNA1) mutation in hereditary diffuse gastric cancer. J Pathol. 2013 Mar;229(4):621–9. PMID:23208944
2013. Majewski JT, Wilson SD. The MEA-I syndrome: an all or none phenomenon? Surgery. 1979 Sep;86(3):475–84. PMID:38521
2014. Makhlouf HR, Abdul-Al HM, Wang G, et al. Calcifying nested stromal-epithelial tumors of the liver: a clinicopathologic, immunohistochemical, and molecular genetic study of 9 cases with a long-term follow-up. Am J Surg Pathol. 2009 Jul;33(7):976–83. PMID:19363442
2015. Makhlouf HR, Burke AP, Sobin LH. Carcinoid tumors of the ampulla of Vater: a comparison with duodenal carcinoid tumors. Cancer. 1999 Mar 15;85(6):1241–9. PMID:10189128
2016. Makhlouf HR, Ishak KG, Goodman ZD. Epithelioid hemangioendothelioma of the liver: a clinicopathologic study of 137 cases. Cancer. 1999 Feb 1;85(3):562–82. PMID:10091730
2017. Makhlouf HR, Ishak KG, Shekar R, et al. Melanoma markers in angiomyolipoma of the liver and kidney: a comparative study. Arch Pathol Lab Med. 2002 Jan;126(1):49–55. PMID:11800647
2018. Makhlouf HR, Remotti HE, Ishak KG. Expression of KIT (CD117) in angiomyolipoma. Am J Surg Pathol. 2002 Apr;26(4):493–7. PMID:11914628
2019. Makhlouf HR, Sobin LH. Inflammatory myofibroblastic tumors (inflammatory pseudotumors) of the gastrointestinal tract: how closely are they related to inflammatory fibroid polyps? Hum Pathol. 2002 Mar;33(3):307–15. PMID:11979371
2020. Maki M, Kaneko Y, Ohta Y, et al. Somatostatinoma of the pancreas associated with von Hippel-Lindau disease. Intern Med. 1995 Jul;34(7):661–5. PMID:7496080
2021. Makino H, Miyashita M, Nomura T, et al. Solitary fibrous tumor of the cervical esophagus. Dig Dis Sci. 2007 Sep;52(9):2195–200. PMID:17429725
2022. Makuuchi R, Terashima M, Kusuhara M, et al. Comprehensive analysis of gene mutation and expression profiles in neuroendocrine carcinomas of the stomach. Biomed Res. 2017;38(1):19–27. PMID:28239029
2023. Malaguarnera G, Madeddu R, Catania VE, et al. Anorectal mucosal melanoma. Oncotarget. 2018 Jan 2;9(9):8785–800. PMID:29492238
2024. Malamut G, Afchain P, Verkarre V, et al. Presentation and long-term follow-up of refractory celiac disease: comparison of type I with type II. Gastroenterology. 2009 Jan;136(1):81–90. PMID:19014942
2025. Malamut G, Chandesris O, Verkarre V, et al. Enteropathy associated T cell lymphoma in celiac disease: a large retrospective study. Dig Liver Dis. 2013 May;45(5):377–84. PMID:23313469
2026. Malamut G, El Machhour R, Montcuquet N, et al. IL-15 triggers an antiapoptotic pathway in human intraepithelial lymphocytes that is a potential new target in celiac disease-associated inflammation and lymphomagenesis. J Clin Invest. 2010 Jun;120(6):2131–43. PMID:20440074
2027. Malamut G, Meresse B, Cellier C, et al. Refractory celiac disease: from bench to bedside. Semin Immunopathol. 2012 Jul;34(4):601–13. PMID:22810901
2028. Malamut G, Verkarre V, Callens C, et al. Enteropathy-associated T-cell lymphoma complicating an autoimmune enteropathy. Gastroenterology. 2012 Apr;142(4):726–9.e3, quiz e13–4. PMID:22226659
2029. Malanga D, De Gisi S, Riccardi M, et al. Functional characterization of a rare germline mutation in the gene encoding the cyclin-dependent kinase inhibitor p27Kip1 (CDKN1B) in a Spanish patient with multiple endocrine neoplasia-like phenotype. Eur J Endocrinol. 2012 Mar;166(3):551–60. PMID:22129891
2030. Malek-Hosseini SA, Baezzat SR, Shamsaie A, et al. Huge immature teratoma of the liver in an adult: a case report and review of the literature. Clin J Gastroenterol. 2010 Dec;3(6):332–6. PMID:26190492
2031. Malfertheiner P, Megraud F, O'Morain CA, et al. Management of Helicobacter pylori infection-the Maastricht V/Florence Consensus Report. Gut. 2017 Jan;66(1):6–30. PMID:27707777
2032. Malogolowkin MH, Katzenstein HM, Meyers RL, et al. Complete surgical resection is curative for children with hepatoblastoma with pure fetal histology: a report from the Children's Oncology Group. J Clin Oncol. 2011 Aug 20;29(24):3301–6. PMID:21768450
2033. Malowany JI, Merritt NH, Chan NG, et al. Nested stromal epithelial tumor of the liver in Beckwith-Wiedemann syndrome. Pediatr Dev Pathol. 2013 Jul-Aug;16(4):312–7. PMID:23570373
2034. Mamessier E, Song JY, Eberle FC, et al. Early lesions of follicular lymphoma: a genetic perspective. Haematologica. 2014 Mar;99(3):481–8. PMID:24162788
2035. Mamone G, Caruso S, Cortis K, et al. Complete spontaneous regression of giant focal nodular hyperplasia of the liver: magnetic resonance imaging evaluation with hepatobiliary contrast media. World J Gastroenterol. 2016 Dec 21;22(47):10461–4. PMID:28058027
2036. Mandard AM, Dalibard F, Mandard JC, et al. Pathologic assessment of tumor regression after preoperative chemoradiotherapy of esophageal carcinoma. Clinicopathologic correlations. Cancer. 1994 Jun 1;73(11):2680–6. PMID:8194005
2037. Mandell JW, Gulley ML, Williams ME, et al. Recurrent Epstein-Barr virus-associated post-transplant lymphoproliferative disorder: report of a patient with histologically similar but clonally distinct metachronous abdominal and brain lesions. Hum Pathol. 1999 Oct;30(10):1262–5. PMID:10534178
2038. Manguso N, Johnson J, Harit A, et al. Prognostic factors associated with outcomes in small bowel neuroendocrine tumors. Am Surg. 2017 Oct 1;83(10):1174–8. PMID:29391119

2039. Mani H, Climent F, Colomo L, et al. Gall bladder and extrahepatic bile duct lymphomas: clinicopathological observations and biological implications. Am J Surg Pathol. 2010 Sep;34(9):1277–86. PMID:20679881

2040. Manley PN, Abu-Abed S, Kirsch R, et al. Familial PDGFRA-mutation syndrome: somatic and gastrointestinal phenotype. Hum Pathol. 2018 Jun;76:52–7. PMID:29486293

2041. Mannath J, Ragunath K. Role of endoscopy in early oesophageal cancer. Nat Rev Gastroenterol Hepatol. 2016 Dec;13(12):720–30. PMID:27807370

2042. Mansoor A, Pittaluga S, Beck PL, et al. NK-cell enteropathy: a benign NK-cell lymphoproliferative disease mimicking intestinal lymphoma: clinicopathologic features and follow-up in a unique case series. Blood. 2011 Feb 3;117(5):1447–52. PMID:20966166

2043. Mantoo S, Sanaka MR, Chute DJ. Cytologic features of tubular adenoma of ampulla causing distal common bile duct stricture: a case report and review of the literature. Cytojournal. 2017 Aug 22;14:19. PMID:28900465

2044. Mao C, Shah A, Hanson DJ, et al. Von Recklinghausen's disease associated with duodenal somatostatinoma: contrast of duodenal versus pancreatic somatostatinomas. J Surg Oncol. 1995 May;59(1):67–73. PMID:7745981

2045. Maragliano R, Vanoli A, Albarello L, et al. ACTH-secreting pancreatic neoplasms associated with Cushing syndrome: clinicopathologic study of 11 cases and review of the literature. Am J Surg Pathol. 2015 Mar;39(3):374–82. PMID:25353285

2046. Marchegiani G, Andrianello S, Malleo G, et al. Does size matter in pancreatic cancer?: Reappraisal of tumour dimension as a predictor of outcome beyond the TNM. Ann Surg. 2017 Jul;266(1):142–8. PMID:27322188

2047. Marchegiani G, Andrianello S, Massignani M, et al. Solid pseudopapillary tumors of the pancreas: specific pathological features predict the likelihood of postoperative recurrence. J Surg Oncol. 2016 Oct;114(5):597–601. PMID:27471041

2048. Marchegiani G, Mino-Kenudson M, Ferrone CR, et al. Oncocytic-type intraductal papillary mucinous neoplasms: a unique malignant pancreatic tumor with good long-term prognosis. J Am Coll Surg. 2015 May;220(5):839–44. PMID:25840549

2049. Marchio A, Terris B, Meddeb M, et al. Chromosomal abnormalities in liver cell dysplasia detected by comparative genomic hybridisation. Mol Pathol. 2001 Aug;54(4):270–4. PMID:11477144

2050. Marcus DM, Edgar MA, Hawk NN, et al. Small cell carcinoma of the anus in the setting of prior squamous dysplasia and carcinoma in situ. J Gastrointest Oncol. 2013 Jun;4(2):E1–4. PMID:23730521

2051. Marcus R, Maitra A, Roszik J. Recent advances in genomic profiling of adenosquamous carcinoma of the pancreas. J Pathol. 2017 Nov;243(3):271–2. PMID:28816351

2052. Margolskee E, Jobanputra V, Lewis SK, et al. Indolent small intestinal CD4+ T-cell lymphoma is a distinct entity with unique biologic and clinical features. PLoS One. 2013 Jul 4;8(7):e68343. PMID:23861889

2052A. Mariette C, Carneiro F, Grabsch HI, et al. Consensus on the pathological definition and classification of poorly cohesive gastric carcinoma. Gastric Cancer. 2019 Jan;22(1):1–9. PMID:30167905

2053. Marinoni I, Kurrer AS, Vassella E, et al. Loss of DAXX and ATRX are associated with chromosome instability and reduced survival of patients with pancreatic neuroendocrine tumors. Gastroenterology. 2014 Feb;146(2):453–60.e5. PMID:24148618

2054. Mariño-Enríquez A, Dal Cin P. ALK as a paradigm of oncogenic promiscuity: different mechanisms of activation and different fusion partners drive tumors of different lineages. Cancer Genet. 2013 Nov;206(11):357–73. PMID:24091028

2055. Mariño-Enríquez A, Wang WL, Roy A, et al. Epithelioid inflammatory myofibroblastic sarcoma: an aggressive intra-abdominal variant of inflammatory myofibroblastic tumor with nuclear membrane or perinuclear ALK. Am J Surg Pathol. 2011 Jan;35(1):135–44. PMID:21164297

2056. Marks E, Shi Y. Duodenal-type follicular lymphoma: a clinicopathologic review. Arch Pathol Lab Med. 2018 Apr;142(4):542–7. PMID:29565210

2057. Marquardt JU, Seo D, Andersen JB, et al. Sequential transcriptome analysis of human liver cancer indicates late stage acquisition of malignant traits. J Hepatol. 2014 Feb;60(2):346–53. PMID:24512821

2058. Marrelli D, Polom K, de Manzoni G, et al. Multimodal treatment of gastric cancer in the west: Where are we going? World J Gastroenterol. 2015 Jul 14;21(26):7954–69. PMID:26185368

2059. Marrero JA, Ahn J, Rajender Reddy K. ACG clinical guideline: the diagnosis and management of focal liver lesions. Am J Gastroenterol. 2014 Sep;109(9):1328–47, quiz 1348. PMID:25135008

2060. Martignoni ME, Friess H, Lübke D, et al. Study of a primary gastrinoma in the common hepatic duct - a case report. Digestion. 1999 Mar-Apr;60(2):187–90. PMID:10095161

2061. Martin FC, Chenevix-Trench G, Yeomans ND. Systematic review with meta-analysis: fundic gland polyps and proton pump inhibitors. Aliment Pharmacol Ther. 2016 Nov;44(9):915–25. PMID:27634363

2062. Martin JA, Haber GB. Ampullary adenoma: clinical manifestations, diagnosis, and treatment. Gastrointest Endosc Clin N Am. 2003 Oct;13(4):649–69. PMID:14986792

2063. Martin-Carbonero L, Barrios A, Saballs P, et al. Pegylated liposomal doxorubicin plus highly active antiretroviral therapy versus highly active antiretroviral therapy alone in HIV patients with Kaposi's sarcoma. AIDS. 2004 Aug 20;18(12):1737–40. PMID:15280789

2064. Martinez D, Valera A, Perez NS, et al. Plasmablastic transformation of low-grade B-cell lymphomas: report on 6 cases. Am J Surg Pathol. 2013 Feb;37(2):272–81. PMID:23282972

2065. Martinez OM, Krams SM. The immune response to Epstein Barr virus and implications for posttransplant lymphoproliferative disorder. Transplantation. 2017 Sep;101(9):2009–16. PMID:28376031

2066. Maru DM, Khurana H, Rashid A, et al. Retrospective study of clinicopathologic features and prognosis of high-grade neuroendocrine carcinoma of the esophagus. Am J Surg Pathol. 2008 Sep;32(9):1404–11. PMID:18670347

2067. Marvin ML, Mazzoni SM, Herron CM, et al. AXIN2-associated autosomal dominant ectodermal dysplasia and neoplastic syndrome. Am J Med Genet A. 2011 Apr;155A(4):898–902. PMID:21416598

2068. Mas-Moya J, Dudley B, Brand RE, et al. Clinicopathological comparison of colorectal and endometrial carcinomas in patients with Lynch-like syndrome versus patients with Lynch syndrome. Hum Pathol. 2015 Nov;46(11):1616–25. PMID:26319271

2069. Masciari S, Dewanwala A, Stoffel EM, et al. Gastric cancer in individuals with Li-Fraumeni syndrome. Genet Med. 2011 Jul;13(7):651–7. PMID:21552135

2070. Mason EF, Hornick JL. Conventional risk stratification fails to predict progression of succinate dehydrogenase-deficient gastrointestinal stromal tumors: a clinicopathologic study of 76 cases. Am J Surg Pathol. 2016 Dec;40(12):1616–21. PMID:27340750

2071. Masoomi H, Ziogas A, Lin BS, et al. Population-based evaluation of adenosquamous carcinoma of the colon and rectum. Dis Colon Rectum. 2012 May;55(5):509–14. PMID:22513428

2072. Massironi S, Rossi RE, Ferrero S, et al. An esophageal gastrointestinal stromal tumor in a patient with MEN1-related pancreatic gastrinoma: an unusual association and review of the literature. J Cancer Res Ther. 2014 Apr-Jun;10(2):443–5. PMID:25022420

2073. Masson EA, MacFarlane IA, Graham D, et al. Spontaneous hypoglycaemia due to a pleural fibroma: role of insulin like growth factors. Thorax. 1991 Dec;46(12):930–1. PMID:1792643

2074. Mastrangelo G, Coindre JM, Ducimetière F, et al. Incidence of soft tissue sarcoma and beyond: a population-based prospective study in 3 European regions. Cancer. 2012 Nov 1;118(21):5339–48. PMID:22517534

2075. Mathias MD, Ambati SR, Chou AJ, et al. A single-center experience with undifferentiated embryonal sarcoma of the liver. Pediatr Blood Cancer. 2016 Dec;63(12):2246–8. PMID:27427850

2076. Mathieu D, Kobeiter H, Maison P, et al. Oral contraceptive use and focal nodular hyperplasia of the liver. Gastroenterology. 2000 Mar;118(3):560–4. PMID:10702207

2077. Matson DR, Xu J, Huffman L, et al. KRAS and GNAS co-mutation in metastatic low-grade appendiceal mucinous neoplasm (LAMN) to the ovaries: a practical role for next-generation sequencing. Am J Case Rep. 2017 May 20;18:558–62. PMID:28526814

2078. Matsubara A, Ogawa R, Suzuki H, et al. Activating GNAS and KRAS mutations in gastric foveolar metaplasia, gastric heterotopia, and adenocarcinoma of the duodenum. Br J Cancer. 2015 Apr 14;112(8):1398–404. PMID:25867268

2079. Matsubara A, Sekine S, Kushima R, et al. Frequent GNAS and KRAS mutations in pyloric gland adenoma of the stomach and duodenum. J Pathol. 2013 Mar;229(4):579–87. PMID:23208952

2080. Matsubayashi H, Takaori K, Morizane C, et al. Familial pancreatic cancer: concept, management and issues. World J Gastroenterol. 2017 Feb 14;23(6):935–48. PMID:28246467

2081. Matsuda A, Higashi M, Nakagawa T, et al. Assessment of tumor characteristics based on glycoform analysis of membrane-tethered MUC1. Lab Invest. 2017 Sep;97(9):1103–13. PMID:28581490

2082. Matsuda Y, Furukawa T, Yachida S, et al. The prevalence and clinicopathological characteristics of high-grade pancreatic intraepithelial neoplasia: autopsy study evaluating the entire pancreatic parenchyma. Pancreas. 2017 May/Jun;46(5):658–64. PMID:28196020

2083. Matsumoto M, Nomiyama T, Nakae J, et al. Combination chemotherapy for a senile patient with adenoid cystic carcinoma of the esophagus: a case report. Jpn J Clin Oncol. 1993 Aug;23(4):258–62. PMID:8411740

2084. Matsumoto T, Imai Y, Inokuma T. Neuroendocrine carcinoma of the gallbladder accompanied by pancreaticobiliary maljunction. Clin Gastroenterol Hepatol. 2016 Mar;14(3):e29–30. PMID:26247168

2085. Matsuno S, Egawa S, Fukuyama S, et al. Pancreatic Cancer Registry in Japan: 20 years of experience. Pancreas. 2004 Apr;28(3):219–30. PMID:15084961

2086. Matsuura S, Aishima S, Taguchi K, et al. 'Scirrhous' type hepatocellular carcinomas: a special reference to expression of cytokeratin 7 and hepatocyte paraffin 1. Histopathology. 2005 Oct;47(4):382–90. PMID:16178893

2087. Matsuzawa G, Shirabe K, Gion T, et al. Surgically resected undifferentiated carcinoma with osteoclast-like giant cells of the periampullary region involving the orifice of the papilla of Vater: report of a case. Surg Today. 2010 Apr;40(4):376–9. PMID:20339995

2088. Matthaei H, Lingohr P, Strässer A, et al. Biliary intraepithelial neoplasia (BilIN) is frequently found in surgical margins of biliary tract cancer resection specimens but has no clinical implications. Virchows Arch. 2015 Feb;466(2):133–41. PMID:25425476

2089. Matthaei H, Wu J, Dal Molin M, et al. GNAS codon 201 mutations are uncommon in intraductal papillary neoplasms of the bile duct. HPB (Oxford). 2012 Oct;14(10):677–83. PMID:22954004

2090. Matthaei H, Wu J, Dal Molin M, et al. GNAS sequencing identifies IPMN-specific mutations in a subgroup of diminutive pancreatic cysts referred to as "incipient IPMNs". Am J Surg Pathol. 2014 Mar;38(3):360–3. PMID:24525507

2091. Maurer CA, Baer HU, Dyong TH, et al. Carcinoid of the pancreas: clinical characteristics and morphological features. Eur J Cancer. 1996 Jun;32A(7):1109–16. PMID:8758239

2092. Mazer LM, Losada HF, Chaudhry RM, et al. Tumor characteristics and survival analysis of incidental versus suspected gallbladder carcinoma. J Gastrointest Surg. 2012 Jul;16(7):1311–7. PMID:22570074

2093. Mazzaferro V, Regalia E, Doci R, et al. Liver transplantation for the treatment of small hepatocellular carcinomas in patients with cirrhosis. N Engl J Med. 1996 Mar 14;334(11):693–9. PMID:8594428

2094. Mazzoni SM, Fearon ER. AXIN1 and AXIN2 variants in gastrointestinal cancers. Cancer Lett. 2014 Dec 1;355(1):1–8. PMID:25236910

2095. Mbulaiteye SM, Anderson WF, Ferlay J, et al. Pediatric, elderly, and emerging adult-onset peaks in Burkitt's lymphoma incidence diagnosed in four continents, excluding Africa. Am J Hematol. 2012 Jun;87(6):573–8. PMID:22488262

2096. McCall CM, Shi C, Cornish TC, et al. Grading of well-differentiated pancreatic neuroendocrine tumors is improved by the inclusion of both Ki67 proliferative index and mitotic rate. Am J Surg Pathol. 2013 Nov;37(11):1671–7. PMID:24121170

2097. McCall CM, Shi C, Klein AP, et al. Serotonin expression in pancreatic neuroendocrine tumors correlates with a trabecular histologic pattern and large duct involvement. Hum Pathol. 2012 Aug;43(8):1169–76. PMID:22221702

2098. McCarthy DM, Brat DJ, Wilentz RE, et al. Pancreatic intraepithelial neoplasia and infiltrating adenocarcinoma: analysis of progression and recurrence by DPC4 immunohistochemical labeling. Hum Pathol. 2001 Jun;32(6):638–42. PMID:11431719

2099. McCloskey JC, Kast WM, Flexman JP, et al. Syndemic synergy of HPV and other sexually transmitted pathogens in the development of high-grade anal squamous intraepithelial lesions. Papillomavirus Res. 2017 Dec;4:90–8. PMID:29179876

2100. McCluney S, Wijesuriya N, Sheshappanavar V, et al. Solid pseudopapillary tumour of the pancreas: clinicopathological analysis. ANZ J Surg. 2018 Sep;88(9):891–5. PMID:29316119

2101. McDuffie LA, Sabesan A, Allgäeuer M,

et al. β-Catenin activation in fundic gland polyps, gastric cancer and colonic polyps in families afflicted by 'gastric adenocarcinoma and proximal polyposis of the stomach' (GAPPS). J Clin Pathol. 2016 Sep;69(9):826–33. PMID:27406052
2102. McEvoy MP, Rich B, Klimstra D, et al. Acinar cell cystadenoma of the pancreas in a 9-year-old boy. J Pediatr Surg. 2010 May;45(5):e7–9. PMID:20438912
2103. McFaul CD, Greenhalf W, Earl J, et al. Anticipation in familial pancreatic cancer. Gut. 2006 Feb;55(2):252–8. PMID:15972300
2104. McKenney JK, Heerema-McKenney A, Rouse RV. Extragonadal germ cell tumors: a review with emphasis on pathologic features, clinical prognostic variables, and differential diagnostic considerations. Adv Anat Pathol. 2007 Mar;14(2):69–92. PMID:17471115
2105. McKinney M, Moffitt AB, Gaulard P, et al. The genetic basis of hepatosplenic T-cell lymphoma. Cancer Discov. 2017 Apr;7(4):369–79. PMID:28122867
2106. McLean CA, Pedersen JS. Endocrine cell carcinoma of the gallbladder. Histopathology. 1991 Aug;19(2):173–6. PMID:1661701
2107. McLean MH, El-Omar EM. Genetics of gastric cancer. Nat Rev Gastroenterol Hepatol. 2014 Nov;11(11):664–74. PMID:25134511
2108. McWilliams RR, Matsumoto ME, Burch PA, et al. Obesity adversely affects survival in pancreatic cancer patients. Cancer. 2010 Nov 1;116(21):5054–62. PMID:20665496
2109. Medeiros F, Corless CL, Duensing A, et al. KIT-negative gastrointestinal stromal tumors: proof of concept and therapeutic implications. Am J Surg Pathol. 2004 Jul;28(7):889–94. PMID:15223958
2110. Mehrabi A, Fischer L, Hafezi M, et al. A systematic review of localization, surgical treatment options, and outcome of insulinoma. Pancreas. 2014 Jul;43(5):675–86. PMID:24921202
2111. Mehrabi A, Kashfi A, Fonouni H, et al. Primary malignant hepatic epithelioid hemangioendothelioma: a comprehensive review of the literature with emphasis on the surgical therapy. Cancer. 2006 Nov 1;107(9):2108–21. PMID:17019735
2112. Mehrvarz Sarshekeh A, Advani S, Halperin DM, et al. Regional lymph node involvement and outcomes in appendiceal neuroendocrine tumors: a SEER database analysis. Oncotarget. 2017 Aug 19;8(59):99541–51. PMID:29245922
2113. Meis JM, Enzinger FM. Inflammatory fibrosarcoma of the mesentery and retroperitoneum. A tumor closely simulating inflammatory pseudotumor. Am J Surg Pathol. 1991 Dec;15(12):1146–56. PMID:1746682
2114. Meis-Kindblom JM, Kindblom LG. Angiosarcoma of soft tissue: a study of 80 cases. Am J Surg Pathol. 1998 Jun;22(6):683–97. PMID:9630175
2115. Melck AL, Yip L, Carty SE. The utility of BRAF testing in the management of papillary thyroid cancer. Oncologist. 2010;15(12):1285–93. PMID:21147872
2116. Meletani T, Cantini L, Lanese A, et al. Are liver nested stromal epithelial tumors always low aggressive? World J Gastroenterol. 2017 Dec 14;23(46):8248–55. PMID:29290661
2117. Melo S, Figueiredo J, Fernandes MS, et al. Predicting the functional impact of CDH1 missense mutations in hereditary diffuse gastric cancer. Int J Mol Sci. 2017 Dec 12;18(12):E2687. PMID:29231860
2118. Melson J, Ma K, Arshad S, et al. Presence of small sessile serrated polyps increases rate of advanced neoplasia upon surveillance compared with isolated low-risk tubular adenomas. Gastrointest Endosc. 2016 Aug;84(2):307–14. PMID:26855297
2119. Mendlick MR, Nelson M, Pickering D, et al. Translocation t(1;3)(p36.3;q25) is a nonrandom aberration in epithelioid hemangioendothelioma. Am J Surg Pathol. 2001 May;25(5):684–7. PMID:11342784
2120. Meng Y, Zhang J, Wang H, et al. Poorer prognosis in patients with advanced gastric squamous cell carcinoma compared with adenocarcinoma of the stomach: case report. Medicine (Baltimore). 2017 Dec;96(50):e9224. PMID:29390350
2121. Menko FH, Kneepkens CM, de Leeuw N, et al. Variable phenotypes associated with 10q23 microdeletions involving the PTEN and BMPR1A genes. Clin Genet. 2008 Aug;74(2):145–54. PMID:18510548
2122. Mention JJ, Ben Ahmed M, Bègue B, et al. Interleukin 15: a key to disrupted intraepithelial lymphocyte homeostasis and lymphomagenesis in celiac disease. Gastroenterology. 2003 Sep;125(3):730–45. PMID:12949719
2123. Mera RM, Bravo LE, Camargo MC, et al. Dynamics of Helicobacter pylori infection as a determinant of progression of gastric precancerous lesions: 16-year follow-up of an eradication trial. Gut. 2018 Jul;67(7):1239–46. PMID:28647684
2124. Meriden Z, Montgomery EA. Anal duct carcinoma: a report of 5 cases. Hum Pathol. 2012 Feb;43(2):216–20. PMID:21820151
2125. Mescoli C, Albertoni L, D'incá R, et al. Dysplasia in inflammatory bowel diseases. Dig Liver Dis. 2013 Mar;45(3):186–94. PMID:22974564
2126. Mester J, Eng C. When overgrowth bumps into cancer: the PTEN-opathies. Am J Med Genet C Semin Med Genet. 2013 May;163C(2):114–21. PMID:23613428
2127. Metcalf RA, Monabati A, Vyas M, et al. Myeloid cell nuclear differentiation antigen is expressed in a subset of marginal zone lymphomas and is useful in the differential diagnosis with follicular lymphoma. Hum Pathol. 2014 Aug;45(8):1730–6. PMID:24925224
2128. Metz DC, Cadiot G, Poitras P, et al. Diagnosis of Zollinger-Ellison syndrome in the era of PPIs, faulty gastrin assays, sensitive imaging and limited access to acid secretory testing. Int J Endocr Oncol. 2017;4(4):167–85. PMID:29326808
2129. Mewa Kinoo S, Maharaj K, Singh B, et al. Primary esophageal sclerosing mucoepidermoid carcinoma with "tissue eosinophilia". World J Gastroenterol. 2014 Jun 14;20(22):7055–60. PMID:24944502
2130. Meyer CT, Troncale FJ, Galloway S, et al. Arteriovenous malformations of the bowel: an analysis of 22 cases and a review of the literature. Medicine (Baltimore). 1981 Jan;60(1):36–48. PMID:6969839
2131. Meyers RL, Maibach R, Hiyama E, et al. Risk-stratified staging in paediatric hepatoblastoma: a unified analysis from the Children's Hepatic Tumors International Collaboration. Lancet Oncol. 2017 Jan;18(1):122–31. PMID:27884679
2132. Meza JL, Anderson J, Pappo AS, et al. Analysis of prognostic factors in patients with nonmetastatic rhabdomyosarcoma treated on intergroup rhabdomyosarcoma studies III and IV: the Children's Oncology Group. J Clin Oncol. 2006 Aug 20;24(24):3844–51. PMID:16921036
2133. Micchelli ST, Vivekanandan P, Boitnott JK, et al. Malignant transformation of hepatic adenomas. Mod Pathol. 2008 Apr;21(4):491–7. PMID:18246041
2134. Michaels PJ, Brachtel EF, Bounds BC, et al. Intraductal papillary mucinous neoplasm of the pancreas: cytologic features predict histologic grade. Cancer. 2006 Jun 25;108(3):163–73. PMID:16550572
2135. Michalova K, Michal M, Sedivcova M, et al. Solid pseudopapillary neoplasm (SPN) of the testis: comprehensive mutational analysis of 6 testicular and 8 pancreatic SPNs. Ann Diagn Pathol. 2018 Aug;35:42–7. PMID:29705715
2136. Michopoulos S. Critical appraisal of guidelines for screening and surveillance of Barrett's esophagus. Ann Transl Med. 2018 Jul;6(13):259. PMID:30094245
2137. Middleton SB, Frayling IM, Phillips RK. Desmoids in familial adenomatous polyposis are monoclonal proliferations. Br J Cancer. 2000 Feb;82(4):827–32. PMID:10732754
2138. Miettinen M, Dow N, Lasota J, et al. A distinctive novel epitheliomesenchymal biphasic tumor of the stomach in young adults ("gastroblastoma"): a series of 3 cases. Am J Surg Pathol. 2009 Sep;33(9):1370–7. PMID:19718790
2139. Miettinen M, Felisiak-Golabek A, Wang Z, et al. GIST manifesting as a retroperitoneal tumor: clinicopathologic immunohistochemical, and molecular genetic study of 112 cases. Am J Surg Pathol. 2017 May;41(5):577–85. PMID:28288036
2140. Miettinen M, Fetsch JF, Sobin LH, et al. Gastrointestinal stromal tumors in patients with neurofibromatosis 1: a clinicopathologic and molecular genetic study of 45 cases. Am J Surg Pathol. 2006 Jan;30(1):90–6. PMID:16330947
2141. Miettinen M, Fetsch JF. Distribution of keratins in normal endothelial cells and a spectrum of vascular tumors: implications in tumor diagnosis. Hum Pathol. 2000 Sep;31(9):1062–7. PMID:11014572
2142. Miettinen M, Furlong M, Sarlomo-Rikala M, et al. Gastrointestinal stromal tumors, intramural leiomyomas, and leiomyosarcomas in the rectum and anus: a clinicopathologic, immunohistochemical, and molecular genetic study of 144 cases. Am J Surg Pathol. 2001 Sep;25(9):1121–33. PMID:11688571
2143. Miettinen M, Kopczynski J, Makhlouf HR, et al. Gastrointestinal stromal tumors, intramural leiomyomas, and leiomyosarcomas in the duodenum: a clinicopathologic, immunohistochemical, and molecular genetic study of 167 cases. Am J Surg Pathol. 2003 May;27(5):625–41. PMID:12717247
2144. Miettinen M, Lasota J, Sobin LH. Gastrointestinal stromal tumors of the stomach in children and young adults: a clinicopathologic, immunohistochemical, and molecular genetic study of 44 cases with long-term follow-up and review of the literature. Am J Surg Pathol. 2005 Oct;29(10):1373–81. PMID:16160481
2145. Miettinen M, Lasota J. Gastrointestinal stromal tumors. Gastroenterol Clin North Am. 2013 Jun;42(2):399–415. PMID:23639648
2146. Miettinen M, Lasota J. Gastrointestinal stromal tumors: pathology and prognosis at different sites. Semin Diagn Pathol. 2006 May;23(2):70–83. PMID:17193820
2147. Miettinen M, Lindenmayer AE, Chaubal A. Endothelial cell markers CD31, CD34, and BNH9 antibody to H- and Y-antigens–evaluation of their specificity and sensitivity in the diagnosis of vascular tumors and comparison with von Willebrand factor. Mod Pathol. 1994 Jan;7(1):82–90. PMID:7512718
2148. Miettinen M, Makhlouf H, Sobin LH, et al. Gastrointestinal stromal tumors of the jejunum and ileum: a clinicopathologic, immunohistochemical, and molecular genetic study of 906 cases before imatinib with long-term follow-up. Am J Surg Pathol. 2006 Apr;30(4):477–89. PMID:16625094
2149. Miettinen M, Makhlouf HR, Sobin LH, et al. Plexiform fibromyxoma: a distinctive benign gastric antral neoplasm not to be confused with a myxoid GIST. Am J Surg Pathol. 2009 Nov;33(11):1624–32. PMID:19675452
2150. Miettinen M, Paal E, Lasota J, et al. Gastrointestinal glomus tumors: a clinicopathologic, immunohistochemical, and molecular genetic study of 32 cases. Am J Surg Pathol. 2002 Mar;26(3):301–11. PMID:11859201
2151. Miettinen M, Sarlomo-Rikala M, Sobin LH, et al. Esophageal stromal tumors: a clinicopathologic, immunohistochemical, and molecular genetic study of 17 cases and comparison with esophageal leiomyomas and leiomyosarcomas. Am J Surg Pathol. 2000 Feb;24(2):211–22. PMID:10680889
2152. Miettinen M, Sarlomo-Rikala M, Sobin LH, et al. Gastrointestinal stromal tumors and leiomyosarcomas in the colon: a clinicopathologic, immunohistochemical, and molecular genetic study of 44 cases. Am J Surg Pathol. 2000 Oct;24(10):1339–52. PMID:11023095
2153. Miettinen M, Shekitka KM, Sobin LH. Schwannomas in the colon and rectum: a clinicopathologic and immunohistochemical study of 20 cases. Am J Surg Pathol. 2001 Jul;25(7):846–55. PMID:11420455
2154. Miettinen M, Sobin LH, Lasota J. Gastrointestinal stromal tumors of the stomach: a clinicopathologic, immunohistochemical, and molecular genetic study of 1765 cases with long-term follow-up. Am J Surg Pathol. 2005 Jan;29(1):52–68. PMID:15613856
2155. Miettinen M, Sobin LH, Lasota J. True smooth muscle tumors of the small intestine: a clinicopathologic, immunhistochemical, and molecular genetic study of 25 cases. Am J Surg Pathol. 2009 Mar;33(3):430–6. PMID:18971781
2156. Miettinen M, Wang ZF, Lasota J. DOG1 antibody in the differential diagnosis of gastrointestinal stromal tumors: a study of 1840 cases. Am J Surg Pathol. 2009 Sep;33(9):1401–8. PMID:19606013
2157. Miettinen M, Wang ZF, Paetau A, et al. ERG transcription factor as an immunohistochemical marker for vascular endothelial tumors and prostatic carcinoma. Am J Surg Pathol. 2011 Mar;35(3):432–41. PMID:21317715
2158. Miettinen M, Wang ZF, Sarlomo-Rikala M, et al. Succinate dehydrogenase-deficient GISTs: a clinicopathologic, immunohistochemical, and molecular genetic study of 66 gastric GISTs with predilection to young age. Am J Surg Pathol. 2011 Nov;35(11):1712–21. PMID:21997692
2159. Miftahussurur M, Yamaoka Y, Graham DY. Helicobacter pylori as an oncogenic pathogen, revisited. Expert Rev Mol Med. 2017 Mar 21;19:e4. PMID:28322182
2160. Mihaylova VT, Bindra RS, Yuan J, et al. Decreased expression of the DNA mismatch repair gene Mlh1 under hypoxic stress in mammalian cells. Mol Cell Biol. 2003 May;23(9):3265–73. PMID:12697826
2161. Miki K. Gastric cancer screening using the serum pepsinogen test method. Gastric Cancer. 2006;9(4):245–53. PMID:17235625
2162. Miles RR, Arnold S, Cairo MS. Risk factors and treatment of childhood and adolescent Burkitt lymphoma/leukaemia. Br J Haematol. 2012 Mar;156(6):730–43. PMID:22260323
2163. Milione M, Maisonneuve P, Pellegrinelli A, et al. Ki67 proliferative index of the neuroendocrine component drives MANEC prognosis. Endocr Relat Cancer. 2018 May;25(5):583–93. PMID:29592868
2164. Milione M, Maisonneuve P, Spada F, et al. The clinicopathologic heterogeneity of grade 3 gastroenteropancreatic neuroendocrine neoplasms: morphological differentiation and proliferation identify different prognostic categories. Neuroendocrinology. 2017;104(1):85–93. PMID:26943788
2165. Mills SE, Allen MS Jr, Cohen AR. Small-cell undifferentiated carcinoma of the colon. A clinicopathological study of five cases and their association with colonic adenomas. Am J Surg

Pathol. 1983 Oct;7(7):643–51. PMID:6314828
2166. Mills SE, Greenson JK, Hornick JL, et al., editors. Sternberg's diagnostic surgical pathology. 6th ed. Philadelphia (PA): Lippincott Williams & Wilkins; 2015.
2167. Min BH, Hwang J, Kim NK, et al. Dysregulated Wnt signalling and recurrent mutations of the tumour suppressor RNF43 in early gastric carcinogenesis. J Pathol. 2016 Nov;240(3):304–14. PMID:27514024
2168. Minatsuki S, Miura I, Yao A, et al. Platelet-derived growth factor receptor-tyrosine kinase inhibitor, imatinib, is effective for treating pulmonary hypertension induced by pulmonary tumor thrombotic microangiopathy. Int Heart J. 2015;56(2):245–8. PMID:25740390
2169. Ming SC. Gastric carcinoma. A pathobiological classification. Cancer. 1977 Jun;39(6):2475–85. PMID:872047
2170. Mingazzini PL, Malchiodi Albedi F, Blandamura V. Villous adenoma of the duodenum: cellular composition and histochemical findings. Histopathology. 1982 Mar;6(2):235–44. PMID:7076140
2171. Minicozzi A, Borzellino G, Momo R, et al. Perianal Paget's disease: presentation of six cases and literature review. Int J Colorectal Dis. 2010 Jan;25(1):1–7. PMID:19707774
2172. Mino-Kenudson M, Fernández-del Castillo C, Baba Y, et al. Prognosis of invasive intraductal papillary mucinous neoplasm depends on histological and precursor epithelial subtypes. Gut. 2011 Dec;60(12):1712–20. PMID:21508421
2173. Miranda C, Nucifora M, Molinari F, et al. KRAS and BRAF mutations predict primary resistance to imatinib in gastrointestinal stromal tumors. Clin Cancer Res. 2012 Mar 15;18(6):1769–76. PMID:22282465
2174. Misdraji J, Burgart LJ, Lauwers GY. Defective mismatch repair in the pathogenesis of low-grade appendiceal mucinous neoplasms and adenocarcinomas. Mod Pathol. 2004 Dec;17(12):1447–54. PMID:15354187
2175. Misdraji J, Yantiss RK, Graeme-Cook FM, et al. Appendiceal mucinous neoplasms: a clinicopathologic analysis of 107 cases. Am J Surg Pathol. 2003 Aug;27(8):1089–103. PMID:12883241
2176. Mishra MV, Keith SW, Shen X, et al. Primary pancreatic lymphoma: a population-based analysis using the SEER program. Am J Clin Oncol. 2013 Feb;36(1):38–43. PMID:22134518
2177. Missiaglia E, Dalai I, Barbi S, et al. Pancreatic endocrine tumors: expression profiling evidences a role for AKT-mTOR pathway. J Clin Oncol. 2010 Jan 10;28(2):245–55. PMID:19917848
2178. Mitsunaga S, Hasebe T, Kinoshita T, et al. Detail histologic analysis of nerve plexus invasion in invasive ductal carcinoma of the pancreas and its prognostic impact. Am J Surg Pathol. 2007 Nov;31(11):1636–44. PMID:18059219
2180. Miyazaki K, Yamaguchi M, Suzuki R, et al. CD5-positive diffuse large B-cell lymphoma: a retrospective study in 337 patients treated by chemotherapy with or without rituximab. Ann Oncol. 2011 Jul;22(7):1601–7. PMID:21199885
2181. Miyazawa M, Matsuda M, Yano M, et al. Gastric adenocarcinoma of fundic gland type: five cases treated with endoscopic resection. World J Gastroenterol. 2015 Jul 14;21(26):8208–14. PMID:26185396
2182. Mizobuchi S, Tachimori Y, Kato H, et al. Metastatic esophageal tumors from distant primary lesions: report of three esophagectomies and study of 1835 autopsy cases. Jpn J Clin Oncol. 1997 Dec;27(6):410–4. PMID:9438004
2183. Mo JQ, Dimashkieh HH, Bove KE. GLUT1 endothelial reactivity distinguishes hepatic infantile hemangioma from congenital hepatic vascular malformation with associated capillary proliferation. Hum Pathol. 2004 Feb;35(2):200–9. PMID:14991538
2184. Moch H, Humphrey PA, Ulbright TM, et al., editors. WHO classification of tumours of the urinary system and male genital organs. Lyon (France): International Agency for Research on Cancer; 2016. (WHO classification of tumours series, 4th ed.; vol. 8). http://publications.iarc.fr/540.
2185. Modlin IM, Lye KD, Kidd M. A 5-decade analysis of 13,715 carcinoid tumors. Cancer. 2003 Feb 15;97(4):934–59. PMID:12569593
2186. Modlin IM, Lye KD, Kidd M. Carcinoid tumors of the stomach. Surg Oncol. 2003 Aug;12(2):153–72. PMID:12946486
2187. Modlin IM, Sandor A. An analysis of 8305 cases of carcinoid tumors. Cancer. 1997 Feb 15;79(4):813–29. PMID:9024720
2188. Modlin IM, Shapiro MD, Kidd M. An analysis of rare carcinoid tumors: clarifying these clinical conundrums. World J Surg. 2005 Jan;29(1):92–101. PMID:15599742
2189. Moeini A, Sia D, Zhang Z, et al. Mixed hepatocellular cholangiocarcinoma tumors: cholangiolocellular carcinoma is a distinct molecular entity. J Hepatol. 2017 May;66(5):952–61. PMID:28126467
2190. Moertel CG, Weiland LH, Nagorney DM, et al. Carcinoid tumor of the appendix: treatment and prognosis. N Engl J Med. 1987 Dec 31;317(27):1699–701. PMID:3696178
2191. Moffitt AB, Ondrejka SL, McKinney M, et al. Enteropathy-associated T cell lymphoma subtypes are characterized by loss of function of SETD2. J Exp Med. 2017 May 1;214(5):1371–86. PMID:28424246
2192. Moffitt RA, Marayati R, Flate EL, et al. Virtual microdissection identifies distinct tumor- and stroma-specific subtypes of pancreatic ductal adenocarcinoma. Nat Genet. 2015 Oct;47(10):1168–78. PMID:26343385
2193. Mohajeri A, Tayebwa J, Collin A, et al. Comprehensive genetic analysis identifies a pathognomonic NAB2/STAT6 fusion gene, nonrandom secondary genomic imbalances, and a characteristic gene expression profile in solitary fibrous tumor. Genes Chromosomes Cancer. 2013 Oct;52(10):873–86. PMID:23761323
2194. Mohammadkhani Shali S, Schmitt V, Behrendt FF, et al. Metabolic tumour volume of anal carcinoma on (18)FDG PET/CT before combined radiochemotherapy is the only independant determinant of recurrence free survival. Eur J Radiol. 2016 Aug;85(8):1390–4. PMID:27423677
2195. Mohr VH, Vortmeyer AO, Zhuang Z, et al. Histopathology and molecular genetics of multiple cysts and microcystic (serous) adenomas of the pancreas in von Hippel-Lindau patients. Am J Pathol. 2000 Nov;157(5):1615–21. PMID:11073821
2196. Mohri D, Asaoka Y, Ijichi H, et al. Different subtypes of intraductal papillary mucinous neoplasm in the pancreas have distinct pathways to pancreatic cancer progression. J Gastroenterol. 2012 Feb;47(2):203–13. PMID:22041919
2197. Moinzadeh P, Breuhahn K, Stützer H, et al. Chromosome alterations in human hepatocellular carcinomas correlate with aetiology and histological grade–results of an explorative CGH meta-analysis. Br J Cancer. 2005 Mar 14;92(5):935–41. PMID:15756261
2198. Molberg KH, Heffess C, Delgado R, et al. Undifferentiated carcinoma with osteoclast-like giant cells of the pancreas and periampullary region. Cancer. 1998 Apr 1;82(7):1279–87. PMID:9529019
2199. Moldovan GL, D'Andrea AD. How the Fanconi anemia pathway guards the genome. Annu Rev Genet. 2009;43:223–49. PMID:19686080
2200. Molin MD, Matthaei H, Wu J, et al. Clinicopathological correlates of activating GNAS mutations in intraductal papillary mucinous neoplasm (IPMN) of the pancreas. Ann Surg Oncol. 2013 Nov;20(12):3802–8. PMID:23846778
2201. Molyneux EM, Rochford R, Griffin B, et al. Burkitt's lymphoma. Lancet. 2012 Mar 31;379(9822):1234–44. PMID:22333947
2202. Montes-Moreno S, Gonzalez-Medina AR, Rodriguez-Pinilla SM, et al. Aggressive large B-cell lymphoma with plasma cell differentiation: immunohistochemical characterization of plasmablastic lymphoma and diffuse large B-cell lymphoma with partial plasmablastic phenotype. Haematologica. 2010 Aug;95(8):1342–9. PMID:20418245
2203. Montes-Moreno S, Martinez-Magunacelaya N, Zecchini-Barrese T, et al. Plasmablastic lymphoma phenotype is determined by genetic alterations in MYC and PRDM1. Mod Pathol. 2017 Jan;30(1):85–94. PMID:27687004
2204. Montgomery E, Bronner MP, Greenson JK, et al. Are ulcers a marker for invasive carcinoma in Barrett's esophagus? Data from a diagnostic variability study with clinical follow-up. Am J Gastroenterol. 2002 Jan;97(1):27–31. PMID:11808966
2205. Monzen M, Shimizu K, Hatori T, et al. Usefulness of cell block cytology for preoperative grading and typing of intraductal papillary mucinous neoplasms. Pancreatology. 2013 Jul-Aug;13(4):369–78. PMID:23890135
2206. Moore PS, Chang Y. Detection of herpesvirus-like DNA sequences in Kaposi's sarcoma in patients with and those without HIV infection. N Engl J Med. 1995 May 4;332(18):1181–5. PMID:7700310
2207. Moore PS, Zamboni G, Brighenti A, et al. Molecular characterization of pancreatic serous microcystic adenomas: evidence for a tumor suppressor gene on chromosome 10q. Am J Pathol. 2001 Jan;158(1):317–21. PMID:11141506
2208. Morais DJ, Yamanaka A, Zeitune JM, et al. Gastric polyps: a retrospective analysis of 26,000 digestive endoscopies. Arq Gastroenterol. 2007 Jan-Mar;44(1):14–7. PMID:17639176
2209. Morak M, Koehler U, Schackert HK, et al. Biallelic MLH1 SNP cDNA expression or constitutional promoter methylation can hide genomic rearrangements causing Lynch syndrome. J Med Genet. 2011 Aug;48(8):513–9. PMID:21712435
2210. Morak M, Massdorf T, Sykora H, et al. First evidence for digenic inheritance in hereditary colorectal cancer by mutations in the base excision repair genes. Eur J Cancer. 2011 May;47(7):1046–55. PMID:21195604
2211. Moran CA, Ishak KG, Goodman ZD. Solitary fibrous tumor of the liver: a clinicopathologic and immunohistochemical study of nine cases. Ann Diagn Pathol. 1998 Feb;2(1):19–24. PMID:9845719
2212. Moran S, Martínez-Cardús A, Sayols S, et al. Epigenetic profiling to classify cancer of unknown primary: a multicentre, retrospective analysis. Lancet Oncol. 2016 Oct;17(10):1386–95. PMID:27575023
2213. Mori M, Iwashita A, Enjoji M. Adenosquamous carcinoma of the stomach. A clinicopathologic analysis of 28 cases. Cancer. 1986 Jan 15;57(2):333–9. PMID:3942965
2214. Mori Y, Sato N, Taniguchi R, et al. Pancreatic somatostatinoma diagnosed preoperatively: report of a case. JOP. 2014 Jan 10;15(1):66–71. PMID:24413789
2215. Morikawa T, Okabayashi T, Shima Y, et al. Adenomyomatosis concomitant with primary gallbladder carcinoma. Acta Med Okayama. 2017 Apr;71(2):113–8. PMID:28420892
2216. Morin PJ, Sparks AB, Korinek V, et al. Activation of beta-catenin-Tcf signaling in colon cancer by mutations in beta-catenin or APC. Science. 1997 Mar 21;275(5307):1787–90. PMID:9065402
2217. Morinaga S, Tsumuraya M, Nakajima T, et al. Ciliated-cell adenocarcinoma of the pancreas. Acta Pathol Jpn. 1986 Dec;36(12):1905–10. PMID:3825537
2218. Moris D, Ntanasis-Stathopoulos I, Tsilimigras DI, et al. Update on surgical management of small bowel neuroendocrine tumors. Anticancer Res. 2018 Mar;38(3):1267–78. PMID:29491050
2219. Moris D, Tsilimigras DI, Vagios S, et al. Neuroendocrine neoplasms of the appendix: a review of the literature. Anticancer Res. 2018 Feb;38(2):601–11. PMID:29374682
2220. Morita FH, Bernardo WM, Ide E, et al. Narrow band imaging versus lugol chromoendoscopy to diagnose squamous cell carcinoma of the esophagus: a systematic review and meta-analysis. BMC Cancer. 2017 Jan 13;17(1):54. PMID:28086818
2221. Moriya K, Tamura H, Nakamura K, et al. A primary esophageal MALT lymphoma patient with Helicobacter pylori infection achieved complete remission after H. pylori eradication without anti-lymphoma treatment. Leuk Res Rep. 2016 Dec 20;7:2–5. PMID:28053856
2222. Morris-Stiff G, Falk GA, El-Hayek K, et al. Jejunal cavernous lymphangioma. BMJ Case Rep. 2011 May 12;2011. PMID:22696733
2223. Morris-Stiff G, Lentz G, Chalikonda S, et al. Pancreatic cyst aspiration analysis for cystic neoplasms: mucin or carcinoembryonic antigen–which is better? Surgery. 2010 Oct;148(4):638–44, discussion 644–5. PMID:20797749
2224. Morscio J, Dierickx D, Ferreiro JF, et al. Gene expression profiling reveals clear differences between EBV-positive and EBV-negative posttransplant lymphoproliferative disorders. Am J Transplant. 2013 May;13(5):1305–16. PMID:23489474
2225. Morscio J, Dierickx D, Nijs J, et al. Clinicopathologic comparison of plasmablastic lymphoma in HIV-positive, immunocompetent, and posttransplant patients: single-center series of 25 cases and meta-analysis of 277 reported cases. Am J Surg Pathol. 2014 Jul;38(7):875–86. PMID:24832164
2226. Morscio J, Dierickx D, Tousseyn T. Molecular pathogenesis of B-cell posttransplant lymphoproliferative disorder: what do we know so far? Clin Dev Immunol. 2013;2013:150835. PMID:23690819
2227. Morson BC, Sobin LH, Grundmann E, et al. Precancerous conditions and epithelial dysplasia in the stomach. J Clin Pathol. 1980 Aug;33(8):711–21. PMID:7430384
2228. Morton M, Coupes B, Roberts SA, et al. Epidemiology of posttransplantation lymphoproliferative disorder in adult renal transplant recipients. Transplantation. 2013 Feb 15;95(3):470–8. PMID:23222821
2229. Mosquera JM, Sboner A, Zhang L, et al. Novel MIR143-NOTCH fusions in benign and malignant glomus tumors. Genes Chromosomes Cancer. 2013 Nov;52(11):1075–87. PMID:23999936
2230. Mostafa ME, Erbarut-Seven I, Pehlivanoglu B, et al. Pathologic classification of "pancreatic cancers": current concepts and challenges. Chin Clin Oncol. 2017 Dec;6(6):59. PMID:29307199
2231. Motoshima S, Yonemoto K, Kamei H, et al. Prognostic implications of HER2 heterogeneity in gastric cancer. Oncotarget. 2018 Jan 18;9(10):9262–72. PMID:29507688
2232. Motosugi U, Ichikawa T, Morisaka H, et al. Detection of pancreatic carcinoma and liver metastases with gadoxetic acid-enhanced

MR imaging: comparison with contrast-enhanced multi-detector row CT. Radiology. 2011 Aug;260(2):446–53. PMID:21693662

2233. Mounajjed T, Yasir S, Aleff PA, et al. Pigmented hepatocellular adenomas have a high risk of atypia and malignancy. Mod Pathol. 2015 Sep;28(9):1265–74. PMID:26205181

2234. Moussaly E, Atallah JP. A rare case of undifferentiated carcinoma of the colon with rhabdoid features: a case report and review of the literature. Case Rep Oncol Med. 2015;2015:531348. PMID:26064731

2235. Movahedi M, Bishop DT, Macrae F, et al. Obesity, aspirin, and risk of colorectal cancer in carriers of hereditary colorectal cancer: a prospective investigation in the CAPP2 study. J Clin Oncol. 2015 Nov 1;33(31):3591–7. PMID:26282643

2236. Movahedi-Lankarani S, Hruban RH, Westra WH, et al. Primitive neuroectodermal tumors of the pancreas: a report of seven cases of a rare neoplasm. Am J Surg Pathol. 2002 Aug;26(8):1040–7. PMID:12170091

2237. Movassaghian M, Brunner AM, Blonquist TM, et al. Presentation and outcomes among patients with isolated myeloid sarcoma: a Surveillance, Epidemiology, and End Results database analysis. Leuk Lymphoma. 2015 Jun;56(6):1698–703. PMID:25213180

2238. Moynihan MJ, Bast MA, Chan WC, et al. Lymphomatous polyposis. A neoplasm of either follicular mantle or germinal center cell origin. Am J Surg Pathol. 1996 Apr;20(4):442–52. PMID:8604811

2239. Mukai S, Oue N, Oshima T, et al. Overexpression of PCDHB9 promotes peritoneal metastasis and correlates with poor prognosis in patients with gastric cancer. J Pathol. 2017 Sep;243(1):100–10. PMID:28671736

2240. Mullen JT, Savarese DM. Carcinoid tumors of the appendix: a population-based study. J Surg Oncol. 2011 Jul 1;104(1):41–4. PMID:21294132

2242. Mulligan RM. Histogenesis and biologic behavior of gastric carcinoma. Pathol Annu. 1972;7:349–415. PMID:4557936

2243. Mulrooney DA, Carpenter B, Georgieff M, et al. Hepatic mesenchymal hamartoma in a neonate: a case report and review of the literature. J Pediatr Hematol Oncol. 2001 Jun-Jul;23(5):316–7. PMID:11464991

2244. Mundo L, Ambrosio MR, Picciolini M, et al. Unveiling another missing piece in EBV-driven lymphomagenesis: EBV-encoded microRNAs expression in EBER-negative Burkitt lymphoma cases. Front Microbiol. 2017 Mar 1;8:229. PMID:28298901

2245. Munghate GS, Agarwala S, Bhatnagar V. Primary yolk sac tumor of the common bile duct. J Pediatr Surg. 2011 Jun;46(6):1271–3. PMID:21683236

2246. Muraki T, Memis B, Reid MD, et al. Reflux-associated cholecystopathy: analysis of 76 gallbladders from patients with supra-Oddi union of the pancreatic duct and common bile duct (pancreatobiliary maljunction) elucidates a specific diagnostic pattern of mucosal hyperplasia as a prelude to carcinoma. Am J Surg Pathol. 2017 Sep;41(9):1167–77. PMID:28622182

2247. Muraki T, Pehlivanoglu B, Memis B, et al. Pancreatobiliary maljunction-associated gallbladder cancer is as common in the West as in the East, shows distinct clinicopathologic characteristics and offers an invaluable model for reflux-associated physio-chemical carcinogenesis [abstract]. Lab Invest. 2018 Mar;98(S1):670–94. Abstract no. 1903. PMID:29551802

2248. Muraki T, Reid MD, Basturk O, et al. Undifferentiated carcinoma with osteoclastic giant cells of the pancreas: clinicopathologic

analysis of 38 cases highlights a more protracted clinical course than currently appreciated. Am J Surg Pathol. 2016 Sep;40(9):1203–16. PMID:27508975

2249. Muraki T, Uehara T, Sano K, et al. A case of MUC5AC-positive intraductal neoplasm of the pancreas classified as an intraductal tubulopapillary neoplasm? Pathol Res Pract. 2015 Dec;211(12):1034–9. PMID:26586167

2250. Murali R, Doubrovsky A, Watson GF, et al. Diagnosis of metastatic melanoma by fine-needle biopsy: analysis of 2,204 cases. Am J Clin Pathol. 2007 Mar;127(3):385–97. PMID:17276948

2251. Murata M, Iwao K, Miyoshi Y, et al. Molecular and biological analysis of carcinoma of the small intestine: beta-catenin gene mutation by interstitial deletion involving exon 3 and replication error phenotype. Am J Gastroenterol. 2000 Jun;95(6):1576–80. PMID:10894600

2252. Murphy G, Pfeiffer R, Camargo MC, et al. Meta-analysis shows that prevalence of Epstein-Barr virus-positive gastric cancer differs based on sex and anatomic location. Gastroenterology. 2009 Sep;137(3):824–33. PMID:19445939

2253. Murphy SB, Hustu HO. A randomized trial of combined modality therapy of childhood non-Hodgkin's lymphoma. Cancer. 1980 Feb 15;45(4):630–7. PMID:6986967

2254. Murray SE, Lloyd RV, Sippel RS, et al. Postoperative surveillance of small appendiceal carcinoid tumors. Am J Surg. 2014 Mar;207(3):342–5, discussion 345. PMID:24393285

2255. Mutrie CJ, Donahue DM, Wain JC, et al. Esophageal leiomyoma: a 40-year experience. Ann Thorac Surg. 2005 Apr;79(4):1122–5. PMID:15797036

2256. Myerson RJ, Karnell LH, Menck HR. The National Cancer Data Base report on carcinoma of the anus. Cancer. 1997 Aug 15;80(4):805–15. PMID:9264365

2257. Myhre-Jensen O. A consecutive 7-year series of 1331 benign soft tissue tumours. Clinicopathologic data. Comparison with sarcomas. Acta Orthop Scand. 1981 Jun;52(3):287–93. PMID:7282321

2258. Mylonas KS, Doulamis IP, Tsilimigras DI, et al. Solid pseudopapillary and malignant pancreatic tumors in childhood: a systematic review and evidence quality assessment. Pediatr Blood Cancer. 2018 Oct;65(10):e27114. PMID:29697193

2259. Mylonas KS, Nasioudis D, Tsilimigras DI, et al. A population-based analysis of a rare oncologic entity: malignant pancreatic tumors in children. J Pediatr Surg. 2018 Apr;53(4):647–52. PMID:28693851

2260. Méndez-Martínez R, Rivera-Martínez NE, Crabtree-Ramírez B, et al. Multiple human papillomavirus infections are highly prevalent in the anal canal of human immunodeficiency virus-positive men who have sex with men. BMC Infect Dis. 2014 Dec 16;14:671. PMID:25510243

2261. Møller P, Seppälä T, Bernstein I, et al. Cancer incidence and survival in Lynch syndrome patients receiving colonoscopic and gynaecological surveillance: first report from the prospective Lynch syndrome database. Gut. 2017 Mar;66(3):464–72. PMID:26657901

2262. Møller P, Seppälä T, Bernstein I, et al. Incidence of and survival after subsequent cancers in carriers of pathogenic MMR variants with previous cancer: a report from the prospective Lynch syndrome database. Gut. 2017 Sep;66(9):1657–64. PMID:27261338

2263. Møller P, Seppälä TT, Bernstein I, et al. Cancer risk and survival in path_MMR carriers by gene and gender up to 75 years of age: a report from the Prospective Lynch Syndrome

Database. Gut. 2018 Jul;67(7):1306–16. PMID:28754778

2264. Müller MF, Ibrahim AE, Arends MJ. Molecular pathological classification of colorectal cancer. Virchows Arch. 2016 Aug;469(2):125–34. PMID:27325016

2265. N Kalimuthu S, Serra S, Hafezi-Bakhtiari S, et al. Mucin-rich variant of traditional serrated adenoma: a distinct morphological variant. Histopathology. 2017 Aug;71(2):208–16. PMID:28295534

2266. Nafidi O, Nguyen BN, Roy A. Carcinoid tumor of the common bile duct: a rare complication of von Hippel-Lindau syndrome. World J Gastroenterol. 2008 Feb 28;14(8):1299–301. PMID:18300362

2267. Nagakawa T, Kayahara M, Ueno K, et al. Clinicopathological study on neural invasion to the extrapancreatic nerve plexus in pancreatic cancer. Hepatogastroenterology. 1992 Feb;39(1):51–5. PMID:1314766

2268. Nagami Y, Tominaga K, Machida H, et al. Usefulness of non-magnifying narrow-band imaging in screening of early esophageal squamous cell carcinoma: a prospective comparative study using propensity score matching. Am J Gastroenterol. 2014 Jun;109(6):845–54. PMID:24751580

2269. Nagata K, Horinouchi M, Saitou M, et al. Mucin expression profile in pancreatic cancer and the precursor lesions. J Hepatobiliary Pancreat Surg. 2007;14(3):243–54. PMID:17520199

2270. Nagata N, Shimbo T, Yazaki H, et al. Predictive clinical factors in the diagnosis of gastrointestinal Kaposi's sarcoma and its endoscopic severity. PLoS One. 2012;7(11):e46967. PMID:23226197

2271. Nagtegaal ID, Knijn N, Hugen N, et al. Tumor deposits in colorectal cancer: improving the value of modern staging-a systematic review and meta-analysis. J Clin Oncol. 2017 Apr 1;35(10):1119–27. PMID:28029327

2272. Nagtegaal ID, Quirke P. What is the role for the circumferential margin in the modern treatment of rectal cancer? J Clin Oncol. 2008 Jan 10;26(2):303–12. PMID:18182672

2273. Nagtegaal ID, van de Velde CJ, Marijnen CA, et al. Low rectal cancer: a call for a change of approach in abdominoperineal resection. J Clin Oncol. 2005 Dec 20;23(36):9257–64. PMID:16361623

2274. Nagtegaal ID, van de Velde CJ, van der Worp E, et al. Macroscopic evaluation of rectal cancer resection specimen: clinical significance of the pathologist in quality control. J Clin Oncol. 2002 Apr 1;20(7):1729–34. PMID:11919228

2275. Naguib A, Cooke JC, Happerfield L, et al. Alterations in PTEN and PIK3CA in colorectal cancers in the EPIC Norfolk study: associations with clinicopathological and dietary factors. BMC Cancer. 2011 Apr 7;11:123. PMID:21473780

2276. Naguib A, Mitrou PN, Gay LJ, et al. Dietary, lifestyle and clinicopathological factors associated with BRAF and K-ras mutations arising in distinct subsets of colorectal cancers in the EPIC Norfolk study. BMC Cancer. 2010 Mar 16;10:99. PMID:20233436

2277. Nagula S, Kennedy T, Schattner MA, et al. Evaluation of cyst fluid CEA analysis in the diagnosis of mucinous cysts of the pancreas. J Gastrointest Surg. 2010 Dec;14(12):1997–2003. PMID:20658204

2278. Naini BV, Souza RF, Odze RD. Barrett's esophagus: a comprehensive and contemporary review for pathologists. Am J Surg Pathol. 2016 May;40(5):e45–66. PMID:26813745

2279. Nairismägi ML, Tan J, Lim JQ, et al. JAK-STAT and G-protein-coupled receptor signaling pathways are frequently altered in epitheliotropic intestinal T-cell lymphoma. Leukemia.

2016 Jun;30(6):1311–9. PMID:26854024

2280. Nakahara H, Moriya Y, Shinkai T, et al. Small cell carcinoma of the anus in a human HIV carrier: report of a case. Surg Today. 1993;23(1):85–8. PMID:8384908

2281. Nakajo S, Yamamoto M, Tahara E. Morphometric analysis of gallbladder adenocarcinoma: discrimination between carcinoma and dysplasia. Virchows Arch A Pathol Anat Histopathol. 1989;416(2):133–40. PMID:2512741

2282. Nakamura A, Horinouchi M, Goto M, et al. New classification of pancreatic intraductal papillary-mucinous tumour by mucin expression: its relationship with potential for malignancy. J Pathol. 2002 Jun;197(2):201–10. PMID:12015744

2283. Nakamura H, Arai Y, Totoki Y, et al. Genomic spectra of biliary tract cancer. Nat Genet. 2015 Sep;47(9):1003–10. PMID:26258846

2284. Nakamura K, Sugano H, Takagi K. Carcinoma of the stomach in incipient phase: its histogenesis and histological appearances. Gan. 1968 Jun;59(3):251–8. PMID:5726267

2285. Nakamura S, Akazawa K, Yao T, et al. A clinicopathologic study of 233 cases with special reference to evaluation with the MIB-1 index. Cancer. 1995 Oct 15;76(8):1313–24. PMID:8620403

2286. Nakamura S, Matsumoto T, Kobori Y, et al. Impact of Helicobacter pylori infection and mucosal atrophy on gastric lesions in patients with familial adenomatous polyposis. Gut. 2002 Oct;51(4):485–9. PMID:12235068

2287. Nakamura S, Matsumoto T. Helicobacter pylori and gastric mucosa-associated lymphoid tissue lymphoma: recent progress in pathogenesis and management. World J Gastroenterol. 2013 Dec 7;19(45):8181–7. PMID:24363507

2288. Nakamura S, Sugiyama T, Matsumoto T, et al. Long-term clinical outcome of gastric MALT lymphoma after eradication of Helicobacter pylori: a multicentre cohort follow-up study of 420 patients in Japan. Gut. 2012 Apr;61(4):507–13. PMID:21890816

2289. Nakamura S, Ye H, Bacon CM, et al. Clinical impact of genetic aberrations in gastric MALT lymphoma: a comprehensive analysis using interphase fluorescence in situ hybridisation. Gut. 2007 Oct;56(10):1358–63. PMID:17525089

2290. Nakamura T, Nakamura S, Yonezumi M, et al. Helicobacter pylori and the t(11;18)(q21;q21) translocation in gastric low-grade B-cell lymphoma of mucosa-associated lymphoid tissue type. Jpn J Cancer Res. 2000 Mar;91(3):301–9. PMID:10760689

2291. Nakamura T, Seto M, Tajika M, et al. Clinical features and prognosis of gastric MALT lymphoma with special reference to responsiveness to H. pylori eradication and API2-MALT1 status. Am J Gastroenterol. 2008 Jan;103(1):62–70. PMID:17894851

2292. Nakanishi Y, Kondo S, Zen Y, et al. Impact of residual in situ carcinoma on postoperative survival in 125 patients with extrahepatic bile duct carcinoma. J Hepatobiliary Pancreat Sci. 2010 Mar;17(2):166–73. PMID:19521656

2293. Nakanishi Y, Nakanuma Y, Ohara M, et al. Intraductal papillary neoplasm arising from peribiliary glands connecting with the inferior branch of the bile duct of the anterior segment of the liver. Pathol Int. 2011 Dec;61(12):773–7. PMID:22126388

2294. Nakanishi Y, Zen Y, Kondo S, et al. Expression of cell cycle-related molecules in biliary premalignant lesions: biliary intraepithelial neoplasia and biliary intraductal papillary neoplasm. Hum Pathol. 2008 Aug;39(8):1153–61. PMID:18495210

2295. Nakanuma Y, Jang KT, Fukushima N, et al. A statement by the Japan-Korea expert

pathologists for future clinicopathological and molecular analyses toward consensus building of intraductal papillary neoplasm of the bile duct through several opinions at the present stage. J Hepatobiliary Pancreat Sci. 2018 Mar;25(3):181–7. PMID:29272078
2296. Nakanuma Y, Kakuda Y, Uesaka K, et al. Characterization of intraductal papillary neoplasm of bile duct with respect to histopathologic similarities to pancreatic intraductal papillary mucinous neoplasm. Hum Pathol. 2016 May;51:103–13. PMID:27067788
2297. Nakanuma Y, Kakuda Y. Pathologic classification of cholangiocarcinoma: new concepts. Best Pract Res Clin Gastroenterol. 2015 Apr;29(2):277–93. PMID:25966428
2298. Nakanuma Y, Sato Y, Ikeda H, et al. Intrahepatic cholangiocarcinoma with predominant "ductal plate malformation" pattern: a new subtype. Am J Surg Pathol. 2012 Nov;36(11):1629–35. PMID:23073321
2299. Nakanuma Y, Sato Y. Cystic and papillary neoplasm involving peribiliary glands: a biliary counterpart of branch-type intraductal papillary mucinous [corrected] neoplasm? Hepatology. 2012 Jun;55(6):2040–1. PMID:22262399
2300. Nakanuma Y, Sudo Y. Biliary tumors with pancreatic counterparts. Semin Diagn Pathol. 2017 Mar;34(2):167–75. PMID:28109714
2301. Nakanuma Y, Uchida T, Sato Y, et al. An S100P-positive biliary epithelial field is a preinvasive intraepithelial neoplasm in nodular-sclerosing cholangiocarcinoma. Hum Pathol. 2017 Feb;60:46–57. PMID:27984121
2302. Nakanuma Y, Uesaka K, Miyayama S, et al. Intraductal neoplasms of the bile duct. A new challenge to biliary tract tumor pathology. Histol Histopathol. 2017 Oct;32(10):1001–15. PMID:28337739
2303. Nakao A, Harada A, Nonami T, et al. Clinical significance of carcinoma invasion of the extrapancreatic nerve plexus in pancreatic cancer. Pancreas. 1996 May;12(4):357–61. PMID:8740402
2304. Nakao A, Harada A, Nonami T, et al. Clinical significance of portal invasion by pancreatic head carcinoma. Surgery. 1995 Jan;117(1):50–5. PMID:7809836
2305. Nakasono M, Hirokawa M, Suzuki M, et al. Lymphoepithelioma-like carcinoma of the esophagus: report of a case with non-progressive behavior. J Gastroenterol Hepatol. 2007 Dec;22(12):2344–7. PMID:18031397
2306. Nakata B, Yashiro M, Nishioka N, et al. Very low incidence of microsatellite instability in intraductal papillary-mucinous neoplasm of the pancreas. Int J Cancer. 2002 Dec 20;102(6):655–9. PMID:12448010
2307. Nakken S, Hovig E, Møller P, editors. Prospective Lynch Syndrome Database [Internet]. Edinburgh (UK): European Hereditary Tumour Group & Middlesex (UK): International Society for Gastrointestinal Hereditary Tumours; 2018. Available from: http://www.lscarisk.org.
2308. Nallamothu G, Adler DG. Large colonic lipomas. Gastroenterol Hepatol (N Y). 2011 Jul;7(7):490–2. PMID:22298986
2308A. Nam AR, Kim JW, Cha Y, et al. Therapeutic implication of HER2 in advanced biliary tract cancer. Oncotarget. 2016 Sep 6;7(36):58007–21. PMID:27517322
2309. Namasivayam S, Martin DR, Saini S. Imaging of liver metastases: MRI. Cancer Imaging. 2007;7:2–9. PMID:17293303
2310. Napoléon B, Lemaistre AI, Pujol B, et al. A novel approach to the diagnosis of pancreatic serous cystadenoma: needle-based confocal laser endomicroscopy. Endoscopy. 2015 Jan;47(1):26–32. PMID:25325684
2311. Nara S, Shimada K, Kosuge T, et al. Minimally invasive intraductal papillary-mucinous carcinoma of the pancreas: clinicopathologic study of 104 intraductal papillary-mucinous neoplasms. Am J Surg Pathol. 2008 Feb;32(2):243–55. PMID:18223327
2312. Naresh KN, Ibrahim HA, Lazzi S, et al. Diagnosis of Burkitt lymphoma using an algorithmic approach–applicable in both resource-poor and resource-rich countries. Br J Haematol. 2011 Sep;154(6):770–6. PMID:21718280
2313. Narita T, Moriyama Y, Ito Y. Endodermal sinus (yolk sac) tumour of the liver. A case report and review of the literature. J Pathol. 1988 May;155(1):41–7. PMID:3288736
2314. Nart D, Ertan Y, Yilmaz F, et al. Primary hepatic marginal zone B-cell lymphoma of mucosa-associated lymphoid tissue type in a liver transplant patient with hepatitis B cirrhosis. Transplant Proc. 2005 Dec;37(10):4408–12. PMID:16387133
2315. Nascimbeni R, Villanacci V, Di Fabio F, et al. Solitary microcarcinoid of the rectal stump in ulcerative colitis. Neuroendocrinology. 2005;81(6):400–4. PMID:16276118
2316. Naseem M, Barzi A, Brezden-Masley C, et al. Outlooks on Epstein-Barr virus associated gastric cancer. Cancer Treat Rev. 2018 May;66:15–22. PMID:29631196
2317. Nassar H, Albores-Saavedra J, Klimstra DS. High-grade neuroendocrine carcinoma of the ampulla of Vater: a clinicopathologic and immunohistochemical analysis of 14 cases. Am J Surg Pathol. 2005 May;29(5):588–94. PMID:15832081
2318. Natarajan S, Theise ND, Thung SN, et al. Large-cell change of hepatocytes in cirrhosis may represent a reaction to prolonged cholestasis. Am J Surg Pathol. 1997 Mar;21(3):312–8. PMID:9060601
2319. National Institute for Health and Care Excellence [Internet]. London (UK): National Institute for Health and Care Excellence; 2018. Molecular testing strategies for Lynch syndrome in people with colorectal cancer: Diagnostics guidance [DG27]; published 2017 Feb. Available from: https://www.nice.org.uk/guidance/dg27.
2320. Natkunam Y, Farinha P, Hsi ED, et al. LMO2 protein expression predicts survival in patients with diffuse large B-cell lymphoma treated with anthracycline-based chemotherapy with and without rituximab. J Clin Oncol. 2008 Jan 20;26(3):447–54. PMID:18086797
2321. Natori T, Teshima S, Kikuchi Y, et al. Primary yolk sac tumor of the liver. An autopsy case with ultrastructural and immunopathological studies. Acta Pathol Jpn. 1983 May;33(3):555–64. PMID:6353852
2322. Nault JC, Bioulac-Sage P, Zucman-Rossi J. Hepatocellular benign tumors-from molecular classification to personalized clinical care. Gastroenterology. 2013 May;144(5):888–902. PMID:23485860
2323. Nault JC, Calderaro J, Di Tommaso L, et al. Telomerase reverse transcriptase promoter mutation is an early somatic genetic alteration in the transformation of premalignant nodules in hepatocellular carcinoma on cirrhosis. Hepatology. 2014 Dec;60(6):1983–92. PMID:25123086
2324. Nault JC, Couchy G, Balabaud C, et al. Molecular classification of hepatocellular adenoma associates with risk factors, bleeding, and malignant transformation. Gastroenterology. 2017 Mar;152(4):880–94.e6. PMID:27939373
2325. Nault JC, Galle PR, Marquardt JU. The role of molecular enrichment on future therapies in hepatocellular carcinoma. J Hepatol. 2018 Jul;69(1):237–47. PMID:29505843
2326. Nault JC, Mallet M, Pilati C, et al. High frequency of telomerase reverse-transcriptase promoter somatic mutations in hepatocellular carcinoma and preneoplastic lesions. Nat Commun. 2013;4:2218. PMID:23887712
2327. Navaneethan U, Hasan MK, Lourdusamy V, et al. Single-operator cholangioscopy and targeted biopsies in the diagnosis of indeterminate biliary strictures: a systematic review. Gastrointest Endosc. 2015 Oct;82(4):608–14.e2. PMID:26071061
2328. Nawgiri RS, Nagle JA, Wilbur DC, et al. Cytomorphology and B72.3 labeling of benign and malignant ductal epithelium in pancreatic lesions compared to gastrointestinal epithelium. Diagn Cytopathol. 2007 May;35(5):300–5. PMID:17427224
2329. Nelen MR, Kremer H, Konings IB, et al. Novel PTEN mutations in patients with Cowden disease: absence of clear genotype-phenotype correlations. Eur J Hum Genet. 1999 Apr;7(3):267–73. PMID:10234502
2330. Nelen MR, Padberg GW, Peeters EA, et al. Localization of the gene for Cowden disease to chromosome 10q22-23. Nat Genet. 1996 May;13(1):114–6. PMID:8673088
2331. Nelen MR, van Staveren WC, Peeters EA, et al. Germline mutations in the PTEN/MMAC1 gene in patients with Cowden disease. Hum Mol Genet. 1997 Aug;6(8):1383–7. PMID:9259288
2332. Nelson BP, Wolniak KL, Evens A, et al. Early posttransplant lymphoproliferative disease: clinicopathologic features and correlation with mTOR signaling pathway activation. Am J Clin Pathol. 2012 Oct;138(4):568–78. PMID:23010712
2333. Nelson S, Näthke IS. Interactions and functions of the adenomatous polyposis coli (APC) protein at a glance. J Cell Sci. 2013 Feb 15;126(Pt 4):873–7. PMID:23589686
2334. Neoptolemos JP, Dunn JA, Stocken DD, et al. Adjuvant chemoradiotherapy and chemotherapy in resectable pancreatic cancer: a randomised controlled trial. Lancet. 2001 Nov 10;358(9293):1576–85. PMID:11716884
2335. Neoptolemos JP, Stocken DD, Dunn JA, et al. Influence of resection margins on survival for patients with pancreatic cancer treated by adjuvant chemoradiation and/or chemotherapy in the ESPAC-1 randomized controlled trial. Ann Surg. 2001 Dec;234(6):758–68. PMID:11729382
2336. Neoptolemos JP, Stocken DD, Friess H, et al. A randomized trial of chemoradiotherapy and chemotherapy after resection of pancreatic cancer. N Engl J Med. 2004 Mar 18;350(12):1200–10. PMID:15028824
2337. Nesi G, Marcucci T, Rubio CA, et al. Somatostatinoma: clinico-pathological features of three cases and literature reviewed. J Gastroenterol Hepatol. 2008 Apr;23(4):521–6. PMID:17645474
2338. Neumann WL, Coss E, Rugge M, et al. Autoimmune atrophic gastritis–pathogenesis, pathology and management. Nat Rev Gastroenterol Hepatol. 2013 Sep;10(9):529–41. PMID:23774773
2339. Neuville A, Chibon F, Coindre JM. Grading of soft tissue sarcomas: from histological to molecular assessment. Pathology. 2014 Feb;46(2):113–20. PMID:24378389
2340. Newman DH, Doerhoff CR, Bunt TJ. Villous adenoma of the duodenum. Am Surg. 1984 Jan;50(1):26–8. PMID:6691630
2341. Ng IO, Guan XY, Poon RT, et al. Determination of the molecular relationship between multiple tumour nodules in hepatocellular carcinoma differentiates multicentric origin from intrahepatic metastasis. J Pathol. 2003 Mar;199(3):345–53. PMID:12579536
2342. Ngoma T, Adde M, Durosinmi M, et al. Treatment of Burkitt lymphoma in equatorial Africa using a simple three-drug combination followed by a salvage regimen for patients with persistent or recurrent disease. Br J Haematol. 2012 Sep;158(6):749–62. PMID:22844968
2343. Nguyen BN, Fléjou JF, Terris B, et al. Focal nodular hyperplasia of the liver: a comprehensive pathologic study of 305 lesions and recognition of new histologic forms. Am J Surg Pathol. 1999 Dec;23(12):1441–54. PMID:10584697
2344. Nguyen NQ, Johns AL, Gill AJ, et al. Clinical and immunohistochemical features of 34 solid pseudopapillary tumors of the pancreas. J Gastroenterol Hepatol. 2011 Feb;26(2):267–74. PMID:21261715
2345. Nguyen NT, Harring TR, Holley L, et al. Biliary adenofibroma with carcinoma in situ: a rare case report. Case Reports Hepatol. 2012;2012:793963. PMID:25374710
2346. Nguyen TB, Roncalli M, Di Tommaso L, et al. Combined use of heat-shock protein 70 and glutamine synthetase is useful in the distinction of typical hepatocellular adenoma from atypical hepatocellular neoplasms and well-differentiated hepatocellular carcinoma. Mod Pathol. 2016 Mar;29(3):283–92. PMID:26769138
2347. Nguyen TT, Gorman B, Shields D, et al. Malignant hepatic angiomyolipoma: report of a case and review of literature. Am J Surg Pathol. 2008 May;32(5):793–8. PMID:18391749
2348. Ni PZ, Yang YS, Hu WP, et al. Primary adenosquamous carcinoma of the esophagus: an analysis of 39 cases. J Thorac Dis. 2016 Oct;8(10):2689–96. PMID:27867543
2349. Ni Y, Zbuk KM, Sadler T, et al. Germline mutations and variants in the succinate dehydrogenase genes in Cowden and Cowden-like syndromes. Am J Hum Genet. 2008 Aug;83(2):261–8. PMID:18678321
2350. Nicholson HS, Egeler RM, Nesbit ME. The epidemiology of Langerhans cell histiocytosis. Hematol Oncol Clin North Am. 1998 Apr;12(2):379–84. PMID:9561907
2351. Nicol K, Savell V, Moore J, et al. Distinguishing undifferentiated embryonal sarcoma of the liver from biliary tract rhabdomyosarcoma: a Children's Oncology Group study. Pediatr Dev Pathol. 2007 Mar-Apr;10(2):89–97. PMID:17378682
2352. Nicolae A, Xi L, Pham TH, et al. Mutations in the JAK/STAT and RAS signaling pathways are common in intestinal T-cell lymphomas. Leukemia. 2016 Nov;30(11):2245–7. PMID:27389054
2353. Nicolae A, Xi L, Pittaluga S, et al. Frequent STAT5B mutations in γδ hepatosplenic T-cell lymphomas. Leukemia. 2014 Nov;28(11):2244–8. PMID:24947020
2354. Niederle MB, Hackl M, Kaserer K, et al. Gastroenteropancreatic neuroendocrine tumours: the current incidence and staging based on the WHO and European Neuroendocrine Tumour Society classification: an analysis based on prospectively collected parameters. Endocr Relat Cancer. 2010 Oct 5;17(4):909–18. PMID:20702725
2355. Nielsen GP, Dickersin GR, Provenzal JM, et al. Lipomatous hemangiopericytoma. A histologic, ultrastructural and immunohistochemical study of a unique variant of hemangiopericytoma. Am J Surg Pathol. 1995 Jul;19(7):748–56. PMID:7793472
2356. Nielsen GP, O'Connell JX, Dickersin GR, et al. Solitary fibrous tumor of soft tissue: a report of 15 cases, including 5 malignant examples with light microscopic, immunohistochemical, and ultrastructural data. Mod Pathol. 1997 Oct;10(10):1028–37. PMID:9346183
2357. Nieser M, Henopp T, Brix J, et al. Loss of chromosome 18 in neuroendocrine tumors of the small intestine: the enigma remains. Neuroendocrinology. 2017;104(3):302–12. PMID:27222126
2358. Nieuwenhuis MH, Vogt S, Jones N, et al. Evidence for accelerated colorectal adenoma–carcinoma progression in MUTYH-associated polyposis? Gut. 2012 May;61(5):734–8.

PMID:21846783
2359. Nikfarjam M, Warshaw AL, Axelrod L, et al. Improved contemporary surgical management of insulinomas: a 25-year experience at the Massachusetts General Hospital. Ann Surg. 2008 Jan;247(1):165–72. PMID:18156937
2360. Nikiforova MN, Khalid A, Fasanella KE, et al. Integration of KRAS testing in the diagnosis of pancreatic cystic lesions: a clinical experience of 618 pancreatic cysts. Mod Pathol. 2013 Nov;26(11):1478–87. PMID:23743931
2361. Nikolaisen C, Figenschau Y, Nossent JC. Anemia in early rheumatoid arthritis is associated with interleukin 6-mediated bone marrow suppression, but has no effect on disease course or mortality. J Rheumatol. 2008 Mar;35(3):380–6. PMID:18260177
2362. Nilbert M, Planck M, Fernebro E, et al. Microsatellite instability is rare in rectal carcinomas and signifies hereditary cancer. Eur J Cancer. 1999 Jun;35(6):942–5. PMID:10533476
2363. Nilbert M, Rambech E. Beta-catenin activation through mutation is rare in rectal cancer. Cancer Genet Cytogenet. 2001 Jul 1;128(1):43–5. PMID:11454429
2364. Nilsson B, Bümming P, Meis-Kindblom JM, et al. Gastrointestinal stromal tumors: the incidence, prevalence, clinical course, and prognostication in the preimatinib mesylate era–a population-based study in western Sweden. Cancer. 2005 Feb 15;103(4):821–9. PMID:15648083
2365. Nilsson O. Profiling of ileal carcinoids. Neuroendocrinology. 2013;97(1):7–18. PMID:22986706
2366. Nirmala V, Chopra P, Machado NO. An unusual adult hepatic teratoma. Histopathology. 2003 Sep;43(3):306–8. PMID:12940789
2367. Nishigami T, Kataoka TR, Ikeuchi H, et al. Adenocarcinomas associated with perianal fistulae in Crohn's disease have a rectal, not an anal, immunophenotype. Pathology. 2011 Jan;43(1):36–9. PMID:21240063
2368. Nishihara K, Nagai E, Tsuneyoshi M, et al. Small-cell carcinoma combined with adenocarcinoma of the gallbladder. A case report with immunohistochemical and flow cytometric studies. Arch Pathol Lab Med. 1994 Feb;118(2):177–81. PMID:8311660
2369. Nishihara K, Nagoshi M, Tsuneyoshi M, et al. Papillary cystic tumors of the pancreas. Assessment of their malignant potential. Cancer. 1993 Jan 1;71(1):82–92. PMID:8416730
2370. Nishihara K, Tsuneyoshi M. Undifferentiated spindle cell carcinoma of the gallbladder: a clinicopathologic, immunohistochemical, and flow cytometric study of 11 cases. Hum Pathol. 1993 Dec;24(12):1298–305. PMID:8276377
2371. Nishihara K, Yamaguchi K, Hashimoto H, et al. Tubular adenoma of the gallbladder with squamoid spindle cell metaplasia. Report of three cases with immunohistochemical study. Acta Pathol Jpn. 1991 Jan;41(1):41–5. PMID:1709553
2372. Nishikawa G, Sekine S, Ogawa R, et al. Frequent GNAS mutations in low-grade appendiceal mucinous neoplasms. Br J Cancer. 2013 Mar 5;108(4):951–8. PMID:23403822
2373. Nishino H, Hatano E, Seo S, et al. Histological features of mixed neuroendocrine carcinoma and hepatocellular carcinoma in the liver: a case report and literature review. Clin J Gastroenterol. 2016 Aug;9(4):272–9. PMID:27384317
2374. Nitecki SS, Wolff BG, Schlinkert R, et al. The natural history of surgically treated primary adenocarcinoma of the appendix. Ann Surg. 1994 Jan;219(1):51–7. PMID:8297177
2375. Niwa A, Kuwano S, Tomita H, et al. The different pathogeneses of sporadic adenoma and adenocarcinoma in non-ampullary lesions of the proximal and distal duodenum. Oncotarget. 2017 Jun 20;8(25):41078–90. PMID:28467793
2376. Noble F, Lloyd MA, Turkington R, et al. Multicentre cohort study to define and validate pathological assessment of response to neoadjuvant therapy in oesophagogastric adenocarcinoma. Br J Surg. 2017 Dec;104(13):1816–28. PMID:28944954
2377. Noble F, Nolan L, Bateman AC, et al. Refining pathological evaluation of neoadjuvant therapy for adenocarcinoma of the esophagus. World J Gastroenterol. 2013 Dec 28;19(48):9282–93. PMID:24409055
2378. Noda Y, Fujita N, Kobayashi G, et al. Histological study of gallbladder and bile duct epithelia in patients with anomalous arrangement of the pancreaticobiliary ductal system: comparison between those with and without a dilated common bile duct. J Gastroenterol. 2007 Mar;42(3):211–8. PMID:17380279
2379. Noguchi R, Yano H, Gohda Y, et al. Molecular profiles of high-grade and low-grade pseudomyxoma peritonei. Cancer Med. 2015 Dec;4(12):1809–16. PMID:26475379
2380. Nojima T, Nakamura F, Ishikura M, et al. Pleomorphic carcinoma of the pancreas with osteoclast-like giant cells. Int J Pancreatol. 1993 Dec;14(3):275–81. PMID:8113629
2381. Nomura R, Saito T, Mitomi H, et al. GNAS mutation as an alternative mechanism of activation of the Wnt/β-catenin signaling pathway in gastric adenocarcinoma of the fundic gland type. Hum Pathol. 2014 Dec;45(12):2488–96. PMID:25288233
2382. Nomura Y, Nakashima O, Akiba J, et al. Clinicopathological features of neoplasms with neuroendocrine differentiation occurring in the liver. J Clin Pathol. 2017 Jul;70(7):563–70. PMID:27881473
2383. Nonaka D, Wang BY, Edmondson D, et al. A study of gata3 and phox2b expression in tumors of the autonomic nervous system. Am J Surg Pathol. 2013 Aug;37(8):1236–41. PMID:23715162
2384. Nonomura A, Mizukami Y, Takayanagi N, et al. Immunohistochemical study of hepatic angiomyolipoma. Pathol Int. 1996 Jan;46(1):24–32. PMID:10846546
2385. Noorani A, Bornschein J, Lynch AG, et al. A comparative analysis of whole genome sequencing of esophageal adenocarcinoma pre- and post-chemotherapy. Genome Res. 2017 Jun;27(6):902–12. PMID:28465312
2386. Norlén O, Stålberg P, Öberg K, et al. Long-term results of surgery for small intestinal neuroendocrine tumors at a tertiary referral center. World J Surg. 2012 Jun;36(6):1419–31. PMID:21984144
2387. Noronha V, Shafi NQ, Obando JA, et al. Primary non-Hodgkin's lymphoma of the liver. Crit Rev Oncol Hematol. 2005 Mar;53(3):199–207. PMID:15718146
2388. Norris AL, Roberts NJ, Jones S, et al. Familial and sporadic pancreatic cancer share the same molecular pathogenesis. Fam Cancer. 2015 Mar;14(1):95–103. PMID:25240578
2389. Norsworthy KJ, Bhatnagar B, Singh ZN, et al. Myeloid sarcoma of the hepatobiliary system: a case series and review of the literature. Acta Haematol. 2016;135(4):241–51. PMID:27007946
2390. Notta F, Chan-Seng-Yue M, Lemire M, et al. A renewed model of pancreatic cancer evolution based on genomic rearrangement patterns. Nature. 2016 Oct 20;538(7625):378–82. PMID:27732578
2391. Novelli M, Rossi S, Rodriguez-Justo M, et al. DOG1 and CD117 are the antibodies of choice in the diagnosis of gastrointestinal stromal tumours. Histopathology. 2010 Aug;57(2):259–70. PMID:20716168
2392. Noë M, Pea A, Luchini C, et al. Whole-exome sequencing of duodenal neuroendocrine tumors in patients with neurofibromatosis type 1. Mod Pathol. 2018 Oct;31(10):1532–8. PMID:29849115
2393. Noë M, Rezaee N, Asrani K, et al. Immunolabeling of cleared human pancreata provides insights into three-dimensional pancreatic anatomy and pathology. Am J Pathol. 2018 Jul;188(7):1530–5. PMID:29684363
2394. Nugent KP, Spigelman AD, Phillips RK. Life expectancy after colectomy and ileorectal anastomosis for familial adenomatous polyposis. Dis Colon Rectum. 1993 Nov;36(11):1059–62. PMID:8223060
2395. Nummela P, Saarinen L, Thiel A, et al. Genomic profile of pseudomyxoma peritonei analyzed using next-generation sequencing and immunohistochemistry. Int J Cancer. 2015 Mar 1;136(5):E282–9. PMID:25274248
2396. Nunes G, Coelho H, Patita M, et al. Pancreatoblastoma: an unusual diagnosis in an adult patient. Clin J Gastroenterol. 2018 Apr;11(2):161–6. PMID:29285688
2397. Nusse R, Clevers H. Wnt/β-catenin signaling, disease, and emerging therapeutic modalities. Cell. 2017 Jun 1;169(6):985–99. PMID:28575679
2398. Nyström-Lahti M, Kristo P, Nicolaides NC, et al. Founding mutations and Alu-mediated recombination in hereditary colon cancer. Nat Med. 1995 Nov;1(11):1203–6. PMID:7584997
2399. Nzeako UC, Goodman ZD, Ishak KG. Comparison of tumor pathology with duration of survival of North American patients with hepatocellular carcinoma. Cancer. 1995 Aug 15;76(4):579–88. PMID:8625150
2400. O'Brien MJ, Yang S, Clebanoff JL, et al. Hyperplastic (serrated) polyps of the colorectum: relationship of CpG island methylator phenotype and K-ras mutation to location and histologic subtype. Am J Surg Pathol. 2004 Apr;28(4):423–34. PMID:15087661
2401. O'Brien MJ, Zhao Q, Yang S. Colorectal serrated pathway cancers and precursors. Histopathology. 2015 Jan;66(1):49–65. PMID:25263173
2402. O'Connell JB, Maggard MA, Manunga J Jr, et al. Survival after resection of ampullary carcinoma: a national population-based study. Ann Surg Oncol. 2008 Jul;15(7):1820–7. PMID:18369675
2404. O'Farrelly C, Feighery C, O'Briain DS, et al. Humoral response to wheat protein in patients with coeliac disease and enteropathy associated T cell lymphoma. Br Med J (Clin Res Ed). 1986 Oct 11;293(6552):908–10. PMID:3094712
2405. O'Sullivan MJ, Swanson PE, Knoll J, et al. Undifferentiated embryonal sarcoma with unusual features arising within mesenchymal hamartoma of the liver: report of a case and review of the literature. Pediatr Dev Pathol. 2001 Sep-Oct;4(5):482–9. PMID:11779051
2406. Oda, Kondo H, Yamao T, et al. Metastatic tumors to the stomach: analysis of 54 patients diagnosed at endoscopy and 347 autopsy cases. Endoscopy. 2001 Jun;33(6):507–10. PMID:11437044
2407. Odeh M, Misselevich I, Oliven A, et al. Small intestinal carcinoma with osteoclast-like giant cells. Am J Gastroenterol. 1995 Jul;90(7):1177–9. PMID:7611227
2408. Odze R, Antonioli D, Shocket D, et al. Esophageal squamous papillomas. A clinicopathologic study of 38 lesions and analysis for human papillomavirus by the polymerase chain reaction. Am J Surg Pathol. 1993 Aug;17(8):803–12. PMID:8393303
2409. Odze RD, Farraye FA, Hecht JL, et al. Long-term follow-up after polypectomy treatment for adenoma-like dysplastic lesions in ulcerative colitis. Clin Gastroenterol Hepatol. 2004 Jul;2(7):534–41. PMID:15224277
2410. Odze RD, Goldblum JR, editors. Odze and Goldblum surgical pathology of the GI tract, liver, biliary tract and pancreas. 3rd ed. Philadelphia (PA): Saunders; 2015.
2411. Oehler-Jänne C, Huguet F, Provencher S, et al. HIV-specific differences in outcome of squamous cell carcinoma of the anal canal: a multicentric cohort study of HIV-positive patients receiving highly active antiretroviral therapy. J Clin Oncol. 2008 May 20;26(15):2550–7. PMID:18427149
2412. Oettle H, Post S, Neuhaus P, et al. Adjuvant chemotherapy with gemcitabine vs observation in patients undergoing curative-intent resection of pancreatic cancer: a randomized controlled trial. JAMA. 2007 Jan 17;297(3):267–77. PMID:17227978
2413. Offerhaus GJ, Giardiello FM, Krush AJ, et al. The risk of upper gastrointestinal cancer in familial adenomatous polyposis. Gastroenterology. 1992 Jun;102(6):1980–2. PMID:1316858
2414. Offerhaus GJ, Giardiello FM, Moore GW, et al. Partial gastrectomy: a risk factor for carcinoma of the pancreas? Hum Pathol. 1987 Mar;18(3):285–8. PMID:3028929
2415. Offman J, Muldrew B, O'Donovan M, et al. Barrett's oESophagus trial 3 (BEST3): study protocol for a randomised controlled trial comparing the Cytosponge-TFF3 test with usual care to facilitate the diagnosis of oesophageal pre-cancer in primary care patients with chronic acid reflux. BMC Cancer. 2018 Aug 3;18(1):784. PMID:30075763
2416. Ogawa H, Haneda S, Shibata C, et al. Adenocarcinoma associated with perianal fistulas in Crohn's disease. Anticancer Res. 2013 Feb;33(2):685–9. PMID:23393368
2417. Ogiwara H, Sugimoto M, Ohno T, et al. Role of deletion located between the intermediate and middle regions of the Helicobacter pylori vacA gene in cases of gastroduodenal diseases. J Clin Microbiol. 2009 Nov;47(11):3493–500. PMID:19726606
2418. Ogwang MD, Bhatia K, Biggar RJ, et al. Incidence and geographic distribution of endemic Burkitt lymphoma in northern Uganda revisited. Int J Cancer. 2008 Dec 1;123(11):2658–63. PMID:18767045
2419. Oh D, Yi NJ, Song S, et al. Split liver transplantation for retroperitoneal immature teratoma masquerading as hepatoblastoma. Pediatr Transplant. 2017 Nov;21(7). PMID:28714114
2420. Ohashi S, Miyamoto S, Kikuchi O, et al. Recent advances from basic and clinical studies of esophageal squamous cell carcinoma. Gastroenterology. 2015 Dec;149(7):1700–15. PMID:26376349
2421. Ohike N, Coban I, Kim GE, et al. Tumor budding as a strong prognostic indicator in invasive ampullary adenocarcinomas. Am J Surg Pathol. 2010 Oct;34(10):1417–24. PMID:20871215
2422. Ohike N, Jürgensen A, Pipeleers-Marichal M, et al. Mixed ductal-endocrine carcinomas of the pancreas and ductal adenocarcinomas with scattered endocrine cells: characterization of the endocrine cells. Virchows Arch. 2003 Mar;442(3):258–65. PMID:12647216
2423. Ohike N, Kim GE, Tajiri T, et al. Intra-ampullary papillary-tubular neoplasm (IAPN): characterization of tumoral intraepithelial neoplasia occurring within the ampulla: a clinicopathologic analysis of 82 cases. Am J Surg Pathol. 2010 Dec;34(12):1731–48. PMID:21084962
2424. Ohike N, Kosmahl M, Klöppel G. Mixed acinar-endocrine carcinoma of the pancreas. A clinicopathological study and comparison with acinar-cell carcinoma. Virchows Arch. 2004 Sep;445(3):231–5. PMID:15517367
2425. Ohike N, Morohoshi T. Exocrine

pancreatic neoplasms of nonductal origin: acinar cell carcinoma, pancreatoblastoma, and solid-pseudopapillary neoplasm. Surg Pathol Clin. 2011 Jun;4(2):579–88. PMID:26837489
2426. Ohmoto T, Yoshitani N, Nishitsuji K, et al. CD44-expressing undifferentiated carcinoma with rhabdoid features of the pancreas: molecular analysis of aggressive invasion and metastasis. Pathol Int. 2015 May;65(5):264–70. PMID:25753521
2427. Ohnishi N, Takata K, Miyata-Takata T, et al. CD10 down expression in follicular lymphoma correlates with gastrointestinal lesion involving the stomach and large intestine. Cancer Sci. 2016 Nov;107(11):1687–95. PMID:27513891
2428. Ohnishi T, Tomita N, Monden T, et al. A detailed analysis of the role of K-ras gene mutation in the progression of colorectal adenoma. Br J Cancer. 1997;75(3):341–7. PMID:9020477
2429. Ohsawa M, Aozasa K, Horiuchi K, et al. Malignant lymphoma of the liver. Report of five cases and review of the literature. Dig Dis Sci. 1992 Jul;37(7):1105–9. PMID:1618060
2430. Ohtomo R, Sekine S, Taniguchi H, et al. Anal canal neuroendocrine carcinoma associated with squamous intraepithelial neoplasia: a human papillomavirus 18-related lesion. Pathol Int. 2012 May;62(5):356–9. PMID:22524667
2431. Ohuchida K, Mizumoto K, Miyasaka Y, et al. Over-expression of S100A2 in pancreatic cancer correlates with progression and poor prognosis. J Pathol. 2007 Nov;213(3):275–82. PMID:17940995
2432. Oikawa T, Ojima H, Yamasaki S, et al. Multistep and multicentric development of hepatocellular carcinoma: histological analysis of 980 resected nodules. J Hepatol. 2005 Feb;42(2):225–9. PMID:15664248
2433. Okabayashi T, Hanazaki K. Surgical outcome of adenosquamous carcinoma of the pancreas. World J Gastroenterol. 2008 Nov 28;14(44):6765–70. PMID:19058301
2434. Okada K, Fujisaki J, Kasuga A, et al. Sporadic nonampullary duodenal adenoma in the natural history of duodenal cancer: a study of follow-up surveillance. Am J Gastroenterol. 2011 Feb;106(2):357–64. PMID:21139577
2435. Okamoto N, Kawachi H, Yoshida T, et al. "Crawling-type" adenocarcinoma of the stomach: a distinct entity preceding poorly differentiated adenocarcinoma. Gastric Cancer. 2013 Apr;16(2):220–32. PMID:22865191
2436. Oku T, Ono K, Nagamachi Y, et al. [Pedunculated carcinoid tumor of the gallbladder–analysis of the relationship between location and morphology in carcinoid tumor of the gallbladder]. Nihon Shokakibyo Gakkai Zasshi. 2008 Mar;105(3):397–403. Japanese. PMID:18332605
2437. Okumura K, Ikebe M, Shimokama T, et al. An unusual enteropathy-associated T-cell lymphoma with MYC translocation arising in a Japanese patient: a case report. World J Gastroenterol. 2012 May 21;18(19):2434–7. PMID:22654438
2438. Okumura Y, Kohashi K, Wang H, et al. Combined primary hepatic neuroendocrine carcinoma and hepatocellular carcinoma with aggressive biological behavior (adverse clinical course): a case report. Pathol Res Pract. 2017 Oct;213(10):1322–6. PMID:28647212
2439. Oliveira C, Pinheiro H, Figueiredo J, et al. Familial gastric cancer: genetic susceptibility, pathology, and implications for management. Lancet Oncol. 2015 Feb;16(2):e60–70. PMID:25638682
2440. Oliveira C, Senz J, Kaurah P, et al. Germline CDH1 deletions in hereditary diffuse gastric cancer families. Hum Mol Genet. 2009 May 1;18(9):1545–55. PMID:19168852
2441. Oliveira C, Sousa S, Pinheiro H, et al. Quantification of epigenetic and genetic 2nd hits in CDH1 during hereditary diffuse gastric cancer syndrome progression. Gastroenterology. 2009 Jun;136(7):2137–48. PMID:19269290
2442. Oliver RL, Davis JR, White A. Characterisation of ACTH related peptides in ectopic Cushing's syndrome. Pituitary. 2003;6(3):119–26. PMID:14971736
2444. Omland LH, Jepsen P, Krarup H, et al. Liver cancer and non-Hodgkin lymphoma in hepatitis C virus-infected patients: results from the DANVIR cohort study. Int J Cancer. 2012 May 15;130(10):2310–7. PMID:21780099
2445. Ong CK, Subimerb C, Pairojkul C, et al. Exome sequencing of liver fluke-associated cholangiocarcinoma. Nat Genet. 2012 May 6;44(6):690–3. PMID:22561520
2446. Ong EJ, Wang LM, Darby J. Synchronous Merkel cell and squamous cell carcinoma of the anal canal in an HIV-positive patient: a case report. Colorectal Dis. 2012 Dec;14(12):e819–20. PMID:22329967
2447. Ong JJ, Fairley CK, Carroll S, et al. Cost-effectiveness of screening for anal cancer using regular digital ano-rectal examinations in men who have sex with men living with HIV. J Int AIDS Soc. 2016 Mar 1;19(1):20514. PMID:26942721
2448. Ong JJ, Fairley CK, Read TRH, et al. Age-specific pattern of anogenital wart in men who have sex with men. Sex Transm Dis. 2018 Mar;45(3):186–8. PMID:29420447
2449. Onkendi EO, Boostrom SY, Sarr MG, et al. 15-year experience with surgical treatment of duodenal carcinoma: a comparison of periampullary and extra-ampullary duodenal carcinomas. J Gastrointest Surg. 2012 Apr;16(4):682–91. PMID:22350721
2450. Online Mendelian Inheritance in Man. OMIM [Internet]. Baltimore (MD): Johns Hopkins University; 2016. MIM Number: 175100. Available from: https://omim.org/entry/175100.
2451. Onnis A, De Falco G, Antonicelli G, et al. Alteration of microRNAs regulated by c-Myc in Burkitt lymphoma. PLoS One. 2010 Sep 24;5(9):e12960. PMID:20930934
2452. Ono H, Yao K, Fujishiro M, et al. Guidelines for endoscopic submucosal dissection and endoscopic mucosal resection for early gastric cancer. Dig Endosc. 2016 Jan;28(1):3–15. PMID:26234303
2453. Oohashi Y, Watanabe H, Ajioka Y, et al. p53 immunostaining distinguishes malignant from benign lesions of the gall-bladder. Pathol Int. 1995 Jan;45(1):58–65. PMID:7704245
2454. Ooi A, Nakanishi I, Itoh T, et al. Predominant Paneth cell differentiation in an intestinal type gastric cancer. Pathol Res Pract. 1991 Mar;187(2-3):220–5. PMID:2068003
2455. Ooi A, Ota M, Katsuda S, et al. An unusual case of multiple gastric carcinoids associated with diffuse endocrine cell hyperplasia and parietal cell hypertrophy. Endocr Pathol. 1995 Autumn;6(3):229–37. PMID:12114744
2456. Oono Y, Fu K, Nagahisa E, et al. Primary gastric squamous cell carcinoma in situ originating from gastric squamous metaplasia. Endoscopy. 2010;42 Suppl 2:E290–1. PMID:21113875
2459. Orloff MS, Eng C. Genetic and phenotypic heterogeneity in the PTEN hamartoma tumour syndrome. Oncogene. 2008 Sep 18;27(41):5387–97. PMID:18794875
2460. Orosey M, Amin M, Cappell MSA. A 14-year study of 398 esophageal adenocarcinomas diagnosed among 156,256 EGDs performed at two large hospitals: an inlet patch is proposed as a significant risk factor for proximal esophageal adenocarcinoma. Dig Dis Sci. 2018 Feb;63(2):452–65. PMID:29249048
2461. Osborn NK, Keate RF, Trastek VF, et al. Verrucous carcinoma of the esophagus: clinicopathophysiologic features and treatment of a rare entity. Dig Dis Sci. 2003 Mar;48(3):465–74. PMID:12757157
2462. Osborne BM, Butler JJ, Guarda LA. Primary lymphoma of the liver. Ten cases and a review of the literature. Cancer. 1985 Dec 15;56(12):2902–10. PMID:3840404
2463. Osmond A, Li-Chang H, Kirsch R, et al. Interobserver variability in assessing dysplasia and architecture in colorectal adenomas: a multicentre Canadian study. J Clin Pathol. 2014 Sep;67(9):781–6. PMID:25004943
2464. Ota H, Yamaguchi D, Iwaya M, et al. Principal cells in gastric neoplasia of fundic gland (chief cell predominant) type show characteristics of immature chief cells. Pathol Int. 2015 Apr;65(4):202–4. PMID:25597649
2465. Ott PA, Piha-Paul SA, Munster P, et al. Safety and antitumor activity of the anti-PD-1 antibody pembrolizumab in patients with recurrent carcinoma of the anal canal. Ann Oncol. 2017 May 1;28(5):1036–41. PMID:28453692
2466. Otter R, Gerrits WB, vd Sandt MM, et al. Primary extranodal and nodal non-Hodgkin's lymphoma. A survey of a population-based registry. Eur J Cancer Clin Oncol. 1989 Aug;25(8):1203–10. PMID:2767109
2467. Otter R, Willemze R. Extranodal non-Hodgkin's lymphoma. Neth J Med. 1988 Aug;33(1-2):49–51. PMID:3247010
2468. Ouansafi I, He B, Fraser C, et al. Transformation of follicular lymphoma to plasmablastic lymphoma with c-myc gene rearrangement. Am J Clin Pathol. 2010 Dec;134(6):972–81. PMID:21088162
2469. Oue N, Naito Y, Hayashi T, et al. Signal peptidase complex 18, encoded by SEC11A, contributes to progression via TGF-α secretion in gastric cancer. Oncogene. 2014 Jul 24;33(30):3918–26. PMID:23995782
2470. Overman MJ, Fournier K, Hu CY, et al. Improving the AJCC/TNM staging for adenocarcinomas of the appendix: the prognostic impact of histological grade. Ann Surg. 2013 Jun;257(6):1072–8. PMID:23001080
2471. Overman MJ, Hu CY, Kopetz S, et al. A population-based comparison of adenocarcinoma of the large and small intestine: insights into a rare disease. Ann Surg Oncol. 2012 May;19(5):1439–45. PMID:22187121
2472. Overman MJ, Hu CY, Wolff RA, et al. Prognostic value of lymph node evaluation in small bowel adenocarcinoma: analysis of the Surveillance, Epidemiology, and End Results database. Cancer. 2010 Dec 1;116(23):5374–82. PMID:20715162
2473. Overman MJ, Kunitake H. UpToDate [Internet]. Waltham (MA): UpToDate Inc.; 2018. Epidemiology, clinical features, and types of small bowel neoplasms; updated 2018 May 4 [cited 2018 Jan 4]. Available from: https://www.uptodate.com/contents/epidemiology-clinical-features-and-types-of-small-bowel-neoplasms.
2474. Overman MJ, Pozadzides J, Kopetz S, et al. Immunophenotype and molecular characterisation of adenocarcinoma of the small intestine. Br J Cancer. 2010 Jan 5;102(1):144–50. PMID:19935793
2475. Overman MJ, Soifer HS, Schueneman AJ, et al. Performance and prognostic utility of the 92-gene assay in the molecular subclassification of ampullary adenocarcinoma. BMC Cancer. 2016 Aug 22;16:668. PMID:27549176
2476. Owosho AA, Chen S, Kashikar S, et al. Clinical and molecular heterogeneity of head and neck spindle cell and sclerosing rhabdomyosarcoma. Oral Oncol. 2016 Jul;58:e6–11. PMID:27261172
2477. Oyama T, Inoue H, Arima M, et al. Prediction of the invasion depth of superficial squamous cell carcinoma based on microvessel morphology: magnifying endoscopic classification of the Japan Esophageal Society. Esophagus. 2017;14(2):105–12. PMID:28386209
2478. Ozaki H, Hiraoka T, Mizumoto R, et al. The prognostic significance of lymph node metastasis and intrapancreatic perineural invasion in pancreatic cancer after curative resection. Surg Today. 1999;29(1):16–22. PMID:9934826
2479. Ozaki Y, Miura Y, Koganemaru S, et al. Ewing sarcoma of the liver with multilocular cystic mass formation: a case report. BMC Cancer. 2015 Jan 22;15:16. PMID:25608963
2480. Ozawa K, Kinoshita M, Kagata Y, et al. A case of double carcinoid tumors of the gallbladder. Dig Dis Sci. 2003 Sep;48(9):1760–1. PMID:14560997
2481. Ozçelik H, Schmocker B, Di Nicola N, et al. Germline BRCA2 6174delT mutations in Ashkenazi Jewish pancreatic cancer patients. Nat Genet. 1997 May;16(1):17–8. PMID:9140390
2482. Paal E, Thompson LD, Frommelt RA, et al. A clinicopathologic and immunohistochemical study of 35 anaplastic carcinomas of the pancreas with a review of the literature. Ann Diagn Pathol. 2001 Jun;5(3):129–40. PMID:11436166
2483. Padmanabhan N, Ushijima T, Tan P. How to stomach an epigenetic insult: the gastric cancer epigenome. Nat Rev Gastroenterol Hepatol. 2017 Aug;14(8):467–78. PMID:28513632
2484. Pagès F, Mlecnik B, Marliot F, et al. International validation of the consensus Immunoscore for the classification of colon cancer: a prognostic and accuracy study. Lancet. 2018 May 26;391(10135):2128–39. PMID:29754777
2485. Pahlman L, Bujko K, Rutkowski A, et al. Altering the therapeutic paradigm towards a distal bowel margin of < 1 cm in patients with low-lying rectal cancer: a systematic review and commentary. Colorectal Dis. 2013 Apr;15(4):e166–74. PMID:23331717
2486. Pai RK, Beck AH, Norton JA, et al. Appendiceal mucinous neoplasms: clinicopathologic study of 116 cases with analysis of factors predicting recurrence. Am J Surg Pathol. 2009 Oct;33(10):1425–39. PMID:19641451
2487. Pai RK, Hart J, Noffsinger AE. Sessile serrated adenomas strongly predispose to synchronous serrated polyps in non-syndromic patients. Histopathology. 2010 Apr;56(5):581–8. PMID:20459568
2488. Pai RK, Hartman DJ, Gonzalo DH, et al. Serrated lesions of the appendix frequently harbor KRAS mutations and not BRAF mutations indicating a distinctly different serrated neoplastic pathway in the appendix. Hum Pathol. 2014 Feb;45(2):227–35. PMID:24439221
2489. Pai RK, Mojtahed A, Rouse RV, et al. Histologic and molecular analyses of colonic perineurial-like proliferations in serrated polyps: perineurial-like stromal proliferations are seen in sessile serrated adenomas. Am J Surg Pathol. 2011 Sep;35(9):1373–80. PMID:21836484
2490. Pai RK, Mojtahed K, Pai RK. Mutations in the RAS/RAF/MAP kinase pathway commonly occur in gallbladder adenomas but are uncommon in gallbladder adenocarcinomas. Appl Immunohistochem Mol Morphol. 2011 Mar;19(2):133–40. PMID:21307665
2491. Palazzo JP, Edmonston TB, Chaille-Arnold LM, et al. Invasive papillary adenocarcinoma of the colon. Hum Pathol. 2002 Mar;33(3):372–5. PMID:11979380
2492. Palefsky JM, Holly EA, Hogeboom CJ, et al. Anal cytology as a screening tool for anal squamous intraepithelial lesions. J Acquir Immune Defic Syndr Hum Retrovirol. 1997 Apr 15;14(5):415–22. PMID:9170415
2493. Palles C, Cazier JB, Howarth KM, et

al. Germline mutations affecting the proofreading domains of POLE and POLD1 predispose to colorectal adenomas and carcinomas. Nat Genet. 2013 Feb;45(2):136–44. PMID:23263490
2494. Pan CC, Chung MY, Ng KF, et al. Constant allelic alteration on chromosome 16p (TSC2 gene) in perivascular epithelioid cell tumour (PEComa): genetic evidence for the relationship of PEComa with angiomyolipoma. J Pathol. 2008 Feb;214(3):387–93. PMID:18085521
2495. Pan ST, Cheng CY, Lee NS, et al. Follicular dendritic cell sarcoma of the inflammatory pseudotumor-like variant presenting as a colonic polyp. Korean J Pathol. 2014 Apr;48(2):140–5. PMID:24868227
2496. Pan SY, Morrison H. Epidemiology of cancer of the small intestine. World J Gastrointest Oncol. 2011 Mar 15;3(3):33–42. PMID:21461167
2497. Pan Z, Xie Q, Repertinger S, et al. Plasmablastic transformation of low-grade CD5+ B-cell lymphoproliferative disorder with MYC gene rearrangements. Hum Pathol. 2013 Oct;44(10):2139–48. PMID:23791008
2498. Pandalai PK, Lauwers GY, Chung DC, et al. Prophylactic total gastrectomy for individuals with germline CDH1 mutation. Surgery. 2011 Mar;149(3):347–55. PMID:20719348
2499. Pande M, Lynch PM, Hopper JL, et al. Smoking and colorectal cancer in Lynch syndrome: results from the Colon Cancer Family Registry and the University of Texas M.D. Anderson Cancer Center. Clin Cancer Res. 2010 Feb 15;16(4):1331–9. PMID:20145170
2500. Pandilla R, Kotapalli V, Gowrishankar S, et al. Distinct genetic aberrations in oesophageal adeno and squamous carcinoma. Eur J Clin Invest. 2013 Dec;43(12):1233–9. PMID:24102414
2501. Paner GP, Thompson KS, Reyes CV. Hepatoid carcinoma of the pancreas. Cancer. 2000 Apr 1;88(7):1582–9. PMID:10738216
2502. Pantham G, Ganesan S, Einstadter D, et al. Assessment of the incidence of squamous cell papilloma of the esophagus and the presence of high-risk human papilloma virus. Dis Esophagus. 2017 Jan 1;30(1):1–5. PMID:27001250
2503. Papadaki L, Wotherspoon AC, Isaacson PG. The lymphoepithelial lesion of gastric low-grade B-cell lymphoma of mucosa-associated lymphoid tissue (MALT): an ultrastructural study. Histopathology. 1992 Nov;21(5):415–21. PMID:1452124
2504. Pape UF, Perren A, Niederle B, et al. ENETS Consensus Guidelines for the management of patients with neuroendocrine neoplasms from the jejuno-ileum and the appendix including goblet cell carcinomas. Neuroendocrinology. 2012;95(2):135–56. PMID:22262080
2505. Papotti M, Bongiovanni M, Volante M, et al. Expression of somatostatin receptor types 1-5 in 81 cases of gastrointestinal and pancreatic endocrine tumors. A correlative immunohistochemical and reverse-transcriptase polymerase chain reaction analysis. Virchows Arch. 2002 May;440(5):461–75. PMID:12021920
2506. Papotti M, Cassoni P, Sapino A, et al. Large cell neuroendocrine carcinoma of the gallbladder: report of two cases. Am J Surg Pathol. 2000 Oct;24(10):1424–8. PMID:11023106
2507. Papotti M, Cassoni P, Taraglio S, et al. Oncocytic and oncocytoid tumors of the exocrine pancreas, liver, and gastrointestinal tract. Semin Diagn Pathol. 1999 May;16(2):126–34. PMID:10452578
2508. Papotti M, Cassoni P, Volante M, et al. Ghrelin-producing endocrine tumors of the stomach and intestine. J Clin Endocrinol Metab. 2001 Oct;86(10):5052–9. PMID:11600584
2509. Paradis V, Benzekri A, Dargère D, et al. Telangiectatic focal nodular hyperplasia: a variant of hepatocellular adenoma. Gastroenterology. 2004 May;126(5):1323–9. PMID:15131793
2510. Paradis V, Bièche I, Dargère D, et al. A quantitative gene expression study suggests a role for angiopoietins in focal nodular hyperplasia. Gastroenterology. 2003 Mar;124(3):651–9. PMID:12612904
2511. Paradis V, Champault A, Ronot M, et al. Telangiectatic adenoma: an entity associated with increased body mass index and inflammation. Hepatology. 2007 Jul;46(1):140–6. PMID:17596890
2512. Paradis V, Laurent A, Flejou JF, et al. Evidence for the polyclonal nature of focal nodular hyperplasia of the liver by the study of X-chromosome inactivation. Hepatology. 1997 Oct;26(4):891–5. PMID:9328310
2513. Paradis V, Zalinski S, Chelbi E, et al. Hepatocellular carcinomas in patients with metabolic syndrome often develop without significant liver fibrosis: a pathological analysis. Hepatology. 2009 Mar;49(3):851–9. PMID:19115377
2513A. Pareja F, Brandes AH, Basili T, et al. Loss-of-function mutations in ATP6AP1 and ATP6AP2 in granular cell tumors. Nat Commun. 2018 Aug 30;9(1):3533. PMID:30166553
2514. Parente F, Cernuschi M, Orlando G, et al. Kaposi's sarcoma and AIDS: frequency of gastrointestinal involvement and its effect on survival. A prospective study in a heterogeneous population. Scand J Gastroenterol. 1991 Oct;26(10):1007–12. PMID:1947766
2515. Parfitt JR, McLean CA, Joseph MG, et al. Granular cell tumours of the gastrointestinal tract: expression of nestin and clinicopathological evaluation of 11 patients. Histopathology. 2006 Mar;48(4):424–30. PMID:16487364
2516. Parfitt JR, Rodriguez-Justo M, Feakins R, et al. Gastrointestinal Kaposi's sarcoma: CD117 expression and the potential for misdiagnosis as gastrointestinal stromal tumour. Histopathology. 2008 Jun;52(7):816–23. PMID:18494611
2517. Parfitt JR, Shepherd NA. Polypoid mucosal prolapse complicating low rectal adenomas: beware the inflammatory cloacogenic polyp! Histopathology. 2008 Jul;53(1):91–6. PMID:18484980
2518. Parham DM, Barr FG. Classification of rhabdomyosarcoma and its molecular basis. Adv Anat Pathol. 2013 Nov;20(6):387–97. PMID:24113309
2519. Parham DM, Fisher C. Angiosarcomas of the breast developing post radiotherapy. Histopathology. 1997 Aug;31(2):189–95. PMID:9279573
2520. Parikh U, Marcus C, Sarangi R, et al. FDG PET/CT in pancreatic and hepatobiliary carcinomas: value to patient management and patient outcomes. PET Clin. 2015 Jul;10(3):327–43. PMID:26099670
2521. Park C, Ha SY, Kim ST, et al. Identification of the BRAF V600E mutation in gastroenteropancreatic neuroendocrine tumors. Oncotarget. 2016 Jan 26;7(4):4024–35. PMID:26684240
2522. Park DY, Srivastava A, Kim GH, et al. Adenomatous and foveolar gastric dysplasia: distinct patterns of mucin expression and background intestinal metaplasia. Am J Surg Pathol. 2008 Apr;32(4):524–33. PMID:18300795
2523. Park DY, Srivastava A, Kim GH, et al. CDX2 expression in the intestinal-type gastric epithelial neoplasia: frequency and significance. Mod Pathol. 2010 Jan;23(1):54–61. PMID:19820687
2524. Park HJ, Kim SY, Kim HJ, et al. Intraductal papillary neoplasm of the bile duct: clinical, imaging, and pathologic features. AJR Am J Roentgenol. 2018 Jul;211(1):67–75. PMID:29629808
2525. Park IU, Introcaso C, Dunne EF. Human papillomavirus and genital warts: a review of the evidence for the 2015 Centers for Disease Control and Prevention sexually transmitted diseases treatment guidelines. Clin Infect Dis. 2015 Dec 15;61 Suppl 8:S849–55. PMID:26602622
2526. Park JG, Park KJ, Ahn YO, et al. Risk of gastric cancer among Korean familial adenomatous polyposis patients. Report of three cases. Dis Colon Rectum. 1992 Oct;35(10):996–8. PMID:1327683
2527. Park JK, Paik WH, Lee K, et al. DAXX/ATRX and MEN1 genes are strong prognostic markers in pancreatic neuroendocrine tumors. Oncotarget. 2017 Jul 25;8(30):49796–806. PMID:28591701
2528. Park JY, Cornish TC, Lam-Himlin D, et al. Gastric lesions in patients with autoimmune metaplastic atrophic gastritis (AMAG) in a tertiary care setting. Am J Surg Pathol. 2010 Nov;34(11):1591–8. PMID:20975338
2529. Park S, Ko YH. Peripheral T cell lymphoma in Asia. Int J Hematol. 2014 Mar;99(3):227–39. PMID:24481942
2530. Park SK, Andreotti G, Rashid A, et al. Polymorphisms of estrogen receptors and risk of biliary tract cancers and gallstones: a population-based study in Shanghai, China. Carcinogenesis. 2010 May;31(5):842–6. PMID:20172949
2531. Park SK, Andreotti G, Sakoda LC, et al. Variants in hormone-related genes and the risk of biliary tract cancers and stones: a population-based study in China. Carcinogenesis. 2009 Apr;30(4):606–14. PMID:19168589
2532. Park SY, Rhee Y, Youn JC, et al. Ectopic Cushing's syndrome due to concurrent corticotropin-releasing hormone (CRH) and adrenocorticotropic hormone (ACTH) secreted by malignant gastrinoma. Exp Clin Endocrinol Diabetes. 2007 Jan;115(1):13–6. PMID:17286228
2533. Park YN, Kojiro M, Di Tommaso L, et al. Ductular reaction is helpful in defining early stromal invasion, small hepatocellular carcinomas, and dysplastic nodules. Cancer. 2007 Mar 1;109(5):915–23. PMID:17279586
2534. Park YN, Roncalli M. Large liver cell dysplasia: a controversial entity. J Hepatol. 2006 Nov;45(5):734–43. PMID:16982109
2535. Park YN, Yang CP, Fernandez GJ, et al. Neoangiogenesis and sinusoidal "capillarization" in dysplastic nodules of the liver. Am J Surg Pathol. 1998 Jun;22(6):656–62. PMID:9630172
2536. Parry S, Burt RW, Win AK, et al. Reducing the polyp burden in serrated polyposis by serial colonoscopy: the impact of nationally coordinated community surveillance. N Z Med J. 2017 Mar 3;130(1451):57–67. PMID:28253245
2537. Parwani AV, Geradts J, Caspers E, et al. Immunohistochemical and genetic analysis of non-small cell and small cell gallbladder carcinoma and their precursor lesions. Mod Pathol. 2003 Apr;16(4):299–308. PMID:12692194
2538. Pasini B, McWhinney SR, Bei T, et al. Clinical and molecular genetics of patients with the Carney-Stratakis syndrome and germline mutations of the genes coding for the succinate dehydrogenase subunits SDHB, SDHC, and SDHD. Eur J Hum Genet. 2008 Jan;16(1):79–88. PMID:17667967
2539. Pasini FS, Zilberstein B, Snitcovsky I, et al. A gene expression profile related to immune dampening in the tumor microenvironment is associated with poor prognosis in gastric adenocarcinoma. J Gastroenterol. 2014 Nov;49(11):1453–66. PMID:24217965
2540. Pasman EA, Heifert TA, Nylund CM. Esophageal squamous papillomas with focal dermal hypoplasia and eosinophilic esophagitis. World J Gastroenterol. 2017 Mar 28;23(12):2246–50. PMID:28405153
2541. Pasqualucci L, Dalla-Favera R. Genetics of diffuse large B-cell lymphoma. Blood. 2018 May 24;131(21):2307–19. PMID:29666115
2542. Passmore SJ, Berry PJ, Oakhill A. Recurrent pancreatoblastoma with inappropriate adrenocorticotrophic hormone secretion. Arch Dis Child. 1988 Dec;63(12):1494–6. PMID:2852926
2543. Pasternak S, Carter MD, Ly TY, et al. Immunohistochemical profiles of different subsets of Merkel cell carcinoma. Hum Pathol. 2018 Dec;82:232–8. PMID:30067951
2544. Patel HS, Silver AR, Levine T, et al. Human papillomavirus infection and anal dysplasia in renal transplant recipients. Br J Surg. 2010 Nov;97(11):1716–21. PMID:20730855
2545. Patel NR, Salim AA, Sayeed H, et al. Molecular characterization of epithelioid haemangioendotheliomas identifies novel WWTR1-CAMTA1 fusion variants. Histopathology. 2015 Nov;67(5):699–708. PMID:25817592
2546. Patel P, De P. Trends in colorectal cancer incidence and related lifestyle risk factors in 15-49-year-olds in Canada, 1969-2010. Cancer Epidemiol. 2016 Jun;42:90–100. PMID:27060626
2547. Patel R, Varadarajulu S, Wilcox CM. Endoscopic ampullectomy: techniques and outcomes. J Clin Gastroenterol. 2012 Jan;46(1):8–15. PMID:22064552
2548. Patel RM, Goldblum JR, Hsi ED. Immunohistochemical detection of human herpes virus-8 latent nuclear antigen-1 is useful in the diagnosis of Kaposi sarcoma. Mod Pathol. 2004 Apr;17(4):456–60. PMID:14990970
2549. Patel S, Roa JC, Tapia O, et al. Hyalinizing cholecystitis and associated carcinomas: clinicopathologic analysis of a distinctive variant of cholecystitis with porcelain-like features and accompanying diagnostically challenging carcinomas. Am J Surg Pathol. 2011 Aug;35(8):1104–13. PMID:21716080
2550. Patel SG, Prasad ML, Escrig M, et al. Primary mucosal malignant melanoma of the head and neck. Head Neck. 2002 Mar;24(3):247–57. PMID:11891956
2551. Paterson C, Musselman L, Chorneyko K, et al. Merkel cell (neuroendocrine) carcinoma of the anal canal: report of a case. Dis Colon Rectum. 2003 May;46(5):676–8. PMID:12792446
2552. Patil DT, Goldblum JR, Billings SD. Clinicopathological analysis of basal cell carcinoma of the anal region and its distinction from basaloid squamous cell carcinoma. Mod Pathol. 2013 Oct;26(10):1382–9. PMID:23599161
2553. Pawa N, Clift AK, Osmani H, et al. Surgical management of patients with neuroendocrine neoplasms of the appendix: appendectomy or more. Neuroendocrinology. 2018;106(3):242–51. PMID:28641291
2554. Pawlik TM, Gleisner AL, Cameron JL, et al. Prognostic relevance of lymph node ratio following pancreaticoduodenectomy for pancreatic cancer. Surgery. 2007 May;141(5):610–8. PMID:17462460
2555. Pea A, Hruban RH, Wood LD. Genetics of pancreatic neuroendocrine tumors: implications for the clinic. Expert Rev Gastroenterol Hepatol. 2015;9(11):1407–19. PMID:26413978
2557. Pedrazzani C, Marrelli D, Pacelli F, et al. Gastric linitis plastica: which role for surgical resection? Gastric Cancer. 2012 Jan;15(1):56–60. PMID:21717092
2558. Peifer M, Fernández-Cuesta L, Sos ML, et al. Integrative genome analyses identify key somatic driver mutations of small-cell lung cancer. Nat Genet. 2012 Oct;44(10):1104–10. PMID:22941188
2559. Peifer M, Polakis P. Wnt signaling in oncogenesis and embryogenesis–a look

outside the nucleus. Science. 2000 Mar 3;287(5458):1606–9. PMID:10733430

2560. Pelaez-Luna M, Chari ST, Smyrk TC, et al. Do consensus indications for resection in branch duct intraductal papillary mucinous neoplasm predict malignancy? A study of 147 patients. Am J Gastroenterol. 2007 Aug;102(8):1759–64. PMID:17686073

2562. Pelletier G, Cortot A, Launay JM, et al. Serotonin-secreting and insulin-secreting ileal carcinoid tumor and the use of in vitro culture of tumoral cells. Cancer. 1984 Jul 15;54(2):319–22. PMID:6372987

2563. Pelosi G, Bresaola E, Bogina G, et al. Endocrine tumors of the pancreas: Ki 67 immunoreactivity on paraffin sections is an independent predictor for malignancy: a comparative study with proliferating-cell nuclear antigen and progesterone receptor protein immunostaining, mitotic index, and other clinicopathologic variables. Hum Pathol. 1996 Nov;27(11):1124–34. PMID:8912819

2564. Penel N, Chibon F, Salas S. Adult desmoid tumors: biology, management and ongoing trials. Curr Opin Oncol. 2017 Jul;29(4):268–74. PMID:28489620

2565. Pengelly RJ, Rowaiye B, Pickard K, et al. Analysis of mutation and loss of heterozygosity by whole-exome sequencing yields insights into pseudomyxoma peritonei. J Mol Diagn. 2018 Sep;20(5):635–42. PMID:29936255

2566. Penn I. Kaposi's sarcoma in transplant recipients. Transplantation. 1997 Sep 15;64(5):669–73. PMID:9311700

2567. Pereira P, Aho V, Arola J, et al. Bile microbiota in primary sclerosing cholangitis: impact on disease progression and development of biliary dysplasia. PLoS One. 2017 Aug 10;12(8):e0182924. PMID:28796833

2568. Perez-Montiel MD, Frankel WL, Suster S. Neuroendocrine carcinomas of the pancreas with 'rhabdoid' features. Am J Surg Pathol. 2003 May;27(5):642–9. PMID:12717248

2569. Pernot S, Voron T, Perkins G, et al. Signet-ring cell carcinoma of the stomach: impact on prognosis and specific therapeutic challenge. World J Gastroenterol. 2015 Oct 28;21(40):11428–38. PMID:26523107

2570. Perry AM, Alvarado-Bernal Y, Laurini JA, et al. MYC and BCL2 protein expression predicts survival in patients with diffuse large B-cell lymphoma treated with rituximab. Br J Haematol. 2014 May;165(3):382–91. PMID:24506200

2571. Perry AM, Warnke RA, Hu Q, et al. Indolent T-cell lymphoproliferative disease of the gastrointestinal tract. Blood. 2013 Nov 21;122(22):3599–606. PMID:24009234

2572. Perzin KH, Bridge MF. Adenomas of the small intestine: a clinicopathologic review of 51 cases and a study of their relationship to carcinoma. Cancer. 1981 Aug 1;48(3):799–819. PMID:7248908

2573. Peters AC, Akinwumi MS, Cervera C, et al. The changing epidemiology of posttransplant lymphoproliferative disorder in adult solid organ transplant recipients over 30 years: a single-center experience. Transplantation. 2018 Sep;102(9):1553–62. PMID:29485513

2574. Petersen GM. Familial pancreatic cancer. Semin Oncol. 2016 Oct;43(5):548–53. PMID:27899186

2575. Petrara MR, Giunco S, Serraino D, et al. Post-transplant lymphoproliferative disorders: from epidemiology to pathogenesis-driven treatment. Cancer Lett. 2015 Dec 1;369(1):37–44. PMID:26279520

2576. Petrick JL, Falk RT, Hyland PL, et al. Association between circulating levels of sex steroid hormones and esophageal adenocarcinoma in the FINBAR Study. PLoS One. 2018 Jan 17;13(1):e0190325. PMID:29342161

2577. Petrick JL, Yang B, Altekruse SF, et al.

Risk factors for intrahepatic and extrahepatic cholangiocarcinoma in the United States: a population-based study in SEER-Medicare. PLoS One. 2017 Oct 19;12(10):e0186643. PMID:29049401

2578. Petursson SR. Adenoid cystic carcinoma of the esophagus. Complete response to combination chemotherapy. Cancer. 1986 Apr 15;57(8):1464–7. PMID:3004692

2579. Piccaluga PP, De Falco G, Kustagi M, et al. Gene expression analysis uncovers similarity and differences among Burkitt lymphoma subtypes. Blood. 2011 Mar 31;117(13):3596–608. PMID:21245480

2580. Piccaluga PP, Navari M, De Falco G, et al. Virus-encoded microRNA contributes to the molecular profile of EBV-positive Burkitt lymphomas. Oncotarget. 2016 Jan 5;7(1):224–40. PMID:26325594

2581. Pihlak R, Valle JW, McNamara MG. Germline mutations in pancreatic cancer and potential new therapeutic options. Oncotarget. 2017 Apr 20;8(42):73240–57. PMID:29069866

2582. Pilarski R, Burt R, Kohlman W, et al. Cowden syndrome and the PTEN hamartoma tumor syndrome: systematic review and revised diagnostic criteria. J Natl Cancer Inst. 2013 Nov 6;105(21):1607–16. PMID:24136893

2583. Pilati C, Letouzé E, Nault JC, et al. Genomic profiling of hepatocellular adenomas reveals recurrent FRK-activating mutations and the mechanisms of malignant transformation. Cancer Cell. 2014 Apr 14;25(4):428–41. PMID:24735922

2584. Pileri SA, Grogan TM, Harris NL, et al. Tumours of histiocytes and accessory dendritic cells: an immunohistochemical approach to classification from the International Lymphoma Study Group based on 61 cases. Histopathology. 2002 Jul;41(1):1–29. PMID:12121233

2585. Pillai S, Gopalan V, Lam AK. DNA genome sequencing in esophageal adenocarcinoma. Methods Mol Biol. 2018;1756:231–46. PMID:29600374

2586. Pimentel-Nunes P, Dinis-Ribeiro M, Ponchon T, et al. Endoscopic submucosal dissection: European Society of Gastrointestinal Endoscopy (ESGE) Guideline. Endoscopy. 2015 Sep;47(9):829–54. PMID:26317585

2587. Pinho AC, Melo RB, Oliveira M, et al. Adenoma-carcinoma sequence in intrahepatic cholangiocarcinoma. Int J Surg Case Rep. 2012;3(4):131–3. PMID:22326450

2588. Pink A, Anzengruber F, Navarini AA. Acne and hidradenitis suppurativa. Br J Dermatol. 2018 Mar;178(3):619–31. PMID:29380349

2589. Piro G, Carbone C, Santoro R, et al. Predictive biomarkers for the treatment of resectable esophageal and esophago-gastric junction adenocarcinoma: from hypothesis generation to clinical validation. Expert Rev Mol Diagn. 2018 Apr;18(4):357–70. PMID:29544370

2591. Pitman MB, Centeno BA, Daglilar ES, et al. Cytological criteria of high-grade epithelial atypia in the cyst fluid of pancreatic intraductal papillary mucinous neoplasms. Cancer Cytopathol. 2014 Jan;122(1):40–7. PMID:23939829

2593. Pitman MB, Layfield LJ. The Papanicolaou Society of Cytopathology system for reporting pancreaticobiliary cytology: definitions, criteria and explanatory notes. Cham (Switzerland): Springer International Publishing; 2015.

2594. Pitman MB, Lewandrowski K, Shen J, et al. Pancreatic cysts: preoperative diagnosis and clinical management. Cancer Cytopathol. 2010 Feb 25;118(1):1–13. PMID:20043327

2595. Pitman MB, Michaels PJ, Deshpande V, et al. Cytological and cyst fluid analysis of small (< or =3 cm) branch duct intraductal papillary mucinous neoplasms adds value to patient management decisions. Pancreatology.

2008;8(3):277–84. PMID:18497541

2596. Pittman ME, Rao R, Hruban RH. Classification, morphology, molecular pathogenesis, and outcome of premalignant lesions of the pancreas. Arch Pathol Lab Med. 2017 Dec;141(12):1606–14. PMID:29189063

2597. Pizzi S, Azzoni C, Bassi D, et al. Genetic alterations in poorly differentiated endocrine carcinomas of the gastrointestinal tract. Cancer. 2003 Sep 15;98(6):1273–82. PMID:12973852

2597A. Pizzi S, D'Adda T, Azzoni C, et al. Malignancy-associated allelic losses on the X-chromosome in foregut but not in midgut endocrine tumours. J Pathol. 2002 Apr;196(4):401–7. PMID:11920735

2598. Planck M, Ericson K, Piotrowska Z, et al. Microsatellite instability and expression of MLH1 and MSH2 in carcinomas of the small intestine. Cancer. 2003 Mar 15;97(6):1551–7. PMID:12627520

2599. Plebani M, Basso D, Cassaro M, et al. Helicobacter pylori serology in patients with chronic gastritis. Am J Gastroenterol. 1996 May;91(5):954–8. PMID:8633587

2600. Plentz RR, Park YN, Lechel A, et al. Telomere shortening and inactivation of cell cycle checkpoints characterize human hepatocarcinogenesis. Hepatology. 2007 Apr;45(4):968–76. PMID:17393506

2601. Pohl H, Srivastava A, Bensen SP, et al. Incomplete polyp resection during colonoscopy-results of the complete adenoma resection (CARE) study. Gastroenterology. 2013 Jan;144(1):74–80.e1. PMID:23022496

2602. Polom K, Marano L, Marrelli D, et al. Meta-analysis of microsatellite instability in relation to clinicopathological characteristics and overall survival in gastric cancer. Br J Surg. 2018 Feb;105(3):159–67. PMID:29091259

2603. Polydorides AD, Harpaz N. Serrated lesions in inflammatory bowel disease. Gastrointest Endosc. 2017 Feb;85(2):461. PMID:27424192

2604. Poon KK, Mills S, Booth IW, et al. Inflammatory cloacogenic polyp: an unrecognized cause of hematochezia and tenesmus in childhood. J Pediatr. 1997 Feb;130(2):327–9. PMID:9042143

2605. Portela-Gomes GM, Grimelius L, Stridsberg M. Secretogranin III in human neuroendocrine tumours: a comparative immunohistochemical study with chromogranins A and B and secretogranin II. Regul Pept. 2010 Nov 30;165(1):30–5. PMID:20550951

2606. Poruk KE, Gay DZ, Brown K, et al. The clinical utility of CA 19-9 in pancreatic adenocarcinoma: diagnostic and prognostic updates. Curr Mol Med. 2013 Mar;13(3):340–51. PMID:23331006

2607. Posner S, Colletti L, Knol J, et al. Safety and long-term efficacy of transduodenal excision for tumors of the ampulla of Vater. Surgery. 2000 Oct;128(4):694–701. PMID:11015104

2609. Potter DD, Murray JA, Donohue JH, et al. The role of defective mismatch repair in small bowel adenocarcinoma in celiac disease. Cancer Res. 2004 Oct 1;64(19):7073–7. PMID:15466202

2610. Poulogiannis G, Frayling IM, Arends MJ. DNA mismatch repair deficiency in sporadic colorectal cancer and Lynch syndrome. Histopathology. 2010 Jan;56(2):167–79. PMID:20102395

2611. Poulogiannis G, Ichimura K, Hamoudi RA, et al. Prognostic relevance of DNA copy number changes in colorectal cancer. J Pathol. 2010 Feb;220(3):338–47. PMID:19911421

2612. Poultsides GA, Reddy S, Cameron JL, et al. Histopathologic basis for the favorable survival after resection of intraductal papillary mucinous neoplasm-associated invasive adenocarcinoma of the pancreas. Ann Surg. 2010

Mar;251(3):470–6. PMID:20142731

2613. Prasad ML, Busam KJ, Patel SG, et al. Clinicopathologic differences in malignant melanoma arising in oral squamous and sinonasal respiratory mucosa of the upper aerodigestive tract. Arch Pathol Lab Med. 2003 Aug;127(8):997–1002. PMID:12873174

2614. Prenen H, De Schutter J, Jacobs B, et al. PIK3CA mutations are not a major determinant of resistance to the epidermal growth factor receptor inhibitor cetuximab in metastatic colorectal cancer. Clin Cancer Res. 2009 May 1;15(9):3184–8. PMID:19366826

2615. Prezzi D, Mandegaran R, Gourtsoyianni S, et al. The impact of MRI sequence on tumour staging and gross tumour volume delineation in squamous cell carcinoma of the anal canal. Eur Radiol. 2018 Apr;28(4):1512–9. PMID:29134349

2616. Price TN, Thompson GB, Lewis JT, et al. Zollinger-Ellison syndrome due to primary gastrinoma of the extrahepatic biliary tree: three case reports and review of literature. Endocr Pract. 2009 Nov-Dec;15(7):737–49. PMID:19491075

2617. Puente XS, Jares P, Campo E. Chronic lymphocytic leukemia and mantle cell lymphoma: crossroads of genetic and microenvironment interactions. Blood. 2018 May 24;131(21):2283–96. PMID:29666114

2618. Puglisi F, Damante G, Pizzolitto S, et al. Combined yolk sac tumor and adenocarcinoma in a gastric stump: molecular evidence of clonality. Cancer. 1999 May 1;85(9):1910–6. PMID:10223229

2619. Pujals A, Amaddeo G, Castain C, et al. BRAF V600E mutations in bile duct adenomas. Hepatology. 2015 Jan;61(1):403–5. PMID:24634053

2620. Pujals A, Bioulac-Sage P, Castain C, et al. BRAF V600E mutational status in bile duct adenomas and hamartomas. Histopathology. 2015 Oct;67(4):562–7. PMID:25704541

2621. Pulitzer DR, Martin PC, Reed RJ. Epithelioid glomus tumor. Hum Pathol. 1995 Sep;26(9):1022–7. PMID:7672784

2622. Pyo JS, Sohn JH, Kang G. Medullary carcinoma in the colorectum: a systematic review and meta-analysis. Hum Pathol. 2016 Jul;53:91–6. PMID:27001432

2623. Périgny M, Hammel P, Corcos O, et al. Pancreatic endocrine microadenomatosis in patients with von Hippel-Lindau disease: characterization by VHL/HIF pathway proteins expression. Am J Surg Pathol. 2009 May;33(5):739–48. PMID:19238077

2624. Qazi TM, O'Brien MJ, Farraye FA, et al. Epidemiology of goblet cell and microvesicular hyperplastic polyps. Am J Gastroenterol. 2014 Dec;109(12):1922–32. PMID:25350766

2625. Qizilbash AH. Mucoceles of the appendix. Their relationship to hyperplastic polyps, mucinous cystadenomas, and cystadenocarcinomas. Arch Pathol. 1975 Oct;99(10):548–55. PMID:1191124

2626. Quante M, Graham TA, Jansen M. Insights into the pathophysiology of esophageal adenocarcinoma. Gastroenterology. 2018 Jan;154(2):406–20. PMID:29037468

2627. Quartey B. Primary hepatic neuroendocrine tumor: what do we know now? World J Oncol. 2011 Oct;2(5):209–16. PMID:29147250

2628. Quigley B, Reid MD, Pehlivanoglu B, et al. Hepatobiliary mucinous cystic neoplasms with ovarian type stroma (so-called "hepatobiliary cystadenoma/cystadenocarcinoma"): clinicopathologic analysis of 36 cases illustrates rarity of carcinomatous change. Am J Surg Pathol. 2018 Jan;42(1):95–102. PMID:29016404

2629. Quinn AM, Farraye FA, Naini BV, et al. Polypectomy is adequate treatment for adenoma-like dysplastic lesions (DALMs) in

Crohn's disease. Inflamm Bowel Dis. 2013 May;19(6):1186–93. PMID:23567776

2630. Quintana I, Mejías-Luque R, Terradas M, et al. Evidence suggests that germline RNF43 mutations are a rare cause of serrated polyposis. Gut. 2018 Dec;67(12):2230–2. PMID:29330307

2631. Qunaj L, Castillo JJ, Olszewski AJ. Survival of patients with CD20-negative variants of large B-cell lymphoma: an analysis of the National Cancer Data Base. Leuk Lymphoma. 2018 Jun;59(6):1375–83. PMID:29019447

2632. Qureshi SS, Bhagat M, Kurkure PA, et al. Ectopic Cushing syndrome secondary to recurrent pancreatoblastoma in a child: lessons learnt. J Cancer Res Ther. 2015 Oct-Dec;11(4):1027. PMID:26881602

2633. Radaszkiewicz T, Dragosics B, Bauer P. Gastrointestinal malignant lymphomas of the mucosa-associated lymphoid tissue: factors relevant to prognosis. Gastroenterology. 1992 May;102(5):1628–38. PMID:1568573

2634. Raddatz D, Horstmann O, Basenau D, et al. Cushing's syndrome due to ectopic adreno-corticotropic hormone production by a non-metastatic gastrinoma after long-term conservative treatment of Zollinger-Ellison syndrome. Ital J Gastroenterol Hepatol. 1998 Dec;30(6):636–40. PMID:10076790

2635. Raderer M, Streubel B, Woehrer S, et al. High relapse rate in patients with MALT lymphoma warrants lifelong follow-up. Clin Cancer Res. 2005 May 1;11(9):3349–52. PMID:15867234

2636. Radojkovic M, Ilic D, Ilic I. Primary signet ring cell carcinoma of the pancreas with a good response to chemotherapy: case report and literature review. Tumori. 2017 Nov 15;103(Suppl 1):e50–2. PMID:28708232

2637. Radomski M, Pai RK, Shuai Y, et al. Curative surgical resection as a component of multimodality therapy for peritoneal metastases from goblet cell carcinoids. Ann Surg Oncol. 2016 Dec;23(13):4338–43. PMID:27401448

2638. Radu OM, Nikiforova MN, Farkas LM, et al. Challenging cases encountered in colorectal cancer screening for Lynch syndrome reveal novel findings: nucleolar MSH6 staining and impact of prior chemoradiation therapy. Hum Pathol. 2011 Sep;42(9):1247–58. PMID:21334712

2639. Radyk MD, Burclaff J, Willet SG, et al. Metaplastic cells in the stomach arise, independently of stem cells, via dedifferentiation or transdifferentiation of chief cells. Gastroenterology. 2018 Mar;154(4):839–43.e2. PMID:29248442

2640. Rahemtullah A, Misdraji J, Pitman MB. Adenosquamous carcinoma of the pancreas: cytologic features in 14 cases. Cancer. 2003 Dec 25;99(6):372–8. PMID:14681946

2641. Rahib L, Smith BD, Aizenberg R, et al. Projecting cancer incidence and deaths to 2030: the unexpected burden of thyroid, liver, and pancreas cancers in the United States. Cancer Res. 2014 Jun 1;74(11):2913–21. PMID:24840647

2642. Rahmat K, Vijayananthan A, Abdullah B, et al. Benign teratoma of the liver: a rare cause of cholangitis. Biomed Imaging Interv J. 2006 Jul;2(3):e20. PMID:21614237

2643. Raimondi S, Bruno S, Mondelli MU, et al. Hepatitis C virus genotype 1b as a risk factor for hepatocellular carcinoma development: a meta-analysis. J Hepatol. 2009 Jun;50(6):1142–54. PMID:19395111

2644. Raimondi S, Lowenfels AB, Morselli-Labate AM, et al. Pancreatic cancer in chronic pancreatitis; aetiology, incidence, and early detection. Best Pract Res Clin Gastroenterol. 2010 Jun;24(3):349–58. PMID:20510834

2645. Rainey JJ, Omenah D, Sumba PO, et al. Spatial clustering of endemic Burkitt's lymphoma in high-risk regions of Kenya. Int J Cancer. 2007 Jan 1;120(1):121–7. PMID:17019706

2646. Rajaram V, Knezevich S, Bove KE, et al. DNA sequence of the translocation break-points in undifferentiated embryonal sarcoma arising in mesenchymal hamartoma of the liver harboring the t(11;19)(q11;q13.4) translocation. Genes Chromosomes Cancer. 2007 May;46(5):508–13. PMID:17311249

2647. Rajpal S, Warren RS, Alexander M, et al. Pancreatoblastoma in an adult: case report and review of the literature. J Gastrointest Surg. 2006 Jun;10(6):829–36. PMID:16769539

2648. Ramalingam P, Hart WR, Goldblum JR. Cytokeratin subset immunostaining in rectal adenocarcinoma and normal anal glands. Arch Pathol Lab Med. 2001 Aug;125(8):1074–7. PMID:11473461

2649. Ramanujam TM, Ramesh JC, Goh DW, et al. Malignant transformation of mesenchymal hamartoma of the liver: case report and review of the literature. J Pediatr Surg. 1999 Nov;34(11):1684–6. PMID:10591570

2650. Ramezani M, Sadeghi M. Carcinoid tumour of the oesophagus: a systematic review. Prz Gastroenterol. 2018;13(3):196–9. PMID:30302162

2651. Ramnani DM, Wistuba II, Behrens C, et al. K-ras and p53 mutations in the pathogenesis of classical and goblet cell carcinoids of the appendix. Cancer. 1999 Jul 1;86(1):14–21. PMID:10391558

2652. Rampado S, Ruol A, Guido M, et al. Mediastinal carcinosis involving the esophagus in breast cancer: the "breast-esophagus" syndrome: report on 25 cases and guidelines for diagnosis and treatment. Ann Surg. 2007 Aug;246(2):316–22. PMID:17667512

2652A. Raney RB, Maurer HM, Anderson JR, et al. The Intergroup Rhabdomyosarcoma Study Group (IRSG): major lessons from the IRS-I through IRS-IV studies as background for the current IRS-V treatment protocols. Sarcoma. 2001;5(1):9–15. PMID:18521303

2653. Ranheim EA, Jones C, Zehnder JL, et al. Spontaneously relapsing clonal, mucosal cytotoxic T-cell lymphoproliferative disorder: case report and review of the literature. Am J Surg Pathol. 2000 Feb;24(2):296–301. PMID:10680899

2654. Rantshabeng PS, Moyo S, Moraka NO, et al. Prevalence of oncogenic human papillomavirus genotypes in patients diagnosed with anogenital malignancies in Botswana. BMC Infect Dis. 2017 Nov 25;17(1):731. PMID:29178840

2655. Raphael M, Gentilhomme O, Tulliez M, et al. Histopathologic features of high-grade non-Hodgkin's lymphomas in acquired immunodeficiency syndrome. Arch Pathol Lab Med. 1991 Jan;115(1):15–20. PMID:1987908

2656. Rascarachi G, Sierra M, Hernando M, et al. Primary liver carcinoid tumour with a Zollinger Ellison syndrome - an unusual diagnosis: a case report. Cases J. 2009 Aug 7;2:6346. PMID:19918579

2657. Rashid A, Gao YT, Bhakta S, et al. Beta-catenin mutations in biliary tract cancers: a population-based study in China. Cancer Res. 2001 Apr 15;61(8):3406–9. PMID:11309300

2658. Rault-Petit B, Do Cao C, Guyétant S, et al. Current management and predictive factors of lymph node metastasis of appendix neuroendocrine tumors: a national study from the French Group of Endocrine Tumors (GTE). Ann Surg. 2018 Mar 19. PMID:29557879

2659. Raut CP, Miceli R, Strauss DC, et al. External validation of a multi-institutional retroperitoneal sarcoma nomogram. Cancer. 2016 May 1;122(9):1417–24. PMID:26916507

2660. Ray S, Saluja SS, Gupta R, et al. Esophageal leiomyomatosis – an unusual cause of pseudoachalasia. Can J Gastroenterol. 2008 Feb;22(2):187–9. PMID:18299739

2661. Rayner E, van Gool IC, Palles C, et al. A panoply of errors: polymerase proofreading domain mutations in cancer. Nat Rev Cancer. 2016 Feb;16(2):71–81. PMID:26822575

2662. Raza MA, Mazzara PF. Sarcomatoid carcinoma of esophagus. Arch Pathol Lab Med. 2011 Jul;135(7):945–8. PMID:21732788

2663. Ready E, Chernushkin K, Partovi N, et al. Posttransplant lymphoproliferative disorder in adults receiving kidney transplantation in British Columbia: a retrospective cohort analysis. Can J Kidney Health Dis. 2018 Apr 1;5:2054358118760831. PMID:29636980

2664. Real FXA. A "catastrophic hypothesis" for pancreas cancer progression. Gastroenterology. 2003 Jun;124(7):1958–64. PMID:12806629

2665. Rebouissou S, Amessou M, Couchy G, et al. Frequent in-frame somatic deletions activate gp130 in inflammatory hepatocellular tumours. Nature. 2009 Jan 8;457(7226):200–4. PMID:19020503

2666. Rebouissou S, Bioulac-Sage P, Zucman-Rossi J. Molecular pathogenesis of focal nodular hyperplasia and hepatocellular adenoma. J Hepatol. 2008 Jan;48(1):163–70. PMID:17997499

2667. Rebouissou S, Couchy G, Libbrecht L, et al. The beta-catenin pathway is activated in focal nodular hyperplasia but not in cirrhotic FNH-like nodules. J Hepatol. 2008 Jul;49(1):61–71. PMID:18466996

2668. Rebouissou S, Franconi A, Calderaro J, et al. Genotype-phenotype correlation of CTNNB1 mutations reveals different ß-catenin activity associated with liver tumor progression. Hepatology. 2016 Dec;64(6):2047–61. PMID:27177928

2669. Rebours V, Gaujoux S, d'Assignies G, et al. Obesity and fatty pancreatic infiltration are risk factors for pancreatic precancerous lesions (PanIN). Clin Cancer Res. 2015 Aug 1;21(15):3522–8. PMID:25700304

2670. Recine M, Kaw M, Evans DB, et al. Fine-needle aspiration cytology of mucinous tumors of the pancreas. Cancer. 2004 Apr 25;102(2):92–9. PMID:15098253

2671. Reddy A, Zhang J, Davis NS, et al. Genetic and functional drivers of diffuse large B cell lymphoma. Cell. 2017 Oct 5;171(2):481–94.e15. PMID:28985567

2672. Reddy RP, Smyrk TC, Zapiach M, et al. Pancreatic mucinous cystic neoplasm defined by ovarian stroma: demographics, clinical features, and prevalence of cancer. Clin Gastroenterol Hepatol. 2004 Nov;2(11):1026–31. PMID:15551256

2673. Reddy S, Cameron JL, Scudiere J, et al. Surgical management of solid-pseudopapillary neoplasms of the pancreas (Franz or Hamoudi tumors): a large single-institutional series. J Am Coll Surg. 2009 May;208(5):950–7, discussion 957–9. PMID:19476869

2674. Redston MS, Caldas C, Seymour AB, et al. p53 mutations in pancreatic carcinoma and evidence of common involvement of homocopolymer tracts in DNA microdeletions. Cancer Res. 1994 Jun 1;54(11):3025–33. PMID:8187092

2675. Reed RC, Beischel L, Schoof J, et al. Androgenetic/biparental mosaicism in an infant with hepatic mesenchymal hamartoma and placental mesenchymal dysplasia. Pediatr Dev Pathol. 2008 Sep-Oct;11(5):377–83. PMID:18260692

2676. Reggiani S, Cosso L, Adriani A, et al. A case of intestinal mastocytosis misdiagnosed as Crohn's disease. Case Rep Gastroenterol. 2015 Jun 3;9(2):188–93. PMID:26120300

2677. Reginelli A, Granata V, Fusco R, et al. Diagnostic performance of magnetic resonance imaging and 3D endoanal ultrasound in detection, staging and assessment post treatment, in anal cancer. Oncotarget. 2017 Apr 4;8(14):22980–90. PMID:28152518

2678. Rehfeld JF, Federspiel B, Bardram L. A neuroendocrine tumor syndrome from cholecystokinin secretion. N Engl J Med. 2013 Mar 21;368(12):1165–6. PMID:23514309

2679. Reid BJ, Haggitt RC, Rubin CE, et al. Observer variation in the diagnosis of dysplasia in Barrett's esophagus. Hum Pathol. 1988 Feb;19(2):166–78. PMID:3343032

2680. Reid BJ, Levine DS, Longton G, et al. Predictors of progression to cancer in Barrett's esophagus: baseline histology and flow cytometry identify low- and high-risk patient subsets. Am J Gastroenterol. 2000 Jul;95(7):1669–76. PMID:10925966

2681. Reid M. Cytology of the pancreas: a practical review for cytopathologists. Surg Pathol Clin. 2011 Jun;4(2):651–91. PMID:26837492

2682. Reid MD, Bagci P, Adsay NV. Histopathologic assessment of pancreatic cancer: does one size fit all? J Surg Oncol. 2013 Jan;107(1):67–77. PMID:22711682

2683. Reid MD, Balci S, Ohike N, et al. Ampullary carcinoma is often of mixed or hybrid histologic type: an analysis of reproducibility and clinical relevance of classification as pancreatobiliary versus intestinal in 232 cases. Mod Pathol. 2016 Dec;29(12):1575–85. PMID:27586202

2684. Reid MD, Balci S, Saka B, et al. Neuroendocrine tumors of the pancreas: current concepts and controversies. Endocr Pathol. 2014 Mar;25(1):65–79. PMID:24430597

2685. Reid MD, Basturk O, Shaib WL, et al. Adenocarcinoma ex-goblet cell carcinoid (appendiceal-type crypt cell adenocarcinoma) is a morphologically distinct entity with highly aggressive behavior and frequent association with peritoneal/intra-abdominal dissemination: an analysis of 77 cases. Mod Pathol. 2016 Oct;29(10):1243–53. PMID:27338636

2686. Reid MD, Choi HJ, Memis B, et al. Serous neoplasms of the pancreas: a clinicopathologic analysis of 193 cases and literature review with new insights on macrocystic and solid variants and critical reappraisal of so-called "serous cystadenocarcinoma". Am J Surg Pathol. 2015 Dec;39(12):1597–610. PMID:26559376

2687. Reid MD, Lewis MM, Willingham FF, et al. The evolving role of pathology in new developments, classification, terminology, and diagnosis of pancreatobiliary neoplasms. Arch Pathol Lab Med. 2017 Mar;141(3):366–80. PMID:28055239

2688. Reid MD, Muraki T, HooKim K, et al. Cytologic features and clinical implications of undifferentiated carcinoma with osteoclastic giant cells of the pancreas: an analysis of 15 cases. Cancer Cytopathol. 2017 Jul;125(7):563–75. PMID:28371566

2689. Reid MD, Roa JC, Memis B, et al. Neuroendocrine neoplasms of the gallbladder. An immunohistochemical and clinicopathologic analysis of 29 cases [abstract]. Mod Pathol. 2017 Feb;30(S2):157–210. Abstract no. 784. PMID:28134903

2690. Reid MD, Stallworth CR, Lewis MM, et al. Cytopathologic diagnosis of oncocytic type intraductal papillary mucinous neoplasm: criteria and clinical implications of accurate diagnosis. Cancer Cytopathol. 2016 Feb;124(2):122–34. PMID:26415076

2692. Reiman A, Kikuchi H, Scocchia D, et al. Validation of an NGS mutation detection panel for melanoma. BMC Cancer. 2017 Feb 22;17(1):150. PMID:28228113

2693. Relles D, Baek J, Witkiewicz A, et al. Periampullary and duodenal neoplasms in

neurofibromatosis type 1: two cases and an updated 20-year review of the literature yielding 76 cases. J Gastrointest Surg. 2010 Jun;14(6):1052–61. PMID:20300877
2694. Remstein ED, Dogan A, Einerson RR, et al. The incidence and anatomic site specificity of chromosomal translocations in primary extranodal marginal zone B-cell lymphoma of mucosa-associated lymphoid tissue (MALT lymphoma) in North America. Am J Surg Pathol. 2006 Dec;30(12):1546–53. PMID:17122510
2694A. Ren M, Lu Y, Lv J, et al. Prognostic factors in primary anorectal melanoma: a clinicopathological study of 60 cases in China. Hum Pathol. 2018 Sep;79:77–85. PMID:29763716
2695. Rengifo-Cam W, Jasperson K, Garrido-Laguna I, et al. A 30-year-old man with three primary malignancies: a case of constitutional mismatch repair deficiency. ACG Case Rep J. 2017 Mar 1;4:e34. PMID:28286799
2696. Renzulli M, Biselli M, Brocchi S, et al. New hallmark of hepatocellular carcinoma, early hepatocellular carcinoma and high grade dysplastic nodules on Gd-EOB-DTPA MRI in patients with cirrhosis: a new diagnostic algorithm. Gut. 2018 Sep;67(9):1674–82. PMID:29437912
2697. Repak R, Kohoutova D, Podhola M, et al. The first European family with gastric adenocarcinoma and proximal polyposis of the stomach: case report and review of the literature. Gastrointest Endosc. 2016 Oct;84(4):718–25. PMID:27343414
2698. Reuschenbach M, Kloor M, Morak M, et al. Serum antibodies against frameshift peptides in microsatellite unstable colorectal cancer patients with Lynch syndrome. Fam Cancer. 2010 Jun;9(2):173–9. PMID:19957108
2699. Rex DK, Ahnen DJ, Baron JA, et al. Serrated lesions of the colorectum: review and recommendations from an expert panel. Am J Gastroenterol. 2012 Sep;107(9):1315–29, quiz 1314, 1330. PMID:22710576
2700. Reyes CV, Wang T. Undifferentiated small cell carcinoma of the pancreas: a report of five cases. Cancer. 1981 May 15;47(10):2500–2. PMID:6268272
2701. Reynoso J, Davis RE, Daniels WW, et al. Esophageal papillomatosis complicated by squamous cell carcinoma in situ. Dis Esophagus. 2004;17(4):345–7. PMID:15569375
2702. Rhee H, Ko JE, Chung T, et al. Transcriptomic and histopathological analysis of cholangiolocellular differentiation trait in intrahepatic cholangiocarcinoma. Liver Int. 2018 Jan;38(1):113–24. PMID:28608943
2703. Rhee H, Nahm JH, Kim H, et al. Poor outcome of hepatocellular carcinoma with stemness marker under hypoxia: resistance to transarterial chemoembolization. Mod Pathol. 2016 Sep;29(9):1038–49. PMID:27312064
2704. Ribeiro MA Jr, Papaiordanou F, Gonçalves JM, et al. Spontaneous rupture of hepatic hemangiomas: a review of the literature. World J Hepatol. 2010 Dec 27;2(12):428–33. PMID:21191518
2705. Ricci R, Martini M, Cenci T, et al. PDGFRA-mutant syndrome. Mod Pathol. 2015 Jul;28(7):954–64. PMID:25975287
2706. Ricci R. Syndromic gastrointestinal stromal tumors. Hered Cancer Clin Pract. 2016 Jul 19;14:15. PMID:27437068
2707. Rice TW, Gress DM, Patil DT, et al. Cancer of the esophagus and esophagogastric junction-Major changes in the American Joint Committee on Cancer eighth edition cancer staging manual. CA Cancer J Clin. 2017 Jul 8;67(4):304–17. PMID:28556024
2708. Rice TW, Patil DT, Blackstone EH. 8th edition AJCC/UICC staging of cancers of the esophagus and esophagogastric junction: application to clinical practice. Ann Cardiothorac Surg. 2017 Mar;6(2):119–30. PMID:28447000
2709. Rice TW, Rusch VW, Apperson-Hansen C, et al. Worldwide esophageal cancer collaboration. Dis Esophagus. 2009;22(1):1–8. PMID:19196264
2710. Richard S, Gardie B, Couvé S, et al. Von Hippel-Lindau: how a rare disease illuminates cancer biology. Semin Cancer Biol. 2013 Feb;23(1):26–37. PMID:22659535
2711. Richter J, Schlesner M, Hoffmann S, et al. Recurrent mutation of the ID3 gene in Burkitt lymphoma identified by integrated genome, exome and transcriptome sequencing. Nat Genet. 2012 Dec;44(12):1316–20. PMID:23143595
2712. Riddell RH, Goldman H, Ransohoff DF, et al. Dysplasia in inflammatory bowel disease: standardized classification with provisional clinical applications. Hum Pathol. 1983 Nov;14(11):931–68. PMID:6629368
2713. Rieker RJ, Quentmeier A, Weiss C, et al. Cystic lymphangioma of the small-bowel mesentery: case report and a review of the literature. Pathol Oncol Res. 2000;6(2):146–8. PMID:10936792
2714. Rindi G, Azzoni C, La Rosa S, et al. ECL cell tumor and poorly differentiated endocrine carcinoma of the stomach: prognostic evaluation by pathological analysis. Gastroenterology. 1999 Mar;116(3):532–42. PMID:10029611
2715. Rindi G, Bordi C, Rappel S, et al. Gastric carcinoids and neuroendocrine carcinomas: pathogenesis, pathology, and behavior. World J Surg. 1996 Feb;20(2):168–72. PMID:8661813
2716. Rindi G, Falconi M, Klersy C, et al. TNM staging of neoplasms of the endocrine pancreas: results from a large international cohort study. J Natl Cancer Inst. 2012 May 16;104(10):764–77. PMID:22525418
2716A. Rindi G, Klersy C, Albarello L, et al. Competitive testing of the WHO 2010 versus the WHO 2017 grading of pancreatic neuroendocrine neoplasms: data from a large international cohort study. Neuroendocrinology. 2018;107(4):375–86. PMID:30300897
2717. Rindi G, Klimstra DS, Abedi-Ardekani B, et al. A common classification framework for neuroendocrine neoplasms: an International Agency for Research on Cancer (IARC) and World Health Organization (WHO) expert consensus proposal. Mod Pathol. 2018 Dec;31(12):1770–86. PMID:30140036
2718. Rindi G, Klöppel G, Alhman H, et al. TNM staging of foregut (neuro)endocrine tumors: a consensus proposal including a grading system. Virchows Arch. 2006 Oct;449(4):395–401. PMID:16967267
2719. Rindi G, Klöppel G, Couvelard A, et al. TNM staging of midgut and hindgut (neuro) endocrine tumors: a consensus proposal including a grading system. Virchows Arch. 2007 Oct;451(4):757–62. PMID:17674042
2720. Rindi G, Luinetti O, Cornaggia M, et al. Three subtypes of gastric argyrophil carcinoid and the gastric neuroendocrine carcinoma: a clinicopathologic study. Gastroenterology. 1993 Apr;104(4):994–1006. PMID:7681798
2721. Rindi G, Solcia E. Endocrine hyperplasia and dysplasia in the pathogenesis of gastrointestinal and pancreatic endocrine tumors. Gastroenterol Clin North Am. 2007 Dec;36(4):851–65, vi. PMID:17996794
2722. Rivera B, Castellsagué E, Bah I, et al. Biallelic NTHL1 mutations in a woman with multiple primary tumors. N Engl J Med. 2015 Nov 12;373(20):1985–6. PMID:26559593
2723. Rivera B, Perea J, Sánchez E, et al. A novel AXIN2 germline variant associated with attenuated FAP without signs of oligondontia or ectodermal dysplasia. Eur J Hum Genet. 2014 Mar;22(3):423–6. PMID:23838596
2724. Rivero-Sanchez L, Lopez-Ceron M, Carballal S, et al. Reassessment colonoscopy to diagnose serrated polyposis syndrome in a colorectal cancer screening population. Endoscopy. 2017 Jan;49(1):44–53. PMID:27741536
2725. Roa EI, Muñoz NS, Ibacache SG, et al. [Natural history of gallbladder cancer. Analysis of biopsy specimens]. Rev Med Chil. 2009 Jul;137(7):873–80. Spanish. PMID:19802413
2726. Roa I, Araya JC, Villaseca M, et al. Gallbladder cancer in a high risk area: morphological features and spread patterns. Hepatogastroenterology. 1999 May-Jun;46(27):1540–6. PMID:10430291
2727. Roa I, de Aretxabala X, Araya JC, et al. Preneoplastic lesions in gallbladder cancer. J Surg Oncol. 2006 Jun 15;93(8):615–23. PMID:16724345
2728. Roa I, de Aretxabala X, Morgan R, et al. [Clinicopathological features of gallbladder polyps and adenomas]. Rev Med Chil. 2004 Jun;132(6):673–9. Spanish. PMID:15332368
2729. Roa I, Ibacache G, Muñoz S, et al. Gallbladder cancer in Chile: pathologic characteristics of survival and prognostic factors: analysis of 1,366 cases. Am J Clin Pathol. 2014 May;141(5):675–82. PMID:24713738
2730. Roa JC, Roa I, Correa P, et al. Microsatellite instability in preneoplastic and neoplastic lesions of the gallbladder. J Gastroenterol. 2005 Jan;40(1):79–86. PMID:15692793
2731. Roa JC, Tapia O, Cakir A, et al. Squamous cell and adenosquamous carcinomas of the gallbladder: clinicopathological analysis of 34 cases identified in 606 carcinomas. Mod Pathol. 2011 Aug;24(8):1069–78. PMID:21532545
2732. Roa JC, Tapia O, Manterola C, et al. Early gallbladder carcinoma has a favorable outcome but Rokitansky-Aschoff sinus involvement is an adverse prognostic factor. Virchows Arch. 2013 Nov;463(5):651–61. PMID:24022828
2733. Robberecht P, Conlon TP, Gardner JD. Interaction of porcine vasoactive intestinal peptide with dispersed pancreatic acinar cells from the guinea pig. Structural requirements for effects of vasoactive intestinal peptide and secretin on cellular adenosine 3':5'-monophosphate. J Biol Chem. 1976 Aug 10;251(15):4635–9. PMID:181379
2734. Robbiani DF, Deroubaix S, Feldhahn N, et al. Plasmodium infection promotes genomic instability and AID-dependent B cell lymphoma. Cell. 2015 Aug 13;162(4):727–37. PMID:26276629
2735. Roberti A, Dobay MP, Bisig B, et al. Type II enteropathy-associated T-cell lymphoma features a unique genomic profile with highly recurrent SETD2 alterations. Nat Commun. 2016 Sep 7;7:12602. PMID:27600764
2736. Roberts NJ, Norris AL, Petersen GM, et al. Whole genome sequencing defines the genetic heterogeneity of familial pancreatic cancer. Cancer Discov. 2016 Feb;6(2):166–75. PMID:26658419
2737. Robinson DR, Wu YM, Kalyana-Sundaram S, et al. Identification of recurrent NAB2-STAT6 gene fusions in solitary fibrous tumor by integrative sequencing. Nat Genet. 2013 Feb;45(2):180–5. PMID:23313952
2738. Robison K, Cronin B, Bregar A, et al. Anal cytology and human papillomavirus genotyping in women with a history of lower genital tract neoplasia compared with low-risk women. Obstet Gynecol. 2015 Dec;126(6):1294–300. PMID:26551180
2739. Robles AI, Traverso G, Zhang M, et al. Whole-exome sequencing analyses of inflammatory bowel disease-associated colorectal cancers. Gastroenterology. 2016 Apr;150(4):931–43. PMID:26764183
2740. Rocha FG, Lee H, Katabi N, et al. Intraductal papillary neoplasm of the bile duct: a biliary equivalent to intraductal papillary mucinous neoplasm of the pancreas? Hepatology. 2012 Oct;56(4):1352–60. PMID:22504729
2741. Rodriguez JR, Salvia R, Crippa S, et al. Branch-duct intraductal papillary mucinous neoplasms: observations in 145 patients who underwent resection. Gastroenterology. 2007 Jul;133(1):72–9, quiz 309–10. PMID:17631133
2742. Rodríguez-Alcalde D, Carballal S, Moreira L, et al. High incidence of advanced colorectal neoplasia during endoscopic surveillance in serrated polyposis syndrome. Endoscopy. 2019 Feb;51(2):142–51. PMID:30068004
2742A. Rogers AC, Winter DC, Heeney A, et al. Systematic review and meta-analysis of the impact of tumour budding in colorectal cancer. Br J Cancer. 2016 Sep 27;115(7):831–40. PMID:27599041
2743. Rogers WM, Dobo E, Norton JA, et al. Risk-reducing total gastrectomy for germline mutations in E-cadherin (CDH1): pathologic findings with clinical implications. Am J Surg Pathol. 2008 Jun;32(6):799–809. PMID:18391748
2744. Roh JH, Srivastava A, Lauwers GY, et al. Micropapillary carcinoma of stomach: a clinicopathologic and immunohistochemical study of 11 cases. Am J Surg Pathol. 2010 Aug;34(8):1139–46. PMID:20661012
2745. Roithmann S, Toledano M, Tourani JM, et al. HIV-associated non-Hodgkin's lymphomas: clinical characteristics and outcome. The experience of the French Registry of HIV-associated tumors. Ann Oncol. 1991 Apr;2(4):289–95. PMID:1868025
2746. Rokkas T, Pistiolas D, Sechopoulos P, et al. Risk of colorectal neoplasm in patients with acromegaly: a meta-analysis. World J Gastroenterol. 2008 Jun 14;14(22):3484–9. PMID:18567075
2747. Rokutan H, Hosoda F, Hama N, et al. Comprehensive mutation profiling of mucinous gastric carcinoma. J Pathol. 2016 Oct;240(2):137–48. PMID:27313181
2748. Roldo C, Missiaglia E, Hagan JP, et al. MicroRNA expression abnormalities in pancreatic endocrine and acinar tumors are associated with distinctive pathologic features and clinical behavior. J Clin Oncol. 2006 Oct 10;24(29):4677–84. PMID:16966691
2749. Romaguera JE, Medeiros LJ, Hagemeister FB, et al. Frequency of gastrointestinal involvement and its clinical significance in mantle cell lymphoma. Cancer. 2003 Feb 1;97(3):586–91. PMID:12548600
2750. Rombouts AJM, Hugen N, van Beek JJP, et al. Does pelvic radiation increase rectal cancer incidence? - A systematic review and meta-analysis. Cancer Treat Rev. 2018 Jul;68:136–44. PMID:29957373
2751. Rondonotti E, Koulaouzidis A, Georgiou J, et al. Small bowel tumours: update in diagnosis and management. Curr Opin Gastroenterol. 2018 May;34(3):159–64. PMID:29438117
2752. Ronkainen J, Aro P, Storskrubb T, et al. Prevalence of Barrett's esophagus in the general population: an endoscopic study. Gastroenterology. 2005 Dec;129(6):1825–31. PMID:16344051
2753. Ronnett BM, Yan H, Kurman RJ, et al. Patients with pseudomyxoma peritonei associated with disseminated peritoneal adenomucinosis have a significantly more favorable prognosis than patients with peritoneal mucinous carcinomatosis. Cancer. 2001 Jul 1;92(1):85–91. PMID:11443613
2754. Rooks JB, Ory HW, Ishak KG, et al. Epidemiology of hepatocellular adenoma. The role of oral contraceptive use. JAMA. 1979 Aug 17;242(7):644–8. PMID:221698
2755. Rooney SL, Shi J. Intraductal tubulopapillary neoplasm of the pancreas: an

update from a pathologist's perspective. Arch Pathol Lab Med. 2016 Oct;140(10):1068–73. PMID:27684978
2756. Rose DM, Hochwald SN, Klimstra DS, et al. Primary duodenal adenocarcinoma: a ten-year experience with 79 patients. J Am Coll Surg. 1996 Aug;183(2):89–96. PMID:8696551
2757. Rosenberg JM, Welch JP. Carcinoid tumors of the colon. A study of 72 patients. Am J Surg. 1985 Jun;149(6):775–9. PMID:2409828
2758. Rosolen A, Perkins SL, Pinkerton CR, et al. Revised international pediatric non-hodgkin lymphoma staging system. J Clin Oncol. 2015 Jun 20;33(18):2112–8. PMID:25940716
2759. Ross-Innes CS, Becq J, Warren A, et al. Whole-genome sequencing provides new insights into the clonal architecture of Barrett's esophagus and esophageal adenocarcinoma. Nat Genet. 2015 Sep;47(9):1038–46. PMID:26192915
2760. Rossi S, Gasparotto D, Cacciatore M, et al. Neurofibromin C terminus-specific antibody (clone NFC) is a valuable tool for the identification of NF1-inactivated GISTs. Mod Pathol. 2018 Jan;31(1):160–8. PMID:28862263
2761. Rossi S, Gasparotto D, Miceli R, et al. KIT, PDGFRA, and BRAF mutational spectrum impacts on the natural history of imatinib-naive localized GIST: a population-based study. Am J Surg Pathol. 2015 Jul;39(7):922–30. PMID:25970686
2762. Rossi S, Miceli R, Messerini L, et al. Natural history of imatinib-naive GISTs: a retrospective analysis of 929 cases with long-term follow-up and development of a survival nomogram based on mitotic index and size as continuous variables. Am J Surg Pathol. 2011 Nov;35(11):1646–56. PMID:21997685
2763. Rossidis G, Arroyo MR, Abbitt PL, et al. Malignant transformation of a pancreatic serous cystadenoma. Am Surg. 2012 Feb;78(2):260–3. PMID:22369840
2764. Rosty C, Buchanan DD, Walsh MD, et al. Phenotype and polyp landscape in serrated polyposis syndrome: a series of 100 patients from genetics clinics. Am J Surg Pathol. 2012 Jun;36(6):876–82. PMID:22510757
2765. Rosty C, Hewett DG, Brown IS, et al. Serrated polyps of the large intestine: current understanding of diagnosis, pathogenesis, and clinical management. J Gastroenterol. 2013 Mar;48(3):287–302. PMID:23208018
2766. Rosty C, Walsh MD, Walters RJ, et al. Multiplicity and molecular heterogeneity of colorectal carcinomas in individuals with serrated polyposis. Am J Surg Pathol. 2013 Mar;37(3):434–42. PMID:23211288
2767. Rottenburger C, Papantoniou D, Mandair D, et al. A case series of molecular imaging of glucagonoma after initial therapy-68Ga-DOTATATE PET/CT reveals similar results as in neuroendocrine tumors of other origin in follow-up and re-evaluation. Clin Nucl Med. 2018 Apr;43(4):252–5. PMID:29432346
2768. Rowe PS, Read AP, Mountford R, et al. Three DNA markers for hypophosphataemic rickets. Hum Genet. 1992 Jul;89(5):539–42. PMID:1353055
2769. Roy AC, Wattchow D, Astill D, et al. Uncommon anal neoplasms. Surg Oncol Clin N Am. 2017 Jan;26(1):143–61. PMID:27889033
2770. Roy N, Malik S, Villanueva KE, et al. Brg1 promotes both tumor-suppressive and oncogenic activities at distinct stages of pancreatic cancer formation. Genes Dev. 2015 Mar 15;29(6):658–71. PMID:25792600
2771. Roy S, LaFramboise WA, Liu TC, et al. Loss of chromatin-remodeling proteins and/or CDKN2A associates with metastasis of pancreatic neuroendocrine tumors and reduced patient survival times. Gastroenterology. 2018 Jun;154(8):2060–3.e8. PMID:29486199
2772. Rozek LS, Schmit SL, Greenson JK, et al. Tumor-infiltrating lymphocytes, Crohn's-like lymphoid reaction, and survival from colorectal cancer. J Natl Cancer Inst. 2016 May 12;108(8). PMID:27172903
2773. Rubenstein JH, Shaheen NJ. Epidemiology, diagnosis, and management of esophageal adenocarcinoma. Gastroenterology. 2015 Aug;149(2):302–17.e1. PMID:25957861
2774. Rubin BP, Singer S, Tsao C, et al. KIT activation is a ubiquitous feature of gastrointestinal stromal tumors. Cancer Res. 2001 Nov 15;61(22):8118–21. PMID:11719439
2775. Rubin DT, Huo D, Kinnucan JA, et al. Inflammation is an independent risk factor for colonic neoplasia in patients with ulcerative colitis: a case-control study. Clin Gastroenterol Hepatol. 2013 Dec;11(12):1601–8.e1, 4. PMID:23872237
2776. Rubio CA. Serrated adenomas of the appendix. J Clin Pathol. 2004 Sep;57(9):946–9. PMID:15333655
2777. Rubio CA. Traditional serrated adenomas of the upper digestive tract. J Clin Pathol. 2016 Jan;69(1):1–5. PMID:26468393
2778. Rubio-Tapia A, Kelly DG, Lahr BD, et al. Clinical staging and survival in refractory celiac disease: a single center experience. Gastroenterology. 2009 Jan;136(1):99–107, quiz 352–3. PMID:18996383
2779. Ruel J, Ko HM, Roda G, et al. Anal neoplasia in inflammatory bowel disease is associated with HPV and perianal disease. Clin Transl Gastroenterol. 2016 Mar 3;7:e148. PMID:26938479
2780. Rugge M, Bersani G, Bertorelle R, et al. Microsatellite instability and gastric non-invasive neoplasia in a high risk population in Cesena, Italy. J Clin Pathol. 2005 Aug;58(8):805–10. PMID:16049280
2781. Rugge M, Capelle LG, Cappellesso R, et al. Precancerous lesions in the stomach: from biology to clinical patient management. Best Pract Res Clin Gastroenterol. 2013 Apr;27(2):205–23. PMID:23809241
2782. Rugge M, Cassaro M, Di Mario F, et al. The long term outcome of gastric non-invasive neoplasia. Gut. 2003 Aug;52(8):1111–6. PMID:12865267
2783. Rugge M, Correa P, Dixon MF, et al. Gastric dysplasia: the Padova international classification. Am J Surg Pathol. 2000 Feb;24(2):167–76. PMID:10680883
2784. Rugge M, Correa P, Dixon MF, et al. Gastric mucosal atrophy: interobserver consistency using new criteria for classification and grading. Aliment Pharmacol Ther. 2002 Jul;16(7):1249–59. PMID:12144574
2785. Rugge M, de Boni M, Pennelli G, et al. Gastritis OLGA-staging and gastric cancer risk: a twelve-year clinico-pathological follow-up study. Aliment Pharmacol Ther. 2010 May;31(10):1104–11. PMID:20180784
2786. Rugge M, Farinati F, Di Mario F, et al. Gastric epithelial dysplasia: a prospective multicenter follow-up study from the Interdisciplinary Group on Gastric Epithelial Dysplasia. Hum Pathol. 1991 Oct;22(10):1002–8. PMID:1842372
2787. Rugge M, Fassan M, Cavallin F, et al. Re: Risk of malignant progression in Barrett's esophagus patients: results from a large population-based study. J Natl Cancer Inst. 2012 Nov 21;104(22):1771–2. PMID:23042934
2788. Rugge M, Fassan M, Graham DY. Clinical guidelines: secondary prevention of gastric cancer. Nat Rev Gastroenterol Hepatol. 2012 Feb 14;9(3):128–9. PMID:22330815
2789. Rugge M, Fassan M, Pizzi M, et al. Autoimmune gastritis: histology phenotype and OLGA staging. Aliment Pharmacol Ther. 2012 Jun;35(12):1460–6. PMID:22519568
2790. Rugge M, Fassan M, Pizzi M, et al. Operative Link for Gastritis Assessment gastritis staging incorporates intestinal metaplasia subtyping. Hum Pathol. 2011 Oct;42(10):1539–44. PMID:21481917
2791. Rugge M, Genta RM, Di Mario F, et al. Gastric cancer as preventable disease. Clin Gastroenterol Hepatol. 2017 Dec;15(12):1833–43. PMID:28532700
2792. Rugge M, Genta RM, Graham DY, et al. Chronicles of a cancer foretold: 35 years of gastric cancer risk assessment. Gut. 2016 May;65(5):721–5. PMID:26927528
2793. Rugge M, Genta RM. Staging gastritis: an international proposal. Gastroenterology. 2005 Nov;129(5):1807–8. PMID:16285989
2794. Rugge M, Genta RM. Staging and grading of chronic gastritis. Hum Pathol. 2005 Mar;36(3):228–33. PMID:15791566
2795. Rugge M, Leandro G, Farinati F, et al. Gastric epithelial dysplasia. How clinicopathologic background relates to management. Cancer. 1995 Aug 1;76(3):376–82. PMID:8625116
2796. Rugge M, Meggio A, Pennelli G, et al. Gastritis staging in clinical practice: the OLGA staging system. Gut. 2007 May;56(5):631–6. PMID:17142647
2797. Rugge M, Meggio A, Pravadelli C, et al. Gastritis staging in the endoscopic follow-up for the secondary prevention of gastric cancer: a 5-year prospective study of 1755 patients. Gut. 2019 Jan;68(1):11–7. PMID:29306868
2798. Rugge M, Sonego F, Militello C, et al. Primary carcinoid tumor of the cystic and common bile ducts. Am J Surg Pathol. 1992 Aug;16(8):802–7. PMID:1497121
2799. Rugge M. Gastric cancer risk in patients with Helicobacter pylori infection and following its eradication. Gastroenterol Clin North Am. 2015 Sep;44(3):609–24. PMID:26314671
2800. Ruijs MW, Verhoef S, Rookus MA, et al. TP53 germline mutation testing in 180 families suspected of Li-Fraumeni syndrome: mutation detection rate and relative frequency of cancers in different familial phenotypes. J Med Genet. 2010 Jun;47(6):421–8. PMID:20522432
2801. Ruiz B, Garay J, Johnson W, et al. Morphometric assessment of gastric antral atrophy: comparison with visual evaluation. Histopathology. 2001 Sep;39(3):235–42. PMID:11532033
2802. Ruo L, Coit DG, Brennan MF, et al. Long-term follow-up of patients with familial adenomatous polyposis undergoing pancreaticoduodenal surgery. J Gastrointest Surg. 2002 Sep-Oct;6(5):671–5. PMID:12399055
2802A. Ruskoné-Fourmestraux A, Dragosics B, Morgner A, et al. Paris staging system for primary gastrointestinal lymphomas. Gut. 2003 Jun;52(6):912–3. PMID:12740354
2803. Rustagi T, Gleeson FC, Chari ST, et al. Endoscopic ultrasound fine-needle aspiration diagnosis of synchronous primary pancreatic adenocarcinoma and effects on staging and resectability. Clin Gastroenterol Hepatol. 2017 Feb;15(2):299–302.e4. PMID:27539084
2804. Rutter M, Saunders B, Wilkinson K, et al. Severity of inflammation is a risk factor for colorectal neoplasia in ulcerative colitis. Gastroenterology. 2004 Feb;126(2):451–9. PMID:14762782
2805. Rutter MD, Saunders BP, Wilkinson KH, et al. Thirty-year analysis of a colonoscopic surveillance program for neoplasia in ulcerative colitis. Gastroenterology. 2006 Apr;130(4):1030–8. PMID:16618396
2806. Saad RS, Mahood LK, Clary KM, et al. Role of cytology in the diagnosis of Barrett's esophagus and associated neoplasia. Diagn Cytopathol. 2003 Sep;29(3):130–5. PMID:12951679
2807. Sachatello CR, Griffen WO Jr. Hereditary polypoid diseases of the gastrointestinal tract: a working classification. Am J Surg. 1975 Feb;129(2):198–203. PMID:1091175
2808. Sacher AG, Gandhi L. Biomarkers for the clinical use of PD-1/PD-L1 inhibitors in non-small-cell lung cancer: a review. JAMA Oncol. 2016 Sep 1;2(9):1217–22. PMID:27310809
2809. Sadanandam A, Wullschleger S, Lyssiotis CA, et al. A cross-species analysis in pancreatic neuroendocrine tumors reveals molecular subtypes with distinctive clinical, metastatic, developmental, and metabolic characteristics. Cancer Discov. 2015 Dec;5(12):1296–313. PMID:26446169
2811. Saeki N, Saito A, Choi IJ, et al. A functional single nucleotide polymorphism in mucin 1, at chromosome 1q22, determines susceptibility to diffuse-type gastric cancer. Gastroenterology. 2011 Mar;140(3):892–902. PMID:21070779
2812. Safari MT, Shahrokh S, Miri MB, et al. Biliary mucinous cystic neoplasm: a case report and review of the literature. Gastroenterol Hepatol Bed Bench. 2016 Dec;9 Suppl1:S88–92. PMID:28224034
2813. Sagar J, Sagar B, Patel AF, et al. Ciliated median raphe cyst of perineum presenting as perianal polyp: a case report with immunohistochemical study, review of literature, and pathogenesis. ScientificWorldJournal. 2006 Mar 5;6:2339–44. PMID:17619701
2814. Saha SK, Parachoniak CA, Ghanta KS, et al. Mutant IDH inhibits HNF-4α to block hepatocyte differentiation and promote biliary cancer. Nature. 2014 Sep 4;513(7516):110–4. PMID:25043045
2815. Saha SK, Zhu AX, Fuchs CS, et al. Forty-year trends in cholangiocarcinoma incidence in the U.S.: intrahepatic disease on the rise. Oncologist. 2016 May;21(5):594–9. PMID:27000463
2816. Sahani DV, Kadavigere R, Blake M, et al. Intraductal papillary mucinous neoplasm of pancreas: multi-detector row CT with 2D curved reformations–correlation with MRCP. Radiology. 2006 Feb;238(2):560–9. PMID:16436817
2817. Sahin IH, Lowery MA, Stadler ZK, et al. Genomic instability in pancreatic adenocarcinoma: a new step towards precision medicine and novel therapeutic approaches. Expert Rev Gastroenterol Hepatol. 2016 Aug;10(8):893–905. PMID:26881472
2818. Saito R, Abe H, Kunita A, et al. Overexpression and gene amplification of PD-L1 in cancer cells and PD-L1+ immune cells in Epstein-Barr virus-associated gastric cancer: the prognostic implications. Mod Pathol. 2017 Mar;30(3):427–39. PMID:27934877
2819. Saito S, Azumi M, Muneoka Y, et al. Cost-effectiveness of combined serum anti-Helicobacter pylori IgG antibody and serum pepsinogen concentrations for screening for gastric cancer risk in Japan. Eur J Health Econ. 2018 May;19(4):545–55. PMID:28550494
2820. Saito S, Hosoya Y, Morishima K, et al. A clinicopathological and immunohistochemical study of gastric cancer with squamous cell carcinoma components: a clinically aggressive tumor. J Dig Dis. 2012 Aug;13(8):407–13. PMID:22788926
2821. Saito Y, Hinoi T, Ueno H, et al. Risk factors for the development of desmoid tumor after colectomy in patients with familial adenomatous polyposis: multicenter retrospective cohort study in Japan. Ann Surg Oncol. 2016 Aug;23 Suppl 4:559–65. PMID:27387679
2822. Saka B, Balci S, Basturk O, et al. Pancreatic ductal adenocarcinoma is spread to the peripancreatic soft tissue in the majority of resected cases, rendering the AJCC T-stage protocol (7th edition) inapplicable and insignificant: a size-based staging system (pT1: ≤2, pT2: >2-≤4, pT3: >4 cm) is more valid

and clinically relevant. Ann Surg Oncol. 2016 Jun;23(6):2010–8. PMID:26832882
2823. Sakai Y, Kupelioglu AA, Yanagisawa A, et al. Origin of giant cells in osteoclast-like giant cell tumors of the pancreas. Hum Pathol. 2000 Oct;31(10):1223–9. PMID:11070115
2824. Sakamoto H, Kuboki Y, Hatori T, et al. Clinicopathological significance of somatic RNF43 mutation and aberrant expression of ring finger protein 43 in intraductal papillary mucinous neoplasms of the pancreas. Mod Pathol. 2015 Feb;28(2):261–7. PMID:25081753
2825. Sakamoto LH, DE Camargo B, Cajaiba M, et al. MT1G hypermethylation: a potential prognostic marker for hepatoblastoma. Pediatr Res. 2010 Apr;67(4):387–93. PMID:20032811
2827. Sakurai U, Lauwers GY, Vieth M, et al. Gastric high-grade dysplasia can be associated with submucosal invasion: evaluation of its prevalence in a series of 121 endoscopically resected specimens. Am J Surg Pathol. 2014 Nov;38(11):1545–50. PMID:25310837
2828. Salar A, Juanpere N, Bellosillo B, et al. Gastrointestinal involvement in mantle cell lymphoma: a prospective clinic, endoscopic, and pathologic study. Am J Surg Pathol. 2006 Oct;30(10):1274–80. PMID:17001159
2829. Salas S, Brulard C, Terrier P, et al. Gene expression profiling of desmoid tumors by cDNA microarrays and correlation with progression-free survival. Clin Cancer Res. 2015 Sep 15;21(18):4194–200. PMID:25878329
2830. Salaverria I, Martin-Guerrero I, Wagener R, et al. A recurrent 11q aberration pattern characterizes a subset of MYC-negative high-grade B-cell lymphomas resembling Burkitt lymphoma. Blood. 2014 Feb 20;123(8):1187–98. PMID:24398325
2831. Salaverria I, Royo C, Carvajal-Cuenca A, et al. CCND2 rearrangements are the most frequent genetic events in cyclin D1(-) mantle cell lymphoma. Blood. 2013 Feb 21;121(8):1394–402. PMID:23255553
2832. Saleem A. Severe hyponatremia presenting as paraneoplastic syndrome in a patient with small cell carcinoma of gallbladder. J Coll Physicians Surg Pak. 2016 May;26(5):451–2. PMID:27225161
2833. Salmon JS, Thompson MA, Arildsen RC, et al. Non-Hodgkin's lymphoma involving the liver: clinical and therapeutic considerations. Clin Lymphoma Myeloma. 2006 Jan;6(4):273–80. PMID:16507204
2834. Salomao M, Luna AM, Sepulveda JL, et al. Mutational analysis by next generation sequencing of gastric type dysplasia occurring in hyperplastic polyps of the stomach: mutations in gastric hyperplastic polyps. Exp Mol Pathol. 2015 Dec;99(3):468–73. PMID:26325218
2835. Salomao M, Yu WM, Brown RS Jr, et al. Steatohepatitic hepatocellular carcinoma (SH-HCC): a distinctive histological variant of HCC in hepatitis C virus-related cirrhosis with associated NAFLD/NASH. Am J Surg Pathol. 2010 Nov;34(11):1630–6. PMID:20975341
2836. Salotti JA, Nanduri V, Pearce MS, et al. Incidence and clinical features of Langerhans cell histiocytosis in the UK and Ireland. Arch Dis Child. 2009 May;94(5):376–80. PMID:19060008
2837. Salvia R, Fernández-del Castillo C, Bassi C, et al. Main-duct intraductal papillary mucinous neoplasms of the pancreas: clinical predictors of malignancy and long-term survival following resection. Ann Surg. 2004 May;239(5):678–85, discussion 685–7. PMID:15082972
2838. Sampaio MS, Cho YW, Shah T, et al. Association of immunosuppressive maintenance regimens with posttransplant lymphoproliferative disorder in kidney transplant recipients. Transplantation. 2012 Jan 15;93(1):73–81. PMID:22129761
2839. Sanaka MR, Kowalski TE, Brotz C, et al. Solid serous adenoma of the pancreas: a rare form of serous cystadenoma. Dig Dis Sci. 2007 Nov;52(11):3154–6. PMID:17393319
2840. Sander S, Calado DP, Srinivasan L, et al. Synergy between PI3K signaling and MYC in Burkitt lymphomagenesis. Cancer Cell. 2012 Aug 14;22(2):167–79. PMID:22897848
2841. Sano M, Homma T, Hayashi E, et al. Clinicopathological characteristics of anaplastic carcinoma of the pancreas with rhabdoid features. Virchows Arch. 2014 Nov;465(5):531–8. PMID:25031015
2842. Sano T, Coit DG, Kim HH, et al. Proposal of a new stage grouping of gastric cancer for TNM classification: International Gastric Cancer Association staging project. Gastric Cancer. 2017 Mar;20(2):217–25. PMID:26897166
2843. Santarelli R, De Marco R, Masala MV, et al. Direct correlation between human herpesvirus-8 seroprevalence and classic Kaposi's sarcoma incidence in Northern Sardinia. J Med Virol. 2001 Oct;65(2):368–72. PMID:11536246
2844. Santoro E, Sacchi M, Scutari F, et al. Primary adenocarcinoma of the duodenum: treatment and survival in 89 patients. Hepatogastroenterology. 1997 Jul-Aug;44(16):1157–63. PMID:9261617
2845. Sanyal AJ, Yoon SK, Lencioni R. The etiology of hepatocellular carcinoma and consequences for treatment. Oncologist. 2010;15 Suppl 4:14–22. PMID:21115577
2846. Sarbia M, Verreet P, Bittinger F, et al. Basaloid squamous cell carcinoma of the esophagus: diagnosis and prognosis. Cancer. 1997 May 15;79(10):1871–8. PMID:9149011
2847. Sarlomo-Rikala M, Miettinen M. Gastric schwannoma–a clinicopathological analysis of six cases. Histopathology. 1995 Oct;27(4):355–60. PMID:8847066
2848. Sarr MG, Carpenter HA, Prabhakar LP, et al. Clinical and pathologic correlation of 84 mucinous cystic neoplasms of the pancreas: can one reliably differentiate benign from malignant (or premalignant) neoplasms? Ann Surg. 2000 Feb;231(2):205–12. PMID:10674612
2849. Sartore-Bianchi A, Martini M, Molinari F, et al. PIK3CA mutations in colorectal cancer are associated with clinical resistance to EGFR-targeted monoclonal antibodies. Cancer Res. 2009 Mar 1;69(5):1851–7. PMID:19223544
2850. Sasaki A, Nakajima T, Egashira H, et al. Condyloma acuminatum of the anal canal, treated with endoscopic submucosal dissection. World J Gastroenterol. 2016 Feb 28;22(8):2636–41. PMID:26937152
2851. Sasaki M, Matsubara T, Kakuda Y, et al. Immunostaining for polycomb group protein EZH2 and senescent marker p16INK4a may be useful to differentiate cholangiolocellular carcinoma from ductular reaction and bile duct adenoma. Am J Surg Pathol. 2014 Mar;38(3):364–9. PMID:24487593
2852. Sasaki M, Matsubara T, Nitta T, et al. GNAS and KRAS mutations are common in intraductal papillary neoplasms of the bile duct. PLoS One. 2013 12 2;8(12):e81706. PMID:24312577
2853. Sasaki M, Matsubara T, Yoneda N, et al. Overexpression of enhancer of zeste homolog 2 and MUC1 may be related to malignant behaviour in intraductal papillary neoplasm of the bile duct. Histopathology. 2013 Feb;62(3):446–57. PMID:23163606
2854. Sasaki M, Nitta T, Sato Y, et al. Autophagy may occur at an early stage of cholangiocarcinogenesis via biliary intraepithelial neoplasia. Hum Pathol. 2015 Feb;46(2):202–9. PMID:25466963
2855. Sasaki M, Sato H, Kakuda Y, et al. Clinicopathological significance of 'subtypes with stem-cell feature' in combined hepatocellular-cholangiocarcinoma. Liver Int. 2015 Mar;35(3):1024–35. PMID:24712771
2856. Sasaki M, Sato Y, Nakanuma Y. Mutational landscape of combined hepatocellular carcinoma and cholangiocarcinoma, and its clinicopathological significance. Histopathology. 2017 Feb;70(3):423–34. PMID:27634656
2857. Sasaki M, Sato Y. Insulin-like growth factor II mRNA-binding protein 3 (IMP3) is a marker that predicts presence of invasion in papillary biliary tumors. Hum Pathol. 2017 Apr;62:152–9. PMID:28089541
2858. Sasaki M, Yoneda N, Sawai Y, et al. Clinicopathological characteristics of serum amyloid A-positive hepatocellular neoplasms/nodules arising in alcoholic cirrhosis. Histopathology. 2015 May;66(6):836–45. PMID:25318388
2859. Sasi OA, Sathiapalan R, Rifai A, et al. Colonic neuroendocrine carcinoma in a child. Pediatr Radiol. 2005 Mar;35(3):339–43. PMID:15565344
2860. Sato H, Maeda K, Maruta M, et al. Mucinous adenocarcinoma associated with chronic anal fistula reconstructed by gracilis myocutaneous flaps. Tech Coloproctol. 2006 Oct;10(3):249–52. PMID:16969607
2861. Sato T, Konishi K, Kimura H, et al. Adenoma and tiny carcinoma in adenoma of the papilla of Vater–p53 and PCNA. Hepatogastroenterology. 1999 May-Jun;46(27):1959–62. PMID:10430377
2862. Sato Y, Harada K, Sasaki M, et al. Clinicopathological significance of S100 protein expression in cholangiocarcinoma. J Gastroenterol Hepatol. 2013 Aug;28(8):1422–9. PMID:23621473
2863. Sato Y, Harada K, Sasaki M, et al. Histological characteristics of biliary intraepithelial neoplasia-3 and intraepithelial spread of cholangiocarcinoma. Virchows Arch. 2013 Apr;462(4):421–7. PMID:23446751
2864. Satou A, Asano N, Nakazawa A, et al. Epstein-Barr virus (EBV)-positive sporadic Burkitt lymphoma: an age-related lymphoproliferative disorder? Am J Surg Pathol. 2015 Feb;39(2):227–35. PMID:25321330
2866. Saul SH. Inflammatory cloacogenic polyp: relationship to solitary rectal ulcer syndrome/mucosal prolapse and other bowel disorders. Hum Pathol. 1987 Nov;18(11):1120–5. PMID:3500106
2867. Saurin JC, Gutknecht C, Napoleon B, et al. Surveillance of duodenal adenomas in familial adenomatous polyposis reveals high cumulative risk of advanced disease. J Clin Oncol. 2004 Feb 1;22(3):493–8. PMID:14752072
2868. Sauter M, Keilholz G, Kranzbühler H, et al. Presenting symptoms predict local staging of anal cancer: a retrospective analysis of 86 patients. BMC Gastroenterol. 2016 Apr 6;16:46. PMID:27048435
2869. Savant D, Lee L, Das K. Intraductal tubulopapillary neoplasm of the pancreas masquerading as pancreatic neuroendocrine carcinoma: review of the literature with a case report. Acta Cytol. 2016;60(3):267–74. PMID:27459312
2870. Saw EC, Yu GS, Wagner G, et al. Synchronous primary neuroendocrine carcinoma and adenocarcinoma in Barrett's esophagus. J Clin Gastroenterol. 1997 Mar;24(2):116–9. PMID:9077732
2871. Sawada G, Moon J, Saito A, et al. A case of adenoid cystic carcinoma of the esophagus. Surg Case Rep. 2015 Dec;1(1):119. PMID:26943443
2872. Sawada T, Yashiro M, Sentani K, et al. New molecular staging with G-factor supplements TNM classification in gastric cancer: a multicenter collaborative research by the Japan Society for Gastroenterological Carcinogenesis G-Project committee. Gastric Cancer. 2015 Jan;18(1):119–28. PMID:24488015
2873. Sawey ET, Chanrion M, Cai C, et al. Identification of a therapeutic strategy targeting amplified FGF19 in liver cancer by oncogenomic screening. Cancer Cell. 2011 Mar 8;19(3):347–58. PMID:21397858
2874. Sawhney MS, Dickstein J, LeClair J, et al. Adenomas with high-grade dysplasia and early adenocarcinoma are more likely to be sessile in the proximal colon. Colorectal Dis. 2015 Aug;17(8):682–8. PMID:25619115
2875. Sayed MG, Ahmed AF, Ringold JR, et al. Germline SMAD4 or BMPR1A mutations and phenotype of juvenile polyposis. Ann Surg Oncol. 2002 Nov;9(9):901–6. PMID:12417513
2876. Saygin C, Uzunaslan D, Ozguroglu M, et al. Dendritic cell sarcoma: a pooled analysis including 462 cases with presentation of our case series. Crit Rev Oncol Hematol. 2013 Nov;88(2):253–71. PMID:23755890
2877. Scardoni M, Vittoria E, Volante M, et al. Mixed adenoneuroendocrine carcinomas of the gastrointestinal tract: targeted next-generation sequencing suggests a monoclonal origin of the two components. Neuroendocrinology. 2014;100(4):310–6. PMID:25342539
2878. Scarpa A, Chang DK, Nones K, et al. Whole-genome landscape of pancreatic neuroendocrine tumours. Nature. 2017 Mar 2;543(7643):65–71. PMID:28199314
2879. Scarpa A, Mantovani W, Capelli P, et al. Pancreatic endocrine tumors: improved TNM staging and histopathological grading permit a clinically efficient prognostic stratification of patients. Mod Pathol. 2010 Jun;23(6):824–33. PMID:20305616
2880. Scarpa M, Castagliuolo I, Castoro C, et al. Inflammatory colonic carcinogenesis: a review on pathogenesis and immunosurveillance mechanisms in ulcerative colitis. World J Gastroenterol. 2014 Jun 14;20(22):6774–85. PMID:24944468
2881. Schaefer IM, Mariño-Enríquez A, Fletcher JA. What is new in gastrointestinal stromal tumor? Adv Anat Pathol. 2017 Sep;24(5):259–67. PMID:28632504
2882. Schaefer IM, Wang Y, Liang CW, et al. MAX inactivation is an early event in GIST development that regulates p16 and cell proliferation. Nat Commun. 2017 Mar 8;8:14674. PMID:28270683
2883. Schildhaus HU, Cavlar T, Binot E, et al. Inflammatory fibroid polyps harbour mutations in the platelet-derived growth factor receptor alpha (PDGFRA) gene. J Pathol. 2008 Oct;216(2):176–82. PMID:18686281
2884. Schizas D, Mastoraki A, Kirkilesis GI, et al. Neuroendocrine tumors of the esophagus: state of the art in diagnostic and therapeutic management. J Gastrointest Cancer. 2017 Dec;48(4):299–304. PMID:28656561
2885. Schlemper RJ, Kato Y, Stolte M. Review of histological classifications of gastrointestinal epithelial neoplasia: differences in diagnosis of early carcinomas between Japanese and Western pathologists. J Gastroenterol. 2001 Jul;36(7):445–56. PMID:11480788
2886. Schlemper RJ, Riddell RH, Kato Y, et al. The Vienna classification of gastrointestinal epithelial neoplasia. Gut. 2000 Aug;47(2):251–5. PMID:10896917
2887. Schlesinger S, Aleksandrova K, Pischon T, et al. Diabetes mellitus, insulin treatment, diabetes duration, and risk of biliary tract cancer and hepatocellular carcinoma in a European cohort. Ann Oncol. 2013 Sep;24(9):2449–55. PMID:23720454
2888. Schlitter AM, Born D, Bettstetter M, et al. Intraductal papillary neoplasms of the bile duct: stepwise progression to carcinoma involves common molecular pathways. Mod Pathol. 2014 Jan;27(1):73–86. PMID:23828315

2889. Schlitter AM, Esposito I. Definition of microscopic tumor clearance (r0) in pancreatic cancer resections. Cancers (Basel). 2010 Nov 25;2(4):2001–10. PMID:24281214
2890. Schlitter AM, Jang KT, Klöppel G, et al. Intraductal tubulopapillary neoplasms of the bile ducts: clinicopathologic, immunohistochemical, and molecular analysis of 20 cases. Mod Pathol. 2015 Sep;28(9):1249–64. PMID:26111977
2891. Schlitter AM, Jesinghaus M, Jäger C, et al. pT but not pN stage of the 8th TNM classification significantly improves prognostication in pancreatic ductal adenocarcinoma. Eur J Cancer. 2017 Oct;84:121–9. PMID:28802189
2892. Schlitter AM, Konukiewitz B, Kleeff J, et al. [Recurrent duodenal ulcer bleeding as the first manifestation of a solid pseudopapillary neoplasm of the pancreas with hepatic metastases]. Dtsch Med Wochenschr. 2013 May;138(20):1050–3. German. PMID:23670260
2893. Schlitter AM, Segler A, Steiger K, et al. Molecular, morphological and survival analysis of 177 resected pancreatic ductal adenocarcinomas (PDACs): identification of prognostic subtypes. Sci Rep. 2017 Feb 1;7:41064. PMID:28145465
2894. Schmatz AI, Streubel B, Kretschmer-Chott E, et al. Primary follicular lymphoma of the duodenum is a distinct mucosal/submucosal variant of follicular lymphoma: a retrospective study of 63 cases. J Clin Oncol. 2011 Apr 10;29(11):1445–51. PMID:21383289
2895. Schmelz M, Montes-Moreno S, Piris M, et al. Lack and/or aberrant localization of major histocompatibility class II (MHCII) protein in plasmablastic lymphoma. Haematologica. 2012 Oct;97(10):1614–6. PMID:22689685
2896. Schmitt AM, Anlauf M, Rousson V, et al. WHO 2004 criteria and CK19 are reliable prognostic markers in pancreatic endocrine tumors. Am J Surg Pathol. 2007 Nov;31(11):1677–82. PMID:18059224
2897. Schmitt AM, Schmid S, Rudolph T, et al. VHL inactivation is an important pathway for the development of malignant sporadic pancreatic endocrine tumors. Endocr Relat Cancer. 2009 Dec;16(4):1219–27. PMID:19690016
2898. Schmitz F, Tjon JM, Lai Y, et al. Identification of a potential physiological precursor of aberrant cells in refractory coeliac disease type II. Gut. 2013 Apr;62(4):509–19. PMID:22760007
2899. Schmitz R, Wright GW, Huang DW, et al. Genetics and pathogenesis of diffuse large B-cell lymphoma. N Engl J Med. 2018 Apr 12;378(15):1396–407. PMID:29641966
2900. Schmitz R, Young RM, Ceribelli M, et al. Burkitt lymphoma pathogenesis and therapeutic targets from structural and functional genomics. Nature. 2012 Oct 4;490(7418):116–20. PMID:22885699
2901. Schneider-Stock R, Boltze C, Lasota J, et al. High prognostic value of p16INK4 alterations in gastrointestinal stromal tumors. J Clin Oncol. 2003 May 1;21(9):1688–97. PMID:12721243
2902. Schnelldorfer T, Sarr MG, Nagorney DM, et al. Experience with 208 resections for intraductal papillary mucinous neoplasm of the pancreas. Arch Surg. 2008 Jul;143(7):639–46, discussion 646. PMID:18645105
2903. Schnelldorfer T, Ware AL, Sarr MG, et al. Long-term survival after pancreatoduodenectomy for pancreatic adenocarcinoma: is cure possible? Ann Surg. 2008 Mar;247(3):456–62. PMID:18376190
2904. Schoenmakers EF, Wanschura S, Mols R, et al. Recurrent rearrangements in the high mobility group protein gene, HMGI-C, in benign mesenchymal tumours. Nat Genet. 1995 Aug;10(4):436–44. PMID:7670494
2905. Scholtysik R, Kreuz M, Klapper W, et al. Detection of genomic aberrations in molecularly defined Burkitt's lymphoma by array-based, high resolution, single nucleotide polymorphism analysis. Haematologica. 2010 Dec;95(12):2047–55. PMID:20823134
2906. Schoonhoven LM, Sparnaay T, van Wissen W, et al. Seven-week persistence of an oviposition-deterrent pheromone. J Chem Ecol. 1981 May;7(3):583–8. PMID:24420597
2907. Schottenfeld D, Beebe-Dimmer JL, Vigneau FD. The epidemiology and pathogenesis of neoplasia in the small intestine. Ann Epidemiol. 2009 Jan;19(1):58–69. PMID:19064190
2908. Schrader KA, Nelson TN, De Luca A, et al. Multiple granular cell tumors are an associated feature of LEOPARD syndrome caused by mutation in PTPN11. Clin Genet. 2009 Feb;75(2):185–9. PMID:19054014
2909. Schreuder MI, van den Brand M, Hebeda KM, et al. Novel developments in the pathogenesis and diagnosis of extranodal marginal zone lymphoma. J Hematop. 2017 Sep 25;10(3-4):91–107. PMID:29225710
2911. Schulze K, Imbeaud S, Letouzé E, et al. Exome sequencing of hepatocellular carcinomas identifies new mutational signatures and potential therapeutic targets. Nat Genet. 2015 May;47(5):505–11. PMID:25822088
2912. Schutte M, Hruban RH, Geradts J, et al. Abrogation of the Rb/p16 tumor-suppressive pathway in virtually all pancreatic carcinomas. Cancer Res. 1997 Aug 1;57(15):3126–30. PMID:9242437
2913. Schwartz AM, Henson DE. Familial and sporadic pancreatic carcinoma, epidemiologic concordance. Am J Surg Pathol. 2007 Apr;31(4):645–6. PMID:17414117
2914. Schwartz G, Colanta A, Gaetz H, et al. Primary carcinoid tumors of the liver. World J Surg Oncol. 2008 Aug 27;6:91. PMID:18727836
2915. Schwartz RA, Torre DP. The Muir-Torre syndrome: a 25-year retrospect. J Am Acad Dermatol. 1995 Jul;33(1):90–104. PMID:7601953
2916. Schwarz RE, Smith DD. Extent of lymph node retrieval and pancreatic cancer survival: information from a large US population database. Ann Surg Oncol. 2006 Sep;13(9):1189–200. PMID:16955385
2917. Schwarzkopf G, Pfisterer J. [Metastasizing gastrinoma and tuberous sclerosis complex. Association or coincidence?]. Zentralbl Pathol. 1994 Feb;139(6):477–81. German. PMID:8161496
2918. Schweizer L, Koelsche C, Sahm F, et al. Meningeal hemangiopericytoma and solitary fibrous tumors carry the NAB2-STAT6 fusion and can be diagnosed by nuclear expression of STAT6 protein. Acta Neuropathol. 2013 May;125(5):651–8. PMID:23575898
2919. Schönleben F, Qiu W, Bruckman KC, et al. BRAF and KRAS gene mutations in intraductal papillary mucinous neoplasm/carcinoma (IPMN/IPMC) of the pancreas. Cancer Lett. 2007 May 8;249(2):242–8. PMID:17097223
2919A. Sciarra A, Di Tommaso L, Nakano M, et al. Morphophenotypic changes in human multistep hepatocarcinogenesis with translational implications. J Hepatol. 2016 Jan;64(1):87–93. PMID:26343958
2920. Scoazec JY, Degott C, Brousse N, et al. Non-Hodgkin's lymphoma presenting as a primary tumor of the liver: presentation, diagnosis and outcome in eight patients. Hepatology. 1991 May;13(5):870–5. PMID:2029991
2921. Scott DW, Wright GW, Williams PM, et al. Determining cell-of-origin subtypes of diffuse large B-cell lymphoma using gene expression in formalin-fixed paraffin-embedded tissue. Blood. 2014 Feb 20;123(8):1214–7. PMID:24398326
2922. Scott N, Jamali A, Verbeke C, et al. Retroperitoneal margin involvement by adenocarcinoma of the caecum and ascending colon: what does it mean? Colorectal Dis. 2008 Mar;10(3):289–93. PMID:17764533
2923. Secrier M, Li X, de Silva N, et al. Mutational signatures in esophageal adenocarcinoma define etiologically distinct subgroups with therapeutic relevance. Nat Genet. 2016 Oct;48(10):1131–41. PMID:27595477
2924. Seevaratnam R, Cardoso R, McGregor C, et al. How useful is preoperative imaging for tumor, node, metastasis (TNM) staging of gastric cancer? A meta-analysis. Gastric Cancer. 2012 Sep;15 Suppl 1:S3–18. PMID:21837458
2925. Segura S, Muthukumarana V, West J, et al. Primary hepatic neuroendocrine carcinoma: case reports and review of the literature. Conn Med. 2016 Jan;80(1):19–23. PMID:26882787
2926. Seguí N, Mina LB, Lázaro C, et al. Germline mutations in FAN1 cause hereditary colorectal cancer by impairing DNA repair. Gastroenterology. 2015 Sep;149(3):563–6. PMID:26052075
2927. Sei CA, Glembotski CC. Calcium dependence of phenylephrine-, endothelin-, and potassium chloride-stimulated atrial natriuretic factor secretion from long term primary neonatal rat atrial cardiocytes. J Biol Chem. 1990 May 5;265(13):7166–72. PMID:2158988
2928. Sei Y, Feng J, Zhao X, et al. Polyclonal crypt genesis and development of familial small intestinal neuroendocrine tumors. Gastroenterology. 2016 Jul;151(1):140–51. PMID:27003604
2929. Sei Y, Zhao X, Forbes J, et al. A hereditary form of small intestinal carcinoid associated with a germline mutation in inositol polyphosphate multikinase. Gastroenterology. 2015 Jul;149(1):67–78. PMID:25865046
2930. Seidel G, Zahurak M, Iacobuzio-Donahue C, et al. Almost all infiltrating colloid carcinomas of the pancreas and periampullary region arise from in situ papillary neoplasms: a study of 39 cases. Am J Surg Pathol. 2002 Jan;26(1):56–63. PMID:11756769
2931. Seket B, Saurin JC, Scoazec JY, et al. [Pancreatic acinar cell carcinoma in a patient with familial adenomatous polyposis]. Gastroenterol Clin Biol. 2003 Aug-Sep;27(8-9):818–20. French. PMID:14586255
2932. Seki S, Sakaguchi H, Kitada T, et al. Outcomes of dysplastic nodules in human cirrhotic liver: a clinicopathological study. Clin Cancer Res. 2000 Sep;6(9):3469–73. PMID:10999730
2933. Sekine S, Ogawa R, Hashimoto T, et al. Comprehensive characterization of RSPO fusions in colorectal traditional serrated adenomas. Histopathology. 2017 Oct;71(4):601–9. PMID:28543708
2934. Sekine S, Ogawa R, Saito S, et al. Cytoplasmic MSH2 immunoreactivity in a patient with Lynch syndrome with an EPCAM-MSH2 fusion. Histopathology. 2017 Mar;70(4):664–9. PMID:27896849
2935. Sekine S, Shibata T, Yamauchi Y, et al. Beta-catenin mutations in sporadic fundic gland polyps. Virchows Arch. 2002 Apr;440(4):381–6. PMID:11956818
2936. Sekine S, Yamashita S, Tanabe T, et al. Frequent PTPRK-RSPO3 fusions and RNF43 mutations in colorectal traditional serrated adenoma. J Pathol. 2016 Jun;239(2):133–8. PMID:26924569
2937. Sekine S, Yoshida H, Jansen M, et al. The Japanese viewpoint on the histopathology of early gastric cancer. Adv Exp Med Biol. 2016;908:331–46. PMID:27573779
2938. Sekiya S, Suzuki A. Intrahepatic cholangiocarcinoma can arise from Notch-mediated conversion of hepatocytes. J Clin Invest. 2012 Nov;122(11):3914–8. PMID:23023701
2939. Selby DM, Stocker JT, Ishak KG. Angiosarcoma of the liver in childhood: a clinicopathologic and follow-up study of 10 cases. Pediatr Pathol. 1992 Jul-Aug;12(4):485–98. PMID:1409148
2940. Selby DM, Stocker JT, Waclawiw MA, et al. Infantile hemangioendothelioma of the liver. Hepatology. 1994 Jul;20(1 Pt 1):39–45. PMID:8020903
2941. Sellner F. Investigations on the significance of the adenoma-carcinoma sequence in the small bowel. Cancer. 1990 Aug 15;66(4):702–15. PMID:2167140
2942. Selves J, Meggetto F, Brousset P, et al. Inflammatory pseudotumor of the liver. Evidence for follicular dendritic reticulum cell proliferation associated with clonal Epstein-Barr virus. Am J Surg Pathol. 1996 Jun;20(6):747–53. PMID:8651355
2944. Sempoux C, Balabaud C, Bioulac-Sage P. Malignant transformation of hepatocellular adenoma. Hepat Oncol. 2014 Oct;1(4):421–31. PMID:30190977
2945. Sempoux C, Balabaud C, Bioulac-Sage P. Pictures of focal nodular hyperplasia and hepatocellular adenomas. World J Hepatol. 2014 Aug 27;6(8):580–95. PMID:25232451
2946. Sempoux C, Balabaud C, Paradis V, et al. Hepatocellular nodules in vascular liver diseases. Virchows Arch. 2018 Jul;473(1):33–44. PMID:29804132
2947. Sempoux C, Fan C, Singh P, et al. Cholangiolocellular carcinoma: an innocent-looking malignant liver tumor mimicking ductular reaction. Semin Liver Dis. 2011 Feb;31(1):104–10. PMID:21344355
2948. Sempoux C, Paradis V, Komuta M, et al. Hepatocellular nodules expressing markers of hepatocellular adenomas in Budd-Chiari syndrome and other rare hepatic vascular disorders. J Hepatol. 2015 Nov;63(5):1173–80. PMID:26119687
2949. Sempoux C, Paradis V, Saxena R. Variant differentiation patterns in primary liver carcinoma. Semin Diagn Pathol. 2017 Mar;34(2):176–82. PMID:28256363
2950. Sena Teixeira Mendes L, D Attygalle A, C Wotherspoon A. Helicobacter pylori infection in gastric extranodal marginal zone lymphoma of mucosa-associated lymphoid tissue (MALT) lymphoma: a re-evaluation. Gut. 2014 Sep;63(9):1526–7. PMID:24951256
2951. Sendagorta E, Herranz P, Guadalajara H, et al. Prevalence of abnormal anal cytology and high-grade squamous intraepithelial lesions among a cohort of HIV-infected men who have sex with men. Dis Colon Rectum. 2014 Apr;57(4):475–81. PMID:24608304
2952. Sener SF, Fremgen A, Menck HR, et al. Pancreatic cancer: a report of treatment and survival trends for 100,313 patients diagnosed from 1985-1995, using the National Cancer Database. J Am Coll Surg. 1999 Jul;189(1):1–7. PMID:10401733
2953. Seok JY, Na DC, Woo HG, et al. A fibrous stromal component in hepatocellular carcinoma reveals a cholangiocarcinoma-like gene expression trait and epithelial-mesenchymal transition. Hepatology. 2012 Jun;55(6):1776–86. PMID:22234953
2954. Seppälä T, Pylvänäinen K, Evans DG, et al. Colorectal cancer incidence in path_MLH1 carriers subjected to different follow-up protocols: a Prospective Lynch Syndrome Database report. Hered Cancer Clin Pract. 2017 Oct 10;15:18. PMID:29046738
2955. Sepulveda AR, Hamilton SR, Allegra CJ, et al. Molecular biomarkers for the evaluation of colorectal cancer: guideline summary from the American Society for Clinical Pathology, College of American Pathologists, Association for Molecular Pathology, and American Society of Clinical Oncology. J Oncol Pract. 2017

May;13(5):333–7. PMID:28350513

2956. Service FJ, McMahon MM, O'Brien PC, et al. Functioning insulinoma–incidence, recurrence, and long-term survival of patients: a 60-year study. Mayo Clin Proc. 1991 Jul;66(7):711–9. PMID:1677058

2957. Service FJ. Diagnostic approach to adults with hypoglycemic disorders. Endocrinol Metab Clin North Am. 1999 Sep;28(3):519–32, vi. PMID:10500929

2958. Seshachalam VP, Sekar K, Hui KM. Insights into the etiology-associated gene regulatory networks in hepatocellular carcinoma from The Cancer Genome Atlas. J Gastroenterol Hepatol. 2018 Dec;33(12):2037–47. PMID:29672926

2959. Sessa F, Bonato M, Frigerio B, et al. Ductal cancers of the pancreas frequently express markers of gastrointestinal epithelial cells. Gastroenterology. 1990 Jun;98(6):1655–65. PMID:1692551

2960. Setia N, Agoston AT, Han HS, et al. A protein and mRNA expression-based classification of gastric cancer. Mod Pathol. 2016 Jul;29(7):772–84. PMID:27032689

2961. Shaco-Levy R, Jasperson KW, Martin K, et al. Gastrointestinal polyposis in Cowden syndrome. J Clin Gastroenterol. 2017 Aug;51(7):e60–7. PMID:27661969

2962. Shaco-Levy R, Jasperson KW, Martin K, et al. Morphologic characterization of hamartomatous gastrointestinal polyps in Cowden syndrome, Peutz-Jeghers syndrome, and juvenile polyposis syndrome. Hum Pathol. 2016 Mar;49:39–48. PMID:26826408

2963. Shafqat H, Ali S, Salhab M, et al. Survival of patients with neuroendocrine carcinoma of the colon and rectum: a population-based analysis. Dis Colon Rectum. 2015 Mar;58(3):294–303. PMID:25664707

2964. Shah NA, Urusova IA, D'Agnolo A, et al. Primary hepatic carcinoid tumor presenting as Cushing's syndrome. J Endocrinol Invest. 2007 Apr;30(4):327–33. PMID:17556871

2965. Shah SB, Pickham D, Araya H, et al. Prevalence of anal dysplasia in patients with inflammatory bowel disease. Clin Gastroenterol Hepatol. 2015 Nov;13(11):1955–61.e1. PMID:26044314

2966. Shaheen NJ, Falk GW, Iyer PG, et al. ACG clinical guideline: diagnosis and management of Barrett's esophagus. Am J Gastroenterol. 2016 Jan;111(1):30–50, quiz 51. PMID:26526079

2967. Shaib WL, Nammour JP, Gill H, et al. The future prospects of immune therapy in gastric and esophageal adenocarcinoma. J Clin Med. 2016 Nov 14;5(11):E100. PMID:27854242

2968. Shaib YH, Rugge M, Graham DY, et al. Management of gastric polyps: an endoscopy-based approach. Clin Gastroenterol Hepatol. 2013 Nov;11(11):1374–84. PMID:23583466

2969. Shaikh F, Murray MJ, Amatruda JF, et al. Paediatric extracranial germ-cell tumours. Lancet Oncol. 2016 Apr;17(4):e149–62. PMID:27300675

2970. Shames JM, Dhurandhar NR, Blackard WG. Insulin-secreting bronchial carcinoid tumor with widespread metastases. Am J Med. 1968 Apr;44(4):632–7. PMID:4296076

2971. Shao Y, Yu ZL, Ji M, et al. Lugol chromoendoscopic screening for esophageal dysplasia/early squamous cell carcinoma in patients with esophageal symptoms in low-risk region in China. Oncol Lett. 2015 Jul;10(1):45–50. PMID:26170975

2972. Sharif K, Ramani P, Lochbühler H, et al. Recurrent mesenchymal hamartoma associated with 19q translocation. A call for more radical surgical resection. Eur J Pediatr Surg. 2006 Feb;16(1):64–7. PMID:16544232

2973. Sharma A, Mukewar S, Vege SS. Clinical profile of pancreatic cystic lesions in von Hippel-Lindau disease: a series of 48 patients seen at a tertiary institution. Pancreas. 2017 Aug;46(7):948–52. PMID:28697137

2974. Sharma A, Oishi N, Boddicker RL, et al. Recurrent STAT3-JAK2 fusions in indolent T-cell lymphoproliferative disorder of the gastrointestinal tract. Blood. 2018 May 17;131(20):2262–6. PMID:29592893

2975. Sharma A, Smyrk TC, Levy MJ, et al. Fasting blood glucose levels provide estimate of duration and progression of pancreatic cancer before diagnosis. Gastroenterology. 2018 Aug;155(2):490–500.e2. PMID:29723506

2976. Sharma P, Falk GW, Weston AP, et al. Dysplasia and cancer in a large multicenter cohort of patients with Barrett's esophagus. Clin Gastroenterol Hepatol. 2006 May;4(5):566–72. PMID:16630761

2977. Shastri A, Msaouel P, Montagna C, et al. Primary hepatic small cell carcinoma: two case reports, molecular characterization and pooled analysis of known clinical data. Anticancer Res. 2016 Jan;36(1):271–7. PMID:26722053

2978. Shehata BM, Gupta NA, Katzenstein HM, et al. Undifferentiated embryonal sarcoma of the liver is associated with mesenchymal hamartoma and multiple chromosomal abnormalities: a review of eleven cases. Pediatr Dev Pathol. 2011 Mar-Apr;14(2):111–6. PMID:20925497

2979. Shek TW, Luk IS, Loong F, et al. Inflammatory cell-rich gastrointestinal autonomic nerve tumor. An expansion of its histologic spectrum. Am J Surg Pathol. 1996 Mar;20(3):325–31. PMID:8772786

2980. Shen J, Gibson JA, Schulte S, et al. Clinical, pathologic, and outcome study of hyperplastic and sessile serrated polyps in inflammatory bowel disease. Hum Pathol. 2015 Oct;46(10):1548–56. PMID:26297256

2981. Shen SC, Wu CC, Ng KF, et al. Follicular dendritic cell sarcoma mimicking giant cell carcinoma of the pancreas. Pathol Int. 2006 Aug;56(8):466–70. PMID:16872443

2982. Shepherd NA, Hall PA. Epithelial-mesenchymal interactions can influence the phenotype of carcinoma metastases in the mucosa of the intestine. J Pathol. 1990 Feb;160(2):103–9. PMID:2319390

2983. Shetty S, Natarajan B, Thomas P, et al. Proposed classification of pseudomyxoma peritonei: influence of signet ring cells on survival. Am Surg. 2013 Nov;79(11):1171–6. PMID:24165252

2984. Shetty T, Chase TN. Central monoamines and hyperkinase of childhood. Neurology. 1976 Oct;26(10):1000–2. PMID:986582

2985. Shi C, Hong SM, Lim P, et al. KRAS2 mutations in human pancreatic acinar-ductal metaplastic lesions are limited to those with PanIN: implications for the human pancreatic cancer cell of origin. Mol Cancer Res. 2009 Feb;7(2):230–6. PMID:19208745

2986. Shi C, Hruban RH, Klein AP. Familial pancreatic cancer. Arch Pathol Lab Med. 2009 Mar;133(3):365–74. PMID:19260742

2987. Shi C, Klein AP, Goggins M, et al. Increased prevalence of precursor lesions in familial pancreatic cancer patients. Clin Cancer Res. 2009 Dec 15;15(24):7737–43. PMID:19996207

2988. Shi C, Klimstra DS. Pancreatic neuroendocrine tumors: pathologic and molecular characteristics. Semin Diagn Pathol. 2014 Nov;31(6):498–511. PMID:25441311

2989. Shi C, Zhao Q, Dai B, et al. Primary hepatic neuroendocrine neoplasm: long-time surgical outcome and prognosis. Medicine (Baltimore). 2018 Aug;97(31):e11764. PMID:30075602

2990. Shi E, Chmielecki J, Tang CM, et al. FGFR1 and NTRK3 actionable alterations in "wild-type" gastrointestinal stromal tumors. J Transl Med. 2016 Dec 14;14(1):339. PMID:27974047

2991. Shi H, Cao D, Wei L, et al. Inflammatory angiomyolipomas of the liver: a clinicopathologic and immunohistochemical analysis of 5 cases. Ann Diagn Pathol. 2010 Aug;14(4):240–6. PMID:20637427

2992. Shi Y, Rojas Y, Zhang W, et al. Characteristics and outcomes in children with undifferentiated embryonal sarcoma of the liver: a report from the National Cancer Database. Pediatr Blood Cancer. 2017 Apr;64(4). PMID:27781381

2993. Shia J, Guillem JG, Moore HG, et al. Patterns of morphologic alteration in residual rectal carcinoma following preoperative chemoradiation and their association with long-term outcome. Am J Surg Pathol. 2004 Feb;28(2):215–23. PMID:15043311

2994. Shia J, Holck S, Depetris G, et al. Lynch syndrome-associated neoplasms: a discussion on histopathology and immunohistochemistry. Fam Cancer. 2013 Jun;12(2):241–60. PMID:23435936

2995. Shia J, Tang LH, Weiser MR, et al. Is nonsmall cell type high-grade neuroendocrine carcinoma of the tubular gastrointestinal tract a distinct disease entity? Am J Surg Pathol. 2008 May;32(5):719–31. PMID:18360283

2996. Shia J, Tickoo SK, Guillem JG, et al. Increased endocrine cells in treated rectal adenocarcinomas: a possible reflection of endocrine differentiation in tumor cells induced by chemotherapy and radiotherapy. Am J Surg Pathol. 2002 Jul;26(7):863–72. PMID:12131153

2997. Shia J, Zhang L, Shike M, et al. Secondary mutation in a coding mononucleotide tract in MSH6 causes loss of immunoexpression of MSH6 in colorectal carcinomas with MLH1/PMS2 deficiency. Mod Pathol. 2013 Jan;26(1):131–8. PMID:22918162

2998. Shia J. An update on tumors of the anal canal. Arch Pathol Lab Med. 2010 Nov;134(11):1601–11. PMID:21043813

2999. Shibahara H, Tamada S, Goto M, et al. Pathologic features of mucin-producing bile duct tumors: two histopathologic categories as counterparts of pancreatic intraductal papillary-mucinous neoplasms. Am J Surg Pathol. 2004 Mar;28(3):327–38. PMID:15104295

3000. Shibata H, Toyama K, Shioya H, et al. Rapid colorectal adenoma formation initiated by conditional targeting of the Apc gene. Science. 1997 Oct 3;278(5335):120–3. PMID:9311916

3001. Shibata T, Arai Y, Totoki Y. Molecular genomic landscapes of hepatobiliary cancer. Cancer Sci. 2018 May;109(5):1282–91. PMID:29573058

3002. Shibuya R, Matsuyama A, Shiba E, et al. CAMTA1 is a useful immunohistochemical marker for diagnosing epithelioid haemangioendothelioma. Histopathology. 2015 Dec;67(6):827–35. PMID:25879300

3003. Shichijo S, Hirata Y, Niikura R, et al. Histologic intestinal metaplasia and endoscopic atrophy are predictors of gastric cancer development after Helicobacter pylori eradication. Gastrointest Endosc. 2016 Oct;84(4):618–24. PMID:26995689

3004. Shida T, Kishimoto T, Furuya M, et al. Expression of an activated mammalian target of rapamycin (mTOR) in gastroenteropancreatic neuroendocrine tumors. Cancer Chemother Pharmacol. 2010 Apr;65(5):889–93. PMID:19657638

3005. Shiels MS, Kreimer AR, Coghill AE, et al. Anal cancer incidence in the United States, 1977-2011: distinct patterns by histology and behavior. Cancer Epidemiol Biomarkers Prev. 2015 Oct;24(10):1548–56. PMID:26224796

3006. Shiels MS, Pfeiffer RM, Chaturvedi AK, et al. Impact of the HIV epidemic on the incidence rates of anal cancer in the United States. J Natl Cancer Inst. 2012 Oct 17;104(20):1591–8. PMID:23042932

3007. Shih A, Lauwers GY, Balabaud C, et al. Simultaneous occurrence of focal nodular hyperplasia and HNF1A-inactivated hepatocellular adenoma: a collision tumor simulating a composite FNH-HCA. Am J Surg Pathol. 2015 Sep;39(9):1296–300. PMID:26274031

3008. Shim KN, Yang SK, Myung SJ, et al. Atypical endoscopic features of rectal carcinoids. Endoscopy. 2004 Apr;36(4):313–6. PMID:15057680

3009. Shim YH, Park HJ, Choi MS, et al. Hypermethylation of the p16 gene and lack of p16 expression in hepatoblastoma. Mod Pathol. 2003 May;16(5):430–6. PMID:12748249

3010. Shimada H, Matsubara H, Okazumi S, et al. Improved surgical results in thoracic esophageal squamous cell carcinoma: a 40-year analysis of 792 patients. J Gastrointest Surg. 2008 Mar;12(3):518–26. PMID:17823842

3011. Shimada K, Sakamoto Y, Sano T, et al. Invasive carcinoma originating in an intraductal papillary mucinous neoplasm of the pancreas: a clinicopathologic comparison with a common type of invasive ductal carcinoma. Pancreas. 2006 Apr;32(3):281–7. PMID:16628084

3012. Shimada K, Sakamoto Y, Sano T, et al. Prognostic factors after distal pancreatectomy with extended lymphadenectomy for invasive pancreatic adenocarcinoma of the body and tail. Surgery. 2006 Mar;139(3):288–95. PMID:16546491

3013. Shimada K, Sakamoto Y, Sano T, et al. Reappraisal of the clinical significance of tumor size in patients with pancreatic ductal carcinoma. Pancreas. 2006 Oct;33(3):233–9. PMID:17003643

3014. Shimizu T, Marusawa H, Matsumoto Y, et al. Accumulation of somatic mutations in TP53 in gastric epithelium with Helicobacter pylori infection. Gastroenterology. 2014 Aug;147(2):407–17.e3. PMID:24786892

3015. Shimizu Y, Yamaue H, Maguchi H, et al. Predictors of malignancy in intraductal papillary mucinous neoplasm of the pancreas: analysis of 310 pancreatic resection patients at multiple high-volume centers. Pancreas. 2013 Jul;42(5):883–8. PMID:23508017

3016. Shin DH, Lee JH, Kang HJ, et al. Novel epitheliomesenchymal biphasic stomach tumour (gastroblastoma) in a 9-year-old: morphological, ultrastructural and immunohistochemical findings. J Clin Pathol. 2010 Mar;63(3):270–4. PMID:20203230

3017. Shin HR, Oh JK, Lim MK, et al. Descriptive epidemiology of cholangiocarcinoma and clonorchiasis in Korea. J Korean Med Sci. 2010 Jul;25(7):1011–6. PMID:20592891

3018. Shin N, Jo HJ, Kim WK, et al. Gastric pit dysplasia in adjacent gastric mucosa in 414 gastric cancers: prevalence and characteristics. Am J Surg Pathol. 2011 Jul;35(7):1021–9. PMID:21677540

3019. Shindo K, Yu J, Suenaga M, et al. Deleterious germline mutations in patients with apparently sporadic pancreatic adenocarcinoma. J Clin Oncol. 2017 Oct 20;35(30):3382–90. PMID:28767289

3020. Shindoh J, de Aretxabala X, Aloia TA, et al. Tumor location is a strong predictor of tumor progression and survival in T2 gallbladder cancer: an international multicenter study. Ann Surg. 2015 Apr;261(4):733–9. PMID:24854451

3021. Shinozaki-Ushiku A, Kunita A, Fukayama M. Update on Epstein-Barr virus and gastric cancer (review). Int J Oncol. 2015 Apr;46(4):1421–34. PMID:25633561

3022. Shiono S, Suda K, Nobukawa B, et al. Pancreatic, hepatic, splenic, and mesenteric mucinous cystic neoplasms (MCN) are lumped

together as extra ovarian MCN. Pathol Int. 2006 Feb;56(2):71–7. PMID:16445818
3023. Shiraki T, Kuroda H, Takada A, et al. Intraoperative frozen section diagnosis of bile duct margin for extrahepatic cholangiocarcinoma. World J Gastroenterol. 2018 Mar 28;24(12):1332–42. PMID:29599608
3024. Shorter NA, Glick RD, Klimstra DS, et al. Malignant pancreatic tumors in childhood and adolescence: the Memorial Sloan-Kettering experience, 1967 to present. J Pediatr Surg. 2002 Jun;37(6):887–92. PMID:12037756
3025. Shoushtari AN, Munhoz RR, Kuk D, et al. The efficacy of anti-PD-1 agents in acral and mucosal melanoma. Cancer. 2016 Nov 15;122(21):3354–62. PMID:27533633
3026. Shu X, Sundquist K, Sundquist J, et al. Time trends in incidence, causes of death, and survival of cancer of unknown primary in Sweden. Eur J Cancer Prev. 2012 May;21(3):281–8. PMID:21968687
3027. Sia D, Hoshida Y, Villanueva A, et al. Integrative molecular analysis of intrahepatic cholangiocarcinoma reveals 2 classes that have different outcomes. Gastroenterology. 2013 Apr;144(4):829–40. PMID:23295441
3028. Sia D, Villanueva A, Friedman SL, et al. Liver cancer cell of origin, molecular class, and effects on patient prognosis. Gastroenterology. 2017 Mar;152(4):745–61. PMID:28043904
3029. Sie AS, Mensenkamp AR, Adang EM, et al. Fourfold increased detection of Lynch syndrome by raising age limit for tumour genetic testing from 50 to 70 years is cost-effective. Ann Oncol. 2014 Oct;25(10):2001–7. PMID:25081898
3030. Sieber OM, Lipton L, Crabtree M, et al. Multiple colorectal adenomas, classic adenomatous polyposis, and germ-line mutations in MYH. N Engl J Med. 2003 Feb 27;348(9):791–9. PMID:12606733
3031. Sieber OM, Segditsas S, Knudsen AL, et al. Disease severity and genetic pathways in attenuated familial adenomatous polyposis vary greatly but depend on the site of the germline mutation. Gut. 2006 Oct;55(10):1440–8. PMID:16461775
3032. Siegel RL, Fedewa SA, Anderson WF, et al. Colorectal cancer incidence patterns in the United States, 1974-2013. J Natl Cancer Inst. 2017 Aug 1;109(8). PMID:28376186
3033. Siegel RL, Miller KD, Jemal A. Cancer statistics, 2017. CA Cancer J Clin. 2017 Jan;67(1):7–30. PMID:28055103
3034. Siegel RL, Miller KD, Jemal A. Cancer statistics, 2018. CA Cancer J Clin. 2018 Jan;68(1):7–30. PMID:29313949
3035. Siegenbeek van Heukelom ML, Richel O, de Vries HJ, et al. Low- and high-risk human papillomavirus genotype infections in intra-anal warts in HIV-positive men who have sex with men. Br J Dermatol. 2016 Oct;175(4):735–43. PMID:26994411
3036. Sieniawski M, Angamuthu N, Boyd K, et al. Evaluation of enteropathy-associated T-cell lymphoma comparing standard therapies with a novel regimen including autologous stem cell transplantation. Blood. 2010 May 6;115(18):3664–70. PMID:20197551
3037. Sierra EM, Villanueva Saenz E, Martínez PH, et al. Mucinous adenocarcinoma associated with fistula in ano: report of a case. Tech Coloproctol. 2006 Mar;10(1):51–3. PMID:16528482
3038. Sierzega M, Bobrzyński Ł, Matyja A, et al. Factors predicting adequate lymph node yield in patients undergoing pancreatoduodenectomy for malignancy. World J Surg Oncol. 2016 Sep 20;14(1):248. PMID:27644962
3040. Siewert JR, Stein HJ. Classification of adenocarcinoma of the oesophagogastric junction. Br J Surg. 1998 Nov;85(11):1457–9. PMID:9823902
3041. Sigel CS, Klimstra DS. Cytomorphologic and immunophenotypical features of acinar cell neoplasms of the pancreas. Cancer Cytopathol. 2013 Aug;121(8):459–70. PMID:23408736
3042. Sigel CS, Krauss Silva VW, Reid MD, et al. Assessment of cytologic differentiation in high-grade pancreatic neuroendocrine neoplasms: a multi-institutional study. Cancer Cytopathol. 2018 Jan;126(1):44–53. PMID:29044913
3043. Sigel JE, Petras RE, Lashner BA, et al. Intestinal adenocarcinoma in Crohn's disease: a report of 30 cases with a focus on coexisting dysplasia. Am J Surg Pathol. 1999 Jun;23(6):651–5. PMID:10366146
3044. Silva VW, Askan G, Daniel TD, et al. Biliary carcinomas: pathology and the role of DNA mismatch repair deficiency. Chin Clin Oncol. 2016 Oct;5(5):62. PMID:27829276
3045. Simard G, Loiseau D, Girault A, et al. Reactivity of HDL subfractions towards lecithin-cholesterol acyltransferase. Modulation by their content in free cholesterol. Biochim Biophys Acta. 1989 Oct 17;1005(3):245–52. PMID:2804054
3046. Simchuk EJ, Low DE. Direct esophageal metastasis from a distant primary tumor is a submucosal process: a review of six cases. Dis Esophagus. 2001;14(3-4):247–50. PMID:11869331
3047. Singh K, Patel N, Patil P, et al. Primary ovarian solid pseudopapillary neoplasm with CTNNB1 c.98C>G (p.S33C) point mutation. Int J Gynecol Pathol. 2018 Mar;37(2):110–6. PMID:28463908
3048. Singh R, Basturk O, Klimstra DS, et al. Lipid-rich variant of pancreatic endocrine neoplasms. Am J Surg Pathol. 2006 Feb;30(2):194–200. PMID:16434893
3049. Singh S, Manickam P, Amin AV, et al. Incidence of esophageal adenocarcinoma in Barrett's esophagus with low-grade dysplasia: a systematic review and meta-analysis. Gastrointest Endosc. 2014 Jun;79(6):897–909.e4, quiz 983.e1, 983.e3. PMID:24556051
3050. Singhal S, Baker RD, Khan A, et al. A rare case of esophageal papilloma due to human papillomavirus with uncommon presentation of dysphagia in a 2-year-old child. Clin Pediatr (Phila). 2016 Oct;55(12):1168–70. PMID:26538585
3051. Singhi AD, Adsay NV, Swierczynski SL, et al. Hyperplastic Luschka ducts: a mimic of adenocarcinoma in the gallbladder fossa. Am J Surg Pathol. 2011 Jun;35(6):883–90. PMID:21566517
3052. Singhi AD, Chu LC, Tatsas AD, et al. Cystic pancreatic neuroendocrine tumors: a clinicopathologic study. Am J Surg Pathol. 2012 Nov;36(11):1666–73. PMID:23073325
3053. Singhi AD, Davison JM, Choudry HA, et al. GNAS is frequently mutated in both low-grade and high-grade disseminated appendiceal mucinous neoplasms but does not affect survival. Hum Pathol. 2014 Aug;45(8):1737–43. PMID:24925222
3054. Singhi AD, Ishida H, Ali SZ, et al. A histomorphologic comparison of familial and sporadic pancreatic cancers. Pancreatology. 2015 Jul-Aug;15(4):387–91. PMID:25959245
3055. Singhi AD, Klimstra DS. Well-differentiated pancreatic neuroendocrine tumours (PanNETs) and poorly differentiated pancreatic neuroendocrine carcinomas (PanNECs): concepts, issues and a practical diagnostic approach to high-grade (G3) cases. Histopathology. 2018 Jan;72(1):168–77. PMID:29239037
3056. Singhi AD, Lazenby AJ, Montgomery EA. Gastric adenocarcinoma with chief cell differentiation: a proposal for reclassification as oxyntic gland polyp/adenoma. Am J Surg Pathol. 2012 Jul;36(7):1030–5. PMID:22472957
3057. Singhi AD, Liu TC, Roncaioli JL, et al. Alternative lengthening of telomeres and loss of DAXX/ATRX expression predicts metastatic disease and poor survival in patients with pancreatic neuroendocrine tumors. Clin Cancer Res. 2017 Jan 15;23(2):600–9. PMID:27407094
3058. Singhi AD, McGrath K, Brand RE, et al. Preoperative next-generation sequencing of pancreatic cyst fluid is highly accurate in cyst classification and detection of advanced neoplasia. Gut. 2018 Dec;67(12):2131–41. PMID:28970292
3059. Singhi AD, Montgomery EA. Colorectal granular cell tumor: a clinicopathologic study of 26 cases. Am J Surg Pathol. 2010 Aug;34(8):1186–92. PMID:20661017
3060. Singhi AD, Montgomery EA. Gastrointestinal tract langerhans cell histiocytosis: a clinicopathologic study of 12 patients. Am J Surg Pathol. 2011 Feb;35(2):305–10. PMID:21263252
3061. Singhi AD, Norwood S, Liu TC, et al. Acinar cell cystadenoma of the pancreas: a benign neoplasm or non-neoplastic ballooning of acinar and ductal epithelium? Am J Surg Pathol. 2013 Sep;37(9):1329–35. PMID:24076773
3062. Singhi AD, Pai RK, Kant JA, et al. The histopathology of PRSS1 hereditary pancreatitis. Am J Surg Pathol. 2014 Mar;38(3):346–53. PMID:24525505
3063. Singhi AD, Seethala RR, Nason K, et al. Undifferentiated carcinoma of the esophagus: a clinicopathological study of 16 cases. Hum Pathol. 2015 Mar;46(3):366–75. PMID:25582499
3064. Sinkre PA, Murakata L, Rabin L, et al. Clear cell carcinoid tumor of the gallbladder: another distinctive manifestation of von Hippel-Lindau disease. Am J Surg Pathol. 2001 Oct;25(10):1334–9. PMID:11688471
3065. Sipos B, Frank S, Gress T, et al. Pancreatic intraepithelial neoplasia revisited and updated. Pancreatology. 2009;9(1-2):45–54. PMID:19077454
3066. Sipos B, Sperveslage J, Anlauf M, et al. Glucagon cell hyperplasia and neoplasia with and without glucagon receptor mutations. J Clin Endocrinol Metab. 2015 May;100(5):E783–8. PMID:25695890
3067. Sjödahl RI, Myrelid P, Söderholm JD. Anal and rectal cancer in Crohn's disease. Colorectal Dis. 2003 Sep;5(5):490–5. PMID:12925087
3068. Skubitz KM. Biology and treatment of aggressive fibromatosis or desmoid tumor. Mayo Clin Proc. 2017 Jun;92(6):947–64. PMID:28578783
3069. Slater DN, Cotton DW, Azzopardi JG. Oncocytic glomus tumour: a new variant. Histopathology. 1987 May;11(5):523–31. PMID:3038728
3070. Slowik V, Attard T, Dai H, et al. Desmoid tumors complicating familial adenomatous polyposis: a meta-analysis mutation spectrum of affected individuals. BMC Gastroenterol. 2015 Jul 16;15:84. PMID:26179480
3071. Slukvin II, Hafez GR, Niederhuber JE, et al. Combined serous microcystic adenoma and well-differentiated endocrine pancreatic neoplasm: a case report and review of the literature. Arch Pathol Lab Med. 2003 Oct;127(10):1369–72. PMID:14521452
3072. Smit VT, Boot AJ, Smits AM, et al. KRAS codon 12 mutations occur very frequently in pancreatic adenocarcinomas. Nucleic Acids Res. 1988 Aug 25;16(16):7773–82. PMID:3047672
3073. Smith JD, Reidy DL, Goodman KA, et al. A retrospective review of 126 high-grade neuroendocrine carcinomas of the colon and rectum. Ann Surg Oncol. 2014 Sep;21(9):2956–62. PMID:24763982
3074. Smith SL, Branton SA, Avino AJ, et al. Vasoactive intestinal polypeptide secreting islet cell tumors: a 15-year experience and review of the literature. Surgery. 1998 Dec;124(6):1050–5. PMID:9854582
3075. Smyrk TC, Watson P, Kaul K, et al. Tumor-infiltrating lymphocytes are a marker for microsatellite instability in colorectal carcinoma. Cancer. 2001 Jun 15;91(12):2417–22. PMID:11413533
3076. Smyth EC, Fassan M, Cunningham D, et al. Effect of pathologic tumor response and nodal status on survival in the Medical Research Council adjuvant gastric infusional chemotherapy trial. J Clin Oncol. 2016 Aug 10;34(23):2721–7. PMID:27298411
3077. Snowsill T, Coelho H, Huxley N, et al. Molecular testing for Lynch syndrome in people with colorectal cancer: systematic reviews and economic evaluation. Health Technol Assess. 2017 Sep;21(51):1–238. PMID:28895526
3078. Snowsill T, Huxley N, Hoyle M, et al. A systematic review and economic evaluation of diagnostic strategies for Lynch syndrome. Health Technol Assess. 2014 Sep;18(58):1–406. PMID:25244061
3079. Soeberg MJ, Rogers K, Currow DC, et al. Trends in incidence and survival for anal cancer in New South Wales, Australia, 1972-2009. Cancer Epidemiol. 2015 Dec;39(6):842–7. PMID:26651444
3080. Soetikno RM, Lin OS, Heidenreich PA, et al. Increased risk of colorectal neoplasia in patients with primary sclerosing cholangitis and ulcerative colitis: a meta-analysis. Gastrointest Endosc. 2002 Jul;56(1):48–54. PMID:12085034
3081. Soga J, Tazawa K. Pathologic analysis of carcinoids. Histologic reevaluation of 62 cases. Cancer. 1971 Oct;28(4):990–8. PMID:4106849
3082. Soga J, Yakuwa Y. Glucagonomas/diabetico-dermatogenic syndrome (DDS): a statistical evaluation of 407 reported cases. J Hepatobiliary Pancreat Surg. 1998;5(3):312–9. PMID:9880781
3083. Soga J, Yakuwa Y. Somatostatinoma/inhibitory syndrome: a statistical evaluation of 173 reported cases as compared to other pancreatic endocrinomas. J Exp Clin Cancer Res. 1999 Mar;18(1):13–22. PMID:10374671
3084. Soga J, Yakuwa Y. The gastrinoma/Zollinger-Ellison syndrome: statistical evaluation of a Japanese series of 359 cases. J Hepatobiliary Pancreat Surg. 1998;5(1):77–85. PMID:9683758
3085. Soga J, Yakuwa Y. Vipoma/diarrheogenic syndrome: a statistical evaluation of 241 reported cases. J Exp Clin Cancer Res. 1998 Dec;17(4):389–400. PMID:10089056
3086. Soga J. Carcinoids of the pancreas: an analysis of 156 cases. Cancer. 2005 Sep 15;104(6):1180–7. PMID:16104045
3087. Soga J. Endocrinocarcinomas (carcinoids and their variants) of the duodenum. An evaluation of 927 cases. J Exp Clin Cancer Res. 2003 Sep;22(3):349–63. PMID:14582691
3088. Soga J. Primary endocrinomas (carcinoids and variant neoplasms) of the gallbladder. A statistical evaluation of 138 reported cases. J Exp Clin Cancer Res. 2003 Mar;22(1):5–15. PMID:12725316
3089. Soga J. Primary hepatic endocrinomas (carcinoids and variant neoplasms). A statistical evaluation of 126 reported cases. J Exp Clin Cancer Res. 2002 Dec;21(4):457–68. PMID:12636090
3090. Sogabe M, Taniki T, Fukui Y, et al. A patient with esophageal hemangioma treated by endoscopic mucosal resection: a case report and review of the literature. J Med Invest. 2006 Feb;53(1-2):177–82. PMID:16538013

3091. Sohn TA, Yeo CJ, Cameron JL, et al. Intraductal papillary mucinous neoplasms of the pancreas: an updated experience. Ann Surg. 2004 Jun;239(6):788–97, discussion 797–9. PMID:15166958
3092. Sohn TA, Yeo CJ, Cameron JL, et al. Resected adenocarcinoma of the pancreas-616 patients: results, outcomes, and prognostic indicators. J Gastrointest Surg. 2000 Nov-Dec;4(6):567–79. PMID:11307091
3093. Soini Y, Welsh JA, Ishak KG, et al. p53 mutations in primary hepatic angiosarcomas not associated with vinyl chloride exposure. Carcinogenesis. 1995 Nov;16(11):2879–81. PMID:7586214
3094. Solcia E, Capella C, Fiocca R, et al. Disorders of the endocrine system. In: Ming SC, Goldman H, editors. Pathology of the gastrointestinal tract. 2nd ed. Philadelphia (PA): Williams and Wilkins; 1998. pp. 295–322.
3095. Solcia E, Capella C, Klöppel G. Tumors of the pancreas. Washington, DC: Armed Forces Institute of Pathology; 1997. (AFIP atlas of tumor pathology, series 3; fascicle 20).
3096. Solcia E, Capella C, Riva C, et al. The morphology and neuroendocrine profile of pancreatic epithelial VIPomas and extrapancreatic, VIP-producing, neurogenic tumors. Ann N Y Acad Sci. 1988;527:508–17. PMID:2839087
3097. Song HG, Yoo KS, Ju NR, et al. [A case of adenosquamous carcinoma of the papilla of Vater]. Korean J Gastroenterol. 2006 Aug;48(2):132–6. Korean. PMID:16929159
3098. Song X, Zheng S, Yang G, et al. Glucagonoma and the glucagonoma syndrome. Oncol Lett. 2018 Mar;15(3):2749–55. PMID:29435000
3099. Song Y, Li L, Ou Y, et al. Identification of genomic alterations in oesophageal squamous cell cancer. Nature. 2014 May 1;509(7498):91–5. PMID:24670651
3100. Sonnenberg A, Genta RM. Prevalence of benign gastric polyps in a large pathology database. Dig Liver Dis. 2015 Feb;47(2):164–9. PMID:25458775
3101. Sonoda Y, Yamaguchi K, Nagai E, et al. Small cell carcinoma of the cystic duct: a case report. J Gastrointest Surg. 2003 Jul-Aug;7(5):631–4. PMID:12850675
3102. Sorahan T, Lancashire RJ. Parental cigarette smoking and childhood risks of hepatoblastoma: OSCC data. Br J Cancer. 2004 Mar 8;90(5):1016–8. PMID:14997199
3103. Sorbye H, Strosberg J, Baudin E, et al. Gastroenteropancreatic high-grade neuroendocrine carcinoma. Cancer. 2014 Sep 15;120(18):2814–23. PMID:24771552
3104. Sorbye H, Welin S, Langer SW, et al. Predictive and prognostic factors for treatment and survival in 305 patients with advanced gastrointestinal neuroendocrine carcinoma (WHO G3): the NORDIC NEC study. Ann Oncol. 2013 Jan;24(1):152–60. PMID:22967994
3105. Sowery RD, Jensen C, Morrison KB, et al. Comparative genomic hybridization detects multiple chromosomal amplifications and deletions in undifferentiated embryonal sarcoma of the liver. Cancer Genet Cytogenet. 2001 Apr 15;126(2):128–33. PMID:11376805
3106. Spans L, Fletcher CD, Antonescu CR, et al. Recurrent MALAT1-GLI1 oncogenic fusion and GLI1 up-regulation define a subset of plexiform fibromyxoma. J Pathol. 2016 Jul;239(3):335–43. PMID:27101025
3107. Spechler SJ, Merchant JL, Wang TC, et al. A summary of the 2016 James W. Freston Conference of the American Gastroenterological Association: intestinal metaplasia in the esophagus and stomach: origins, differences, similarities and significance. Gastroenterology. 2017 Jul;153(1):e6–13. PMID:28583825
3108. Spector LG, Ross JA. Smoking and hepatoblastoma: confounding by birth weight? Br J Cancer. 2003 Aug 4;89(3):602, author reply 603. PMID:12888836
3109. Speel EJ, Richter J, Moch H, et al. Genetic differences in endocrine pancreatic tumor subtypes detected by comparative genomic hybridization. Am J Pathol. 1999 Dec;155(6):1787–94. PMID:10595906
3110. Speisky D, Duces A, Bièche I, et al. Molecular profiling of pancreatic neuroendocrine tumors in sporadic and Von Hippel-Lindau patients. Clin Cancer Res. 2012 May 15;18(10):2838–49. PMID:22461457
3111. Spence RW, Burns-Cox CJ. ACTH-secreting 'apudoma' of gallbladder. Gut. 1975 Jun;16(6):473–6. PMID:168130
3112. Sperti C, Pasquali C, Pedrazzoli S. Ductal adenocarcinoma of the body and tail of the pancreas. J Am Coll Surg. 1997 Sep;185(3):255–9. PMID:9291403
3113. Spier I, Holzapfel S, Altmüller J, et al. Frequency and phenotypic spectrum of germline mutations in POLE and seven other polymerase genes in 266 patients with colorectal adenomas and carcinomas. Int J Cancer. 2015 Jul 15;137(2):320–31. PMID:25529843
3114. Spigelman AD, Williams CB, Talbot IC, et al. Upper gastrointestinal cancer in patients with familial adenomatous polyposis. Lancet. 1989 Sep 30;2(8666):783–5. PMID:2571019
3116. Spiridakis KG, Sfakianakis EE, Flamourakis ME, et al. Synchronous mucinous adenocarcinoma of the recto sigmoid revealed by and seeding an anal fistula. (A case report and review of the literature). Int J Surg Case Rep. 2017;37:48–51. PMID:28641190
3117. Spring KJ, Zhao ZZ, Karamatic R, et al. High prevalence of sessile serrated adenomas with BRAF mutations: a prospective study of patients undergoing colonoscopy. Gastroenterology. 2006 Nov;131(5):1400–7. PMID:17101316
3118. Springer S, Wang Y, Dal Molin M, et al. A combination of molecular markers and clinical features improve the classification of pancreatic cysts. Gastroenterology. 2015 Nov;149(6):1501–10. PMID:26253305
3119. Srinivasan N, Teo JY, Chin YK, et al. Systematic review of the clinical utility and validity of the Sendai and Fukuoka Consensus Guidelines for the management of intraductal papillary mucinous neoplasms of the pancreas. HPB (Oxford). 2018 Jun;20(6):497–504. PMID:29486917
3120. Srivastava A, Hornick JL, Li X, et al. Extent of low-grade dysplasia is a risk factor for the development of esophageal adenocarcinoma in Barrett's esophagus. Am J Gastroenterol. 2007 Mar;102(3):483–93, quiz 694. PMID:17338734
3121. Srouji MN, Chatten J, Schulman WM, et al. Mesenchymal hamartoma of the liver in infants. Cancer. 1978 Nov;42(5):2483–9. PMID:363258
3122. Stachler MD, Taylor-Weiner A, Peng S, et al. Paired exome analysis of Barrett's esophagus and adenocarcinoma. Nat Genet. 2015 Sep;47(9):1047–55. PMID:26192918
3123. Stahl TJ, Schoetz DJ Jr, Roberts PL, et al. Crohn's disease and carcinoma: increasing justification for surveillance? Dis Colon Rectum. 1992 Sep;35(9):850–6. PMID:1511645
3124. Stancu M, Wu TT, Wallace C, et al. Genetic alterations in goblet cell carcinoids of the vermiform appendix and comparison with gastrointestinal carcinoid tumors. Mod Pathol. 2003 Dec;16(12):1189–98. PMID:14681318
3125. Adler DG, Qureshi W, Davila R, et al. The role of endoscopy in ampullary and duodenal adenomas. Gastrointest Endosc. 2006 Dec;64(6):849–54. PMID:17140885
3126. Stang A, Kluttig A. Etiologic insights from surface adjustment of colorectal carcinoma incidences: an analysis of the U.S. SEER data 2000-2004. Am J Gastroenterol. 2008 Nov;103(11):2853–61. PMID:18759825
3127. Starker LF, Carling T. Molecular genetics of gastroenteropancreatic neuroendocrine tumors. Curr Opin Oncol. 2009 Jan;21(1):29–33. PMID:19125015
3128. Stebbing J, Sanitt A, Nelson M, et al. A prognostic index for AIDS-associated Kaposi's sarcoma in the era of highly active antiretroviral therapy. Lancet. 2006 May 6;367(9521):1495–502. PMID:16679162
3129. Steele SR, Mullenix PS, Martin MJ, et al. Heterotopic gastric mucosa of the anus: a case report and review of the literature. Am Surg. 2004 Aug;70(8):715–9. PMID:15328807
3130. Steiner R, Kridel R, Giostra E, et al. Low 5-year cumulative incidence of post-transplant lymphoproliferative disorders after solid organ transplantation in Switzerland. Swiss Med Wkly. 2018 Mar 8;148:w14596. PMID:29518251
3131. Steinmüller T, Kianmanesh R, Falconi M, et al. Consensus guidelines for the management of patients with liver metastases from digestive (neuro)endocrine tumors: foregut, midgut, hindgut, and unknown primary. Neuroendocrinology. 2008;87(1):47–62. PMID:18097131
3132. Stelow EB, Murad FM, Debol SM, et al. A limited immunocytochemical panel for the distinction of subepithelial gastrointestinal mesenchymal neoplasms sampled by endoscopic ultrasound-guided fine-needle aspiration. Am J Clin Pathol. 2008 Feb;129(2):219–25. PMID:18208801
3133. Stelow EB, Shaco-Levy R, Bao F, et al. Pancreatic acinar cell carcinomas with prominent ductal differentiation: mixed acinar ductal carcinoma and mixed acinar endocrine ductal carcinoma. Am J Surg Pathol. 2010 Apr;34(4):510–8. PMID:20182344
3134. Stelow EB, Shami VM, Abbott TE, et al. The use of fine needle aspiration cytology for the distinction of pancreatic mucinous neoplasia. Am J Clin Pathol. 2008 Jan;129(1):67–74. PMID:18089490
3135. Stelzner S, Emmrich P. The mixed type in Laurén's classification of gastric carcinoma. Histologic description and biologic behavior. Gen Diagn Pathol. 1997 Jul;143(1):39–48. PMID:9269907
3136. Stephen AE, Berger DL. Carcinoma in the porcelain gallbladder: a relationship revisited. Surgery. 2001 Jun;129(6):699–703. PMID:11391368
3137. Stewart CJ, Mills PR, Carter R, et al. Brush cytology in the assessment of pancreatico-biliary strictures: a review of 406 cases. J Clin Pathol. 2001 Jun;54(6):449–55. PMID:11376018
3138. Stiles ZE, Behrman SW, Deneve JL, et al. Ampullary adenocarcinoma: defining predictors of survival and the impact of adjuvant therapy following surgical resection for stage I disease. J Surg Oncol. 2018 Jun;117(7):1500–8. PMID:29518820
3139. Stinner B, Kisker O, Zielke A, et al. Surgical management for carcinoid tumors of small bowel, appendix, colon, and rectum. World J Surg. 1996 Feb;20(2):183–8. PMID:8661815
3140. Stinner B, Rothmund M. Neuroendocrine tumours (carcinoids) of the appendix. Best Pract Res Clin Gastroenterol. 2005 Oct;19(5):729–38. PMID:16253897
3141. Stock N, Chibon F, Binh MB, et al. Adult-type rhabdomyosarcoma: analysis of 57 cases with clinicopathologic description, identification of 3 morphologic patterns and prognosis. Am J Surg Pathol. 2009 Dec;33(12):1850–9. PMID:19898221
3142. Stocker JT, Ishak KG. Undifferentiated (embryonal) sarcoma of the liver: report of 31 cases. Cancer. 1978 Jul;42(1):336–48. PMID:208754
3143. Stolte M. The new Vienna classification of epithelial neoplasia of the gastrointestinal tract: advantages and disadvantages. Virchows Arch. 2003 Feb;442(2):99–106. PMID:12596058
3144. Stolzenberg-Solomon RZ, Schairer C, Moore S, et al. Lifetime adiposity and risk of pancreatic cancer in the NIH-AARP Diet and Health Study cohort. Am J Clin Nutr. 2013 Oct;98(4):1057–65. PMID:23985810
3145. Stratakis CA, Carney JA. The triad of paragangliomas, gastric stromal tumours and pulmonary chondromas (Carney triad), and the dyad of paragangliomas and gastric stromal sarcomas (Carney-Stratakis syndrome): molecular genetics and clinical implications. J Intern Med. 2009 Jul;266(1):43–52. PMID:19522824
3146. Streubel B, Huber D, Wöhrer S, et al. Frequency of chromosomal aberrations involving MALT1 in mucosa-associated lymphoid tissue lymphoma in patients with Sjögren's syndrome. Clin Cancer Res. 2004 Jan 15;10(2):476–80. PMID:14760068
3147. Streubel B, Lamprecht A, Dierlamm J, et al. t(14;18)(q32;q21) involving IGH and MALT1 is a frequent chromosomal aberration in MALT lymphoma. Blood. 2003 Mar 15;101(6):2335–9. PMID:12406890
3148. Streubel B, Seitz G, Stolte M, et al. MALT lymphoma associated genetic aberrations occur at different frequencies in primary and secondary intestinal MALT lymphomas. Gut. 2006 Nov;55(11):1581–5. PMID:16556668
3149. Streubel B, Vinatzer U, Lamprecht A, et al. t(3;14)(p14.1;q32) involving IGH and FOXP1 is a novel recurrent chromosomal aberration in MALT lymphoma. Leukemia. 2005 Apr;19(4):652–8. PMID:15703784
3150. Strobel O, Hank T, Hinz U, et al. Pancreatic cancer surgery: the new R-status counts. Ann Surg. 2017 Mar;265(3):565–73. PMID:27918310
3151. Strobel O, Hartwig W, Bergmann F, et al. Anaplastic pancreatic cancer: presentation, surgical management, and outcome. Surgery. 2011 Feb;149(2):200–8. PMID:20542529
3152. Strobel O, Z'graggen K, Schmitz-Winnenthal FH, et al. Risk of malignancy in serous cystic neoplasms of the pancreas. Digestion. 2003;68(1):24–33. PMID:12949436
3153. Strosberg JR, Coppola D, Klimstra DS, et al. The NANETS consensus guidelines for the diagnosis and management of poorly differentiated (high-grade) extrapulmonary neuroendocrine carcinomas. Pancreas. 2010 Aug;39(6):799–800. PMID:20664477
3154. Sakamoto H, Yoshimura K, Saeki N, et al. Genetic variation in PSCA is associated with susceptibility to diffuse-type gastric cancer. Nat Genet. 2008 Jun;40(6):730–40. PMID:18488030
3156. Stålberg P, Westin G, Thirlwell C. Genetics and epigenetics in small intestinal neuroendocrine tumours. J Intern Med. 2016 Dec;280(6):584–94. PMID:27306880
3157. Su GH, Bansal R, Murphy KM, et al. ACVR1B (ALK4, activin receptor type 1B) gene mutations in pancreatic carcinoma. Proc Natl Acad Sci U S A. 2001 Mar 13;98(6):3254–7. PMID:11248065
3158. Su GH, Hruban RH, Bansal RK, et al. Germline and somatic mutations of the STK11/LKB1 Peutz-Jeghers gene in pancreatic and biliary cancers. Am J Pathol. 1999 Jun;154(6):1835–40. PMID:10362809
3159. Subramaniam K, Yeung D, Grimpen F, et al. Hepatosplenic T-cell lymphoma, immunosuppressive agents and biologicals: what are the risks? Intern Med J. 2014 Mar;44(3):287–90. PMID:24621284

3160. Suda K, Hirai S, Matsumoto Y, et al. Variant of intraductal carcinoma (with scant mucin production) is of main pancreatic duct origin: a clinicopathological study of four patients. Am J Gastroenterol. 1996 Apr;91(4):798–800. PMID:8677955
3161. Sugai T, Sugimoto R, Habano W, et al. Genetic differences stratified by PCR-based microsatellite analysis in gastric intramucosal neoplasia. Gastric Cancer. 2017 Mar;20(2):286–96. PMID:27236438
3162. Sugano K, Tack J, Kuipers EJ, et al. Kyoto global consensus report on Helicobacter pylori gastritis. Gut. 2015 Sep;64(9):1353–67. PMID:26187502
3163. Sugarbaker PH, Chang D. Results of treatment of 385 patients with peritoneal surface spread of appendiceal malignancy. Ann Surg Oncol. 1999 Dec;6(8):727–31. PMID:10622499
3164. Sugawara G, Yamaguchi A, Isogai M, et al. Small cell neuroendocrine carcinoma of the ampulla of Vater with foci of squamous differentiation: a case report. J Hepatobiliary Pancreat Surg. 2004;11(1):56–60. PMID:15747032
3164A. Sugawara S, Hirai I, Watanabe T, et al. A case of mucinous cystic neoplasm of the gallbladder. Clin J Gastroenterol. 2018 Oct;11(5):428–32. PMID:29536429
3165. Sugawara W, Haruta M, Sasaki F, et al. Promoter hypermethylation of the RASSF1A gene predicts the poor outcome of patients with hepatoblastoma. Pediatr Blood Cancer. 2007 Sep;49(3):240–9. PMID:16937357
3166. Sugihara A, Nakasho K, Ikuta S, et al. Oncocytic non-functioning endocrine tumor of the pancreas. Pathol Int. 2006 Dec;56(12):755–9. PMID:17096734
3167. Sugimoto S, Komatsu H, Morohoshi Y, et al. Recognition of and recent issues in hereditary diffuse gastric cancer. J Gastroenterol. 2015 Aug;50(8):831–43. PMID:26049741
3168. Sugimoto S, Yamada H, Takahashi M, et al. Early-onset diffuse gastric cancer associated with a de novo large genomic deletion of CDH1 gene. Gastric Cancer. 2014 Oct;17(4):745–9. PMID:23812922
3169. Sugiura T, Uesaka K, Kanemoto H, et al. Serum CA19-9 is a significant predictor among preoperative parameters for early recurrence after resection of pancreatic adenocarcinoma. J Gastrointest Surg. 2012 May;16(5):977–85. PMID:22411488
3170. Sugiyama M, Izumisato Y, Abe N, et al. Predictive factors for malignancy in intraductal papillary-mucinous tumours of the pancreas. Br J Surg. 2003 Oct;90(10):1244–9. PMID:14515294
3170A. Sulas P, Di Tommaso L, Novello C, et al. A large set of miRNAs is dysregulated from the earliest steps of human hepatocellular carcinoma development. Am J Pathol. 2018 Mar;188(3):785–94. PMID:29248455
3171. Sumazin P, Chen Y, Treviño LR, et al. Genomic analysis of hepatoblastoma identifies distinct molecular and prognostic subgroups. Hepatology. 2017 Jan;65(1):104–21. PMID:27775819
3172. Sumiyama K. Past and current trends in endoscopic diagnosis for early stage gastric cancer in Japan. Gastric Cancer. 2017 Mar;20 Suppl 1:20–7. PMID:27734273
3173. Sun J, Lu Z, Yang D, et al. Primary intestinal T-cell and NK-cell lymphomas: a clinicopathological and molecular study from China focused on type II enteropathy-associated T-cell lymphoma and primary intestinal NK-cell lymphoma. Mod Pathol. 2011 Jul;24(7):983–92. PMID:21423155
3174. Sun J, Yang Q, Lu Z, et al. Distribution of lymphoid neoplasms in China: analysis of 4,638 cases according to the World Health Organization classification. Am J Clin Pathol. 2012 Sep;138(3):429–34. PMID:22912361
3175. Sun P, Li YH, Wang W, et al. Malignancies of the anal canal: a multi-center retrospective analysis in South China population. J BUON. 2014 Jan-Mar;19(1):103–8. PMID:24659650
3176. Sun Y, Deng D, You WC, et al. Methylation of p16 CpG islands associated with malignant transformation of gastric dysplasia in a population-based study. Clin Cancer Res. 2004 Aug 1;10(15):5087–93. PMID:15297411
3177. Sun Y, Lu X, Xu Y, et al. Spontaneous rupture of a giant hepatobiliary serous cystadenoma: report of a case and literature review. Hepatol Int. 2010 Oct 12;5(1):603–6. PMID:21442059
3178. Sundaram V, Schuster DP, Falko JM. Unusual manifestations of Cushing's syndrome in a multiple endocrine neoplasia type I kindred. Endocr Pract. 1998 Jul-Aug;4(4):190–4. PMID:15251731
3179. Sundaresan S, Kang AJ, Merchant JL. Pathophysiology of gastric NETs: role of gastrin and menin. Curr Gastroenterol Rep. 2017 Jul;19(7):32. PMID:28608155
3180. Sundin A, Vullierme MP, Kaltsas G, et al. ENETS Consensus Guidelines for the Standards of Care in Neuroendocrine Tumors: radiological examinations. Neuroendocrinology. 2009;90(2):167–83. PMID:19077417
3181. Sunesen KG, Nørgaard M, Thorlacius-Ussing O, et al. Immunosuppressive disorders and risk of anal squamous cell carcinoma: a nationwide cohort study in Denmark, 1978-2005. Int J Cancer. 2010 Aug 1;127(3):675–84. PMID:19960431
3182. Sung JK. Diagnosis and management of gastric dysplasia. Korean J Intern Med. 2016 Mar;31(2):201–9. PMID:26932397
3183. Surveillance, Epidemiology, and End Results Program [Internet]. Bethesda (MD): National Cancer Institute; 2018. Cancer Stat Facts. Available from: https://seer.cancer.gov/statfacts/.
3184. Suster S, Huszar M, Herczeg E, et al. Adenosquamous carcinoma of the gallbladder with spindle cell features. A light microscopic and immunocytochemical study of a case. Histopathology. 1987 Feb;11(2):209–14. PMID:2437004
3185. Suzuki Y, Atomi Y, Sugiyama M, et al. Cystic neoplasm of the pancreas: a Japanese multiinstitutional study of intraductal papillary mucinous tumor and mucinous cystic tumor. Pancreas. 2004 Apr;28(3):241–6. PMID:15084964
3186. Suzuki Y, Mori T, Yokoyama M, et al. Hepatolithiasis: analysis of Japanese nationwide surveys over a period of 40 years. J Hepatobiliary Pancreat Sci. 2014 Sep;21(9):617–22. PMID:24824191
3187. Sveen A, Bruun J, Eide PW, et al. Colorectal cancer consensus molecular subtypes translated to preclinical models uncover potentially targetable cancer cell dependencies. Clin Cancer Res. 2018 Feb 15;24(4):794–806. PMID:29242316
3188. Svrcek M, Piton G, Cosnes J, et al. Small bowel adenocarcinomas complicating Crohn's disease are associated with dysplasia: a pathological and molecular study. Inflamm Bowel Dis. 2014 Sep;20(9):1584–92. PMID:25029614
3189. Swerdlow SH, Campo E, Harris NL, et al., editors. WHO classification of tumours of haematopoietic and lymphoid tissues. Lyon (France): International Agency for Research on Cancer; 2017. (WHO classification of tumours series, 4th rev. ed.; vol. 2). http://publications.iarc.fr/556.
3190. Swerdlow SH, Campo E, Pileri SA, et al. The 2016 revision of the World Health Organization classification of lymphoid neoplasms. Blood. 2016 May 19;127(20):2375–90. PMID:26980727
3191. Swerdlow SH, Campo E, Seto M, et al. Mantle cell lymphoma. In: Swerdlow SH, Campo E, Harris NL, et al., editors. WHO classification of tumours of haematopoietic and lymphoid tissues. Lyon (France): International Agency for Research on Cancer; 2017. pp. 285–90. (WHO classification of tumours series, 4th rev. ed.; vol. 2). http://publications.iarc.fr/556.
3192. Swerdlow SH, Webber SA, Chadburn A, et al. Post-transplant lymphoproliferative disorders. In: Swerdlow SH, Campo E, Harris NL, et al., editors. WHO classification of tumours of haematopoietic and lymphoid tissues. Lyon (France): International Agency for Research on Cancer; 2017. pp. 453–62. (WHO classification of tumours series, 4th rev. ed.; vol. 2). http://publications.iarc.fr/556.
3193. Syngal S, Brand RE, Church JM, et al. ACG clinical guideline: genetic testing and management of hereditary gastrointestinal cancer syndromes. Am J Gastroenterol. 2015 Feb;110(2):223–62, quiz 263. PMID:25645574
3194. Szucs Z, Thway K, Fisher C, et al. Molecular subtypes of gastrointestinal stromal tumors and their prognostic and therapeutic implications. Future Oncol. 2017 Jan;13(1):93–107. PMID:27600498
3195. Szántó I, Szentirmay Z, Banai J, et al. [Squamous papilloma of the esophagus. Clinical and pathological observations based on 172 papillomas in 155 patients]. Orv Hetil. 2005 Mar 20;146(12):547–52. Hungarian. PMID:15853063
3196. Tabatabaei SA, Moghadam NA, Ahmadinejad M, et al. Giant esophageal squamous papilloma: a case report. J Dig Dis. 2009 Aug;10(3):228–30. PMID:19659792
3197. Tachimori Y, Ozawa S, Numasaki H, et al. Comprehensive registry of esophageal cancer in Japan, 2010. Esophagus. 2017;14(3):189–214. PMID:28725168
3198. Tack GJ, van Wanrooij RL, Langerak AW, et al. Origin and immunophenotype of aberrant IEL in RCDII patients. Mol Immunol. 2012 Apr;50(4):262–70. PMID:22364936
3199. Taddesse-Heath L, Meloni-Ehrig A, Scheerle J, et al. Plasmablastic lymphoma with MYC translocation: evidence for a common pathway in the generation of plasmablastic features. Mod Pathol. 2010 Jul;23(7):991–9. PMID:20348882
3200. Tadepalli US, Feihel D, Miller KM, et al. A morphologic analysis of sessile serrated polyps observed during routine colonoscopy (with video). Gastrointest Endosc. 2011 Dec;74(6):1360–8. PMID:22018553
3201. Taefi A, Matsukuma K, Chak E. Massive epithelioid hemangioendothelioma causing noncirrhotic portal hypertension. Clin Gastroenterol Hepatol. 2018 Mar 31;S1542-3565(18)30334-3. PMID:29609064
3202. Taggart MW, Abraham SC, Overman MJ, et al. Goblet cell carcinoid tumor, mixed goblet cell carcinoid-adenocarcinoma, and adenocarcinoma of the appendix: comparison of clinicopathologic features and prognosis. Arch Pathol Lab Med. 2015 Jun;139(6):782–90. PMID:26030247
3203. Taggart MW, Galbincea J, Mansfield PF, et al. High-level microsatellite instability in appendiceal carcinomas. Am J Surg Pathol. 2013 Aug;37(8):1192–200. PMID:23648460
3204. Taghavi N, Biramijamal F, Sotoudeh M, et al. p16INK4a hypermethylation and p53, p16 and MDM2 protein expression in esophageal squamous cell carcinoma. BMC Cancer. 2010 Apr 13;10:138. PMID:20388212
3205. Tai CC, Curtis JL, Szmuszkovicz JR, et al. Abdominal involvement in pediatric heart and lung transplant recipients with posttransplant lymphoproliferative disease increases the risk of mortality. J Pediatr Surg. 2008 Dec;43(12):2174–7. PMID:19040929
3206. Taira N, Kawasaki H, Koja A, et al. Giant pedunclated lipoma of the esophagus: a case report. Int J Surg Case Rep. 2017;30:55–7. PMID:27902957
3207. Tajima S. Intraductal tubulopapillary neoplasm of the pancreas suspected by endoscopic ultrasonography-fine-needle aspiration cytology: report of a case confirmed by surgical specimen histology. Diagn Cytopathol. 2015 Dec;43(12):1003–6. PMID:26390029
3208. Tajiri T, Tate G, Inagaki T, et al. Intraductal tubular neoplasms of the pancreas: histogenesis and differentiation. Pancreas. 2005 Mar;30(2):115–21. PMID:15714133
3209. Tajiri T, Tate G, Kunimura T, et al. Histologic and immunohistochemical comparison of intraductal tubular carcinoma, intraductal papillary-mucinous carcinoma, and ductal adenocarcinoma of the pancreas. Pancreas. 2004 Aug;29(2):116–22. PMID:15257103
3210. Takahashi Y, Shimizu S, Ishida T, et al. Plexiform angiomyxoid myofibroblastic tumor of the stomach. Am J Surg Pathol. 2007 May;31(5):724–8. PMID:17460456
3211. Takahashi Y, Suzuki M, Fukusato T. Plexiform angiomyxoid myofibroblastic tumor of the stomach. World J Gastroenterol. 2010 Jun 21;16(23):2835–40. PMID:20556828
3212. Takano A, Hirotsu Y, Amemiya K, et al. Genetic basis of a common tumor origin in the development of pancreatic mixed acinar-neuroendocrine-ductal carcinoma: a case report. Oncol Lett. 2017 Oct;14(4):4428–32. PMID:29085438
3213. Takashima M, Ueki T, Nagai E, et al. Carcinoma of the ampulla of Vater associated with or without adenoma: a clinicopathologic analysis of 198 cases with reference to p53 and Ki-67 immunohistochemical expressions. Mod Pathol. 2000 Dec;13(12):1300–7. PMID:11144926
3214. Takata K, Miyata-Takata T, Sato Y, et al. Gastrointestinal follicular lymphoma: current knowledge and future challenges. Pathol Int. 2018 Jan;68(1):1–6. PMID:29292593
3215. Takata K, Noujima-Harada M, Miyata-Takata T, et al. Clinicopathologic analysis of 6 lymphomatoid gastropathy cases: expanding the disease spectrum to CD4-CD8+ cases. Am J Surg Pathol. 2015 Sep;39(9):1259–66. PMID:25929350
3216. Takata K, Okada H, Ohmiya N, et al. Primary gastrointestinal follicular lymphoma involving the duodenal second portion is a distinct entity: a multicenter, retrospective analysis in Japan. Cancer Sci. 2011 Aug;102(8):1532–6. PMID:21561531
3217. Takata K, Sato Y, Nakamura N, et al. Duodenal and nodal follicular lymphomas are distinct: the former lacks activation-induced cytidine deaminase and follicular dendritic cells despite ongoing somatic hypermutations. Mod Pathol. 2009 Jul;22(7):940–9. PMID:19396151
3218. Takata K, Sato Y, Nakamura N, et al. Duodenal follicular lymphoma lacks AID but expresses BACH2 and has memory B-cell characteristics. Mod Pathol. 2013 Jan;26(1):22–31. PMID:22899287
3219. Takata K, Tanino M, Ennishi D, et al. Duodenal follicular lymphoma: comprehensive gene expression analysis with insights into pathogenesis. Cancer Sci. 2014 May;105(5):608–15. PMID:24602001
3220. Takenaka A, Kaji I, Kasugai H, et al. Usefulness of diagnostic criteria for aspiration cytology of hepatocellular carcinoma. Acta Cytol. 1999 Jul-Aug;43(4):610–6. PMID:10432883
3221. Takeno A, Takemasa I, Seno S, et al.

Gene expression profile prospectively predicts peritoneal relapse after curative surgery of gastric cancer. Ann Surg Oncol. 2010 Apr;17(4):1033–42. PMID:20012501
3222. Takeuchi K, Yokoyama M, Ishizawa S, et al. Lymphomatoid gastropathy: a distinct clinicopathologic entity of self-limited pseudomalignant NK-cell proliferation. Blood. 2010 Dec 16;116(25):5631–7. PMID:20829373
3223. Takiff H, Calabria R, Yin L, et al. Mesenteric cysts and intra-abdominal cystic lymphangiomas. Arch Surg. 1985 Nov;120(11):1266–9. PMID:4051731
3224. Takubo K, Aida J, Sawabe M, et al. Early squamous cell carcinoma of the oesophagus: the Japanese viewpoint. Histopathology. 2007 Dec;51(6):733–42. PMID:17617215
3225. Takubo K, Nakagawa H, Tsuchiya S, et al. Seedling leiomyoma of the esophagus and esophagogastric junction zone. Hum Pathol. 1981 Nov;12(11):1006–10. PMID:7319487
3226. Talamonti MS, Goetz LH, Rao S, et al. Primary cancers of the small bowel: analysis of prognostic factors and results of surgical management. Arch Surg. 2002 May;137(5):564–70, discussion 570–1. PMID:11982470
3227. Talmon GA, Cohen SM. Mesenchymal hamartoma of the liver with an interstitial deletion involving chromosome band 19q13.4: a theory as to pathogenesis? Arch Pathol Lab Med. 2006 Aug;130(8):1216–8. PMID:16879027
3228. Tamura A, Ogasawara T, Fujii Y, et al. Glucagonoma with necrolytic migratory erythema: metabolic profile and detection of biallelic inactivation of DAXX gene. J Clin Endocrinol Metab. 2018 Jul 1;103(7):2417–23. PMID:29688432
3229. Tamura K, Yu J, Hata T, et al. Mutations in the pancreatic secretory enzymes CPA1 and CPB1 are associated with pancreatic cancer. Proc Natl Acad Sci U S A. 2018 May 1;115(18):4767–72. PMID:29669919
3230. Tan D, Lynch HT, editors. Principles of molecular diagnostics and personalized cancer medicine. Philadelphia (PA): Lippincott Williams & Wilkins; 2013.
3231. Tan MC, Basturk O, Brannon AR, et al. GNAS and KRAS mutations define separate progression pathways in intraductal papillary mucinous neoplasm-associated carcinoma. J Am Coll Surg. 2015 May;220(5):845–54.e1. PMID:25840541
3232. Tan MH, Mester J, Peterson C, et al. A clinical scoring system for selection of patients for PTEN mutation testing is proposed on the basis of a prospective study of 3042 probands. Am J Hum Genet. 2011 Jan 7;88(1):42–56. PMID:21194675
3233. Tan MH, Mester JL, Ngeow J, et al. Lifetime cancer risks in individuals with germline PTEN mutations. Clin Cancer Res. 2012 Jan 15;18(2):400–7. PMID:22252256
3234. Tan P, Yeoh KG. Genetics and molecular pathogenesis of gastric adenocarcinoma. Gastroenterology. 2015 Oct;149(5):1153–62.e3. PMID:26073375
3235. Tan SY, Chuang SS, Tang T, et al. Type II EATL (epitheliotropic intestinal T-cell lymphoma): a neoplasm of intra-epithelial T-cells with predominant CD8αα phenotype. Leukemia. 2013 Aug;27(8):1688–96. PMID:23399895
3236. Tan SY, Ooi AS, Ang MK, et al. Nuclear expression of MATK is a novel marker of type II enteropathy-associated T-cell lymphoma. Leukemia. 2011 Mar;25(3):555–7. PMID:21233830
3237. Tanabe S, Hirabayashi S, Oda I, et al. Gastric cancer treated by endoscopic submucosal dissection or endoscopic mucosal resection in Japan from 2004 through 2006: JGCA nationwide registry conducted in 2013. Gastric Cancer. 2017 Sep;20(5):834–42. PMID:28205058
3238. Tanaka M, Chari S, Adsay V, et al. International consensus guidelines for management of intraductal papillary mucinous neoplasms and mucinous cystic neoplasms of the pancreas. Pancreatology. 2006;6(1-2):17–32. PMID:16327281
3239. Tanaka M, Fernández-del Castillo C, Adsay V, et al. International consensus guidelines 2012 for the management of IPMN and MCN of the pancreas. Pancreatology. 2012 May-Jun;12(3):183–97. PMID:22687371
3240. Tanaka M, Fernández-Del Castillo C, Kamisawa T, et al. Revisions of international consensus Fukuoka guidelines for the management of IPMN of the pancreas. Pancreatology. 2017 Sep-Oct;17(5):738–53. PMID:28735806
3241. Tanaka M, Sawai H, Okada Y, et al. Clinicopathologic study of intraductal papillary-mucinous tumors and mucinous cystic tumors of the pancreas. Hepatogastroenterology. 2006 Sep-Oct;53(71):783–7. PMID:17086889
3242. Tanaka M, Wanless IR. Pathology of the liver in Budd-Chiari syndrome: portal vein thrombosis and the histogenesis of veno-centric cirrhosis, veno-portal cirrhosis, and large regenerative nodules. Hepatology. 1998 Feb;27(2):488–96. PMID:9462648
3243. Tanaka M. Intraductal papillary mucinous neoplasm of the pancreas as the main focus for early detection of pancreatic adenocarcinoma. Pancreas. 2018 May/Jun;47(5):544–50. PMID:29702531
3244. Tanaka T, Megahed N, Takata K, et al. A case of lymphomatoid gastropathy: an indolent CD56-positive atypical gastric lymphoid proliferation, mimicking aggressive NK/T cell lymphomas. Pathol Res Pract. 2011 Dec 15;207(12):786–9. PMID:22078056
3245. Tanaka Y, Ijiri R, Yamanaka S, et al. Pancreatoblastoma: optically clear nuclei in squamoid corpuscles are rich in biotin. Mod Pathol. 1998 Oct;11(10):945–9. PMID:9796720
3246. Tanaka Y, Kato K, Notohara K, et al. Frequent beta-catenin mutation and cytoplasmic/nuclear accumulation in pancreatic solid-pseudopapillary neoplasm. Cancer Res. 2001 Dec 1;61(23):8401–4. PMID:11731417
3247. Tanaka Y, Kato K, Notohara K, et al. Significance of aberrant (cytoplasmic/nuclear) expression of beta-catenin in pancreatoblastoma. J Pathol. 2003 Feb;199(2):185–90. PMID:12533831
3248. Tanaka Y, Notohara K, Kato K, et al. Usefulness of beta-catenin immunostaining for the differential diagnosis of solid-pseudopapillary neoplasm of the pancreas. Am J Surg Pathol. 2002 Jun;26(6):818–20. PMID:12023593
3249. Tanas MR, Sboner A, Oliveira AM, et al. Identification of a disease-defining gene fusion in epithelioid hemangioendothelioma. Sci Transl Med. 2011 Aug 31;3(98):98ra82. PMID:21885404
3250. Tanase A, Schmitz N, Stein H, et al. Allogeneic and autologous stem cell transplantation for hepatosplenic T-cell lymphoma: a retrospective study of the EBMT Lymphoma Working Party. Leukemia. 2015 Mar;29(3):686–8. PMID:25234166
3251. Tanase H, Suda K, Yamasaki S, et al. Intraductal low papillary histological pattern of carcinoma component shows intraductal spread in invasive carcinoma of the pancreas. J Hepatobiliary Pancreat Surg. 2006;13(3):235–8. PMID:16708301
3252. Tang LH, Aydin H, Brennan MF, et al. Clinically aggressive solid pseudopapillary tumors of the pancreas: a report of two cases with components of undifferentiated carcinoma and a comparative clinicopathologic analysis of 34 conventional cases. Am J Surg Pathol. 2005 Apr;29(4):512–9. PMID:15767807
3253. Tang LH, Basturk O, Sue JJ, et al. A practical approach to the classification of WHO grade 3 (G3) well-differentiated neuroendocrine tumor (WD-NET) and poorly differentiated neuroendocrine carcinoma (PD-NEC) of the pancreas. Am J Surg Pathol. 2016 Sep;40(9):1192–202. PMID:27259015
3254. Tang LH, Contractor T, Clausen R, et al. Attenuation of the retinoblastoma pathway in pancreatic neuroendocrine tumors due to increased Cdk4/Cdk6. Clin Cancer Res. 2012 Sep 1;18(17):4612–20. PMID:22761470
3255. Tang LH, Shia J, Soslow RA, et al. Pathologic classification and clinical behavior of the spectrum of goblet cell carcinoid tumors of the appendix. Am J Surg Pathol. 2008 Oct;32(10):1429–43. PMID:18685490
3256. Tang LH, Untch BR, Reidy DL, et al. Well-differentiated neuroendocrine tumors with a morphologically apparent high-grade component: a pathway distinct from poorly differentiated neuroendocrine carcinomas. Clin Cancer Res. 2016 Feb 15;22(4):1011–7. PMID:26482044
3257. Tang M, Deng Z, Li B, et al. Circulating tumor DNA is effective for detection of KRAS mutation in colorectal cancer: a meta-analysis. Int J Biol Markers. 2017 Oct 31;32(4):e421–7. PMID:28885658
3258. Taniere P, Borghi-Scoazec G, Saurin JC, et al. Cytokeratin expression in adenocarcinomas of the esophagogastric junction: a comparative study of adenocarcinomas of the distal esophagus and of the proximal stomach. Am J Surg Pathol. 2002 Sep;26(9):1213–21. PMID:12218578
3259. Taniguchi K, Roberts LR, Aderca IN, et al. Mutational spectrum of beta-catenin, AXIN1, and AXIN2 in hepatocellular carcinomas and hepatoblastomas. Oncogene. 2002 Jul 18;21(31):4863–71. PMID:12101426
3260. Tanimura A, Yamamoto H, Shibata H, et al. Carcinoma in heterotopic gastric pancreas. Acta Pathol Jpn. 1979 Mar;29(2):251–7. PMID:552797
3261. Tanno S, Obara T, Fujii T, et al. Alpha-fetoprotein-producing adenocarcinoma of the pancreas presenting focal hepatoid differentiation. Int J Pancreatol. 1999 Aug;26(1):43–7. PMID:10566157
3262. Tari A, Asaoku H, Takata K, et al. The role of "watch and wait" in intestinal follicular lymphoma in rituximab era. Scand J Gastroenterol. 2016 Mar;51(3):321–8. PMID:26382560
3263. Tari A, Kitadai Y, Mouri R, et al. Watch-and-wait policy versus rituximab-combined chemotherapy in Japanese patients with intestinal follicular lymphoma. J Gastroenterol Hepatol. 2018 Aug;33(8):1461–8. PMID:29377265
3264. Taruscio D, Paradisi S, Zamboni G, et al. Pancreatic acinar carcinoma shows a distinct pattern of chromosomal imbalances by comparative genomic hybridization. Genes Chromosomes Cancer. 2000 Jul;28(3):294–9. PMID:10862035
3265. Tateishi R, Taniguchi H, Wada A, et al. Argyrophil cells and melanocytes in esophageal mucosa. Arch Pathol. 1974 Aug;98(2):87–9. PMID:4134908
3266. Taylor PR, Abnet CC, Dawsey SM. Squamous dysplasia–the precursor lesion for esophageal squamous cell carcinoma. Cancer Epidemiol Biomarkers Prev. 2013 Apr;22(4):540–52. PMID:23549398
3267. Techavichit P, Masand PM, Himes RW, et al. Undifferentiated embryonal sarcoma of the liver (UESL): a single-center experience and review of the literature. J Pediatr Hematol Oncol. 2016 May;38(4):261–8. PMID:26925712
3268. Tekin K, Sungurtekin U, Aytekin FO, et al. Ectopic prostatic tissue of the anal canal presenting with rectal bleeding: report of a case. Dis Colon Rectum. 2002 Jul;45(7):979–80. PMID:12130891
3269. Temellini F, Bavosi M, Lamarra M, et al. Pancreatic metastasis 25 years after nephrectomy for renal cancer. Tumori. 1989 Oct 31;75(5):503–4. PMID:2603224
3270. Terada T, Matsunaga Y, Maeta H, et al. Mixed ductal-endocrine carcinoma of the pancreas presenting as gastrinoma with Zollinger-Ellison syndrome: an autopsy case with a 24 year survival period. Virchows Arch. 1999 Dec;435(6):606–11. PMID:10628803
3271. Terada T, Ohta T, Kitamura Y, et al. Cell proliferative activity in intraductal papillary-mucinous neoplasms and invasive ductal adenocarcinomas of the pancreas: an immunohistochemical study. Arch Pathol Lab Med. 1998 Jan;122(1):42–6. PMID:9448015
3272. Terada T, Ohta T, Nakanuma Y. Expression of oncogene products, anti-oncogene products and oncofetal antigens in intraductal papillary-mucinous neoplasm of the pancreas. Histopathology. 1996 Oct;29(4):355–61. PMID:8910043
3273. Terada T. Epstein-Barr virus associated lymphoepithelial carcinoma of the esophagus. Int J Clin Exp Med. 2013;6(3):219–26. PMID:23573354
3274. Terada T. Primary combined adenoid cystic carcinoma, basaloid squamous cell carcinoma, and squamous cell carcinoma of the esophagus. Endoscopy. 2012;44 Suppl 2 UCTN:E102–3. PMID:22473577
3275. Terada T. Primary signet-ring cell carcinoma of the pancreas diagnosed by endoscopic retrograde pancreatic duct biopsy: a case report with an immunohistochemical study. Endoscopy. 2012;44 Suppl 2 UCTN:E141–2. PMID:22619039
3276. Terada T. Small cell carcinoma of the ileum that developed 10 years after total gastrectomy for gastric signet-ring cell carcinoma. Appl Immunohistochem Mol Morphol. 2012 Dec;20(6):618–9. PMID:22417855
3277. Terai T, Sugimoto M, Uozaki H, et al. Lymphomatoidgastropathy mimicking extranodal NK/T cell lymphoma, nasal type: a case report. World J Gastroenterol. 2012 May 7;18(17):2140–4. PMID:22563204
3278. Terashima M, Kitada K, Ochiai A, et al. Impact of expression of human epidermal growth factor receptors EGFR and ERBB2 on survival in stage II/III gastric cancer. Clin Cancer Res. 2012 Nov 1;18(21):5992–6000. PMID:22977193
3279. Terris B, Cavard C. Diagnosis and molecular aspects of solid-pseudopapillary neoplasms of the pancreas. Semin Diagn Pathol. 2014 Nov;31(6):484–90. PMID:25524568
3280. Terris B, Dubois S, Buisine MP, et al. Mucin gene expression in intraductal papillary-mucinous pancreatic tumours and related lesions. J Pathol. 2002 Aug;197(5):632–7. PMID:12210083
3281. Tessier Cloutier B, Costa FD, Tazelaar HD, et al. Aberrant expression of neuroendocrine markers in angiosarcoma: a potential diagnostic pitfall. Hum Pathol. 2014 Aug;45(8):1618–24. PMID:24846674
3282. Testini M, Gurrado A, Lissidini G, et al. Management of mucinous cystic neoplasms of the pancreas. World J Gastroenterol. 2010 Dec 7;16(45):5682–92. PMID:21128317
3283. Tezuka K, Yamakawa M, Jingu A, et al. An unusual case of undifferentiated carcinoma in situ with osteoclast-like giant cells of the pancreas. Pancreas. 2006 Oct;33(3):304–10. PMID:17003654
3284. Thai E, Dalla Valle R, Evaristi F, et al. A case of biliary adenofibroma with malignant transformation. Pathol Res Pract. 2016 May;212(5):468–70. PMID:26778388
3285. The Cancer of the Liver Italian Program

(CLIP) investigators. A new prognostic system for hepatocellular carcinoma: a retrospective study of 435 patients. Hepatology. 1998 Sep;28(3):751–5. PMID:9731568
3286. The Non-Hodgkin's Lymphoma Classification Project. A clinical evaluation of the International Lymphoma Study Group classification of non-Hodgkin's lymphoma. Blood. 1997 Jun 1;89(11):3909–18. PMID:9166827
3287. The Paris endoscopic classification of superficial neoplastic lesions: esophagus, stomach, and colon: November 30 to December 1, 2002. Gastrointest Endosc. 2003 Dec;58(6 Suppl):S3–43. PMID:14652541
3288. Theegarten D, Reinacher A, Graeven U, et al. Mixed malignant germ cell tumour of the liver. Virchows Arch. 1998 Jul;433(1):93–6. PMID:9692832
3289. Thieblemont C, Bastion Y, Berger F, et al. Mucosa-associated lymphoid tissue gastrointestinal and nongastrointestinal lymphoma behavior: analysis of 108 patients. J Clin Oncol. 1997 Apr;15(4):1624–30. PMID:9193362
3290. Thieblemont C, Berger F, Dumontet C, et al. Mucosa-associated lymphoid tissue lymphoma is a disseminated disease in one third of 158 patients analyzed. Blood. 2000 Feb 1;95(3):802–6. PMID:10648389
3291. Thieblemont C, Bertoni F, Copie-Bergman C, et al. Chronic inflammation and extranodal marginal-zone lymphomas of MALT-type. Semin Cancer Biol. 2014 Feb;24:33–42. PMID:24333758
3292. Thierry AR, Mouliere F, El Messaoudi S, et al. Clinical validation of the detection of KRAS and BRAF mutations from circulating tumor DNA. Nat Med. 2014 Apr;20(4):430–5. PMID:24658074
3293. Thies S, Guldener L, Slotta-Huspenina J, et al. Impact of peritumoral and intratumoral budding in esophageal adenocarcinomas. Hum Pathol. 2016 Jun;52:1–8. PMID:26980046
3294. Thies S, Langer R. Tumor regression grading of gastrointestinal carcinomas after neoadjuvant treatment. Front Oncol. 2013 Oct 7;3:262. PMID:24109590
3295. Thirabanjasak D, Basturk O, Altinel D, et al. Is serous cystadenoma of the pancreas a model of clear-cell-associated angiogenesis and tumorigenesis? Pancreatology. 2009;9(1-2):182–8. PMID:19077470
3296. Thirunavukarasu P, Sathaiah M, Singla S, et al. Medullary carcinoma of the large intestine: a population based analysis. Int J Oncol. 2010 Oct;37(4):901–7. PMID:20811712
3297. Thomas de Montpréville V, Le Pavec J, Le Roy Ladurie F, et al. Lymphoproliferative disorders after lung transplantation: clinicopathological characterization of 16 cases with identification of very-late-onset forms. Respiration. 2015;90(6):451–9. PMID:26506523
3298. Thomas M, Bienkowski R, Vandermeer TJ, et al. Malignant transformation in perianal fistulas of Crohn's disease: a systematic review of literature. J Gastrointest Surg. 2010 Jan;14(1):66–73. PMID:19826882
3299. Thomas RM, Sobin LH. Gastrointestinal cancer. Cancer. 1995 Jan 1;75(1 Suppl):154–70. PMID:8000994
3300. Thompson BA, Spurdle AB, Plazzer JP, et al. Application of a 5-tiered scheme for standardized classification of 2,360 unique mismatch repair gene variants in the InSiGHT locus-specific database. Nat Genet. 2014 Feb;46(2):107–15. PMID:24362816
3301. Thompson K, Castelli MJ, Gattuso P. Metastatic papillary oncocytic carcinoma of the pancreas to the liver diagnosed by fine-needle aspiration. Diagn Cytopathol. 1998 Apr;18(4):291–6. PMID:9557266
3302. Thompson LD, Becker RC, Przygodzki RM, et al. Mucinous cystic neoplasm (mucinous cystadenocarcinoma of low-grade malignant potential) of the pancreas: a clinicopathologic study of 130 cases. Am J Surg Pathol. 1999 Jan;23(1):1–16. PMID:9888699
3303. Thompson SM, Zendejas-Mummert B, Hartgers ML, et al. Malignant transformation of biliary adenofibroma: a rare biliary cystic tumor. J Gastrointest Oncol. 2016 Dec;7(6):E107–12. PMID:28078134
3304. Thonhofer R, Siegel C, Trummer M, et al. Mastocytic enterocolitis as a rare cause of chronic diarrhea in a patient with rheumatoid arthritis. Wien Klin Wochenschr. 2011 May;123(9-10):297–8. PMID:21499916
3305. Thrift AP. Barrett's esophagus and esophageal adenocarcinoma: how common are they really? Dig Dis Sci. 2018 Aug;63(8):1988–96. PMID:29671158
3306. Thrift AP. The epidemic of oesophageal carcinoma: Where are we now? Cancer Epidemiol. 2016 Apr;41:88–95. PMID:26851752
3307. Thurberg BL, Duray PH, Odze RD. Polypoid dysplasia in Barrett's esophagus: a clinicopathologic, immunohistochemical, and molecular study of five cases. Hum Pathol. 1999 Jul;30(7):745–52. PMID:10414492
3308. Thway K, Fisher C. Diffuse ganglioneuromatosis in small intestine associated with neurofibromatosis type 1. Ann Diagn Pathol. 2009 Feb;13(1):50–4. PMID:19118783
3309. Tickoo SK, Zee SY, Obiekwe S, et al. Combined hepatocellular-cholangiocarcinoma: a histopathologic, immunohistochemical, and in situ hybridization study. Am J Surg Pathol. 2002 Aug;26(8):989–97. PMID:12170085
3310. Tiemann K, Heitling U, Kosmahl M, et al. Solid pseudopapillary neoplasms of the pancreas show an interruption of the Wnt-signaling pathway and express gene products of 11q. Mod Pathol. 2007 Sep;20(9):955–60. PMID:17632456
3311. Tierney RJ, Shannon-Lowe CD, Fitzsimmons L, et al. Unexpected patterns of Epstein-Barr virus transcription revealed by a high throughput PCR array for absolute quantification of viral mRNA. Virology. 2015 Jan 1;474:117–30. PMID:25463610
3312. Tjon JM, Verbeek WH, Kooy-Winkelaar YM, et al. Defective synthesis or association of T-cell receptor chains underlies loss of surface T-cell receptor-CD3 expression in enteropathy-associated T-cell lymphoma. Blood. 2008 Dec 15;112(13):5103–10. PMID:18815285
3313. Toba T, Inoshita N, Kaise M, et al. Clinicopathological features of superficial non-ampurally duodenal epithelial tumor; gastric phenotype of histology correlates to higher malignant potency. J Gastroenterol. 2018 Jan;53(1):64–70. PMID:28321513
3314. Todoroki T, Sano T, Yamada S, et al. Clear cell carcinoid tumor of the distal common bile duct. World J Surg Oncol. 2007 Jan 17;5:6. PMID:17227590
3315. Tohda G, Osawa T, Asada Y, et al. Gastric adenocarcinoma of fundic gland type: endoscopic and clinicopathological features. World J Gastrointest Endosc. 2016 Feb 25;8(4):244–51. PMID:26962407
3316. Tomasetti C, Marchionni L, Nowak MA, et al. Only three driver gene mutations are required for the development of lung and colorectal cancers. Proc Natl Acad Sci U S A. 2015 Jan 6;112(1):118–23. PMID:25535351
3317. Tomasetti C, Vogelstein B, Parmigiani G. Half or more of the somatic mutations in cancers of self-renewing tissues originate prior to tumor initiation. Proc Natl Acad Sci U S A. 2013 Feb 5;110(6):1999–2004. PMID:23345422
3319. Tomioka K, Fukoe Y, Lee Y, et al. Primary neuroendocrine carcinoma of the appendix: a case report and review of the literature. Anticancer Res. 2013 Jun;33(6):2635–8. PMID:23749920
3320. Tomita S, Kikuti YY, Carreras J, et al. Genomic and immunohistochemical profiles of enteropathy-associated T-cell lymphoma in Japan. Mod Pathol. 2015 Oct;28(10):1286–96. PMID:26226842
3321. Tomizawa M, Saisho H. Insulin-like growth factor (IGF)-II regulates CCAAT/enhancer binding protein alpha expression via phosphatidyl-inositol 3 kinase in human hepatoblastoma cell lines. J Cell Biochem. 2007 Sep 1;102(1):161–70. PMID:17372916
3322. Tomlinson JS, Jain S, Bentrem DJ, et al. Accuracy of staging node-negative pancreas cancer: a potential quality measure. Arch Surg. 2007 Aug;142(8):767–73, discussion 773–4. PMID:17709731
3323. Tomlinson JS, Jarnagin WR, DeMatteo RP, et al. Actual 10-year survival after resection of colorectal liver metastases defines cure. J Clin Oncol. 2007 Oct 10;25(29):4575–80. PMID:17925551
3324. Topalian SL, Taube JM, Anders RA, et al. Mechanism-driven biomarkers to guide immune checkpoint blockade in cancer therapy. Nat Rev Cancer. 2016 May;16(5):275–87. PMID:27079802
3325. Torbenson M. Fibrolamellar carcinoma: 2012 update. Scientifica (Cairo). 2012;2012:743790. PMID:24278737
3326. Torbenson M. Hepatic adenomas: classification, controversies, and consensus. Surg Pathol Clin. 2018 Jun;11(2):351–66. PMID:29751879
3327. Torbenson MS. Morphologic subtypes of hepatocellular carcinoma. Gastroenterol Clin North Am. 2017 Jun;46(2):365–91. PMID:28506370
3328. Torlakovic E, Skovlund E, Snover DC, et al. Morphologic reappraisal of serrated colorectal polyps. Am J Surg Pathol. 2003 Jan;27(1):65–81. PMID:12502929
3329. Torlakovic EE, Gomez JD, Driman DK, et al. Sessile serrated adenoma (SSA) vs. traditional serrated adenoma (TSA). Am J Surg Pathol. 2008 Jan;32(1):21–9. PMID:18162766
3330. Tornesello ML, Biryahwaho B, Downing R, et al. Human herpesvirus type 8 variants circulating in Europe, Africa and North America in classic, endemic and epidemic Kaposi's sarcoma lesions during pre-AIDS and AIDS era. Virology. 2010 Mar 15;398(2):280–9. PMID:20079510
3331. Torre LA, Siegel RL, Ward EM, et al. Global cancer incidence and mortality rates and trends–an update. Cancer Epidemiol Biomarkers Prev. 2016 Jan;25(1):16–27. PMID:26667886
3331A. Torrecilla S, Sia D, Harrington AN, et al. Trunk mutational events present minimal intra- and inter-tumoral heterogeneity in hepatocellular carcinoma. J Hepatol. 2017 Dec;67(6):1222–31. PMID:28843658
3332. Toumi O, Ammar H, Korbi I, et al. Gastroblastoma, a biphasic neoplasm of stomach: a case report. Int J Surg Case Rep. 2017;39:72–6. PMID:28822310
3333. Towbin AJ, Meyers RL, Woodley H, et al. 2017 PRETEXT: radiologic staging system for primary hepatic malignancies of childhood revised for the Paediatric Hepatic International Tumour Trial (PHITT). Pediatr Radiol. 2018 Apr;48(4):536–54. PMID:29427028
3334. Tracey KJ, O'Brien MJ, Williams LF, et al. Signet ring carcinoma of the pancreas, a rare variant with very high CEA values. Immunohistologic comparison with adenocarcinoma. Dig Dis Sci. 1984 Jun;29(6):573–6. PMID:6327210
3335. Trakarnsanga A, Gönen M, Shia J, et al. Comparison of tumor regression grade systems for locally advanced rectal cancer after multimodality treatment. J Natl Cancer Inst. 2014 Sep 22;106(10):dju248. PMID:25249540
3336. Tran-Duy A, Spaetgens B, Hoes AW, et al. Use of proton pump inhibitors and risks of fundic gland polyps and gastric cancer: systematic review and meta-analysis. Clin Gastroenterol Hepatol. 2016 Dec;14(12):1706–19.e5. PMID:27211501
3337. Trappe RU, Choquet S, Dierickx D, et al. International prognostic index, type of transplant and response to rituximab are key parameters to tailor treatment in adults with CD20-positive B cell PTLD: clues from the PTLD-1 trial. Am J Transplant. 2015 Apr;15(4):1091–100. PMID:25736912
3338. Traverso LW, Peralta EA, Ryan JA Jr, et al. Intraductal neoplasms of the pancreas. Am J Surg. 1998 May;175(5):426–32. PMID:9600293
3339. Travert M, Huang Y, de Leval L, et al. Molecular features of hepatosplenic T-cell lymphoma unravels potential novel therapeutic targets. Blood. 2012 Jun 14;119(24):5795–806. PMID:22510872
3340. Trikudanathan G, Navaneethan U, Njei B, et al. Diagnostic yield of bile duct brushings for cholangiocarcinoma in primary sclerosing cholangitis: a systematic review and meta-analysis. Gastrointest Endosc. 2014 May;79(5):783–9. PMID:24140129
3341. Tripathi M, Swanson PE. Rare tumors of esophageal squamous mucosa. Ann N Y Acad Sci. 2016 Oct;1381(1):122–32. PMID:27310830
3342. Trobaugh-Lotrario AD, Tomlinson GE, Finegold MJ, et al. Small cell undifferentiated variant of hepatoblastoma: adverse clinical and molecular features similar to rhabdoid tumors. Pediatr Blood Cancer. 2009 Mar;52(3):328–34. PMID:18985717
3343. Trovik CS, Bauer HC, Alvegård TA, et al. Surgical margins, local recurrence and metastasis in soft tissue sarcomas: 559 surgically-treated patients from the Scandinavian Sarcoma Group Register. Eur J Cancer. 2000 Apr;36(6):710–6. PMID:10762742
3344. Truta B, Chen YY, Blanco AM, et al. Tumor histology helps to identify Lynch syndrome among colorectal cancer patients. Fam Cancer. 2008;7(3):267–74. PMID:18283560
3345. Tsai DE, Bagley S, Reshef R, et al. The changing face of adult posttransplant lymphoproliferative disorder: changes in histology between 1999 and 2013. Am J Hematol. 2018 Jul;93(7):874–81. PMID:29659047
3346. Tsai JH, Liau JY, Lin YL, et al. Traditional serrated adenoma has two pathways of neoplastic progression that are distinct from the sessile serrated pathway of colorectal carcinogenesis. Mod Pathol. 2014 Oct;27(10):1375–85. PMID:24603588
3347. Tsai JH, Liau JY, Yuan CT, et al. RNF43 is an early and specific mutated gene in the serrated pathway, with increased frequency in traditional serrated adenoma and its associated malignancy. Am J Surg Pathol. 2016 Oct;40(10):1352–9. PMID:27305845
3348. Tsai JH, Liau JY, Yuan CT, et al. RNF43 mutation frequently occurs with GNAS mutation and mucin hypersecretion in intraductal papillary neoplasms of the bile duct. Histopathology. 2017 Apr;70(5):756–65. PMID:27864998
3349. Tsai JH, Yuan RH, Chen YL, et al. GNAS is frequently mutated in a specific subgroup of intraductal papillary neoplasms of the bile duct. Am J Surg Pathol. 2013 Dec;37(12):1862–70. PMID:24061513
3350. Tsang ES, McConnell YJ, Schaeffer DF, et al. Prognostic factors for locoregional recurrence in neuroendocrine tumors of the rectum. Dis Colon Rectum. 2018 Feb;61(2):187–92. PMID:29337773
3351. Tschang TP, Garza-Garza R, Kissane JM. Pleomorphic carcinoma of the

pancreas: an analysis of 15 cases. Cancer. 1977 May;39(5):2114–26. PMID:870168
3352. Tse E, Gill H, Loong F, et al. Type II enteropathy-associated T-cell lymphoma: a multicenter analysis from the Asia Lymphoma Study Group. Am J Hematol. 2012 Jul;87(7):663–8. PMID:22641357
3353. Tseng HF, Morgenstern H, Mack TM, et al. Risk factors for anal cancer: results of a population-based case–control study. Cancer Causes Control. 2003 Nov;14(9):837–46. PMID:14682441
3354. Tseng JF, Warshaw AL, Sahani DV, et al. Serous cystadenoma of the pancreas: tumor growth rates and recommendations for treatment. Ann Surg. 2005 Sep;242(3):413–9, discussion 419–21. PMID:16135927
3355. Tsokos CG, Krings G, Yilmaz F, et al. Proliferative index facilitates distinction between benign biliary lesions and intrahepatic cholangiocarcinoma. Hum Pathol. 2016 Nov;57:61–7. PMID:27396933
3356. Tsoukalas N, Chatzellis E, Rontogianni D, et al. Pancreatic carcinoids (serotonin-producing pancreatic neuroendocrine neoplasms): report of 5 cases and review of the literature. Medicine (Baltimore). 2017 Apr;96(16):e6201. PMID:28422824
3357. Tsuboniwa N, Miki T, Kuroda M, et al. Primary adenocarcinoma in an ileal conduit. Int J Urol. 1996 Jan;3(1):64–6. PMID:8646603
3358. Tsuchiya K, Komuta M, Yasui Y, et al. Expression of keratin 19 is related to high recurrence of hepatocellular carcinoma after radiofrequency ablation. Oncology. 2011;80(3-4):278–88. PMID:21734420
3359. Tsuda M, Asaka M, Kato M, et al. Effect on Helicobacter pylori eradication therapy against gastric cancer in Japan. Helicobacter. 2017 Oct;22(5). PMID:28771894
3360. Tsui WM, Colombari R, Portmann BC, et al. Hepatic angiomyolipoma: a clinicopathologic study of 30 cases and delineation of unusual morphologic variants. Am J Surg Pathol. 1999 Jan;23(1):34–48. PMID:9888702
3361. Tsui WM, Lam PW, Mak CK, et al. Fine-needle aspiration cytologic diagnosis of intrahepatic biliary papillomatosis (intraductal papillary tumor): report of three cases and comparative study with cholangiocarcinoma. Diagn Cytopathol. 2000 May;22(5):293–8. PMID:10790236
3362. Tsui WM, Loo KT, Chow LT, et al. Biliary adenofibroma. A heretofore unrecognized benign biliary tumor of the liver. Am J Surg Pathol. 1993 Feb;17(2):186–92. PMID:8422113
3363. Tsukashita S, Kushima R, Bamba M, et al. MUC gene expression and histogenesis of adenocarcinoma of the stomach. Int J Cancer. 2001 Oct 15;94(2):166–70. PMID:11668493
3364. Tsutsui A, Bando Y, Sato Y, et al. Biliary adenofibroma with ominous features of imminent malignant changes. Clin J Gastroenterol. 2014 Oct;7(5):441–8. PMID:26184026
3365. Tuncel D, Roa JC, Araya JC, et al. Poorly cohesive cell (diffuse-infiltrative/signet ring cell) carcinomas of the gallbladder: clinicopathological analysis of 24 cases identified in 628 gallbladder carcinomas. Hum Pathol. 2017 Feb;60:24–31. PMID:27666767
3366. Turaga KK, Kvols LK. Recent progress in the understanding, diagnosis, and treatment of gastroenteropancreatic neuroendocrine tumors. CA Cancer J Clin. 2011 Mar-Apr;61(2):113–32. PMID:21388967
3367. Turcot J, Despres JP, St Pierre F. Malignant tumors of the central nervous system associated with familial polyposis of the colon: report of two cases. Dis Colon Rectum. 1959 Sep-Oct;2:465–8. PMID:13839882
3368. Turner JK, Williams GT, Morgan M, et al. Interobserver agreement in the reporting of colorectal polyp pathology among bowel cancer screening pathologists in Wales. Histopathology. 2013 May;62(6):916–24. PMID:23611360
3369. Turner JR, Odze RD. Proliferative characteristics of differentiated cells in familial adenomatous polyposis-associated duodenal adenomas. Hum Pathol. 1996 Jan;27(1):63–9. PMID:8543313
3370. Turner KO, Genta RM, Sonnenberg A. Oesophageal signet ring cell carcinoma as complication of gastro-oesophageal reflux disease. Aliment Pharmacol Ther. 2015 Nov;42(10):1222–31. PMID:26345286
3371. Tustumi F, Takeda FR, Uema RH, et al. Primary neuroendocrine neoplasm of the esophagus - report of 14 cases from a single institute and review of the literature. Arq Gastroenterol. 2017 Jan-Mar;54(1):4–10. PMID:28079231
3372. Tuttle R, Kane JM 3rd. Biopsy techniques for soft tissue and bowel sarcomas. J Surg Oncol. 2015 Apr;111(5):504–12. PMID:25663366
3373. Tyson GL, El-Serag HB. Risk factors for cholangiocarcinoma. Hepatology. 2011 Jul;54(1):173–84. PMID:21488076
3374. Tyson GL, Ilyas JA, Duan Z, et al. Secular trends in the incidence of cholangiocarcinoma in the USA and the impact of misclassification. Dig Dis Sci. 2014 Dec;59(12):3103–10. PMID:25204668
3375. Tzeng CW, Balachandran A, Ahmad M, et al. Serum carbohydrate antigen 19-9 represents a marker of response to neoadjuvant therapy in patients with borderline resectable pancreatic cancer. HPB (Oxford). 2014 May;16(5):430–8. PMID:23991810
3376. Ubiali A, Benetti A, Papotti M, et al. Genetic alterations in poorly differentiated endocrine colon carcinomas developing in tubulo-villous adenomas: a report of two cases. Virchows Arch. 2001 Dec;439(6):776–81. PMID:11787850
3377. Uccella S, Blank A, Maragliano R, et al. Calcitonin-producing neuroendocrine neoplasms of the pancreas: clinicopathological study of 25 cases and review of the literature. Endocr Pathol. 2017 Dec;28(4):351–61. PMID:29063495
3378. Uccella S, La Rosa S, Volante M, et al. Immunohistochemical biomarkers of gastrointestinal, pancreatic, pulmonary, and thymic neuroendocrine neoplasms. Endocr Pathol. 2018 Jun;29(2):150–68. PMID:29520563
3379. Uchida N, Kamada H, Tsutsui K, et al. Utility of pancreatic duct brushing for diagnosis of pancreatic carcinoma. J Gastroenterol. 2007 Aug;42(8):657–62. PMID:17701129
3380. Ueda T, Volinia S, Okumura H, et al. Relation between microRNA expression and progression and prognosis of gastric cancer: a microRNA expression analysis. Lancet Oncol. 2010 Feb;11(2):136–46. PMID:20022810
3381. Ueno H, Mochizuki H, Hashiguchi Y, et al. Histological grading of colorectal cancer: a simple and objective method. Ann Surg. 2008 May;247(5):811–8. PMID:18438118
3382. Ueo T, Kashima K, Daa T, et al. Immunohistochemical analysis of morules in colonic neoplasms: morules are morphologically and qualitatively different from squamous metaplasia. Pathobiology. 2005;72(5):269–78. PMID:16374071
3383. Ueyama H, Matsumoto K, Nagahara A, et al. Gastric adenocarcinoma of the fundic gland type (chief cell predominant type). Endoscopy. 2014 Feb;46(2):153–7. PMID:24338239
3384. Ueyama H, Yao T, Nakashima Y, et al. Gastric adenocarcinoma of fundic gland type (chief cell predominant type): proposal for a new entity of gastric adenocarcinoma. Am J Surg Pathol. 2010 May;34(5):609–19. PMID:20410811
3385. Ueyama T, Nagai E, Yao T, et al. Vimentin-positive gastric carcinomas with rhabdoid features. A clinicopathologic and immunohistochemical study. Am J Surg Pathol. 1993 Aug;17(8):813–9. PMID:7687828
3385A. UICC [Internet]. Geneva (Switzerland): Union for International Cancer Control; 2019. TNM Publications and Resources; updated 2019 Feb 4. Available from: https://www.uicc.org/resources/tnm/publications-resources.
3385B. Um TH, Kim H, Oh BK, et al. Aberrant CpG island hypermethylation in dysplastic nodules and early HCC of hepatitis B virus-related human multistep hepatocarcinogenesis. J Hepatol. 2011 May;54(5):939–47. PMID:21145824
3386. Umar SB, Fleischer DE. Esophageal cancer: epidemiology, pathogenesis and prevention. Nat Clin Pract Gastroenterol Hepatol. 2008 Sep;5(9):517–26. PMID:18679388
3387. Uncu H, Erdem E, Kuterdem E. Lymphangiomas of the ileum: a report of two cases and a review of the literature. Surg Today. 1997;27(6):542–5. PMID:9306548
3389. Urganci N, Genc DB, Kose G, et al. Colorectal cancer due to constitutional mismatch repair deficiency mimicking neurofibromatosis I. Pediatrics. 2015 Oct;136(4):e1047–50. PMID:26391938
3390. Uribe-Uribe NO, Jimenez-Garduño AM, Henson DE, et al. Paraneoplastic sensory neuropathy associated with small cell carcinoma of the gallbladder. Ann Diagn Pathol. 2009 Apr;13(2):124–6. PMID:19302962
3391. Ushiku T, Arnason T, Ban S, et al. Very well-differentiated gastric carcinoma of intestinal type: analysis of diagnostic criteria. Mod Pathol. 2013 Dec;26(12):1620–31. PMID:23723017
3392. Ushiku T, Arnason T, Fukayama M, et al. Extra-ampullary duodenal adenocarcinoma. Am J Surg Pathol. 2014 Nov;38(11):1484–93. PMID:25310836
3393. Ushiku T, Ishikawa S, Kakiuchi M, et al. RHOA mutation in diffuse-type gastric cancer: a comparative clinicopathology analysis of 87 cases. Gastric Cancer. 2016 Apr;19(2):403–11. PMID:25823974
3394. Ushiku T, Matsusaka K, Iwasaki Y, et al. Gastric carcinoma with invasive micropapillary pattern and its association with lymph node metastasis. Histopathology. 2011 Dec;59(6):1081–9. PMID:22175888
3395. Ushiku T, Shinozaki A, Shibahara J, et al. SALL4 represents fetal gut differentiation of gastric cancer, and is diagnostically useful in distinguishing hepatoid gastric carcinoma from hepatocellular carcinoma. Am J Surg Pathol. 2010 Apr;34(4):533–40. PMID:20182341
3396. Ushiku T, Shinozaki-Ushiku A, Maeda D, et al. Distinct expression pattern of claudin-6, a primitive phenotypic tight junction molecule, in germ cell tumours and visceral carcinomas. Histopathology. 2012 Dec;61(6):1043–56. PMID:22803571
3397. Ushiku T, Uozaki H, Shinozaki A, et al. Glypican 3-expressing gastric carcinoma: distinct subgroup unifying hepatoid, clear-cell, and alpha-fetoprotein-producing gastric carcinomas. Cancer Sci. 2009 Apr;100(4):626–32. PMID:19243386
3398. Utsunomiya T, Yao T, Masuda K, et al. Vimentin-positive adenocarcinomas of the stomach: co-expression of vimentin and cytokeratin. Histopathology. 1996 Dec;29(6):507–16. PMID:8971557
3399. Vakiani E, Nandula SV, Subramaniyam S, et al. Cytogenetic analysis of B-cell post-transplant lymphoproliferations validates the World Health Organization classification and suggests inclusion of florid follicular hyperplasia as a precursor lesion. Hum Pathol. 2007 Feb;38(2):315–25. PMID:17134734
3400. Valente P, Garrido M, Gullo I, et al. Epithelial dysplasia of the stomach with gastric immunophenotype shows features of biological aggressiveness. Gastric Cancer. 2015 Oct;18(4):720–8. PMID:25146833
3401. Valera A, Balagué O, Colomo L, et al. IG/MYC rearrangements are the main cytogenetic alteration in plasmablastic lymphomas. Am J Surg Pathol. 2010 Nov;34(11):1686–94. PMID:20962620
3402. Vallat-Decouvelaere AV, Dry SM, Fletcher CD. Atypical and malignant solitary fibrous tumors in extrathoracic locations: evidence of their comparability to intra-thoracic tumors. Am J Surg Pathol. 1998 Dec;22(12):1501–11. PMID:9850176
3403. Valle L. Recent discoveries in the genetics of familial colorectal cancer and polyposis. Clin Gastroenterol Hepatol. 2017 Jun;15(6):809–19. PMID:27712984
3404. Valsangkar NP, Morales-Oyarvide V, Thayer SP, et al. 851 resected cystic tumors of the pancreas: a 33-year experience at the Massachusetts General Hospital. Surgery. 2012 Sep;152(3 Suppl 1):S4–12. PMID:22770958
3405. Van Baeten C, Van Dorpe J. Splenic Epstein-Barr virus-associated inflammatory pseudotumor. Arch Pathol Lab Med. 2017 May;141(5):722–7. PMID:28447898
3406. Van Cutsem E, Bang YJ, Feng-Yi F, et al. HER2 screening data from ToGA: targeting HER2 in gastric and gastroesophageal junction cancer. Gastric Cancer. 2015 Jul;18(3):476–84. PMID:25038874
3407. Van Cutsem E, Lenz HJ, Köhne CH, et al. Fluorouracil, leucovorin, and irinotecan plus cetuximab treatment and RAS mutations in colorectal cancer. J Clin Oncol. 2015 Mar 1;33(7):692–700. PMID:25605843
3408. van de Wouw AJ, Janssen-Heijnen ML, Coebergh JW, et al. Epidemiology of unknown primary tumours; incidence and population-based survival of 1285 patients in Southeast Netherlands, 1984-1992. Eur J Cancer. 2002 Feb;38(3):409–13. PMID:11818207
3409. van den Berg W, Tascilar M, Offerhaus GJ, et al. Pancreatic mucinous cystic neoplasms with sarcomatous stroma: molecular evidence for monoclonal origin with subsequent divergence of the epithelial and sarcomatous components. Mod Pathol. 2000 Jan;13(1):86–91. PMID:10658914
3411. Van den Broeck A, Sergeant G, Ectors N, et al. Patterns of recurrence after curative resection of pancreatic ductal adenocarcinoma. Eur J Surg Oncol. 2009 Jun;35(6):600–4. PMID:19131205
3412. van der Meer JW, Weening RS, Schellekens PT, et al. Colorectal cancer in patients with X-linked agammaglobulinaemia. Lancet. 1993 Jun 5;341(8858):1439–40. PMID:8099142
3413. van der Paardt MP, Zagers MB, Beets-Tan RG, et al. Patients who undergo preoperative chemoradiotherapy for locally advanced rectal cancer restaged by using diagnostic MR imaging: a systematic review and meta-analysis. Radiology. 2013 Oct;269(1):101–12. PMID:23801777
3414. van der Post RS, Gullo I, Oliveira C, et al. Histopathological, molecular, and genetic profile of hereditary diffuse gastric cancer: current knowledge and challenges for the future. Adv Exp Med Biol. 2016;908:371–91. PMID:27573781
3415. van der Post RS, Vogelaar IP, Carneiro F, et al. Hereditary diffuse gastric cancer: updated clinical guidelines with an emphasis on germline CDH1 mutation carriers. J Med Genet. 2015 Jun;52(6):361–74. PMID:25979631
3416. van der Post RS, Vogelaar IP, Manders

P, et al. Accuracy of hereditary diffuse gastric cancer testing criteria and outcomes in patients with a germline mutation in CDH1. Gastroenterology. 2015 Oct;149(4):897–906.e19. PMID:26072394
3417. van der Zee RP, Richel O, de Vries HJ, et al. The increasing incidence of anal cancer: can it be explained by trends in risk groups? Neth J Med. 2013 Oct;71(8):401–11. PMID:24127500
3418. Van Dyke TJ, Johlin FC, Bellizzi AM, et al. Serous cystadenocarcinoma of the pancreas: clinical features and management of a rare tumor. Dig Surg. 2016;33(3):240–8. PMID:26998825
3419. van Eeden S, de Leng WW, Offerhaus GJ, et al. Ductuloinsular tumors of the pancreas: endocrine tumors with entrapped nonneoplastic ductules. Am J Surg Pathol. 2004 Jun;28(6):813–20. PMID:15166675
3420. van Gils T, Nijeboer P, van Wanrooij RL, et al. Mechanisms and management of refractory coeliac disease. Nat Rev Gastroenterol Hepatol. 2015 Oct;12(10):572–9. PMID:26347156
3421. van Hattem WA, Brosens LA, de Leng WW, et al. Large genomic deletions of SMAD4, BMPR1A and PTEN in juvenile polyposis. Gut. 2008 May;57(5):623–7. PMID:18178612
3422. van Hattem WA, Langeveld D, de Leng WW, et al. Histologic variations in juvenile polyp phenotype correlate with genetic defect underlying juvenile polyposis. Am J Surg Pathol. 2011 Apr;35(4):530–6. PMID:21412070
3423. van Herwaarden YJ, Verstegen MH, Dura P, et al. Low prevalence of serrated polyposis syndrome in screening populations: a systematic review. Endoscopy. 2015 Nov;47(11):1043–9. PMID:26126164
3424. Van Leer-Greenberg B, Kole A, Chawla S. Hepatic Kaposi sarcoma: a case report and review of the literature. World J Hepatol. 2017 Feb 8;9(4):171–9. PMID:28217255
3425. van Lier MG, Leenen CH, Wagner A, et al. Yield of routine molecular analyses in colorectal cancer patients ≤70 years to detect underlying Lynch syndrome. J Pathol. 2012 Apr;226(5):764–74. PMID:22081473
3426. van Lier MG, Westerman AM, Wagner A, et al. High cancer risk and increased mortality in patients with Peutz-Jeghers syndrome. Gut. 2011 Feb;60(2):141–7. PMID:21205875
3427. van Meerten E, Eskens FA, van Gameren EC, et al. First-line treatment with oxaliplatin and capecitabine in patients with advanced or metastatic oesophageal cancer: a phase II study. Br J Cancer. 2007 May 7;96(9):1348–52. PMID:17437008
3428. van Putten PG, Hol L, van Dekken H, et al. Inter-observer variation in the histological diagnosis of polyps in colorectal cancer screening. Histopathology. 2011 May;58(6):974–81. PMID:21585430
3429. van Rees BP, Rouse RW, de Wit MJ, et al. Molecular evidence for the same clonal origin of both components of an adenosquamous Barrett carcinoma. Gastroenterology. 2002 Mar;122(3):784–8. PMID:11875011
3430. van Roessel S, Kasumova GG, Tabatabaie O, et al. Pathological margin clearance and survival after pancreaticoduodenectomy in a US and European pancreatic center. Ann Surg Oncol. 2018 Jun;25(6):1760–7. PMID:29651577
3431. van Velthuysen ML, Groen EJ, van der Noort V, et al. Grading of neuroendocrine neoplasms: mitoses and Ki-67 are both essential. Neuroendocrinology. 2014;100(2-3):221–7. PMID:25358267
3432. van Vugt LJ, van der Vleuten CJM, Flucke U, et al. The utility of GLUT1 as a diagnostic marker in cutaneous vascular anomalies: a review of literature and recommendations for daily practice. Pathol Res Pract. 2017 Jun;213(6):591–7. PMID:28552538
3433. van Wanrooij RL, de Jong D, Langerak AW, et al. Novel variant of EATL evolving from mucosal γδ-T-cells in a patient with type I RCD. BMJ Open Gastroenterol. 2015 Jun 9;2(1):e000026. PMID:26462278
3434. van Wanrooij RL, Müller DM, Neefjes-Borst EA, et al. Optimal strategies to identify aberrant intra-epithelial lymphocytes in refractory coeliac disease. J Clin Immunol. 2014 Oct;34(7):828–35. PMID:25062848
3435. Vanacker L, Smeets D, Hoorens A, et al. Mixed adenoneuroendocrine carcinoma of the colon: molecular pathogenesis and treatment. Anticancer Res. 2014 Oct;34(10):5517–21. PMID:25275049
3436. VandenBussche CJ, Allison DB, Graham MK, et al. Alternative lengthening of telomeres and ATRX/DAXX loss can be reliably detected in FNAs of pancreatic neuroendocrine tumors. Cancer Cytopathol. 2017 Jul;125(7):544–51. PMID:28371511
3437. Vanoli A, Argenti F, Vinci A, et al. Hepatoid carcinoma of the pancreas with lymphoid stroma: first description of the clinical, morphological, immunohistochemical, and molecular characteristics of an unusual pancreatic carcinoma. Virchows Arch. 2015 Aug;467(2):237–45. PMID:25989715
3438. Vanoli A, Di Sabatino A, Martino M, et al. Epstein-Barr virus-positive ileal carcinomas associated with Crohn's disease. Virchows Arch. 2017 Oct;471(4):549–52. PMID:28752215
3439. Vanoli A, La Rosa S, Klersy C, et al. Four neuroendocrine tumor types and neuroendocrine carcinoma of the duodenum: analysis of 203 cases. Neuroendocrinology. 2017;104(2):112–25. PMID:26910321
3440. Vanoli A, La Rosa S, Luinetti O, et al. Histologic changes in type A chronic atrophic gastritis indicating increased risk of neuroendocrine tumor development: the predictive role of dysplastic and severely hyperplastic enterochromaffin-like cell lesions. Hum Pathol. 2013 Sep;44(9):1827–37. PMID:23642738
3441. Vanoli A, La Rosa S, Miceli E, et al. Prognostic evaluations tailored to specific gastric neuroendocrine neoplasms: analysis of 200 cases with extended follow-up. Neuroendocrinology. 2018;107(2):114–26. PMID:29895024
3442. Vardaman C, Albores-Saavedra J. Clear cell carcinomas of the gallbladder and extrahepatic bile ducts. Am J Surg Pathol. 1995 Jan;19(1):91–9. PMID:7802141
3443. Vargas-Parra GM, González-Acosta M, Thompson BA, et al. Elucidating the molecular basis of MSH2-deficient tumors by combined germline and somatic analysis. Int J Cancer. 2017 Oct 1;141(7):1365–80. PMID:28577310
3444. Varghese S, Lao-Sirieix P, Fitzgerald RC. Identification and clinical implementation of biomarkers for Barrett's esophagus. Gastroenterology. 2012 Mar;142(3):435–41.e2. PMID:22266150
3445. Varley JM, McGown G, Thorncroft M, et al. An extended Li-Fraumeni kindred with gastric carcinoma and a codon 175 mutation in TP53. J Med Genet. 1995 Dec;32(12):942–5. PMID:8825920
3446. Varma JD, Hill MC, Harvey LA. Hemangioma of the small intestine manifesting as gastrointestinal bleeding. Radiographics. 1998 Jul-Aug;18(4):1029–33. PMID:9672985
3447. Varnholt H, Vauthey JN, Dal Cin P, et al. Biliary adenofibroma: a rare neoplasm of bile duct origin with an indolent behavior. Am J Surg Pathol. 2003 May;27(5):693–8. PMID:12717255
3448. Vasen HF, Blanco I, Aktan-Collan K, et al. Revised guidelines for the clinical management of Lynch syndrome (HNPCC): recommendations by a group of European experts. Gut. 2013 Jun;62(6):812–23. PMID:23408351
3449. Vasen HF, Bülow S, Myrhøj T, et al. Decision analysis in the management of duodenal adenomatosis in familial adenomatous polyposis. Gut. 1997 Jun;40(6):716–9. PMID:9245923
3450. Vasen HF, Ghorbanoghli Z, Bourdeaut F, et al. Guidelines for surveillance of individuals with constitutional mismatch repair-deficiency proposed by the European Consortium "Care for CMMR-D" (C4CMMR-D). J Med Genet. 2014 May;51(5):283–93. PMID:24556086
3451. Vasen HF, Möslein G, Alonso A, et al. Guidelines for the clinical management of familial adenomatous polyposis (FAP). Gut. 2008 May;57(5):704–13. PMID:18194984
3452. Vega F, Chang CC, Schwartz MR, et al. Atypical NK-cell proliferation of the gastrointestinal tract in a patient with antigliadin antibodies but not celiac disease. Am J Surg Pathol. 2006 Apr;30(4):539–44. PMID:16625103
3453. Vega F, Medeiros LJ, Bueso-Ramos C, et al. Hepatosplenic gamma/delta T-cell lymphoma in bone marrow. A sinusoidal neoplasm with blastic cytologic features. Am J Clin Pathol. 2001 Sep;116(3):410–9. PMID:11554170
3454. Vega F, Medeiros LJ, Gaulard P. Hepatosplenic and other gammadelta T-cell lymphomas. Am J Clin Pathol. 2007 Jun;127(6):869–80. PMID:17509984
3455. Velazquez I, Alter BP. Androgens and liver tumors: Fanconi's anemia and non-Fanconi's conditions. Am J Hematol. 2004 Nov;77(3):257–67. PMID:15495253
3456. Venesio T, Balsamo A, Errichiello E, et al. Oxidative DNA damage drives carcinogenesis in MUTYH-associated-polyposis by specific mutations of mitochondrial and MAPK genes. Mod Pathol. 2013 Oct;26(10):1371–81. PMID:23599153
3457. Venkatesh S, Ordonez NG, Ajani J, et al. Islet cell carcinoma of the pancreas. A study of 98 patients. Cancer. 1990 Jan 15;65(2):354–7. PMID:2153046
3458. Verbeek WH, Goerres MS, von Blomberg BM, et al. Flow cytometric determination of aberrant intra-epithelial lymphocytes predicts T-cell lymphoma development more accurately than T-cell clonality analysis in refractory celiac disease. Clin Immunol. 2008 Jan;126(1):48–56. PMID:18024205
3459. Verbeek WH, von Blomberg BM, Coupe VM, et al. Aberrant T-lymphocytes in refractory coeliac disease are not strictly confined to a small intestinal intraepithelial localization. Cytometry B Clin Cytom. 2009 Nov;76(6):367–74. PMID:19444812
3460. Verbeke CS, Gladhaug IP. Resection margin involvement and tumour origin in pancreatic head cancer. Br J Surg. 2012 Aug;99(8):1036–49. PMID:22517199
3461. Verbeke SL, de Jong D, Bertoni F, et al. Array CGH analysis identifies two distinct subgroups of primary angiosarcoma of bone. Genes Chromosomes Cancer. 2015 Feb;54(2):72–81. PMID:25231439
3462. Verdú M, Román R, Calvo M, et al. Clinicopathological and molecular characterization of colorectal micropapillary carcinoma. Mod Pathol. 2011 May;24(5):729–38. PMID:21336262
3463. Vereide DT, Seto E, Chiu YF, et al. Epstein-Barr virus maintains lymphomas via its miRNAs. Oncogene. 2014 Mar 6;33(10):1258–64. PMID:23503461
3464. Verhulst J, Ferdinande L, Demetter P, et al. Mucinous subtype as prognostic factor in colorectal cancer: a systematic review and meta-analysis. J Clin Pathol. 2012 May;65(5):381–8. PMID:22259177
3465. Verkarre V, Asnafi V, Lecomte T, et al. Refractory coeliac sprue is a diffuse gastrointestinal disease. Gut. 2003 Feb;52(2):205–11. PMID:12524401
3466. Verma M, Agarwal S, Mohta A. Primary mixed germ cell tumour of the liver–a case report. Indian J Pathol Microbiol. 2003 Oct;46(4):658–9. PMID:15025371
3467. Verma R, Sharma PC. Next generation sequencing-based emerging trends in molecular biology of gastric cancer. Am J Cancer Res. 2018 Feb 1;8(2):207–25. PMID:29511593
3468. Verner JV, Morrison AB. Islet cell tumor and a syndrome of refractory watery diarrhea and hypokalemia. Am J Med. 1958 Sep;25(3):374–80. PMID:13571250
3469. Vernerey D, Huguet F, Vienot A, et al. Prognostic nomogram and score to predict overall survival in locally advanced untreated pancreatic cancer (PROLAP). Br J Cancer. 2016 Jul 26;115(3):281–9. PMID:27404456
3470. Verschoor AJ, Bovée JVMG, Overbeek LIH, et al. The incidence, mutational status, risk classification and referral pattern of gastro-intestinal stromal tumours in the Netherlands: a nationwide pathology registry (PALGA) study. Virchows Arch. 2018 Feb;472(2):221–9. PMID:29308530
3471. Verset L, Arvanitakis M, Loi P, et al. TTF-1 positive small cell cancers: Don't think they're always primary pulmonary! World J Gastrointest Oncol. 2011 Oct 15;3(10):144–7. PMID:22046491
3472. Veteläinen R, Erdogan D, de Graaf W, et al. Liver adenomatosis: re-evaluation of aetiology and management. Liver Int. 2008 Apr;28(4):499–508. PMID:18339077
3473. Vieira AR, Abar L, Chan DSM, et al. Foods and beverages and colorectal cancer risk: a systematic review and meta-analysis of cohort studies, an update of the evidence of the WCRF-AICR Continuous Update Project. Ann Oncol. 2017 Aug 1;28(8):1788–802. PMID:28407090
3474. Vieth M, Kushima R, Borchard F, et al. Pyloric gland adenoma: a clinico-pathological analysis of 90 cases. Virchows Arch. 2003 Apr;442(4):317–21. PMID:12715167
3475. Vieth M, Kushima R, Mukaisho K, et al. Immunohistochemical analysis of pyloric gland adenomas using a series of mucin 2, mucin 5ac, mucin 6, CD10, Ki67 and p53. Virchows Arch. 2010 Nov;457(5):529–36. PMID:20827489
3476. Vieth M, Montgomery EA, Riddell RH. Observations of different patterns of dysplasia in barretts esophagus - a first step to harmonize grading. Cesk Patol. 2016;52(3):154–63. PMID:27526016
3477. Vieth M, Montgomery EA. Some observations on pyloric gland adenoma: an uncommon and long ignored entity! J Clin Pathol. 2014 Oct;67(10):883–90. PMID:25092673
3478. Vinayek R, Capurso G, Larghi A. Grading of EUS-FNA cytologic specimens from patients with pancreatic neuroendocrine neoplasms: it is time move to tissue core biopsy? Gland Surg. 2014 Nov;3(4):222–5. PMID:25493252
3479. Vinik AI, Strodel WE, Eckhauser FE, et al. Somatostatinomas, PPomas, neurotensinomas. Semin Oncol. 1987 Sep;14(3):263–81. PMID:2820062
3480. Vishnevsky VA, Mohan VS, Pomelov VS, et al. Surgical treatment of giant cavernous hemangioma liver. HPB Surg. 1991 May;4(1):69–78, discussion 78–9. PMID:1911479
3481. Vlajnic T, Brisse HJ, Aerts I, et al. Fine needle aspiration in the diagnosis and classification of hepatoblastoma: analysis of 21 new cases. Diagn Cytopathol. 2017 Feb;45(2):91–100. PMID:27933740
3482. Vogelaar IP, van der Post RS, van Krieken JHJ, et al. Unraveling genetic

predisposition to familial or early onset gastric cancer using germline whole-exome sequencing. Eur J Hum Genet. 2017 Nov;25(11):1246–52. PMID:28875981
3483. Volante M, Brizzi MP, Faggiano A, et al. Somatostatin receptor type 2A immunohistochemistry in neuroendocrine tumors: a proposal of scoring system correlated with somatostatin receptor scintigraphy. Mod Pathol. 2007 Nov;20(11):1172–82. PMID:17873898
3484. Volante M, Daniele L, Asioli S, et al. Tumor staging but not grading is associated with adverse clinical outcome in neuroendocrine tumors of the appendix: a retrospective clinical pathologic analysis of 138 cases. Am J Surg Pathol. 2013 Apr;37(4):606–12. PMID:23426123
3485. Volante M, La Rosa S, Castellano I, et al. Clinico-pathological features of a series of 11 oncocytic endocrine tumours of the pancreas. Virchows Arch. 2006 May;448(5):545–51. PMID:16491376
3486. Volante M, Monica V, Birocco N, et al. Expression analysis of genes involved in DNA repair or synthesis in mixed neuroendocrine/nonneuroendocrine carcinomas. Neuroendocrinology. 2015;101(2):151–60. PMID:25633872
3487. Volkan Adsay N. Cystic lesions of the pancreas. Mod Pathol. 2007 Feb;20 Suppl 1:S71–93. PMID:17486054
3488. Voltaggio L, Murray R, Lasota J, et al. Gastric schwannoma: a clinicopathologic study of 51 cases and critical review of the literature. Hum Pathol. 2012 May;43(5):650–9. PMID:22137423
3489. von Horn H, Tally M, Hall K, et al. Expression levels of insulin-like growth factor binding proteins and insulin receptor isoforms in hepatoblastomas. Cancer Lett. 2001 Jan 26;162(2):253–60. PMID:11146233
3490. von Roon AC, Reese G, Teare J, et al. The risk of cancer in patients with Crohn's disease. Dis Colon Rectum. 2007 Jun;50(6):839–55. PMID:17308939
3491. von Salomé J, Liu T, Keihäs M, et al. Haplotype analysis suggest that the MLH1 c.2059C > T mutation is a Swedish founder mutation. Fam Cancer. 2018 Oct;17(4):531–7. PMID:29288294
3492. Vonderheide RH. Tumor-promoting inflammatory networks in pancreatic neoplasia: another reason to loathe Kras. Cancer Cell. 2014 May 12;25(5):553–4. PMID:24823632
3493. Voong KR, Davison J, Pawlik TM, et al. Resected pancreatic adenosquamous carcinoma: clinicopathologic review and evaluation of adjuvant chemotherapy and radiation in 38 patients. Hum Pathol. 2010 Jan;41(1):113–22. PMID:19801164
3494. Voong KR, Rashid A, Crane CH, et al. Chemoradiation for high-grade neuroendocrine carcinoma of the rectum and anal canal. Am J Clin Oncol. 2017 Dec;40(6):555–60. PMID:26237193
3495. Vortmeyer AO, Lubensky IA, Fogt F, et al. Allelic deletion and mutation of the von Hippel-Lindau (VHL) tumor suppressor gene in pancreatic microcystic adenomas. Am J Pathol. 1997 Oct;151(4):951–6. PMID:9327728
3496. Vortmeyer AO, Lubensky IA, Merino MJ, et al. Concordance of genetic alterations in poorly differentiated colorectal neuroendocrine carcinomas and associated adenocarcinomas. J Natl Cancer Inst. 1997 Oct 1;89(19):1448–53. PMID:9326914
3497. Vose J, Armitage J, Weisenburger D. International peripheral T-cell and natural killer/T-cell lymphoma study: pathology findings and clinical outcomes. J Clin Oncol. 2008 Sep 1;26(25):4124–30. PMID:18626005
3498. Voss MH, Lunning MA, Maragulia JC, et al. Intensive induction chemotherapy followed by early high-dose therapy and hematopoietic stem cell transplantation results in improved outcome for patients with hepatosplenic T-cell lymphoma: a single institution experience. Clin Lymphoma Myeloma Leuk. 2013 Feb;13(1):8–14. PMID:23107915
3499. Vrieling A, Bueno-de-Mesquita HB, Boshuizen HC, et al. Cigarette smoking, environmental tobacco smoke exposure and pancreatic cancer risk in the European Prospective Investigation into Cancer and Nutrition. Int J Cancer. 2010 May 15;126(10):2394–403. PMID:19790196
3500. Waddell N, Pajic M, Patch AM, et al. Whole genomes redefine the mutational landscape of pancreatic cancer. Nature. 2015 Feb 26;518(7540):495–501. PMID:25719666
3501. Wagner AJ, Remillard SP, Zhang YX, et al. Loss of expression of SDHA predicts SDHA mutations in gastrointestinal stromal tumors. Mod Pathol. 2013 Feb;26(2):289–94. PMID:22955521
3502. Wagner PL, Chen YT, Yantiss RK. Immunohistochemical and molecular features of sporadic and FAP-associated duodenal adenomas of the ampullary and nonampullary mucosa. Am J Surg Pathol. 2008 Sep;32(9):1388–95. PMID:18670349
3503. Wakabayashi H, Matsutani T, Fujita I, et al. A rare case of primary squamous cell carcinoma of the stomach and a review of the 56 cases reported in Japan. J Gastric Cancer. 2014 Mar;14(1):58–62. PMID:24765539
3504. Wakasugi M, Tanemura M, Furukawa K, et al. Signet ring cell carcinoma of the ampulla of Vater: report of a case and a review of the literature. Int J Surg Case Rep. 2015;12:108–11. PMID:26057354
3505. Walter FM, Mills K, Mendonça SC, et al. Symptoms and patient factors associated with diagnostic intervals for pancreatic cancer (SYMPTOM pancreatic study): a prospective cohort study. Lancet Gastroenterol Hepatol. 2016 Dec;1(4):298–306. PMID:28404200
3506. Walter T, Hervieu V, Adham M, et al. Primary neuroendocrine tumors of the main pancreatic duct: a rare entity. Virchows Arch. 2011 May;458(5):537–46. PMID:21431402
3507. Wan XS, Xu YY, Qian JY, et al. Intraductal papillary neoplasm of the bile duct. World J Gastroenterol. 2013 Dec 14;19(46):8595–604. PMID:24379576
3508. Wang F, Liu DB, Zhao Q, et al. The genomic landscape of small cell carcinoma of the esophagus. Cell Res. 2018 Jul;28(7):771–4. PMID:29728688
3509. Wang G, Ji L, Qu FZ, et al. Acinar cell cystadenoma of the pancreas: a retrospective analysis of ten-year experience from a single academic institution. Pancreatology. 2016 Jul-Aug;16(4):625–31. PMID:27086062
3510. Wang GG, Yao JC, Worah S, et al. Comparison of genetic alterations in neuroendocrine tumors: frequent loss of chromosome 18 in ileal carcinoid tumors. Mod Pathol. 2005 Aug;18(8):1079–87. PMID:15920555
3511. Wang GQ, Abnet CC, Shen Q, et al. Histological precursors of oesophageal squamous cell carcinoma: results from a 13 year prospective follow up study in a high risk population. Gut. 2005 Feb;54(2):187–92. PMID:15647178
3512. Wang HH, Doria MI Jr, Purohit-Buch S, et al. Barrett's esophagus. The cytology of dysplasia in comparison to benign and malignant lesions. Acta Cytol. 1992 Jan-Feb;36(1):60–4. PMID:1546513
3513. Wang HH, Wu MS, Shun CT, et al. Lymphoepithelioma-like carcinoma of the stomach: a subset of gastric carcinoma with distinct clinicopathological features and high prevalence of Epstein-Barr virus infection. Hepatogastroenterology. 1999 Mar-Apr;46(26):1214–9. PMID:10370694
3514. Wang J, Thway K. Clear cell sarcoma-like tumor of the gastrointestinal tract: an evolving entity. Arch Pathol Lab Med. 2015 Mar;139(3):407–12. PMID:25724038
3515. Wang KL, Yang Q, Cleary KR, et al. The significance of neuroendocrine differentiation in adenocarcinoma of the esophagus and esophagogastric junction after preoperative chemoradiation. Cancer. 2006 Oct 1;107(7):1467–74. PMID:16955509
3516. Wang L, Basturk O, Wang J, et al. A FISH assay efficiently screens for BRAF gene rearrangements in pancreatic acinar-type neoplasms. Mod Pathol. 2018 Jan;31(1):132–40. PMID:28884748
3517. Wang L, Yang M, Zhang Y, et al. Prognostic validation of the WHO 2010 grading system in pancreatic insulinoma patients. Neoplasma. 2015;62(3):484–90. PMID:25866230
3518. Wang LD, Yang HH, Fan ZM, et al. Cytological screening and 15 years' follow-up (1986-2001) for early esophageal squamous cell carcinoma and precancerous lesions in a high-risk population in Anyang County, Henan Province, Northern China. Cancer Detect Prev. 2005;29(4):317–22. PMID:16118042
3519. Wang Q, Luan W, Villanueva GA, et al. Clinical prognostic variables in young patients (under 40 years) with hepatitis B virus-associated hepatocellular carcinoma. J Dig Dis. 2012 Apr;13(4):214–8. PMID:22435506
3520. Wang T, Askan G, Adsay V, et al. Reappraisal of the clinical-pathological characteristics of intraductal oncocytic papillary neoplasms: an analysis of 25 cases. Am J Surg Pathol. Forthcoming 2019.
3521. Wang Y, Liu YY, Han GP. Hepatoid adenocarcinoma of the extrahepatic duct. World J Gastroenterol. 2013 Jun 14;19(22):3524–7. PMID:23801851
3522. Wang Y, Marino-Enriquez A, Bennett RR, et al. Dystrophin is a tumor suppressor in human cancers with myogenic programs. Nat Genet. 2014 Jun;46(6):601–6. PMID:24793134
3523. Wangjam T, Zhang Z, Zhou XC, et al. Resected pancreatic ductal adenocarcinomas with recurrence limited in lung have a significantly better prognosis than those with other recurrence patterns. Oncotarget. 2015 Nov 3;6(34):36903–10. PMID:26372811
3524. Wanless IR, Albrecht S, Bilbao J, et al. Multiple focal nodular hyperplasia of the liver associated with vascular malformations of various organs and neoplasia of the brain: a new syndrome. Mod Pathol. 1989 Sep;2(5):456–62. PMID:2813344
3525. Wanless IR, Mawdsley C, Adams R. On the pathogenesis of focal nodular hyperplasia of the liver. Hepatology. 1985 Nov-Dec;5(6):1194–200. PMID:4065824
3526. Wanless IR. Benign liver tumors. Clin Liver Dis. 2002 May;6(2):513–26, ix. PMID:12122868
3527. Ward SC, Huang J, Tickoo SK, et al. Fibrolamellar carcinoma of the liver exhibits immunohistochemical evidence of both hepatocyte and bile duct differentiation. Mod Pathol. 2010 Sep;23(9):1180–90. PMID:20495535
3528. Wardell CP, Fujita M, Yamada T, et al. Genomic characterization of biliary tract cancers identifies driver genes and predisposing mutations. J Hepatol. 2018 May;68(5):959–69. PMID:29360550
3530. Warren M, Thompson KS. Two cases of primary yolk sac tumor of the liver in childhood: case reports and literature review. Pediatr Dev Pathol. 2009 Sep-Oct;12(5):410–6. PMID:19284801
3531. Warthin AS. Classics in oncology. Heredity with reference to carcinoma as shown by the study of the cases examined in the pathological laboratory of the University of Michigan, 1895-1913. By Aldred Scott Warthin. 1913. CA Cancer J Clin. 1985 Nov-Dec;35(6):348–59. PMID:3931868
3532. Wasel BA, Keough V, Huang WY, et al. Histological percutaneous diagnosis of stage IV microcystic serous cystadenocarcinoma of the pancreas. BMJ Case Rep. 2013 Jan 30;2013. PMID:23370947
3533. Washington K, McDonagh D. Secondary tumors of the gastrointestinal tract: surgical pathologic findings and comparison with autopsy survey. Mod Pathol. 1995 May;8(4):427–33. PMID:7567944
3534. Washington K, Rourk MH Jr, McDonagh D, et al. Inflammatory cloacogenic polyp in a child: part of the spectrum of solitary rectal ulcer syndrome. Pediatr Pathol. 1993 Jul-Aug;13(4):409–14. PMID:8372025
3535. Wassef M, Blei F, Adams D, et al. Vascular anomalies classification: recommendations from the International Society for the Study of Vascular Anomalies. Pediatrics. 2015 Jul;136(1):e203–14. PMID:26055853
3536. Watanabe H, Enjoji M, Imai T. Gastric carcinoma with lymphoid stroma. Its morphologic characteristics and prognostic correlations. Cancer. 1976 Jul;38(1):232–43. PMID:947518
3537. Watanabe I, Kasai M, Suzuki S. True teratoma of the liver–report of a case and review of the literature–. Acta Hepatogastroenterol (Stuttg). 1978 Feb;25(1):40–4. PMID:636740
3538. Waters AM, Der CJ. KRAS: the critical driver and therapeutic target for pancreatic cancer. Cold Spring Harb Perspect Med. 2018 Sep 4;8(9):a031435. PMID:29229669
3539. Weaver JMJ, Ross-Innes CS, Shannon N, et al. Ordering of mutations in preinvasive disease stages of esophageal carcinogenesis. Nat Genet. 2014 Aug;46(8):837–43. PMID:24952744
3540. Webber SA. Post-transplant lymphoproliferative disorders: a preventable complication of solid organ transplantation? Pediatr Transplant. 1999 May;3(2):95–9. PMID:10389129
3541. Wee A, Nilsson B. Combined hepatocellular-cholangiocarcinoma. Diagnostic challenge in hepatic fine needle aspiration biopsy. Acta Cytol. 1999 Mar-Apr;43(2):131–8. PMID:10097699
3542. Weilert F, Bhat YM, Binmoeller KF, et al. EUS-FNA is superior to ERCP-based tissue sampling in suspected malignant biliary obstruction: results of a prospective, single-blind, comparative study. Gastrointest Endosc. 2014 Jul;80(1):97–104. PMID:24559784
3543. Weinberg BA, Xiu J, Hwang JJ, et al. Immuno-oncology biomarkers for gastric and gastroesophageal junction adenocarcinoma: why pd-l1 testing may not be enough. Oncologist. 2018 Oct;23(10):1171–7. PMID:29703766
3544. Weisbrod AB, Zhang L, Jain M, et al. Altered PTEN, ATRX, CHGA, CHGB, and TP53 expression are associated with aggressive VHL-associated pancreatic neuroendocrine tumors. Horm Cancer. 2013 Jun;4(3):165–75. PMID:23361940
3545. Wen KW, Grenert JP, Joseph NM, et al. Genomic profile of appendiceal goblet cell carcinoid is distinct compared to appendiceal neuroendocrine tumor and conventional adenocarcinoma. Hum Pathol. 2018 Jul;77:166–74. PMID:29634977
3546. Wen KW, Rabinovitch PS, Huang D, et al. Use of DNA flow cytometry in the diagnosis, risk stratification, and management of gastric epithelial dysplasia. Mod Pathol. 2018 Oct;31(10):1578–87. PMID:29789650
3547. Wen X, Wu W, Wang B, et al. Signet ring cell carcinoma of the ampulla of Vater: immunophenotype and differentiation. Oncol Lett. 2014 Oct;8(4):1687–92. PMID:25202392

3548. Weren RD, Ligtenberg MJ, Geurts van Kessel A, et al. NTHL1 and MUTYH polyposis syndromes: two sides of the same coin? J Pathol. 2018 Feb;244(2):135–42. PMID:29105096
3549. Weren RD, Ligtenberg MJ, Kets CM, et al. A germline homozygous mutation in the base-excision repair gene NTHL1 causes adenomatous polyposis and colorectal cancer. Nat Genet. 2015 Jun;47(6):668–71. PMID:25938944
3550. Weren RDA, van der Post RS, Vogelaar IP, et al. Role of germline aberrations affecting CTNNA1, MAP3K6 and MYD88 in gastric cancer susceptibility. J Med Genet. 2018 Oct;55(10):669–74. PMID:29330337
3551. Wermers RA, Fatourechi V, Wynne AG, et al. The glucagonoma syndrome. Clinical and pathologic features in 21 patients. Medicine (Baltimore). 1996 Mar;75(2):53–63. PMID:8606627
3552. West NP, Morris EJ, Rotimi O, ct al. Pathology grading of colon cancer surgical resection and its association with survival: a retrospective observational study. Lancet Oncol. 2008 Sep;9(9):857–65. PMID:18667357
3553. West RB, Corless CL, Chen X, et al. The novel marker, DOG1, is expressed ubiquitously in gastrointestinal stromal tumors irrespective of KIT or PDGFRA mutation status. Am J Pathol. 2004 Jul;165(1):107–13. PMID:15215166
3554. Westerman AM, Entius MM, de Baar E, et al. Peutz-Jeghers syndrome: 78-year follow-up of the original family. Lancet. 1999 Apr 10;353(9160):1211–5. PMID:10217080
3555. Westra WH, Sturm P, Drillenburg P, et al. K-ras oncogene mutations in osteoclast-like giant cell tumors of the pancreas and liver: genetic evidence to support origin from the duct epithelium. Am J Surg Pathol. 1998 Oct;22(10):1247–54. PMID:9777987
3556. Wey EA, Britton AJ, Sferra JJ, et al. Gastroblastoma in a 28-year-old man with nodal metastasis: proof of the malignant potential. Arch Pathol Lab Med. 2012 Aug;136(8):961–4. PMID:22849746
3557. Wheeler JM, Warren BF, Mortensen NJ, et al. An insight into the genetic pathway of adenocarcinoma of the small intestine. Gut. 2002 Feb;50(2):218–23. PMID:11788563
3558. White R, D'Angelica M, Katabi N, et al. Fate of the remnant pancreas after resection of noninvasive intraductal papillary mucinous neoplasm. J Am Coll Surg. 2007 May;204(5):987–93, discussion 993–5. PMID:17481526
3559. Whitworth J, Skytte AB, Sunde L, et al. Multilocus inherited neoplasia alleles syndrome: a case series and review. JAMA Oncol. 2016 Mar;2(3):373–9. PMID:26659639
3559A. Wiegand S, Eivazi B, Barth PJ, et al. Pathogenesis of lymphangiomas. Virchows Arch. 2008 Jul;453(1):1–8. PMID:18500536
3560. Wiland HO 4th, Shadrach B, Allende D, et al. Morphologic and molecular characterization of traditional serrated adenomas of the distal colon and rectum. Am J Surg Pathol. 2014 Sep;38(9):1290–7. PMID:25127095
3561. Wilentz RE, Albores-Saavedra J, Zahurak M, et al. Pathologic examination accurately predicts prognosis in mucinous cystic neoplasms of the pancreas. Am J Surg Pathol. 1999 Nov;23(11):1320–7. PMID:10555000
3562. Wilentz RE, Goggins M, Redston M, et al. Genetic, immunohistochemical, and clinical features of medullary carcinoma of the pancreas: a newly described and characterized entity. Am J Pathol. 2000 May;156(5):1641–51. PMID:10793075
3563. Wilentz RE, Iacobuzio-Donahue CA, Argani P, et al. Loss of expression of Dpc4 in pancreatic intraepithelial neoplasia: evidence that DPC4 inactivation occurs late in neoplastic progression. Cancer Res. 2000 Apr 1;60(7):2002–6. PMID:10766191
3564. Wilentz RE, Su GH, Dai JL, et al. Immunohistochemical labeling for dpc4 mirrors genetic status in pancreatic adenocarcinomas: a new marker of DPC4 inactivation. Am J Pathol. 2000 Jan;156(1):37–43. PMID:10623651
3565. Wilhelm A, Müller SA, Steffen T, et al. Patients with adenocarcinoma of the small intestine with 9 or more regional lymph nodes retrieved have a higher rate of positive lymph nodes and improved survival. J Gastrointest Surg. 2016 Feb;20(2):401–10. PMID:26487334
3566. Wilkinson JR, Morris EJ, Downing A, et al. The rising incidence of anal cancer in England 1990-2010: a population-based study. Colorectal Dis. 2014 Jul;16(7):O234–9. PMID:24410872
3567. Willems S, Carneiro F, Geboes K. Gastric carcinoma with osteoclast-like giant cells and lymphoepithelioma-like carcinoma of the stomach: two of a kind? Histopathology. 2005 Sep;47(3):331–3. PMID:16115241
3568. Williams RF, Fernandez-Pineda I, Gosain A. Pediatric sarcomas. Surg Clin North Am. 2016 Oct;96(5):1107–25. PMID:27542645
3569. Wilson AL, Swerdlow SH, Przybylski GK, et al. Intestinal γδ T-cell lymphomas are most frequently of type II enteropathy-associated T-cell type. Hum Pathol. 2013 Jun;44(6):1131–45. PMID:23332928
3570. Wilson PM, Labonte MJ, Lenz HJ. Molecular markers in the treatment of metastatic colorectal cancer. Cancer J. 2010 May-Jun;16(3):262–72. PMID:20526105
3571. Wilson WH, Young RM, Schmitz R, et al. Targeting B cell receptor signaling with ibrutinib in diffuse large B cell lymphoma. Nat Med. 2015 Aug;21(8):922–6. PMID:26193343
3572. Wimmer K, Kratz CP, Vasen HF, et al. Diagnostic criteria for constitutional mismatch repair deficiency syndrome: suggestions of the European consortium 'care for CMMRD' (C4CMMRD). J Med Genet. 2014 Jun;51(6):355–65. PMID:24737826
3573. Win AK, Dowty JG, English DR, et al. Body mass index in early adulthood and colorectal cancer risk for carriers and non-carriers of germline mutations in DNA mismatch repair genes. Br J Cancer. 2011 Jun 28;105(1):162–9. PMID:21559014
3574. Win AK, Jenkins MA, Dowty JG, et al. Prevalence and penetrance of major genes and polygenes for colorectal cancer. Cancer Epidemiol Biomarkers Prev. 2017 Mar;26(3):404–12. PMID:27799157
3575. Win AK, Walters RJ, Buchanan DD, et al. Cancer risks for relatives of patients with serrated polyposis. Am J Gastroenterol. 2012 May;107(5):770–8. PMID:22525305
3576. Winawer SJ, Zauber AG, Fletcher RH, et al. Guidelines for colonoscopy surveillance after polypectomy: a consensus update by the US Multi-Society Task Force on Colorectal Cancer and the American Cancer Society. CA Cancer J Clin. 2006 May-Jun;56(3):143–59, quiz 184–5. PMID:16737947
3577. Wincewicz A, Kowalik A, Zięba S, et al. Morphology with immunohistochemical and genetic profiling of high-grade neuroendocrine carcinoma of colon - a case report with review of literature. Rom J Morphol Embryol. 2017;58(2):655–63. PMID:28730258
3578. Winter JM, Cameron JL, Campbell KA, et al. 1423 pancreaticoduodenectomies for pancreatic cancer: a single-institution experience. J Gastrointest Surg. 2006 Nov;10(9):1199–210, discussion 1210–1. PMID:17114007
3579. Winter JM, Tang LH, Klimstra DS, et al. Failure patterns in resected pancreas adenocarcinoma: lack of predicted benefit to SMAD4 expression. Ann Surg. 2013 Aug;258(2):331–5. PMID:23360922
3580. Winter JM, Ting AH, Vilardell F, et al. Absence of E-cadherin expression distinguishes noncohesive from cohesive pancreatic cancer. Clin Cancer Res. 2008 Jan 15;14(2):412–8. PMID:18223216
3581. Winter TC 3rd, Freeny P. Hepatic teratoma in an adult. Case report with a review of the literature. J Clin Gastroenterol. 1993 Dec;17(4):308–10. PMID:8308217
3582. Wistuba II, Gazdar AF, Roa I, et al. p53 protein overexpression in gallbladder carcinoma and its precursor lesions: an immunohistochemical study. Hum Pathol. 1996 Apr;27(4):360–5. PMID:8617479
3583. Wistuba II, Miquel JF, Gazdar AF, et al. Gallbladder adenomas have molecular abnormalities different from those present in gallbladder carcinomas. Hum Pathol. 1999 Jan;30(1):21–5. PMID:9923922
3584. Witte DP, Kissane JM, Askin FB. Hepatic teratomas in children. Pediatr Pathol. 1983 Jan-Mar;1(1):81–92. PMID:6208545
3585. Witteman BJ, Janssens AR, Terpstra JL, et al. Villous tumors of the duodenum. Presentation of five cases. Hepatogastroenterology. 1991 Dec;38(6):550–3. PMID:1778589
3586. Wlodarska I, Martin-Garcia N, Achten R, et al. Fluorescence in situ hybridization study of chromosome 7 aberrations in hepatosplenic T-cell lymphoma: isochromosome 7q as a common abnormality accumulating in forms with features of cytologic progression. Genes Chromosomes Cancer. 2002 Mar;33(3):243–51. PMID:11807981
3587. Woischke C, Schaaf CW, Yang HM, et al. In-depth mutational analyses of colorectal neuroendocrine carcinomas with adenoma or adenocarcinoma components. Mod Pathol. 2017 Jan;30(1):95–103. PMID:27586204
3588. Wolf AM, Shirley LA, Winter JM, et al. Acinar cell cystadenoma of the pancreas: report of three cases and literature review. J Gastrointest Surg. 2013 Jul;17(7):1322–6. PMID:23605178
3589. Wolfgang CL, Herman JM, Laheru DA, et al. Recent progress in pancreatic cancer. CA Cancer J Clin. 2013 Sep;63(5):318–48. PMID:23856911
3590. Wolpin BM, Chan AT, Hartge P, et al. ABO blood group and the risk of pancreatic cancer. J Natl Cancer Inst. 2009 Mar 18;101(6):424–31. PMID:19276450
3591. Wong AK, Chan RC, Aggarwal N, et al. Human papillomavirus genotypes in anal intraepithelial neoplasia and anal carcinoma as detected in tissue biopsies. Mod Pathol. 2010 Jan;23(1):144–50. PMID:19838162
3592. Wong AY, Rahilly MA, Adams W, et al. Mucinous anal gland carcinoma with perianal Pagetoid spread. Pathology. 1998 Feb;30(1):1–3. PMID:9534198
3593. Wong MCS, Jiang JY, Liang M, et al. Global temporal patterns of pancreatic cancer and association with socioeconomic development. Sci Rep. 2017 Jun 9;7(1):3165. PMID:28600530
3594. Wong MW, Bair MJ, Shih SC, et al. Using typical endoscopic features to diagnose esophageal squamous papilloma. World J Gastroenterol. 2016 Feb 21;22(7):2349–56. PMID:26900297
3595. Wong NA, D'Costa H, Barry RE, et al. Primary yolk sac tumour of the liver in adulthood. J Clin Pathol. 1998 Dec;51(12):939–40. PMID:10070339
3596. Wong NA, Gonzalez D, Salto-Tellez M, et al. RAS testing of colorectal carcinoma—a guidance document from the Association of Clinical Pathologists Molecular Pathology and Diagnostics Group. J Clin Pathol. 2014 Sep;67(9):751–7. PMID:24996433
3597. Wong NA, Shirazi T, Hamer-Hodges DW, et al. Adenocarcinoma arising within a Crohn's-related anorectal fistula: a form of anal gland carcinoma? Histopathology. 2002 Mar;40(3):302–4. PMID:11895502
3598. Wong P, Verselis SJ, Garber JE, et al. Prevalence of early onset colorectal cancer in 397 patients with classic Li-Fraumeni syndrome. Gastroenterology. 2006 Jan;130(1):73–9. PMID:16401470
3599. Wood BP, Putnam TC, Chacko AK. Infantile hepatic hemangioendotheliomas associated with hemihypertrophy. Pediatr Radiol. 1977;5(4):242–5. PMID:263514
3600. Wood LD, Heaphy CM, Daniel HD, et al. Chromophobe hepatocellular carcinoma with abrupt anaplasia: a proposal for a new subtype of hepatocellular carcinoma with unique morphological and molecular features. Mod Pathol. 2013 Dec;26(12):1586–93. PMID:23640129
3601. Wood LD, Klimstra DS. Pathology and genetics of pancreatic neoplasms with acinar differentiation. Semin Diagn Pathol. 2014 Nov;31(6):491–7. PMID:25441307
3602. Wood LD, Noë M, Hackeng W, et al. Patients with McCune-Albright syndrome have a broad spectrum of abnormalities in the gastrointestinal tract and pancreas. Virchows Arch. 2017 Apr;470(4):391–400. PMID:28188442
3603. Wood LD, Parsons DW, Jones S, et al. The genomic landscapes of human breast and colorectal cancers. Science. 2007 Nov 16;318(5853):1108–13. PMID:17932254
3604. Wood LD, Salaria SN, Cruise MW, et al. Upper GI tract lesions in familial adenomatous polyposis (FAP): enrichment of pyloric gland adenomas and other gastric and duodenal neoplasms. Am J Surg Pathol. 2014 Mar;38(3):389–93. PMID:24525509
3605. Woodford-Richens K, Bevan S, Churchman M, et al. Analysis of genetic and phenotypic heterogeneity in juvenile polyposis. Gut. 2000 May;46(5):656–60. PMID:10764709
3606. Woodford-Richens K, Williamson J, Bevan S, et al. Allelic loss at SMAD4 in polyps from juvenile polyposis patients and use of fluorescence in situ hybridization to demonstrate clonal origin of the epithelium. Cancer Res. 2000 May 1;60(9):2477–82. PMID:10811127
3607. Worthley DL, Phillips KD, Wayte N, et al. Gastric adenocarcinoma and proximal polyposis of the stomach (GAPPS): a new autosomal dominant syndrome. Gut. 2012 May;61(5):774–9. PMID:21813476
3608. Wotherspoon AC, Doglioni C, Diss TC, et al. Regression of primary low-grade B-cell gastric lymphoma of mucosa-associated lymphoid tissue type after eradication of Helicobacter pylori. Lancet. 1993 Sep 4;342(8871):575–7. PMID:8102719
3609. Wotherspoon AC, Ortiz-Hidalgo C, Falzon MR, et al. Helicobacter pylori-associated gastritis and primary B-cell gastric lymphoma. Lancet. 1991 Nov 9;338(8776):1175–6. PMID:1682595
3610. Wright DH. Burkitt's lymphoma: a review of the pathology, immunology, and possible etiologic factors. Pathol Annu. 1971;6:337–63. PMID:4342309
3611. Wu AH, Yu MC, Mack TM. Smoking, alcohol use, dietary factors and risk of small intestinal adenocarcinoma. Int J Cancer. 1997 Mar 4;70(5):512–7. PMID:9052748
3612. Wu CM, Fishman EK, Hruban RK, et al. Serous cystic neoplasm involving the pancreas and liver: an unusual clinical entity. Abdom Imaging. 1999 Jan-Feb;24(1):75–7. PMID:9933679
3613. Wu F, Yuan G, Chen J, et al. Network analysis based on TCGA reveals hub genes in colon cancer. Contemp Oncol (Pozn). 2017;21(2):136–44. PMID:28947883
3615. Wu H, Wasik MA, Przybylski G, et al.

Hepatosplenic gamma-delta T-cell lymphoma as a late-onset posttransplant lymphoproliferative disorder in renal transplant recipients. Am J Clin Pathol. 2000 Apr;113(4):487–96. PMID:10761449
3616. Wu J, Jiao Y, Dal Molin M, et al. Whole-exome sequencing of neoplastic cysts of the pancreas reveals recurrent mutations in components of ubiquitin-dependent pathways. Proc Natl Acad Sci U S A. 2011 Dec 27;108(52):21188–93. PMID:22158988
3617. Wu J, Matthaei H, Maitra A, et al. Recurrent GNAS mutations define an unexpected pathway for pancreatic cyst development. Sci Transl Med. 2011 Jul 20;3(92):92ra66. PMID:21775669
3618. Wu SG, Zhang WW, He ZY, et al. Sites of metastasis and overall survival in esophageal cancer: a population-based study. Cancer Manag Res. 2017 Dec 6;9:781–8. PMID:29255373
3619. Wu X, Renuse S, Sahasrabuddhe NA, et al. Activation of diverse signalling pathways by oncogenic PIK3CA mutations. Nat Commun. 2014 Sep 23;5:4961. PMID:25247763
3620. Xia M, Singhi AD, Dudley B, et al. Small bowel adenocarcinoma frequently exhibits Lynch syndrome-associated mismatch repair protein deficiency but does not harbor sporadic MLH1 deficiency. Appl Immunohistochem Mol Morphol. 2017 Jul;25(6):399–406. PMID:27258561
3621. Xiao C, Wu F, Jiang H, et al. Hepatoid adenocarcinoma of the stomach: nine case reports and treatment outcomes. Oncol Lett. 2015 Sep;10(3):1605–9. PMID:26622718
3622. Xiao HD, Yamaguchi H, Dias-Santagata D, et al. Molecular characteristics and biological behaviours of the oncocytic and pancreatobiliary subtypes of intraductal papillary mucinous neoplasms. J Pathol. 2011 Aug;224(4):508–16. PMID:21547907
3623. Xiao Y, Qiu HZ, Zhou JL, et al. [Diagnosis and surgical treatment of colorectal cavernous hemangioma: a report of 4 cases and review of Chinese literatures]. Zhonghua Wei Chang Wai Ke Za Zhi. 2008 Jul;11(4):312–6. Chinese. PMID:18636349
3624. Xie J, Itzkowitz SH. Cancer in inflammatory bowel disease. World J Gastroenterol. 2008 Jan 21;14(3):378–89. PMID:18200660
3625. Xu AM, Gong SJ, Song WH, et al. Primary mixed germ cell tumor of the liver with sarcomatous components. World J Gastroenterol. 2010 Feb 7;16(5):652–6. PMID:20128038
3626. Xu-Monette ZY, Dabaja BS, Wang X, et al. Clinical features, tumor biology, and prognosis associated with MYC rearrangement and Myc overexpression in diffuse large B-cell lymphoma patients treated with rituximab-CHOP. Mod Pathol. 2015 Dec;28(12):1555–73. PMID:26541272
3627. Xu-Monette ZY, Wu L, Visco C, et al. Mutational profile and prognostic significance of TP53 in diffuse large B-cell lymphoma patients treated with R-CHOP: report from an International DLBCL Rituximab-CHOP Consortium Program Study. Blood. 2012 Nov 8;120(19):3986–96. PMID:22955915
3628. Xue Y, Reid MD, Balci S, et al. Immunohistochemical classification of ampullary carcinomas: critical reappraisal fails to confirm prognostic relevance for recently proposed panels, and highlights MUC5AC as a strong prognosticator. Am J Surg Pathol. 2017 Jul;41(7):865–76. PMID:28505002
3629. Xue Y, Vanoli A, Balci S, et al. Non-ampullary-duodenal carcinomas: clinicopathologic analysis of 47 cases and comparison with ampullary and pancreatic adenocarcinomas. Mod Pathol. 2017 Feb;30(2):255–66. PMID:27739441
3630. Yabe M, Medeiros LJ, Daneshbod Y, et al. Hepatosplenic T-cell lymphoma arising in patients with immunodysregulatory disorders: a study of 7 patients who did not receive tumor necrosis factor-α inhibitor therapy and literature review. Ann Diagn Pathol. 2017 Feb;26:16–22. PMID:28038706
3631. Yachida S, Iacobuzio-Donahue CA. The pathology and genetics of metastatic pancreatic cancer. Arch Pathol Lab Med. 2009 Mar;133(3):413–22. PMID:19260747
3632. Yachida S, Vakiani E, White CM, et al. Small cell and large cell neuroendocrine carcinomas of the pancreas are genetically similar and distinct from well-differentiated pancreatic neuroendocrine tumors. Am J Surg Pathol. 2012 Feb;36(2):173–84. PMID:22251937
3633. Yadav D, Lowenfels AB. The epidemiology of pancreatitis and pancreatic cancer. Gastroenterology. 2013 Jun;144(6):1252–61. PMID:23622135
3634. Yadav R, Jain D, Mathur SR, et al. Cytomorphology of neuroendocrine tumours of the gallbladder. Cytopathology. 2016 Apr;27(2):97–102. PMID:25689921
3635. Yadav R, Jain D, Mathur SR, et al. Gallbladder carcinoma: an attempt of WHO histological classification on fine needle aspiration material. Cytojournal. 2013 Jun 18;10:12. PMID:23858322
3636. Yaeger R, Shah MA, Miller VA, et al. Genomic alterations observed in colitis-associated cancers are distinct from those found in sporadic colorectal cancers and vary by type of inflammatory bowel disease. Gastroenterology. 2016 Aug;151(2):278–87.e6. PMID:27063727
3637. Yamada M, Fukagawa T, Nakajima T, et al. Hereditary diffuse gastric cancer in a Japanese family with a large deletion involving CDH1. Gastric Cancer. 2014 Oct;17(4):750–6. PMID:24037103
3638. Yamada S, Ohira M, Horie H, et al. Expression profiling and differential screening between hepatoblastomas and the corresponding normal livers: identification of high expression of the PLK1 oncogene as a poor-prognostic indicator of hepatoblastomas. Oncogene. 2004 Aug 5;23(35):5901–11. PMID:15221005
3639. Yamada T, Yoshikawa T, Taguri M, et al. The survival difference between gastric cancer patients from the UK and Japan remains after weighted propensity score analysis considering all background factors. Gastric Cancer. 2016 Apr;19(2):479–89. PMID:25761964
3640. Yamaguchi H, Goldenring JR, Kaminishi M, et al. Identification of spasmolytic polypeptide expressing metaplasia (SPEM) in remnant gastric cancer and surveillance postgastrectomy biopsies. Dig Dis Sci. 2002 Mar;47(3):573–8. PMID:11911345
3641. Yamaguchi H, Kuboki Y, Hatori T, et al. Somatic mutations in PIK3CA and activation of AKT in intraductal tubulopapillary neoplasms of the pancreas. Am J Surg Pathol. 2011 Dec;35(12):1812–7. PMID:21945955
3642. Yamaguchi H, Kuboki Y, Hatori T, et al. The discrete nature and distinguishing molecular features of pancreatic intraductal tubulopapillary neoplasms and intraductal papillary mucinous neoplasms of the gastric type, pyloric gland variant. J Pathol. 2013 Nov;231(3):335–41. PMID:23893889
3643. Yamaguchi H, Shimizu M, Ban S, et al. Intraductal tubulopapillary neoplasms of the pancreas distinct from pancreatic intraepithelial neoplasia and intraductal papillary mucinous neoplasms. Am J Surg Pathol. 2009 Aug;33(8):1164–72. PMID:19440145
3644. Yamaguchi K, Kanemitsu S, Hatori T, et al. Pancreatic ductal adenocarcinoma derived from IPMN and pancreatic ductal adenocarcinoma concomitant with IPMN. Pancreas. 2011 May;40(4):571–80. PMID:21499212
3645. Yamaguchi K, Ohuchida J, Ohtsuka T, et al. Intraductal papillary-mucinous tumor of the pancreas concomitant with ductal carcinoma of the pancreas. Pancreatology. 2002;2(5):484–90. PMID:12378117
3646. Yamaguchi K, Tanaka M. Mucin-hypersecreting tumor of the pancreas with mucin extrusion through an enlarged papilla. Am J Gastroenterol. 1991 Jul;86(7):835–9. PMID:2058624
3647. Yamaguchi S, Fujii T, Izumi Y, et al. Identification and characterization of a novel adenomatous polyposis coli mutation in adult pancreatoblastoma. Oncotarget. 2018 Jan 6;9(12):10818–27. PMID:29535845
3648. Yamamoto H, Handa M, Tobo T, et al. Clinicopathological features of primary leiomyosarcoma of the gastrointestinal tract following recognition of gastrointestinal stromal tumours. Histopathology. 2013 Aug;63(2):194–207. PMID:23763337
3649. Yamamoto H, Itoh F, Nakamura H, et al. Genetic and clinical features of human pancreatic ductal adenocarcinomas with widespread microsatellite instability. Cancer Res. 2001 Apr 1;61(7):3139–44. PMID:11306499
3650. Yamamoto H, Yoshida A, Taguchi K, et al. ALK, ROS1 and NTRK3 gene rearrangements in inflammatory myofibroblastic tumours. Histopathology. 2016 Jul;69(1):72–83. PMID:26647767
3651. Yamamoto J, Fujishima F, Ichinohasama R, et al. A case of benign natural killer cell proliferative disorder of the stomach (gastric manifestation of natural killer cell lymphomatoid gastroenteropathy) mimicking extranodal natural killer/T-cell lymphoma. Leuk Lymphoma. 2011 Sep;52(9):1803–5. PMID:21649544
3652. Yamamoto M, Nakajo S, Miyoshi N, et al. Endocrine cell carcinoma (carcinoid) of the gallbladder. Am J Surg Pathol. 1989 Apr;13(4):292–302. PMID:2648878
3653. Yamanaka T, Oki E, Yamazaki K, et al. 12-gene recurrence score assay stratifies the recurrence risk in stage ii/iii colon cancer with surgery alone: the SUNRISE study. J Clin Oncol. 2016 Aug 20;34(24):2906–13. PMID:27325854
3654. Yamane L, Scapulatempo-Neto C, Reis RM, et al. Serrated pathway in colorectal carcinogenesis. World J Gastroenterol. 2014 Mar 14;20(10):2634–40. PMID:24627599
3655. Yamao K, Yanagisawa A, Takahashi K, et al. Clinicopathological features and prognosis of mucinous cystic neoplasm with ovarian-type stroma: a multi-institutional study of the Japan Pancreas Society. Pancreas. 2011 Jan;40(1):67–71. PMID:20924309
3656. Yamao T, Hayashi H, Higashi T, et al. Colon cancer metastasis mimicking intraductal papillary neoplasm of the extra-hepatic bile duct. Int J Surg Case Rep. 2015;10:91–3. PMID:25818370
3657. Yamashita K, Sakuramoto S, Katada N, et al. Diffuse type advanced gastric cancer showing dismal prognosis is characterized by deeper invasion and emerging peritoneal cancer cell: the latest comparative study to intestinal advanced gastric cancer. Hepatogastroenterology. 2009 Jan-Feb;56(89):276–81. PMID:19453074
3658. Yamashita K, Sakuramoto S, Watanabe M. Genomic and epigenetic profiles of gastric cancer: potential diagnostic and therapeutic applications. Surg Today. 2011 Jan;41(1):24–38. PMID:21191688
3659. Yamashita S, Kishino T, Takahashi T, et al. Genetic and epigenetic alterations in normal tissues have differential impacts on cancer risk among tissues. Proc Natl Acad Sci U S A. 2018 Feb 6;115(6):1328–33. PMID:29358395
3660. Yamazaki K, Eyden B. An immunohistochemical and ultrastructural study of pancreatic microcystic serous cyst adenoma with special reference to tumor-associated microvasculature and vascular endothelial growth factor in tumor cells. Ultrastruct Pathol. 2006 Jan-Feb;30(1):119–28. PMID:16517478
3661. Yamazawa S, Ushiku T, Shinozaki-Ushiku A, et al. Gastric cancer with primitive enterocyte phenotype: an aggressive subgroup of intestinal-type adenocarcinoma. Am J Surg Pathol. 2017 Jul;41(7):989–97. PMID:28505005
3662. Yan BC, Gong C, Song J, et al. Arginase-1: a new immunohistochemical marker of hepatocytes and hepatocellular neoplasms. Am J Surg Pathol. 2010 Aug;34(8):1147–54. PMID:20661013
3663. Yan HHN, Lai JCW, Ho SL, et al. RNF43 germline and somatic mutation in serrated neoplasia pathway and its association with BRAF mutation. Gut. 2017 Sep;66(9):1645–56. PMID:27329244
3664. Yan Z, Grenert JP, Joseph NM, et al. Hepatic angiomyolipoma: mutation analysis and immunohistochemical pitfalls in diagnosis. Histopathology. 2018 Jul;73(1):101–8. PMID:29512829
3665. Yanagisawa N, Mikami T, Saegusa M, et al. More frequent beta-catenin exon 3 mutations in gallbladder adenomas than in carcinomas indicate different lineages. Cancer Res. 2001 Jan 1;61(1):19–22. PMID:11196159
3666. Yanaru-Fujisawa R, Nakamura S, Moriyama T, et al. Familial fundic gland polyposis with gastric cancer. Gut. 2012 Jul;61(7):1103–4. PMID:22027476
3667. Yang A, Sisson R, Gupta A, et al. Germline APC mutations in hepatoblastoma. Pediatr Blood Cancer. 2018 Apr;65(4). PMID:29251405
3668. Yang BL, Shao WJ, Sun GD, et al. Perianal mucinous adenocarcinoma arising from chronic anorectal fistulae: a review from single institution. Int J Colorectal Dis. 2009 Sep;24(9):1001–6. PMID:19205706
3669. Yang D, Duckworth LV, Draganov PV. More than meets the eye: esophageal invasive mucinous adenocarcinoma masquerading as a submucosal lipoma on endoscopic ultrasound. Endoscopy. 2014;46 Suppl 1 UCTN:E502–3. PMID:25314219
3670. Yang JF, Tang SJ, Lash RH, et al. Anatomic distribution of sessile serrated adenoma/polyp with and without cytologic dysplasia. Arch Pathol Lab Med. 2015 Mar;139(3):388–93. PMID:25724036
3671. Yang K, Yun SP, Kim S, et al. Clinicopathological features and surgical outcomes of neuroendocrine tumors of ampulla of Vater. BMC Gastroenterol. 2017 May 31;17(1):70. PMID:28569146
3672. Yang SJ, Ooyang CH, Wang SY, et al. Adenosquamous carcinoma of the ampulla of Vater - a rare disease at unusual location. World J Surg Oncol. 2013 May 31;11:124. PMID:23721111
3673. Yang X, Li A, Wu M. Hepatic angiomyolipoma: clinical, imaging and pathological features in 178 cases. Med Oncol. 2013 Mar;30(1):416. PMID:23292871
3674. Yang Z, Klimstra DS, Hruban RH, et al. Immunohistochemical characterization of the origins of metastatic well-differentiated neuroendocrine tumors to the liver. Am J Surg Pathol. 2017 Jul;41(7):915–22. PMID:28498280
3675. Yang Z, Tang LH, Klimstra DS. Effect of tumor heterogeneity on the assessment of Ki67 labeling index in well-differentiated neuroendocrine tumors metastatic to the liver: implications for prognostic stratification. Am J Surg Pathol. 2011 Jun;35(6):853–60. PMID:21566513
3676. Yanik EL, Kaunitz GJ, Cottrell TR, et al.

Association of HIV status with local immune response to anal squamous cell carcinoma: implications for immunotherapy. JAMA Oncol. 2017 Jul 1;3(7):974–8. PMID:28334399

3677. Yano T, Ishikura H, Wada T, et al. Hepatoid adenocarcinoma of the pancreas. Histopathology. 1999 Jul;35(1):90–2. PMID:10383723

3678. Yantiss RK, Chang HK, Farraye FA, et al. Prevalence and prognostic significance of acinar cell differentiation in pancreatic endocrine tumors. Am J Surg Pathol. 2002 Jul;26(7):893–901. PMID:12131156

3679. Yantiss RK, Panczykowski A, Misdraji J, et al. A comprehensive study of nondysplastic and dysplastic serrated polyps of the vermiform appendix. Am J Surg Pathol. 2007 Nov;31(11):1742–53. PMID:18059232

3680. Yantiss RK, Shia J, Klimstra DS, et al. Prognostic significance of localized extra-appendiceal mucin deposition in appendiceal mucinous neoplasms. Am J Surg Pathol. 2009 Feb;33(2):248–55. PMID:18852679

3681. Yantiss RK, Woda BA, Fanger GR, et al. KOC (K homology domain containing protein overexpressed in cancer): a novel molecular marker that distinguishes between benign and malignant lesions of the pancreas. Am J Surg Pathol. 2005 Feb;29(2):188–95. PMID:15644775

3682. Yao FY, Xiao L, Bass NM, et al. Liver transplantation for hepatocellular carcinoma: validation of the UCSF-expanded criteria based on preoperative imaging. Am J Transplant. 2007 Nov;7(11):2587–96. PMID:17868066

3683. Yao JC, Eisner MP, Leary C, et al. Population-based study of islet cell carcinoma. Ann Surg Oncol. 2007 Dec;14(12):3492–500. PMID:17896148

3684. Yao JC, Hassan M, Phan A, et al. One hundred years after "carcinoid": epidemiology of and prognostic factors for neuroendocrine tumors in 35,825 cases in the United States. J Clin Oncol. 2008 Jun 20;26(18):3063–72. PMID:18565894

3685. Yao K. Clinical application of magnifying endoscopy with narrow-band imaging in the stomach. Clin Endosc. 2015 Nov;48(6):481–90. PMID:26668793

3686. Yao T, Kajiwara M, Kuroiwa S, et al. Malignant transformation of gastric hyperplastic polyps: alteration of phenotypes, proliferative activity, and p53 expression. Hum Pathol. 2002 Oct;33(10):1016–22. PMID:12395375

3687. Yasuda H, Takada T, Amano H, et al. Surgery for mucin-producing pancreatic tumor. Hepatogastroenterology. 1998 Nov-Dec;45(24):2009–15. PMID:9951855

3688. Yasuda K, Adachi Y, Shiraishi N, et al. Papillary adenocarcinoma of the stomach. Gastric Cancer. 2000 Aug 4;3(1):33–8. PMID:11984707

3689. Yasui W, Oue N, Aung PP, et al. Molecular-pathological prognostic factors of gastric cancer: a review. Gastric Cancer. 2005;8(2):86–94. PMID:15864715

3690. Yasui W, Oue N, Sentani K, et al. Transcriptome dissection of gastric cancer: identification of novel diagnostic and therapeutic targets from pathology specimens. Pathol Int. 2009 Mar;59(3):121–36. PMID:19261089

3691. Yasui W, Sentani K, Sakamoto N, et al. Molecular pathology of gastric cancer: research and practice. Pathol Res Pract. 2011 Oct 15;207(10):608–12. PMID:22005013

3691A. Yau T, Tang VY, Yao TJ, et al. Development of Hong Kong Liver Cancer staging system with treatment stratification for patients with hepatocellular carcinoma. Gastroenterology. 2014 Jun;146(7):1691–700.e3. PMID:24583061

3692. Yeh CN, Jan YY, Yeh TS, et al. Hepatic

resection of the intraductal papillary type of peripheral cholangiocarcinoma. Ann Surg Oncol. 2004 Jun;11(6):606–11. PMID:15172934

3693. Yeh JM, Hur C, Ward Z, et al. Gastric adenocarcinoma screening and prevention in the era of new biomarker and endoscopic technologies: a cost-effectiveness analysis. Gut. 2016 Apr;65(4):563–74. PMID:25779597

3694. Yeh YC, Lei HJ, Chen MH, et al. C-reactive protein (CRP) is a promising diagnostic immunohistochemical marker for intrahepatic cholangiocarcinoma and is associated with better prognosis. Am J Surg Pathol. 2017 Dec;41(12):1630–41. PMID:28945626

3695. Yen JB, Kong MS, Lin JN. Hepatic mesenchymal hamartoma. J Paediatr Child Health. 2003 Nov;39(8):632–4. PMID:14629534

3696. Yendamuri S, Huang M, Malhotra U, et al. Prognostic implications of signet ring cell histology in esophageal adenocarcinoma. Cancer. 2013 Sep 1;119(17):3156–61. PMID:23719932

3697. Yendamuri S, Malhotra U, Hennon M, et al. Clinical characteristics of adenosquamous esophageal carcinoma. J Gastrointest Oncol. 2017 Feb;8(1):89–95. PMID:28280613

3698. Yeong ML, Wood KP, Scott B, et al. Synchronous squamous and glandular neoplasia of the anal canal. J Clin Pathol. 1992 Mar;45(3):261–3. PMID:1313454

3699. Yerci O, Sehitoglu I, Ugras N, et al. Somatostatin receptor 2 and 5 expressions in gastroenteropancreatic neuroendocrine tumors in Turkey. Asian Pac J Cancer Prev. 2015;16(10):4377–81. PMID:26028102

3700. Yergiyev O, Krishnamurti U, Mohanty A, et al. Fine needle aspiration cytology of acinar cell cystadenoma of the pancreas. Acta Cytol. 2014;58(3):297–302. PMID:24852936

3701. Yesim G, Gupse T, Zafer U, et al. Mesenchymal hamartoma of the liver in adulthood: immunohistochemical profiles, clinical and histopathological features in two patients. J Hepatobiliary Pancreat Surg. 2005;12(6):502–7. PMID:16365828

3702. Yettimis E, Trompetas V, Varsamidakis N, et al. Pathologic splenic rupture: an unusual presentation of pancreatic cancer. Pancreas. 2003 Oct;27(3):273–4. PMID:14508136

3703. Ying H, Kimmelman AC, Lyssiotis CA, et al. Oncogenic Kras maintains pancreatic tumors through regulation of anabolic glucose metabolism. Cell. 2012 Apr 27;149(3):656–70. PMID:22541435

3704. Ylagan LR, Liu LH, Maluf HM. Endoscopic bile duct brushing of malignant pancreatic biliary strictures: retrospective study with comparison of conventional smear and ThinPrep techniques. Diagn Cytopathol. 2003 Apr;28(4):196–204. PMID:12672095

3705. Yokode M, Akita M, Fujikura K, et al. High-grade PanIN presenting with localised stricture of the main pancreatic duct: a clinicopathological and molecular study of 10 cases suggests a clue for the early detection of pancreatic cancer. Histopathology. 2018 Aug;73(2):247–58. PMID:29660164

3706. Yokoyama A, Hirota T, Omori T, et al. Development of squamous neoplasia in esophageal iodine-unstained lesions and the alcohol and aldehyde dehydrogenase genotypes of Japanese alcoholic men. Int J Cancer. 2012 Jun 15;130(12):2949–60. PMID:21796615

3707. Yoo S. GI-associated hemangiomas and vascular malformations. Clin Colon Rectal Surg. 2011 Sep;24(3):193–200. PMID:22942801

3708. Yoon H, Kim N. Diagnosis and management of high risk group for gastric cancer. Gut Liver. 2015 Jan;9(1):5–17. PMID:25547086

3709. Yoon HH, Khan M, Shi Q, et al. The prognostic value of clinical and pathologic factors in esophageal adenocarcinoma: a mayo cohort of 796 patients with extended follow-up

after surgical resection. Mayo Clin Proc. 2010 Dec;85(12):1080–9. PMID:21123634

3710. Yoon WJ, Lee JK, Lee KH, et al. Cystic neoplasms of the exocrine pancreas: an update of a nationwide survey in Korea. Pancreas. 2008 Oct;37(3):254–8. PMID:18815545

3711. Yoshida T, Tajika M, Tanaka T, et al. The features of colorectal tumors in a patient with Li-Fraumeni syndrome. Intern Med. 2017;56(3):295–300. PMID:28154273

3712. Yoshida Y, Endo T, Tanaka E, et al. Oncocytic type intraductal papillary mucinous neoplasm of the pancreas with unusually low mucin production mimicking intraductal tubulopapillary neoplasm: a report of a case diagnosed by a preoperative endoscopic biopsy. Intern Med. 2017 Dec 1;56(23):3183–8. PMID:29021473

3713. Yoshikawa D, Ojima H, Iwasaki M, et al. Clinicopathological and prognostic significance of EGFR, VEGF, and HER2 expression in cholangiocarcinoma. Br J Cancer. 2008 Jan 29;98(2):418–25. PMID:18087285

3714. Yoshikawa K, Kinoshita A, Hirose Y, et al. Endoscopic submucosal dissection in a patient with esophageal adenoid cystic carcinoma. World J Gastroenterol. 2017 Dec 7;23(45):8097–103. PMID:29259386

3715. Yoshimi N, Sugie S, Tanaka T, et al. A rare case of serous cystadenocarcinoma of the pancreas. Cancer. 1992 May 15;69(10):2449–53. PMID:1568167

3716. Yoshizawa T, Toyoki Y, Hirai H, et al. Invasive micropapillary carcinoma of the extrahepatic bile duct and its malignant potential. Oncol Rep. 2014 Oct;32(4):1355–61. PMID:25109922

3717. Young AL, Igami T, Senda Y, et al. Evolution of the surgical management of perihilar cholangiocarcinoma in a Western centre demonstrates improved survival with endoscopic biliary drainage and reduced use of blood transfusion. HPB (Oxford). 2011 Jul;13(7):483–93. PMID:21689232

3718. Young JP, Win AK, Rosty C, et al. Rising incidence of early-onset colorectal cancer in Australia over two decades: report and review. J Gastroenterol Hepatol. 2015 Jan;30(1):6–13. PMID:25251195

3719. Young RJ, Brown NJ, Reed MW, et al. Angiosarcoma. Lancet Oncol. 2010 Oct;11(10):983–91. PMID:20537949

3720. Youssef H, Newman C, Chandrakumaran K, et al. Operative findings, early complications, and long-term survival in 456 patients with pseudomyxoma peritonei syndrome of appendiceal origin. Dis Colon Rectum. 2011 Mar;54(3):293–9. PMID:21304299

3721. Yozu M, Johncilla ME, Srivastava A, et al. Histologic and outcome study supports reclassifying appendiceal goblet cell carcinoids as goblet cell adenocarcinomas, and grading and staging similarly to colonic adenocarcinomas. Am J Surg Pathol. 2018 Jul;42(7):898–910. PMID:29579011

3722. Yu GH, Nayar R, Furth EE. Adenocarcinoma in colonic brushing cytology: high-grade dysplasia as a diagnostic pitfall. Diagn Cytopathol. 2001 May;24(5):364–8. PMID:11335971

3723. Yu H, Fang C, Chen L, et al. Worse prognosis in papillary, compared to tubular, early gastric carcinoma. J Cancer. 2017 Jan 1;8(1):117–23. PMID:28123605

3724. Yu Y, Demierre MF, Mahalingam M. Anaplastic Kaposi's sarcoma: an uncommon histologic phenotype with an aggressive clinical course. J Cutan Pathol. 2010 Oct;37(10):1088–91. PMID:19638066

3725. Yuan H, Dong Q, Zheng B, et al. Lymphovascular invasion is a high risk factor for stage I/II colorectal cancer: a systematic review and meta-analysis. Oncotarget. 2017 Jul 11;8(28):46565–79. PMID:28430621

3726. Yuan L, Luo X, Lu X, et al. Comparison

of clinicopathological characteristics between cirrhotic and non-cirrhotic patients with intrahepatic cholangiocarcinoma: a large-scale retrospective study. Mol Clin Oncol. 2017 Oct;7(4):615–22. PMID:29046795

3727. Yurgelun MB, Kulke MH, Fuchs CS, et al. Cancer susceptibility gene mutations in individuals with colorectal cancer. J Clin Oncol. 2017 Apr 1;35(10):1086–95. PMID:28135145

3728. Zagari RM, Rabitti S, Greenwood DC, et al. Systematic review with meta-analysis: diagnostic performance of the combination of pepsinogen, gastrin-17 and anti-Helicobacter pylori antibodies serum assays for the diagnosis of atrophic gastritis. Aliment Pharmacol Ther. 2017 Oct;46(7):657–67. PMID:28782119

3729. Zagars GK, Ballo MT, Pisters PW, et al. Prognostic factors for patients with localized soft-tissue sarcoma treated with conservation surgery and radiation therapy: an analysis of 1225 patients. Cancer. 2003 May 15;97(10):2530–43. PMID:12733153

3730. Zaidel-Bar R. Cadherin adhesome at a glance. J Cell Sci. 2013 Jan 15;126(Pt 2):373–8. PMID:23547085

3731. Zaman S, Mistry P, Hendrickse C, et al. Cloacogenic polyps in an adolescent: a rare cause of rectal bleeding. J Pediatr Surg. 2013 Aug;48(8):e5–7. PMID:23932634

3732. Zamboni G, Bonetti F, Scarpa A, et al. Expression of progesterone receptors in solid-cystic tumour of the pancreas: a clinicopathological and immunohistochemical study of ten cases. Virchows Arch A Pathol Anat Histopathol. 1993;423(6):425–31. PMID:8291215

3733. Zamboni G, Scarpa A, Bogina G, et al. Mucinous cystic tumors of the pancreas: clinicopathological features, prognosis, and relationship to other mucinous cystic tumors. Am J Surg Pathol. 1999 Apr;23(4):410–22. PMID:10199470

3734. Zamboni G, Terris B, Scarpa A, et al. Acinar cell cystadenoma of the pancreas: a new entity? Am J Surg Pathol. 2002 Jun;26(6):698–704. PMID:12023573

3735. Zarandi A, Irani S, Savabkar S, et al. Evaluation of promoter methylation status of MLH1 gene in Iranian patients with colorectal tumors and adenoma polyps. Gastroenterol Hepatol Bed Bench. 2017 Winter;10(Suppl1):S117–21. PMID:29511481

3736. Zatkova A, Rouillard JM, Hartmann W, et al. Amplification and overexpression of the IGF2 regulator PLAG1 in hepatoblastoma. Genes Chromosomes Cancer. 2004 Feb;39(2):126–37. PMID:14695992

3737. Zauber P, Berman E, Marotta S, et al. Ki-ras gene mutations are invariably present in low-grade mucinous tumors of the vermiform appendix. Scand J Gastroenterol. 2011 Jul;46(7-8):869–74. PMID:21443421

3738. Zavras N, Schizas D, Machairas N, et al. Carcinoid syndrome from a carcinoid tumor of the pancreas without liver metastases: a case report and literature review. Oncol Lett. 2017 Apr;13(4):2373–6. PMID:28454406

3739. Zea-Iriarte WL, Sekine I, Itsuno M, et al. Carcinoma in gastric hyperplastic polyps. A phenotypic study. Dig Dis Sci. 1996 Feb;41(2):377–86. PMID:8601386

3740. Zee SY, Hochwald SN, Conlon KC, et al. Pleomorphic pancreatic endocrine neoplasms: a variant commonly confused with adenocarcinoma. Am J Surg Pathol. 2005 Sep;29(9):1194–200. PMID:16096409

3741. Zeiton MA, Knight BC, Khaled YN, et al. Carcinoma arising within an anal gland. BMJ Case Rep. 2011 Feb 15;2011. PMID:22707467

3742. Zeki S, Fitzgerald RC. The use of molecular markers in predicting dysplasia and guiding treatment. Best Pract Res Clin Gastroenterol. 2015 Feb;29(1):113–24. PMID:25743460

3743. Zen C, Zen Y, Mitry RR, et al. Mixed phenotype hepatocellular carcinoma after transarterial chemoembolization and liver transplantation. Liver Transpl. 2011 Aug;17(8):943–54. PMID:21491582

3744. Zen Y, Adsay NV, Bardadin K, et al. Biliary intraepithelial neoplasia: an international interobserver agreement study and proposal for diagnostic criteria. Mod Pathol. 2007 Jun;20(6):701–9. PMID:17431410

3745. Zen Y, Aishima S, Ajioka Y, et al. Proposal of histological criteria for intraepithelial atypical/proliferative biliary epithelial lesions of the bile duct in hepatolithiasis with respect to cholangiocarcinoma: preliminary report based on interobserver agreement. Pathol Int. 2005 Apr;55(4):180–8. PMID:15826244

3746. Zen Y, Fujii T, Itatsu K, et al. Biliary papillary tumors share pathological features with intraductal papillary mucinous neoplasm of the pancreas. Hepatology. 2006 Nov;44(5):1333–43. PMID:17058219

3747. Zen Y, Jang KT, Ahn S, et al. Intraductal papillary neoplasms and mucinous cystic neoplasms of the hepatobiliary system: demographic differences between Asian and Western populations, and comparison with pancreatic counterparts. Histopathology. 2014 Aug;65(2):164–73. PMID:24456415

3748. Zen Y, Pedica F, Patcha VR, et al. Mucinous cystic neoplasms of the liver: a clinicopathological study and comparison with intraductal papillary neoplasms of the bile duct. Mod Pathol. 2011 Aug;24(8):1079–89. PMID:21516077

3749. Zen Y, Sasaki M, Fujii T, et al. Different expression patterns of mucin core proteins and cytokeratins during intrahepatic cholangiocarcinogenesis from biliary intraepithelial neoplasia and intraductal papillary neoplasm of the bile duct–an immunohistochemical study of 110 cases of hepatolithiasis. J Hepatol. 2006 Feb;44(2):350–8. PMID:16360234

3750. Zenali M, Overman MJ, Rashid A, et al. Clinicopathologic features and prognosis of duodenal adenocarcinoma and comparison with ampullary and pancreatic ductal adenocarcinoma. Hum Pathol. 2013 Dec;44(12):2792–8. PMID:24139211

3750A. Zevallos Quiroz JC, Jiménez Agüero R, Garmendi Irizar M, et al. Mucinous cystic neoplasm of the gallbladder obstructing the common bile duct, a rare entity with a new name. Cir Esp. 2014 Oct;92(8):567–9. PMID:23827932

3751. Zhang B, Xie QP, Gao SL, et al. Pancreatic somatostatinoma with obscure inhibitory syndrome and mixed pathological pattern. J Zhejiang Univ Sci B. 2010 Jan;11(1):22–6. PMID:20043348

3752. Zhang G, Cai YZ, Xu GH. Diagnostic accuracy of MRI for assessment of T category and circumferential resection margin involvement in patients with rectal cancer: a meta-analysis. Dis Colon Rectum. 2016 Aug;59(8):789–99. PMID:27384098

3753. Zhang GJ, Li RT, Zhou Y, et al. Solitary fibrous tumor of small bowel mesentery with postoperative bowel obstruction: a case report and review of literature. Int J Clin Exp Pathol. 2015 Sep 1;8(9):11691–7. PMID:26617912

3754. Zhang L, Sanderson SO, Lloyd RV, et al. Pancreatic intraepithelial neoplasia in heterotopic pancreas: evidence for the progression model of pancreatic ductal adenocarcinoma. Am J Surg Pathol. 2007 Aug;31(8):1191–5. PMID:17667542

3754A. Zhang L, Smyrk TC, Oliveira AM, et al. KIT is an independent prognostic marker for pancreatic endocrine tumors: a finding derived from analysis of islet cell differentiation markers. Am J Surg Pathol. 2009 Oct;33(10):1562–9. PMID:19574886

3755. Zhang L, Smyrk TC, Young WF Jr, et al. Gastric stromal tumors in Carney triad are different clinically, pathologically, and behaviorally from sporadic gastric gastrointestinal stromal tumors: findings in 104 cases. Am J Surg Pathol. 2010 Jan;34(1):53–64. PMID:19935059

3756. Zhang L, Zhou Y, Cheng C, et al. Genomic analyses reveal mutational signatures and frequently altered genes in esophageal squamous cell carcinoma. Am J Hum Genet. 2015 Apr 2;96(4):597–611. PMID:25839328

3757. Zhang Q, Ming J, Zhang S, et al. Micropapillary component in gastric adenocarcinoma: an aggressive variant associated with poor prognosis. Gastric Cancer. 2015 Jan;18(1):93–9. PMID:24562421

3758. Zhang W, Wang DH. Origins of metaplasia in Barrett's esophagus: is this an esophageal stem or progenitor cell disease? Dig Dis Sci. 2018 Aug;63(8):2005–12. PMID:29675663

3759. Zhang X, Zhu H, Yang X, et al. Post-obstructive cyst formation in pancreas and cystic acinar transformation: Are they same? Pathol Res Pract. 2017 Aug;213(8):997–1001. PMID:28599853

3760. Zhang XY, Zhang WH. An unusual case of aggressive systemic mastocytosis mimicking hepatic cirrhosis. Cancer Biol Med. 2014 Jun;11(2):134–8. PMID:25009756

3761. Zhang Y, Guan DH, Bi RX, et al. Prognostic value of microRNAs in gastric cancer: a meta-analysis. Oncotarget. 2017 Jun 21;8(33):55489–510. PMID:28903436

3762. Zhao H, Davydova L, Mandich D, et al. S100A4 protein and mesothelin expression in dysplasia and carcinoma of the extrahepatic bile duct. Am J Clin Pathol. 2007 Mar;127(3):374–9. PMID:17276942

3763. Zhao Q, Rashid A, Gong Y, et al. Pathologic complete response to neoadjuvant therapy in patients with pancreatic ductal adenocarcinoma is associated with a better prognosis. Ann Diagn Pathol. 2012 Jan;16(1):29–37. PMID:22050964

3764. Zhao S, Xue Q, Ye B, et al. Synchronous primary carcinosarcoma and adenosquamous carcinoma of the esophagus. Ann Thorac Surg. 2011 Mar;91(3):926–8. PMID:21353036

3765. Zhao ZM, Wang J, Ugwuowo UC, et al. Primary hepatic neuroendocrine carcinoma: report of two cases and literature review. BMC Clin Pathol. 2018 Mar 1;18:3. PMID:29507528

3766. Zhelnin K, Xue Y, Quigley B, et al. Nonmucinous biliary epithelium is a frequent finding and is often the predominant epithelial type in mucinous cystic neoplasms of the pancreas and liver. Am J Surg Pathol. 2017 Jan;41(1):116–20. PMID:27673548

3767. Zheng DJ, Cooke DT. A survival comparison of mucin-producing adenocarcinoma of the esophagus to conventional adenocarcinoma after esophagectomy. Am Surg. 2013 Jan;79(1):49–53. PMID:23317610

3768. Zheng H, Takahashi H, Murai Y, et al. Pathobiological characteristics of intestinal and diffuse-type gastric carcinoma in Japan: an immunostaining study on the tissue microarray. J Clin Pathol. 2007 Mar;60(3):273–7. PMID:16714395

3769. Zheng HC, Li XH, Hara T, et al. Mixed-type gastric carcinomas exhibit more aggressive features and indicate the histogenesis of carcinomas. Virchows Arch. 2008 May;452(5):525–34. PMID:18266006

3770. Zheng S, Zhu Y, Zhao Z, et al. Liver fluke infection and cholangiocarcinoma: a review. Parasitol Res. 2017 Jan;116(1):11–9. PMID:27718017

3771. Zheng SL, Yip VS, Pedica F, et al. Intrahepatic bile duct mixed adenoneuroendocrine carcinoma: a case report and review of the literature. Diagn Pathol. 2015 Nov 20;10:204. PMID:26589730

3772. Zhong L. Magnetic resonance imaging in the detection of pancreatic neoplasms. J Dig Dis. 2007 Aug;8(3):128–32. PMID:17650223

3773. Zhou C, Dhall D, Nissen NN, et al. Homozygous P86S mutation of the human glucagon receptor is associated with hyperglucagonemia, alpha cell hyperplasia, and islet cell tumor. Pancreas. 2009 Nov;38(8):941–6. PMID:19657311

3774. Zhou H, Schaefer N, Wolff M, et al. Carcinoma of the ampulla of Vater: comparative histologic/immunohistochemical classification and follow-up. Am J Surg Pathol. 2004 Jul;28(7):875–82. PMID:15223956

3775. Zhou H, Shen Z, Zhao J, et al. [Distribution characteristics and risk factors of colorectal adenomas]. Zhonghua Wei Chang Wai Ke Za Zhi. 2018 Jun 25;21(6):678–84. Chinese. PMID:29968244

3776. Zhou II, Wang H, Zhou D, et al. Hepatitis B virus-associated intrahepatic cholangiocarcinoma and hepatocellular carcinoma may hold common disease process for carcinogenesis. Eur J Cancer. 2010 Apr;46(6):1056–61. PMID:20202823

3777. Zhou L, Rui JA, Wang SB, et al. Outcomes and prognostic factors of cirrhotic patients with hepatocellular carcinoma after radical major hepatectomy. World J Surg. 2007 Sep;31(9):1782–7. PMID:17610113

3778. Zhou Y, Shao W, Lu W. Diagnostic value of endorectal ultrasonography for rectal carcinoma: a meta-analysis. J Cancer Res Ther. 2014 Dec;10 Suppl:319–22. PMID:25693944

3779. Zhou Y, Zang Y, Xiang J, et al. Adenoid cystic carcinoma of the cardia: report of a rare case and review of the Chinese literature. Oncol Lett. 2014 Aug;8(2):726–30. PMID:25013491

3780. Zhu H, Qin L, Zhong M, et al. Carcinoma ex microcystic adenoma of the pancreas: a report of a novel form of malignancy in serous neoplasms. Am J Surg Pathol. 2012 Feb;36(2):305–10. PMID:22189969

3781. Zhu L, Li Z, Wang Y, et al. Microsatellite instability and survival in gastric cancer: a systematic review and meta-analysis. Mol Clin Oncol. 2015 May;3(3):699–705. PMID:26137290

3782. Zhuang Z, Vortmeyer AO, Pack S, et al. Somatic mutations of the MEN1 tumor suppressor gene in sporadic gastrinomas and insulinomas. Cancer Res. 1997 Nov 1;57(21):4682–6. PMID:9354421

3783. Ziarkiewicz-Wroblewska B, Gornicka B, Suleiman W, et al. Primary lymphoma of the liver – morphological and clinical analysis of 6 cases. Success of aggressive treatment. Neoplasma. 2005;52(3):267–72. PMID:15875091

3784. Zidar N, Langner C, Odar K, et al. Anal verrucous carcinoma is not related to infection with human papillomaviruses and should be distinguished from giant condyloma (Buschke-Löwenstein tumour). Histopathology. 2017 May;70(6):938–45. PMID:28012208

3785. Zimmermann H, Babel N, Dierickx D, et al. Immunosuppression is associated with clinical features and relapse risk of B cell posttransplant lymphoproliferative disorder: a retrospective analysis based on the prospective, international, multicenter PTLD-1 trials. Transplantation. 2018 Nov;102(11):1914–23. PMID:29757894

3786. Zlobec I, Lugli A. Epithelial mesenchymal transition and tumor budding in aggressive colorectal cancer: tumor budding as oncotarget. Oncotarget. 2010 Nov;1(7):651–61. PMID:21317460

3787. Zou S, Li J, Zhou H, et al. Mutational landscape of intrahepatic cholangiocarcinoma. Nat Commun. 2014 Dec 15;5:5696. PMID:25526346

3788. Zucca E, Bertoni F. The spectrum of MALT lymphoma at different sites: biological and therapeutic relevance. Blood. 2016 Apr 28;127(17):2082–92. PMID:26989205

3789. Zucman-Rossi J, Jeannot E, Nhieu JT, et al. Genotype-phenotype correlation in hepatocellular adenoma: new classification and relationship with HCC. Hepatology. 2006 Mar;43(3):515–24. PMID:16496320

3790. Zucman-Rossi J, Villanueva A, Nault JC, et al. Genetic landscape and biomarkers of hepatocellular carcinoma. Gastroenterology. 2015 Oct;149(5):1226–39.e4. PMID:26099527

3791. Zuo M, Rashid A, Wang Y, et al. RNA sequencing-based analysis of gallbladder cancer reveals the importance of the liver X receptor and lipid metabolism in gallbladder cancer. Oncotarget. 2016 Jun 7;7(23):35302–12. PMID:27167107

Subject index

Bold page numbers indicate the main discussion(s) of the topic.

Numbers and symbols

1p   186, 333, 351, 443, 513
1q   186, 333, 388, 391, 412
2p   241, 411, 413, 444, 513, 514, 519
3p   191, 304, 327, 333, 351, 358, 514, 519
3q   418, 514
4p   391
4q   186, 442
5q   186, 333, 388, 391, 447, 513, 523
6q   333, 351, 358, 412, 418, 447
7p   186, 391, 513, 519
7q   186, 391, 398
8p   186, 333, 391
8q   186, 241, 333, 411, 413
9p   324, 333
9q   388, 391, 418, 514
10q   304, 514, 542, 543, 548
11p   241, 339
11q   358, 412, 414, 418, 514
12p   324, 391, 504, 514
12q   186, 448, 451, 513
13q   186, 412, 513
14q   186, 411, 413, 443, 514
15q   186, 443, 513
16p   513, 514
16q   388, 391, 513, 535
17p   186, 324, 333, 351, 412, 513, 514
17q   48, 186, 333, 360, 513, 514, 533
18p   186
18q   179, 186, 191, 324, 333, 513
19p   513, 514
19q   186, 489
20p   186, 514
20q   186, 333, 447
22q   186, 242, 411, 351, 413, 443
1F6   245–246
5-HIAA   365
α1-antitrypsin   341–342, 350
α-catenin   536
α-hCG   108
α-inhibin   251–252, 320
β-catenin   67, 79, 82, 84, 118, 125, 170, 179,
    216, 222–225, 227–228, 231, 241, 243,
    271, 285, 330, 334, 336, 338–342, 350,
    371, 446–447, 490–491, 505, 513, 517,
    524–525, 527, 531
β-endorphin   363–364
βF1   387, 394
β-hCG   504
β-thalassaemia   224
γ-radiation   86
γδ T cell   397

A

ABC   403–405
ABCB1   398
ABCG8   284
ABO   323, 540
achalasia   48, 52
acinar cell carcinoma   19, 295–296, 298,
    302, 316, 330, **333–336**, 339, 345, 350,
    367–368, 370–371, 540
acinar cystic transformation of the
    pancreas   300
ACTH   337, 343, 362–364
ACTH-producing neuroendocrine
    tumour   295, 363
activating mutations   132, 164, 171,
    179–180, 225, 227, 307–308, 319, 391,
    395, 437, 442, 446–447, 452
activation-induced cytidine deaminase   175,
    412
ACVR2A   186
ACVRL1   550
ADAM9   See disintegrin and
    metalloproteinase domain–containing
    protein 9 (ADAM9)
adenocarcinoma, intestinal type   112,
    127–128, 266, 283, 286
adenocarcinoma, metastatic   43, 150, 245,
    258, 500, 506
adenocarcinoma with mixed subtypes   60,
    85
adenofibroma   215–216, 245–246, 248–249,
    256
adenoid cystic carcinoma   23–24, 44–45, 52
adenoma–carcinoma pathway   179, 534
adenoma-like adenocarcinoma   158, 177,
    180–181
adenomatous polyp   60, 79, 81, 83, 112,
    118, 121, 158, 170
adenomatous polyposis   67, 77–81, 118,
    121–122, 125, 128, 171, 178, 187,
    240–241, 271, 273, 284, 311, 333,
    337, 339–340, 436, 446–447, 511–513,
    516–517, 522–524, 526, 528–531, 550
adenosquamous carcinoma   15, 24, 46–47,
    59–60, 89, 98, 126–127, 129, 158, 177,
    181, 266, 286, 289–290, 296, 320, 322,
    327, 330
advanced adenoma   158, 170, 172
AE1/AE3   133, 293, 358
aFGF   365
AFP   91, 230, 232, 239–244, 261, 328, 330,
    333–334, 337–339, 488, 498, 504–505

Africa   49, 231, 322–323, 379, 411, 414
aggressive systemic mastocytosis   374, 423
AGR2   254
AIDS   468
AKT1   125, 144, 514
AKT/mTOR   207, 403, 442, 472, 514
Alcian blue   42, 44, 77, 79, 325, 335
alcohol   14, 30, 48, 57, 116, 125, 178, 189,
    224–225, 230–231, 323, 344, 517
ALDH1A1   48
ALDH2   48
ALK   388, 416, 444–445, 455, 550
Alport syndrome   456
alveolar rhabdomyosarcoma   185–186, 434,
    460–461
AMACR   32, 34
AMER1   186
amphicrine   149
ampulla   19, 111–114, 116–118, **121–125,
    127–131**, 134, 201, 250, 270–271, 273,
    276, 311, 324–325, 328, 361, 506
ampullary adenocarcinoma   111, 116, 122,
    124, 126–128, 130
ampullary adenoma   111, 116, 121–123, 125
anabolic steroids   224
anal adenocarcinoma   197, 208
anal canal   19, 193–197, 200–202, 204–205,
    208–213
anal condyloma   200–201
anal neuroendocrine neoplasm   212–213
anal squamous dysplasia   202, 207
anaplastic carcinoma   100–101, 322
anastomosing haemangioma   434, 462–463
aneuploidy   32, 49–50, 75, 174–175, 258,
    351
angiodysplasia   434, 462, 464
angiolipoma   434, 450–451
angiomyolipoma   225, 238, 433–434,
    485–487
angiopoietin   222
angiosarcoma   238, 433–434, 436, **463–464,
    467–468**, 471–472
ANGPT1   222
ANGPT2   222
ANO1   441, 445, 453
antrum   61, 64–65, 69, 71, 77, 85, 102–104,
    452, 454, 473, 526–527
anus   196, 198, 200, 202, 204–205, 207–208,
    212, 506, 542
ANXA8   326
APC   67, 72, 75–77, 79, 81, 84, 86, 122,
    144, 149, 170–171, 175, 179, 185–187,

191, 241, 334, 336, 339, 371, 436–437, 446–447, 512–513, 516–517, **522–526**, 528–529, 531

apoptosis 32, 50, 171, 242, 244, 294, 388, 412, 420, 512, 514, 517, 548

appendiceal adenocarcinoma 146–147, 151

appendiceal goblet cell adenocarcinoma 149, 151–152

appendiceal mucinous neoplasm 136–137, 140, 143–145, 148

appendiceal neuroendocrine neoplasm 140, 152–155

appendiceal serrated lesions 141–142

appendicitis 141, 144, 147, 149, 153

AR 187, 513–514

ARG1 232, 261, 487

ARHGAP 315

ARID1A 75, 88, 94, 101, 130, 149, 182, 231, 258, 285, 290, 324, 336, 346, 412

ARID1B 231, 290

ARID2 75, 77, 149, 230–231, 502

ascending colon 159, 162, 177, 411, 450

ascites 229, 292, 322, 423–424, 466, 471

ASH1L 109

ASS1 227

ASXL1 315

ATF1 494

ATM 230, 324, 408, 411, 536, 539–540

ATP 443

ATP4A 106

ATP6AP1 479

ATP6AP2 479

atrophic gastritis 39, 65, 76–77, 86, 104–106, 108, 523

atrophic gastropathy 65

atrophy 14, 43, 64–65, 71, 79, 86, 284, 307–308, 324–325, 382, 386–389, 398, 523, 540

ATRX 17, 293, 298, 335, 344, 346, 350–351, 354, 367, 371, 502

autoimmune 65, 76, 81–82, 86, 104, 106, 108, 377, 379, 393, 415, 463

AXIN 241, 524

AXIN1 84, 222, 230–231, 241

AXIN2 84, 187, 513, 525, 531

B

B72.3 245, 308, 326

BAP1 258, 317

BARD1 540

Barrett dysplasia 23, 28, 32–34, 40

basaloid squamous cell carcinoma 24, 44, 49, 52–53, 57

BAX 171, 179

B-cell receptor 403, 411–412, 416

BCL2 381, 384–385, 403–407, 413–414, 416

BCL6 381–382, 384, 403–404, 407, 409, 413–414, 416, 418

BCL9 191

BCL10 298, 302, 326, 334, 336, 338, 342,

345, 350, 380–381

BCOR 420

Beckwith–Wiedemann syndrome 240–241, 337, 339, 490

BerEP4 205

bFGF 106

biallelic 67, 79, 185, 225, 307, 360, 398, 487, 513, 515–518, 530–531

bile duct adenoma 215–216, 245–246

biliary adenofibroma 215, 245–246, 248–249, 256

biliary intraepithelial neoplasia 215–216, 245, 254, 256–257, 265–266, 270, 273–275, 281, 290

Billroth 70

BIRC3-MALT1 378–382

BLM 411

BMP 513, 531

BMPR1A 187, 514, 542–544, 550

Borrmann 88

botryoid 460–461

BRAF 122, 141–142, 144, 147, 163–165, 179–181, 184–187, 191, 246, 258, 336, 371, 427, 443, 473–474, 482, 502–503, 517–518, 520, 534

BRCA1 367, 513–514, 539–540

BRCA2 17, 324, 346, 513, 536, 539–540

BTG3-CCDC40 292

BTK 405, 513, 531

BUB1 518, 521, 525

BUB1B 540

BUB3 518, 521, 540

Budd–Chiari syndrome 221, 466

Burkitt lymphoma 373–374, 376–377, 411–413, 418

C

C19MC 489

CA125 326, 399

CA19-9 245, 249–250, 255, 258, 298, 304, 311–312, 319, 322, 326, 332, 350, 367

caecum 159, 162, 177, 402, 450

CAIX 350

calcification 41–42, 50–51, 144–145, 240, 252, 284, 303, 320, 340–341, 348, 360, 362, 440, 463–464, 473, 490–491

calcifying nested stromal-epithelial tumour 433–434, 490, 505

caldesmon 456, 459, 474, 545

calponin 44, 456, 459

CAM5.2 103, 133, 293

Campylobacter jejuni 379

CAMTA1 467

Cancer Genome Atlas 40, 64, 87–88, 94–95, 184, 186, 323

carcinoid syndrome 17, 56, 104–105, 132, 153, 188, 212, 263, 345, 365

carcinoid tumour 16–17, 20, 22, 263

carcinoma of the extrahepatic bile ducts 253, 265, 289–290

carcinoma of the gallbladder 265, 283–284, 287

carcinoma, undifferentiated 23–24, 29, 42, 52, 54–55, 59–60, 89, 100–101, 126–127, 129, 136, 147, 158, 177, 181–182, 216, 260, 262, 266, 283, 287–290, 296, 320, 322, 328–330, 367

carcinoma with osteoclast-like giant cells 60, 100–101, 129, 290, 296, 320, 322, 329

carcinoma with sarcomatoid component 158, 177

cardia 25, 32, 61, 64, 85, 89

Carney complex 333

Caroli disease 255–256, 289

CASP8 186

CBLN2 57

CCK 343

CCL20 384

CCND1 32, 49, 230, 249, 338, 341, 408–409

CCND2 408, 410

CCND3 408, 412

CCR6 384

CD1a 426–427, 429–430

CD2 392, 421

CD3 183, 386–388, 391–392, 396–398, 421

CD3ε 387

CD4 388–389, 392–396, 398, 411, 421

CD5 381–382, 388, 392, 398, 405, 408–409, 413, 421

CD7 387–388, 392, 421

CD8 95, 183, 185, 386–389, 391–394, 396, 398, 421

CD8a 392

CD10 74, 103, 232, 251, 328, 342, 350, 381–382, 384–385, 404, 407, 409, 413, 416, 527

CD11c 381

CD13 430

CD15 418

CD16 421

CD19 404, 407, 412

CD20 381, 384–385, 392, 403–404, 407, 409, 412, 416, 418–419

CD21 383–384, 400, 429–430

CD22 412

CD23 381–382, 400, 409, 413, 429

CD25 425

CD30 387–389, 393–394, 405, 416, 418, 472, 505

CD31 464, 467, 470, 472, 476

CD34 103, 223, 225, 227, 237, 442, 445, 449, 453, 455–457, 459, 461, 464, 467, 470, 472, 474, 476, 478, 482, 496

CD35 400, 429–430

CD38 413, 416

CD43 381, 409, 413

CD44 95, 326, 346

CD45 205, 416

CD56 55, 84, 103, 191, 254, 262, 342, 349–350, 368, 388, 391–392, 396, 398,

416, 421–422, 474, 491, 496
CD57 349, 421, 480
CD68 129, 429–430, 480
CD77 413
CD79a 381, 404, 409, 412, 416
CD99 342, 346
CD103 388, 396
CD133 262
CD138 413, 416
CD163 430
CD200 409
CD207 426–427, 430
CD274 88, 94
CDC27 186
CDH1 86, 90, 94, 125, 149, 512–513, 535–538
CDH10 292
CDK4 49, 367
CDK6 49, 367
CDKN1B 106, 134, 241, 514
CDKN2A 36, 49–50, 94, 231, 241, 249, 271, 285, 300, 305, 307, 324, 326–327, 335–336, 346, 371, 405, 408, 443, 539–540
CDKN2B 285, 336
CDX2 74, 80, 82, 108, 119, 122–123, 128–129, 133, 181, 191, 205, 209, 211, 245, 277, 313, 328, 350, 365, 368, 504, 527
CEA 44, 205, 232, 245, 250, 252, 298, 304, 308, 311–312, 319–320, 322, 326, 328, 330, 337, 342, 345, 350, 371, 491
cell adhesion molecules 87
cell-cycle regulators 32, 49, 87, 106, 346
CHEK1 49
CHEK2 17, 49, 324, 346, 540
CHN2 125
cholangiocarcinoma 15, 215–216, 218, 220, 230–231, 237, 245–246, **253–258**, 260, **263–264**, 266, 280, 282–284, 289–291, 466
cholelithiasis 270–271, 284, 289, 361
cholestasis 127, 222, 255, 426
choriocarcinoma 330, 504–505
chromatin remodelling 17, 87, 149, 231, 317, 346
chromogranin 16–19, 55, 57, 84, 103, 106–109, 129, 133–134, 149, 153–154, 189–191, 205, 212–213, 264, 293, 298, 326, 330, 335, 338, 342–343, 345, 348–350, 356–358, 360, 362–363, 367–368, 370–371, 472, 474, 491, 496
cirrhosis 217, 222–224, 229, 231–232, 239, 246, 252, 254–255, 260, 377, 379, 509
CK5/6 42, 57, 209
CK7 41–42, 47, 119, 122–123, 126, 133, 209–211, 213, 222–223, 226, 235, 237, 243, 245–247, 249, 251–252, 254, 258, 271, 277, 312–313, 318, 320, 326, 330, 334, 350, 527
CK8 133, 252, 313, 320, 326, 330, 358, 467
CK18 133, 252, 313, 320, 326, 330, 442, 467

CK19 41, 222, 237, 239, 241, 243, 245–247, 249, 252, 254, 258, 261–262, 301–302, 312–313, 318, 320, 326, 330, 334, 346, 351, 358
CK20 41, 119, 122–123, 129, 181, 205, 209–211, 213, 245, 277, 313, 527
CLDN18 94
clear cell adenocarcinoma 266, 283
clear cell neuroendocrine tumour 296, 347
clear cell sarcoma 14, 433–434, 436, 494–495
cloacogenic zone 196
Clonorchis sinensis 290
clusterin 400
c-Met 95, 184, 187, 238, 258
CNA.42 400
CNS 414, 417, 419, 477, 522
coeliac disease 116, 125, 386–392
COL4A5 456
COL4A6 456
collision tumour 19, 57, 260, 304, 370–371
colloid carcinoma 281, 287, 296, 299, 312–313, 320, 322, 328
colonoscopy 67, 163, 172, 176, 447, 532–534, 548
colorectal adenocarcinoma 126, 147, 149, 162, 164, 170, 173, **177–178**, 209, 245, 518, 522, 524–525
colorectal adenomas 77, 142, 173, 516, 518, 520, 522–524, 529–531
colorectal neuroendocrine neoplasm 162, **188–191**
colorectal serrated lesion 119, 163–164, 533
combined hepatocellular-cholangiocarcinoma 15, 215, 220, 235, 237–238, **260–262**
combined small cell–squamous cell carcinomas 24, 56
COMPASS-like complex 324
condyloma 193, 197, 200–204, 206–207
congestive heart failure 462, 465
consumptive coagulopathy 463, 465
corpus 61, 64–65, 85, 104, 107, 424
Correa's cascade 64, 86
Cowden syndrome 70, 187, 436, 450, 483, 511, 514, 533, **547–550**
COX-2 230, 258
CPA1 539–540
CPB1 539–540
CpG 67, 94, 134, 163–165, 180, 185
CPS1 487, 491, 498
C-reactive protein 223–225, 227, 228, 230, 254, 259, 399
CREB1 494
CRH 363
Crohn disease 116, 125–126, 174, 176, 178, 197, 206, 209, 396–397
CT 38, 44, 49, 86, 124, 144, 178, 200, 229, 240, 283, 300, 303, 310, 322–323, 337, 340, 348, 353, 357, 359, 361, 437, 439,

477, 486, 494
CTNNA1 149, 536, 538
CTNNB1 64, 67, 77, 79, 84, 125, 149, 185–186, 222, 225, 227–228, 230–231, 241, 260, 271, 285, 336, 339–340, 342, 437, 446–447, 490, 517
Cushing syndrome 263, 292, 337, 363–364, 490
CXCL13 400, 429
cyclin D1 241, 273, 342, 382, 408–410
CYP1A1 284
CYP17A1 284
CYP1B1 225
cystadenocarcinoma 140, 144, 147, 250, 289, 296, 303–306, 319, 330, 333
cystadenoma 140, 144, 245, 250–251, 296, 300, 303–306, 319
cytokine 39, 174–175, 209, 258, 284, 388, 419, 424, 475

D
D10 245–246
D2-40 400, 467, 476, 504
DAXX 17, 293, 298, 335, 344, 346, 350–351, 354, 360, 367, 371
DCC 106, 191, 284, 334
D cell 104, 108, 132, 361
DCP 239
DDX3X 420
dentate line 195–197, 205
dermoid cyst 500, 504
descending colon 159, 162
desmin 103, 198, 320, 442, 445, 447, 449, 453, 455–457, 459, 461, 474, 478, 487, 491, 496–497
desmoid fibromatosis 433, 436–437, 446–447, 522
Dieulafoy lesion 434, 462, 464
diffuse large B-cell lymphoma 373–374, 376–377, 380–382, **402–405**, 413, 418–419
disintegrin and metalloproteinase domain-containing protein 9 (ADAM9) 326
DLK1 241
DMD 443
DNAJB1 15, 220, 230, 238
DNMT1 280
DOG1 103, 441, 443, 445, 453, 455–457, 459, 474, 478, 493, 496
duct adenocarcinoma 208, 296, 322
ductal plate malformation 254, 257–258, 488–489
DUPAN-2 326

E
E6 206–207
E7 206
EBER 88, 91–92, 95, 395, 400–401, 404, 416–417, 421, 459
EBV 55, 86, 91, 95, 287, 328, 373, 376, 391,

398–401, 404, 411, 416–420, 422, 428, 436

E-cadherin 88, 90, 95, 125, 328, 342, 513, 535–537

ECL-cell carcinoid 60, 104–109, 132–133, 153, 189–191

ectopic breast tissue 197

EGF 95, 326

EGFR (HER1) 43, 49–50, 53, 88, 95, 134, 184, 186, 258

EGR1 448

EIF5A2 50

ELF3 290

EMA 65, 101, 119, 122–123, 126, 128–129, 249, 252–254, 257, 259, 277, 281–282, 298, 308, 313, 316, 318, 320, 326, 330, 338–339, 345, 350, 371, 388, 429, 445, 449, 461, 472, 482, 491–493, 498

embryonal carcinoma 500, 504

embryonal rhabdomyosarcoma 434, 460–461

embryonal sarcoma 433–434, 436, 460, 489, 497–498

endometriosis 197

ENG 543, 550

enteropathy 116, 394, 421–422, 426

enteropathy-associated T-cell lymphoma 116, 373–374, 376, **386–389**, 391, 393–394

eosinophilic granuloma 426

EPAS1 132

EpCAM 241, 262, 513, 516, 519

EPHA8 315

epigenetic 32, 40, 49, 64, 67, 76–77, 86–87, 133–134, 164, 175, 178, 180, 258, 324, 331, 367, 403, 513, 516, 520

epithelial–mesenchymal transition 50, 88, 182–183, 185, 538

epithelial misplacement 173, 546

epithelioid angiosarcoma 434, 471

epithelioid haemangioendothelioma 433–434, 466–467

ER 251–253, 320–321, 464

ERBB2 (HER2) 28, 41, 43, 64, 77, 88, 93, 95, 101, 125, 249, 285, 288, 326

ERBB4 125, 292, 315

ERCC2 284

ERG 464, 467, 469–470, 472

estrogen exposure 463

European Neuroendocrine Tumor Society 154, 299, 346, 351, 354, 356, 358, 360, 362–363, 366

EUS 38, 44, 49, 86, 289, 303, 307, 322, 348, 353, 357, 361

EWSR1 14, 494, 496

extra-adrenal paraganglioma 112, 131

extramedullary haematopoiesis 242, 463–464, 487, 489, 497

extranodal marginal zone lymphoma of mucosa-associated lymphoid tissue 373–374, 378–382, 384, 404

extranodal NK/T-cell lymphoma 373–374, 376, 393–394, 420–421

EZH2 246, 280

F

FABP1 226

factor VIII–related antigen 464, 472

faecal occult blood 177–178, 532

familial adenomatous polyposis 1 79, 171, 511–512, 522

familial pancreatic cancer 323, 511–513, 539–540

FAN1 518, 525

FAT1 57

FAT4 144

FRXW7 57, 186

FDG PET 18, 49

FGF19 230–231, 238–239

FGFR1 443

FGFR2 88, 125, 258, 317

FGFR4 231, 238

FHIT 106, 191

fibroepithelial polyp 197, 201

fibrolamellar carcinoma 15, 220, 230, 233, 238

fibromatosis 433–434, 436–437, 446–447, 522, 524

field effect 121, 174, 275, 278, 288

FISH 41, 86, 133, 258, 291, 328, 330, 351, 413–414, 504

fistula 126, 208–210

FLI1 464, 472

FLT1 472

FLT3 125

FLT4 472

FNA 38, 86, 109, 126, 130, 184, 253, 258, 282, 288, 302, 305, 313, 330, 339, 342, 350, 412, 457, 503

focal dermal hypoplasia 30

focal nodular hyperplasia 215, 220–225, 238, 464

follicular dendritic cell sarcoma 373–374, 376–377, 399–400, **428–429**

follicular lymphoma 373–374, 376–377, **382–384**, 406, 415–416

follicular lymphoma, duodenal type 374, 383

foveolar-type adenoma 59, 77, 79–80, 523, 527

foveolar-type dysplasia 33, 74, 118

FOXA2 360

FOXN3 355

FOXO1 461

FOXP1 380, 404

FOXP2 191

Frantz tumour 340

FRK 225

fundic gland polyp 59, 64, 67–70, 73–74, 76, 80–81, 522–524, 526, 528

fundus 61, 64, 79, 81, 85, 102, 104, 107, 283, 285–286, 292, 424, 526, 528

FZD3 186

G

gain-of-function mutations 427, 440, 442

galactosaemia 224

ganglioneuroblastoma 357

ganglioneuroma 357, 433–434, 436, 483–484, 548

ganglioneuromatosis 433–434, 436, 483–484

GAPPS 67–68, 79, 81, 86, 511–513, 522, 526–528

gastric adenocarcinoma 42, 64, 67, 71, 73, 79, 81, 83, **85–95**, 101, 103, 512–513, 522, 526–528, 531

gastric antral vascular ectasia 434, 462, 464

gastric dysplasia 66, 71–75, 83

gastric neuroendocrine neoplasm 106, 109

gastric pit/crypt dysplasia 60, 71, 74

gastric pyloric gland adenoma 81–82, 523

gastric squamous cell carcinoma 96–97

gastric undifferentiated carcinoma 100–101

gastrin 57, 65–66, 106, 108, 132–133, 292, 355–356, 362–363

gastrinoma 17, 60, 104–106, 108, 112, 131, 295–296, 345, **355–356**, 359

gastritis 39, 59, 64–65, 67, 69–70, 76–77, 79–82, 86, 104–106, 108, 408, 523

gastroblastoma 14, 59–60, 64, 102–103

gastrointestinal stromal tumour **433–443**, 456, 458–459, 477, 487, 493, 496

gastro-oesophageal reflux 14, 30, 32, 39, 54, 355, 458

GCDFP-15 205, 211

G cell 104, 105, 107, 108, 132

GCET1 404

GCGR 346, 359–360

G-CSF 230

gene expression profiling 185, 239, 241, 384, 398, 416, 419

genetic susceptibility 86, 512, 535

germ cell tumour 499–500, 504–506, 508

germinoma 500, 504

GFAP 478, 482

ghrelin 108

GHRH 343

giant cell angiofibroma 434, 448–449

glandular intraepithelial neoplasia 60, 71, 158, 174, 296, 307

GLI1 227, 454

glicentin 190

GLMN 473

glomangiomatosis 434, 473

glomus tumour 433–434, 436, 473–474

GLP 353

GLP-1 153, 191

GLP-2 191

glucagon-like peptide-producing tumour 136, 152, 158, 188

glucagonoma 17, 295–296, 343, 345,

359–360

GLUT1   304, 464, 482

gluten enteropathy   116

glycogenosis   224

GNAI2   391

GNAQ   464

GNAS   64, 81, 84, 118–119, 144, 147, 225, 253, 258, 278, 280, 290, 298, 300, 305, 308, 311, 313, 315, 335

goblet cell   14, 21, 32, 77, 98, 135–137, 140, 145, 148–154, 158, 163–164, 166, 168, 176, 198, 286

goblet cell adenocarcinoma   14, 135–136, 140, 145, 148–153

Goltz–Gorlin syndrome   30

gp130   225

GPC3   92, 225, 235–238, 243, 334, 498, 504–505

G protein–coupled receptor   358

granular cell tumour   207, 433–434, 436, 479–480

GREM1   187, 513, 531, 533

GS   222–225, 227–228, 235–236, 238, 243, 487

GTP   179

GTPase   179

H

H⁺/K⁺ ATPase   84, 92

haemangioendothelioma   433–434, 462, 464, **466–467**, 471–472

haemangioma   221–222, 433–434, 436, 462–465, 488

haematemesis   393, 473, 507

haemophagocytosis   430

haemorrhoids   197–198, 502

hamartoma   245–246, 433–434, 436, 450, 477, 483, 488, 497–498, 533, 547–548

HBsAg   258

HBV   231, 255, 377, 379

hCG   505

HCV   231, 255, 377, 379

HDC   108

Helicobacter heilmannii   379

Helicobacter pylori   14, 39, 64–65, 67, 69, 76, 78, 81, 83, 86, 106, 378–382, 408, 523, 537

hepatic flexure   159, 162

hepatic haemangiomatosis   434, 462, 464

hepatic neuroendocrine neoplasm   215, 263–264

hepatoblastoma   215–216, 240–244, 488, 505, 522

hepatocellular adenoma   215–216, 220–221, 223–228, 231, 235, 237

hepatocellular carcinoma   15, 19, 91–92, 215–217, 220, 223–225, 227–239, 242–244, 255–256, 258–264, 284, 287, 328, 334, 350, 505, 507, 509

hepatoid adenocarcinoma   60, 85, 89, 91–92

hepatoid carcinoma   89, 91, 287, 296, 322, 328

hepatosplenic T-cell lymphoma   373–374, 377, 397–398, 418

hepatosplenomegaly   397, 423–424

Hep Par-1   232, 243, 287, 316, 328, 334, 486–487, 491, 498, 504

HER1   See EGFR (HER1)

HER2   See ERBB2 (HER2)

hereditary diffuse gastric cancer   86, 511–512, **535–538**

hereditary haemorrhagic telangiectasia   221, 462, 512, 514, 542, 550

HERPUD1   336

HES staining   360

HHV8   416, 436, 468–470

hidradenoma papilliferum   197

HIF   304, 346, 514

HIF1α   346, 350

HIF2α   132

histamine   423–424

histiocytic sarcoma   373–374, 376–377, 430–431

histone modification   87, 231

HIV   200, 204, 206–207, 209, 212, 377, 411, 415, 468–469

HLA-DPB1   420

HLA-DQ2   387

HLA-E   388

HMB45   205, 478, 486–487, 495–496

HMCN1   292

HMGA2   451

HNF1A   225–226

HPV   14, 30, 48, 52, 196, 200, 202–207, 209, 212

HPV6   200

HPV11   50, 200

HPV16   202, 206, 209

HPV18   209, 212

HPV51   50

HRAS   292

HSP70   225, 235–236, 238

hyalinizing cholecystitis   274, 284, 287

hypergastrinaemia   18, 104–108, 131

hypermutated   185–186

hyperplastic polyp   69, 73, 136, 140–142, 158, 163–166, 169, 176, 532–533

hypoglycaemia   353, 448

I

ID3   336, 412

IDH   258

IDH1   125, 254, 258, 260, 464

IDH2   254, 258, 260, 464

IG   408, 411, 416, 428, 430

IgA   76–77, 381–382

IgD   381

IGF   241

IGF2   448

IGF2BP3   32

IgG   381

IgG4   399

IGH   406–409, 411, 413, 418

IGHV   382, 384, 406, 416

IGK   408, 411, 413

IGL   408, 411, 413

IgM   381, 412

IL-1β   86, 174

IL-6   174, 225, 227, 230, 258, 419

IL-10   258, 419

IL-15   388

IL-21   388

IL6ST   225

ileum   17–18, 20–21, 113, 116, 118, 124–126, 131, 137, 353, 377, 383, 386, 390, 393, 396, 402, 435, 450, 452, 494

immunodeficiency   206, 377, 402, 411, 415, 531

immunoglobulin   380, 382, 384, 404, 408, 411, 416, 428, 430

immunoproliferative small intestinal disease   374, 376, 378–380, 382

IMP3   34, 280

inactivating mutations   57, 179, 225, 308, 442–443, 446, 473, 479, 533

indolent T-cell lymphoproliferative disorder   373–374, 376, 395–396

infantile haemangioma   434, 462, 464–465, 488

inflammatory bowel disease–associated dysplasia   157, 162, 174, 178–179, 209

inflammatory cloacogenic polyp   193, 197–198

inflammatory fibroid polyp   433, 436, 452–453

inflammatory myofibroblastic tumour   433–434, 436, 444

INHBE   227

INSM1   205

insulin gene enhancer protein ISL1   344, 350, 368

insulinoma   17, 295–296, 345, **353–354**, 359, 363–364

International Cancer Genome Consortium   323

intestinal metaplasia   34, 40, 56–57, 65, 75–79, 86, 105, 537

intestinal T-cell lymphoma   373–374, 376, 386, 388, 390–393

intestinal-type adenoma   59–60, 76–79, 112, 118–119, 121–122, 128

intestinal-type dysplasia   60, 71, 74

intra-ampullary papillary-tubular neoplasm   112, 116–117, 121–123, 127

intracholecystic papillary neoplasm   265, 270, 276–277, 288

intracystic papillary neoplasm   81, 266, 276, 283

intraductal oncocytic papillary neoplasm   15, 295–296, 298, 308, 313, 315, 328

intraductal papillary mucinous
  neoplasm 122, 280, 282, 295–296, 298–
  299, 308, 310–315, 317–318, 325–326,
  328, 365, 540
intraductal tubulopapillary neoplasm 15,
  281–282, 295–296, 313, 317–318
intramucosal carcinoma 36, 70, 72, 86, 176,
  535, 537
intussusception 118, 411, 417, 451–452,
  462, 471, 475, 494, 542, 545–546
IPMK 132
IRF4 403–404, 416
IRTA1 381
islet amyloid polypeptide 354
islet cell tumour 17, 347, 357

J

JAK1 225, 388, 420
JAK2 395
JAK3 144, 391, 420
JAK/STAT 225, 230, 388, 394, 398, 419
JAK/STAT3 227
jejunum 20–21, 113, 116, 118, 124–126,
  353, 383, 386, 388, 390, 393, 402, 404,
  435, 452
juvenile polyposis syndrome 187, 511–512,
  514, 542–544, 550

K

Kaposi sarcoma 433–434, 436, 468–470
Kasabach–Merritt syndrome 463
KDM6A 149, 324
KDR 472
KEAP1 230–231
K homology domain containing protein
  overexpressed in cancer 326
Ki-67 16–18, 32, 58, 84, 105–109, 134, 154,
  191, 198, 212, 245–246, 249, 264, 273,
  308, 329, 344–346, 350–352, 356, 358,
  360, 362, 364, 366–369, 384, 396, 404,
  410, 413, 416, 464, 472, 527, 538
KIT 44–45, 103, 125, 262, 342, 346, 351,
  363, 424–425, 436–437, 440–443, 445,
  453, 455–457, 459, 472, 474, 478, 482,
  487, 491, 493, 496, 502–504
Klippel–Trénaunay syndrome 462
KLLN 514
KMT2A 231, 317
KMT2B 317
KMT2C 231, 317, 324
KMT2D 149, 231, 408
koilocytotic atypia 203–204
KRAS 77, 79, 81, 107, 118, 122, 125, 130,
  141–142, 144, 147, 149, 163–165, 170–
  171, 175, 179–181, 184–186, 191, 211,
  253–254, 258, 260, 273, 278, 280, 285,
  290–292, 300, 305, 307, 311, 315, 317,
  319, 324, 327–329, 335, 339, 345–346,
  367, 371, 443, 524, 529, 534
Krukenberg tumour 92

L

Langerhans cell histiocytosis 373–374, 376,
  426–427
langerin 426, 429
large cell carcinoma with rhabdoid
  phenotype 60, 100, 296, 322
large cell neuroendocrine carcinoma 16,
  18–19, 24, 56–58, 60, 104, 106–108, 112,
  131, 133, 136, 152, 158, 188–190, 194,
  212, 216, 263–264, 266, 292–293, 296, 367
large duct intrahepatic
  cholangiocarcinoma 216
latency-associated nuclear antigen 468, 470
L-cell tumour 136, 152, 158, 188
LDH 386, 414, 419
LEF1 382, 409
leiomyoma 433–434, 436, 456
leiomyomatosis 434, 456
leiomyosarcoma 433–434, 436–437,
  457–459
Li–Fraumeni syndrome 187, 512, 514, 550
linitis plastica 88, 94, 286, 506, 536
lipoma 433–434, 436, 450, 486
liver fatty-acid binding protein 225–226, 487
LMO2 404–405
LMP1 399, 400, 416, 419
LMP2A 411
LRRFIP2 516–517
lymphangioma 433–434, 436, 475–476
lymphangiomatosis 433, 436, 475–476
lymphangitic carcinomatosis 92
lymphatic invasion 91, 137, 154, 159,
  181–183, 185, 254, 256, 325, 508
lymphoedema 436
lymphoepithelial lesions 380–382, 421
lymphoepithelioma-like carcinoma 24,
  54–55, 91, 254
lymphomatoid gastropathy 421–422
lymphomatous polyposis 395, 406–408
Lynch syndrome 81, 125, 128, 171, 180,
  185–187, 284, 328, 333, 336, 511–513,
  515–522, 529–531, 539–540, 550

M

MAFA 346, 353
Maffucci syndrome 436, 462, 464
Mahvash disease 359
malabsorption 391, 393, 424, 507
malaria 411
MALAT1 14, 103, 454
MALT lymphoma See *extranodal marginal
  zone lymphoma of mucosa-associated
  lymphoid tissue*
mantle cell lymphoma 373–374, 376–377,
  382, 408–410
MAP2K1 427
MAP7 186
MAPK 125, 171, 179, 185, 231, 258, 394,
  419, 427, 442, 479
mastocytosis 373–374, 376–377, **423–425**

MATK 391–392
MAX 443
McCune–Albright syndrome 81, 311
McKittrick–Wheelock syndrome 170
MDM2 49, 290
Meckel diverticulum 116, 125, 132
medullary carcinoma 60, 85, 91, 112, 124,
  126–129, 180–182, 287, 296, 322, 328,
  518, 540
MEK 336, 443
melanoma 55, 101, 186, 197, 205, 212–213,
  237, 368, 472, 496, 499–500, 502–503,
  506, 539, 548
MEN1 17–18, 106, 132, 191, 298, 335, 346,
  351, 353–355, 358, 367, 371, 514
menin 346, 355, 514
Merkel cell 20, 106, 213
merlin 477
mesenchymal hamartoma 433, 436, 488,
  497–498
MET 88, 125, 144, 187, 258
metabolic syndrome 224–225, 230–231,
  255, 284
metaplasia 14, 32, 34, 40, 56–57, 59, 64–65,
  75–79, 81, 86, 96, 105, 107, 118–119, 125,
  172, 175, 196, 252, 271–272, 284, 307,
  537
methylation 49, 67, 72, 75, 87–88, 94–95,
  163–165, 241, 285, 420, 442, 516–521, 536
MHC 388, 416
MIB1 413
MIC-A 388
microadenoma 296, 347, 523
microbiota 175, 290
micropapillary carcinoma 60, 85, 92, 180,
  286, 299, 328
microsatellite instability 43, 72, 75, 87–88,
  91, 93–95, 125–126, 130, 144, 147,
  164, 179–186, 211, 238, 241, 285, 288,
  292–293, 328, 336, 508–509, 517–521,
  529–531
microscopic colitis 424
MIER3 186
MiNEN See *mixed neuroendocrine–non-
  neuroendocrine neoplasm*
miR-141 230
miR-200f 230
miR-375 230
miR-429 230
MIR143 474
missense 49, 84, 311, 346, 518, 520, 536
MITF 487, 496
mixed acinar-ductal carcinoma 296, 333
mixed acinar-endocrine-ductal
  carcinoma 296, 333, 370
mixed acinar-neuroendocrine
  carcinoma 296, 333, 335, 345, 370–371
mixed germ cell tumour 500, 504
mixed neuroendocrine–non-neuroendocrine
  neoplasm 15–19, 24, 56–58, 60, 104–106,

108–109, 112, 126, 131–134, 136, 152–155, 158, 188–191, 194, 212–213, 216, 262–264, 266, 292–293, 295–296, 299, 335, 345–346, 370–372

mixed serous-neuroendocrine neoplasm 296, 303–304

MLH1 72, 88, 94–95, 163, 165, 167–168, 171, 175, 179–181, 185, 187, 513, 515–521, 529–530, 550

MMP1 95

MMP7 95, 254

MMP10 95

MNDA1 381

monomorphic epitheliotropic intestinal T-cell lymphoma 373–374, 376, 388, 390–394

MRI 38, 44, 86, 178, 200, 205, 221–222, 225–226, 229, 289, 303, 322–323, 340, 348, 353, 357, 359, 361, 437, 466, 486, 548

mRNA 206, 222, 227, 334, 404, 408, 412

MSA 320, 459, 497

MSH 363

MSH2 171, 179, 181, 187, 513, 515–516, 518–520, 529–530, 536, 539–540

MSH3 186–187, 517, 525, 529, 531

MSH6 171, 181, 186–187, 513, 515–516, 518–520, 529–530

mTOR 134, 207, 346, 351, 369, 403, 442, 472, 487, 514

MUC1 65, 87, 119, 122–123, 126, 128–129, 253–254, 259, 277, 281–282, 298, 308, 313, 316, 318, 320, 326, 330, 345, 350, 371

MUC2 65, 74, 80, 82, 119, 122–123, 128–129, 210, 245, 253, 277, 281, 298, 308, 313, 316, 318, 326, 328, 330, 371, 527

MUC4 308

MUC5AC 65, 73–75, 80, 82, 119, 123, 126, 128–130, 209, 245–246, 252–254, 275, 277, 281, 298, 308, 313, 316, 318, 320, 326, 527

MUC6 65, 80, 82, 84, 92, 119, 123, 126, 245–246, 254, 271, 277, 281, 298, 304–305, 308, 313, 316, 318, 527

mucinous adenocarcinoma 60, 85, 90, 108, 112, 124–127, 129, 136, 145, 147–148, 158, 177, 179–180, 209, 266, 283, 286

mucinous cystic neoplasm 144, 215–216, 250–253, 265–266, 282–283, 295–296, 298, 302, 304, 313, 319–321, 330

mucoepidermoid carcinoma 15, 24, 42, 46–47, 60, 85, 92, 206, 254

mucosal melanoma 499, 502–503

mucosal prolapse syndrome 199

mucosal Schwann cell hamartoma 434, 477

multilocus inherited neoplasia alleles syndrome 512, 514, 521, 550

MUM1 403–404, 416

MUTYH 17, 187, 346, 513, 516, 518, 529

MYC 175, 230, 241, 333, 341, 371, 391,

403–405, 411–414, 416, 418

myeloid sarcoma 376–377

MYO1B 186

MYOD1 461, 498

myofibroblast 171, 249, 325, 447, 455

myogenin 461, 498

N

NAB2 448

NANOG 504–505

NB84 496

NCAM 191, 254, 292

NCOA2 461

necrolytic migratory erythema 359

neoadjuvant therapy 19, 26, 38, 42–43, 62, 93, 184, 520

neuroectodermal 14, 243, 433, 479, 494–495, 506

neuroendocrine carcinoma 15–22, 24, 52, 55–58, 60, 104–109, 112, 129, 131–134, 136–137, 152–155, 158, 188–191, 194, 197, 205, 212–213, 216, 263–264, 266, 277, 292–297, 299, 343–345, 347, 350, 367–372, 508, 531

neuroendocrine tumour 15–20, 22, 24, 56–58, 60, 62, 69, 84, 104–109, 112–114, 131–134, 136, 138, 140, 152–155, 158, 160, 188–191, 194, 197, 212–213, 216, 237, 263–264, 266, 270, 292–299, 304, 330, 334–335, 343–351, 353–367, 369, 371–372, 474, 508, 512, 540, 550

neurofibromatosis 132, 346, 355, 361, 437, 440, 477, 479, 483, 514, 516, 531, 550

neurofibromin 442, 514

neuron-specific enolase 191, 342, 348–349, 484, 491, 548

NF1 346, 437, 440, 442–443, 514

NF2 477, 482

NF-κB 174, 380, 403, 419

NFE2L2 49, 230–231

NK cell 376, 395, 418, 421–422

NKG2D 388

NKp46 388

NKX3-1 205

nodular melanoma 500, 502

non-ampullary adenocarcinoma 111, 124–125

non-ampullary adenoma 111, 116, 118, 121, 125

non-functioning pancreatic neuroendocrine tumour 347–352

non-hypermutated 185–186

nonsense 84, 391, 518, 536

Notch 25, 241, 341, 473–474

NOTCH1 49, 57, 125, 149, 408

NOTCH2 408, 474

NOTCH3 49

NPM1 125

NRAS 184, 186, 211

NRG1 292

NS5A 231

NSAID 39, 178

NTHL1 187, 513, 518, 529

NTRK 238, 443–444

O

obstruction 69, 105, 121, 127–128, 131–132, 141, 147, 212, 222, 255, 279, 282, 289, 292, 300–301, 303, 325, 349, 386, 391, 402, 406, 417, 430, 444, 451–452, 454, 458, 460, 462, 471, 473, 483, 494, 507

OCT3/4 504–505

oesophageal adenocarcinoma 32, **38–43**, 44–49

oesophageal adenoid cystic carcinoma 44–45

oesophageal glandular dysplasia 24, 32

oesophageal neuroendocrine neoplasm 56–58, 189

oesophageal squamous cell carcinoma 14, 28, 36–37, 39, **48–53**, 55, 97

oesophageal squamous dysplasia 36–37

oesophageal squamous intraepithelial neoplasia 24, 36

oesophageal squamous papilloma 30, 96

oesophageal undifferentiated carcinoma 54–55

OGG1 284

oncocytic neuroendocrine tumour 296, 347

oncogene 49, 87, 171, 186, 258, 307, 341, 418, 440, 442, 517

Opisthorchis viverrini 256, 290

oral contraceptive 222, 224, 517

ORF73 468

oxyntic gland adenoma 59, 83–84, 92

P

p16 35, 49, 75, 200, 203–206, 230, 241, 246, 273, 280, 292, 307, 324, 326–327, 367, 371, 538

p21 171, 179, 273, 341

p27 106, 134, 241, 341, 346, 514

p40 42, 55, 57, 98, 129, 205, 327

p53 34–36, 49, 69, 72–75, 88, 106, 129, 133, 171, 179, 185, 198, 206–207, 245–246, 273, 275, 292–293, 308, 311, 326–327, 339, 344, 350, 513–514, 527, 538

p63 42, 44–45, 47, 55, 57, 98, 129, 209, 213, 327

Paget disease 197, 205, 210–211

PALB2 324, 536, 539–540

pancreatic acinar cell carcinoma 333, 336, 368, 371, 540

pancreatic ductal adenocarcinoma 130, 285, 290, 300, 305, 307–309, 311–312, 314, 321, **322–331**, 339, 367, 539–540

pancreatic intraductal oncocytic papillary neoplasm 315

pancreatic intraductal papillary mucinous neoplasm 15, **310–314** pancreatic intraductal tubulopapillary neoplasm **317–318**

pancreatic intraepithelial neoplasia 298, 307–309, 311, 313, 318, 322, 324–325, 335, 540

pancreatic mixed neuroendocrine–non-neuroendocrine neoplasm 188, 335, 345–346, 370, 372

pancreatic neuroendocrine carcinoma 343–347, 350, 352, 367–369

pancreatic neuroendocrine neoplasm 299, 304, 316, 343–366

pancreatitis 121, 131, 290, 310, 315, 322–324, 326–327, 330–331, 539–540

pancreatobiliary-type carcinoma 112, 127

pancreatoblastoma 295–296, 330, 334, **337–339**, 350

pancreatoduodenectomy 121, 127

Paneth cells 40, 74, 78, 172, 271

PAP 89, 189, 191

papillary adenocarcinoma 60, 85, 87, 89, 181

papillomatosis 24, 30–31, 276, 279

Papua New Guinea 411

paraganglioma 112, 131–134, 440

paraneoplastic syndrome 56, 292

parietal cells 68, 83, 92, 104, 106, 108

PARP 324, 541

PAS 42, 77, 79–80, 251, 304, 325, 370, 409, 536–537

PASD 304, 346

PAX3 461

PAX5 205, 404, 407, 412, 416

PAX7 461

PAX8 350

PBRM1 324

PCNA 32

PCR 204, 249, 470

PDCD1LG2 94

PDE3A 57

PDGFA 326, 442

PDGFB 326

PDGFR 134

PDGFRA 436–437, 440–443, 452–453, 459

PDGFRB 444

PD-L1 88, 94

PDX1 334, 350, 358, 368

PEComa 101, 433–434, 476, 485–486

pepsinogen 65–66, 84, 92

perforation 61, 113, 144, 147, 181, 217, 386, 391, 402, 417, 420, 422, 439, 446, 451, 462, 471, 507

perianal skin 195–196, 203, 207, 210, 213

perineurioma 433–434, 436, 481–482

PET 18, 44, 49, 205, 289, 322, 348, 353, 361

PET-CT 18, 38, 86, 178, 357, 359

Peutz–Jeghers syndrome 125, 128, 187, 271, 311, 511–512, 514, 539, **545–546**

Peyer patch 380

phaeochromocytoma 133, 357

PHOX2B 484

PI3K 171, 179, 185, 187, 317, 351, 403, 412, 442, 514, 548

PI3K/AKT 403, 442, 548

PIK3CA 88, 94, 107, 144, 171, 179, 184, 186–187, 207, 253, 258, 285, 317, 472, 514

PKA 230

PLAG1 241

PLAP 504

plasmablastic lymphoma 373–374, 376, 415–416

Plasmodium falciparum 411

PLCG1 472

pleomorphic carcinoma 60, 100

plexiform fibromyxoma 103, 433–434, 436, 454–455

PLK1 241

Plummer–Vinson syndrome 48

PMS2 181, 187, 513, 515–516, 518–520, 529–530

PNL2 487

podoplanin 464, 467, 470, 472, 504

POLD1 185, 187, 518, 521, 529–531

POLE 17, 93, 127, 175, 179–180, 185, 187, 513, 518, 521, 529–531

polycystic ovary syndrome 224

polymorphism 49, 87, 174, 284, 540

polyomavirus 106

POMC 363

poorly cohesive carcinoma 60, 85, 89–90, 92, 94, 124, 127, 158, 177, 266, 283, 286, 296, 322, 538

portal vein thrombosis 221

postgastrectomy 69

posttransplant lymphoproliferative disorders 373, 417–419

PP 57, 136, 152, 158, 188, 343, 349, 354, 356, 358, 360, 362

PPARA 241

PP/PYY-producing tumour 136, 152, 158, 188

PR 251–253, 320–321, 342, 351, 464, 491

PRDM1 403, 416

predictive biomarker 75, 95, 184, 186–187

primary biliary cirrhosis 377, 379

PRKACA 290

PRKACB 290

prolapse 69, 173, 197–199, 546

PRSS1 539–540

PSA 205

psammomatous 362, 490–491

PSAP 205

PSCA 87

pseudomyxoma peritonei 143, 145

psoriasis 397

PTEN 125, 171, 179, 187, 317, 346, 351, 354, 358, 450, 472, 483, 514, 533, 543, 547–548

PTGDS 227

PTHrP 343

PTK2 230, 538

PTPN12 186

PTPRB 472

PTPRM 57

pyloric gland adenoma 59, 81–82, 116, 119, 265, 270–272, 277, 523

pylorus 61, 64, 85, 107, 124–125

PYY 190

R

RAD51 324

RAF 125, 186, 443

RAF1 336

RANBP2 444, 445

RAS 49, 125, 184, 186–187, 230, 258, 324, 442–443, 472, 479, 514

RAS-RAF-MEK-ERK 179

RASSF1 241, 334

RASSF1A 230

RB1 17–18, 49, 57, 106–107, 109, 133, 144, 191, 206, 230–231, 292–293, 344–346, 350, 367, 371, 443, 459

receptor tyrosine kinase 87–88, 94–95, 187, 442

RECQL5 536

rectosigmoid junction 159, 162, 435

rectum 19, 22, 119, 153, 157–160, 162–163, 183, 188–191, 195–196, 198, 210, 264, 402, 435, 439, 456, 462, 477, 483, 515–516, 532

Reed–Sternberg 387, 400, 417–418

renal cell carcinoma 287, 350, 506, 547

resection margin 181, 183–184, 243, 331–332

RET 125, 444, 483, 514

rhabdoid 54, 60, 64, 100–101, 125, 129–130, 181–182, 242, 244, 296, 322, 329, 349

rhabdomyosarcoma 433–434, 436, 460–461

RHBDF2 48–49

rheumatoid arthritis 397

RHO 88

RHOA 88, 94, 149, 412

Riddell system 175

RNA 49, 88, 92, 184–185, 327, 354, 395, 400–401, 404, 416–417, 421, 459

RNA expression profiling 185

RNF43 72, 75, 165, 175, 253, 281, 298, 300, 308, 311, 315, 320, 335, 513, 533

Rokitansky–Aschoff sinus 274–276, 287–288

ROS1 444–445

RPL22 175

RPS6KA3 230–231

RRBP1 444

RSPO 165

S

S100 44, 103, 134, 205, 254, 273, 275, 426–427, 429–430, 442, 445, 453, 456, 459,

474, 478, 480, 482, 484, 487, 493–496

S100A4 326

S100A6 326

S100P 326

SALL4 92, 260, 504–505

Salmonella typhi 284

sarcomatoid carcinoma 48, 60, 100, 287, 322

SATB2 205

SCENIC classification 174

schwannoma 433–434, 436–437, 459, 477–479

scirrhous carcinoma 88, 94

serum amyloid A 223–225, 227

SDHA 442–443

SDHB 441–443

SDHC 442–443

SDHD 443

SEC23B 514

seedling leiomyomas 434, 456

SEER 147, 153–154, 439

serotonin 57, 108, 133, 153, 190, 343, 365–366

serotonin-producing neuroendocrine tumour 295, 349, 365

serous cystadenocarcinoma 296, 303–306

serous cystadenoma 245, 251, 296, 303–306

serous neoplasm of the pancreas 303

serrated adenocarcinoma 158, 177, 180–181

serrated dysplasia 60, 71, 74–75, 112, 118, 136, 141–142, 158, 163, 167, 175–176

serrated polyposis 187, 511–513, 531–534

sessile serrated lesion with dysplasia 163–165, 167–169

sessile serrated lesion without dysplasia 136, 141–142

SETD2 351, 391, 398, 502, 518

SF3B1 502

SGCZ 292

SH2D1A 411

sigmoid 159, 162, 177, 403, 512, 515–516

sigmoidoscopy 172

signet-ring cell carcinoma 60, 85, 87, 89, 112, 124, 127, 158, 177, 179–180, 182, 254, 296, 322, 328, 535–538

SIRT1 474

Sjögren syndrome 379

SMA 44, 103, 320, 442, 445, 447, 449, 453, 455–457, 459, 461, 474, 476, 478, 482, 487, 491, 496

SMAD2 144, 186

SMAD4 40, 106–107, 125, 144, 149, 170–171, 179, 186–187, 191, 274, 290, 292, 300, 305, 307–309, 311, 320, 324, 326–327, 330, 332, 335–336, 339, 350, 358, 367–368, 371, 512, 514, 524, 542–544, 550

small cell neuroendocrine carcinoma 16–19,

24, 56–58, 60, 104, 106, 108–109, 112, 131, 133, 136, 152, 158, 188–190, 194, 212–213, 216, 263, 266, 292–294, 296, 367

small duct intrahepatic cholangiocarcinoma 15, 216, 220, 254–259

SMARC 125

SMARCA2 130, 181

SMARCA4 101, 130, 181, 191, 324, 412

SMARCB1 100–101, 129–130, 181, 242–244

smoking 30, 39, 48, 57, 86, 125, 178, 189, 206, 209, 240, 255, 290, 323, 344, 367, 507, 517, 532

SND1 336

SNP 39, 49, 86, 87, 284

SOCS1 230, 388

solid pseudopapillary neoplasm 295–296, 298, 330, 340–342, 350

solitary fibrous tumour 433–434, 436, 448–449

solitary rectal ulcer syndrome 199

somatostatin 18, 108, 133, 343, 348–350, 354, 356, 361–363, 367

somatostatinoma 60, 112, 131–132, 295–296, 345, 361–362

sonic hedgehog 227

SOX10 205, 445, 453, 487, 494–496, 503

SOX11 382, 409–410

SPC18 95

SPINK1 539–540

splenic flexure 159, 162, 177, 534

squamous cell carcinoma 14, 17–19, 23–24, 26, 28–29, 31, 36–37, 39, 42, 44, 46–57, 59–60, 89, 96–99, 126, 129, 181, 190, 193–194, 197, 200, 202, 204–209, 211–213, 237, 266, 283, 286–287, 289, 327, 507–508

squamous cell carcinoma, spindle cell 24, 48–49, 51, 53

squamous cell papilloma 24, 30

squamous hyperplasia 207, 480

squamous intraepithelial neoplasia 24, 36, 194, 202, 212

squamous papillomatosis 24, 30–31

SRC 538

SS18 103

SSTR2 18, 356, 367

SSTR2A 108, 133, 189, 191, 345, 350, 357–358, 363–365

SSTR5 367

SSX 492, 493

STAT3 225, 227, 258, 388, 395, 398, 420, 538

STAT5 395

STAT5B 388, 391, 398, 420

STAT6 448–449

stem cell 40, 46, 96, 170, 174, 178, 258, 260–262, 389, 398, 417, 419, 442

Stewart–Treves syndrome 436

STK11 144, 187, 513–514, 539–540, 546

stricture 35, 49, 308, 386

succinate dehydrogenase 434, 437, 439–442, 548

surveillance 14, 28, 65, 168–169, 172, 231, 239, 263, 327, 509, 532, 534, 544

survivin 241

SWI/SNF 101, 129–130, 181–182, 324, 329

synaptophysin 16–19, 55, 57, 84, 103, 107–109, 129, 133–134, 149, 153–154, 189–191, 205, 212–213, 264, 293, 298, 326, 330, 335, 338, 342–343, 345–346, 349–350, 356, 358, 360, 362–363, 368, 370–371, 472, 474, 478, 484, 491, 496

synovial sarcoma 103, 433–434, 436–437, 492–493

systemic lupus erythematosus 377

T

T-cell receptor 386–388, 392, 394, 396, 398, 421

TCERG1 186

TCF3 412

TCF7L2 186

TCRαβ 394, 396, 398

TCRβ 387, 392

TCRγ 392

TCRγδ 388, 396, 398

TdT 413

TEK 472

teratoma 197, 500, 504–505

TERT 227–228, 230–232, 241, 540

TFE3 467, 487

TFF1 254

TFF2 65, 245–246

TGFB1 241

TGFBR2 186

TGF-α 95, 106, 326

TGF-β 134, 171, 179, 185, 230, 241, 326

Thorotrast 255, 472

thrombosis 221, 359, 462–464

TIA1 388, 392, 394, 396, 398, 421

TIE1 472

tingible-body macrophages 383–384, 406–407, 412

TLE1 493

TNF 86, 397

TNFAIP3 379

TP53 17–18, 32, 40, 49–50, 57, 64, 69, 72, 75, 94, 106–107, 109, 125, 144, 149, 163, 165, 170–171, 175, 179, 185–187, 191, 207, 230–231, 241, 258, 270–271, 273, 278, 280, 285, 290–292, 300, 307, 311, 320, 324, 327, 329, 336, 344, 346, 367, 371, 403, 405, 408, 412, 418, 437, 443, 459, 472, 502, 513–514, 524, 540, 550

transarterial embolization 465

transitional epithelium 195–198

transplantation 200, 235, 239, 389, 397–398, 415, 418–419, 436, 465, 468, 491

transverse colon 61, 159, 162, 177

TRB   386–388, 395, 398
TRD   398
TRG   43, 50, 93, 183–184, 386–388, 395, 398
TRRAP   149
TSC1   230, 351, 487, 514
TSC2   346, 354, 487, 514
TTF1   57, 109, 191, 213, 293, 368, 504
TTN   186
tubular adenocarcinoma   60, 85, 87, 89, 112,
    127, 129, 249, 256–257, 277, 281, 322
tubular adenoma   76, 81, 158, 170–172, 277
tubulovillous adenoma   108, 158, 170–172
tumour budding   41, 130, 181–183, 185
tumour suppressor gene   179, 281, 304, 324,
    443, 482, 523, 546, 550
tyrosinaemia   224, 231
tyrosinase   487

U

ubiquitin   311, 513
ulcerative colitis   174, 178
ultramutated   185–186
uncertain malignant potential   140, 144, 434,
    436, 473–474, 487
undifferentiated carcinoma with osteoclast-
    like giant cells   101, 129, 290, 296, 320,
    322, 329
UPF1   327
USP9X   149

V

VEGF   326
VEGFA   230
VEGF-A   95
VEGFR3   470
Verner–Morrison syndrome   357

verrucous squamous cell carcinoma   24,
    49–51, 194, 205
VGLL2   461
VHL   292–293, 303–305, 345–346, 348–350,
    358, 514
villous adenocarcinoma   181
villous adenoma   158, 170–172, 312, 524
villous atrophy   386–389
vimentin   101, 326, 328, 342, 350
VIP   357–358
VIPoma   295–296, 345, 357–359
VMAT1   365
VMAT2   57, 105, 108, 365
von Hippel–Lindau syndrome   292–293, 296,
    303–305, 345–346, 348–350, 358, 361,
    363, 367, 514, 550
VS38c   416

W

WNT   84, 118, 122, 149, 163, 165, 170, 179,
    185, 227, 231, 241, 243, 341, 446–447,
    513, 517, 524, 531, 533
WNT/β-catenin   84, 118, 231, 241, 243, 341,
    446
WT1   491
WWTR1   466, 467

X

xanthogranulomatous   476
XBP1   416
XPA   550

Y

YAP1   466, 467
yolk sac tumour   500, 504–505
YY1   354, 526, 528

The World Health Organization Classification of Tumours

Breast
Lakhani SR, Ellis IO, Schnitt SJ, et al., editors. WHO classification of tumours of the breast. Lyon (France): International Agency for Research on Cancer; 2012. (WHO classification of tumours series, 4th ed.; vol. 4).
http://publications.iarc.fr/14.

Soft tissue and bone
Fletcher CDM, Bridge JA, Hogendoorn PCW, et al., editors. WHO classification of tumours of soft tissue and bone. Lyon (France): International Agency for Research on Cancer; 2013. (WHO classification of tumours series, 4th ed.; vol. 5).
http://publications.iarc.fr/15.

Female reproductive organs
Kurman RJ, Carcangiu ML, Herrington CS, et al., editors. WHO classification of tumours of female reproductive organs. Lyon (France): International Agency for Research on Cancer; 2014. (WHO classification of tumours series, 4th ed.; vol. 6).
http://publications.iarc.fr/16.

Lung, pleura, thymus and heart
Travis WD, Brambilla E, Burke AP, et al., editors. WHO classification of tumours of the lung, pleura, thymus and heart. Lyon (France): International Agency for Research on Cancer; 2015. (WHO classification of tumours series, 4th ed.; vol. 7).
http://publications.iarc.fr/17.

Urinary system and male genital organs
Moch H, Humphrey PA, Ulbright TM, et al., editors. WHO classification of tumours of the urinary system and male genital organs. Lyon (France): International Agency for Research on Cancer; 2016. (WHO classification of tumours series, 4th ed.; vol. 8).
http://publications.iarc.fr/540.

Central nervous system
Louis DN, Ohgaki H, Wiestler OD, et al., editors. WHO classification of tumours of the central nervous system. Lyon (France): International Agency for Research on Cancer; 2016. (WHO classification of tumours series, 4th rev. ed.; vol. 1).
http://publications.iarc.fr/543.

Head and neck
El-Naggar AK, Chan JKC, Grandis JR, et al., editors. WHO classification of head and neck tumours. Lyon (France): International Agency for Research on Cancer; 2017. (WHO classification of tumours series, 4th ed.; vol. 9).
http://publications.iarc.fr/548.

Endocrine organs
Lloyd RV, Osamura RY, Klöppel G, et al., editors. WHO classification of tumours of endocrine organs. Lyon (France): International Agency for Research on Cancer; 2017. (WHO classification of tumours series, 4th ed.; vol. 10).
http://publications.iarc.fr/554.

Haematopoietic and lymphoid tissues
Swerdlow SH, Campo E, Harris NL, et al., editors. WHO classification of tumours of haematopoietic and lymphoid tissues. Lyon (France): International Agency for Research on Cancer; 2017. (WHO classification of tumours series, 4th rev. ed.; vol. 2).
http://publications.iarc.fr/556.

Skin
Elder DE, Massi D, Scolyer RA, et al., editors. WHO classification of skin tumours. Lyon (France): International Agency for Research on Cancer; 2018. (WHO classification of tumours series, 4th ed.; vol. 11).
http://publications.iarc.fr/560.

Eye
Grossniklaus HE, Eberhart CG, Kivelä TT, editors. WHO classification of tumours of the eye. Lyon (France): International Agency for Research on Cancer; 2018. (WHO classification of tumours series, 4th ed.; vol. 12).
http://publications.iarc.fr/561.

Digestive system
WHO Classification of Tumours Editorial Board. Digestive system tumours. Lyon (France): International Agency for Research on Cancer; 2019. (WHO classification of tumours series, 5th ed.; vol. 1).
http://publications.iarc.fr/579.